Anatomy

DEVELOPMENT

FUNCTION

CLINICAL CORRELATIONS

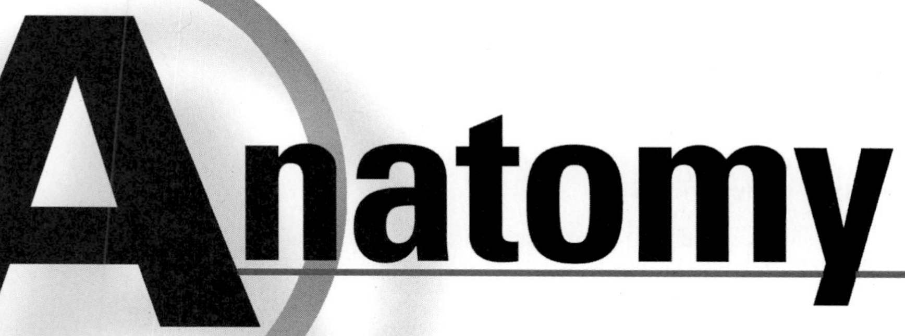

Anatomy

Development
Function
Clinical Correlations

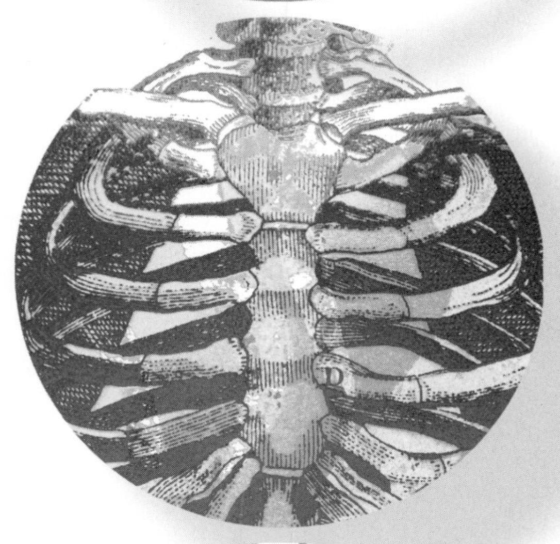

WILLIAM J. LARSEN, PhD
Professor, Department of Cell Biology,
Neurobiology, and Anatomy
Faculty Member, Molecular and Developmental
Biology Graduate Program
University of Cincinnati College of Medicine
Research Faculty, Perinatal Research Institute
Children's Hospital and University of Cincinnati
College of Medicine
Cincinnati, Ohio

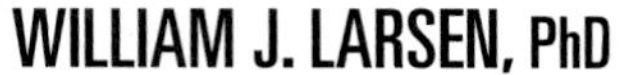

SAUNDERS
An Imprint of Elsevier Science
Philadelphia London New York St. Louis Sydney Toronto

SAUNDERS
An Imprint of Elsevier Science

The Curtis Center
Independence Square West
Philadelphia, Pennsylvania 19106

NOTICE

Pharmacology is an ever-changing field. Standard safety precautions must be followed, but as new research and clinical experience broaden our knowledge, changes in treatment and drug therapy may become necessary or appropriate. Readers are advised to check the most current product information provided by the manufacturer of each drug to be administered to verify the recommended dose, the method and duration of administration, and contraindications. It is the responsibility of the treating physician, relying on experience and knowledge of the patient, to determine dosages and the best treatment for each individual patient. Neither the publisher nor the editor assumes any liability for any injury and/or damage to persons or property arising from this publication.

The Publisher

Library of Congress Cataloging-in-Publication Data

Larsen, William J. (William James)
Anatomy : development, function, clinical correlations / William J. Larsen.
p. ; cm.
Includes bibliographical references and index.
ISBN 0-7216-4646-8 (alk. paper)
1. Human anatomy. I. Title.
[DNLM: 1. Anatomy. 2. Physiology. QS 4 L334a 2002]
QM23.2 .L37 2002
611—dc21

2002021165

Acquisitions Editor: William Schmitt
Developmental Editor: Anne-Marie Shaw
Publishing Services Manager: Patricia Tannian
Senior Project Manager: Suzanne C. Fannin
Book Design Manager: Gail Morey Hudson
Cover Design: Teresa Breckwoldt

ANATOMY: DEVELOPMENT, FUNCTION, CLINICAL CORRELATIONS ISBN: 0-7216-4646-8

GW/QWK

Printed in the United States of America

Last digit is the print number 9 8 7 6 5 4 3 2 1

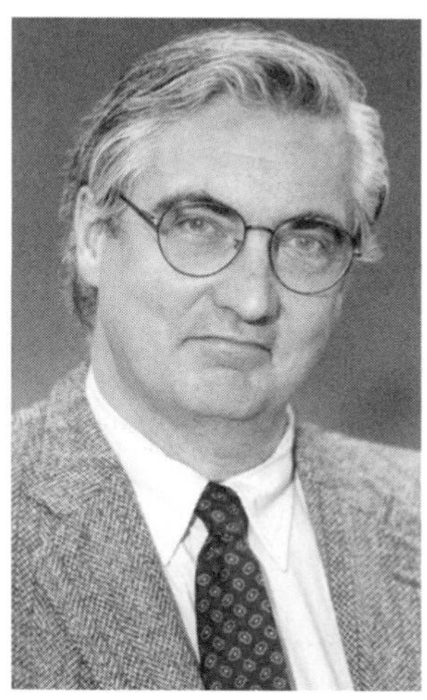

William J. Larsen, PhD
1942–2000

DEDICATION

William J. Larsen was devoted to both research and teaching. His research career addressed many fundamental questions in cell and developmental biology. His papers established the fact that mitochondria divide, demonstrated gap junction endocytosis, and discovered the role of inter-α-inhibitor in cells. Areas of research included studies of adrenal cortical tumor cells, ovarian carcinomas, preterm labor, cumulus expansion, oocyte maturation, ovulation, folliculogenesis, and in vitro fertilization, culminating in over 70 papers and invited reviews, 50 abstracts, several book chapters, and three textbooks. He took great pride in the 12 graduate students and postdoctoral fellows who were trained in his laboratory.

Dr. Larsen's teaching career spanned 25 years. In addition to lecturing in gross anatomy and teaching in anatomy dissection laboratories, he was co-director of a developmental biology course for developmental biology and genetic counseling graduate students—receiving four teaching awards during his time at the University of Cincinnati College of Medicine. He was proud of serving on the Developmental Biology and Human Genetics Task Force and his appointment to the NBME Anatomy Test Committee that develops the questions for the medical boards.

Dr. Larsen felt a great responsibility to medical education and to his students. In fact, he had prepared a lecture for his current medical students class about his own medical case, detailing all the diagnostic tools used in assessing his condition—beginning with a surface anatomical examination and oral patient history, followed by use of a chemical pharmaceutical test, x-rays, surgery, MRI, chemotherapy, and experimental vaccine as part of a third-stage trial to emphasize how all aspects of medical training are important—most of all human compassion. During his illness, he was gratified by the excellent and personal care he received from many of his own former students at every step along the way.

My life with Bill started over 40 years ago when we were both biology majors at Carleton College studying comparative anatomy together. He was a great storyteller and humorist and had a zest for life that was contagious—including a love of travel, gourmet cooking, old maps, Hopi and Zuni cultures, and Native American art. Although he died suddenly of complications from colon cancer and did not see the book in its final stages of production, a host of colleagues and professionals in both the clinical and academic fields helped bring the book through the production process to publication under my direction, a natural extension of our lifetime collaboration.

For Bill, with all my love,
Judith Larsen

PREFACE

What sets this gross anatomy textbook apart from all the rest? No other book presently available combines an organized, logical explanation of anatomical concepts with illustrations that clearly show the spatial and functional relationships of structures as well as detailed views. Anatomy is one of the most difficult subjects to learn because of the many facts and unfamiliar names that must be absorbed. The guiding principle of this text is to provide a logical framework for every topic that helps organize the information, relating details to larger concepts and making it easier for the student to learn this complex subject. For example, the skeleton serves as a framework for virtually all soft tissues of the body, and the fascial system integrates the function of the muscles and bones and plays a role in understanding the spread of infections and diseases. Embryonic development becomes a framework for classification of structures and understanding both normal function and clinical disorders. Knowledge of the human genome (and the developmental outcomes of genetic information) will play an increasingly important clinical role in the future both for diagnostic purposes and effective healthcare.

The overall organization of this book reflects William Larsen's 25 years of teaching medical students. Correlating the text with the practical demands of the dissection laboratory, he has divided the book into three principal sections. Section I, which includes Chapters 1 through 15, introduces the student to the discipline of anatomy and describes the anatomy of the trunk. Section II, Chapters 16 through 21, describes the anatomy of the extremities. Section III, Chapters 22 through 27, describes the anatomy of the head and neck.

Elements of design interact with the text to create an integrated overview of the subject. Chapters are organized to highlight core ideas; headings within chapters are carefully chosen to reflect the logical structure of the organization; topic sentences are included to provide succinct summaries that further guide the student through the chapter; tables and bulleted lists are formatted for easy access to concisely present information, clinical correlations are integrated into the text on a shaded background for quick identification, and special boxes are included to provide additional, detailed information on selected topics. Finally, section opener pages contain the first- and second-level headings, and the page numbers on which they appear, for each chapter within the section.

Dr. Larsen brought to this text not only a superb knowledge of anatomy, but also his devotion to teaching clearly and giving students the tools to help them learn as efficiently as possible. Throughout his years of teaching, he continually honed and refined his lectures, always with the students' needs in mind. Often, humorous models were a part of each lecture, along with an occasional joke and travel slide to help students get through technical sections. Students were even known to come back the following year to hear a lecture (and see a particular model) again. His lectures may be over, but his teaching skill lives on in this text.

William J. Larsen, PhD
Judith I. Larsen, EdD

ACKNOWLEDGMENTS

My heartfelt thanks is extended to the individuals highlighted in the following paragraph who made this book possible. **Noelle A. Granger,** PhD, Professor of Cell Biology and Anatomy and Director of Anatomy at the University of North Carolina, provided the major editing direction, checking text and figures for accuracy and providing significant editorial suggestions for the final two chapters. Her expertise and encouragement made production of the book possible. **Chantal Prewitt,** PhD, Assistant Professor, Department of Cell Biology, Neurobiology, and Anatomy at the University of Cincinnati College of Medicine, also provided a significant contribution, editing both chapters and figures and verifying clinical information. **Michael Hendrix,** PhD, Associate Professor at Biomedical Science at Southwest Missouri State University, contributed clinical correlations for the book. **Kyuran Ann Choe,** MD, Associate Professor, Director of Radiology Residents, Department of Radiology, University of Cincinnati Medical Center, and **Robert Ernst,** MD, radiologist at Christ Hospital, Cincinnati, provided x-ray films. **Jeffery T. Keller,** PhD, Research Professor of Neurosurgery and Director of the Goodyear Microsurgery Laboratory and Division, Department of Neurosurgery, and **Lyon Gleich,** MD, Specialist in Otolaryngology, both at the University of Cincinnati College of Medicine, reviewed sections that pertained to their special areas of research or medical practice. Additional editing was provided by **O.W. Henson,** PhD, former course director for anatomy at the University of North Carolina. I especially thank **Marjorie L. Toensing,** Development Editor, for her skillful editing, encouragement, and perseverance throughout this 10-year project and **Anne-Marie Shaw,** Development Editor and Manager of Textbook Development, who provided superb professional guidance as well as personal support. The medical artist, **Anthony Pazos,** is an expert surgical illustrator who worked tirelessly to create images that clarify anatomical relationships and bring anatomy to life. Together our combined efforts have produced a book of which Dr. Larsen would have been proud.

There is an ancient Hopi ideal that was suggested to me by a Hopi friend of Bill's, Phil Sekaquaptewa, that describes this book's initial creation to its final production. . . *sumi' nangwa,* which roughly translates to mean 'people coming together to do things for the benefit of all people out of a compelling desire and commitment to contribute something of value to society.'

CONTENTS

SECTION III
THE HEAD AND NECK

SECTION 1 THE TRUNK OF THE BODY

1 A Template for Learning Anatomy

ELEMENTS OF THIS BOOK THAT FACILITATE LEARNING

Anatomy is one of the most difficult subjects to learn because there are so many details and unfamiliar names to absorb. Many of the fine points of anatomic structures must be seen to be understood, and absorbing visual information may be an entirely new type of learning for the student. The student may initially feel somewhat daunted by the thought of memorizing countless details. However, the goal of this text is to aid the learning process by relating details to larger concepts. Specifically, the author has incorporated elements into this book that will help the student learn more easily: design elements visually organize the information, finely rendered anatomic illustrations show spatial and functional relationships, and integrative frameworks introduce every body region and system.

Design elements facilitate learning

Design elements of the book make information accessible when the student first encounters it and also facilitate review later on. Almost every topic in the book begins with an informative introductory statement (set in italics after the heading) that summarizes the content of the discussion. Sentences that catalog numerous features of an anatomic structure have been organized as bulleted lists. Both of these devices are designed to catch the reader's eye and to facilitate quick access to critical information. Much detailed information is organized in tabular form to expedite review. Clinical disorders and other correlations are interspersed throughout the text and are highlighted in color.

Many illustrations are provided in which anatomic details are shown clearly

An attempt has been made to illustrate as much of the anatomic information described in the text as possible. In many cases, unique illustrations have been constructed in a diagrammatic-anatomic style to show clearly the spatial and functional relationships of structures as well as their anatomic details. For example, the entire course of a nerve may be illustrated to show all of its target organs within a certain field and all of its functions. In some cases, functionally related structures are illustrated together to emphasize their interactions. In other cases, figures that depict related structures are grouped in the same figure or are presented on the same page.

Integrative frameworks facilitate the study of anatomy

A major aim of this book is to present anatomic information in an efficient, meaningful fashion. One way this is done is by describing anatomic details concisely and logically. Another way is to give an overall view of a body system (e.g., the nervous system) in a cohesive, integrative way. The system then becomes an organizing, or integrative, framework that can be used as a basis for classifying structures related to it. The frameworks help the student understand the morphologic, spatial, developmental, functional, and clinical relationships of anatomic structures to each other and to the body as a whole. The frameworks also help the student to develop deductive skills, which provides a way of learning anatomic information that is much more efficient than that provided by rote memorization. When students begin to practice medicine, they will find that these deductive skills are crucial in interpreting patient histories, making accurate diagnoses, and choosing which treatment to administer (or choosing to withhold treatment).

Organizing, or integrative, frameworks are used in this book to introduce and describe anatomic details of every body region and system. The story of the embryonic development of a region is one integrative framework. Other frameworks are the major systems of the body, such as the skeletal, muscular, nervous, vascular, and fascial systems.

Embryonic development provides a framework for classifying muscles and understanding muscle function and clinical disorders

In Chapter 2 the story of embryonic development is used to organize back structures, illustrate their relationships to one another, show how their functions mesh and intertwine, and show how clinical disorders affect one or more structures. This framework classifies back muscles into three distinct categories: appendicular muscles, hypomeric muscles (which are more closely related to muscles of the anterior body wall), and epimeric (true deep back) muscles (see Table 2–1). The specific origin of each of these muscle groups is reflected in its innervation and vascularization, its location within a specific layer of back muscles, and its function and clinical significance.

The discussion of back muscle development in Chapter 2 introduces the principle of embryonic segmentation, or metameric organization, of the trunk. All of the hypomeric and epimeric muscles of the body wall arise from somites, which are similar repeating subunits. The structures that develop from each individual somite (or the "descendants" of each somite) are variations on a common theme. As a consequence, these muscles may be simply named for their functional group or for the level at which they are positioned within the trunk.

Similarly, in Chapter 3, it becomes apparent that most of the elements found in one vertebra are found in all 37 vertebrae at all levels of the spine because all vertebrae originate from a part of the somite called the *sclerotome.* Therefore, the description of the vertebrae is organized with respect to their elements (e.g., vertebral bodies, spines, or processes). This gives the reader the opportunity to compare and contrast the structures and functions of vertebrae throughout the vertebral column. In addition, the common origins of vertebrae throughout the vertebral column allow most vertebrae to be named by region and specific level (e.g., the first thoracic vertebra is T1 and the first lumbar vertebra is L1). The few exceptions to this rule are vertebrae that are unusually specialized, such as the atlas, or first cervical vertebra; the axis, or second cervical vertebra; and the fused vertebrae that form the sacrum.

The skeletal system provides a structural framework for virtually all soft tissues of the body

Sections on every body region begin with a discussion of the relevant skeletal structures that underlie and organize the soft tissues. This will be especially useful in the study of the muscles and their actions since the primary function of the muscles is their connection to and movement of the skeleton. Thus, the skeleton is an especially important framework for understanding the anatomy and function of the appendicular muscles. The skeleton is also important, however, for understanding the anatomy and function of the trunk muscles, including those of the neck, back, and abdomen; the respiratory muscles of the thorax; and even the muscles of mastication and facial expression in the head. Skeletal anatomy will also be related to the organization of other soft tissues, including nerves and vessels (e.g., the course of the vertebral artery through the transverse foramina of the cervical vertebrae; the course of the thoracic neurovascular bundles within the costal grooves of the ribs). The anatomy of the skull traditionally serves as an especially pertinent frame of reference for understanding the courses of cranial nerves and vessels of the head and neck (see Chapter 23). The anatomy of the pelvis is used to describe the relationships of soft structures that enter and leave the pelvic cavity (see Chapter 14).

The nervous system organizes and integrates the functions of anatomic structures

The spinal cord and peripheral nerves are introduced in the first section of the book not only because they are located in the back, but also because they integrate the functions and pathologic disorders of many anatomic structures, including bones and muscles. For example, the functional organization of the spinal cord and peripheral nervous system is directly reflected in the metameric organization of the trunk muscles, dermis of the integument, and vertebrae (see Chapters 3 to 5). Thus, each muscle and dermal segment of the trunk is innervated by a specific segmental spinal nerve (see Chapter 4). Learning about the anatomy of the nervous system is obviously important in understanding the clinical disorders that affect this system, but it is also important because the nervous system is the mechanism for referred pain. The physician must understand this mechanism in order to ask the right questions when taking a patient's history and to accurately diagnose diseases of visceral organs (see Chapter 4).

The vasculature and fascia integrate the functions of muscles and bones and play a role in the spread of infections and metastatic disease

An understanding of the arterial, venous, and lymphatic systems is the basis for understanding vascular function and disorders. This is particularly true for blockages and deficits of these systems and for the role these systems play in the spread of cancerous metastases. The fascia, which stabilizes and integrates the functions of muscles and bones, is also emphasized in this textbook. The fasciae form compartments, which are important in the spatial relationships of anatomic structures. The fasciae also integrate the functions of structures and play a role in the spread of infectious disease and metastatic tumor cells.

ANATOMIC CONVENTIONS

The discipline of gross anatomy concerns the large structures of the human body, including all of the macroscopic parts of the body (i.e., parts visible to the naked eye), their relationships to other structures, and their positions within the spaces of the body. In order to organize and describe to others the profuse amount of anatomic information, anatomists have adopted two fundamental conventions: the anatomic position and standardized anatomic nomenclature.

The anatomic position and related coordinates of the human body allow the anatomist to describe the body of a patient or cadaver and locate anatomic structures within it, regardless of the position in which the body has been placed

Anatomists have agreed to consistently describe the body and its parts in a certain position known as the anatomic position. This convention allows anyone to immediately identify the body's right, left, front, and back sides and superior and inferior ends. The anatomic position also makes it possible to define coordinates that indicate where a structure is located in the body with respect to a certain plane of the body, the center of the body, or the surface of the body. A thorough understanding of the anatomic position and related axes, lines, and regions is necessary to describe the anatomy of such structures as the trunk.

In the anatomic position, the body is in an upright, standing position with the upper extremities rotated laterally, or outwardly, to expose the palms of the hands to the front, in a position called *supination* (Fig. 1–1*A* and *C*). The feet are placed with the toes pointing forward. The "front" of the body is the anterior, or ventral, surface, and the "back" of the body is the posterior, or dorsal, surface (Fig. 1–1*C*). The head is located at the superior, or cranial, rostral, or cephalic, end of the body and the feet at the inferior, or caudal, end.

A sagittal plane is any plane defined by the dorsoventral and superoinferior axes of the body. A median, or midsagittal, plane is any plane that divides the body into equal right and left halves (Fig. 1–1*D* and *E*). Any longitudinal line within the midsagittal plane of the body is a midline. Structures located to the left or right "away from" the midsagittal plane of the body are lateral structures, whereas those "closer to" the midsagittal plane are medial structures. Planes parallel and lateral to the midsagittal plane are parasagittal planes. A horizontal plane transecting the body is a transverse, or cross-sectional, plane (Fig. 1–1*E* and *F*), and a plane defined by the superoinferior and mediolateral axes of the body is a coronal, or frontal, plane (Fig. 1–1*G*).

The term *superficial* describes the relative proximity of an anatomic structure to the surface of the body, limb, or head; the term *deep* describes the relative proximity of an anatomic structure to the central axis of the body, limb, or head. These terms are used no matter which surface is chosen as a frame of reference. For long structures such as bones or vessels, the term *proximal* describes the region of the structure closest to the trunk or the origin of the structure, and the term *distal* describes the region of the structure farthest from the trunk or the origin of the structure.

Conventions for the naming of anatomic structures come from common terms, eponyms, and formal names from the Nomina Anatomica

During the course of their general education, students of anatomy usually become familiar with the common names of anatomic structures (e.g., stomach, liver). Anatomic purists, however, may insist on using Latin or Greek terms sanctioned by the *Nomina Anatomica,* the official body of anatomic nomenclature created by the International Congress of Anatomists. For example, the *Nomina Anatomica* uses *"gaster"* rather than *stomach* and *"hepar"* rather than *liver.* To further complicate the matter, many health care professionals (especially those educated in past decades) use eponyms, which are names that typically honor the individual who first described a structure. Because of these three naming conventions, for example, the ligament that courses between the anterior superior iliac spine and the pubic tubercle of the pelvis may be described as the **inguinal ligament,** its common English name; the **ligamentum inguinale,** its official name; or **Poupart's ligament,** its eponym.

The fundamental purpose of anatomic nomenclature is to facilitate communication

Academic or clinical discussions of human anatomy involve students, academicians, physicians, nurses, counselors, laboratory technicians, or patients and their family members. Common names are useful when a health care provider is taking a patient's history or discussing an illness with a patient's relatives or friends. On the other hand, formal Latin or Greek names may be used when the physician is comparing a case with other cases in the anatomic or clinical literature. Because they are still widely used, eponyms are often employed in discussions between health care professionals. The most useful terms, therefore, are those that are best understood by the persons involved in a particular discussion, or that are most suitable for a particular purpose. Although Latin and Greek terms or English translations of *Nomina Anatomica* terms are the most precisely descriptive, more common terms or eponyms may be unavoidable in certain situations. In this textbook, the author has defined as many terms and names as is practicable when each structure is introduced.

The student may find that no reference for anatomic nomenclature is more useful than a good medical dictionary.

The Nomina Anatomica *gives an anatomic structure its original Latin or Greek name or a name derived from Latin or Greek*

The preciseness provided by the Latin and Greek names of the *Nomina Anatomica* for bones, bony specializations, and soft tissues can be seen in the following examples.

Foramen ovale septum secundum:

- **foramen** (Latin for aperture)
- **ovale** (Latin for something relating to an ovum or egg or something resembling the outline of the longitudinal section of an egg) is an oval-shaped hole in the

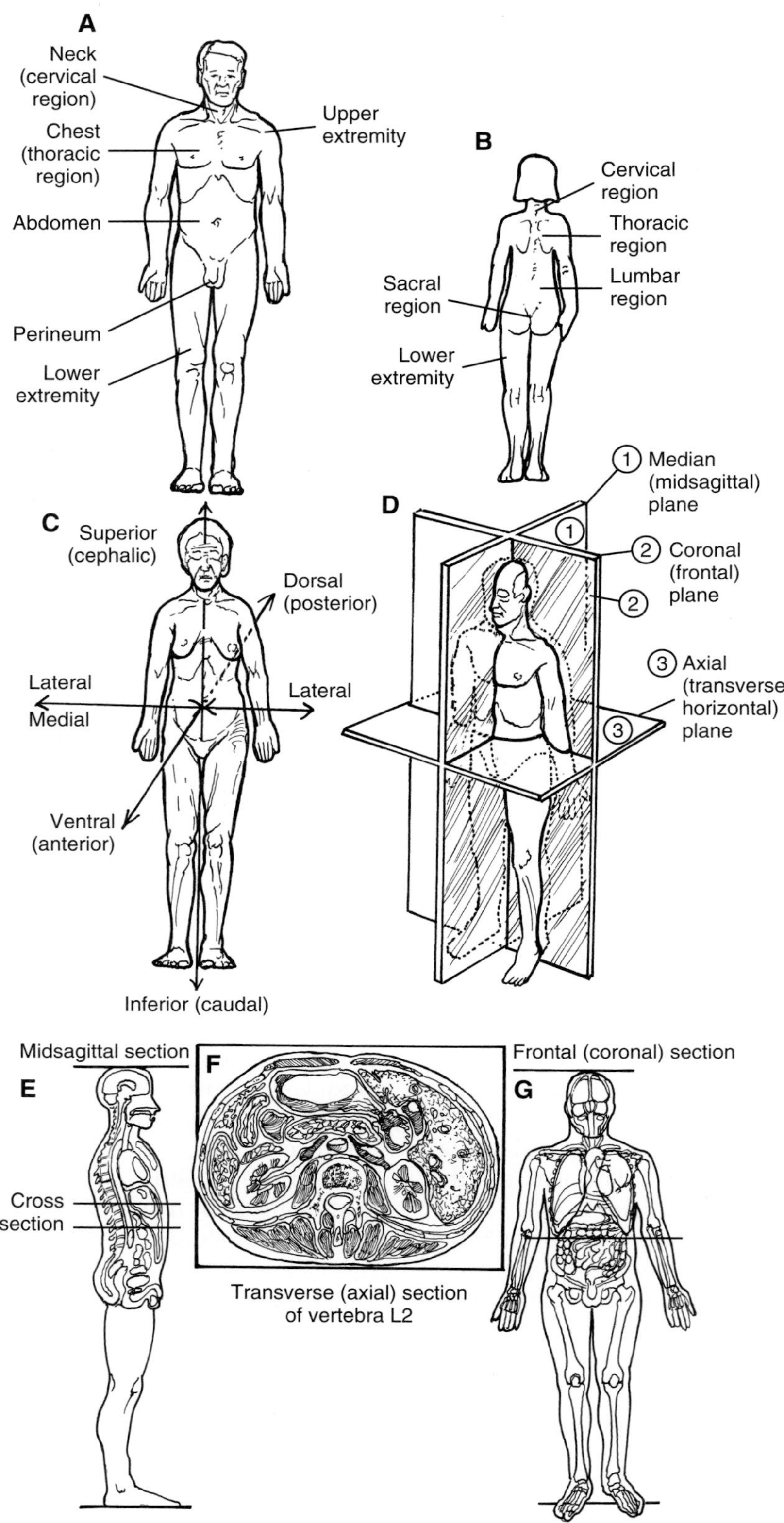

FIGURE 1–1

Anatomic position, axes, and planes. **A.** Anterior aspect of middle-aged man standing in anatomic position. In descriptions of human anatomy, the locations of anatomic structures are designated with reference to this position. Note that hands are supinated (i.e., palms are facing forward). **B.** Posterior aspect of a young girl standing in anatomic position. Note that dorsa of both hands face posteriorly. **C.** Anterior aspect of older woman in anatomic position showing craniocaudal, dorsoventral (posteroanterior), and left and right axes of body. **D.** Anterior and left lateral aspect of older man showing midsagittal, coronal, and transverse planes. **E.** Midsagittal section of human body. **F.** Transverse (axial) section of human body. **G.** Frontal (coronal) section of human body.

- **septum** (Latin for partition) **secundum** (Latin for second or next), which is the second partition formed between the atrial chambers in the heart.

Glenoid fossa humerus:

- **glenoid** (Greek for something resembling a socket)
- **fossa** (Latin for longitudinal depression) of the scapula (Latin for shoulder blade) is the depression with which the head of the
- **humerus** (Latin for shoulder or bone of the arm) articulates.

The conventional anatomic names of muscles are especially revealing. They may reflect the shape, size, or presumed function of a muscle. A complete discussion of muscle nomenclature, using muscles of the back as examples, is provided in Chapter 2.

ANATOMIC IMAGING TECHNIQUES

Visualizing anatomic structures is essential to the study of anatomy

Gross anatomy is a visual science. Therefore, the ability to visualize structures in three dimensions is one of the most useful skills that a student of anatomy can develop. Indeed, it is not surprising that the great anatomists Michelangelo and Leonardo da Vinci were also known as reasonably good artists. The student's goal is to learn the spatial relationships between anatomic structures, and to use this as a basis for understanding the functional interactions between structures and the way in which these interactions may contribute to diseases.

Typically, three main visual resources may be advantageously used in the study of human gross anatomy:

- artistic illustrations in textbooks and atlases;
- a human cadaver, which is dissected in the laboratory; and
- modern imaging techniques such as roentgenography and magnetic resonance imaging (MRI).

Illustrations in Textbooks and Atlases

Textbook illustrations provide a relatively accurate rendering of anatomic structures

The figures in an anatomic atlas tend to be especially accurate. In some cases, these anatomic representations are so accurate that they may partially substitute for the actual dissection of a cadaver or, at least, serve as useful guides for reviewing specific structures during dissection. However, illustrations tend to obscure some of the more general structural and spatial relationships that beginning students must learn and appreciate. Rarely, for example, is the entire course of a nerve shown in a single illustration. In order to understand the "global" function and clinical significance of the nerve, the student must refer to a number of different sources to find the many targets of the nerve and integrate them.

On the other hand, a diagrammatic illustration may depict comprehensive anatomic relationships, providing a larger framework in which to organize anatomic details. Obviously, such diagrammatic representations may not accurately show anatomic structures. They may ignore, for example, certain details or reflect a bias of the illustrator. Nonetheless, illustrations that depict organizing principles of anatomy and interrelate anatomic details are essential for an understanding of many basic anatomic concepts.

Because this textbook is intended to be a primary learning resource for an introductory anatomy course, many of its illustrations have been rendered in a diagrammatic style. Students are encouraged to consult any of the available atlases of human anatomy or to participate in laboratory dissections to learn about the actual appearance of anatomic structures.

Laboratory Dissection

Laboratory dissection provides a wealth of anatomic information

Laboratory dissection is an extremely useful adjunct to the lectures, slides, handouts, atlases, and textbooks commonly used in the teaching of human anatomy. For one thing, drawings in and of themselves cannot provide an adequate sense of the three-dimensional quality of anatomic structures. Dissecting a cadaver provides a more realistic insight into spatial relationships between organs, cavities, and the skeletal framework of the body. Dissection also provides a sense of the true scale, mass, and, to some degree, texture of anatomic structures. Obstructing structures may be cut or removed to reveal the entire or partial course of structures such as arteries and nerves.

Dissection also helps students learn an important concept of human anatomy: variability. While a drawing in a book or an atlas may illustrate the most common configuration of an anatomic structure (with perhaps a few of the most common variations), students in the laboratory can see, with their own eyes, as many variations as there are cadavers. For example, students in the laboratory soon learn that the simple, conventional pattern of coronary vasculature depicted in their textbooks bears only a general similarity to the pattern they are likely to dissect from the wall of a cadaver's heart—a pattern that differs yet again from those in hearts of cadavers at adjacent tables.

Modern Imaging Methods

Imaging methods permit visualization of normal and abnormal structures of the body with little or no physical intervention or disturbance

Noninvasive imaging techniques allow routine visualization of structures that lie deep to the integument, and, in some cases, provide wholly unique images of anatomic structures. Because of this, radiographs and other types of images are useful in the study of human anatomy and in the practice of medicine. Therefore, they will be used to portray anatomic structures and relationships throughout this book.

The visualization of bones with plain x-rays films of the hand was first described in 1895 by Roentgen. Since then, this standard x-ray procedure has been supplemented by several other approaches, each having its particular advantages and limitations. Computerized tomography (CT) scanning produces detailed cross sections of the body by means of x-rays and computer analysis. MRI produces images similar to those of CT scanning but uses magnetic radiation instead of x-rays. MRI can also create sectional images of the body in any plane, not only in the conventional cross-sectional plane. Nuclear medicine methods take advantage of the specific incorporation of radioactive substances to create images of anatomic structures, while ultrasound imaging uses sound waves to portray anatomic structures.

Standard X-Rays

The clarity of images produced with standard radiographic methods depends on how well various structures absorb x-rays

In standard radiographs, an x-ray beam produced by a cathode ray tube is directed at the body part of interest; the x-rays that pass through the structure are recorded on photographic film (Fig. 1–2*A*). X-rays that pass through the body expose the film in a manner analogous to that of light. The image produced on the film is a radiograph. The radiograph reflects the interaction of energy photons in the x-ray band of the photoelectric spectrum with the tissues that the photons encounter as they pass through the body. This interaction depends primarily on the electron density (mass) of the tissues. X-rays pass readily through substances of low electron density, such as air, but tend to be absorbed by substances of high electron density, such as bone or metal. The parts of the film that are exposed to more x-rays are darker than the parts exposed to fewer x-rays. Therefore, air appears black on the film and bone appears white. Water and fat have electron densities between those of bone and air and so they appear as shades of gray. Air is, of course, relevant to anatomic imaging because it is present in several anatomic structures, including the paranasal sinuses, lungs, and regions of the gastrointestinal tract (Fig. 1–2*B*).

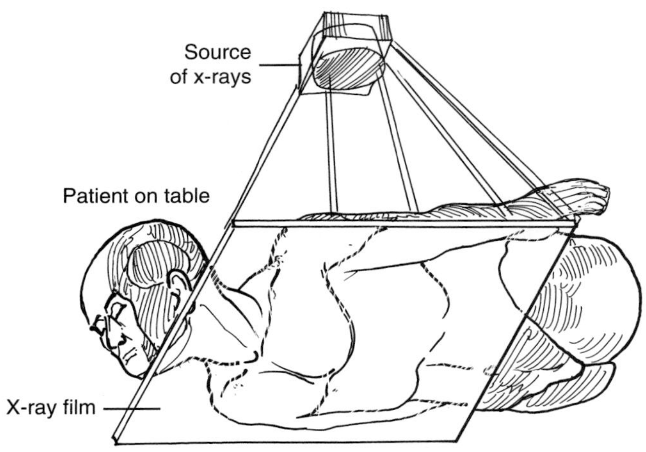

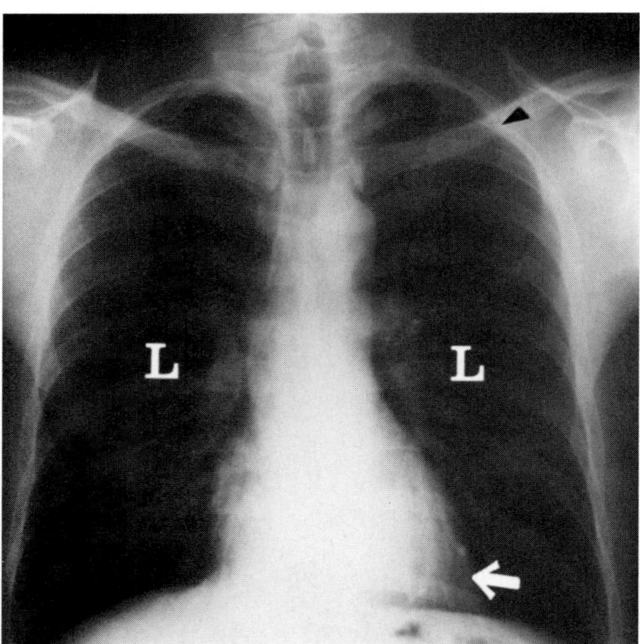

FIGURE 1–2
Thoracic x-rays. **A.** The standard frontal posteroanterior (PA) position for taking a radiograph, showing thorax and abdomen. X-ray is taken from posterior aspect with patient's chest flattened against a canister containing photographic film. **B.** Frontal PA radiograph of chest should be viewed as if one is looking at anterior side of patient. Cardiac apex *(white arrow)* is on the right side of image, which is the left side of patient. Notice that bones, which are dense, appear white *(black arrowhead).* Soft tissues such as the mediastinal structures appear gray. Lungs *(L)* are filled with air and, therefore, are least dense structures and appear nearly black.

Contrast Agents

Contrast agents may enhance differences in adjacent structures that have similar electron densities

Radiographic contrast agents usually contain barium or iodine, both of which have high electron densities. Cavities containing these compounds tend to absorb x-rays and appear white on x-ray film. Barium compounds may be administered into the gastrointestinal tract orally or rectally to increase the x-ray opacity of the gastrointestinal tract (Fig. 1–3). Iodine-based reagents may be given intravascularly or through the gastrointestinal tract. In angiography, these reagents are injected directly into the arterial or venous system to demonstrate the vascular anatomy (Fig. 1–4). Because iodine-based agents are excreted by the kidneys, intravenous urography allows the urinary tract to be visualized. Likewise, the biliary tree can be visualized by endoscopic retrograde cholangiopancreatography (ERCP), which involves endoscopic injection of iodine-based reagents. The lymphatic system can be visualized by

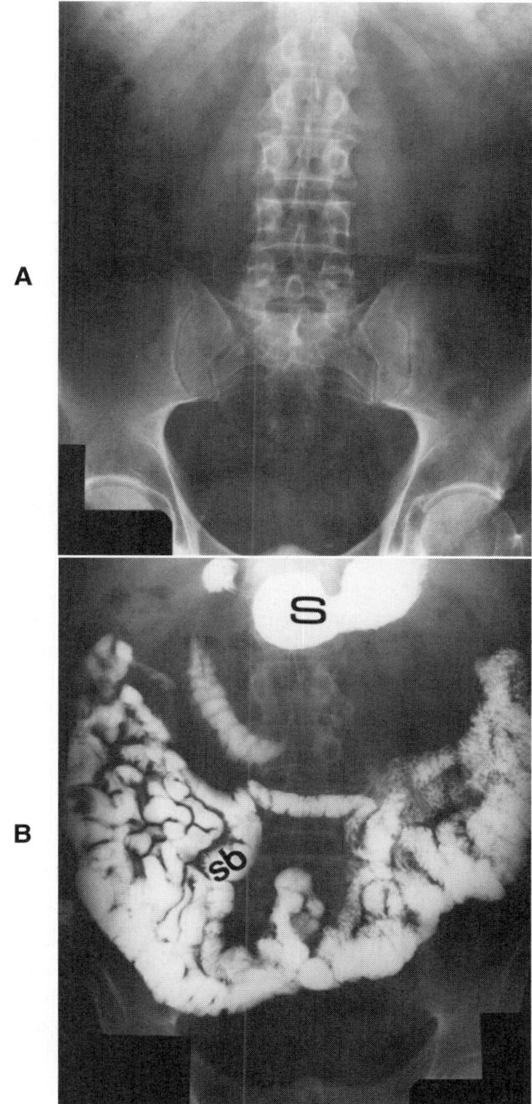

FIGURE 1–3
Frontal radiograph of the abdomen. **A.** As in the chest, bones are dense and seen as white structures. Little contrast is seen in abdomen. **B.** After oral ingestion of barium, stomach *(S)* and small bowel *(SB)* appear white and can be visualized.

lymphangiography. Myelography, which involves direct injection of iodine-based reagents into other anatomic spaces such as the subarachnoid space, allows visualization of the spinal cord. Arthrography, or injection of contrast agents into the synovial cavity, allows visualization of synovial joints.

Analysis of Standard Radiographs

Analysis of standard radiographs is based upon several important conventions

As an x-ray beam passes through the body, it may pass through a number of structures (e.g., skin, subcutaneous fat, bone, and soft tissue). Because the focal plane of a standard radiograph is very deep, it causes structures located virtually anywhere in the body to appear to lie within the same plane. A radiograph is a two-dimensional representation of a three-dimensional anatomic structure and, therefore, is a summation of all of the structures through which the x-ray beam passes. It is impossible to determine whether the radiograph is taken from the front or back of the body, or, in lateral views, from the left or right side of the body. In addition, it may be very difficult to distinguish overlapping or adjacent structures that have similar electron densities.

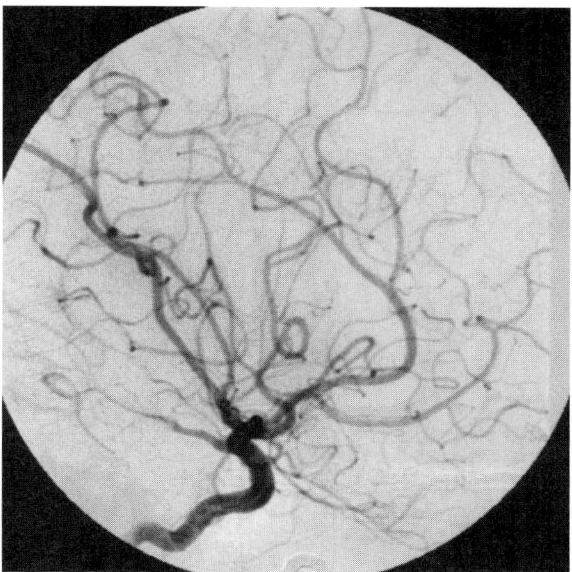

FIGURE 1–4
Conventional angiography. Vessels can be visualized with injection of a contrast material. In conventional angiography, contrast material has an iodine base. This is a carotid angiogram in lateral projection. There is filling of the internal carotid artery and its branches. To visualize this artery, a catheter was placed in the femoral artery and advanced in a retrograde direction through external and common iliac arteries, abdominal aorta, thoracic aorta, common carotid artery, and root of internal carotid artery.

Although typical radiographs of the chest are taken with the x-ray beam passing from the posterior to the anterior side of the patient (PA, view) (see Fig. 1–2*A*), the x-ray should be viewed as if the viewer is looking at the patient from the front. Thus, the micrograph should be positioned so that the patient's right side in the x-ray is to the viewer's left, as if the patient were standing in front of the viewer in anatomic position (see Figs. 1–1 to 1–3).

Mammography

Mammography is a specialized application of the standard radiographic method

Mammography uses lower-energy x-ray beams to evaluate subtle differences in soft tissues of the breast. As the primary screening method for breast cancer,

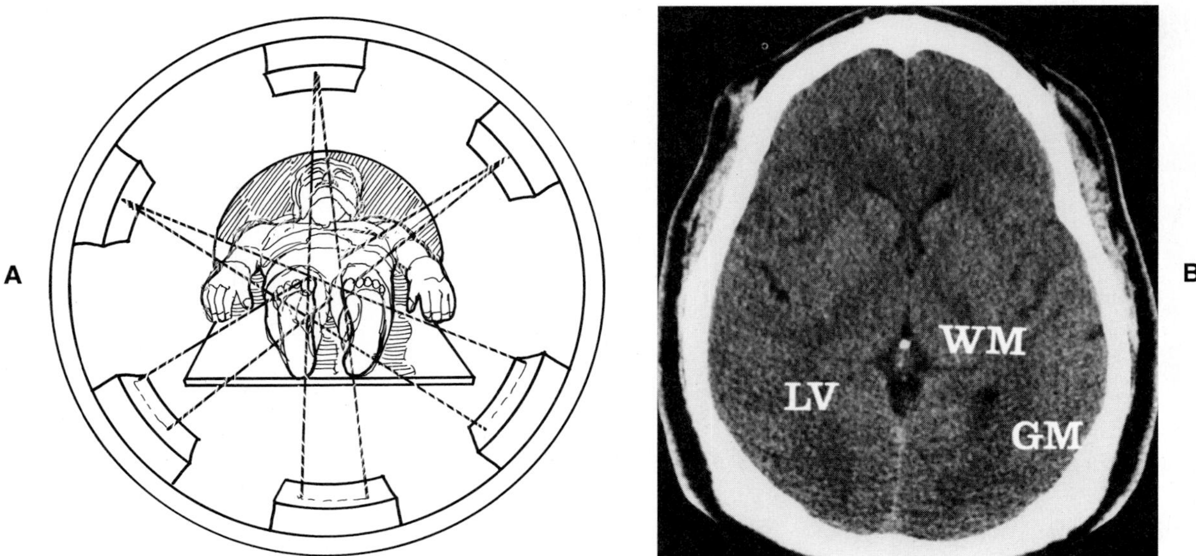

FIGURE 1–5
Computerized tomography (CT) scanning of the head. **A.** In CT scanning, a transverse slice of body is created by rotating an x-ray source 360 degrees around patient. X-rays are detected on opposite side, and a transverse image is reconstructed using a computer algorithm. **B.** CT scan is viewed as if one is standing at patient's feet at the foot of the bed and looking upward toward the head. Therefore, the right side of image is left side of patient (as in a standard x-ray). Notice that calvaria, which is osseous, is white. Brain tissues have different densities, which causes gray matter *(GM)* to appear brighter than white matter *(WM)*. There is fluid in ventricles. Lateral ventricle *(LV)* is less dense than brain tissue and is, therefore, darker.

mammography is used to evaluate palpable lesions detected during a physical examination. In their early stages, cancerous tumors may appear as small dense masses, areas of microcalcification, or architectural distortions of the breast parenchyma, which is the supporting, or connective, tissue of the breast. At present, one in eight women in the United States will be found to have breast cancer, so mammography is a very important diagnostic tool (see Chapter 6).

Computerized Tomography (CT) Scanning

CT scanning minimizes difficulties in the visualization of structures that are superimposed upon one another and allows greater discrimination among tissues with similar densities

There are three significant challenges in the evaluation of plain radiographs. The first challenge is determining the relative positions of superimposed structures. This is because of the extreme depth of focus used in standard radiography. As has been noted, it is difficult to determine which plane of the body overlapping structures occupy. The second challenge is imaging "low-density" soft tissues enclosed within "high-density" bone (e.g., soft tissues of the brain, which are obscured by their encasement within the bony skull). The third challenge is differentiating tissues with similar densities (e.g., the pancreas and kidney, which have similar electron densities).

CT scanning solves these problems by creating a transverse, or axial, "slice" of the body. Although x-rays are used as in standard radiography, the x-ray source is rotated 360 degrees around the body. X-rays passing through the body are picked up by an x-ray detector, and images are digitally reconstructed using a computer algorithm (Fig. 1–5*A*). As in standard radiography, high-density structures such as bone appear white, and low-density structures appear black. Because the images are created as transverse slices, structures are not superimposed upon one another, and their relative positions are therefore apparent. As in standard radiography, contrast agents can be used to distinguish soft tissues of similar density such as the pancreas and kidney. CT scanning is done rapidly and provides details that are particularly useful in assessing the pathologic effects of trauma, infection, and malignant tumors on human anatomy.

As in standard radiographic imaging, certain conventions are followed in viewing a CT scan. When the viewer looks at transverse images, the slice of the body should be positioned so that it is seen as if the viewer is standing at the patient's feet at the foot of the bed. Thus, the viewer is looking toward the patient's head, at the inferior aspect of the slice. The patient's right side should be on the viewer's left side (see Fig. 1–5*B*).

Magnetic Resonance Imaging (MRI)

The technique of MRI is based on the responses of some atomic nuclei to a magnetic field

In the presence of a static magnetic field, certain atomic nuclei have a property known as "spin" (i.e., they orient themselves to the field). When a radiofre-

A

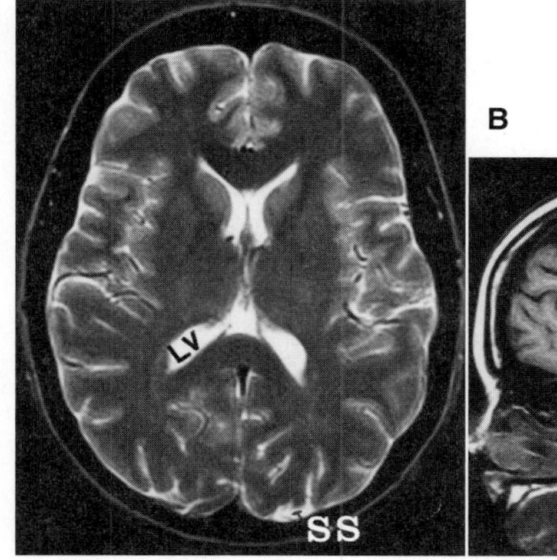

B

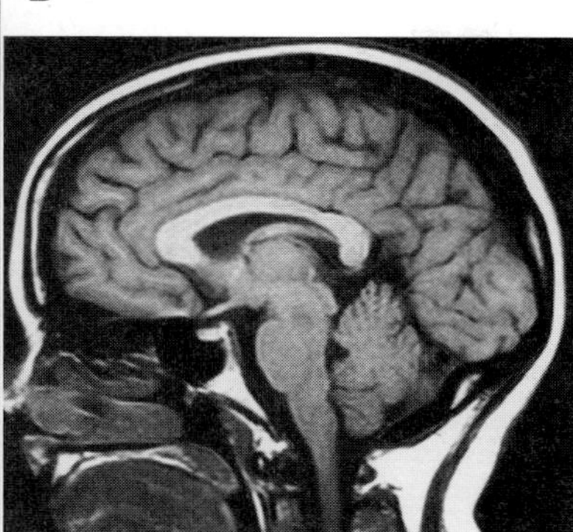

FIGURE 1–6
Magnetic resonance imaging (MRI) scan of the brain. **A.** In this axial image of the brain, note that contrast and resolution between structures is greater than in the CT scan in Fig. 1–5. The MRI scanner has been adjusted so that fluid within the left ventricle *(LV)* and subarachnoid space *(SS)* appears white. **B.** In this sagittal image of the brain, the MRI scanner has been adjusted so that fluid within the basal cisterns and around the cerebellum appears dark gray.

quency pulse is applied, the spin is disturbed; as the nuclei return to their original orientation, a radiofrequency signal is detected and analyzed. These signals are integrated by a computer to produce representations of anatomic structures in a manner similar to that used in CT scanning. However, in addition to producing transverse slices (Fig. 1–6*A*), MRI can produce slices of the body in any plane, including the sagittal (see Fig. 1–6*B*), coronal, and oblique planes (see Chapter 7).

The most common atomic nucleus in the human body that can be used for MRI is the hydrogen atom nucleus. The MRI signal generated by the nucleus not only depends upon the density of the hydrogen atom in its biologic molecule, but also upon its chemical environment. Differences in these factors result in the enhancement of contrast between adjacent soft tissues of similar electron densities. Indeed, the MRI detector can be adjusted so that certain properties of the imaged tissue, such as water content, are accentuated. The detector can also be adjusted to discriminate the movements of hydrogen nuclei. Thus, MRI can be used to great advantage to visualize blood flowing within the heart or vasculature. Because of this property, MRI is used for angiographic imaging without injection of contrast media through intravascular catheters (Fig. 1–7). This capacity does not preclude the use of contrast media in MRI, however. The contrast media are not related to those used in standard radiography or CT scanning.

Because of the strength of the magnetic field used in MRI, safety precautions are paramount. Some clinical systems use magnetic fields as high as 1.5 tesla (T), which equals 15,000 gauss (G). The strength of this field may be appreciated by comparing it with the earth's innate magnetic field, which ranges from 0.1 to 1 G, depending on the geographic location. Thus, the earth's innate magnetic field is four to five orders of magnitude less than that used in MRI. In fact, the strong fields used in MRI may be problematic because they may affect the placement or function of some metallic clinical implants such as electronic pacemakers. Metal

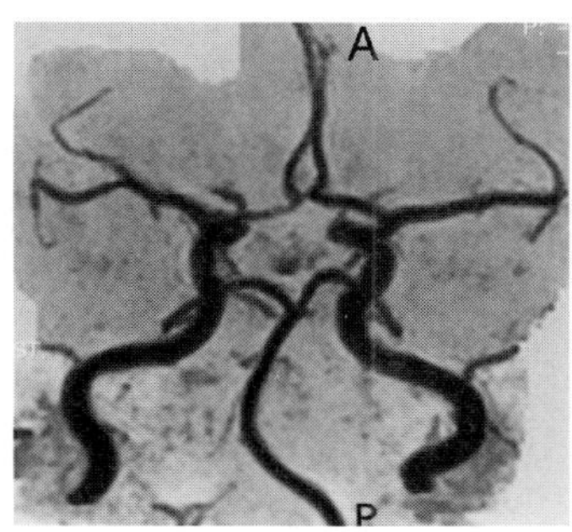

FIGURE 1–7
Magnetic resonance imaging (MRI) angiogram of circle of Willis. MRI scanner has been adjusted to highlight contrast between structures containing moving fluid (i.e., blood) and static surrounding tissues.

clips used to treat brain aneurysms will turn in the direction of these strong magnetic fields and may tear the blood vessel to which they are attached. Obviously, the physician or technician must ascertain whether the patient has such a clip or implanted electronic device before scheduling an MRI scan. Every MRI center uses a screening questionnaire to determine whether a patient has risk factors that might preclude MRI. Conventions for viewing a transverse MRI scan are the same as those described above for CT scans.

Nuclear Medicine

Radioactive materials are used in medicine not only for therapeutic purposes, but also for diagnostic purposes

Certain radioactive elements may be incorporated into biologically active molecules that participate in normal physiologic pathways. These molecules may provide useful anatomic information in addition to insights into physiologic processes.

One such element is iodine, which is used for studies of the thyroid gland. The isotope iodine-123 is generally used in these studies. The human body concentrates iodine-123 in the thyroid gland by incorporating it into thyroid hormone. Once the iodine is adminis-

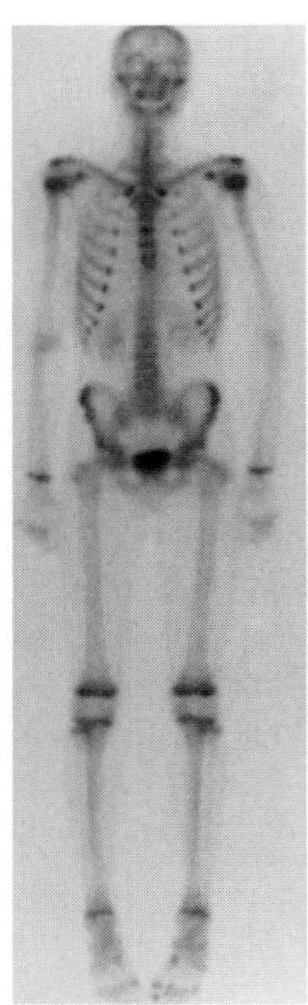

FIGURE 1–8
Nuclear medicine. Skeleton is imaged with a nuclear medicine camera following administration of radiopharmaceutical technetium-99m methylene diphosphonate and its uptake by bone.

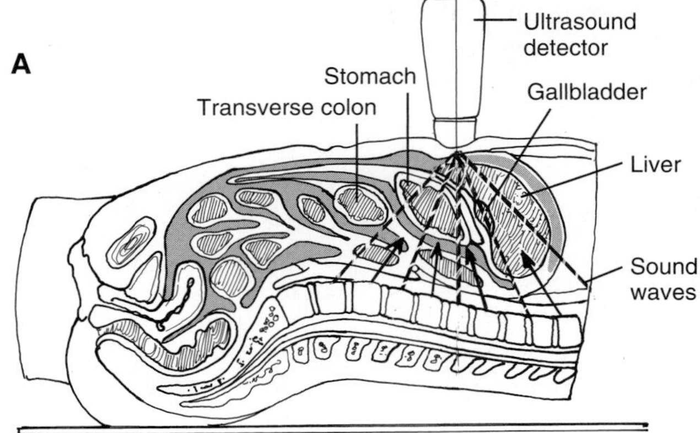

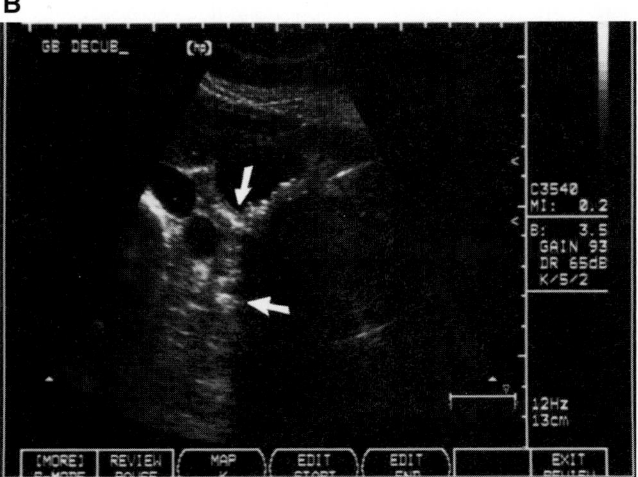

FIGURE 1–9
A. In ultrasonography, body is bombarded with ultrasound waves and a detector senses echoes that are reflected from both soft and hard tissues. **B.** Ultrasound image of gallbladder reveals echoic structures *(arrows)*, which are interpreted as gallstones. Fluid within gallbladder is anechoic (black).

tered and incorporated, the thyroid gland is imaged with a nuclear medicine camera. The appearance of the gland depends on many factors, including the gland's ability to trap iodine and synthesize thyroid hormone and the presence of other tissues within the gland. For example, tumors such as hyperfunctioning adenomas of the thyroid may incorporate more iodine than normal gland tissue. Because some cancerous tumors of the thyroid can incorporate iodine, they can also be treated (killed) with radioactive iodine. Therapeutic approaches use the isotope iodine-131.

Other radioactive agents may be used in a similar manner to image the skeletal system (Fig. 1–8), assess blood flow in the myocardium and brain, record metabolic activity (F18-fluorodeoxyglucose positron emission tomography [F18-FDG PET]), or assess liver function (hepatobiliary imaging). Currently, specific radioactive antibodies are being developed to image specific kinds of tumors.

Ultrasonography

Ultrasound imaging uses sound waves to portray anatomic structures

In ultrasonography, the body is bombarded with ultrasound waves of 3 to 10 MHz. A detector picks up the "echo" returned from reflective anatomic interfaces (Fig. 1–9*A*). (A reflective structure is echoic, and a nonreflective structure is anechoic, or sonolucent.) As in CT scanning and MRI, this information is digitized and integrated to produce images. Water transmits sound and, therefore, has minimal or no reflective properties. As a consequence, water appears black, or sonolucent, on the sonogram. Reflective structures appear white, and very dense materials, such as the calcium deposited in kidney stones, gallstones (see Fig. 1–9*B*), or blood vessels, reflect all of the ultrasound waves that reach them. As a consequence, structures lying deep to such deposits are completely obscured.

Because ionizing radiation is not produced by ultrasonography, this technique is frequently used for pregnant patients and fetuses. It is commonly used to assess gestational age and to diagnose congenital malformations.

Ultrasound can also be used as a dynamic imaging technique to reveal the motions of structures or fluids as they occur in real time. For example, echocardiography is used for real-time imaging of blood flow within the heart and of the motion of atrial or ventricular walls and heart valves.

In your study of anatomy using the organizational study aids, integrative frameworks, and visualizing techniques of this book, it is important to never lose sight of the purpose for this ambitious undertaking.

FUNCTIONAL ANATOMY

Functional anatomy not only reveals what a structure does, but it also provides a basis for understanding clinical problems

A student's first encounter with the academic study of human anatomy, in the absence of a rudimentary understanding of function and pathology, is often limited to an exercise in anatomic cataloging. Although a certain amount of cataloging cannot be escaped, any cataloging for those studying to become medical professionals should serve the higher goal of explaining how pathologic conditions or trauma may interfere with the normal functioning of the body. The brief descriptions of functions and pathologic disorders of many major anatomic structures provide a starting point for the important process of placing human anatomy into a functional and clinical context and provide a basis for exercises in clinical problem solving.

2 Introduction to the Trunk and Back

At the beginning of any medical gross anatomy course, the student, faced with the daunting challenge of learning an awesomely large, apparently cluttered collection of anatomic minutiae, may ask, "Where do I begin? Which facts are more important and which less important? How should I approach all this information? How can I best organize the learning process?"

This chapter provides a quick overview of the trunk and the back, including the general relationships of skeletal elements, nerves, and vessels, and introduces concepts that should prove useful throughout the course for learning anatomy. Chapters 1 and 2, which should be read during the first days of the anatomy course, present the frameworks within which anatomic structures are organized, thereby making the overwhelming clutter of anatomic minutiae more manageable for the student. As the study of the back continues, students will dig deeper into the specific chapters on the axial skeleton, nervous system, and back muscles, which describe the actions and clinical significance of these structures.

Why does this book initiate the study of human anatomy with the back?

Many human anatomy courses begin with the study of the back because it is a relatively simple region in which to initiate dissection. However, another compelling reason for selecting the back is the opportunity it provides for illustrating four pivotal frameworks that organize and streamline the learning process:

- ♦ The back contains the **axial skeleton,** one of the most important structural frames of reference within the human body. The axial skeleton provides names as well as attachment sites for muscles of the back. The axial skeleton consists of the cranium, vertebral column, ribs, and sternum, structures that are critical in organizing much of human anatomy and that also serve as practical references in clinical practice.
- ♦ The framework of **embryonic development,** for example, is particularly evident in descriptions of back anatomy. Development is especially helpful in delineating the common origins and consequent similarities of structures at different levels and in different regions of the back. This framework provides a basis for understanding the general features of the vertebrae at any level of the trunk as well as the innervation, vascularization, and anatomic and functional relationships of three types of muscles of the back: the appendicular muscles, the muscles related to the anterolateral muscles of the trunk, and the true deep back muscles.
- ♦ The back provides an opportunity to study the structure and function of the **nervous system.** The nervous system, in turn, provides a framework for integrating many parts of back anatomy (and, later, the rest of the body) and for understanding several key functional and clinical concepts, including the concepts of **reflex arcs** and **referred pain** (see Chapter 4).
- ♦ Finally, the back muscles can be used to illustrate specific rules of **anatomic nomenclature,** which are useful in naming many other structures of the body.

REGIONS OF THE TRUNK AND BACK

The **trunk** (from the Latin *truncus*), or **torso,** is the body, excluding the head and upper and lower extremities. It includes the **neck, thorax,** and **abdomen** and portions of the **pelvis** and **perineum** (see Fig. 1–1). Skeletal support of the trunk is provided by the **axial skeleton,** which consists of the cranium, vertebral column (spine), ribs, and sternum (see Fig. 3–1). The **body wall** of the trunk, including that of the back, consists of layers of skin, connective tissue, and muscle. All of these tissues are vascularized by a system of **arteries,** which carries blood from the heart to the tissues; a system of **veins,** which returns blood to the heart; and a system of **lymphatic vessels,** which carries interstitial fluid from between the cells back to the venous system in the region of the heart. The trunk body wall is also innervated by **somatic branches of spinal nerves** emanating from the spinal cord, which is enclosed within the vertebral column. Within the trunk, several cavities contain visceral organs: the **pericardial cavity,** which contains the heart; the two **pleural cavities,** which contain the lungs; and the **abdominopelvic cavity,** which contains the gastrointestinal tract, urogenital organs, and other viscera. (*Viscera* is the plural of *viscus,* from the Latin for soft parts or internal organs). The visceral organs are supplied with special systems of arteries, veins, and lymphatic vessels and are innervated by the **autonomic system of visceral nerves** (see Chapter 4).

The region of the **back** includes the posterior cervical, thoracic, lumbar, and sacral regions of the trunk. The back is the posterior body wall of the trunk, which is distinguished from the superior part of the anterior body wall, the **pectoral region,** and the inferior part of the anterolateral body wall, the **abdominal region.**

INTEGUMENT AND FASCIA

The integument and fascia cover and protect the anatomic structures lying beneath them

The skin covers the entire body and accounts for approximately 8% of the total body mass. Its thickness varies from 1.5 to 4 mm. It protects internal tissues from injury, prevents dehydration, and acts as a barrier against penetration by infectious agents. It also contains many sensory organs. Its most superficial layer is the **epidermis,** which is constantly being regenerated (Fig. 2–1). The layer just deep to the epidermis is the **dermis,** which is the deep connective tissue layer of the integument. Blood vessels are located within the dermis. Mechanoreceptors, thermal receptors, and pain receptors are also located within the dermis, as are the sensory endings of the spinal nerves that innervate these receptors.

A fatty layer of **superficial fascia,** the **hypodermis,** is located just deep to the skin (see Fig. 2–1). This layer is protective and is vascularized by the same arteries and veins that supply and drain the overlying dermis. The hypodermis intervenes between the overlying dermis and underlying deep fascia, which tightly invests the musculature. The underlying deep fascia, along with ligaments, tendons, and the axial skeleton, anchors the

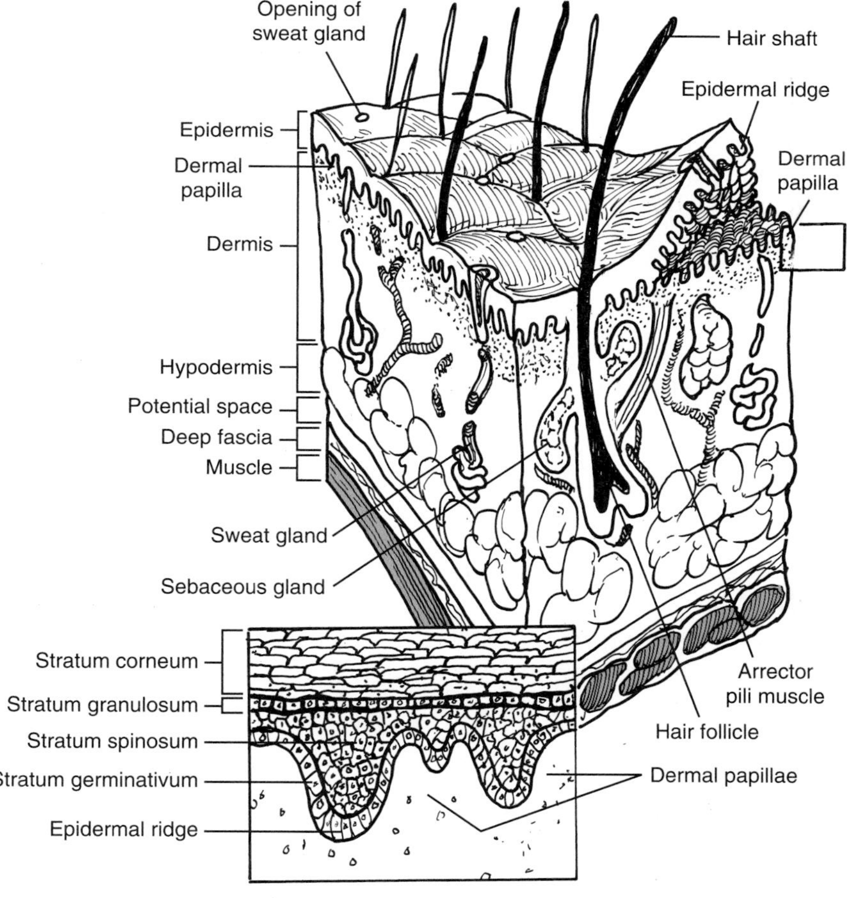

FIGURE 2–1

Integument of the back: the epidermis, dermis, and hypodermis, with the underlying deep fascia and muscle. Sebaceous, sweat, and apocrine glands are formed by downgrowths of epidermis. Hair follicles are composite structures formed by the epidermis and dermis together. Langerhans cells (from bone marrow) and melanocytes (from the neural crest) are also found within the epidermis. Nerves, nerve endings, and blood vessels ramify throughout the dermis.

underlying muscles of the back and contributes to the integration of their actions (see Chapter 5).

SURFACE ANATOMY

Contours and protrusions of the posterior integument of the back provide useful landmarks for localizing underlying structures

Protrusions and topographic landmarks of the body that can be observed at the surface of the skin reveal the location of specific bony structures (Fig. 2–2*A*, and see Chapter 3).

- Major elements of the **axial skeleton** (skull, vertebral column, ribs, and sternum) may be directly observed or **palpated** (felt with the fingers).
- Palpation may locate and identify specialized processes associated with these bones, such as the prominent **occipital protuberance** at the base of the skull.
- **Vertebral spines** of the cervical, thoracic, and lumbar **vertebrae** can be palpated along the entire course of the **vertebral column** from the base of the skull to the pelvis.
- Even the boundary between the cervical and thoracic vertebrae can be deduced from the location of the more prominent spines of vertebrae C6, C7, T1, and T2.
- The 12 thoracic vertebrae progress inferiorly to the inferior limits of the **rib cage,** the general region of which can be located by palpating the **twelfth pair of ribs.**
- All 12 pairs of ribs and the **intercostal spaces** between them can be palpated along the anterolateral aspect of the trunk.
- The five lumbar vertebrae span the interval from the lowest ribs to a level just inferior to the **iliac crests** of the pelvis (which are located at the level of vertebra L4) and superior to the prominent **posterior superior iliac spines.**
- The five sacral vertebrae are fused, forming the **sacrum,** which spans the interval from the lowest lumbar vertebra to the palpable **coccygeal vertebrae (coccyx; tailbone).**

Other prominent landmarks in superolateral regions of the back are the paired **scapular bones,** which, with the anterior clavicles, humerus bones, and bones of the forearms, wrists, hands, and fingers, make up the **appendicular skeleton** of the upper extremities (see Chapter 19). Scapular landmarks that are especially prominent include the **inferior** and **superior scapular angles** (the inferior and superior apices); the **acromial process** laterally and **coracoid process** anteriorly; the lateral, medial, and superior **borders of the scapula;** and the oblique **spine of the scapula** (Fig. 2–2*A* and *B*). The student should attempt to palpate these landmarks on his or her own (or another's) body.

▲ Soft Tissues

Bony landmarks of the back provide clues for localizing soft tissue structures such as muscles

Palpable bony structures of the back serve as landmarks for defining soft tissue structures of the back (Fig. 2–2). The cranium, vertebral column, ribs, and scapulae serve as attachment sites for important stabilizing **ligaments** and for several functional groups of muscles of the back. These muscles include

- two layers of **extrinsic muscles,**
  - the **appendicular muscles** (superficial layer);
  - the so-called **respiratory muscles** (intermediate layer); and
- one layer of **intrinsic muscles,** the **deep back muscles** (deep layer).

Bony landmarks are particularly useful in locating specialized deep back muscles of the **suboccipital region.**

▲ Triangle of Auscultation and Lumbar Triangle

Bony landmarks and muscles are guides to the location of clinically significant "voids" in the back musculature, namely, the triangle of auscultation and the lumbar triangle

The **triangle of auscultation** is bounded medially by the trapezius muscle, laterally by the medial border of the scapula, and inferiorly by the superior border of the latissimus dorsi muscle (Fig. 2–2*B*). When the scapula is rotated laterally (as the inferior angle of the scapula moves laterally), the sixth and seventh ribs and associated intercostal muscles are the only barriers between the superficial fascia and pleural cavities. For this reason, identification of this area is useful in **auscultation** (listening to sounds made by body structures) of the lungs and heart.

The **lumbar triangle** is bounded medially and superiorly by the inferolateral border of the latissimus dorsi muscle, laterally and superiorly by the external abdominis muscle, and inferiorly by the iliac crest of the pelvic bone (Fig. 2–2*B*).

> The location of the lumbar triangle is often revealed by hernias or infections occurring within it.

MUSCLES OF THE BACK AND THEIR RELATION TO SKELETAL AND NEURAL STRUCTURES

Muscles of the back are layered in discrete functional groups

Back muscles of each functional group lie in discrete layers separated by investments of dense **deep fascia** and are associated with skeletal elements that support and mediate their functions (see Chapter 5). From superficial to deep, the layers are

- the appendicular muscles;
- the serratus posterior muscles, which are also designated as so-called respiratory muscles; and

BOX 2–1
NAMING OF THE BACK MUSCLES

Various criteria for the naming of anatomic structures are evident in the names of appendicular muscles. One criterion is that structures may be named for their **shape.** Such muscles include the latissimus dorsi muscles (from the Latin *lat,* which means broad or wide), rhomboid major and minor muscles (from the Greek *rhomb,* which means a parallelogram with equal sides), deltoid muscles (from the Greek letter delta, which has a triangular shape), teres major and teres minor muscles (from the Latin *tere,* which means round and smooth), and serratus anterior muscles (from the Latin for a saw or notched object).

Structures may be named for their **location** in the body. Muscles named for their locations include the latissimus dorsi muscles (from the Latin *dorso,* which means the back); supraspinatus muscle (above the spine of the scapula); infraspinatus muscle (below the spine of the scapula); and subscapularis muscle (under the scapula on its anterior side). The addition of the term *anterior* to the name of a structure (e.g., serratus anterior muscle) implies that a posterior muscle with the same name also exists (e.g., serratus posterior muscle) (see below). The terms *internal* and *external, superior* and *inferior,* and *lateral* and *medial* are also used to designate the relative locations of anatomic structures.

Some anatomic names denote the **relative size** of a structure. For example, the term *major,* as in the rhomboid major, teres major, and pectoralis major muscles, implies that rhomboid minor, teres minor, and pectoralis minor muscles also exist. The terms *maximus* and *minimus, greater* and *lesser,* and *longus* and *brevis* are used in a similar fashion.

Additional criteria for the naming of anatomic structures are evident in the list of deep back muscles. For example, anatomic structures may be named for their **function.** Such muscles include the erector spinae muscles, which hold the spine erect; rotatores muscles, which rotate the spine; and levatores costarum muscles, which are thought to elevate the ribs. Other muscles are named for their **attachment sites.** Included among these are the transversospinal muscles, which connect the transverse process of one vertebra to the spine of another vertebra; interspinales muscles, which connect the spine of one vertebra to the spine of another vertebra; and iliocostalis muscles, which connect the iliac crest to the ribs.

Parts of the deep back muscles may be named for the **region of the trunk** in which they are located. Examples include the iliocostalis cervicis, iliocostalis thoracis, and iliocostalis lumborum muscles and the longissimus cervicis, longissimus thoracis, and longissimus lumborum muscles.

- the deep back muscles, including the suboccipital muscles (see Chapter 5).

Box 2–1 explains the conventions for naming the back muscles. These conventions can also be applied to naming other structures of the body.

▲ Appendicular Muscles

The appendicular muscles lie just deep to the skin and superficial fascia of the back, attaching the mobile clavicle, scapula, and humerus bones to the vertebrae, ribs, and sternum of the axial skeleton (see Fig. 2–2*B* and *C* and Chapters 5 and 20). Appendicular muscles encountered in the back are

- the **trapezius,**
- **levator scapulae,**
- **rhomboid major** and **minor,**
- **teres major** and **minor,**
- **deltoid,**
- **supraspinatus,**
- **infraspinatus,**
- **subscapularis,**
- **latissimus dorsi,** and
- **serratus anterior muscles.**

The **pectoralis major** and **minor** and **subclavius muscles** also belong to this group of appendicular muscles but are located on the ventral body wall.

▲ Intermediate Muscle Layer

Just deep to the appendicular muscles lies an intermediate muscle layer consisting of

- the **serratus posterior superior** and
- **serratus posterior inferior muscles** (see Fig. 2–2*C*)

These muscles are developmentally related to the **anterolateral muscles of the trunk,** such as the thoracic **intercostal muscles** and **abdominal muscles.** Once the serratus posterior muscles have migrated onto the back during embryonic development, they become fixed just deep to the appendicular musculature. The serratus posterior muscles are called **respiratory muscles** by some anatomists because they are attached to the vertebral spines and ribs. This arrangement suggests that the muscles may elevate or depress some of the ribs during respiration. However, from functional evidence, it is unclear whether these muscles actually serve as respiratory muscles in humans (see Chapter 6).

▲ True Deep Back Muscles

Deep to the serratus posterior muscles are the deep muscles of the back, including

- the **erector spinae,**
- **transversospinalis,**
- **interspinales,**
- **intertransverse groups of muscles,** and

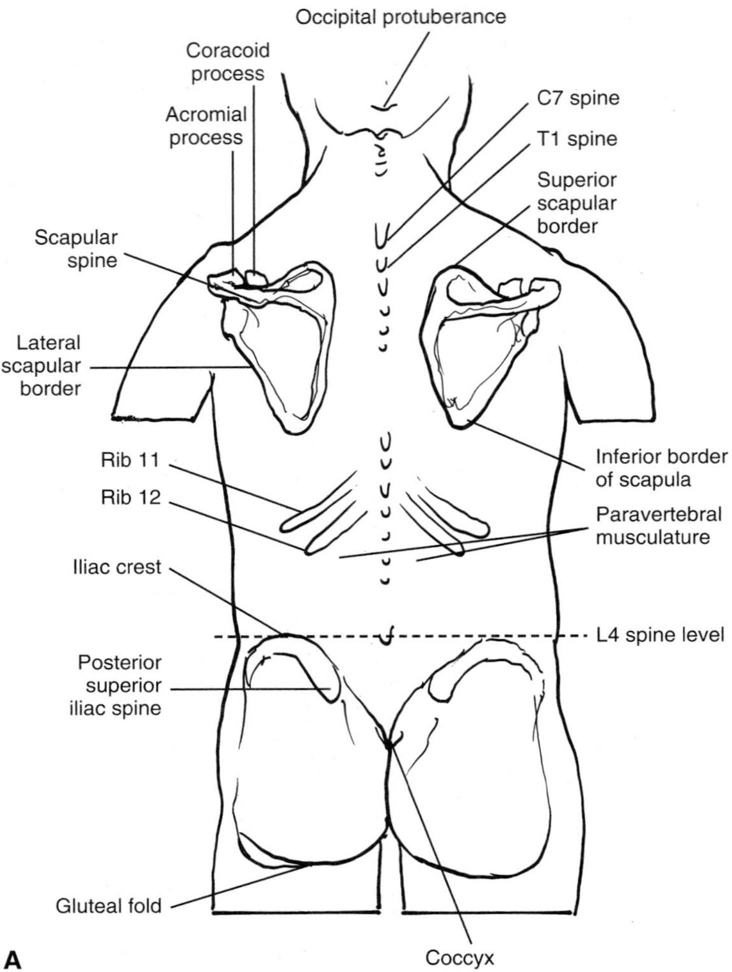

FIGURE 2–2

A. Bony landmarks of the back. Posterior aspect of the back showing its palpable bony landmarks. **B.** Appendicular muscles of the back. The most superficial muscles of the back are the appendicular muscles. These muscles are innervated by named nerves of the brachial plexus and are vascularized by named branches of the subclavian arteries.

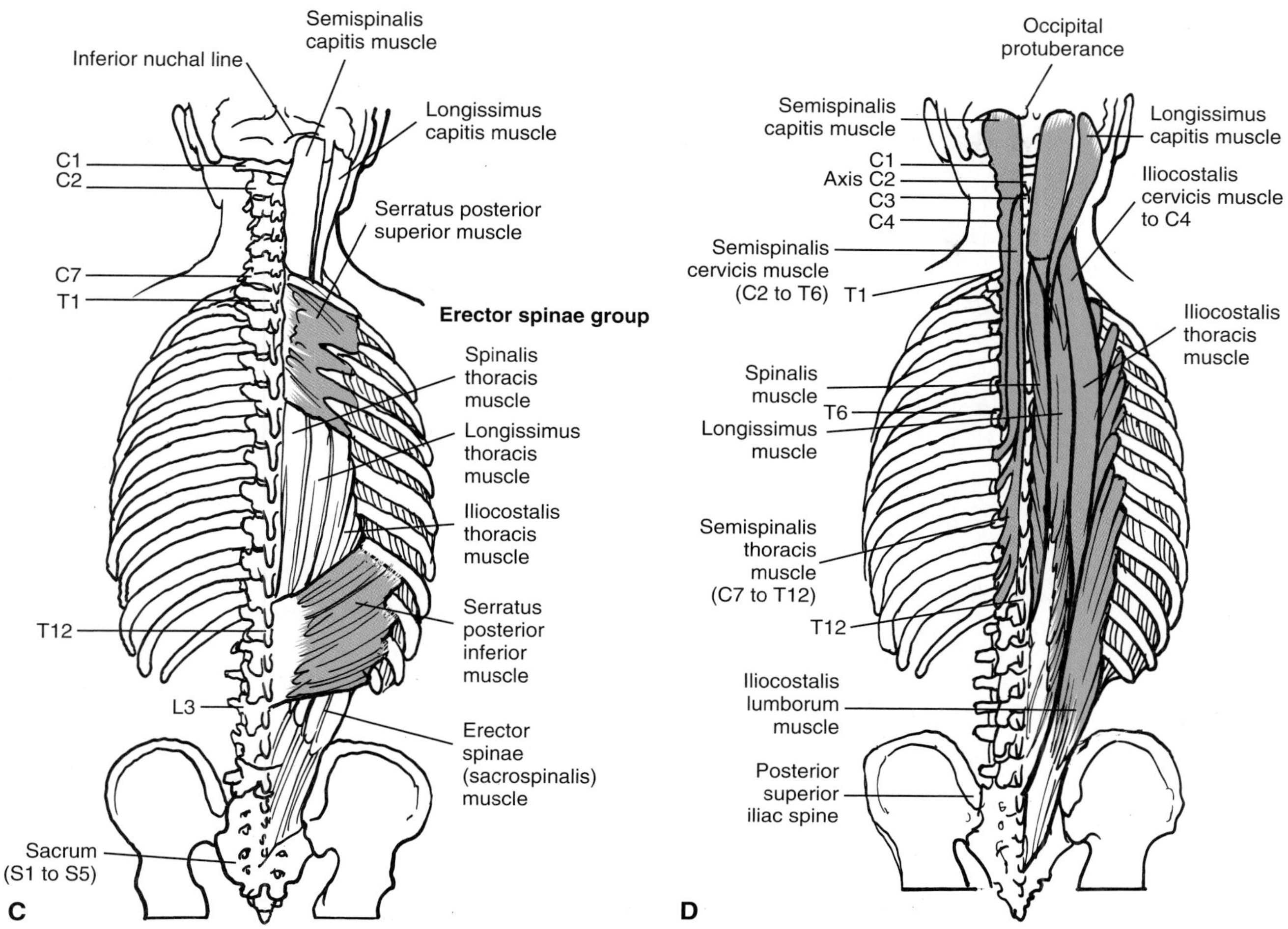

FIGURE 2–2, cont'd

C. Hypomeric so-called respiratory muscles of the back. The serratus posterior superior and serratus posterior inferior muscles are located between the superficial appendicular muscles and the deep back muscles. These muscles are innervated by ventral primary rami and vascularized by repeating intersegmental arteries of the thoracic region. **D.** Erector spinae muscles and deep back muscles. Some of the deep back muscles, the erector spinae muscles, and some of the transversospinalis group of muscles (i.e., the semispinalis muscles) are shown. These muscles are innervated by dorsal primary rami of the cervical, thoracic, and lumbar regions and vascularized by derivatives of intersegmental arteries in the cervical region (see text) and by intersegmental arteries in the thoracic and lumbar regions. *Continued*

- **suboccipital muscles** (see Fig. 2–2*C* to *E* and Chapter 5).

The erector spinae group includes

- the **spinalis,**
- **longissimus,** and
- **iliocostalis muscles** (see Fig. 2–2*C* and *D*).

The transversospinal group includes

- the **rotatores,**
- **multifidus,** and
- **semispinalis muscles** (see Fig. 2–2*D* to *F* and Chapter 5).

In addition

- the **interspinales muscles** connect contiguous spines of the vertebrae, and
- the **posterior proper intertransverse muscles** connect the transverse processes of the vertebrae (see Fig. 2–2*E*).

All of these muscles develop in intimate association with the spines and transverse processes of the vertebrae and become firmly attached to these elements of the axial skeleton. The development of the intertransverse muscles is closely related to the development of another group of so-called respiratory muscles: the **levatores costarum muscles** (see Fig. 2–2*E* and Chapter 5). The levatores costarum muscles are thus best classified as deep back muscles (see discussion of the innervation of so-called respiratory muscles and Fig. 2–8).

The **suboccipital muscles** of the cervical region include

- the **rectus capitis posterior major,**
- **rectus capitis posterior minor,**
- **obliquus capitis superior,** and
- **obliquus capitis inferior muscles.**

Other deep back muscles of the posterior cervical

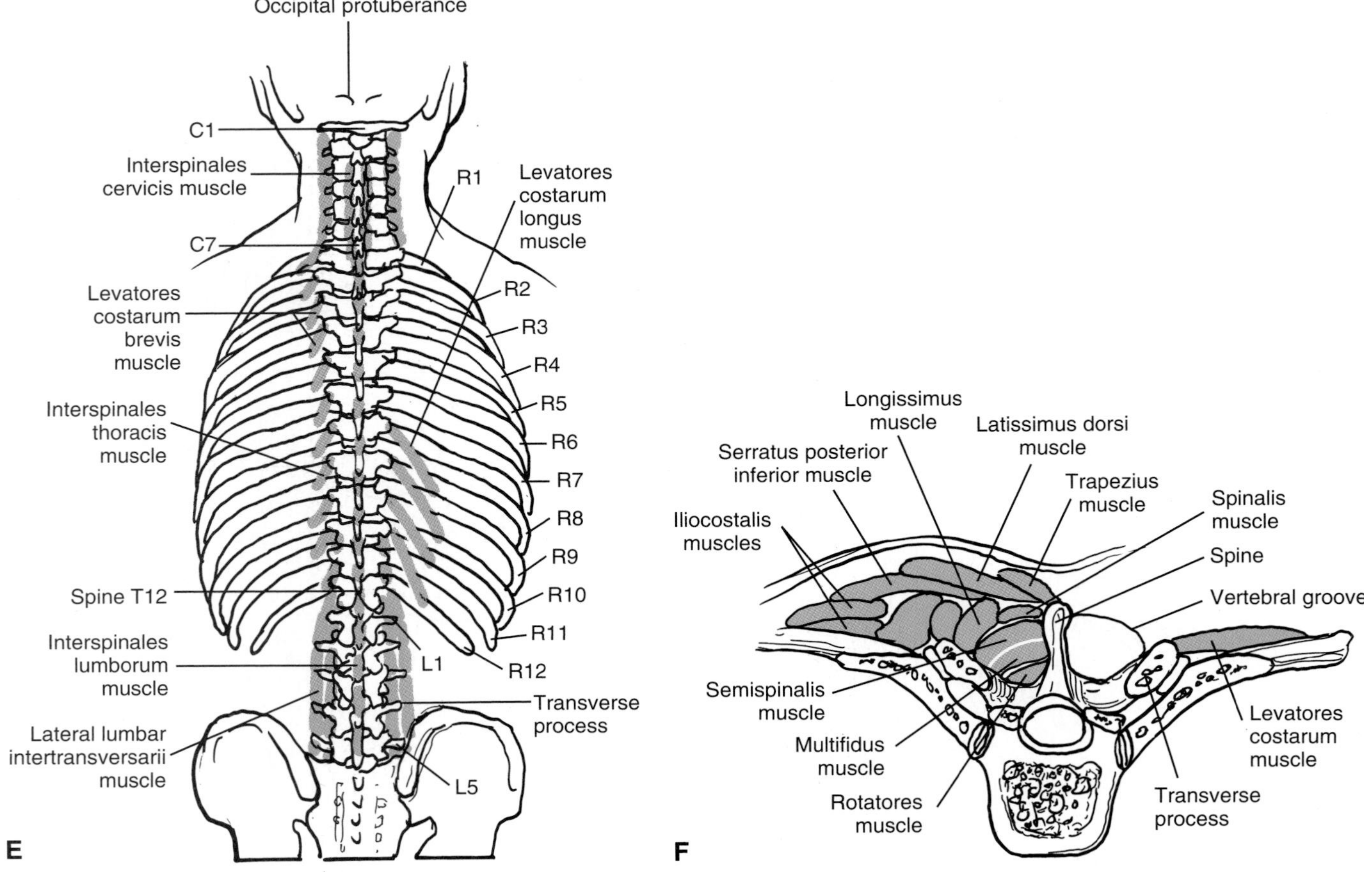

FIGURE 2–2, cont'd

E. Transversospinal muscles, so-called respiratory muscles (i.e., levatores costarum muscles), and deep back muscles. Some of the deep back muscles, including the intertransverse, levatores costarum, and semispinalis muscles. These muscles are innervated by dorsal primary rami and by derivatives of intersegmental arteries in the cervical region and by intersegmental arteries in the thoracic and lumbar regions. **F.** Muscle layers of the back. Cross section of the back musculature showing superficial appendicular muscles (latissimus dorsi and trapezius muscles); the intermediate layer, consisting of the serratus posterior superior and inferior muscles; and the deepest layer, consisting of the deep back muscles (spinalis, longissimus, iliocostalis, semispinalis, multifidus, and rotatores muscles).

region that are not members of the suboccipital, transversospinal, or erector spinae groups are

- the **splenius capitis** and
- **splenius cervicis muscles** (see Chapter 5).

Fig. 2–2*F* shows some of the back muscles and a vertebra in cross section to illustrate the relative positions of the muscles with respect to the surface of the back and the spine.

DEVELOPMENT OF THE TRUNK AND BACK

Definitive muscles and skeletal elements at every level of the back develop from similar segments of tissue called **somites.** This mode of development causes the definitive vertebrae and muscles at each vertebral level to be fundamentally similar. In addition, different groups of back muscles arise from different parts of the somite. This results in predictable differences in the innervation and vascularization of the muscle groups. Thus, the following discussion of back development provides a framework for understanding anatomic and functional relationships of structures of the back.

Paraxial Mesoderm and Somites

Somites are repeating subunits of mesoderm that organize the development and definitive anatomy of the trunk

The development of the axial skeleton, muscles, and parts of the wall of the trunk begins with the formation of solid longitudinal rods of paraxial mesoderm on either side of the developing spinal cord during the third week of embryonic life. The rods become segmented into blocks of mesoderm called **somites** during the fourth week as the basic body plan is established (Fig. 2–3*A* and see Fig. 2–5*A*). All of the segments have similar characteristics. Thirty-three pairs of segmentally arranged somites give rise to definitive structures in the trunk: 8 pairs in the cervical region, 12 pairs in the tho-

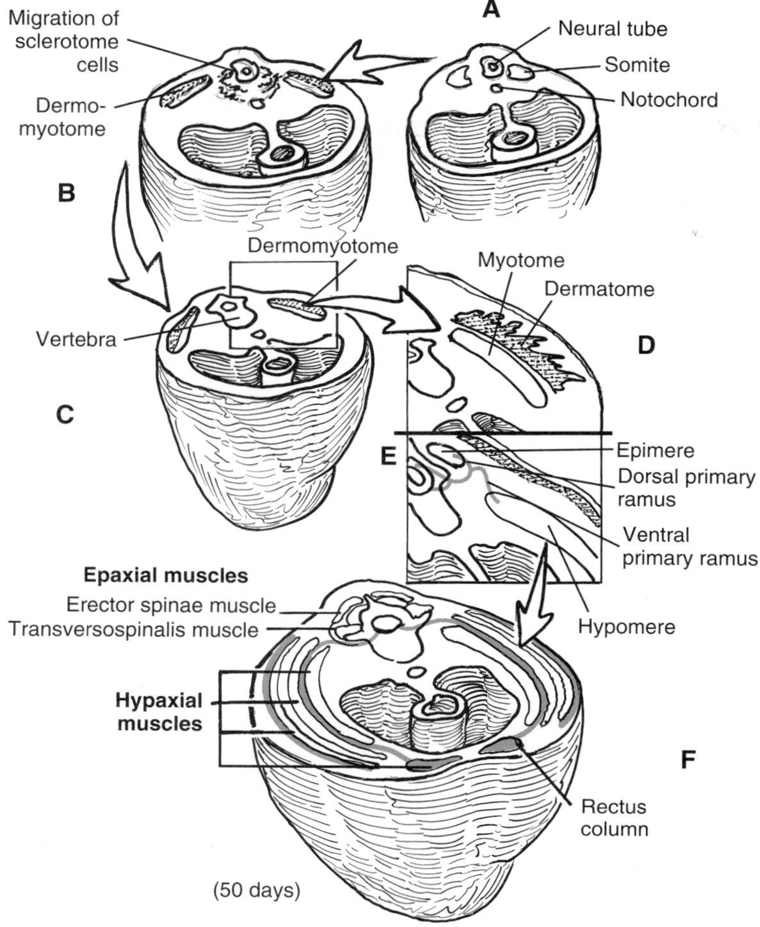

FIGURE 2–3
Derivatives of the somites. Somites give rise to sclerotomes, which form the vertebrae, and dermomyotomes, which form the dermis and the epimeric and hypomeric musculature.

racic region, 5 pairs in the lumbar region, 5 pairs in the sacral region, and 3 pairs in the coccygeal region. Each somite splits into **sclerotomes,** precursors of the vertebrae; **myotomes,** muscles of the body wall; and **dermatomes,** elements of the dermis (Fig. 2–3*B* to *D* and see Fig. 2–4). The myotomes then split to form epimeres and hypomeres. The **epimeres** are precursors of the deep muscles of the back, and the **hypomeres** are precursors of the anterolateral muscles of the trunk (Fig. 2–3*E* and *F*).

The initial segmental organization of the somites is reflected in the organization of the spinal nerves and blood vessels (see below). Each somite induces the outgrowth of a spinal nerve from the neural tube (Fig. 2–4*A*). Each spinal nerve then innervates the vertebral, muscular, and dermal elements that also arise from that somite (Fig. 2–4*B* and see Chapter 4). In addition, successive arteries sprout from longitudinal paired aortas between the somites to vascularize the vertebrae, spinal cord, and body wall (Fig. 2–4*A* and *B* and see Chapter 4). Successive intersegmental veins also sprout from longitudinal veins to form branches that drain the vertebrae, spinal cord, and body wall in the same manner as the intersegmental arteries. It should, therefore, be apparent that the basic plan of the definitive body is **segmental** and that this segmentation begins with the formation of somites (Fig. 2–5).

Because the muscles of the trunk wall originate from the segmental somites, it should not be surprising that they have many characteristics in common. Likewise, the vertebrae at all levels of the trunk can be readily recognized as variations on a common theme (see Chapter 3). Even the sacrum is formed by the fusion of subunits that give rise to individual vertebrae at other levels of the trunk. In addition, the nerves, arteries, and veins within different segments of the trunk have many common anatomic features. An awareness of the common origins of structures at different levels of the trunk simplifies the study of these structures.

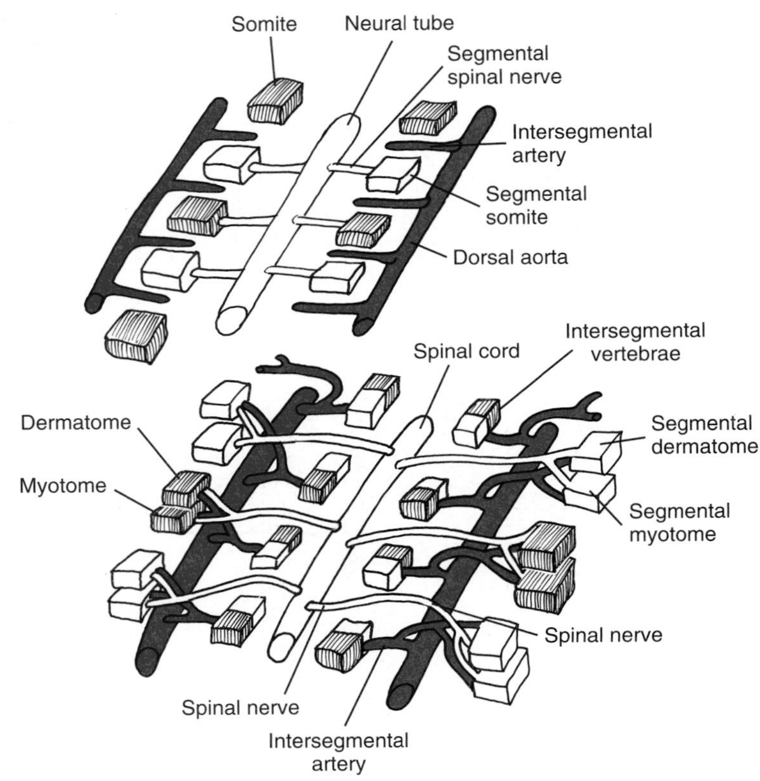

FIGURE 2–4

Nerves and vessels of the back. The segmental spinal nerves and intersegmental vessels innervate and vascularize descendants of the somites.

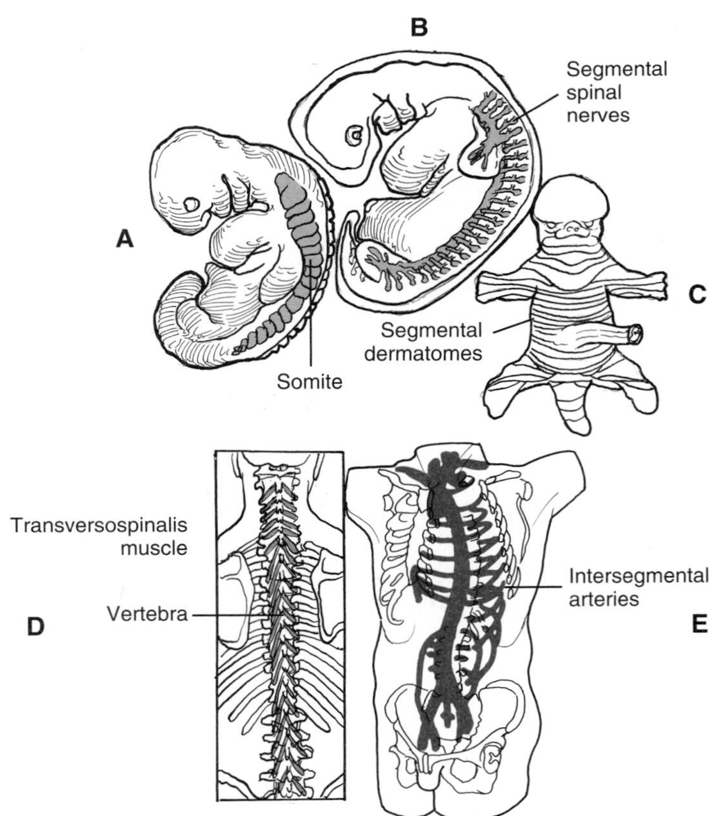

FIGURE 2–5

Segmentation of the trunk. **A.** Segmental somites in a 4-week-old human embryo. **B.** Segmental outgrowth of spinal nerves in a 4-week-old embryo. **C.** Distribution of dermatomes in a 6-week-old embryo. **D.** Posterior view of adult showing segmental vertebrae, ribs, and transversospinalis muscles. **E.** Anterior and left lateral view of trunk of adult showing intersegmental arteries.

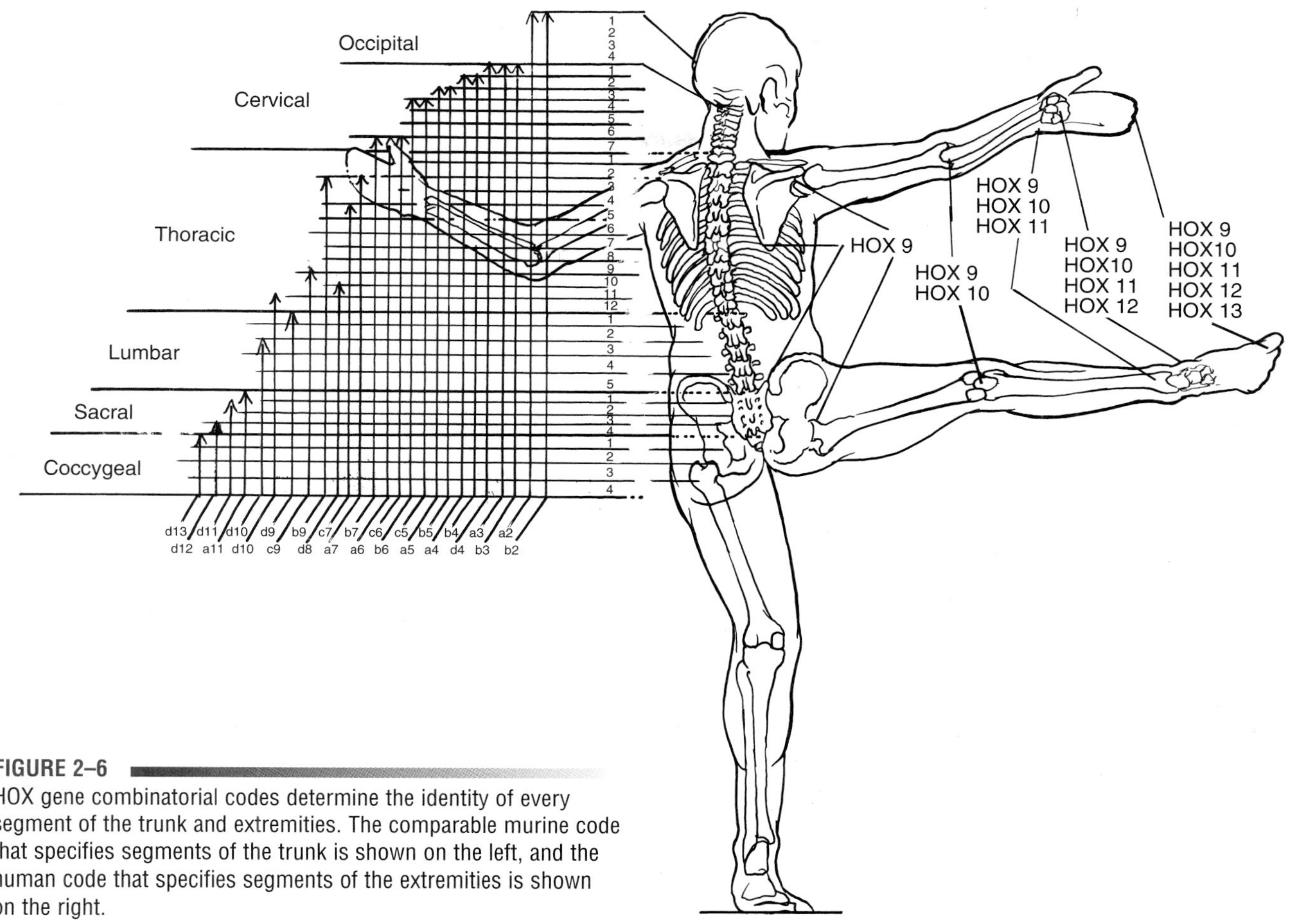

FIGURE 2–6
HOX gene combinatorial codes determine the identity of every segment of the trunk and extremities. The comparable murine code that specifies segments of the trunk is shown on the left, and the human code that specifies segments of the extremities is shown on the right.

▲ Genetic Control of Segmentation of the Trunk and Back

The expression of regulatory genes underlies vertebrate body segmentation and determines the number and identity of body segments

The segmentation of the paraxial mesoderm into somites is controlled by the expression of **regulatory genes.** These genes encode growth factors such as fibroblast growth factor and transcription factors. Although the mechanism is not wholly understood, the factors produced by several of these genes are expressed at the presumptive boundaries of the somites within the paraxial mesoderm, thereby regulating their separation from each other (see Chapter 5). Once the 37 pairs of somites (including 4 pairs of occipital somites) and 7 pairs of cranial somitic precursors called **somitomeres** are formed in the human embryo, each pair specifically differentiates to reflect an identity characteristic of its particular level within the trunk or head (Fig. 2–6). For example, thoracic somites produce vertebrae that bear ribs, whereas cervical and lumbar somites produce vertebrae that lack ribs (see Chapter 3).

The unique differentiation of each segment of the body is under the control of a group of regulatory genes called **HOX genes** (Fig. 2–6). The expression of unique groups of these HOX genes (i.e., a **combinatorial code of HOX genes**) at any given level of the trunk, head, or neck and even along the proximodistal axis of the limbs determines the specific development of the bone and soft tissue structures at that level.

It is now known that mutations or disruptions of some HOX genes alter the identity of structures developing at a given level (e.g., the combinatorial code of HOX gene expression that specifies a cervical vertebra may be changed to a code that more accurately specifies a thoracic vertebra, resulting in development of ribs at the cervical level). Disturbances of HOX gene development explain specific transformations and malformations of limb segments; axial (vertebral column) malformations; and soft tissue anomalies of craniofacial, urinary, and genital structures. Therefore, the concept of segmental development of the human body is not only useful as a tool for learning fundamental anatomy, but also important in understanding certain clinical conditions.

▲ Classification of Trunk and Back Muscles Based on Development

A useful classification of trunk muscles is based on the muscles' developmental origins

All striated (voluntary) muscles of the trunk arise from mesoderm of the somite. However, different functional groups of these muscles arise from different parts of the somite. These muscles, all encountered in the back, are the

- ♦ appendicular muscles associated with the trunk,
- ♦ deep muscles of the back, and
- ♦ anterolateral muscles of the thorax and abdomen.

Before the somite splits into a sclerotome, myotome, and dermatome (see Fig. 2–3), myoblasts within the somite migrate into the developing limb buds to form the **appendicular muscles** of the upper and lower extremities. Once the myotome is produced, it splits into an epimere and a hypomere. Epimeres give rise to the **deep back muscles** and hypomeres to the **anterolateral muscles** of the trunk (see Fig. 2–3). Because these different groups of muscles originate from different parts of the° somite, their innervation and vascularization differ in predictable ways (Table 2–1).

▲ Innervation of Specific Subgroups of Back Muscles

The origins of muscles from different parts of the somite explain their innervation by specific branches of spinal nerves

As has been noted, all of the striated (voluntary) muscles of the trunk arise from somites (see Fig. 2–3). Certain muscle subgroups arise from different parts of the somite and, as a consequence, are innervated by different major branches of the spinal nerves. As the myotomes split into ventral **hypomeres** and dorsal **epimeres,** the outgrowing spinal nerves divide into two major branches, the **ventral primary ramus** and **dorsal primary ramus** (Fig. 2–7*inset* and see Fig. 4–6). Each of these primary branches contains the same mixture of functional motor and sensory axons (see Chapter 4). Developing muscle cells within hypomeres become innervated by nerves that branch from the ventral primary ramus, while epimeric muscles become innervated by nerves that branch from the dorsal primary ramus. Finally, muscles of the upper extremity are innervated by a special group of ventral rami that are organized as a brachial plexus (see Chapter 21).

Innervation of Deep Back Muscles

Deep back muscles are defined by their innervation by branches of dorsal primary rami

Deep muscles of the back arise from epimeres and are, therefore, innervated segmentally by nerves that branch from dorsal primary rami of the spinal nerves, as are the skin and subcutaneous connective tissue overlying these muscles (Fig. 2–7 and see Fig. 4–6 and Table 2–1). After removal of the integument of the back in the laboratory, it may be possible to see the cutaneous branches of the spinal nerves, which penetrate the superficial layer of appendicular muscles. Cutaneous nerves of the cervical and upper thoracic regions are closer to the midline because they are formed by medial branches of dorsal primary rami. Cutaneous nerves in lower regions of the trunk are formed by lateral branches of dorsal primary rami. In contrast, muscles of the lateral and anterior body wall arise from hypomeres and are, therefore, innervated by branches of ventral primary rami of the spinal nerves (Fig. 2–7 and see Fig. 4–6). The skin overlying these anterolateral muscles is also segmentally innervated by branches of ventral primary rami. In addition, deep branches of these ventral rami innervate the thin membrane that lines the pleural cavities (parietal pleura [see Chapter 6]) and the peritoneal cavity (parietal peritoneum; see Chapter 11). Each segment of the body wall innervated by a specific spinal nerve is called a **dermatome** (Fig. 2–7 and see Chapter 4).

As has been noted above, many of the deep back muscles remain distinctly segmental in adults. For example, the small **interspinales muscles** extend from one vertebral spine to the next, and the **posterior intertransversarii muscles** connect adjacent transverse processes. Similarly, each short **rotatores muscle** of the **transversospinal group of muscles** arises from a single epimere and courses from the transverse process of one vertebra to the lateral surface of the lamina of the vertebra immediately superior to it. These muscles are very similar from one level to the next. Each muscle is innervated by a nerve arising from a single dorsal primary ramus, which branches from a single spinal nerve at the same level.

On the other hand, many of the deep back muscles are formed by the fusion of individual epimeres originating from myotomes at two or more segmental levels. The **multifidus muscles** of the transversospinal group form by fusion of epimeres at two to four segmental levels, while the **semispinalis muscles** of the transversospinal group form by fusion of epimeres at as many as six or seven segmental levels. Likewise, the spinalis, iliocostalis, and longissimus muscles of the **erector spinae group** of deep muscles are derived from epimeres arising at many levels of the trunk. Typically, the number of spinal nerves innervating these composite multifidus, semispinalis, and erector spinae muscles is the same as the number of fused epimeres from which the nerves were formed. The **splenius capitis** and **splenius cervicis muscles** are formed by the fusion of several cervical epimeres. Therefore, the splenius capitis muscles are innervated by dorsal rami of the middle cervical nerves, and the splenius cervicis muscles are innervated by dorsal rami of the lower cervical nerves. Like all of the deep back muscles, the **suboccipital muscles** arise from epimeres and are innervated by the dorsal ramus of the first cervical (suboccipital) nerve.

TABLE 2–1
Muscles Encountered in the Superficial Dissection of the Back and Their Innervation and Vascularization

Muscle	Innervation	Vascularization
APPENDICULAR MUSCLES (DERIVED FROM SOMITIC MYOBLASTS)		
Trapezius	Spinal accessory nerve	Superficial branch of transverse cervical vessel
Levator scapulae	Dorsal scapular nerve	Superficial branch of transverse cervical vessel
Rhomboid major	Dorsal scapular nerve	Deep branch of transverse cervical vessel or dorsal scapular vessel
Rhomboid minor	Dorsal scapular nerve	Deep branch of transverse cervical vessel or dorsal scapular vessel
Teres major	Lower subscapular nerve	Deep branch of transverse cervical vessel or dorsal scapular vessel, posterior humeral circumflex vessel
Teres minor	Axillary nerve	Deep branch of transverse cervical vessel or dorsal scapular vessel
Deltoid	Axillary nerve	Deltoid branch of thoracoacromial vessel, subscapular vessel, posterior humeral circumflex vessel
Supraspinatus	Suprascapular nerve	Suprascapular vessel
Infraspinatus	Suprascapular nerve	Suprascapular vessel
Subscapularis	Upper and lower subscapular nerves	Subscapular vessel
Latissimus dorsi	Thoracodorsal nerve	Subscapular vessel
Serratus anterior	Long thoracic nerve	Lateral thoracic vessel
HYPOMERIC MUSCLES		
Serratus posterior	Ventral primary rami of spinal nerves T2 to T5	Superior thoracic intercostal vessels
Serratus posterior inferior	Ventral primary rami of spinal nerves T9 to T12	Inferior thoracic intercostal vessels
Lateral part of intertransversarii	Ventral primary rami of cervical and lumbar spinal nerves	Vertebral, occipital, and deep cervical vessels of cervical region and intersegmental vessels of lumbar region
Intercostal	Ventral primary rami of spinal nerves T1 to T11	Intersegmental vessels of thoracic region (intercostal vessels)

Continued

Innervation of "Respiratory" Muscles

Some of the so-called respiratory muscles arise from epimeres and some arise from hypomeres

The importance of the developmental origins of muscles in understanding muscle innervation is well illustrated by the so-called respiratory muscles of the back. The **levatores costarum muscles** arise from epimeres and are innervated by dorsal rami of the thoracic spinal nerves, while the **serratus posterior superior** and **serratus posterior inferior muscles** arise from hypomeres and are innervated by ventral primary rami of the spinal nerves (see Table 2–1). A brief review of the derivation of the intertransverse muscles provides more details about the relationship between three muscle groups of the trunk: the **intertransverse, levatores costarum,** and **intercostal muscles.**

The cervical, thoracic, and lumbar regions all have **intertransverse muscles,** which connect transverse processes or associated structures of adjacent vertebrae (Fig. 2–8 and see Fig. 2–2*E*). In the cervical region, these intertransverse muscles may be divided into medial and lateral parts. The medial posterior proper intertransver-

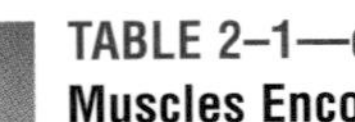

TABLE 2–1—cont'd
Muscles Encountered in the Superficial Dissection of the Back and Their Innervation and Vascularization

Muscle	Innervation	Vascularization
EPIMERIC MUSCLES OF BACK		
Erector spinae Spinalis, longissimus, iliocostalis	Dorsal primary rami of cervical, thoracic, and lumbar spinal nerves	Vertebral, occipital, and deep cervical vessels of cervical region and intersegmental vessels of thoracic and lumbar regions
Transversospinal Rotatores	Dorsal rami of cervical, thoracic, and lumbar spinal nerves	Vertebral, occipital, and deep cervical vessels of cervical region and intersegmental vessels of thoracic and lumbar regions
Multifidus	Dorsal rami of cervical, thoracic, and lumbar spinal nerves	Vertebral, occipital, and deep cervical vessels of cervical region and intersegmental vessels of thoracic and lumbar regions
Semispinalis	Dorsal rami of cervical and thoracic spinal nerves and spinal nerve L1	Vertebral, occipital, and deep cervical vessels of cervical region and intersegmental vessels of thoracic and lumbar regions
Medial part of intertransversarii	Dorsal primary rami of cervical, thoracic, and lumbar spinal nerves	Vertebral, occipital, and deep cervical vessels of cervical region and intersegmental vessels of thoracic and lumbar regions
Levatores costarum	Dorsal primary rami of thoracic spinal nerves	Intercostal vessels
Interspinales	Dorsal primary rami of cervical region; of T1, T2, T11, and T12; and of lumbar spinal nerves	Vertebral, occipital, and deep cervical vessels of cervical region and intersegmental vessels of T1, T2, T11, T12, and lumbar region
Splenius capitis and cervicis	Dorsal primary rami of middle and lower cervical nerves	Vertebral, occipital, and deep cervical vessels of cervical region
Suboccipital		
Rectus capitis posterior major	Dorsal ramus of C1 (suboccipital nerve)	Vertebral and occipital vessels
Rectus capitis posterior minor	Dorsal ramus of C1 (suboccipital nerve)	Vertebral and occipital vessels
Obliquus capitis superior	Dorsal ramus of C1 (suboccipital nerve)	Vertebral and occipital vessels
Obliquus capitis inferior	Dorsal rami of C1 (suboccipital nerve) and of C2 (greater occipital nerve)	Vertebral and occipital vessels

sarii muscles are divided into two slips, but both slips are derived from epimeres and so are innervated by dorsal rami. In contrast, the more lateral intertransversarii muscles are derived from hypomeres and so are innervated by ventral rami (Fig. 2–8 and see Chapter 5).

In the thoracic region the medial part of each intertransverse muscle is also divided into two distinct slips (medial and lateral slips) (Fig. 2–8). The medial slip connects the thoracic transverse processes in the inferior thorax as a **posterior proper intertransverse muscle.** These muscles are poorly developed or absent in more cranial regions of the thorax. The lateral slip of the medial part of the intertransverse muscle, which joins the transverse process of a vertebra with the upper surface of a lower rib, is called a **levatores costarum muscle.** These muscles are found throughout the thoracic region (see Fig. 2–2*E*). Thus, the posterior proper intertransverse and levatores costarum muscles of the thoracic region are innervated by dorsal primary rami. The lateral part of each thoracic intertransverse muscle, however, is elaborated as an **intercostal muscle** (in contrast to the cervical region where it is elaborated as an intertransverse muscle) (see Fig. 5–1). These intercostal muscles, like the lateral parts of the intertransverse muscles of the cervical region, are derived from hypomeres and innervated by ventral primary rami (specifically, the **intercostal nerves**) (Fig. 2–8 and see Fig. 5–1).

In the lumbar region, medial and lateral parts of the intertransverse muscles can also be distinguished. The medial parts are derived from epimeres and are in-

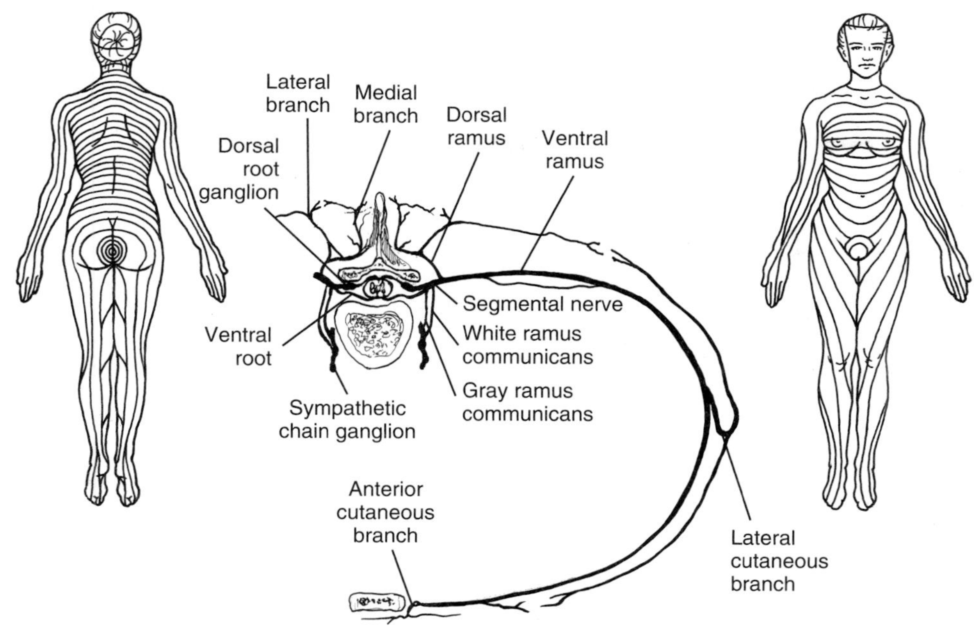

FIGURE 2–7
Dermatomes of the trunk and extremities. Segmental spinal nerves are distributed in beltlike arrays called *dermatomes.* Each dermatome thus represents the primary field of innervation of an individual pair of spinal nerves. However, spinal nerve distributions overlap slightly into adjacent dermatomes. **Inset,** A cross section of a typical spinal nerve. The dorsal root contains sensory fibers, and the ventral root contains motor and autonomic fibers (see Chapter 4). The segmental nerve formed by the joining of the dorsal and ventral roots, therefore, contains all fiber types. This nerve further splits into dorsal and ventral primary rami.

nervated by dorsal primary rami, while the lateral hypomeric muscles are developmentally related to the intercostal muscles of the thoracic region and, thus, are innervated by ventral primary rami (see Figs. 2–2*E,* 2–8, and 5–1). The specific features of these muscles are more completely described and illustrated in Chapter 5.

Innervation of Appendicular Muscles

Appendicular muscles of the back are innervated by special branches of ventral primary rami

Appendicular muscles of the back are associated with elements of the **appendicular skeleton** of the upper extremity and serve to attach the **scapula, clavicle,** and **humerus** to the ribs, sternum, and vertebral column. These muscles will be discussed in detail in Chapter 20, but they will be described briefly here and in Chapter 5 because many of them have such an intimate structural relationship with other muscles of the back.

As has been mentioned, appendicular muscles arise from muscle cells that migrate from the ventrolateral regions of the somites into the developing **limb buds.** Most of these muscles are, therefore, innervated by named nerves that branch from the intermixed ventral primary rami that comprise the **brachial plexus** (see Table 2–1). The only exception to this rule is the **trapezius muscle,** which (along with a ventrolateral muscle of the neck, the **sternocleidomastoid muscle**) receives **motor innervation** from the **eleventh cranial nerve (spinal accessory nerve)** and sensory innervation from spinal nerves C3 and C4 (see Chapter 5).

The **brachial plexus** is a mixture of ventral primary rami arising at spinal cord levels C4 to T1 (see Chapter 21). A similar mixture of ventral primary rami in the lumbar and sacral regions forms the **lumbar** and **sacral plexuses,** which innervate the lower extremities (see Chapter 18).

▲ Vascularization of Specific Subgroups of Back Muscles

Vasculature of the back muscles arises from intersegmental arteries and veins

The vascular pattern within the mesoderm of the developing embryo is initially established by inductive influences of underlying endodermal tissue. It appears that most of the mesodermal tissue forms blood vessels. At first the induction of vascular channels is widespread throughout the embryonic germ disc. Eventually some channels begin to grow much faster than others, giving rise to recognizable arteries and veins of the embryonic and fetal vasculature.

Like the spinal nerves (see Chapter 4), the blood vessels supplying muscles of the back first grow out as re-

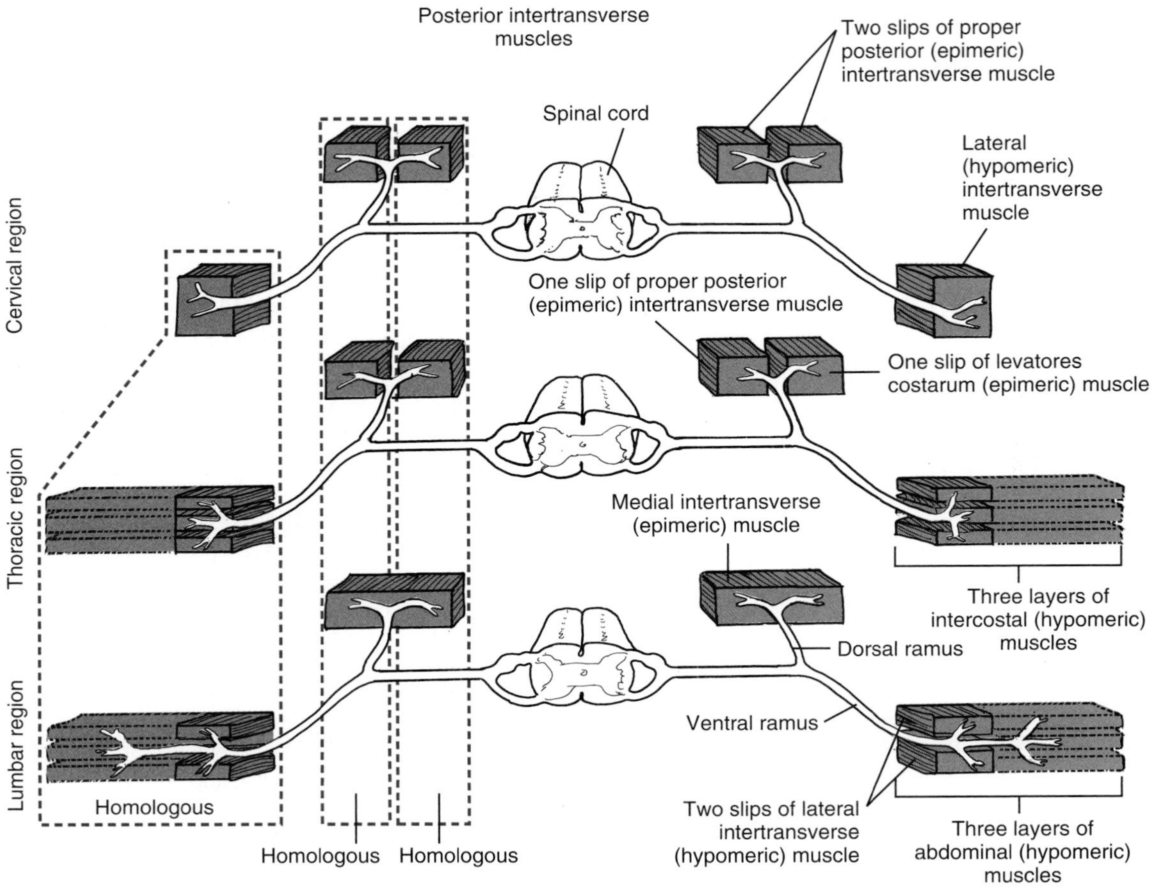

FIGURE 2–8
Origin of the intertransverse, levatores costarum, and intercostal muscles. This diagram illustrates the developmental relationships of intertransverse muscles to the levatores costarum and intercostal muscles. The levatores costarum muscles are homologous to (i.e., have the same embryologic origin as) medial slips of the medial parts of the posterior intertransverse muscles and so are innervated by dorsal primary rami. The intercostal muscles of the thoracic region and anterolateral abdominal muscles are homologous to the more lateral cervical and lumbar intertransverse muscles and so are innervated by ventral primary rami.

peating branches of longitudinally oriented midline structures (see Fig. 2–4). Arteries sprout between developing somites from the paired elongated **dorsal aortas,** which run the length of the trunk. Veins sprout from a paired system of longitudinal veins in the thorax, the presumptive **azygos** and **hemiazygos veins,** and from the longitudinally oriented presumptive **inferior vena cava** in the lumbar region (see Chapters 6 and 10). Because these repeating branches grow out between the developing somites, they are called **intersegmental arteries** and **veins.** Their branches vascularize the vertebral column and spinal cord. It should not be surprising to find that other closely related branches vascularize muscles arising from epimeres and hypomeres that develop in close conjunction with the vertebral column and spinal cord (see Fig. 2–4 and Table 2–1).

Vascularization of Deep Back and So-Called Respiratory Muscles

Most of the deep back muscles and the so-called respiratory muscles are vascularized by intersegmental arteries and veins

However, all of the deep back muscles of the cervical region are vascularized by small branches of the paired **vertebral arteries** and the **occipital** and **deep cervical arteries** (see Table 2–1 and Chapter 21). Nonetheless, these longitudinal arteries are derived from cervical intersegmental arteries, which become connected to each other by longitudinal **anastomoses.** (*Anastomose* means the joining of one vessel directly with another in the absence of an intermediate capillary bed.)

Vascular drainage of the cervical back muscles occurs largely through veins that unite with small tributaries from the vertebral canal. These veins and tributaries form a vessel that becomes a **suboccipital plexus,** which descends with the vertebral artery through the foramina transversaria of vertebrae C2 to C6. The left and right vertebral plexuses condense into the left and right **vertebral veins,** which empty into the left and right brachiocephalic veins. In addition, branches of the vertebral veins anastomose with branches of the **deep cervical vein** to drain into the subclavian vein. The longitudinal vertebral and deep cervical veins (like the vertebral arteries) arise from cervical intersegmental veins, which become connected by longitudinal anastomoses.

The so-called respiratory muscles (i.e., serratus posterior and levatores costarum muscles) and deep back muscles of the thoracic region are vascularized by unnamed **posterior intercostal arteries.** In a similar fashion, deep back muscles of the lumbar region are vascularized by a subcostal artery and branches of the **lumbar arteries.** These vessels are derivatives of the thoracic and lumbar intersegmental arteries, which branch from the originally paired dorsal aortas (see Fig. 2–4 and Chapter 13).

Vascular drainage of the thoracic and lumbar body wall musculature occurs through small branches of the **posterior intercostal, subcostal,** and **lumbar veins** (see Chapter 13).

Vascularization of Appendicular Muscles

Appendicular muscles, including those of the back, are vascularized by branches of a single intersegmental artery and vein

In contrast to the pattern of vasculature of muscles of the body wall, the appendicular muscles of the upper extremity (including the most proximal muscles of the shoulder girdle located in the back) are all vascularized by named branches of the **subclavian arteries** and **veins.** These subclavian vessels arise from the **seventh cervical intersegmental artery** and **vein** (see Table 2–1 and Chapter 21).

3 The Axial Skeleton of the Trunk

The axial skeleton is made up of the **cranium;** the **vertebral column,** which consists of the cervical, thoracic, and lumbar vertebrae, the sacrum, and the coccygeal vertebrae; the **ribs;** and the **sternum.** This chapter focuses on the anatomy and function of the vertebral column only. The ribs and sternum are described in Chapter 6 and the cranium in Chapter 22. The appendicular skeleton, which contains bones of the upper and lower extremities and includes the shoulder girdle (scapula and clavicle) and pelvic girdle (ilia, ischia, and pubes), is discussed in Chapters 16 and 19.

The axial skeleton not only supports and protects soft tissues of the trunk, but it also provides a frame of reference for understanding anatomic relationships of the trunk

The axial skeleton defines the form of the body by serving as the bony substratum to which the soft tissues are attached (Fig. 3–1). Its anatomy is basically the same in all human beings and, therefore, can be used as a frame of reference for understanding the relationships of anatomic structures, a fact that has influenced the organization of this book. Discussions of other regions of the body also begin with a description of the relevant skeletal elements.

The **axial skeleton** of the trunk—specifically, the **vertebral column**—is described in this chapter to lay a foundation for descriptions of the soft tissues of the trunk in the next two chapters, which focus on the **spinal cord** and **spinal nerves** and on the **muscles, nerves,** and **vessels of the back.**

STRUCTURAL UNITS OF THE VERTEBRAL COLUMN: THE VERTEBRAE

Embryonic Development of the Vertebrae

Vertebrae, the building blocks of the vertebral column, arise from the somites

Somites are the precursors of the axial skeleton, muscles, and some of the dermal components of the trunk (see Chapter 2). Somites are paired segments of mesoderm, which split off in a craniocaudal progression from paired solid rods of tissue on both sides of the developing brain and spinal cord. The segmentation continues until 42 to 46 pairs of somites have appeared. Only 37 to 39 pairs survive to form adult structures (i.e., 4 occipital pairs, 8 cervical pairs, 12 thoracic pairs, 5 lumbar pairs, 5 sacral pairs, and 3 to 5 coccygeal pairs). The somites quickly separate further into segments called **dermatomes, myotomes,** and **sclerotomes.**

While the *segmental* myotomes and dermatomes form *segmental* precursors of muscle and dermal tissue (see Chapter 2), the segmental sclerotomes split transversely, and caudal and cranial halves of adjacent sclerotomes fuse together to form the **intersegmental vertebrae.** This process produces 7 cervical, 12 thoracic, 5 lumbar, 5 sacral, and (usually) 3 coccygeal vertebral precursors. The **vertebral column** is formed by the end-to-end association of these repeating vertebral elements. Since precursors to the sacral vertebrae fuse to form the sacrum (see below), the definitive human vertebral column consists of 27 vertebrae and the sacrum (Fig. 3–1).

Basic Features of the Vertebrae

The ventral vertebral body and dorsal vertebral arch are the fundamental elements of a typical vertebra

The basic structure of a vertebra is shown in Fig. 3–2. Most vertebrae have a solid ventral **vertebral body** and a dorsal **vertebral,** or **neural, arch.** Other features may or may not be common to the vertebrae in different regions of the axial skeleton.

The cylindroid vertebral bodies have superior and inferior **junctional surfaces,** which articulate with intervening fibrocartilaginous **intervertebral discs** (see below). The rough central regions of the junctional surfaces are surrounded by a smooth, raised peripheral zone (Fig. 3–2). Foramina (small holes) are located on the anterior, posterior, and lateral surfaces of vertebral bodies. These are sites of penetration by blood vessels. The relatively large foramina on the posterior surfaces of vertebral bodies are orifices for the egress of large **basivertebral veins.**

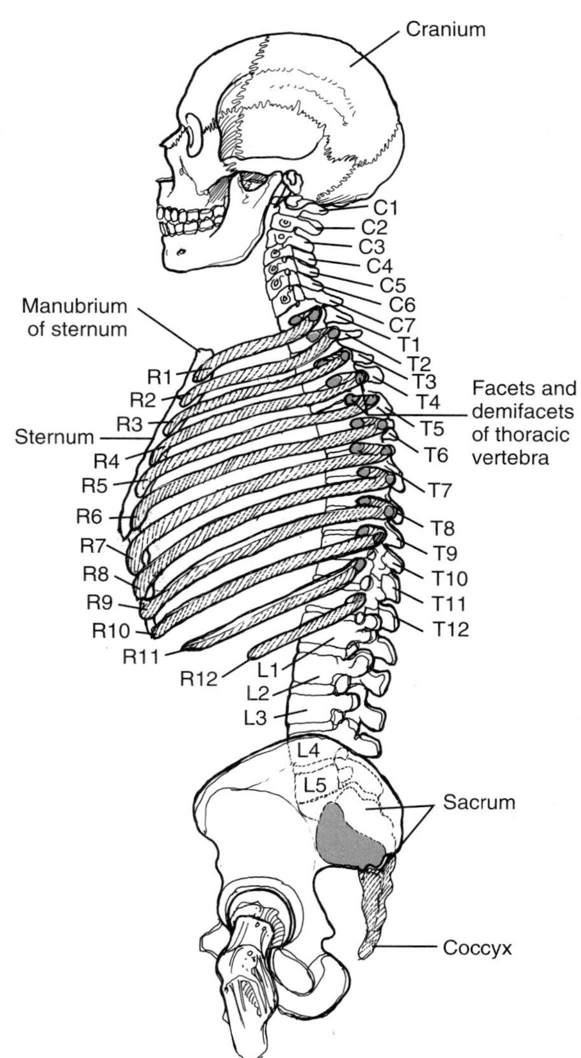

FIGURE 3–1
The axial skeleton includes the cranium, vertebral column, ribs, and sternum (shaded in red). This is in contrast to the appendicular skeleton, which is comprised of the clavicle, scapula, and other bones of the upper extremity (see Chapter 19) and the pelvis and other bones of the lower extremity (see Chapter 16).

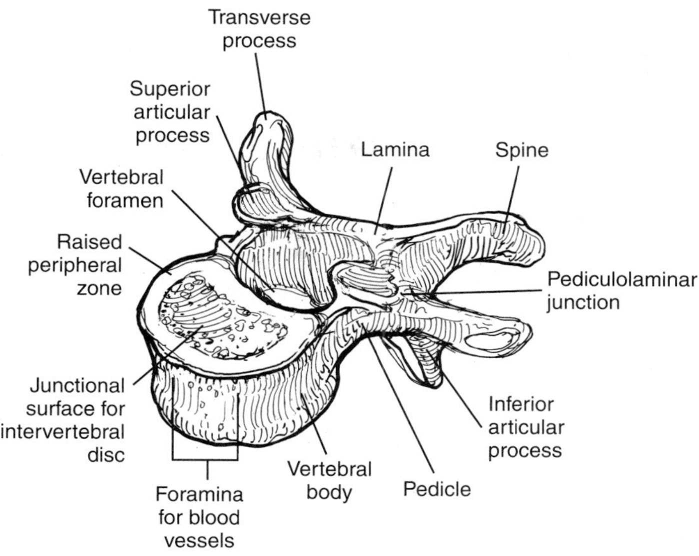

FIGURE 3–2
A typical vertebra, which has a vertebral body, vertebral arch, paired transverse processes, and vertebral spine. However, the first cervical vertebra lacks a spine and the first two cervical vertebrae lack a body. Other vertebrae exhibit other unique features (see Figs. 3–3 to 3–8).

The vertebral arch is made up of paired **pedicles** and **laminae,** which enclose an opening called a **vertebral foramen** (Fig. 3–2). A **transverse process** typically extends laterally from each side of the vertebral arch at the **pediculolaminar junction** (the junction of the pedicles and laminae), and a **vertebral spine** typically extends from the dorsal apex of the arch.

The paired **superior** and **inferior articular processes** also protrude from the pediculolaminar junctions. These processes have **facets,** which are covered with **hyaline articular cartilage.** Each facet forms a **synovial joint** with an apposed facet of an adjacent vertebra (see Figs. 3–19 and 3–20).

A pair of **superior** and **inferior vertebral notches** is located at the superior and inferior boundaries of each of the vertebral pedicles. The superior notch of one vertebra is apposed with the inferior notch of the adjacent vertebra to form an **intervertebral foramen,** which transmits a spinal nerve and associated blood vessels between the vertebral canal and regions exterior to the vertebral column (see Figs. 3–4, 3–20, and 3–22).

▲ Specialized Features of the Vertebrae

Cervical, thoracic, lumbar, sacral, and coccygeal vertebrae have distinctive features that allow them to carry out unique functions

It is useful to know the basic elements of a vertebra, but it must be emphasized that the vertebrae within each region of the trunk differ significantly in structure. These differences allow the vertebrae to perform the unique functions required in each region. Indeed, some components may be highly modified in the vertebrae of one region and entirely absent in the vertebrae of other regions.

Vertebral Bodies. The vertebral bodies are relatively small in the cervical region. They gradually increase in size in a cranial-to-caudal direction along the vertebral column throughout the thoracic and lumbar regions (Fig. 3–3 and see Figs. 3–1, 3–4 and 3–5). In fact, the **first cervical vertebra—vertebra C1** or **atlas**—lacks a definitive vertebral body altogether. In its place, there is a narrow **anterior arch** with a ventrally protruding **anterior tubercle** (Fig. 3–3). The space within the verte-

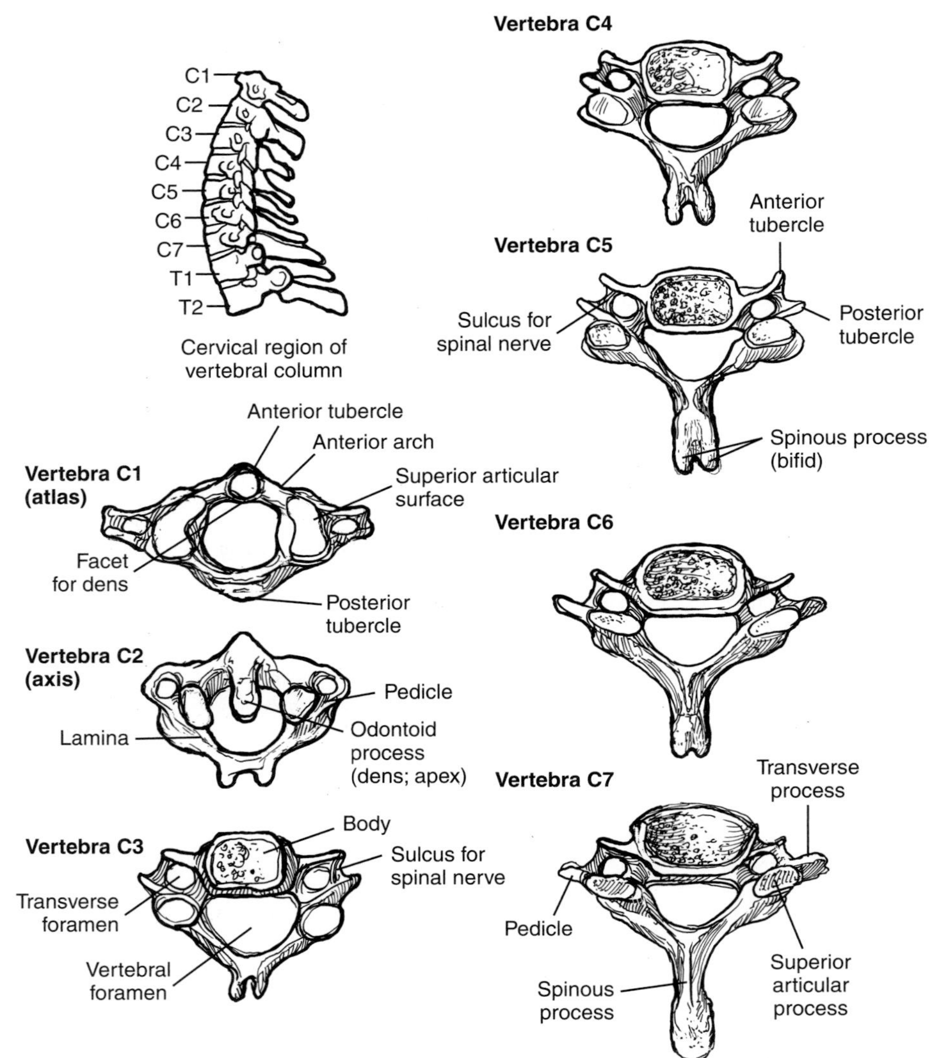

FIGURE 3–3
The first cervical vertebra (atlas) is distinguished by lack of a spine and body. It also has a facet for a unique feature of the second cervical vertebra (the odontoid process, or dens). All of the cervical vertebrae have foramina within their transverse processes to accommodate passage of the vertebral artery and associated veins. The spinous processes of vertebrae C2 to C6 are bifid, whereas the spinous process of vertebra C7 is single.

bral foramen just dorsal to the anterior arch of the atlas is occupied by a bony extension called the **odontoid process,** or **dens** of vertebra C2, or **axis** (see below).

In the thoracic region, the vertebral bodies are larger than they are in the cervical region and are distinguished by small, smooth articulations called **costal facets** on both lateral surfaces (Fig. 3–4). Each facet articulates with the **head** of one of the 12 ribs at a **costovertebral joint.** The facets for ribs 1, 10, 11, and 12 are located wholly upon the surfaces of vertebral bodies T1, T10, T11, and T12, but the facets for ribs 2 through 9 are formed by the association of the **superior demifacet** of one vertebral body with the **inferior demifacet** of the adjacent vertebral body (Fig. 3–4 and see Fig. 3–8*B*).

In the lumbar region, the vertebral bodies are massive and contribute substantially to the functions of support and locomotion (Figs. 3–1 and 3–5).

The bodies (and other elements) of the sacral vertebrae are fused end to end to form a solid bone called the **sacrum** (Fig. 3–6). The most superior sacral vertebral body is the largest, and the bodies of vertebrae S2 to S5 gradually diminish in size. The sacral vertebral bodies are much flatter and wider than the vertebral bodies in other regions. The first sacral vertebral body is easily seen within the pelvis as the **sacral promontory.**

Only the vestiges of vertebral bodies can be identified in the few coccygeal vertebrae remaining in humans (Fig. 3–7). The general structural makeup of the verte-

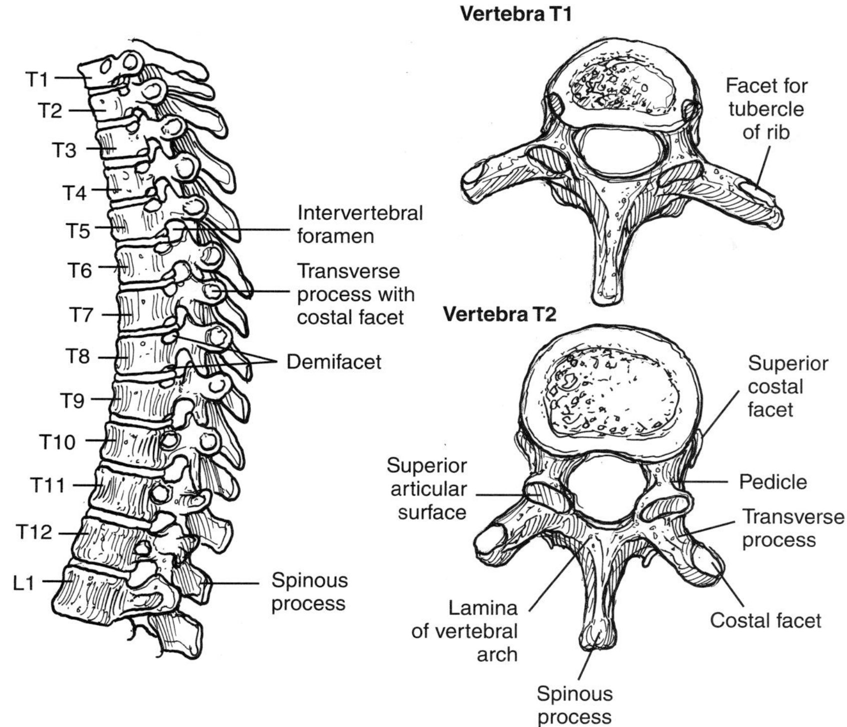

FIGURE 3–4
Thoracic vertebrae. Vertical articular processes and downward-sloping spines contribute to the immobility of this region of the spine.

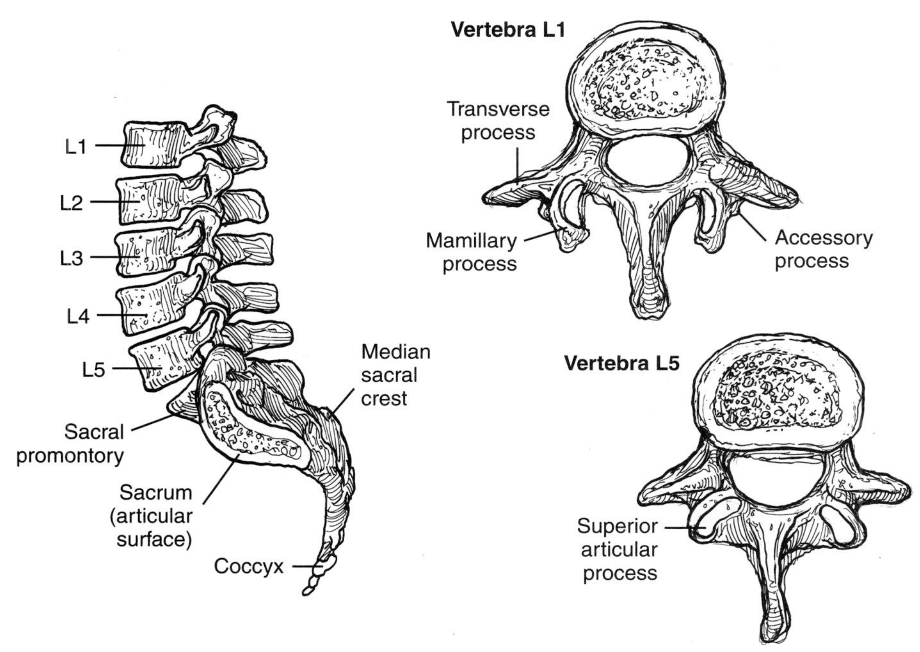

FIGURE 3–5
Lumbar vertebrae. Elements of lumbar vertebrae are massive in keeping with their function of supporting the trunk.

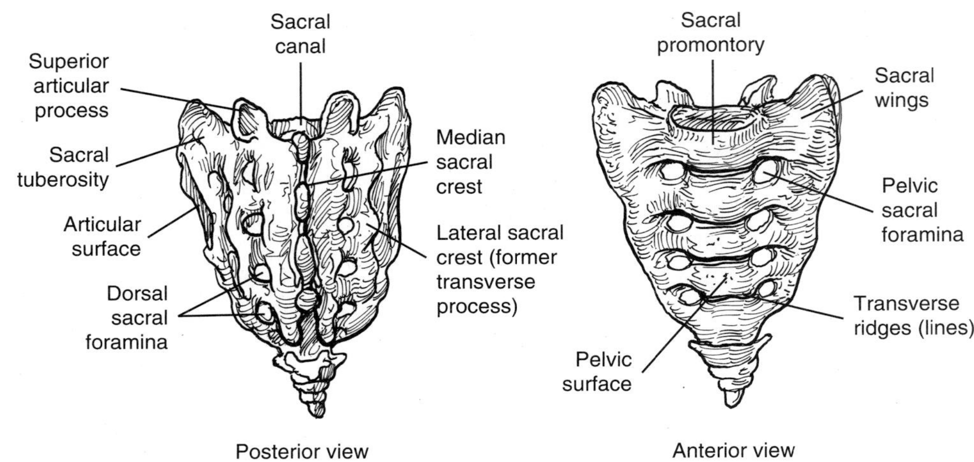

FIGURE 3–6

Sacral vertebrae. The five sacral vertebrae are fused into a single unit (the sacrum). This bone articulates with vertebra L5 above it via an intervertebral joint (symphysis) and iliac bones of the pelvis laterally via a sacroiliac joint (synovial joint).

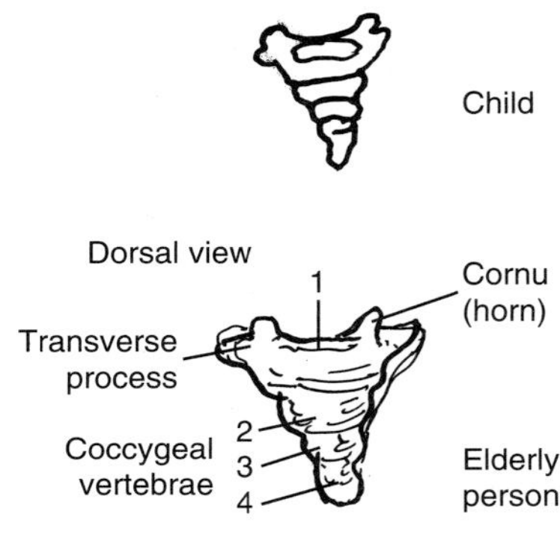

FIGURE 3–7

Coccygeal vertebrae. Three to five highly modified coccygeal vertebrae represent the caudal termination of the spine. By the time a person reaches 30 years of age, these vertebrae have fused into a single unit (the coccyx, or tailbone).

brae is further masked in the coccygeal region during adult life, when the coccygeal vertebrae gradually fuse together to form a single bone, the **coccyx.** However, vertebra Co1 is usually a separate bone until age 30 years.

Vertebral (Neural) Arches. The vertebral arches enclose the spinal cord, spinal nerves and vessels, and investments of the spinal cord. They are present in the vertebrae in all regions except the coccygeal region (Figs. 3–3 to 3–6), where only a vestige of the vertebral arch is apparent on vertebra Co1 (Fig. 3–7). Elsewhere along the vertebral column, the aligned vertebral arches and their enclosed **vertebral foramina** form the **vertebral canal** (see Fig. 3–22). The vertebral foramina are relatively large and triangular in the cervical and lumbar regions and are small and round in the thoracic region. In mature adults the spinal cord usually extends caudally to a level just inferior to vertebra L1. However, the arches of the lower lumbar vertebrae (L2 to L5) and the sacral vertebrae form a caudal extension of the vertebral canal. This caudal region of the vertebral canal contains the lower lumbar, sacral, and coccygeal spinal nerves, or **cauda equina,** and specialized extensions of the spinal cord investments, which anchor the spinal cord to the caudal end of the vertebral canal (see Chapter 4).

Transverse Processes. The transverse processes or their rudiments are apparent in all regions of the vertebral column, except in the lower vertebrae of the coccygeal region (Figs. 3–3 to 3–6). The transverse processes of the cervical vertebrae are unique in that they have **foramina transversaria** for the transmission of the left and right **vertebral arteries** (Fig. 3–8*A* and see Fig. 3–3). These vessels branch from the left and right **subclavian arteries,** course superiorly within the neck through the foramina transversaria of the cervical transverse processes, and enter the cranium via the **foramen magnum,** a large opening through which the spinal cord and lower brainstem are in continuity (see Fig. 3–1 and Chapter 22). The transverse processes of the first 10 thoracic vertebrae can be distinguished by their articular facets, which form **costotransverse joints** with the **tubercles** of the first 10 ribs (see Figs. 3–4 and 3–8*B* and Chapter 6). The transverse processes of vertebrae T11 and T12, however, lack these facets. The transverse processes are extremely well developed in the lumbar region, and the transverse processes of vertebra L5 are especially large in comparison with all of the others (see Figs. 3–5 and 3–8*C*). The large lumbar transverse processes serve as attachments for the massive muscles of the lower back (see Chapter 5). In the sacral region, the transverse processes fuse to form a **lateral sacral crest.** It is studded with short **transverse tuber-**

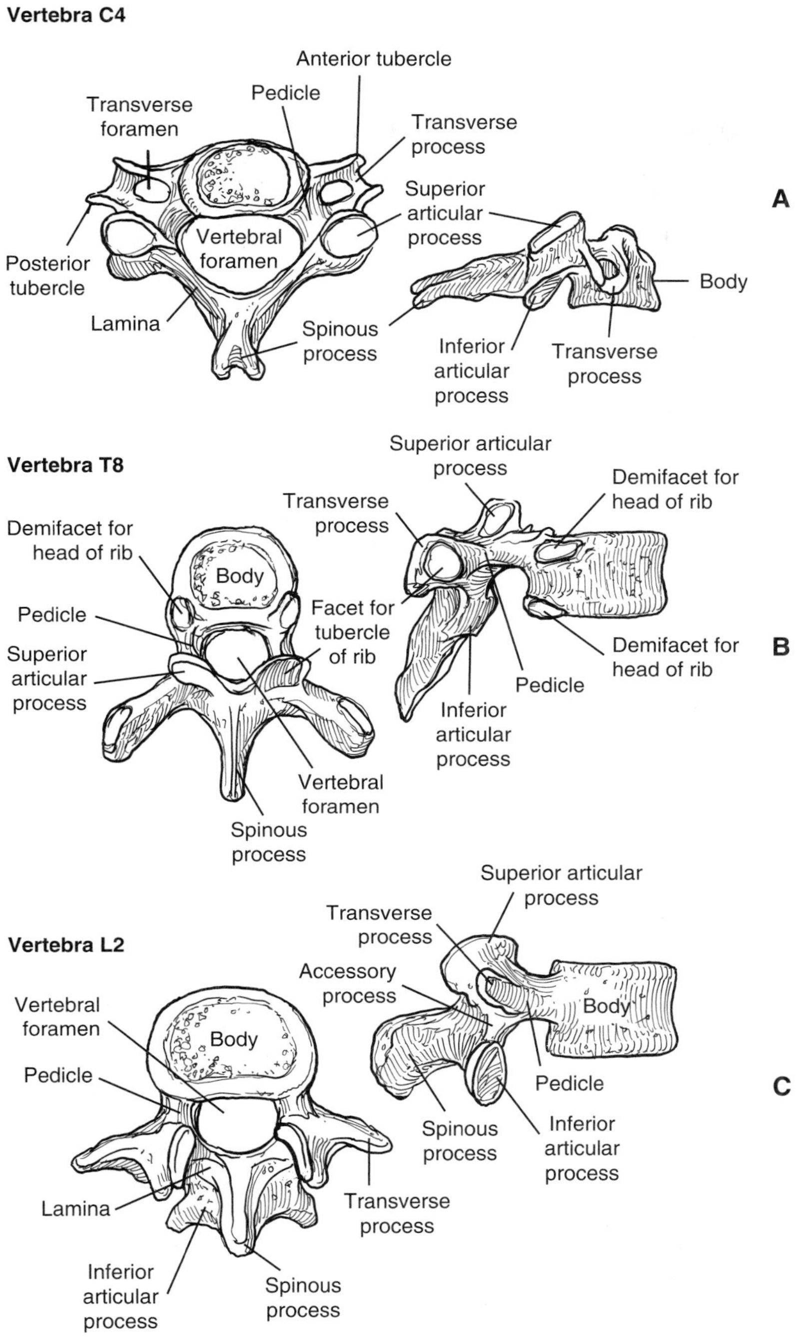

FIGURE 3–8
Comparison of cervical, thoracic, and lumbar vertebrae. These superior and lateral views of the cervical **(A)**, thoracic **(B)**, and lumbar **(C)** vertebrae emphasize major structural differences related to the size of the vertebral foramina, angle of the vertebral spines, and relative size of the transverse processes and spines.

cles, which provide attachment sites for muscles of the lower back and lower extremities (see Fig. 3–6). The lateral part of the sacrum is formed by the fusion of dorsal transverse processes and ventral **costal processes** (see below), which in turn are fused to the lateral margins of the broad, flattened vertebral bodies. The first coccygeal vertebra has a pair of prominent rudimentary transverse processes, which may or may not fuse with vertebra S5 (see Fig. 3–7). The more inferior coccygeal vertebrae lack obvious rudiments of transverse processes.

Vertebral Spines. The first cervical vertebra lacks a **vertebral spine,** but in its place is a small protuberance called a **posterior tubercle** (see Fig. 3–3). The spines of vertebrae C2 to C6 are small and **bifid** (split) (see Figs.

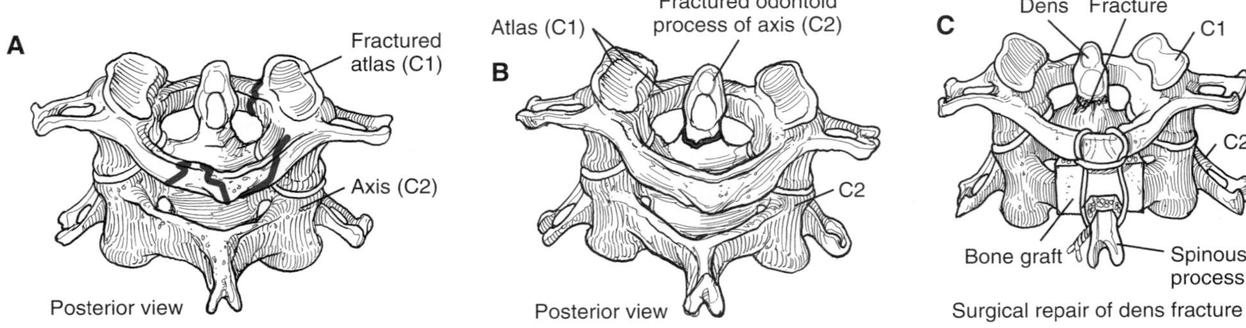

FIGURE 3–9
Fractures of cervical vertebrae. **A.** Common fracture of atlas (C1). Typically, an axial load (as in a diving accident) results in fractures of the anterior and posterior arches of the atlas. **B.** Fracture of the dens of the axis (C2). This common fracture typically results from falls or from automobile accidents. **C.** Fracture of the dens is often treated by wiring or grafting (or both) the atlas and axis together.

3–3 and 3–8*A*). The spine of vertebra C7, however, is larger and single (i.e., not bifid) (see Fig. 3–3). It is similar in size and shape to the long, single spines that typify the vertebrae in the thoracic region. Spines of the superior 10 thoracic vertebrae are exceptionally long and, unlike those of other vertebrae, tend to slant downward (see Figs. 3–4 and 3–8*B*). Spines of the lumbar vertebrae are characterized by their substantial, quadrangular, thickened shape, which helps them anchor the massive muscles of the lower lumbar region (see Figs. 3–5 and 3–8*C*). The rudimentary **spinous tubercles** of the sacral vertebrae are also specialized to assist in anchoring the axial muscles of the lower back (see Fig. 3–6). Vertebrae in the coccygeal region do not have spines (see Fig. 3–7).

Articular Processes. The paired **superior** and **inferior articular processes** are present in all of the vertebrae except those in the sacral and coccygeal regions (see Figs. 3–3 to 3–5 and 3–8). In the cervical region the processes have **facets** that are oriented more horizontally than those in the thoracic and lumbar regions (see Fig. 3–20). The facets of the paired superior articular processes of the first sacral vertebra are also oriented in a vertical plane (see Fig. 3–6). In the coccygeal region, paired rudiments of the superior articular processes fuse with rudimentary pedicles to form the superior **coccygeal cornua** of the first **coccygeal vertebra** (see Fig. 3–7). Articular processes or their rudiments are lacking in the other coccygeal vertebrae.

Dens, or Odontoid Process. The dens is a unique feature of **vertebra C2,** or **axis,** in the cervical region. The dens is a rod of bone that extends into the vertebral foramen of C1 and articulates with a facet on the inner aspect of its anterior arch (see Fig. 3–3 and Fig. 3–9). It is held in place by a **transverse ligament of the atlas.**

Accessory and Mamillary Processes. The accessory processes (at the base of the transverse processes) and mamillary processes (extending superiorly and posteriorly from the articular processes) are specialized structures of the lumbar vertebrae (see Figs. 3–5 and 3–8*C*). They provide attachments for small deep muscles of the lower back (see Chapter 5). The costal processes of the vertebrae are described in Chapter 6.

DISORDERS OF THE VERTEBRAL COLUMN

Clinical disorders of the vertebral column range from those that affect the quality of life to those that are life threatening

Disorders of the axial skeleton that are most commonly encountered by physicians vary widely in severity. Congenital anomalies range from those that are mildly disabling to those that require lifelong care and management to those that are life threatening. The most common injuries and disorders, however, occur after birth and affect 60% to 90% of adults. Injuries of the vertebrae may result in severe disabilities, particularly if neural elements are involved. The most common clinical manifestation of back disorders is lower back pain, which may be caused by disc herniations or chronic degenerative diseases of the vertebrae or intervertebral discs. Although lower back pain does not cause profound changes in lifestyle, it is a significant problem and the most common cause of limited activity in persons under age 45 years.

Disorders of the vertebral column may be related to the patient's age, height, weight, or gender

Disorders of the vertebral column occur in patients of all ages, but certain conditions are more common at certain ages. Newborn infants may suffer from congenital defects of the vertebral column that have developed during embryogenesis. Fractures and dislocations of the vertebral column are most common in young adults. Low back pain resulting from disorders of the vertebral column tends to occur in individuals in the upper 20th percentile of weight and height categories. Osteoporosis, a degenerative disease of the vertebral column, most frequently occurs in postmenopausal women.

Osteoarthritic disease of the vertebral column affects aging males as well as females. Major disorders of the vertebral column are discussed below in association with the structures or functions affected by them.

▲ Congenital Disorders of the Vertebral Column

Parts of the vertebral column may fail to form

The notochord induces ventral cells of the sclerotome to form vertebral bodies. If the induction is defective on one side, the lateral half of the vertebral body may not form. This results in **congenital scoliosis,** which is lateral curvature of the spine. The developing spinal cord and surface ectoderm induce dorsal cells of the sclerotome to form vertebral arches. Failure of development of the spinal cord and vertebral arches results in a spectrum of abnormalities called **spina bifida.** These abnormalities include a relatively mild condition, **spina bifida occulta,** which typically involves a single vertebral arch without affecting the development of the spinal cord. If several arches fail to form, a herniation or sac *(-cele)* may bulge from the surface of the back. The swelling may contain only the meninges **(meningocele)** or the meninges and a segment of the spinal cord and spinal nerves **(meningomyelocele).** These malformations may disrupt neurologic function in the lower part of the body, resulting in **paraplegia** and urinary and sexual dysfunction that require lifelong management. The most serious defect in this series of disorders is **rachischisis,** in which regions of the spinal cord are undifferentiated. This condition is usually life threatening.

▲ Fractures and Dislocations of the Vertebral Column

Vertebral elements may fracture as a result of injury or avulsion at muscle attachments

Injury to the vertebrae may cause fracture of the vertebral body, arch, or processes. Fractures of the vertebral body or arch tend to be serious and may be associated with neurologic complications. Fractures of the spinous or transverse processes are usually relatively minor. Injury of the spinous process of vertebra C7 may result from localized trauma but is more frequently caused by **muscular avulsion,** which occurs when the force exerted by muscles attached to the ligamentum nuchae pulls its bony site of attachment from the rest of the spine. Fractures of the transverse processes, usually the result of direct localized trauma, are most common in the lumbar region.

Fracture of Cervical Vertebrae

Certain fractures and dislocations of the vertebral column tend to be more common at certain sites

Fractures of the atlas (vertebra C1) typically result from an axial load on the top of the head, as would occur in a diving accident. The atlas tends to fracture at its thinnest points, breaking into four pieces (Fig. 3–9*A*). However, this seldom results in neurologic injury. Fractures of the odontoid process of the axis (vertebra C2) are not uncommon (Fig. 3–9*B*) and may be caused by a fall or an automobile accident. They are often repaired by wiring or grafting (or both) the axis and atlas together (Fig. 3–9*C*). **Hangman's fracture,** perhaps the most "infamous" cervical fracture, is that of the pedicle of the axis. This results from hyperextension of the neck, as when the head whips backward in an automobile accident. Despite its sinister-sounding name, the fracture is usually not fatal and tends not to result in neurologic deficits. Fractures of the spinous processes most often occur at the level of vertebra C7 or T1.

Dislocation of Cervical Vertebrae

The lower cervical region (vertebrae C3 to C7) is a common site of dislocation (Fig. 3–10*A* and *B*) partly because of the small size of cervical vertebrae relative to the thoracic and lumbar vertebrae and partly because of the absence of supportive skeletal structures (such as the well-developed lips on

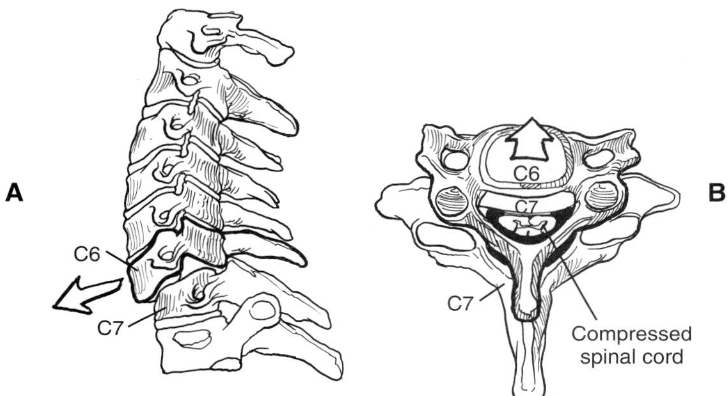

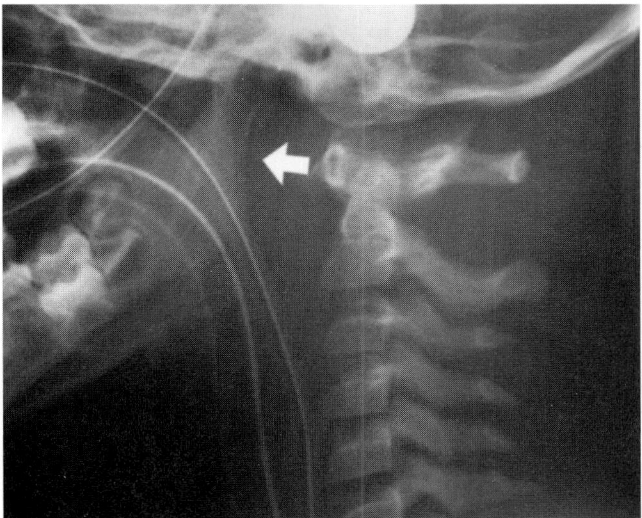

FIGURE 3–10
Dislocation of the spine. **A.** Dislocations of lower cervical vertebrae are the most common. **B.** Dislocations of the spine may compress the spinal cord. **C.** This standard x-ray shows the dislocation of the atlas upon the axis *(arrow),* which is a life-threatening injury but, fortunately, an uncommon one. The patient has been intubated to assist in respiration, which has been impaired because of trauma to the spinal cord superior to levels C3, C4, and C5 (origin of phrenic nerves).

superior edges of junctional surfaces in the upper cervical region and the vertically oriented articulating processes in the thoracic and lumbar regions). The more horizontal orientation of the transverse processes of the cervical vertebrae also predisposes them to dislocation. Dislocation of cervical vertebrae, however, may also occur at higher levels (Fig. 3–10*C*).

Fracture of Thoracic and Lumbar Vertebrae

Axial trauma to the thoracic or lumbar vertebrae frequently causes **burst fractures** in which the vertebral body shatters into fragments (Fig. 3–11). Neurologic damage may result if fragments become dislodged within the vertebral canal and pierce the dura mater, spinal nerves, or spinal cord (Fig. 3–11*B* and *C*). **Shear fractures** and **flexion-distraction injuries** are caused by severe trauma and frequently result in significant neurologic damage, particularly if they occur in the thoracic region. In a shear fracture the vertebral body is torn free of its ligamentous attachments and is displaced in an anteroposterior or lateral direction (Fig. 3–12). Flexion-distraction injuries are similar in that anteroposterior or lateral displacement occurs, but in this type of injury, the vertebral body is shorn in half (Fig. 3–13). This injury commonly occurs in automobile accidents when a person is wearing a lap belt but not a shoulder belt so that the trunk flexes when the vehicle comes to a sudden stop.

▲ Degenerative Diseases of the Vertebral Column

Osteoporosis

The most common underlying cause of vertebral column deformity is osteoporosis

Osteoporosis results from decreased deposition of bone. The process of bone formation and resorption, which occurs throughout life, involves the calcification of a protein matrix. In osteoporosis, there is not enough calcium available and the bone mass shrinks. This process affects the entire skeleton, but the femoral neck, vertebrae, and metacarpals are affected more than other bones. Osteoporosis may result in accentuation of the thoracic kyphosis or in compression fractures of the lumbar vertebral bodies. The disorder most often occurs in postmenopausal women, but it may also occur in patients with endocrine disorders, nutritional deficiencies, and genetic diseases or may be a side effect of drug treatment or abuse.

Osteoarthritis

The vertebral column is a common site of arthritic changes

Osteoarthritis of the vertebral column results in pain similar to that of muscle spasm or inflammation. The pain of osteoarthritis tends to be worse in the morning and results in a decreased range of motion. Degeneration resulting from osteoarthritis of the vertebral column may ultimately involve neurologic elements if the annulus fibrosus becomes com-

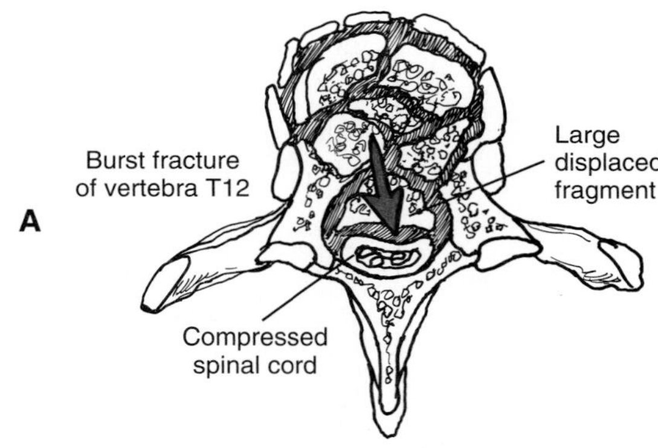

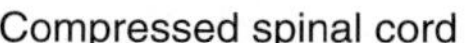

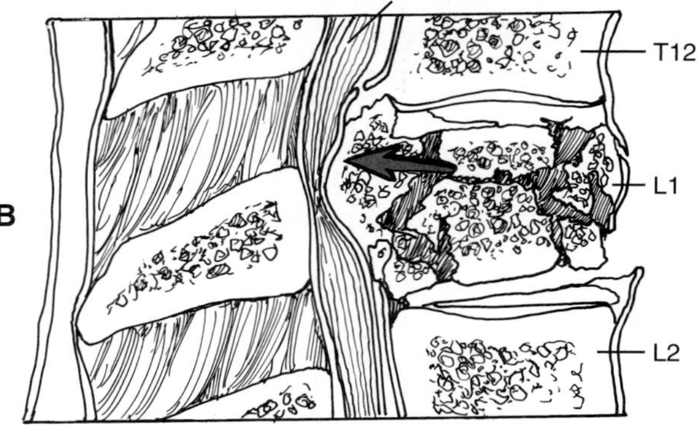

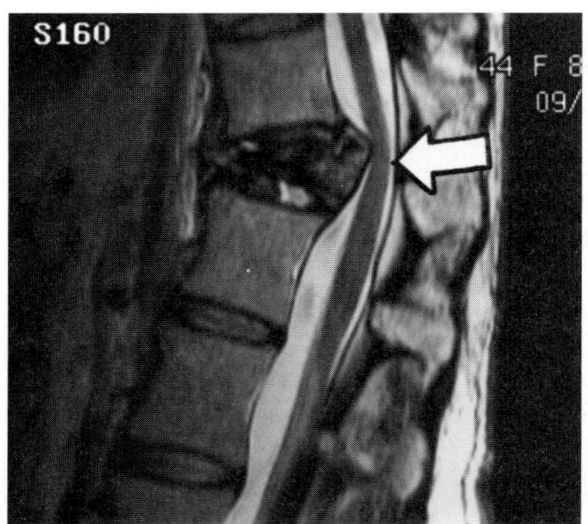

FIGURE 3–11

Burst fracture of a vertebral body. Fragments of the vertebral body may compress the spinal cord. **A.** Burst fracture of vertebra T12. **B.** Midsagittal view of burst fracture of vertebra L1. *Arrows* in **A** and **B,** Direction of movement of dislodged fragments. **C.** In this midsagittal magnetic resonance imaging scan, the shattered vertebral body of T12 *(arrow)* impinges on the vertebral canal, compressing the spinal cord. The vertebral body has been weakened by the invasion of metastases from a carcinoma of the breast.

pressed as the vertebral laminae thicken and bony ridges form on the rims of vertebral bodies and the facets of superior and inferior articulating processes (Fig. 3–14*A*). These bony growths cause narrowing of the vertebral canal and put pressure on the spinal cord, cauda equina, and nerve roots (Fig. 3–14*B*).

▲ Bony Landmarks as Aids in Diagnosis

Prominent bony landmarks may also be observed or palpated to aid in the diagnosis of many disorders of associated soft tissues or underlying viscera

When taking a patient's history or describing a patient's symptoms to others, it is important to establish the location of the disease, trauma, or pain within the body, called **referred pain.** The bony skeleton, particularly the axial skeleton of the trunk, is a useful frame of reference for this purpose.

The most obvious surface landmarks in the posterior region are vertebral spines C7 and T1. These are usually found at the same level as the **acromial spine of the scapula** (see Fig. 2–2). The **inferior angle of the scapula** is at the level of vertebra T7. In the more inferior region of the back, the **iliac crests** can be palpated to locate the level of vertebra L4.

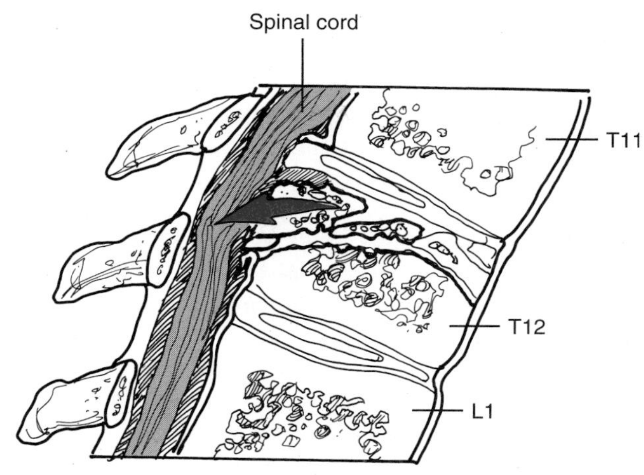

FIGURE 3–13
Flexion-distraction injury of vertebra T12. In this case, fracture of the vertebral body results in posterior displacement of the upper part of the T12 vertebral body into the vertebral canal, resulting in compression of the spinal cord. This type of injury typically results from automobile accidents in which patient was restrained by only a lap belt.

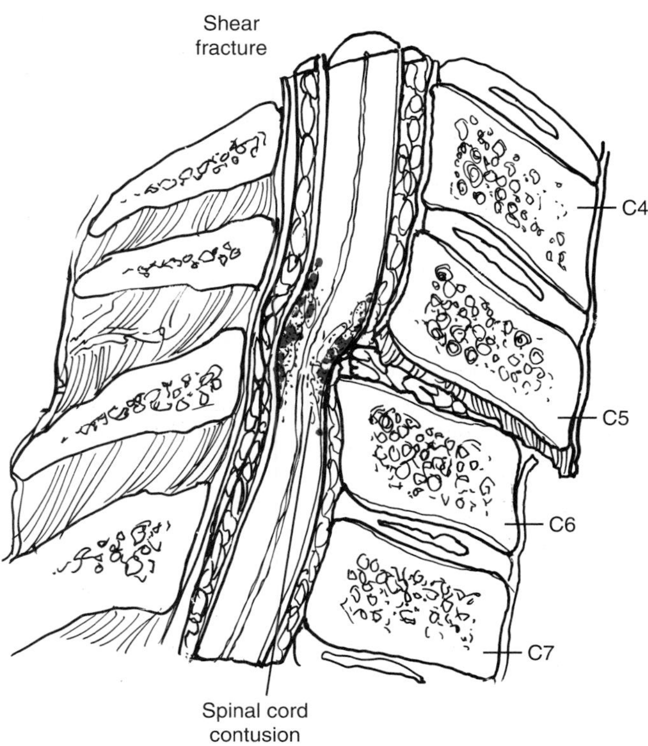

FIGURE 3–12
In this shear fracture, a cervical vertebra is torn from its ligamentous connections to a more superior vertebra, resulting in its posterior displacement and compression of the spinal cord.

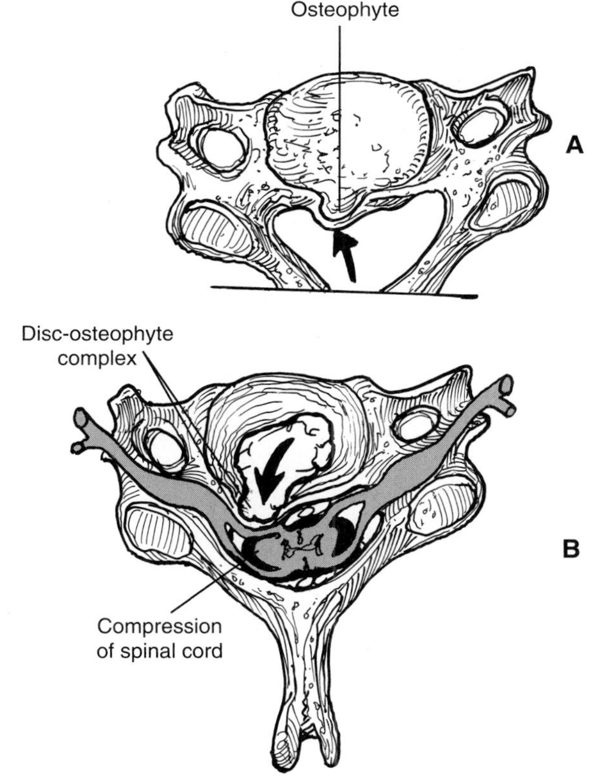

FIGURE 3–14
Degenerative disease of the spine. **A.** An osteophyte *(arrow)* resulting from osteoarthritis impinges on the vertebral canal. **B.** The ventral root of a spinal nerve is compressed by a complex of disc and vertebral tissue that has formed because of osteoarthritis.

INTEGRATION OF THE AXIAL SKELETON OF THE TRUNK: JOINTS, SYMPHYSES, AND CONNECTIVE TISSUES

The strongest joints of the vertebral column form between vertebral bodies via intervertebral discs and accompanying anterior and posterior longitudinal ligaments

Joints of the Vertebral Bodies: The Intervertebral Discs and Anterior and Posterior Longitudinal Ligaments

Each pair of superior and inferior junctional surfaces of the vertebral bodies is bonded to an intervening **intervertebral disc** (Fig. 3–15). This joint is a typical **symphysis,** which is a cartilaginous type of **synarthrosis,** that is, it joins bone to bone via a solid connective tissue element in the following arrangement:

Bone ↔ Hyaline growth cartilage ↔ Fibrocartilaginous disc ↔ Hyaline growth cartilage ↔ Bone

In this scheme the thin layers of **hyaline cartilage** are bonded to the junctional surfaces of the vertebral bodies. The intervening fibrocartilaginous **discs** have two parts: a central gelatinous **nucleus pulposus** and a circumferential ring of concentrically disposed laminae of tougher connective tissue called the **annulus fibrosus** (Fig. 3–15). The nucleus pulposus is initially derived from the embryonic **notochord.** The annulus fibrosus develops from cells of the sclerotome that initially surround the notochord at the level where the sclerotome splits transversely into cranial and caudal halves (see discussion of the development of vertebrae above). The intervertebral disc is, therefore, a *segmental structure,* whereas the definitive vertebrae form at *intersegmental levels.*

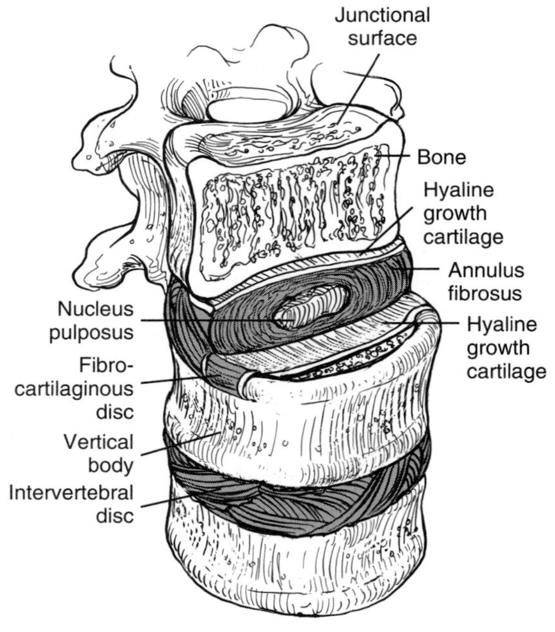

FIGURE 3–15
Intervertebral disc. Coronal section of vertebral body and disc reveals tissue layers of this cartilaginous synarthrosis (symphysis).

> The discs are extremely strong in young persons and not easily damaged. As people grow older, the annulus fibrosus may begin to degenerate and become far more susceptible to injury.

The bond between the vertebral bodies is further strengthened by anterior and posterior longitudinal ligaments, which are commonly classified as components of the intervertebral symphysis (Fig. 3–16). The **anterior longitudinal ligament** is attached to the occipital bone superiorly and to the anterior tubercle of the atlas. It courses along the anterior surfaces of the remaining vertebral bodies and intervertebral discs to the superior part of the sacrum. Its fibers blend with connective tissue of the annulus fibrosus of the intervertebral discs; the periosteum, which is the connective tissue covering of the vertebral bodies; and the perichondrium, the connective tissue covering of the hyaline cartilages (Fig. 3–17 and see Fig. 3–16).

The **posterior longitudinal ligament** lies within the vertebral canal on the posterior surfaces of the vertebral bodies and intervertebral discs (see Figs. 3–16 and 3–17). It is connected superiorly within the cranium to the **tectorial membrane,** which is the connective tissue that covers the base of the brain. It courses inferiorly throughout the vertebral canal to the lower lumbar vertebrae. The fibers of the posterior longitudinal ligament fuse with connective tissues associated with the vertebral bodies, hyaline cartilages, and intervertebral discs in the same way as the fibers of the anterior longitudinal ligament fuse.

All of the joints of the human skeleton classified as symphyses are located within the axial skeleton, except for the **pubic symphysis,** which is a joint of the appendicular skeleton. The pubic symphysis joins the anterior midline articulating facets of the pubic bones (see Chapter 14).

Low Back Pain and the Intervertebral Discs

Herniation of an intervertebral disc may result in chronic low back pain

Back pain, particularly low back pain, occurs in most adults. It may be acute or chronic. **Chronic low back pain** is pain that has lasted for more than 3 months. It usually results from a disorder of the vertebral column such as **disc herniation.** If no orthopedic cause can be detected, muscle spasm or inflammation may be suspected (see Chapter 5).

Two forms of intervertebral disc herniation are now recognized. In the less common type, the nucleus pulposus issues through a ruptured annulus fibrosus, most frequently between vertebrae L4 and L5 or L5 and S1 (Fig. 3–18). The pain is similar to that of muscle disorders of the back. The nucleus pulposus may eventually herniate completely through the annulus in a posterior or posterolateral direction, compressing a spinal nerve or nerve root and resulting in **sciatica** (pain, numbness, or tingling that radiates down the lower limbs). Bladder, bowel, and sexual function may be interrupted in these cases.

The second form of disc herniation frequently occurs in conjunction with **spinal osteoarthritis** (see above). During the aging process the annulus fibrosus is compressed, causing the spaces between adjacent vertebrae to narrow. Although this in itself may not be a major problem, the accompanying osteoarthritis may result in chronic low back pain caused by impingement of the ruptured disc on neural elements (see Fig. 3–14*B*).

▲ Joints and Ligaments of the Vertebral Arches

Vertebral arches are joined by synovial joints of the superior and inferior articular processes and by several ligaments

The facets of the superior and inferior articular processes of two adjacent vertebrae form a **synovial joint,** which is a **diarthrosis** (i.e., a cavitated connective tissue element that joins one bone to another). The matching facets are each covered with a thin layer of hyaline cartilage. A thin **synovial membrane** lines

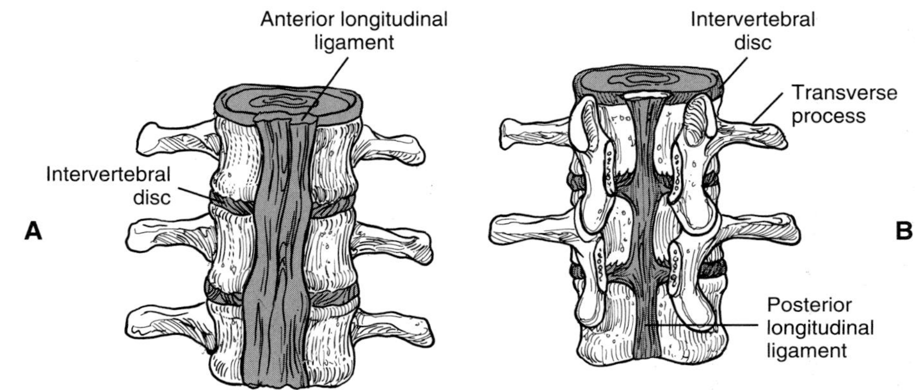

FIGURE 3–16
Anterior and posterior longitudinal ligaments are integral components of the intervertebral symphysis. **A.** Anterior view of vertebral body and anterior longitudinal ligament. **B.** Posterior view of vertebral body with arches cut away to show posterior longitudinal ligament.

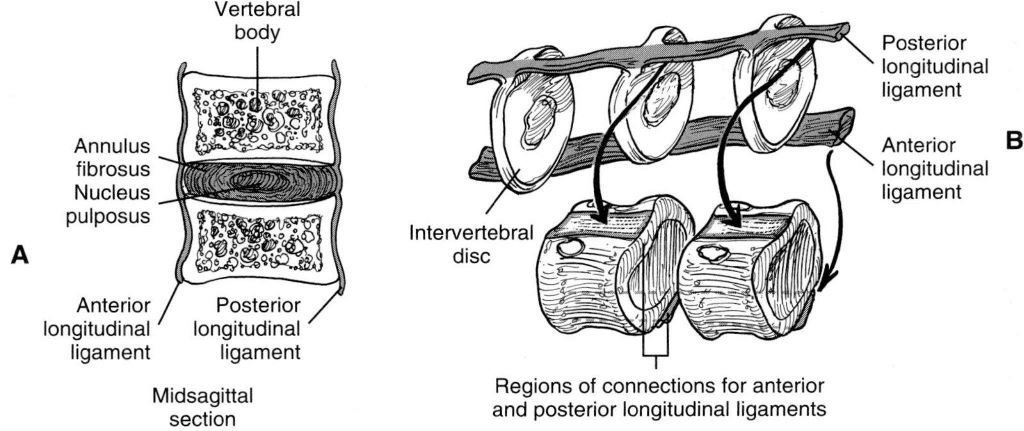

FIGURE 3–17
Anterior and posterior longitudinal ligaments. **A.** Midsagittal section of vertebral column shows connections of anterior and posterior longitudinal ligaments to perichondrium of intervertebral disc. **B.** Removal of the vertebral bodies shows connections of anterior and posterior longitudinal ligaments to the intervertebral discs.

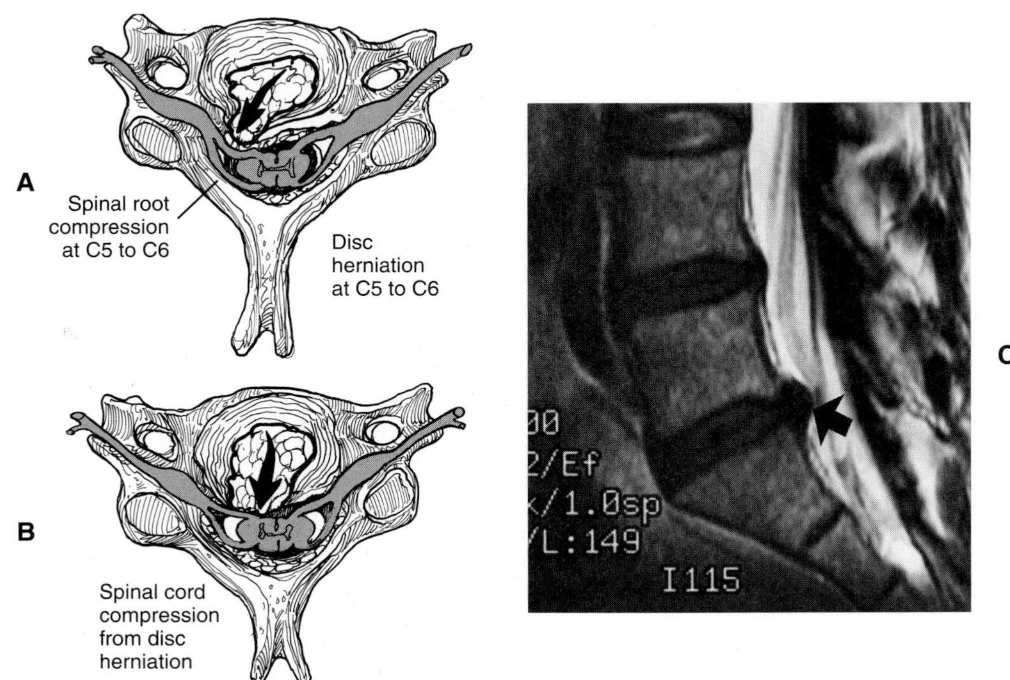

FIGURE 3–18
A. Herniation of an intervertebral disc *(arrow)* compresses the ventral roots of a spinal nerve. **B.** Herniation of an intervertebral disc *(arrow)* compresses the spinal cord. **C.** Midsagittal magnetic resonance imaging scan reveals a herniated disc *(arrow)* between vertebrae L5 and S1 and its impingement on the cauda equina.

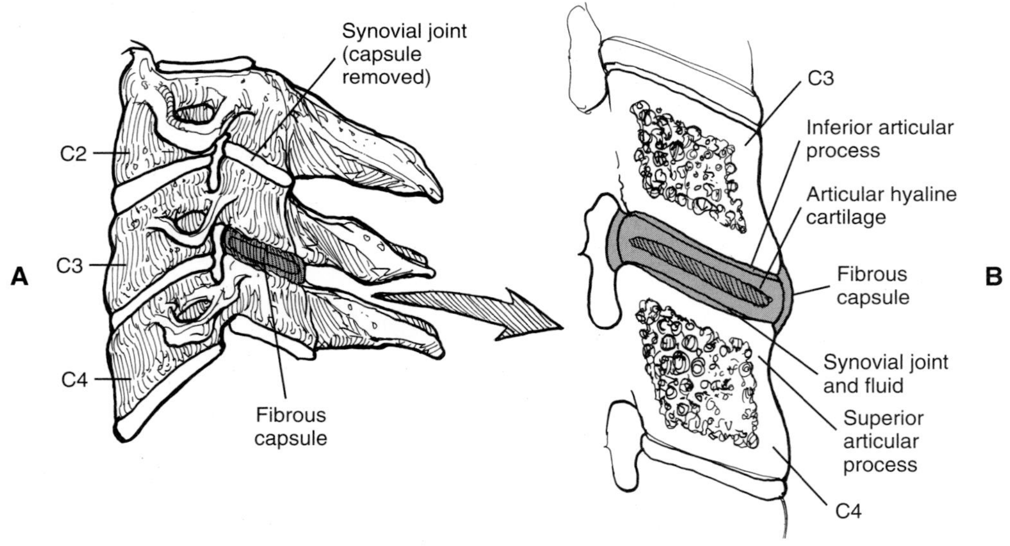

FIGURE 3–19
Synovial joints of articular processes. **A.** Synovial joints connect articular processes of the vertebrae. **B.** Components of the synovial vertebral interarticular joints include a capsule, articular cartilages, a synovial cavity lined with a synovial membrane, and synovial fluid.

all of the nonarticular surfaces within the joint. The synovial membrane secretes a viscous hyaluronic acid-rich dialysate of blood with excellent lubricating properties. The synovial membrane also reabsorbs excess synovial fluid. The entire joint is invested by a loose **fibrous capsule** (Fig. 3–19). The pattern of connections of a synovial joint is illustrated in the following scheme:

Bone ↔ Articular hyaline cartilage ↔ Cavity partially lined by synovial membrane containing synovial fluid ↔ Articular hyaline cartilage ↔ Bone

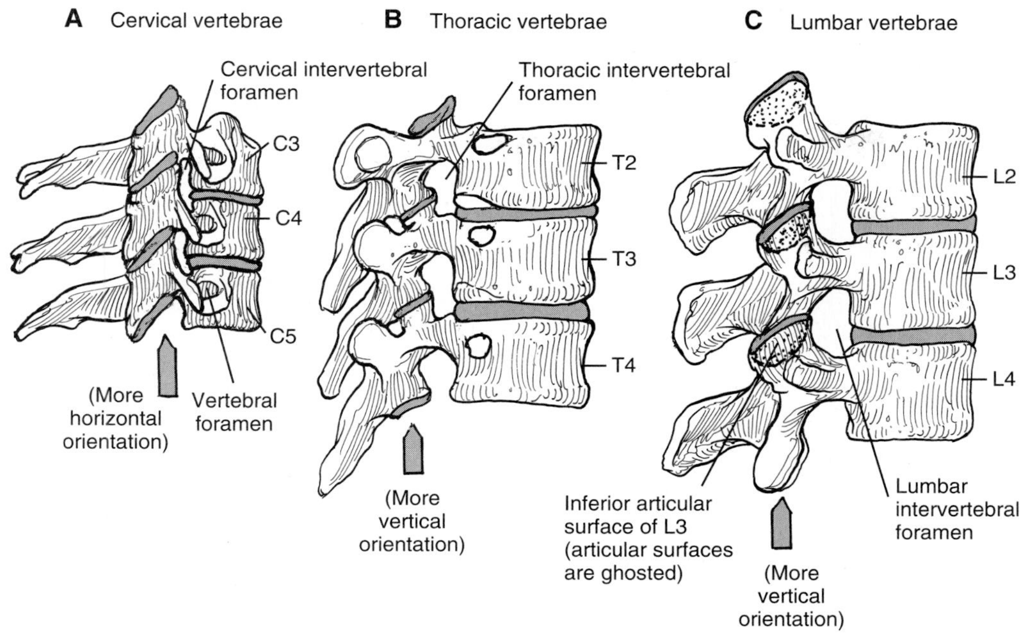

FIGURE 3–20
Anatomic differences in cervical, thoracic, and lumbar regions of the spine affect mobility. Articular facets between cervical vertebrae **(A)** are oriented more horizontally than in other regions, whereas articular facets of the thoracic region **(B)** are oriented more vertically. Articular facets in the lumbar region **(C)** are oriented in a vertical-frontosagittal plane. Intervertebral foramina are smallest in the cervical region and larger in the lumbar region. Vertebral spines of the thoracic region slope downward.

In the cervical region, the facets of the synovial joints are oriented more horizontally than in other regions. This predisposes the vertebrae in this region to dislocation, particularly at inferior cervical levels (see below). The articular facets of the superior and inferior articular processes in the thoracic and lumbar regions are oriented more vertically, and, therefore, they impose limitations on movements between one vertebra and the next (Fig. 3–20 and see Figs. 3–3 to 3–5).

Several ligaments provide additional connections between the vertebral arches and associated processes, including the ligamenta flava, ligamentum nuchae, and supraspinous, interspinous, and intertransverse ligaments (Figs. 3-21 and 3–22). These connections are typically classified as fibrous synarthroses, or **syndesmoses.** A typical pattern of these syndesmoses is illustrated in the following scheme:

Bone ↔ Collagenous interosseous element ↔ Bone

The **ligamenta flava** (yellow ligaments) connect the laminae of adjoining vertebrae on the inside of the vertebral canal (Figs. 3–21 and 3–22). Their color is a consequence of the yellowish elastic tissue of which they are composed. The ligamenta flava limit the separation of vertebral arches and assist in the extension (or straightening) of the vertebral column following flexion (see below).

The **ligamentum nuchae** extends from a bony protuberance of the occipital bone of the cranium called the **occipital protuberance,** or **inion,** to the spine of vertebra C7 (see Fig. 5–14). It is connected to the posterior tubercle of vertebra C1 and to the medial surfaces of the bifid spines of vertebrae C1 to C6. It anchors muscles of the back and neck, including the **trapezius** and other cervical muscles.

The **supraspinous ligaments** connect the apices of vertebral spines from vertebra C7 to the sacrum (Figs. 3–21 and 3–22). The superior extension of this ligament is the ligamentum nuchae.

The **interspinous ligaments** connect adjacent vertebral spines (Figs. 3–21 and 3–22). They are obscure in the cervical region, narrow in the thoracic region, and thicker and broader in the lumbar region. Their more posterior fibers blend with fibers of the supraspinous ligaments, while their more anterior fibers blend with fibers of the ligamenta flava.

The **intertransverse ligaments,** which course between the transverse processes, are not as well developed as the other ligaments just described. In most regions they blend with the intertransverse muscles. Specialized **iliolumbar ligaments** fan out inferiorly and laterally from the large transverse processes of vertebra L5, connecting them to the region of the **sacroiliac joint,** the joint between the sacrum and

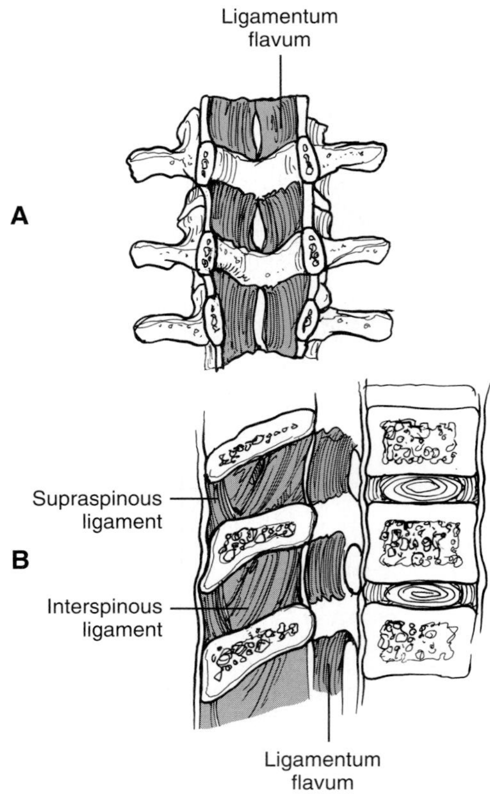

FIGURE 3–21

Ligamenta flava and supraspinous and interspinous ligaments. **A.** Anterior view of the vertebral canal shows the ligamenta flava joining laminae of vertebral arches. **B.** Midsagittal section of the spine shows supraspinous and interspinous ligaments joining vertebral spines.

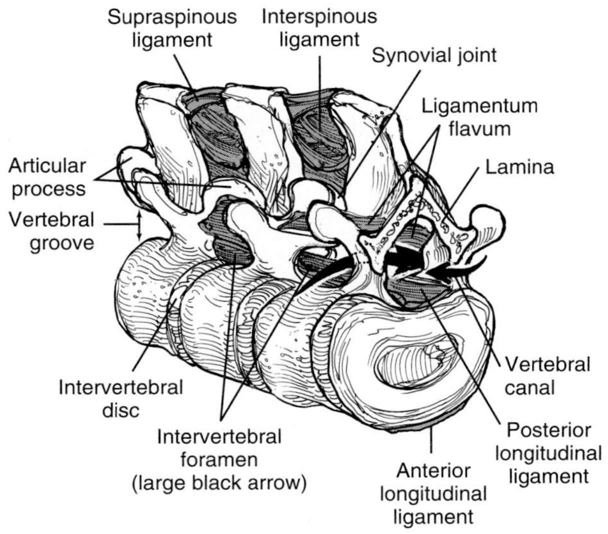

FIGURE 3–22

Vertebral canal. Syndesmoses of the laminae of the vertebral arches (ligamenta flava) and vertebral spines (supraspinous and interspinous ligaments) align individual vertebral foramina to form the vertebral canal.

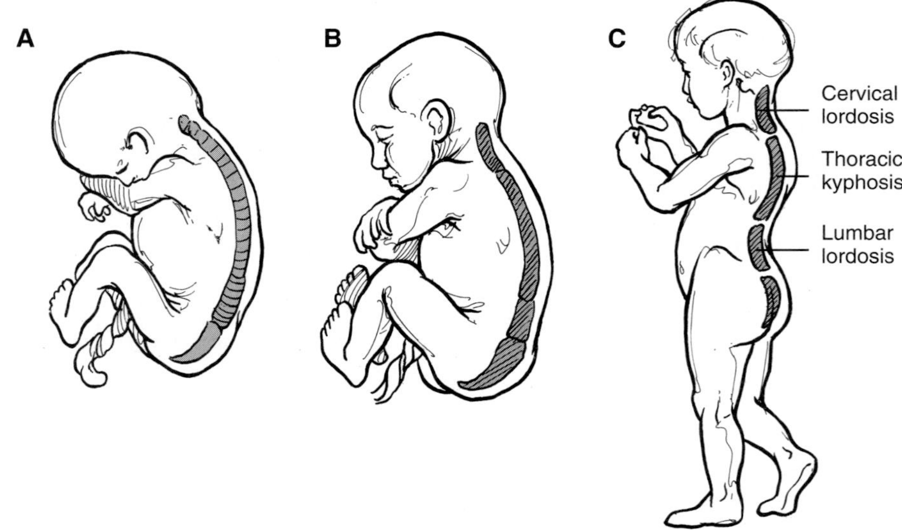

FIGURE 3–23

Development of curvatures of the spinal cord. **A.** Primary curvature (kyphosis) of the spine in a fetus. **B.** Secondary cervical lordosis of the spine in a newborn infant (and up to 9 months of age). **C.** Secondary lumbar lordosis of the spine in a toddler.

iliac bone of the pelvis (see Fig. 5–16 and Chapter 14).

Other specialized ligaments that help anchor the cranium to the superior end of the vertebral column are discussed in Chapter 24.

▲ Curvatures of the Vertebral Column

The end-to-end connections of vertebrae form a vertebral column with characteristic curvatures

During fetal life, the vertebral column develops initially as a C-shaped structure, with its concave side facing anteriorly and its convex side facing posteriorly **(primary curvature of the vertebral column)** (Fig. 3–23*A*). This curvature is called the **primary kyphosis** and is normally retained for life within the thoracic and sacral regions. As development proceeds during late fetal life, however, the cervical region begins to curve in the opposite direction so that the anterior surface is convex and the posterior surface is concave (Fig. 3–23*B*). This **secondary cervical curvature,** or **cervical lordosis,** is accentuated after birth as the infant begins to hold its head up (during the first 3 months of age) and sits upright (at about 9 months of age). Finally, the initial primary curvature of the lumbar region reverses as the infant begins to walk upright at 12 to 18 months of age (see Fig. 3–23*C*). The development of this **secondary lumbar curvature,** or **lumbar lordosis,** is more accentuated in the lower lumbar regions and is generally more pronounced in females than in males.

Scoliosis. **Scoliosis,** a severe lateral curvature of the vertebral column, may be a sign of an underlying congenital malformation of the vertebrae (see above) or a disease process (Fig. 3–24). Normally, however, a slight lateral rightward convexity is apparent in the thoracic region of right-handed individuals and a slight leftward convexity in left-handed individuals.

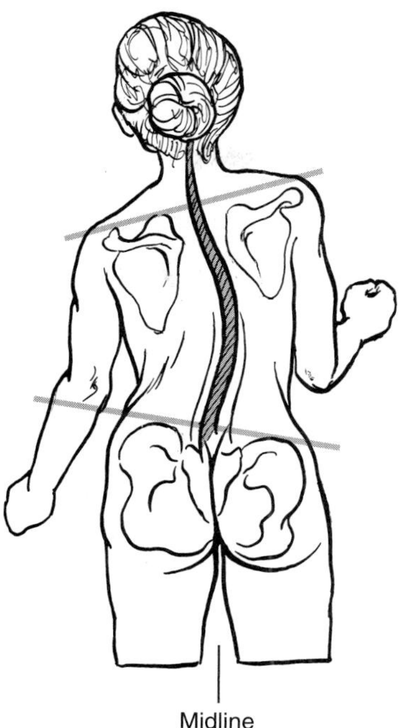

FIGURE 3–24
Vertebral scoliosis. Scoliosis is a lateral curvature of the spine that may be congenital or acquired.

▲ Function of Intervertebral Joints and Ligaments

Movements of the Axial Skeleton

The strength and flexibility of intervertebral joints and ligaments provide the vertebral column with structural integrity and, at the same time, allow a surprisingly extensive range of movement

The range of movement from one vertebra to the next is greatly limited by the well-developed, end-to-end symphyses (at the intervertebral discs), synovial joints between articular processes, and ligamentous connections just discussed. However, the sum total of all of the small movements between vertebrae throughout the entire vertebral column allows for a significant amount of flexion, extension, lateral flexion, rotation, and circumduction of the trunk (Fig. 3–25). These movements maintain the body's posture while a person is sitting, standing, or walking (particularly on uneven terrain) and provide a mechanism for changing the posture when a person is grabbing, bending over, rising from a supine position, or turning. The deformability of the vertebral column also contributes to its ability to protect the spinal cord and thoracic viscera and aids in respiratory movements of the thorax.

Range of Movement of the Axial Skeleton

Movements of the vertebral column are limited by the thickness and flexibility of intervertebral discs, strength and anatomic structure of ligaments, and anatomic structure of articulating bony elements

In general, the range of movement throughout the vertebral column is limited by the properties of intervertebral discs and associated ligaments and by the anatomic structure of the vertebrae. **Flexion** is limited by the tension of the posterior discal fibers (which are connective tissue fibers in the posterior region of the intervertebral disc); the compressibility of the anterior region of the disc; and the tension of the posterior longitudinal ligament, ligamenta flava, interspinous ligaments, and supraspinous ligaments (Fig. 3–25*A*). **Extension** is limited by the tension of the anterior discal fibers, the compressibility of the posterior region of the disc, and the tension of the anterior longitudinal ligament (Fig. 3–25*B*). **Lateral flexion** and **extension** are limited by the compressibility of the lateral edge of the disc and the tension of the discal fibers on the opposite

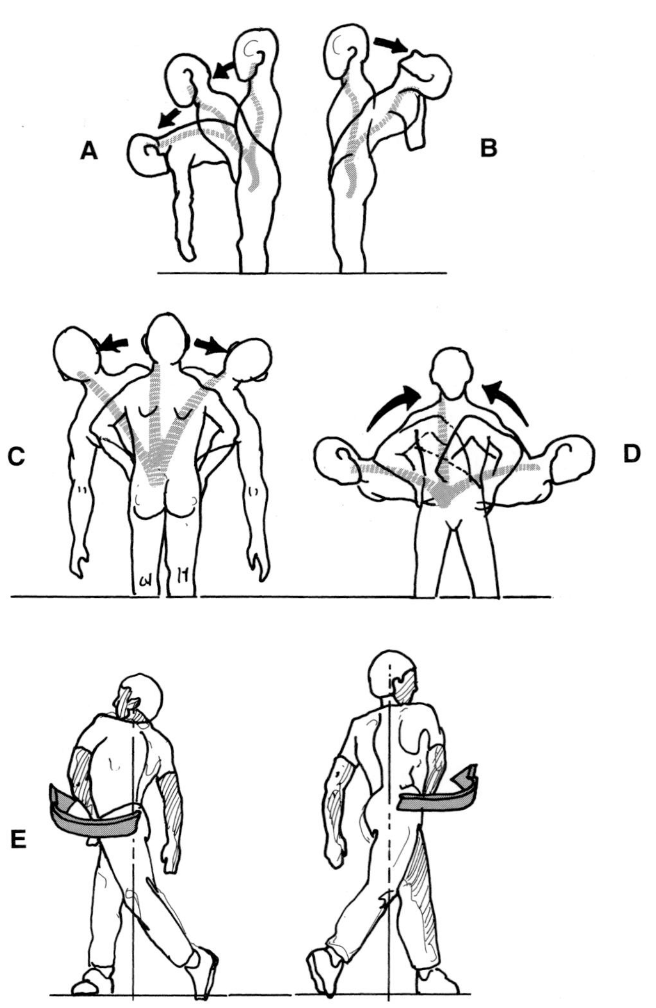

FIGURE 3–25
Movements of spine. **A.** Flexion. **B.** Extension. **C.** Lateral flexion. **D.** Lateral extension. **E.** Rotation.

side (Fig. 3–25*C* and *D*). The degree of compression and tension possible in individual discs, therefore, depends on their innate deformability and thickness. In general, the compression or tension of the intervertebral discs and the resulting range of movement of the vertebral column are greatest in the cervical and lumbar regions, where the discs are thicker. **Rotation** of the vertebral column requires torsional deformation of the discs. Although the movements are minimal at any particular disc, the summation of these movements over the entire length of the vertebral column is extensive (Fig. 3–25*E*).

The horizontal orientation of articular facets in the cervical region allows greater **flexion** in this region than in other regions of the vertebral column. A raised lip at the anterolateral edge of the superior junctional surface of each cervical vertebral body prevents the lower edge of the vertebra immediately above it from sliding too far forward. Flexion of the cervical region is limited by the interference of the sternum (i.e., the chin stops when it touches the sternum). Flexion is limited in the thoracic and lumbar regions by the more vertical orientation of articular facets of the superior and inferior articular processes (see Fig. 3–20). Flexion may be further limited in the lumbar region by subcutaneous abdominal fat and the relative inflexibility of paravertebral muscles.

Extension of the thoracic vertebral column is uniquely limited by physical interference between the long adjacent downward-projecting thoracic vertebral spines (see Fig. 3–20) and by the connections of thoracic vertebrae to the ribs and sternum. The relatively thin thoracic intervertebral discs also tend to restrict extension and other movements in this region.

Although **lateral flexion** is relatively free in the cervical and lumbar regions, it is limited in the thoracic region. This reduces movements that would interfere with respiration. Lateral flexion is limited in the upper part of the thoracic region by the ribs and sternum. The fit of the articulating processes between vertebrae T11 and T12 is so tight that all movements other than flexion are completely prevented at this joint.

Rotational movements are generally slight in the cervical region, except between vertebrae C1 and C2, and they are even more restricted in the lumbar region. Rotation is limited in most areas of the thorax but is relatively free in the superior thoracic region because this movement, unlike flexion, extension, and lateral flexion, does not interfere with respiratory function (see Chapter 6).

■ ANATOMY OF THE VERTEBRAL CANAL

The vertebral canal is continuous throughout the cervical, thoracic, lumbar, and sacral regions of the vertebral column

The vertebral canal is formed by alignment of the individual foramina of the vertebral arches (see Fig. 3–22) and follows the curvatures of the vertebral column. The canal is larger and triangular shaped in the cervical and lumbar regions and smaller and circular shaped in the thoracic region (see Fig. 3–8). These differences are partly related to the relatively large numbers of spinal nerve processes emanating from the spinal cord in the cervical and lumbar regions, which provide the extensive, complex innervation of the upper and lower extremities (see Fig. 4–16). The larger size of the cervical and lumbar vertebral canal may also be related to the vertebral column's need for a greater range of movement in these regions. The contents of the vertebral canal are discussed in Chapter 4.

▲ Function of the Vertebral Canal

The vertebral canal protects the spinal cord and spinal nerves, which are suspended within it

The vertebral canal is an elongated vessel within which the delicate spinal cord and spinal nerve roots and their investments are suspended. The diameter of the spinal cord is significantly less than the diameter of the vertebral canal. The excess space is filled with a specialized dialysate of blood, the **cerebrospinal fluid,** within which the spinal cord floats. The spinal cord is held in place within the center of the canal by **denticulate ligaments,** a **subarachnoidal septum,** and a **filum terminale** (see Figs. 4–22 and 4–23). These structures are specializations of the **pia mater,** which is the innermost connective tissue investment of the spinal cord. (The other two investments are the **arachnoid mater** and **dura mater).** The three coverings are collectively called the **meninges.** The thick bony walls of the vertebral column and the meninges physically protect the spinal cord from penetration by sharp objects. The deformable vertebral column and the cerebrospinal fluid also provide a significant amount of protection by absorbing and dissipating energy from external physical blows or impacts (see Chapter 4 for a more detailed discussion).

▲ Structure and Function of the Intervertebral Foramina

Apposition of adjacent superior and inferior vertebral notches forms the oval intervertebral foramina, which allow spinal nerves and vessels to pass in and out of the vertebral canal

The intervertebral foramina are smallest in the cervical region. They become increasingly larger as they descend from the thoracic to the lumbar region (see Fig. 3–20). These openings allow spinal nerves and their roots to pass from the spinal cord to the motor and sensory target organs of the body wall, viscera, and extremities. These nerves and the spinal cord are discussed in Chapter 4. The intervertebral foramina also provide a channel for the vasculature of the spinal cord and its investments by arteries and veins that branch from vessels outside the vertebral column. These vessels also supply and drain the bones of the vertebral canal (see Fig. 4–24).

▲ Structure and Function of the Vertebral Grooves

Alignment of the vertebrae along the vertebral column provides a continuous surface for attachments of deep longitudinal muscles of the back

The alignment of the vertebrae along the length of the vertebral column results in the formation of long, shallow grooves lateral to the vertebral laminae and dorsal to the transverse processes. The deep muscles of the back lie within these **vertebral grooves.** The grooves are relatively shallow in the cervical and lumbar regions and deep in the thoracic region. They provide a continuous substratum for attachments of the axillary muscles (transversospinal and erector spinae muscles), allowing these muscles to intimately and directly invest and support the vertebral column (see Figs. 2–2 and 3–22).

4 The Spinal Cord and Peripheral Nervous System

The nervous system integrates the structure and functions of the human body and thereby serves as an essential unifying system for the study of all anatomic regions. Moreover, an understanding of the nervous system reveals the mechanism of **referred pain.** This mechanism is a basic tool used by the health care provider in taking patients' histories and making diagnoses. The study of the back, therefore, provides an opportunity to briefly introduce the **central nervous system,** which consists of the brain and spinal cord, and the **peripheral nervous system,** which consists of all of the nerves and ganglia outside of the central nervous system. This chapter will focus on the spinal cord and peripheral nervous system. The brain and cranial nerves are discussed in greater detail in Chapters 23 and 26.

DEVELOPMENT AND ORGANIZATION OF THE SPINAL CORD

Most of the spinal cord and brain arise from surface ectoderm early in development

Neural Plate

During the third week of gestation, cells of the **surface ectoderm** in the dorsal midline of the embryo differentiate into the pseudocolumnar **neuroepithelium of the neural plate** (Fig. 4–1*A*). A widened cranial region of the neural plate forms the **brain,** and a more elongated caudal region will form most of the **spinal cord.** During the fourth week, the lateral edges of the neural plate fold dorsally and medially in the occipitocervical region through a process called **neurulation** (Fig. 4–1*B*). The edges of the resulting **neural folds** continue to come together almost like a zipper superiorly and inferiorly, first closing off the **cranial neuropore** (cranial opening) and then the **caudal neuropore** (caudal opening) to form the hollow **neural tube** (Fig. 4–1*C*). The cavity within the neural tube is the **neural canal,** which becomes the **central canal** of the spinal cord and the **ventricles** of the brain.

As the neural tube forms, it detaches from the surrounding surface ectoderm and sinks into the dorsal body wall. Cells located at the lateral margins of the neural plate become ameboid (i.e., able to migrate) and break away to form a population of cells called the **neural crest.** The neural crest cells migrate from the neural tube to form **neurons** and **neuroglia** (supporting cells) within **peripheral ganglia** of the peripheral nervous system. The surface ectoderm closes over the neural tube to form the precursor of the **epidermis.**

Caudal Eminence

The most caudal segment of the spinal cord arises from a specialized mesodermal structure called the caudal eminence

The most caudal segment of the spinal cord (from vertebra S2 through the coccygeal region) arises from the **caudal eminence** through a process called **secondary neurulation.** This solid mass of mesoderm fuses with the caudal end of the neural tube and then becomes hollowed out as its lumen is made continuous with the more superior neural canal. The caudal eminence also gives rise to the **filum terminale,** an anchoring attachment at the caudal end of the spinal cord (see below).

Neuroblasts, Glioblasts, and Ependymal Cells

As soon as the neural tube forms, its neuroepithelial cells begin to differentiate into neuroblasts, glioblasts, and ependymal cells

As soon as the neural tube is formed, the neuroepithelial cells lining the neural canal elongate and retract in waves, detaching to form **neuroblasts of the mantle layer** (**gray matter** of the spinal cord) or continuing to divide as stem cells within the **ventricular layer.** Subsequent waves of division, elongation, retraction, and detachment of ventricular neuroepithelial cells produce **glioblasts.** Glioblasts also migrate from the ventricular layer into the mantle layer, surrounding the neuroblasts to form supporting **neuroglial cells.** Cells remaining within the ventricular layer form **ependymal cells,** which line the definitive **central canal** of the spinal cord (Fig. 4–2*A*).

As **neuroblasts** differentiate into **neurons** within the mantle layer, they sprout cell processes called **axons.**

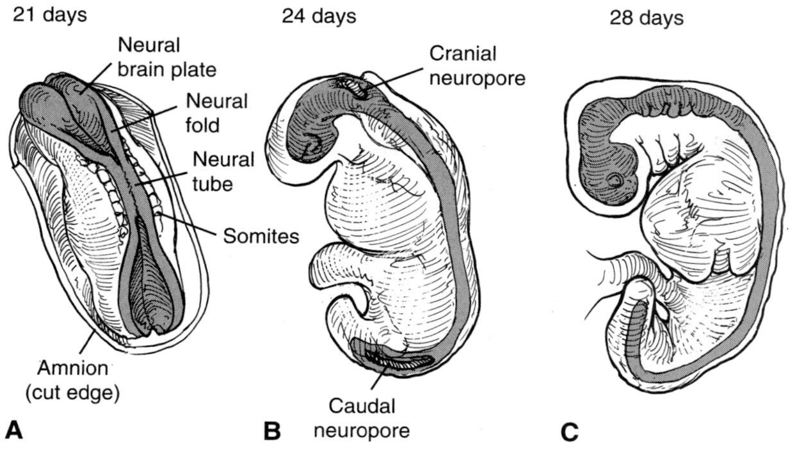

FIGURE 4–1
Neurulation. The central nervous system arises from the surface ectoderm as the neural plate rolls into a neural tube, which sinks into the posterior body wall to form the brain and spinal cord.

Axons elongate through locomotory activity of their distal **growth cones,** which migrate toward their targets through a variety of **path-finding** mechanisms. This proliferation and elongation of axons causes a fiber-filled **marginal layer** to form at the periphery of the mantle layer (Fig. 4–2*A*). The marginal layer is also called the **white matter** of the spinal cord because of the whitish color it assumes as glioblasts give rise to fatty myelin sheaths, which invest the axons in this region. Once the axonal growth cones find their targets (including neurons in the spinal cord, brain, and peripheral nerve ganglia), they form functional connections called **synapses.**

▲ Gray Matter of the Spinal Cord

Neurons of the gray matter become organized into an elongated H-shaped column that extends throughout all regions of the spinal cord

Somatic Motor and Sensory Neurons

Somatic motor neurons of the spinal cord are organized within the ventral gray columns, and sensory neurons are organized within the dorsal gray columns

The spinal cord continues to differentiate as the gray matter forms an elongated column of neurons, which in cross section is shaped like an H (Fig. 4–2*B*). This column extends throughout all regions of the spinal cord. The expanded dorsal arms of the H contain neurons that receive afferent (sensory) impulses from sensory organs, and so these are called **dorsal,** or **sensory, gray columns** of the spinal cord. The larger, expanded ventral arms of the H contain neurons that send out efferent (motor) impulses to peripheral end-organs such as striated muscles, and so these are called **ventral,** or **motor, gray columns** of the spinal cord. The transverse connection between the columns on the right and left sides of the spinal cord (i.e., the crossbar of the H) is the **gray commissure,** which carries nerve impulses between the left and right sides of the spinal cord. The gray commissure encloses the central canal throughout the length of the spinal cord.

Autonomic Motor Neurons

Autonomic motor neurons of the spinal cord are located in intermediolateral gray columns of the cord

Extending from levels T2 to L1 of the spinal cord only is a small, lateral, gray matter projection on each side of the H between the dorsal and ventral columns (Fig. 4–2*C*). These projections, which are called **lateral gray columns** of the spinal cord (along with neurons in this "intermediate" region at T1 to L2), constitute the **intermediolateral gray columns** of the **sympathetic division of the autonomic nervous system** (see Fig. 4–2*C* and below). Neurons situated within the intermediolateral gray columns from spinal cord levels T1 to L2 can be classified as **central motor neurons** of the "two-motor neuron" **sympathetic division** of the autonomic nervous system, which is therefore called the **thoracolumbar system.** The "second" motor neuron in the sympathetic nervous system lies outside the spinal cord within an enlarged knot of nerve cells called a **ganglion.** These ganglia are the **sympathetic chain ganglia** and **prevertebral ganglia** (see Figs. 4–8 to 4–10).

Although there is no obvious lateral gray column in any other region of the spinal cord, intermediate neurons adjacent to the central canal at sacral levels S2, S3, and S4 form short **intermediolateral gray columns.** These neurons can be classified as **central motor neurons** of the two-motor neuron **parasympathetic division** of the autonomic nervous system. Other central neurons of the **parasympathetic nervous system** are located in the **hindbrain** and **midbrain of the brainstem;**

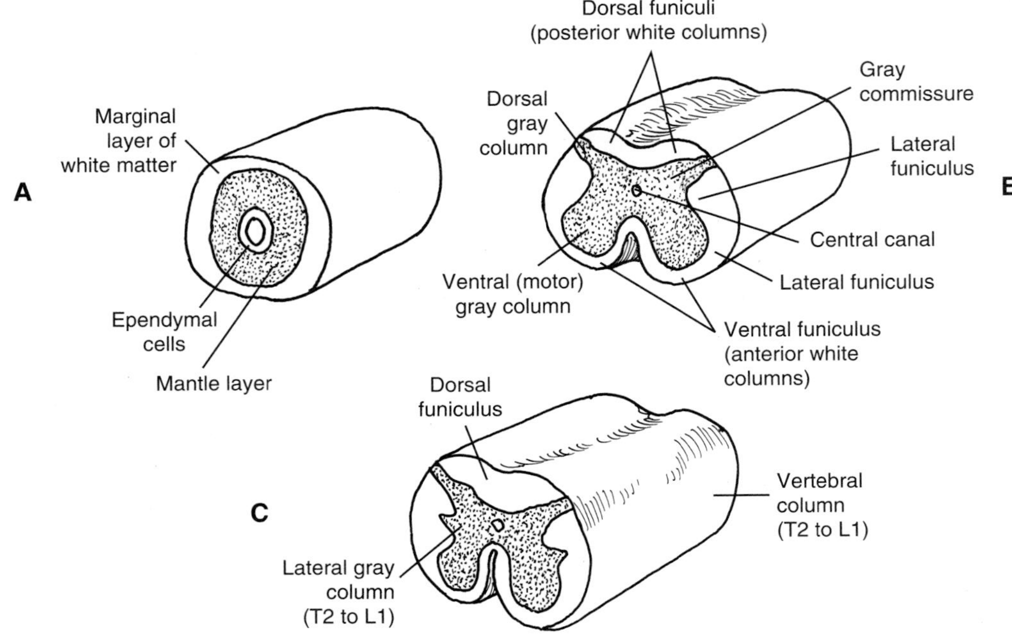

FIGURE 4–2

Differentiation of the neural tube. **A.** At first, the ventricular layer of the neural tube gives rise to neuroblasts and glia, which form the mantle layer. The neuroblasts form neurons, which sprout axons into a surrounding marginal layer. **B.** The mantle layer is shaped like an H (when seen in transverse section). The dorsal horns of the H are elongated sensory columns, which course throughout the length of the spinal cord. The ventral horns of the H are elongated motor columns, which also course throughout the length of the spinal cord. The anterior, posterior, and lateral funiculi contain nerve fiber tracts, which course from one level of the spinal cord to another. **C.** Lateral gray columns are apparent at cord levels T2 to L1. These columns are made up of concentrations of sympathetic neurons in the cord at these levels. Such concentrations of sympathetic neurons also extend into cord levels T1 and L2 but do not create a visible lateral gray column at these levels. Collections of parasympathetic neurons are located at cord levels S2 to S4 but do not produce a visible lateral gray column at these levels.

thus, the parasympathetic system is also called a **craniosacral system.** The second motor neurons of the parasympathetic system are also located in small **ganglia** peripheral to the brain or spinal cord. These ganglia, however, are typically embedded within the walls of the target organ itself (see Fig. 4–11).

White Matter of the Spinal Cord

White matter of the spinal cord contains nerve fiber tracts that serve both the somatic and autonomic nervous systems

Regions of white matter peripheral to and interspersed between the paired ventral and dorsal gray columns form **white columns,** or nerve fiber tracts called **anterior (ventral), posterior (dorsal),** and **lateral funiculi** (Fig. 4–2*B* and *C*). These white columns carry "ascending" and "descending" nerve impulses between different regions of the spinal cord and between the spinal cord and brain. In addition to the neuroglial cells that invest its nerve fibers, the white matter of the spinal cord also contains blood vessels, which vascularize tissues of the spinal cord (Fig. 4–24*A* to *C*).

DEVELOPMENT AND ORGANIZATION OF THE PERIPHERAL NERVOUS SYSTEM

Spinal nerves form at the levels of the segmental somites

Ventral and Dorsal Roots of the Peripheral Spinal Nerves

As the paired somites become segmented from the paraxial mesoderm (see Chapters 1 to 3), they interact with the neural tube, inducing the growth of **motor nerve axons** from both sides of the tube at intervals along the ventrolateral surfaces. Each segmental collection of these outward-growing motor nerve fibers is called a **ventral,** or **motor, root** (Fig. 4–3). Meanwhile, individual groups of **neural crest cells,** which become detached from the lateral edges of the neural plate during neurulation, aggregate adjacent to the dorsolateral region of the neural tube in register with each pair of ventral roots. These aggregations of neural crest cells differentiate into neurons and glioblasts of the paired **sensory dorsal root ganglia** at every somitic level except spinal nerve C1 (Fig. 4–3). Inward-growing nerve fibers of these dorsal root ganglia grow into the spinal cord to

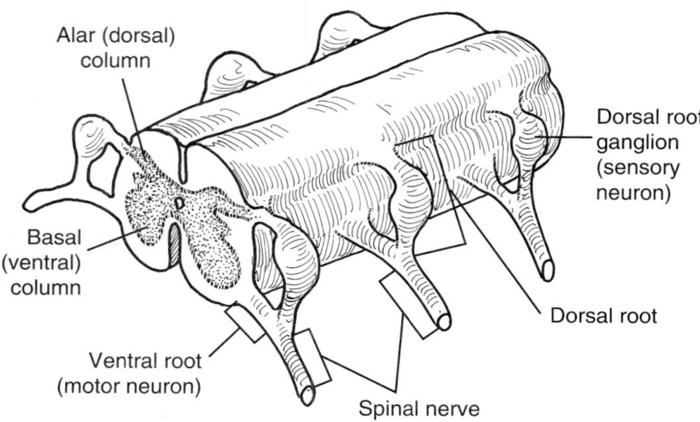

FIGURE 4–3
Dorsal root ganglia. The dorsal roots of all spinal nerves except C1 are characterized by a swelling containing sensory neurons and supporting glia. These are the dorsal root ganglia. Neurons and glia within the dorsal root ganglia arise from neural crest cells. The neurons differentiate into somatic and visceral sensory neurons. The sensory neurons emit centripetal axons, which synapse with association neurons in the dorsal column of the spinal cord. They also emit centrifugal neurons, which grow to the body wall or to the extremities (somatic afferents) and to sensory receptors within the walls of visceral organs (visceral afferents). They function to conduct sensory impulses from the body or the viscera to the spinal cord or brain or both.

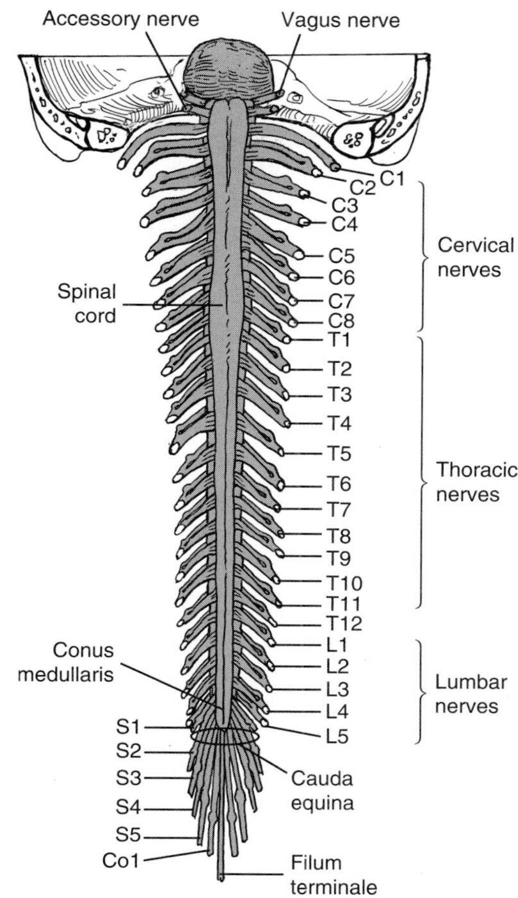

FIGURE 4–4
Spinal cord and spinal nerves. The adult spinal cord extends from vertebra C1 to the disc between vertebrae L1 and L2. There are 8 pairs of spinal nerves in the cervical region, 12 pairs in the thoracic region, 5 pairs in the lumbar region, 5 pairs in the sacral region, and 1 pair in the coccygeal region. Because the spinal cord is much shorter than the vertebral canal, the spinal nerve roots at the lower end of the cord have become elongated to reach the intervertebral foramina that they serve (see Fig. 4–15*C*).

synapse with neurons in the dorsal (sensory) column. Simultaneously, nerve fibers growing outward from dorsal root ganglia join with motor fibers of the ventral root to form a **spinal nerve** (Fig. 4–3). The dorsal root ganglion and its outward-growing and inward-growing fibers are collectively called a **dorsal root** (Fig. 4–3). Altogether, 31 pairs of spinal nerves are formed along the spinal cord: 8 cervical pairs, 12 thoracic pairs, 5 lumbar pairs, 5 sacral pairs, and 1 coccygeal pair (Fig. 4–4).

The fundamental organization of the spinal nerves is segmental (see Figs. 2-7 and 4–4 and Chapter 2). In most cases, each spinal nerve innervates the dermal structures and skeletal muscles that arise from the same somite that induced its growth (Fig. 4–5). As a consequence, the segmental sensory innervation of dermatomes of the integument as well as the segmental motor innervation of muscles of the neck, trunk, and extremities can be used as a basis for the diagnosis of referred pain (see below).

▲ Dorsal and Ventral Primary Rami

Spinal nerves split into two major branches (rami) near their points of origin

Just beyond the point at which the dorsal and ventral roots join together to form a spinal nerve, the nerve splits into a **dorsal primary ramus** and a **ventral primary ramus.** These rami contain the same functional mixture of axons that is present within the spinal nerves from which they branch. Thus the dorsal ramus provides motor innervation to the true back muscles and sensory innervation to the skin of the back, the back of the neck, and the back of the scalp (see Fig. 4–6 and Fig. 2–7). It also contains sympathetic efferent and visceral afferent fibers, which innervate blood vessels and glands (see Fig. 4–10). The ventral primary rami provide motor innervation to the anterolateral musculature of the body wall and neck and to the muscles of the upper and lower extremities (see Fig. 2–7 and 4–6). Their sensory fibers provide sensory innervation to the skin overlying these muscles and to the parietal pericardium (C3 to C5), parietal pleura (T1 to T11), and parietal peritoneum (T12 to L1) of the body cavities (see Fig. 4–6 and Fig. 2–7). These ventral primary rami also contain sympathetic efferent and visceral afferent fibers (see Fig. 4–12).

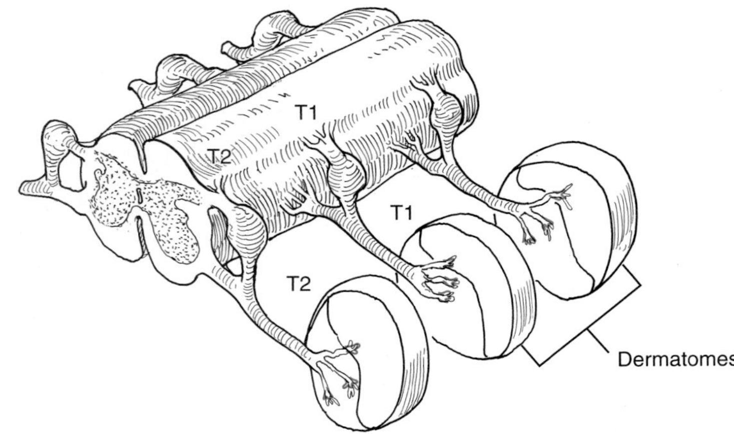

FIGURE 4–5
Somites induce the sprouting of spinal nerves. Derivatives of the somites, including the dermomyotomes, are innervated by the spinal nerve induced by their specific ancestral somite.

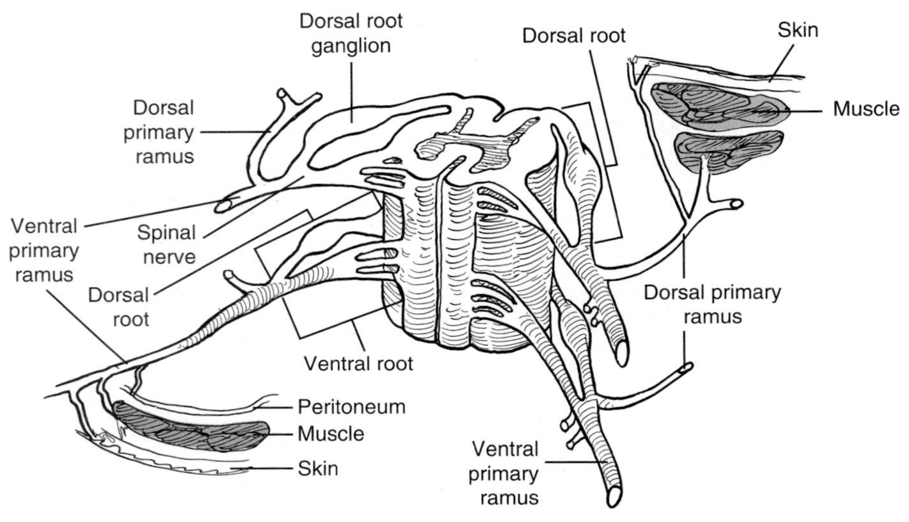

FIGURE 4–6
Dorsal and ventral primary rami. Every spinal nerve branches into a dorsal and a ventral primary ramus. Each of these rami contains all of the elements characteristic of the spinal nerve from which it branches. Dorsal rami innervate dorsal structures, including the deep back muscles and skin of the back. Ventral rami innervate the muscles of the extremities, ventrolateral muscles of the thorax and abdomen, and mesothelial linings of the body cavities.

Brachial and Lumbosacral Plexuses

Spinal nerves serving skeletal muscles of the extremities interconnect to form plexuses of ventral primary rami

Although the distribution of spinal nerves is typically segmental, the ventral rami that innervate muscles and sensory structures of the upper or lower extremities mix together to form the **brachial plexus** (of the upper extremity) and **lumbosacral plexus** (of the lower extremity). The brachial plexus is made up of ventral rami of spinal nerves C4 to T1, while the lumbosacral plexus includes contributions from spinal nerves T12 to S5. Within these plexuses the ventral rami of several spinal nerves may join together and branch from the plexus to form nerves. These plexuses will be described in detail in Chapters 14, 18, and 21.

SPINAL REFLEX ARCS

Basic Elements of Spinal Reflexes

Minimal requirements for a somatic spinal reflex include a peripheral receptor, sensory neuron, motor neuron, and terminal effector organ

In many cases, the actions of striated or smooth muscles are regulated by simple **reflex arcs** involving a single spinal cord segment (Fig. 4–7). A sensory fiber that innervates a peripheral receptor courses to a neuron within the dorsal root ganglion. An inward-directed fiber

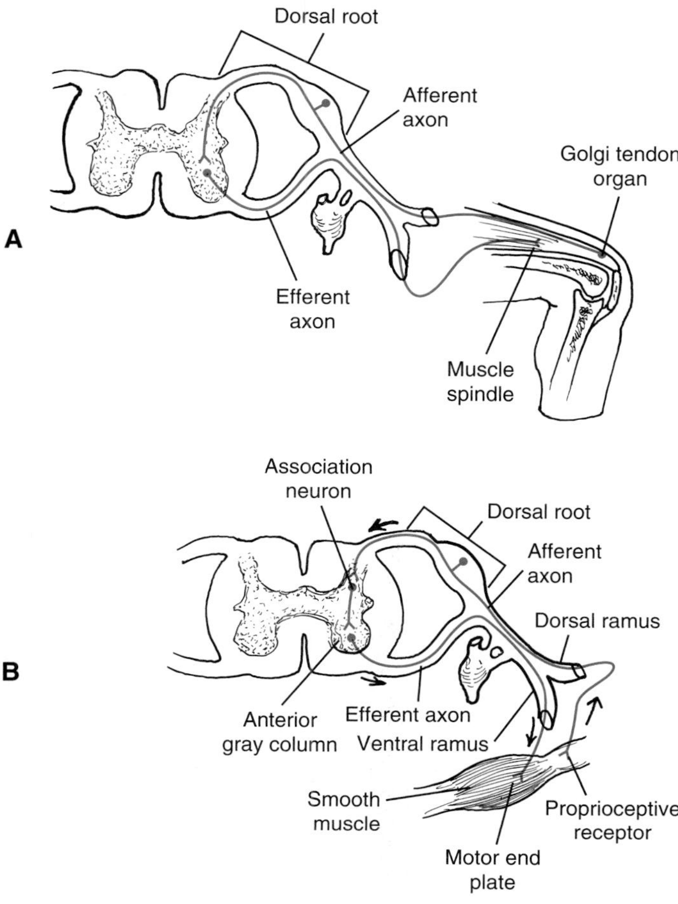

FIGURE 4–7

Reflex arcs. **A.** Monosynaptic reflexes involve direct interactions between a sensory and a motor neuron. **B.** Disynaptic reflexes involve sensory and motor neurons as well as intervening neurons such as association neurons of the dorsal column.

emitted from this neuron enters the spinal cord and passes through the dorsal gray column without synapsing with an association neuron. It directly synapses with a motor neuron within the ventral gray column. An efferent axon emitted from this neuron exits the spinal column via the ventral root to innervate the same organ from which the sensory fiber arises, completing the reflex arc. This is a **monosynaptic reflex arc** (Fig. 4–7*A*). It is the anatomic basis of the simple **patellar tendon reflex,** which can be elicited by abrupt vigorous stretching of the muscle. The consequent mechanical compression of receptors known as **muscle spindles** stimulates the firing of an afferent impulse, which travels through the afferent axon of the dorsal root ganglion, through the dorsal root ganglion, and into the spinal cord, resulting in stimulation of an appropriate motor neuron in the ventral gray column. The motor neuron discharges an efferent motor impulse, which stimulates the same muscle to contract (Fig. 4–7*A*).

Additional Elements of Spinal Reflexes

Many spinal reflexes involve more than the four elements described above; they are modified by additional input from other spinal cord levels or from higher centers within the central nervous system

The preceding description suggests that discharge of a receptor in a reflex arc leads to a single, repeatable, all-or-nothing kind of reflex action, but it is clear that most spinal reflexes are far more complex. In some cases an afferent fiber enters the dorsal gray column and synapses with an association neuron, which, in turn, synapses with a motor neuron within the ventral gray column. Because this arc involves an association neuron within its basic pathway, it is called a **disynaptic reflex arc** (Fig. 4–7*B*). Modification of the receptor's initial signal may occur at the level of the association neuron within the dorsal gray column, possibly through its own characteristic activity or through modification of its activity by other neurons connected to it. Alternatively, the activity of the motor neuron of the reflex arc may be directly modified by input from other neurons whose axons have made synapses with it. Neurons that influence the activity of a spinal reflex may be located at other levels of the spinal cord or on the other side of the spinal cord, and their actions may thus coordinate more complex "reflexes." Other "influential" neurons may be located at higher centers within the central nervous system (e.g., the cerebral cortex), providing conscious modification or stimulation of a spinal reflex (see discussion of sexual reflex activity in Chapter 15).

THE SYMPATHETIC NERVOUS SYSTEM: ELEMENTS AND GENERAL ORGANIZATION

Sympathetic innervation of peripheral structures within the body wall is effected by an efferent sympathetic pathway with two neurons: a central neuron and a peripheral neuron

The intermediolateral gray columns at spinal cord levels T1 to L2 contain central neurons of the two-neuron sympathetic division of the autonomic nervous system, which is known as the **thoracolumbar system** (Fig. 4–8 and see Figs. 4–2*C*, 4–9, and 4–10). As axons grow out from ventral gray columns to form ventral motor roots of the segmental spinal nerves at these levels, axons from the corresponding intermediolateral cell columns also grow out. Each axon follows the course of a ventral root into a spinal nerve (Fig 4–8).

Just after issuing from the intervertebral foramina of the vertebral column, the sympathetic axons exit the spinal nerve through a small branch called a **white ramus communicans,** which is connected to a small ganglion called a **sympathetic chain ganglion** at the same spinal nerve level (Fig. 4–8). Like the dorsal root ganglia, these ganglia arise from neural crest cells, and a pair of them is typically formed in association with every pair of spinal nerves. Chain ganglia in the cervical region, however, fuse into three pairs of ganglia called

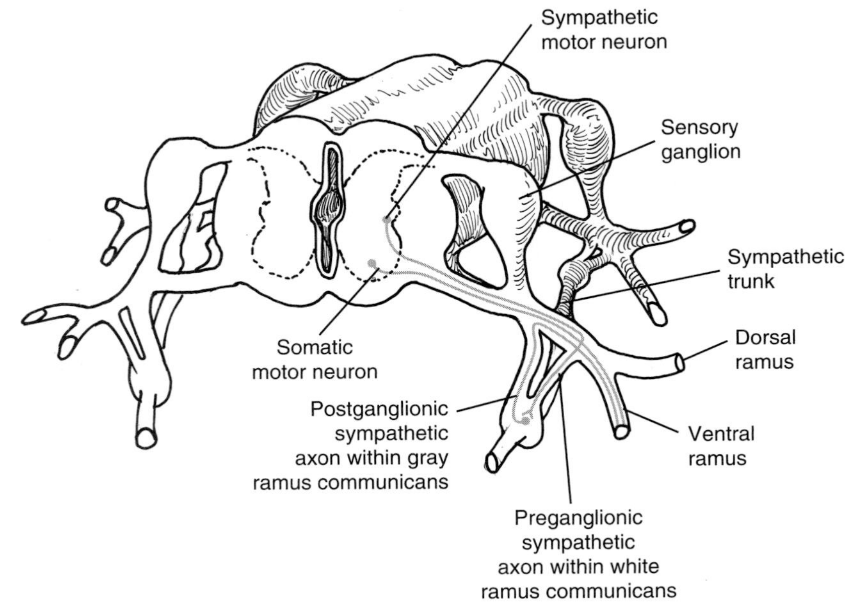

FIGURE 4–8

Preganglionic and postganglionic sympathetic fibers between T1 and L2. A preganglionic axon emitted from the central sympathetic neurons at cord levels T1 to L2 may escape the cord via the ventral root to enter the spinal nerve. It then escapes the spinal nerve via a white ramus to enter the corresponding chain ganglion where it synapses with a peripheral neuron. This postsynaptic neuron then emits an axon, which escapes the chain ganglion via a gray ramus. This postganglionic axon rejoins the spinal nerve for distribution to its target.

the **superior, middle,** and **inferior cervical ganglia** (see Chapter 23). Sometimes the inferior cervical chain ganglion is fused with the first thoracic chain ganglion to form a **stellate ganglion.**

The axon growing into the chain ganglion may synapse with a neuron located within it (Fig. 4–8). In this event, neurons located within this peripheral chain ganglion function as the second motor neuron in the two-neuron sympathetic system. Because the axon that grows from the first (central) sympathetic neuron "comes before" the second (ganglionic) sympathetic neuron in the typical sympathetic pathway, it is called a **preganglionic axon.** The axon growing from the second (ganglionic) neuron is called a **postganglionic axon** (see below).

▲ Sympathetic Innervation of the Body Wall and Extremities

A preganglionic axon growing from the intermediolateral column between spinal nerves T1 and L2 may synapse with a peripheral neuron in a chain ganglion at the same level

Assuming that the preganglionic axon synapses with a second neuron in the associated chain ganglion, an axon growing from this peripheral neuron then exits the ganglion through another small branch called a **gray ramus communicans,** which reconnects the chain ganglion with the spinal nerve (Fig. 4–8). This **postganglionic axon** accompanies somatic motor and sensory fibers of the spinal nerve and is distributed to targets in the body wall and extremities, such as hair follicles and smooth muscle in blood vessels.

Preganglionic axons may also synapse with peripheral neurons in chain ganglia associated with spinal nerves at superior or inferior levels

In some cases, the preganglionic fiber entering a chain ganglion at a given level may not synapse with a neuron within that chain ganglion. Indeed, since all of the central neurons of the sympathetic system are located within intermediolateral columns of spinal nerves T1 to L2, the chain ganglia associated with spinal nerves above T1 must obtain their innervation from preganglionic axons originating at more inferior levels (Fig. 4–9). Likewise, chain ganglia associated with spinal nerves below L2 must obtain their innervation from more superior levels (Fig. 4–9). Preganglionic axons originating from spinal cord level L2, for example, may enter the chain ganglion associated with spinal nerve L2 and, without synapsing there, exit the ganglion through a fiber tract called the **sympathetic trunk** (Fig. 4–9). This preganglionic axon may descend through the sympathetic trunk to enter the chain ganglion associated with the spinal nerve at L3 (or other lower levels) where it synapses with its second neuron. This second neuron, in turn, emits a postganglionic axon via a gray ramus communicans to join with the spinal nerve at L3 for distribution to appropriate end organs within the L3 dermatome (see

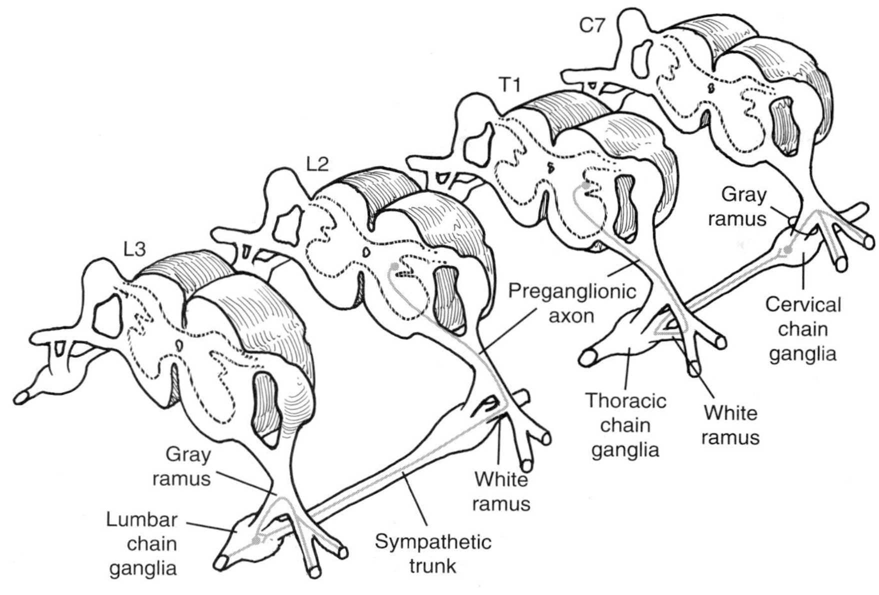

FIGURE 4–9
Sympathetic innervation above T1 and below L2. Chain ganglia above T1 and below L2 must receive their preganglionic fibers from cord levels T1 to L2 via the sympathetic trunk. Note the absence of a white ramus communicans at spinal nerve levels above T1 and below L2.

Fig. 2-7). In the same way, preganglionic axons arising from thoracic levels of the spinal cord may ascend through the sympathetic trunk to innervate peripheral neurons within chain ganglia associated with cervical spinal nerves (see Figs. 4–9 and 4–10).

Because preganglionic fibers enter the cervical chain ganglia or chain ganglia below L2 via the sympathetic trunk, the spinal nerves at these levels lack white rami communicans (note spinal nerves C7 and L3 in Fig. 4–9). Gray rami communicans, however, are found at virtually all levels because postganglionic fibers join the spinal nerves at all levels, whether or not they are innervated by preganglionic fibers that originate from the same level or a different level. It should also be pointed out that postganglionic fibers never enter the sympathetic trunk (Fig. 4–9).

▲ Sympathetic Innervation of the Viscera

Sympathetic visceral nerves innervate viscera of the head, neck, thorax, abdominopelvic cavity, and perineum

Glands and smooth muscle cells of the head and neck as well as the heart, trachea, bronchi, and viscera of the abdominopelvic cavity and the perineum are provided with sympathetic innervation by specialized visceral nerves that emanate from the chain ganglia. These nerves may consist of postganglionic fibers given off by neurons within particular chain ganglia, as in the case of sympathetic nerves to the head, heart, and lungs. In other cases preganglionic fibers pass through the chain ganglia and then synapse with distant ganglia, as in the case of the sympathetic **splanchnic nerves** innervating the prevertebral ganglia that provide sympathetic innervation to the abdominal, pelvic, and perineal viscera (Fig. 4–10 and see Chapters 12, 14, and 15).

▲ Sympathetic Innervation of the Head and Neck

Sympathetic innervation to structures within the head and neck is provided by postganglionic axons arising from the superior cervical ganglion

Preganglionic fibers from the superior five thoracic levels (but mainly from spinal nerves T1 to T3) may ascend through the sympathetic trunk to innervate neurons within inferior, middle, or superior cervical ganglia (Figs. 4–9 and 4–10). These neurons then emit postganglionic sympathetic fibers, which exit directly from their respective ganglia and follow the course of blood vessels to target organs in the head and neck. These target organs include the **dilator pupillae muscles** and the **thyroid, lacrimal,** and **salivary glands** (Fig. 4–10). The innervation of these structures will be described in detail in Chapters 24 and 27.

▲ Sympathetic Innervation of the Heart, Trachea, and Lungs

Sympathetic cardiac and pulmonary nerves consist of postganglionic sympathetic nerve fibers arising from chain ganglia associated with spinal nerves T1 to T5 and from cervical chain ganglia

Preganglionic axons arising from central sympathetic neurons at spinal cord levels T1 to T5 may synapse with neurons within chain ganglia at the same level or rise through the sympathetic trunk to synapse

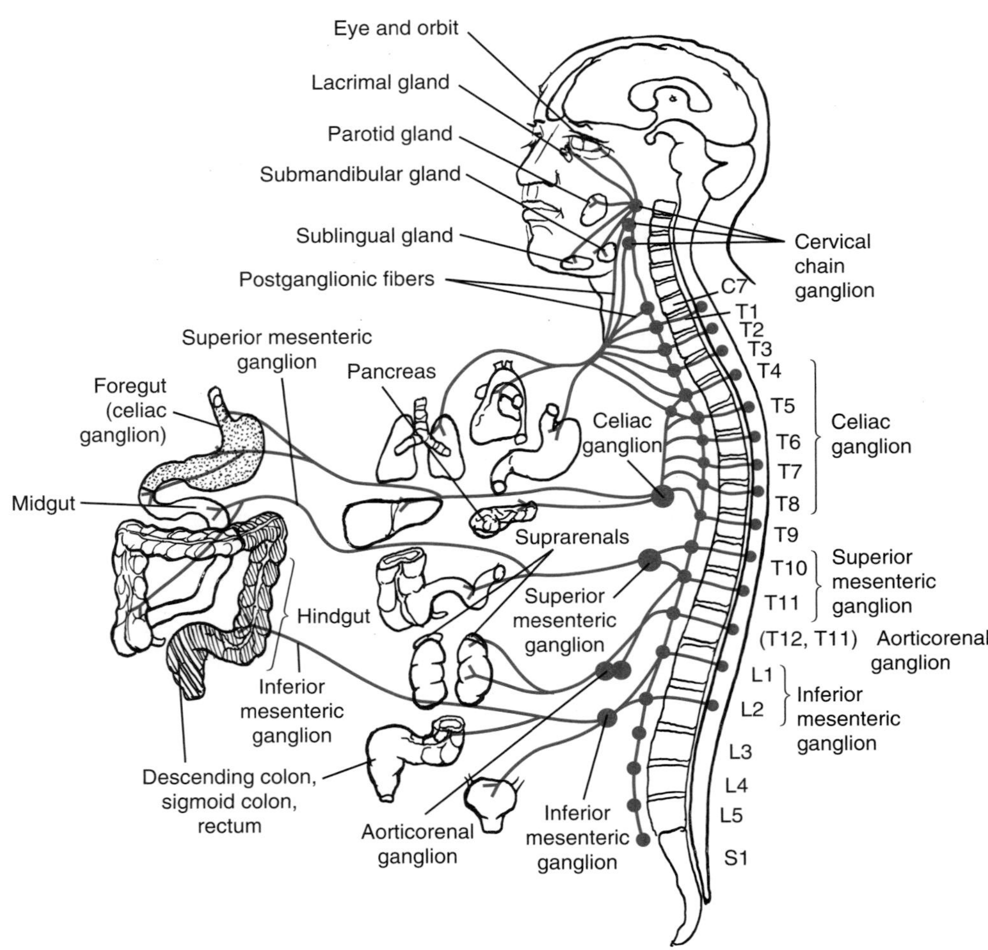

FIGURE 4–10

Sympathetic innervation of viscera. Preganglionic fibers from sympathetic neurons within the cord between levels T1 and L2 are distributed to chain ganglia and to a special group of prevertebral ganglia. Postganglionic fibers emitted by thoracic and cervical chain ganglia innervate the thoracic viscera. Postganglionic fibers emitted by prevertebral ganglia innervate abdominal and pelvic viscera.

with cervical chain ganglia. Postganglionic fibers then directly exit the cervical and thoracic chain ganglia as **sympathetic cardiac** or **pulmonary nerves** to innervate the heart, trachea, or lungs (see Figs. 4–9 and 4–10).

▲ Sympathetic Innervation of the Gastrointestinal and Pelvic Viscera

Gastrointestinal and pelvic viscera are provided with sympathetic innervation via special sympathetic splanchnic nerves

The second (peripheral) neurons in the two-neuron sympathetic motor pathway that innervate the gastrointestinal tract and other viscera of the abdominopelvic cavity and perineum are located within special **prevertebral,** or **preaortic, ganglia.** The neurons and supporting cells within these preaortic ganglia arise from migrating neural crest cells, as in the case of the chain ganglia described above.

Preaortic ganglia are typically described as **celiac, superior mesenteric, aorticorenal,** and **inferior mesenteric ganglia** because they are associated with the main arterial trunks that supply the abdominal viscera (i.e., the celiac, superior mesenteric, and inferior mesenteric and renal arteries). In actuality, peripheral neurons of the more inferior ganglia are more scattered within superior mesenteric, aorticorenal, and inferior mesenteric **plexuses** (see Chapters 13 and 14).

The preaortic ganglia are innervated by preganglionic fibers from special **sympathetic splanchnic nerves,** which exit directly from chain ganglia at the thoracic and lumbar levels, descend along the vertebral column, and pierce the diaphragm to gain entry into the abdominal cavity (Fig. 4–10 and see Chapter 10). The **greater splanchnic nerve** is usually described as consisting of preganglionic fibers arising from neurons located at spinal cord levels T4 or T5 to T9. These fibers exit their chain ganglia and collect into bundles along the lateral surfaces of the thoracic vertebral bodies. The resulting greater splanchnic nerves enter the abdominal cavity through their own foramina within the crura of the diaphragm and innervate peripheral sympathetic neurons within the **celiac ganglia.** Postganglionic axons that issue from celiac ganglia then follow **branches of the celiac artery** to innervate the abdominal esophagus, stomach, superior half of the duodenum, liver, gallbladder, and pancreas (Fig. 4–10). Preganglionic fibers of the **lesser splanchnic nerve** arise from neurons located at spinal cord levels T10 and T11 to innervate peripheral sympathetic neurons within the **superior mesenteric ganglia.** Postganglionic axons arising from these ganglia follow **branches of the superior mesenteric artery** to innervate the inferior half of the duodenum, jejunum, ileum, ascending colon, and about two-thirds of the transverse colon (Fig. 4–10). The **least (lowest) splanchnic nerves** are made up of preganglionic fibers arising from neurons located at spinal cord level T11 or T12 (or both). These fibers innervate peripheral sympathetic neurons within the **aorticorenal ganglia,** which, in turn, give off postganglionic fibers that innervate the kidneys and suprarenal glands **via the arteries to these organs** (Fig. 4–10). Finally, preganglionic fibers arising from neurons located at spinal cord levels L1 and L2 (and sometimes L3) form the **lumbar splanchnic nerves,** which innervate peripheral sympathetic neurons within the **inferior mesenteric ganglia.** These ganglia emit postganglionic fibers, which follow branches of the **inferior mesenteric artery** to innervate the remaining one-third of the transverse colon, the descending and sigmoid colon, the rectum, and the pelvic viscera (Fig. 4–10).

THE PARASYMPATHETIC NERVOUS SYSTEM: ELEMENTS AND GENERAL ORGANIZATION

Parasympathetic innervation of viscera of the head, neck, and trunk is provided by a craniosacral system. Central neurons of the parasympathetic system are located in the brainstem and at spinal cord levels S2 to S4

Like the sympathetic nervous system, the parasympathetic nervous system is a two-neuron motor system. It is made up of central motor neurons, which give off preganglionic axons that innervate peripheral neurons situated in ganglia located outside the central nervous system. Postganglionic axons arising from these peripheral neurons innervate their specific target organs. Although these general features are shared by the sympathetic and parasympathetic systems, the following differences are present in the overall organization of these two systems:

1. Unlike the sympathetic system in which all central neurons are located in intermediolateral columns of the spinal cord in the thoracolumbar regions, the central neurons of the parasympathetic system are located within the brainstem in association with cranial nerves III, VII, IX, and X and within the gray matter of the spinal cord at levels S2 to S4 (Fig. 4–11). Thus, as has been noted above, the parasympathetic system is a **craniosacral system.**
2. Although peripheral neurons of the sympathetic system are localized in discrete ganglia adjacent to the vertebral column (chain ganglia) or in association with the aorta (preaortic ganglia), the ganglia of the parasympathetic system (with the exception of cranial parasympathetic ganglia; see below and Chapter 23]) are typically small, scattered, and embedded within the walls of the many specific target organs.
3. Because of the location of peripheral ganglia in the two systems, the preganglionic axons of the sympathetic system tend to be relatively short and those of the parasympathetic system relatively long. Conversely, postganglionic axons of the sympathetic system tend to be relatively long and those of the parasympathetic system relatively short.

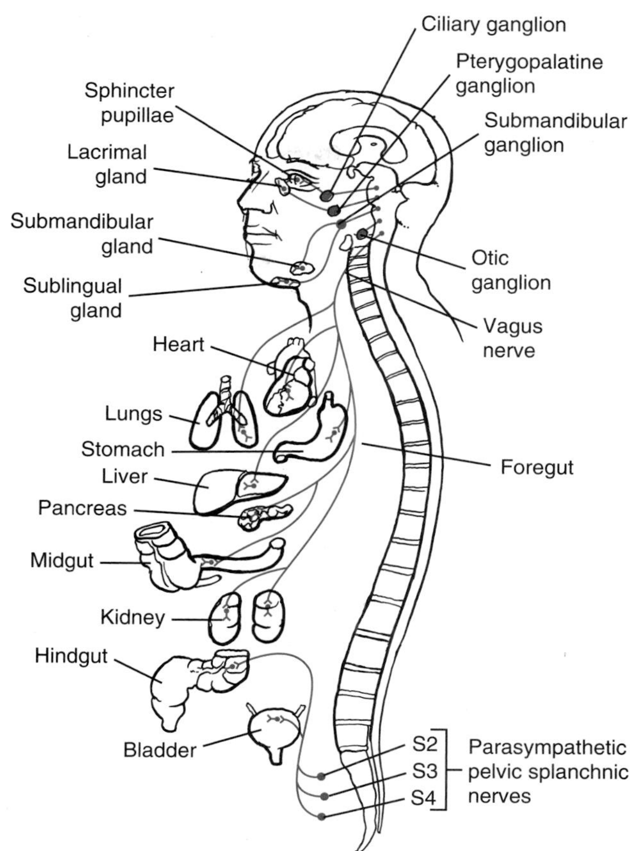

FIGURE 4–11
Parasympathetic innervation of the viscera. The viscera receive parasympathetic innervation via the neurons within the midbrain and hindbrain and in the spinal cord at cord levels S2 to S4. Preganglionic fibers within the vagus nerve and pelvic splanchnic nerves innervate ganglia embedded within the walls of thoracic, abdominal, and pelvic organs. Short postganglionic fibers emitted by these ganglia innervate the specific viscera.

4. Unlike the sympathetic system, the parasympathetic system does not provide innervation to structures within the body wall or extremities such as blood vessels, arrector pili muscles of the hair, or glands. The parasympathetic system innervates structures within the head and neck and the thoracic, abdominopelvic, and perineal viscera only.

▲ Parasympathetic Innervation of the Head and Neck

The cranial part of the parasympathetic nervous system provides parasympathetic innervation to glands and smooth muscle cells of the head and neck

The preganglionic axons emitted from central parasympathetic neurons associated with cranial nerves III, VII, and IX innervate small, discrete peripheral parasympathetic ganglia within the head: the **ciliary, submandibular, pterygopalatine,** and **otic ganglia.** These ganglia, like the sympathetic chain ganglia and the prevertebral ganglia, are formed by neural crest cells. Neurons within these ganglia give rise to postganglionic axons, which innervate the **dilator pupillae muscles; submandibular** and **sublingual salivary glands, lacrimal glands,** and **mucous glands of the nose** and **palate;** and **parotid glands** and **mucous glands of the oral cavity** (Fig. 4–11). This part of the parasympathetic system is described in detail in Chapter 24.

▲ Parasympathetic Innervation of the Thoracic and Abdominal Viscera

Cranial nerve X (vagus nerve [wanderer]) also provides parasympathetic innervation to most of the viscera

Preganglionic axons emitted from central neurons associated with the **vagus nerve** (unlike preganglionic parasympathetic axons associated with nerves III, VII, and IX) exit the head, descend through the neck, and enter the thoracic and abdominal cavities to innervate postganglionic neurons within scattered peripheral ganglia embedded within the walls of the heart, trachea, and bronchi; the gastrointestinal tract to the transverse colon; and the liver, gallbladder, pancreas, and kidney (Fig. 4–11). Like other peripheral ganglia of the autonomic nervous system, these ganglia also arise from neural crest cells. Neurons within these scattered peripheral ganglia, in turn, give off short postganglionic fibers, which immediately innervate structures (primarily smooth muscle cells and glands) within the wall of the organ in which they are embedded.

▲ Parasympathetic Innervation of the Inferior Gastrointestinal Tract and Pelvic Viscera

Central parasympathetic neurons at spinal cord levels S2 to S4 innervate peripheral ganglia associated with the most inferior part of the gastrointestinal tract and with pelvic viscera

Innervation of peripheral parasympathetic neurons within the gastrointestinal tract inferior to the terminal part of the transverse colon and to pelvic and sexual organs is provided by parasympathetic preganglionic fibers that arise from central neurons residing within the spinal cord at cord levels S2 to S4 (Fig. 4–11). The short postganglionic axons arising from these peripheral neurons primarily innervate smooth muscle cells within the walls of the gastrointestinal tract (see Chapter 12), the bladder and its sphincter, the oviducts and uterus, the erectile tissues of the penis or clitoris, and the vasculature of the testes or ovaries (see Chapter 15). This innervation, along with the sympathetic and somatic innervation of these structures, is important for normal **micturition, defecation,** and **sexual function.**

▲ Visceral Afferent Fibers in Autonomic Innervation

Visceral afferent fibers are also associated with autonomic pathways

Although the sympathetic and parasympathetic nervous systems are strictly characterized as two-neuron motor systems, it must be remembered that visceral afferent fibers are also involved in the function of the autonomic nervous system (see Functional Integration of the Spinal Cord and Peripheral Nervous System below). The cell bodies of these visceral afferent fibers are located within dorsal root ganglia, as are the cell bodies of somatic afferent fibers. The visceral afferent fibers travel with the autonomic preganglionic and postganglionic motor fibers from sensory structures (e.g., pressure, stretch, or pain receptors within end-organs) back to the chain ganglia (directly if the fibers are from the viscera or via the gray ramus if the fibers accompany spinal nerves from the body wall), then back to the spinal nerve via the white ramus and into the dorsal root and dorsal root ganglion (Fig. 4–12). From the cell bodies of these visceral afferent pathways, inward-growing axons synapse with sensory neurons within the dorsal gray columns of the spinal cord (see Fig. 4–12).

■ FUNCTIONAL INTEGRATION OF THE SPINAL CORD AND PERIPHERAL NERVOUS SYSTEM

The central and peripheral nervous systems regulate and integrate activities of virtually all of the other tissues and organs of the body. The nervous system accomplishes this feat by transmitting, relaying, and modifying complex chemical and electrical signals through cellular and molecular mechanisms. Therefore, an understanding of the fundamental organization of the central and peripheral nervous systems is crucial to many aspects of clinical history taking, diagnosis, and treatment.

▲ Function of the Somatic Nervous System

Activities of the somatic nervous system are characterized by central voluntary control and conscious movement

In general, neurons within the dorsal and ventral gray columns regulate voluntary activities of the **somatic nervous system.** The ventral gray columns contain mo-

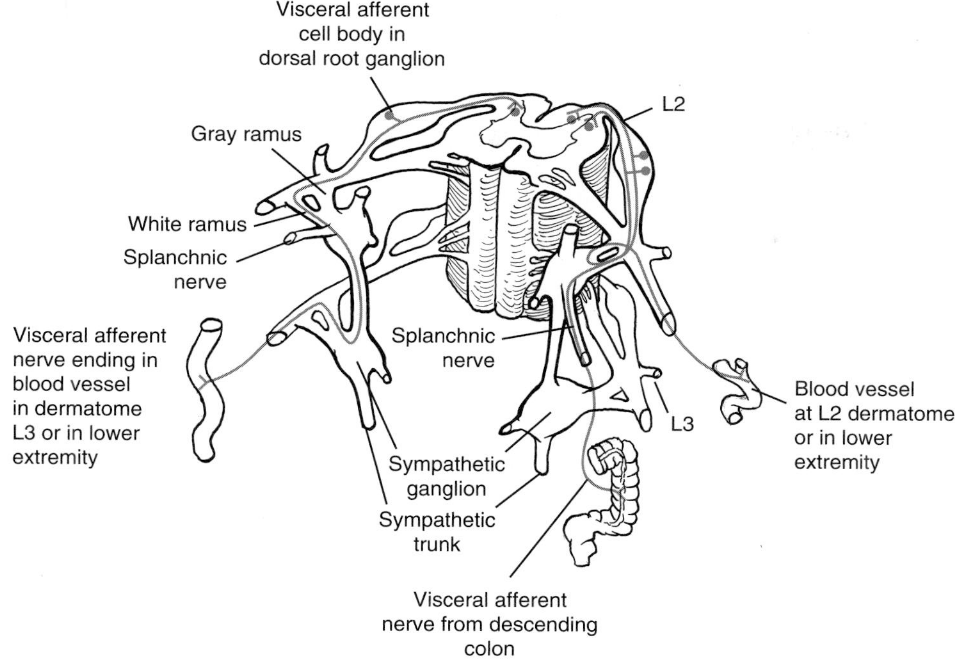

FIGURE 4–12
Visceral afferent fibers accompany both sympathetic and parasympathetic pathways to conduct impulses from pain and pressure (and other) receptors back to the central nervous system.

tor neurons that relay neural impulses from the brain to the striated musculature. For example, neurons in ventral gray columns at spinal cord levels C4 to T1 carry impulses from the brain that result in conscious, coordinated movements of the arms, forearms, wrists, hands, and fingers. Neurons within dorsal root ganglia and dorsal gray columns, on the other hand, relay sensory impulses from the scalp, neck, trunk, and extremities to the brain. For example, neurons within dorsal root ganglia and dorsal gray columns at the level of the lumbosacral cord relay conscious sensations from the lower abdomen, back, and lower extremities to the brain.

While the motor function of the somatic nervous system is limited to stimulating **striated muscle** movements, somatic sensory functions are more varied. Afferent fibers may relay sensations of pain, heat, cold, touch, pressure, tension, or stretching to the spinal cord and higher centers within the central nervous system. One of the most important functions of the sensory part of the somatic nervous system is **proprioceptive function (sense of body position or posture).** This complex sensation involves the initiation of sensory impulses within many tension and pressure receptors in muscles, tendons, and joints; delivery of these impulses to the spinal cord by neurons and processes of the dorsal root ganglia and dorsal gray column; conduction of the impulses to higher centers through the white columns of the spinal cord; and interpretation of the impulses by cortical regions of the brain.

▲ Function of the Autonomic Nervous System

The autonomic nervous system regulates involuntary activities of the viscera

During periods of "peace and relaxation," involuntary visceral body functions are regulated by activities of the parasympathetic nervous system. During periods of relaxation, vagal parasympathetic stimulation causes the heart to beat more slowly and smooth muscle within the walls of the gastrointestinal tract to push digesting food toward the rectum. During periods of "fight and flight," on the other hand, the sympathetic nervous system predominates in the control of visceral body functions. The phrase "fight and flight" provides a clue to the specific effects of this system. It causes the heart to beat faster, peristalsis to cease, and the pupils to open to let in more light and visual information. These responses have been selected for their life-preserving qualities in threatening circumstances.

Because the parasympathetic and sympathetic systems regulate visceral functions during the states of "peace and relaxation" and "fight and flight," one would predict that the effects of one system on a given organ would directly oppose the effects of the other system. This is sometimes true, but at other times the two systems work in a synergistic manner. Opposing effects of the two systems are clearly evident in the heart, where parasympathetic and sympathetic nerves act upon the same organ. In other organs, opposition is achieved in different ways. This is the case with the pupils of the eyes, where the parasympathetic system stimulates constriction of the pupils through its effect on the **constrictor pupillae muscles** and the sympathetic system stimulates dilatation through its effect on the **dilator pupillae muscles.** In yet another scheme, the only mechanism of autonomic innervation of the smooth muscle within blood vessels of the skin is sympathetic innervation. This means that vasoconstriction of the integumental vasculature results from sympathetic stimulation and vasodilatation from the absence of sympathetic stimulation. Finally, it is not unusual to find that the sympathetic and parasympathetic systems act together to coordinate or synergistically affect the sequential steps of many complex physiologic processes. For example, the processes of micturition, defecation, and sexual function are regulated by cooperative interactions between the parasympathetic, sympathetic, and somatic nervous systems (see Chapter 15).

Lesions of the Nervous System

The loss of specific somatic or visceral motor or sensory function may reveal the site of a lesion within the nervous system

The various components of the nervous system described in this chapter have specific functional fibers existing alone or in combination, and so the functional consequences of lesions resulting from trauma or disease processes of particular elements will vary, depending on the fibers involved (Fig. 4–13 and Table 4–1).

▲ Neural and Anatomic Bases of Referred Pain

Disease or injury of viscera may be experienced as pain of the body wall or of an extremity

A common consequence of inflammation, distention, ischemia, or chemical irritation of visceral organs

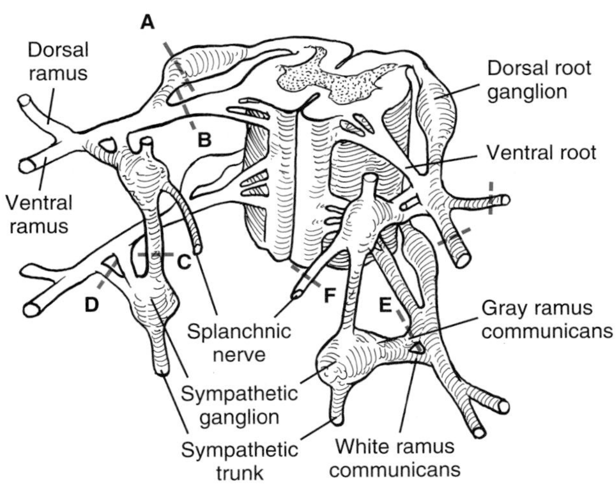

FIGURE 4–13
Functional components of spinal nerves. Lesions of specific neural structures associated with the spinal nerves result in deficits that reflect the specific fiber types within that structure (see Table 4–1). **A.** Dorsal root. **B.** Ventral root. **C.** Sympathetic trunk. **D.** White ramus communicans. **E.** Gray ramus communicans. **F.** Sympathetic splanchnic nerve.

TABLE 4–1
Summary of Neuron and Fiber Types Within Components of the Spinal Central Nervous System and Peripheral Nervous System*

Gross Neural Structure	Functional Cell Bodies or Fibers
Dorsal gray columns of spinal cord	Association neurons of sensory pathway
Intermediolateral gray columns of spinal cord	Central neurons of autonomic nervous system (sympathetic at T1 to L2, parasympathetic at S2 to S4)
Ventral gray columns of spinal cord	Motor neurons
Dorsal roots (see Fig. 4–13*A*)	Dorsal root ganglion containing sensory neuron cell bodies; somatic and visceral afferent (sensory) fibers
Ventral roots (see Fig. 4–13*B*)	Somatic motor fibers; sympathetic preganglionic fibers
Sympathetic trunks (see Fig. 4–13*C*)	Sympathetic preganglionic fibers; visceral afferent fibers
White rami communicans (see Fig. 4–13*D*)	Sympathetic preganglionic fibers; visceral afferent fibers (T5 to L2) associated with splanchnic nerves
Gray rami communicans (see Fig. 4–13*E*)	Sympathetic postganglionic fibers
Splanchnic nerves (see Fig. 4–13*F*)	Sympathetic preganglionic fibers; visceral afferent fibers
Vagus nerves	Parasympathetic preganglionic fibers; afferent visceral fibers; special visceral efferent fibers (see Chapter 23); somatic sensory fibers
Pelvic splanchnic nerves	Parasympathetic preganglionic fibers; visceral afferent fibers

*See Fig. 4–13.

or of torsion or traction of mesenteries is the sensation of pain within the body wall. This phenomenon is called *referred pain.* Examples that should be familiar are heartburn, stomachache, and menstrual cramps. Another clinically relevant example is pain in the shoulder and upper extremity indicating a myocardial infarction ("heart attack"). This visceral pain tends to be slow, aching, and diffuse, unlike true somatic pain, which is usually sharp and localized.

The neurologic basis of referred pain is only partly understood. It has been suggested that constant bombardment of the "viscerosomatic" neurons of the dorsal gray column by afferent impulses from the affected visceral organ may cause the brain to misread these stimuli as pain from the dermatome that also innervates these neurons. Alternatively, it has been suggested that the bombardment of dorsal sensory neurons by input from visceral afferent fibers may "sensitize" nearby somatic association neurons at the same level. These sensitized neurons then send signals to the brain. The signals are then interpreted as somatic pain arising from the dermatomes innervated by the somatic afferents that synapse with the sensitized association neurons (Fig. 4–14).

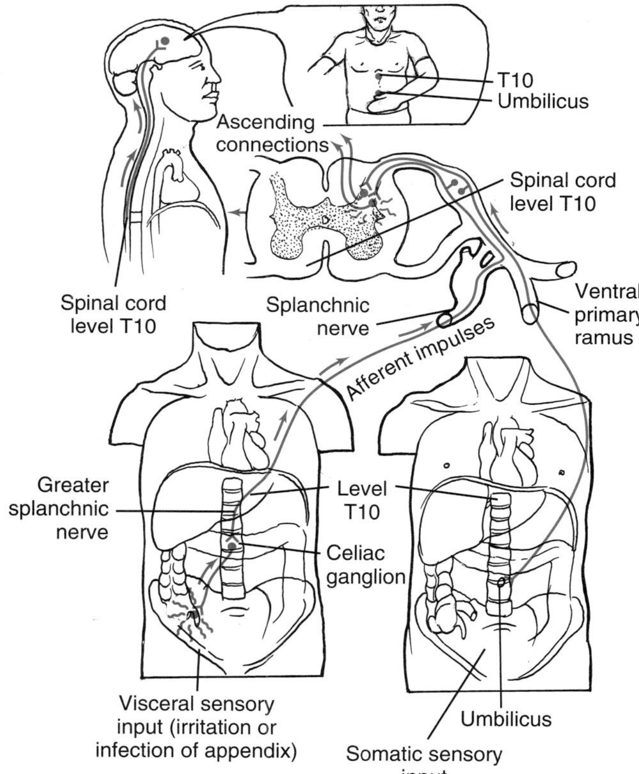

FIGURE 4–14
Referred pain. Impulses from a diseased appendix enter the spinal cord at the level of T10 via the visceral afferent fibers innervating receptors within the appendix. Their activity within the dorsal column may stimulate activity within adjacent somatic association neurons, which normally receive impulses only from dermatome T10 (around the umbilicus). This indirect activity of somatic association neurons at the level of T10 is interpreted by the brain as discomfort around the umbilicus.

Because the visceral afferent fibers that innervate the heart enter the spinal cord at levels T1 to T4, pain is referred to the dermatomes innervated by somatic afferent fibers entering the spinal cord at the levels of the upper chest, shoulder, and anterior arm and forearm (see Fig. 4–10). The knowledge that visceral afferent fibers from different organs enter the spinal cord at different levels can be helpful in making a diagnosis. If a patient gives an accurate description of diffuse pain in the body wall and the health care provider is skillful in relating pain in these tissues to specific dermatomes on the basis of bony landmarks, the provider will be able to more easily make a diagnosis of visceral disease (Fig. 4–14 and see Fig. 5-7).

THE SPINAL CORD AND SPINAL NERVE ROOTS, THEIR INVESTMENTS (MENINGES), AND THEIR VASCULATURE

The anatomy of the spinal cord and its spinal nerve roots and their anatomic relationships to the meningeal investments, vasculature, and bony vertebral canal provide an anatomic basis for clinical diagnosis and treatment

Positioning of the Spinal Cord Within the Vertebral Canal

The spinal cord does not extend the full length of the vertebral canal in adults

The spinal cord is usually about 18 inches long in adults. It extends inferiorly from the base of the brain in the region of the **foramen magnum** (the "large opening" at the base of the skull) to the level of the disc between vertebrae L1 and L2 (Fig. 4–15). In some individuals, its caudal end may reach only to vertebra T12, and in others, it may extend to the disc between vertebrae L2 and L3. The spinal cord is shorter than the vertebral column because of the differential growth of the two structures beginning in the eighth week of development. Until that time, the spinal cord fills the entire vertebral canal (Fig. 4–15*A*). At birth, the spinal cord usually extends to vertebra L3 (Fig. 4–15*B*).

Because the spinal cord in adults usually extends no further inferiorly than the disc between vertebrae L1 and L2, the dorsal and ventral roots of the lower thoracic, lumbar, sacral, and coccygeal spinal nerves must be significantly elongated to reach their appropriate intervertebral foramina and exit the vertebral canal. These elongated nerve roots are gathered in a bunch within a roomy region of the **subarachnoid space (lumbar cistern)** inferior to the caudal end of the spinal cord, forming a **cauda equina** ("horse's tail") (Fig. 4–15*C*). Thus, the lumbar vertebrae can serve as landmarks for making lumbar punctures. This reduces the risk of damage to the spinal cord (see discussion of meningeal structures that anchor and suspend the spinal cord below).

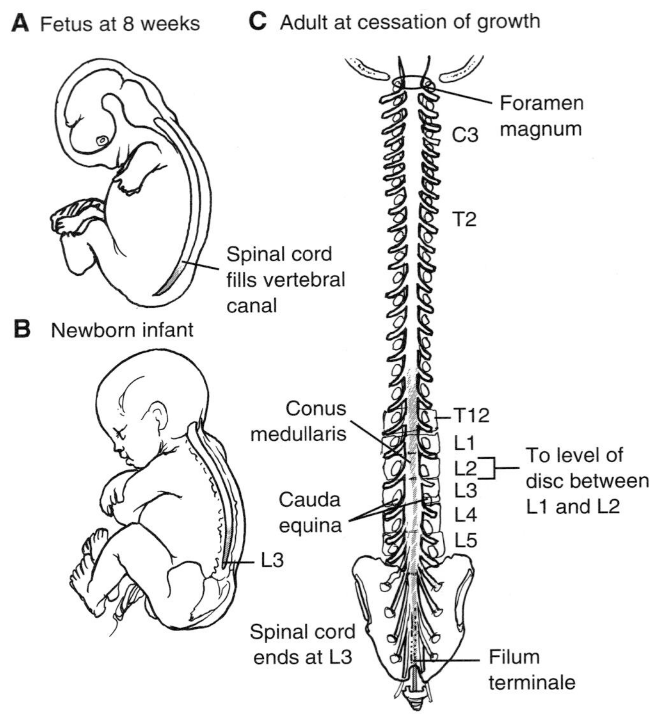

FIGURE 4–15
Spinal cord and vertebral canal. The vertebral column grows faster than the spinal cord. Thus, by adulthood, the spinal cord ends at the level of the disc between vertebrae L1 and L2.

▲ Shape and Surface Features of the Spinal Cord

The spinal cord bulges and tapers, and its surface is inscribed by characteristic sulci, a fissure, and a septum

The spinal cord is somewhat thicker and more oval in the cervicothoracic and lumbosacral regions because of the innervation of the large number of muscles of the upper and lower extremities by nerves issuing from the spinal cord at these levels (see Chapters 2, 18, and 21). The cervicothoracic bulge in the spinal cord extends from vertebrae C3 to T2 and is larger than the lumbosacral bulge, which extends from vertebrae L1 to S3. The tapered inferior end of the spinal cord is the **conus medullaris** (Fig. 4–16 and see Fig. 4–23).

An **anterior median fissure** is apparent along the entire length of the spinal cord, and it extends inward almost to the level of the central canal (Fig. 4–17). A shallow **posterior median sulcus** demarcates the site of a deep **posterior median septum,** which consists of neuroglial cells. This septum extends nearly to the central canal from the posterior surface of the spinal cord (Fig. 4–17). Adjacent to the posterior median sulcus are the shallow **posterior intermediate sulci,** and just lateral to these sulci are the **posterior lateral sulci,** along which the inward-growing axons from dorsal root ganglia enter the spinal cord (Fig. 4–17).

▲ Clinical Disorders of the Spinal Cord

Traumatic injury, vascular disorders, tumor growth, and infectious and degenerative diseases may affect the spinal cord with potentially devastating results. Outcomes range from positive ones, with little or no long-term neurologic deficit, to severe deficit or death.

Traumatic Injury of the Spinal Cord

The most common traumatic injuries to the spinal cord occur in the cervical or upper thoracic region in adolescent or young adult males on summer weekends

Traumatic injury of the spinal cord is most often the result of automobile accidents, falls, recreational activities such as contact sports and diving, or acts of violence. The age group most commonly affected is males 15 to 30 years of age. Injuries most frequently occur in the summer months on weekends. A large proportion of these accidents (possibly more than half) are related to drinking alcohol. All segments of the spinal cord may be involved, but the most common sites of injury are in the cervical region (approximately 50% at the levels of vertebrae C1 to C2 and C4 to C5) and in the lower thoracic and upper lumbar regions (at the levels of vertebrae T11 to L2) (i.e., in the regions of the cervical and lumbar enlargements; see Fig. 4–16). Injuries occur at other levels with less frequency.

The degree of neurologic deficit is greatest immediately following a traumatic spinal cord injury as a consequence of **edema** (collection of fluid within tissue). The deficit may diminish as time passes and as the fluid dissipates. Imaging of the vertebral column and spinal cord and a complete neurologic examination are used to assess the extent of injury (Fig. 4–18). Damage to the spinal cord may be the result of compression by displaced vertebral fragments (see Chapter 3), laceration, or complete transection by bone fragments or foreign materials such as firearm projectiles (Fig. 4–19). Diseases such as metastatic cancer may result in collapse of a vertebra and impingement of its fragments upon the spinal cord (see Fig. 3-11*C*). Vascular damage results in **hemorrhage** (which increases pressure on the cord) (see Fig. 4–25), and deprivation of blood supply **(infarction)** results in cell death and replacement with scar tissue.

The patient who survives the first days following an injury to the upper cervical region of the spinal cord is likely to develop secondary pulmonary **pneumonia** or **atelectasis** (collapse of a portion of a lung). Long-term neurologic deficits include paralysis of the musculature and loss of sensation. When damage occurs in the cervical or upper thoracic region, autonomic dysfunction may also occur. In the latter case the patient will experience problems such as reflex sweating and flushing.

Spinal Cord Tumors

The spinal cord or its vasculature may be compressed by tumors of the meninges or ependymal lining of the central canal

Only 15% of benign and malignant tumors of the central nervous system occur in the spinal cord. Of these, about 70%

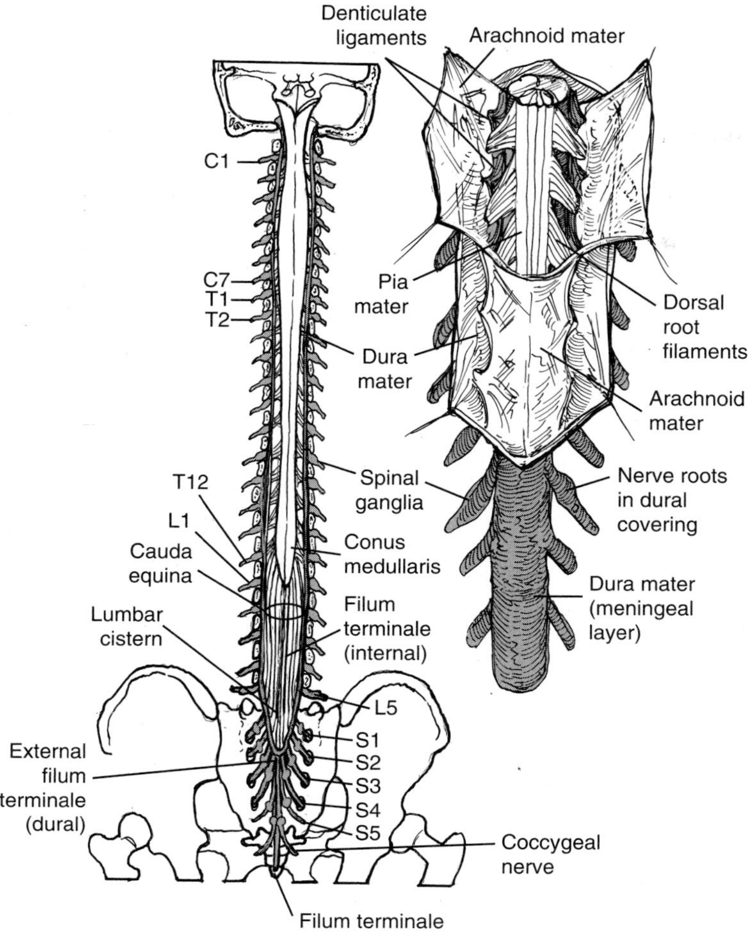

FIGURE 4–16
Shape of the spinal cord. The spinal cord bulges from C3 to T2 (cervicothoracic bulge) and from L1 to S3 (lumbosacral bulge). The cord tapers at its caudal end, which is known as the *conus medullaris.* Because the spinal cord is shorter than the vertebral canal, nerve roots from L1 to Co1 have become elongated to reach the intervertebral foramina. Together these elongated roots are called *cauda equina.*

are **extramedullary tumors,** occurring outside the spinal cord, and about 30% are **intramedullary tumors,** arising within the spinal cord. Spinal cord dysfunction resulting from spinal cord tumors is caused by three factors: direct pressure and eventual destruction of neural elements, pressure on the arterial supply, and, far less frequently, occlusion of venous elements. Symptoms include localized pain and tenderness in the region of the tumor, paresthesia (sensations of burning, "pins and needles," numbness, or tingling), and motor weakness. Motor weakness is usually the last symptom to occur. Many tumors that develop within the spinal cord occur more commonly within the brain (see Chapter 23). Meningiomas and ependymomas, however, are among those that are also common in the spinal cord (see below).

Ependymoma is the most common intramedullary spinal cord tumor (Fig. 4–20). These tumors are derived from cells lining the central canal. They occur in middle age and are usually diagnosed by magnetic resonance imaging (MRI) and computerized tomography (CT) scanning. Although ependymomas are benign and slow growing, their position deep within the spinal cord makes surgical removal difficult or impossible.

Infectious Diseases of the Spinal Cord

Spinal cord function may be compromised by parameningeal infections

An abscess within the epidural space may produce signs similar to those of disc herniation or tumor growth. The patient first reports acute low back pain, which radiates into the affected dermatomes as the disease progresses. Muscle stiffness, fever, headache, and local tenderness usually occur as well. Before antibiotic therapy was available, this condition was always fatal. Recovery following antibiotic therapy depends on the effectiveness of the antibiotic against the causative organism and the extent of neurologic damage and duration of symptoms before the initiation of therapy.

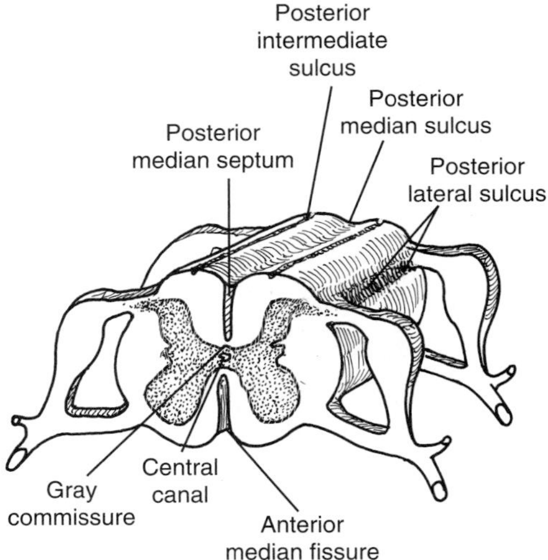

FIGURE 4–17
Surface features of the spinal cord. The spinal cord is marked by an anterior median fissure, a posterior median septum, two posterior intermediate sulci, and two posterior lateral sulci.

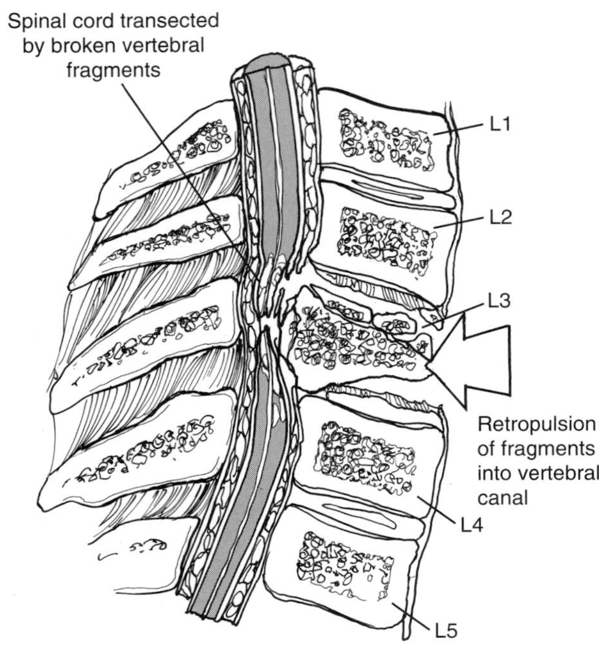

FIGURE 4–19
Damage to the spinal cord. The spinal cord is damaged by the forceful intrusion of vertebral fragments into the vertebral canal (see also Chapter 3).

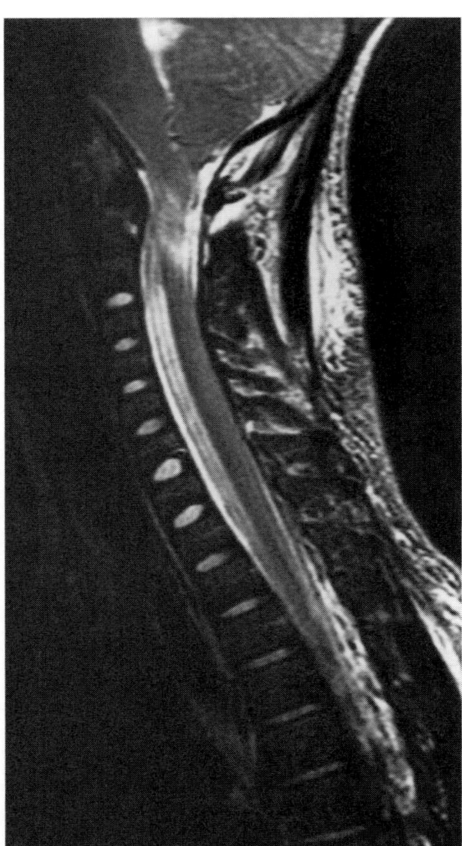

FIGURE 4–18
Imaging the spinal cord. The spinal cord can be readily imaged with magnetic resonance imaging (MRI). This MRI scan shows a midsagittal section of the cervical spinal cord and demonstrates the roominess of the vertebral canal.

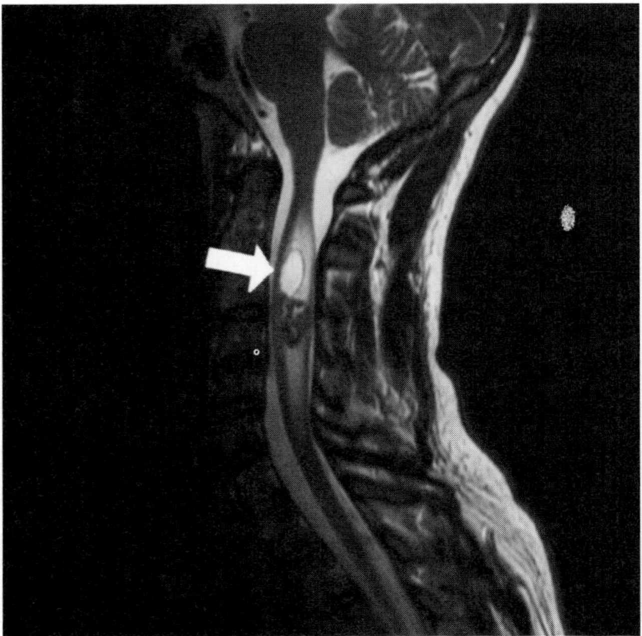

FIGURE 4–20
Midsagittal magnetic resonance imaging (MRI) scan revealing an ependymoma at bright ovoid structure *(arrow)* within the cervical spinal cord. This tumor arises from cells that line the central canal of the spinal cord.

Degenerative Diseases of the Spinal Cord

A variety of degenerative diseases affect spinal cord function

Many degenerative diseases of the central nervous system primarily attack the brain (see Chapter 23). **Amyotrophic lateral sclerosis,** or **Lou Gehrig disease,** is a fatal degenerative disease that may also affect the spinal cord. Because the disease attacks the motor systems of both the brain and spinal cord, it results in progressive paralysis of the skeletal muscles, but sensory functions are not affected. The disease was first described in 1865. There are both familial and nonfamilial variants. Familial forms of the disease appear to result from mutations of the gene encoding the enzyme superoxide dismutase. The onset is usually in late middle age, and males tend to be affected slightly more often than females. The onset is slow, and patients frequently fail to recognize any specific malfunction and attribute the symptoms to "clumsiness." As the disease progresses, patients lose the ability to walk and care for themselves. Death usually results from pulmonary failure within 3 to 10 years after the initial onset of symptoms.

Primary lateral sclerosis is not as common as amyotrophic lateral sclerosis, but both diseases begin with muscular weakness, usually in the lower limbs. The disease progresses quickly, and death results from pulmonary failure.

Syringomyelia is a disease in which a fluid-filled cyst (syrinx) forms within the spinal cord (Fig. 4–21). The cyst may enlarge, destroying neural tissue of the spinal cord and frequently the brainstem as well. The cyst may be present at birth **(congenital syringomyelia)** or develop as the result of trauma, **arachnoiditis** (inflammation of the arachnoid mater), or an intramedullary tumor. Symptoms of the disease include weakness of the upper limbs and muscle wasting, especially in muscles of the hands. Scoliosis (see Chapter 3) frequently develops secondary to loss of innervation to the paravertebral musculature in the thoracic region. Pain and temperature sensations are lost in the affected areas, but proprioception is spared. The onset of symptoms is usually at 25 to 40 years of age, and males are affected more frequently than females. The symptoms grow progressively worse over several years, although in some cases, there may be long periods of stability between periods of progression. Falls, coughing, or sneezing may result in rapid progression of the disease for a short period of time. There are no effective treatments for syringomyelia, although surgical removal of fluid from the cyst is frequently attempted.

▲ Meninges

The spinal cord and its spinal nerve roots are protected by three investments (meninges) within the vertebral canal

From inside to outside, the meninges are the **pia mater** ("tender mother"), **arachnoid mater** ("mother resembling a cobweb"), and **dura mater** ("tough mother") (Fig. 4–22 and see Fig. 4–16).

The pia mater is thin and closely applied to the surface of the spinal cord. The outer membranes of the

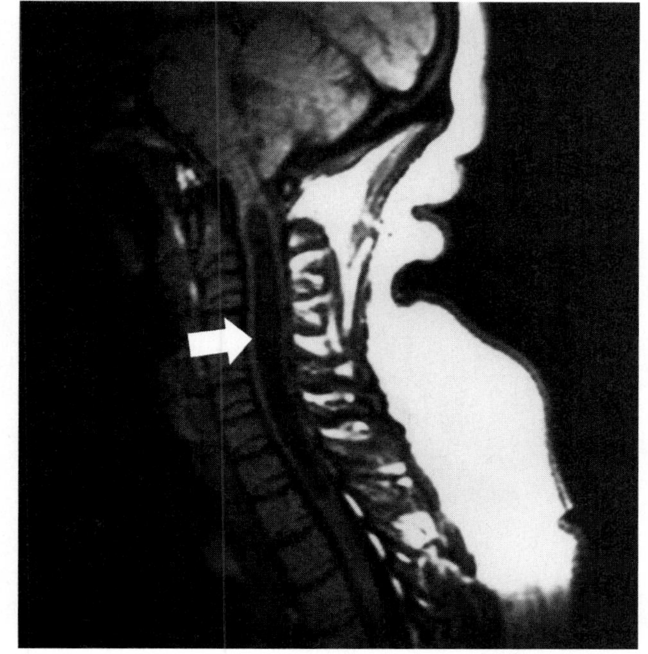

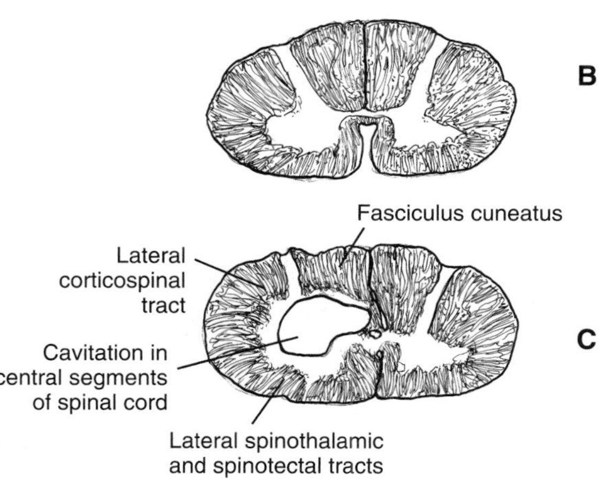

FIGURE 4–21

Syringomyelia. **A.** Midsagittal magnetic resonance imaging (MRI) scan revealing an elongated cyst *(arrow)* within the cervical region of the spinal cord. A transverse section of a normal spinal cord at the level of vertebra C6 **(B)** is compared with a section of a spinal cord with a cavitation characteristic of syringomyelia **(C)**.

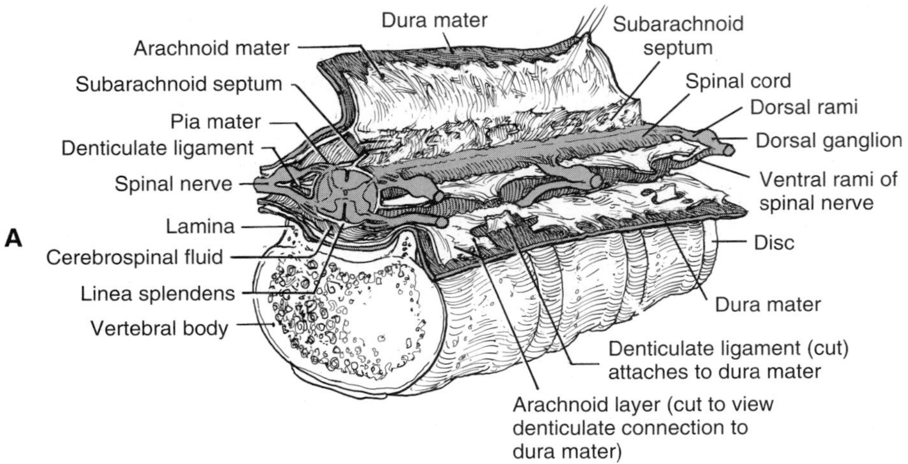

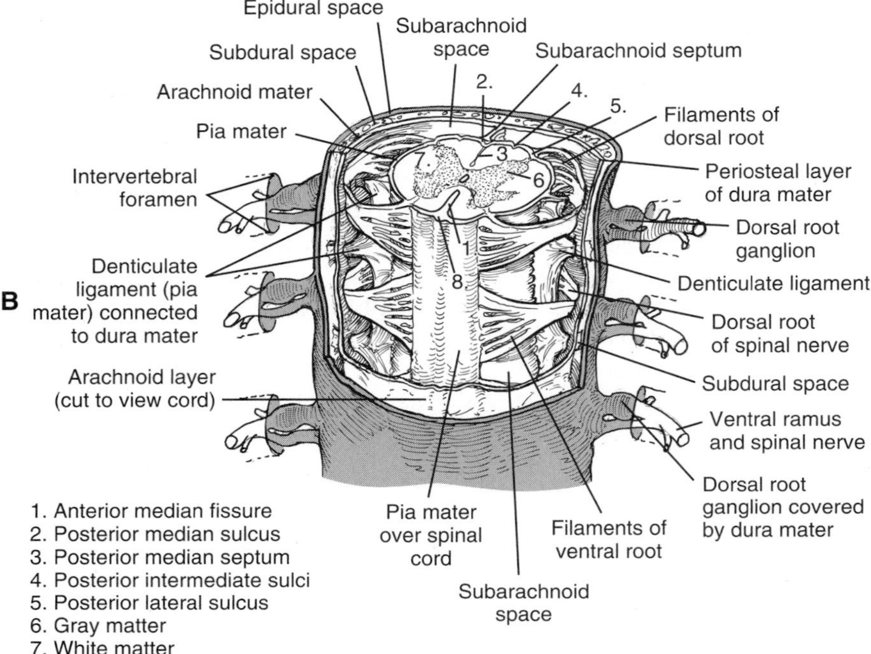

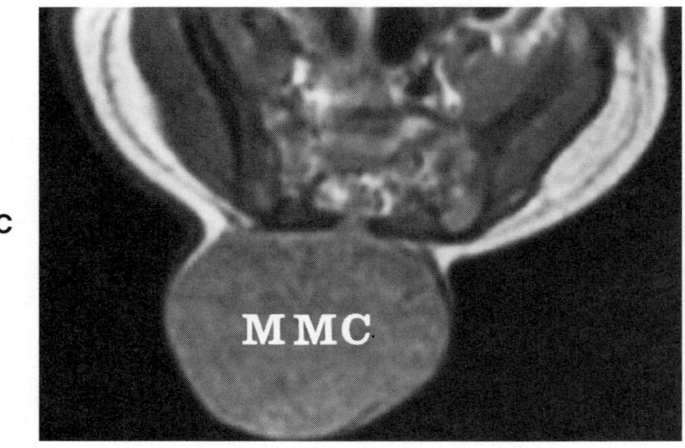

FIGURE 4–22

Meningeal investments of the spinal cord. **A.** Oblique view of the spinal cord with an open vertebral canal showing the dura mater, arachnoid mater, and pia mater. Specializations of the pia mater include the subarachnoid septum, denticulate ligaments, and linea splendens. **B.** Anterior view of spinal cord and associated investments revealing the subarachnoid space and the potential epidural and subdural spaces. **C.** A transverse magnetic resonance imaging (MRI) scan of an infant showing a large sac of dura, or meningomyelocele *(MMC),* protruding from the vertebral column in the sacral region.

arachnoid mater and dura mater are separated from the membrane of the pia mater and lie close to the inner bony surface of the vertebral canal (Fig. 4–22). All of the meningeal coverings enclose the entire spinal cord as well as proximal components of the spinal nerves. The pia mater and arachnoid mater, together called the **leptomeninges,** arise from neural crest cells, and the dura mater is formed from connective tissue associated with the bony vertebral column.

The space between the arachnoid mater and pia mater contains wispy arachnoid connections resembling cobwebs, which give the arachnoid mater its name. The space between the arachnoid mater and pia mater is the **subarachnoid space.** It is filled with a dialysate of blood called **cerebrospinal fluid** (Fig. 4–22). Cerebrospinal fluid is manufactured by specialized areas within ventricles of the brain called **choroid plexuses** (see Chapter 23), and it circulates into the central canal of the spinal cord as well. It reaches the subarachnoid space of the central nervous system by escaping the fourth ventricle (of the hindbrain) through specialized foramina in the pia mater to provide a protective fluid cushion for the spinal cord. The potential space just superficial to the dura mater is the **epidural,** or **peridural, space,** and the potential space between the dura mater and arachnoid mater is the **subdural space** (Figs. 4–22 and 4–23).

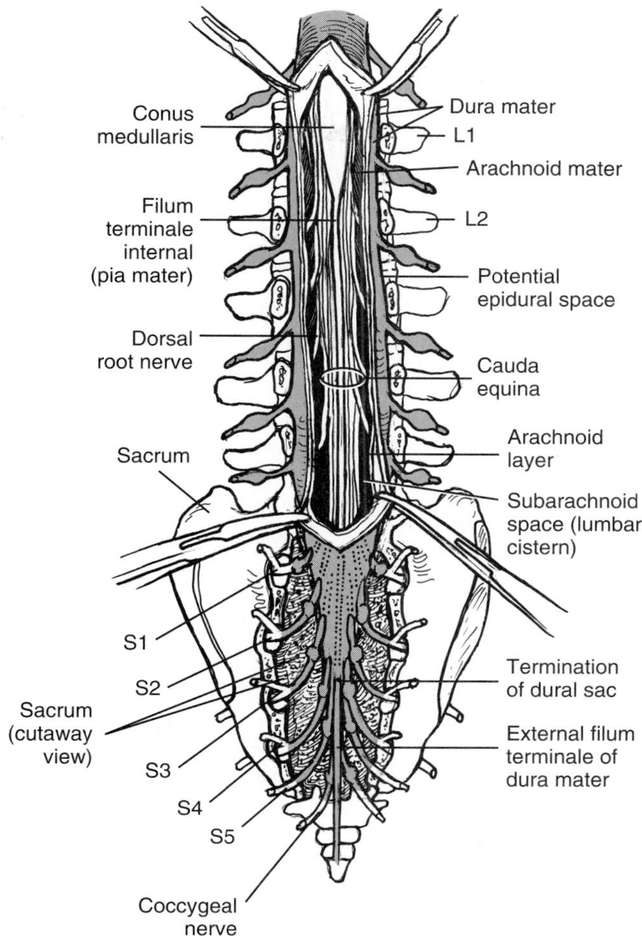

FIGURE 4–23
Opening up the lumbar cistern reveals the filum terminale internum and externum.

Meningeal Structures that Anchor and Suspend the Spinal Cord

Specialized areas of the meninges anchor and suspend the spinal cord within the vertebral canal

The spinal cord is anchored and suspended within the vertebral canal by specialized areas of the meningeal coverings, most notably and somewhat surprisingly, by the delicate pia mater. Although the pia mater tightly ensheathes the spinal cord, it elaborates about 21 pairs of thin projections that extend at intervals from the lateral surface of the spinal cord. These projections, called **denticulate ligaments,** connect the surface of the spinal cord to the dura mater (see Figs. 4–16 and 4–22). The most superior pair of denticulate ligaments is connected to the dura mater immediately superior to the margin of the foramen magnum (within the skull), while the most inferior pair connects the tapered caudal end of the spinal cord with the dura mater in the region of vertebra L1.

The pia mater also projects from the posterior surface of the spinal cord as an elongated sheet of tissue, suspending the spinal cord from the dura mater associated with the midline posterior "roof" of the bony vertebral canal. This **subarachnoid septum** is perforated and incomplete in the cervical region but more complete in the thoracic region of the spinal cord (see Fig. 4–22*A*). The anterior surface of the spinal cord is not directly suspended by specialized meningeal tissues; however, a tough, thickened band of pia mater called the **linea splendens** is located just superficial to the anterior median fissure (see Fig. 4–22*A* and *B*).

Finally, the pia mater and dura mater form a strong tether that projects from the most inferior end of the spinal cord as a **filum terminale** (see Figs. 4–16 and 4–23). The superior part of the filum terminale consists of the pia mater only and is called the **filum terminale internum.** It extends from the tapered caudal conus medullaris at the level of the disc between vertebrae L1 and L2 for about 4 inches to the lower border of vertebra S2. Here, the dura mater tapers and tightly encloses the more inferior extension of the filum terminale to form the **filum terminale externum.** The filum terminale externum extends inferiorly for about 2 inches, attaching to the dorsal surface of the first coccyx vertebra (Co1). The subarachnoid space surrounding the filum terminale internum is especially large and is called the **lumbar cistern.** In addition to the filum terminale internum, it contains elongated dorsal and ventral roots of the cauda equina (see Figs. 4–16 and 4–23). This space is usually

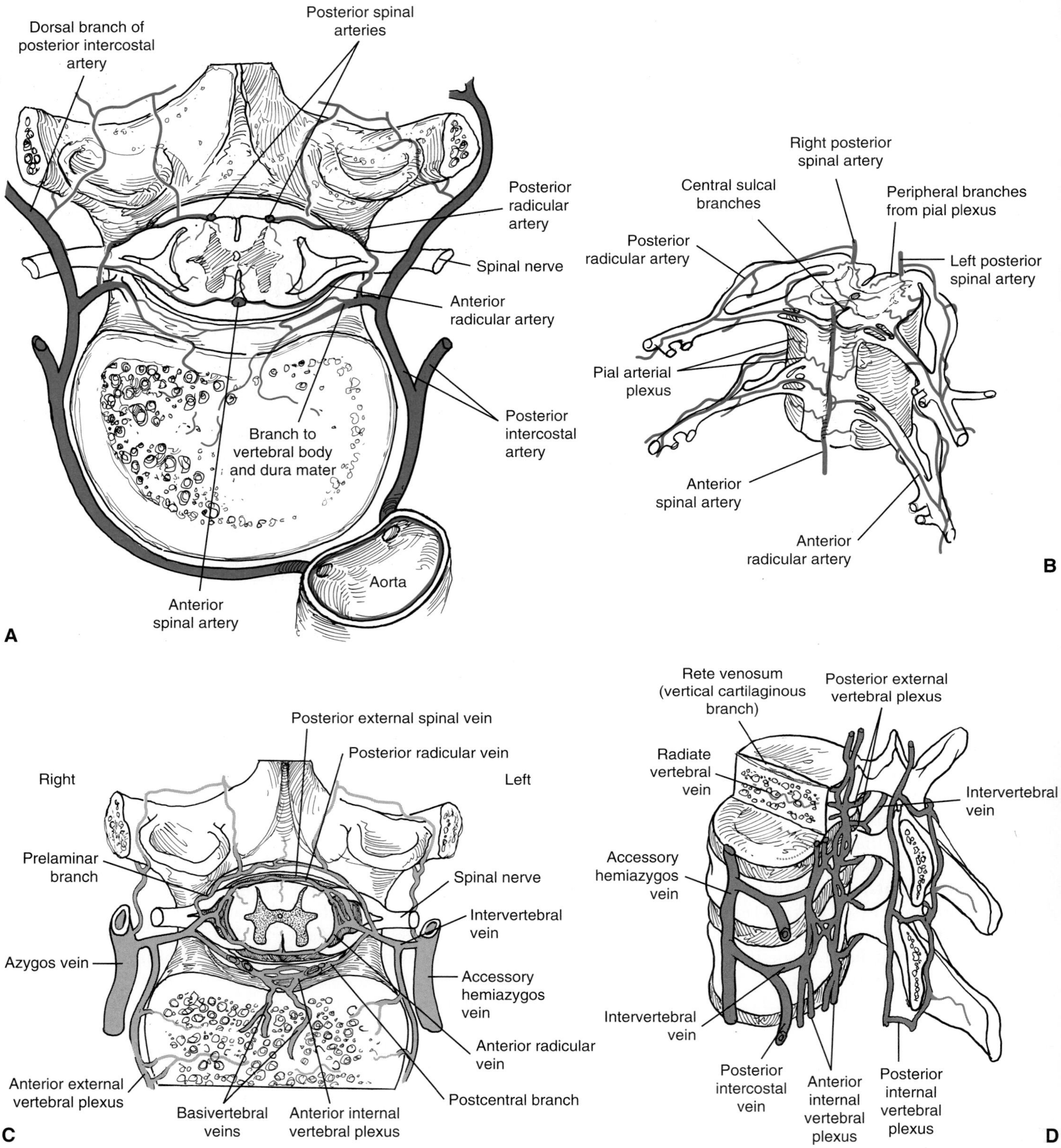

FIGURE 4–24

Vasculature of the spinal cord. **A.** The origin of the spinal arteries from posterior intercostal arteries. **B.** The anterior view of the spinal cord and its vasculature illustrates relationships of the spinal artery branches. **C.** The veins of the spinal cord arise from posterior intercostal veins and ramify throughout the cord and vertebral canal. **D.** Anterior and posterior vertebral plexuses are shown in this cutaway view of the vertebral canal.

used for lumbar puncture if cerebrospinal fluid must be withdrawn for diagnostic tests or if medications such as anesthetics must be injected.

Tumors of Spinal Cord Investments. **Meningioma** is the most common extramedullary spinal cord tumor. The tumors arise from cells of the arachnoid mater and usually occur singly, although multiple meningiomas are reported, especially in association with **von Recklinghausen's disease (neurofibromatosis.)** They tend to occur in mid or late life and are more common in women than men by a ratio of 3 to 2. Growth of these tumors is usually slow, and symptoms vary according to location. In all cases, neurologic symptoms result from the tumor's usurpation of the space within the vertebral canal.

Vasculature of the Spinal Cord

Vasculature of the spinal cord and spinal nerve roots is segmental

Spinal (radicular) arteries originate at different segmental levels from **vertebral, ascending cervical, intercostal,** and **lumbar arteries,** entering the vertebral canal through intervertebral foramina (Fig. 4–24*A*). As the arteries enter the vertebral canal, they branch into **anterior** and **posterior spinal,** or **radicular, arteries,** which course to the spinal cord via ventral and dorsal roots of the various spinal nerves (see Fig. 4–24*A* and *B*). Once they have entered the vertebral canal, these spinal arteries anastomose, forming longitudinal vascular channels within the canal that supply the spinal cord, meninges, and bony and ligamentous elements enclosing the canal. Much of the vasculature within the spinal cord is located in the white matter (see Fig. 4–24*A* to *C*).

A complex **internal vertebral plexus of veins** running throughout the length of the vertebral canal provides drainage for bony elements and ligaments enclosing the canal, the meninges, and the white and gray matter of the spinal cord and spinal nerve roots (see Fig. 4–24*C* and *D*). Most of the plexus is located between the bone and the dura mater. This internal plexus branches into segmental veins called **intervertebral veins,** which exit from the vertebral canal through intervertebral foramina. An **external vertebral plexus** of veins, which drains blood from outer surfaces of the vertebrae, anastomoses with the internal vertebral plexus, both within the vertebral canal and just outside the intervertebral foramina, emptying into intervertebral veins before they join with **vertebral veins, segmental posterior intercostal veins,** or **lumbar veins** (see Fig 4–24*C* and *D*).

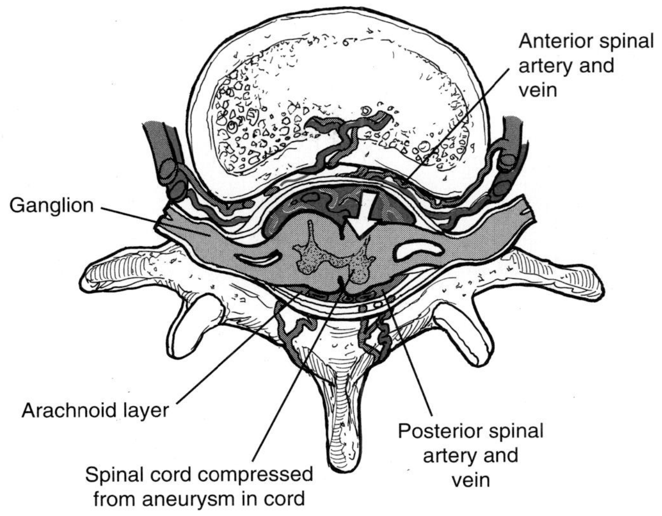

FIGURE 4–25
Hemorrhage of spinal vessels *(arrow).* Extravasation of blood into the vertebral canal may exert traumatic pressure on the spinal cord.

Vascular Disorders of the Spinal Cord

Vascular disorders may compromise the blood supply to the spinal cord

Vascular disorders damage the spinal cord through compression or ischemia. **Aneurysm** (ballooning of the blood vessel wall) or **hemorrhage** results in the compression of neural elements (Fig. 4–25). Conversely, **arteriosclerosis** or **focal hemorrhage** may diminish blood flow via intercostal or lumbar tributaries and results in **localized spinal cord infarction.**

5 Integrating Structure and Function in the Back

The major anatomic elements of the back are the axial skeleton, spinal cord and peripheral nerves, muscles, and blood vessels. This chapter will discuss the relationships between these systems, including the interactions between muscles and bones, integration of various muscle actions, and additional clinical problems that may arise because of abnormalities or injuries of these back structures.

MUSCLE ATTACHMENTS AND MUSCLE ACTIONS

Muscle actions depend upon the sites of muscle attachments

Muscles can contract and shorten, bringing their attachment sites closer together and thereby producing **dynamic movement.** Alternatively, muscles can produce a state of **static tension** simply to resist forces from apposed muscles or from gravity, which tend to pull the points of muscle attachment apart. This static, or isometric, muscle action is integral to the maintenance of the body's stability, posture, and poise.

Muscles usually have an **attachment of origin** (the less movable attachment) and an **attachment of insertion** (the more movable attachment). It may be difficult or impossible to differentiate the two types of attachments in some muscles, when, for example, the muscle action is isometric. In some cases, a given muscle attachment may sometimes be the less movable attachment and at other times the more movable attachment. In the following discussion, references may be made to the origin and insertion of a muscle where these distinctions can be clearly defined; in most cases, however, the general terms *attachment sites* and *attachments* will be used. Qualifying words such as *superior, inferior, proximal,* or *distal* are used where appropriate.

The attachments and actions of three groups of muscles will be described. These are a group of **"true deep back muscles,"** which extend, laterally flex, rotate the vertebral column, and also function in maintaining posture. This group includes the **suboccipital muscles,** two pairs of "intermediate" **so-called respiratory muscles (the serratus posterior muscles),** and the "superficial" **appendicular muscles** of the back. General descriptions of muscle group attachments are given in the text, and specific attachments are listed in accompanying tables. All of these classes of muscles have been introduced and illustrated in Chapter 2.

The description of back structures in Chapter 2 proceeded from superficial to deep to coincide with the order of initial dissection of this region. Because the axial skeleton was introduced in Chapter 3, this chapter will focus on the attachments and functions of intrinsic muscles of the back and therefore will proceed from the deepest to the most superficial structures.

Synergistic Action of Back Muscles

Synergism between deep back muscles is fundamental to their function

While some of the true deep back muscles have been classified as those that either generate movement or simply maintain tension between their points of attachment, nearly all of the muscles of the back can likely perform either of these tasks, depending on need. For example, the massive erector spinae muscles are usually classified as dynamic **extensors** of the back because they are bilaterally active during extension of the trunk. And the concomitant static activity of the shorter **transversospinalis muscles** is thought to maintain tension and stability within the vertebral column by intermittently contracting to force the vertebrae together. The functions of these long and short muscles are not so easily categorized, however. The erector spinae muscles play a static role during **flexion of the trunk,** producing tension that balances the pull of the ventral **rectus abdominis muscles** (see Fig. 5–6), and, although the short **multifidus muscles** act as static muscles, they may also be involved in **extensional and rotational movements** of the vertebral column (see below).

DEEP BACK MUSCLES

Vertebral grooves provide longitudinal paravertebral attachment sites throughout the cervical, thoracic, and lumbar regions for deep muscles of the back

Attachments of the Deep Back Muscles

Vertebral Grooves

Vertebral grooves are formed by articulation of the vertebrae and the connecting **interspinous ligaments** and **ligamenta flava** (see Fig. 3–22). They are sculpted, shallow longitudinal fossae (depressions) just lateral to the vertebral spines and dorsal to the transverse processes (see Figs. 5–4 and 3–22*C*). Thus, the surface of a vertebral groove, which consists of the vertebral spines and interspinous ligaments, vertebral laminae, ligamenta flava, and transverse processes, provides a substratum for attachments of five groups of back muscles: the **intertransversarii muscles, interspinales muscles, transversospinal group of muscles, erector spinae muscles,** and **suboccipital muscles** (see Figs. 5–1 to 5–4 and 5–8).

Intertransversarii Muscle Attachments

Mixed developmental derivations of the intertransversarii muscles are reflected in their specific attachment sites

A complex of intertransversarii muscles connects transverse processes throughout the vertebral column. As was discussed in Chapter 2, the more medial slips of these muscles are derived from epimeres and are innervated by dorsal primary rami (see Fig. 2–8). They are called **posterior proper intertransversarii muscles,** and there are seven pairs of these in the cervical region (Fig. 5–1 and Table 5–1).

Only three pairs of posterior proper intertransversarii muscles are located in the thoracic region. These connect the last three thoracic and first lumbar vertebrae (Fig. 5–1). However, other (somewhat more lateral) slips of the posterior intertransversarii muscles of the thorax are elaborated as levatores costarum muscles (Fig. 5–1). The levatores costarum muscles are so named because each muscle joins the transverse process of one vertebra from C7 to T11 to the upper surface of the rib below the vertebra. For this reason alone, they have been classified as **so-called respiratory muscles.** They are also innervated by dorsal primary rami and clearly arise from epimeres rather than hypomeres (see Fig. 2–8). Although they typically span a single segment, the lower four levatores costarum muscles span two segments (Fig. 5–1).

The vertebrae of the lumbar region are also joined by posterior proper intertransversarii muscles. Each muscle joins the mamillary process of a lumbar vertebra to the accessory process of the adjacent superior vertebra (Fig. 5–1).

More lateral slips of intertransversarii muscles can also be identified in the cervical and lumbar regions (Fig. 5–1). These small muscles, however, are derived from hypomeres and are innervated by ventral primary rami (see Fig. 2–8). These lateral hypomeric intertransversarii muscles connect transverse and costal processes of adjacent vertebrae in the cervical region (Fig. 5–1). In the lumbar spine, the lateral hypomeric intertransversarii muscles are divided into a ventral and a dorsal part (see Fig. 2–8). The ventral parts connect the transverse processes of adjacent vertebrae; the dorsal parts connect the accessory processes of one lumbar vertebra to the transverse processes of the adjacent superior lumbar vertebra (Fig. 5–1).

Lateral hypomeric intertransversarii muscles are lacking in the thoracic region, but homologous hypomeric muscle is elaborated as **intercostal muscles,** which join ribs (see Figs. 5–1 and 2–8 and Chapter 6). Similarly, more lateral hypomeric muscle in the lumbar region is elaborated as the anterolateral musculature of the abdominal body wall (see Fig. 2–8 and Chapter 11). The intercostal and anterolateral abdominal muscles are, therefore, innervated by ventral primary rami.

Interspinales Muscle Attachments

Interspinales muscles connect adjacent vertebral spines

All of the **interspinales muscles** within the cervical, thoracic, and lumbar regions are developmentally related to each other. The muscles arise from epimeres and are innervated by dorsal primary rami (see Tables 2–1 and 5–1). These paired muscles skirt the **interspinous ligament** (see Chapter 3), connecting the spines of adjacent vertebrae (Fig. 5–1).

Six pairs of cervical interspinales muscles connect vertebrae C2 to C7. The upper two and lower two thoracic vertebrae are connected by the thoracic interspinales muscles, and all five lumbar vertebral spines are connected by four pairs of lumbar interspinales muscles (Fig. 5–1).

Transversospinal Muscle Attachments

Some of the muscles of the transversospinal group span a single body segment, and others are longer, spanning two or more segments

All muscles of the transversospinal group are derived from epimeres and are thus innervated by dorsal primary rami. Typically, these muscles originate from an inferior transverse process and insert upon the spine of a more superior vertebra (Fig. 5–2). They may also arise, however, from the cervical articular or lumbar mamillary processes or from the sacrum (Fig. 5–2). The **semispinalis capitis muscles,** rather than inserting on vertebral spines, insert on the occipital bone of the skull between the **superior** and **inferior nuchal lines** (Table 5–2 and see Figs. 5–2*E*, and 5–8).

The transversospinal muscles are of three types, distinguished mainly by their length and distribution along the vertebral column. The shortest and deepest of these are the **rotators (rotatores muscles),** which span a single segment from the lower transverse process of one vertebra to the spine of the adjacent superior vertebra (Fig. 5–2*A*, *C*, and *F*). Irregular and variable in the cervical region (rotatores cervicis muscles), they are best developed in the thoracic region, where there are

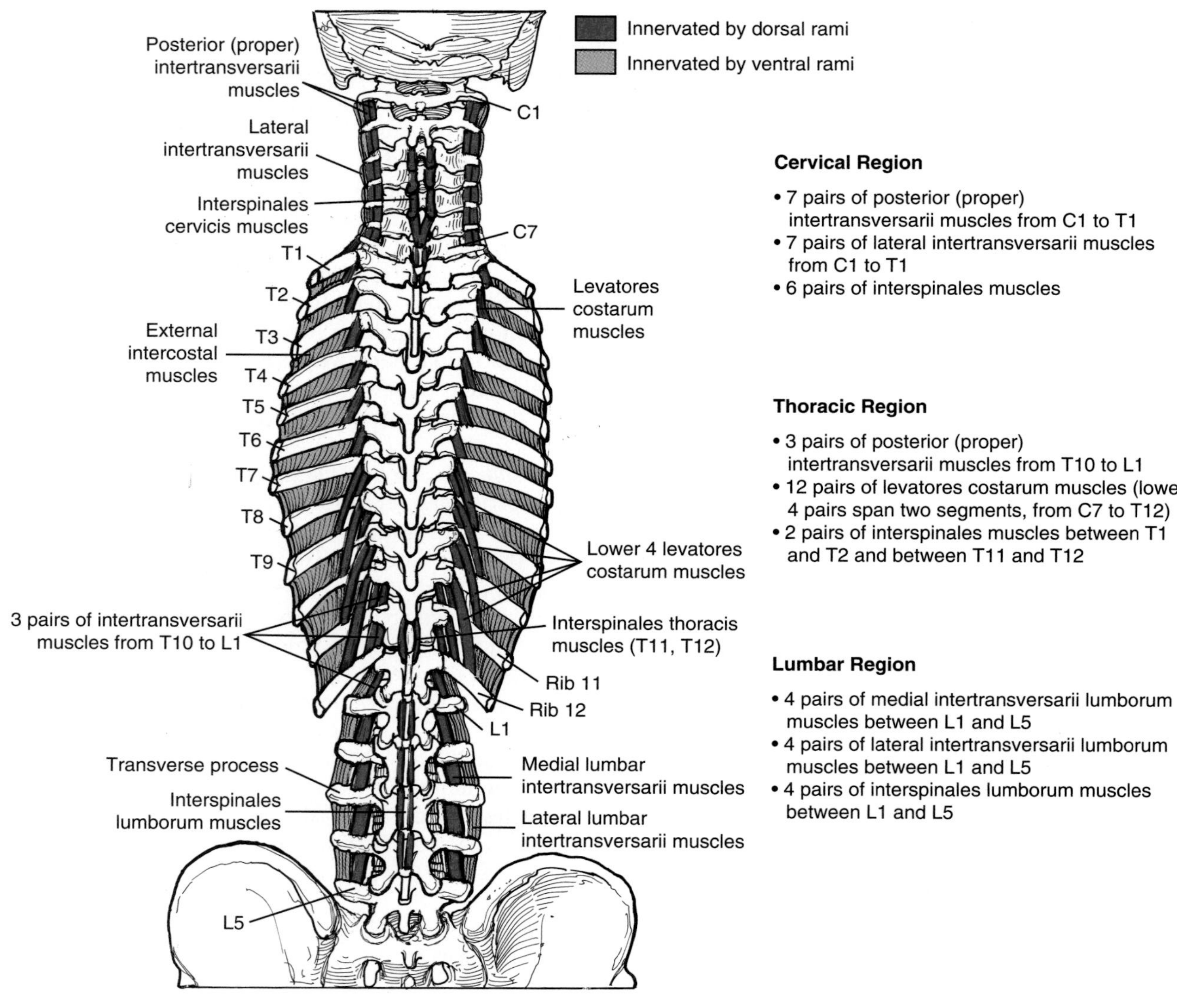

FIGURE 5–1
Attachments of intertransversarii, levatores costarum, intercostal, and interspinales muscles. Posterior proper intertransversarii muscles are distributed throughout the cervical region (seven pairs), within the thoracic region (three pairs from vertebrae T10 to L1), and within the lumbar region (four pairs). Homologous precursors of these muscles in the thoracic region are elaborated as levatores costarum muscles. All of these muscles are derived from epimeres and are innervated by dorsal primary rami. Precursors homologous to the myoblasts that form hypomeric intertransversarii muscles in the cervical and lumbar regions are elaborated as intercostal muscles in the thoracic region. All of these muscles are innervated by ventral primary rami. Finally, the interspinales muscles connect vertebral spines in the cervical, upper and lower thoracic, and lumbar regions. They are true deep back muscles and are innervated by dorsal primary rami.

11 pairs of rotatores thoracis muscles, and are irregular and variable in the lumbar region (rotatores lumborum muscles) (Table 5–2).

The **multifidus muscles,** which are named for their division into many segments, overlie the rotatores muscles. The shortest of these, like the rotatores muscles, span a single segment, whereas successively longer multifidus muscle **fascicles,** which are bundles of muscle fibers, lie in successively superficial layers to span two, three, or four segments (Fig. 5–2*B, D,* and *F*). Multifidus muscles of the cervical region arise from articular processes of the four most inferior cervical vertebrae (Fig. 5–2*B* and *D*). In the thoracic region the multifidus muscles arise from transverse processes, and in the lumbar region they arise from mamillary processes (Fig. 5–2*B*). The lowest multifidus muscles arise from the sacrum (as low as the fourth sacral segment) and associated sacral ligaments and tendons (Table 5–2). Like the rotatores muscles, the multifidus muscles insert upon vertebral spines.

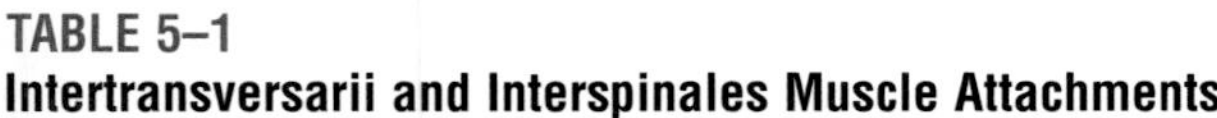

TABLE 5–1
Intertransversarii and Interspinales Muscle Attachments

Muscle	Inferior Attachment	Superior Attachment
EPIMERIC INTERTRANSVERSARII MUSCLES		
Cervical Muscles		
Medial part		
Medial and lateral slips	Transverse processes of vertebrae C2 (axis) to T1	Transverse processes of vertebrae C1 (atlas) to C7
Lateral part	Costal processes of vertebrae C2 to C7	Costal processes of vertebrae C1 to C6
Thoracic Muscles		
Medial part (medial and lateral slips)		
Medial slip	Transverse processes of vertebrae T11 to L1	Transverse processes of vertebrae T10 to T12
Lateral slip (levatores costarum muscles)	Upper surfaces of ribs 1 to 12	Transverse processes of vertebrae C7 to T11
Lateral part (homologous hypomeric intercostal muscles)	Ribs 2 to 12	Ribs 1 to 11
Lumbar Muscles		
Medial part	Mamillary processes of vertebrae L1 to L5	Accessory processes of vertebrae T12 to L4
HYPOMERIC INTERTRANSVERSARII MUSCLES		
Cervical Muscles	Costal processes of vertebrae C2 (axis) to T1	Costal processes of vertebrae C1 (atlas) to C7
Lumbar Muscles		
Lateral part	Costal and accessory processes of vertebrae L2 to L5	Transverse processes of vertebrae T12 to L4
INTERSPINALES MUSCLES		
Cervical Muscles	Spines of vertebrae C3 to T1	Spines of vertebrae C2 to C7
Thoracic Muscles	Spines of vertebrae T2 and T12	Spines of vertebrae T1 and T11
Lumbar Muscles	Spines of vertebrae L1 to L5	Spines of vertebrae T12 to L4

The **semispinalis muscles,** which are named for their incomplete distribution along the vertebral column, are restricted to the cervical and thoracic regions. They are classified in three groups on the basis of their attachments: the **semispinalis capitis muscles, semispinalis cervicis muscles,** and **semispinalis thoracis muscles** (Fig. 5–2*B* and *E*).

Semispinalis muscles typically span five body segments and are located just superficial to the multifidus muscles (Fig. 5–2*B, E,* and *F*). They are attached near the tip of the transverse processes inferiorly and near the apex of the vertebral spines superiorly (Fig. 5–2*E* and *F*).

Specifically, the **semispinalis capitis muscles** arise from transverse processes of the lowest cervical and highest thoracic vertebrae, as well as from articular processes of the lower cervical vertebrae. Superiorly, these muscles are attached to the occipital bone between the **superior** and **inferior nuchal lines** (Fig. 5–2*E* and Table 5–2). The medial fibers of semispinalis capitis muscles are typically blended with the **spinalis capitis muscle of the erector spinae group of muscles** (see below).

The **semispinalis cervicis muscles** arise from transverse processes of the superior thoracic vertebrae and are attached superiorly to spines of the upper cervical vertebrae (Fig. 5–2*B* and *E* and Table 5–2). These muscles are well developed and can be easily palpated in the nape of the neck. (*Nape* comes from the French for "back of the neck.") The attachment of these prominent muscles to the spine of the axis (vertebra C2) provides a useful primary landmark for identification of muscles

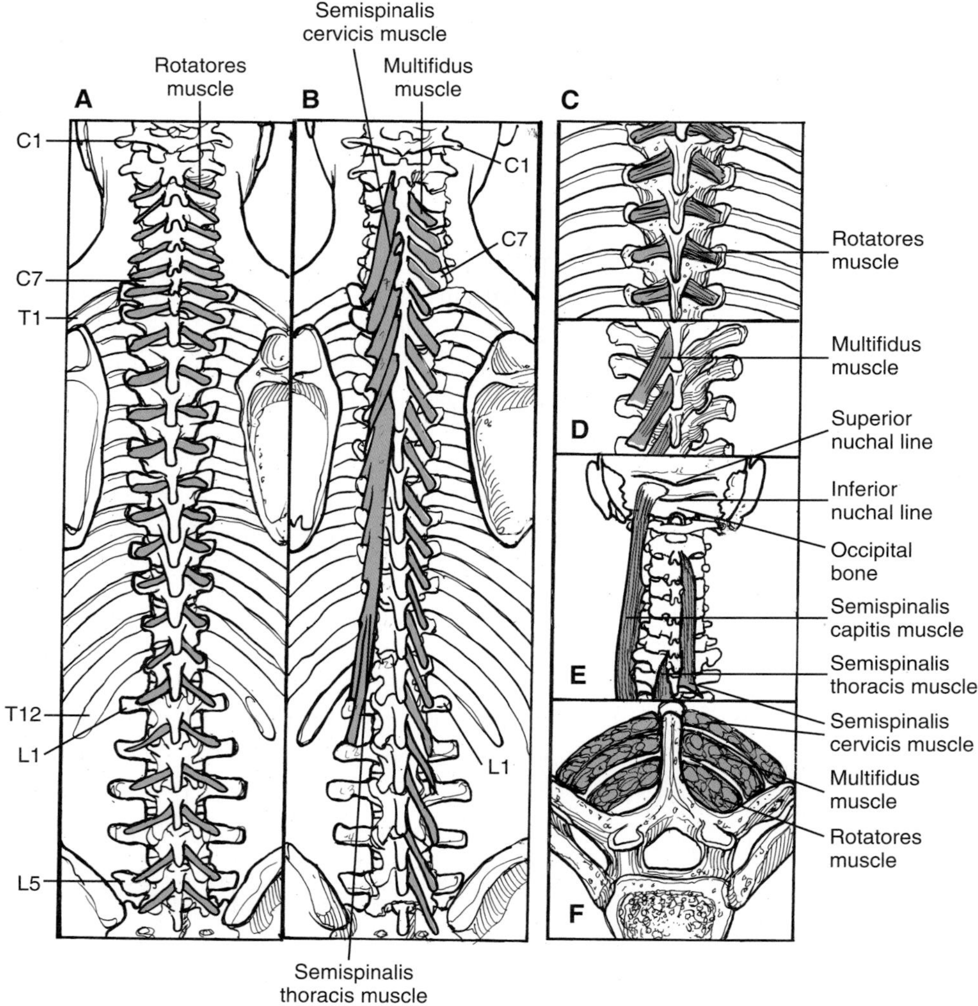

FIGURE 5–2

Attachments of transversospinal muscles. From superficial to deep and from the longest muscles to the shortest muscles, the three types of transversospinal muscles include semispinalis muscles (**B**, **E**, and **F**), which are named for their absence in the lumbar region; multifidus muscles (**B**, **D**, and **F**), which are named for their divisions into many segments; and rotatores muscles (**A**, **C**, and **F**), which are named for their function in rotation of the vertebral column. In all cases their inferior attachments are to transverse processes and their superior attachments are to vertebral spines.

within the suboccipital region (Figs. 5–2*B* and *E* and 5–9). The **semispinalis thoracis muscles** arise from the lower thoracic transverse processes and attach superiorly to the lower cervical and upper thoracic vertebral spines (Fig. 5–2*B* and *E*).

Splenius Cervicis and Splenius Capitis Muscle Attachments

Splenius cervicis and splenius capitis muscles are not transversospinal muscles

Although the **splenius capitis** and **splenius cervicis muscles** (from the Greek *splenion,* meaning "bandage") are not members of the transversospinal muscle group, they are true deep back muscles and are discussed here because they are typically dissected with the superior transversospinal muscles in the laboratory. Like the transversospinal muscles, they arise from epimeres and are innervated by dorsal rami of the cervical spinal nerves. These muscles lie in a plane between the more superficial appendicular muscles in this region (i.e., the trapezius and levator scapulae muscles and the underlying semispinalis muscles) (Fig. 5–3). The **splenius capitis muscle** is attached inferiorly to the lower part of the **ligamentum nuchae** (in the cervical region) and the upper thoracic vertebral spines. Its superior attachment is at the lateral aspect of the base of the skull. The **splenius cervicis muscle** is attached inferiorly to the spines of vertebrae T3 to T6 and superiorly to the transverse processes of the three superior cervical vertebrae (Fig. 5–3*A* and see Table 5–2).

TABLE 5–2
Transversospinal and Splenius Muscle Attachments

Muscle	Inferior Attachment	Superior Attachment
Rotatores muscles	Medial part of transverse processes of vertebrae T2 to T12; poorly developed in cervical and lumbar regions	Anterior part of spines of vertebrae T1 to T11; poorly developed in cervical and lumbar regions
Multifidus muscles	Transverse processes of thoracic vertebrae and articular processes of four inferior cervical vertebrae, mamillary processes of lumbar vertebrae, erector spinae tendon, sacrum, iliolumbar ligament, sacroiliac ligament, posterior superior iliac spine	Spines of vertebrae C1 to L5
Semispinalis capitis muscles	Transverse processes of vertebrae C7 to T6; articular processes of vertebrae C4 to C6	Occipital bone between inferior and superior nuchal lines
Semispinalis cervicis muscles	Transverse processes of vertebrae T2 to T6	Spines of vertebrae C2 to C5
Semispinalis thoracis muscles	Transverse processes of vertebrae T6 to T10	Spines of vertebrae C6 to T4
Splenius capitis muscles	Lower half of ligamentum nuchae and spines of vertebrae C7 to T3	Mastoid process and occipital bone inferior to lateral third of superior nuchal line
Splenius cervicis muscles	Spines of vertebrae T3 to T6	Transverse processes of vertebrae C1 to C3

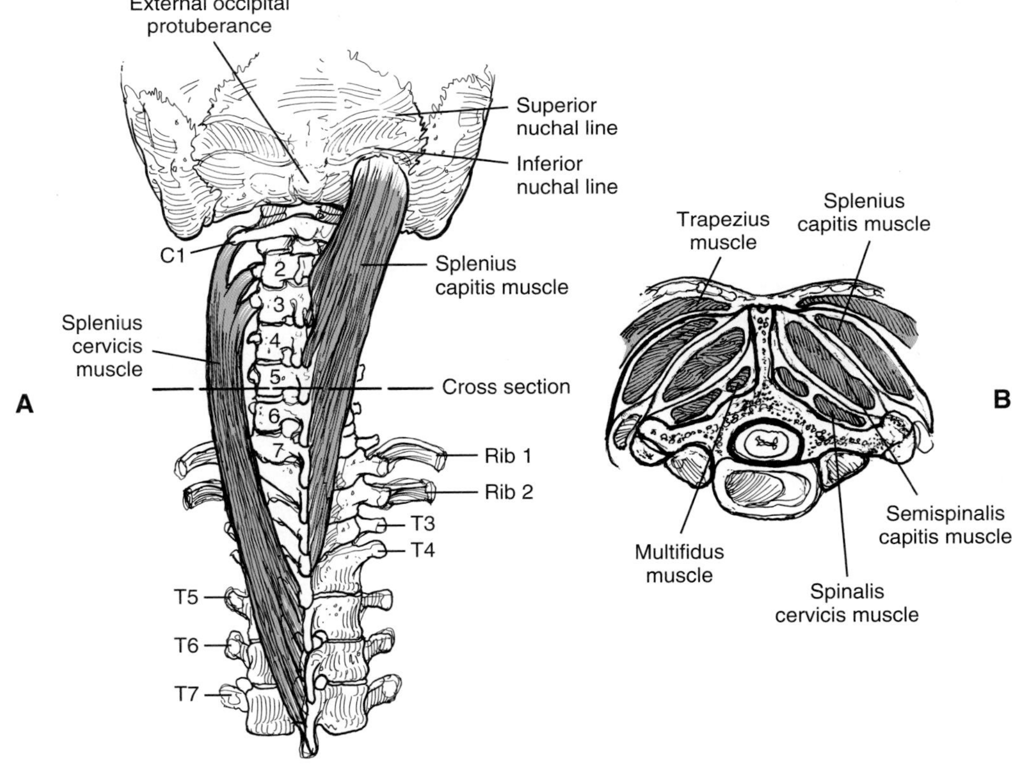

FIGURE 5–3
Attachments of splenius muscles. **A.** Splenius capitis and splenius cervicis muscles are true deep back muscles and are innervated by dorsal primary rami. In contrast to transversospinal muscles, their inferior attachments are to vertebral spines, whereas their lateral attachments are to transverse processes (splenius cervicis muscles) or to lateral regions of the skull base (splenius capitis muscles). **B.** Cross section showing that splenius muscles are superficial to erector spinae muscles but deep to appendicular muscles.

Erector Spinae Muscle Attachments

Erector spinae muscles are massive, elongated muscles extending from the sacrum to the base of the skull

Erector spinae muscles are massive paravertebral muscles which, when considered together, extend from the dorsal surface of the sacrum to the skull, completely filling the vertebral grooves (Fig. 5–4). These bilateral **musculotendinous masses** form an elongated U just superficial to the transversospinal group of muscles (Fig. 5–4*A* and *B*). They can be readily palpated on both sides of the entire length of the vertebral column. Obviously, their length, mass, and distribution throughout the back distinguish them from virtually all of the muscles discussed to this point.

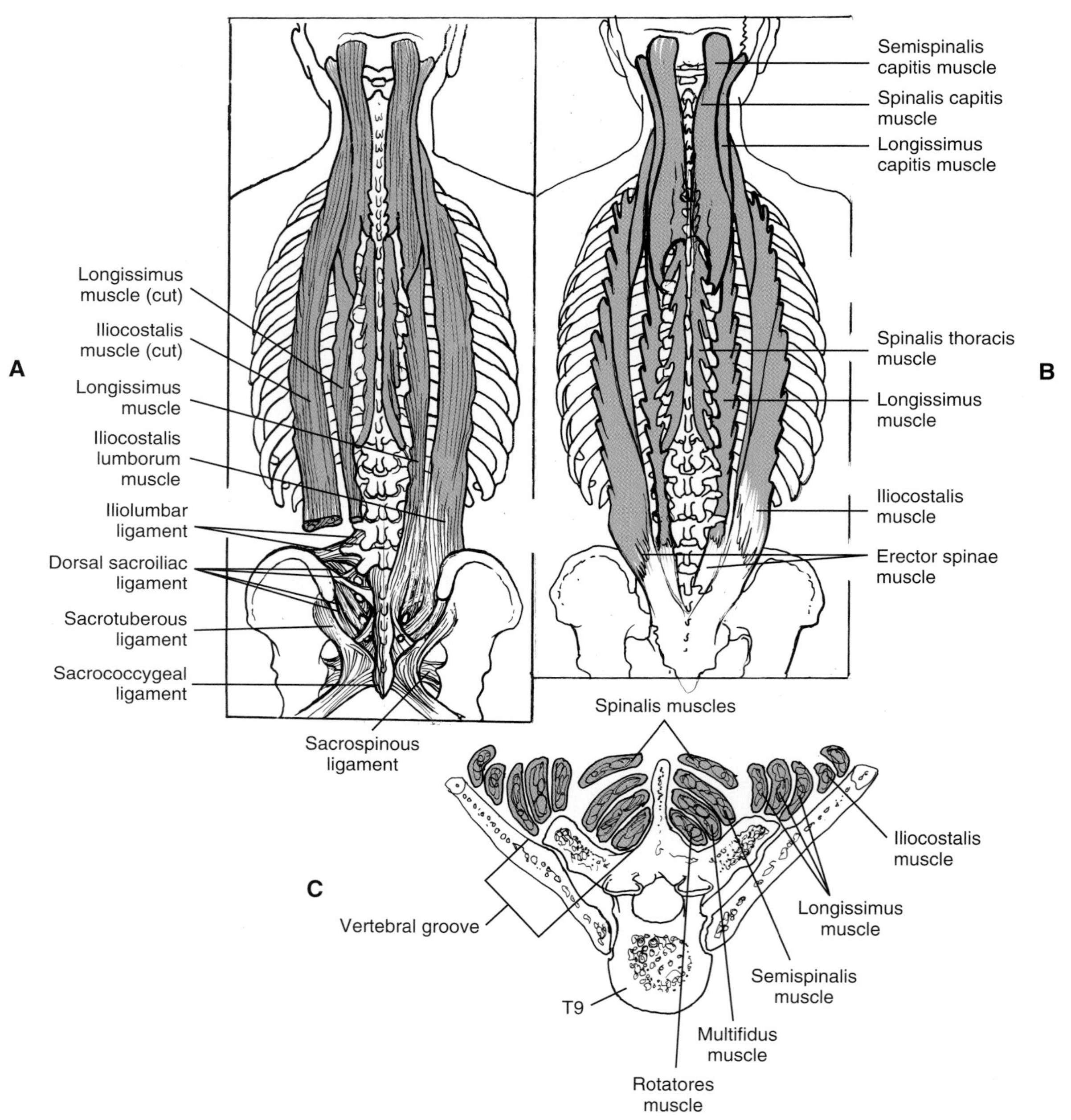

FIGURE 5–4

Attachments of erector spinae muscles. The three groups of erector spinae muscles (from medial to lateral) are spinalis, longissimus, and iliocostalis muscles. **A.** Inferior connections of the erector spinae muscles include the sacrum and a complex of tendons and ligaments, including iliolumbar, dorsal sacroiliac, sacrotuberous, sacrococcygeal, and sacrospinous ligaments (see Fig. 5–16.) **B.** Names of regions of the erector spinae muscles are designated by their locations in the trunk. **C.** Cross section showing relative medial and lateral locations of spinalis, longissimus, and iliocostalis muscles of erector spinae group.

The erector spinae muscles are typically characterized as consisting of three major longitudinal columns: the **iliocostalis muscles** (lateral), **intermediate longissimus muscles,** and **spinalis muscles** (medial) (Fig. 5–4). All of these are true deep back muscles, arising from epimeres and innervated by dorsal rami of the cervical, thoracic, and lumbar spinal nerves. It should be noted that the **spinalis capitis muscle** is typically fused with the **semispinalis capitis muscle** and that the **spinalis cervicis muscles** are frequently absent.

The most inferior parts of the erector spinae muscles arise from a substantial complex of tendons, ligaments, and bones of the lumbar and sacral regions (Fig. 5–4*A* and *B*). The muscle fibers ascend to attach to the vertebrae, ribs, and skull. Each of these longitudinal muscle bundles is further divided into muscle groups based on body region (i.e., cervicis, thoracis, or lumborum) and sites of attachments (Table 5–3 and Fig. 5–4*A* and *C*).

▲ Functions of Deep Back Muscles

Short deep back muscles maintain tension on the vertebral column

The range of movement between adjacent vertebrae is limited and ultimately checked by ligaments (e.g., anterior and posterior longitudinal ligaments, ligamenta flava, and supraspinous ligaments) and intervertebral discs (see Chapter 3). The vertebral column can, therefore, be characterized as a jointed rod of bony elements loosely connected by semiflexible connective tissue ties. In the absence of tension created by the short deep muscles of the back, however, this jointed rod would tend to buckle and collapse. The interspinous, intertransversarii, and transversospinal muscles maintain tension on the vertebral column by intermittently contracting during swaying movements of the body, particularly when a person attempts to maintain an upright standing position or sits in a chair without back support. The actual work performed by these deep back muscles is relatively light when the back is in a vertical position because they contract only to balance the load of the head and trunk upon the vertebral column. Significantly more work is done by these muscles when a person is in a squatting or standing position (e.g., when working at a low table with the back at an oblique angle to vertical).

During active movements of the vertebral column (Fig. 5–5), the short deep muscles may become activated primarily to oppose the longer active extensors, flexors, or rotators of the trunk (see below), thus maintaining rigidity and stability of the vertebral column and contributing to the smoothness of the integrated movements of joints within the vertebral column.

Long deep back muscles may be primarily responsible for dynamic movements of the vertebral column

Back muscles considered to be primarily responsible for dynamic movements of the vertebral column are the longer muscles of the erector spinae group. As has been noted, bilateral contraction of the erector spinae

TABLE 5–3
Erector Spinae Muscle Attachments

Muscle	Inferior Attachment	Superior Attachment
Iliocostalis cervicis muscles	Angles of ribs 3 to 6	Superior 6 ribs and inferior articulating processes of vertebrae C6 and C7
Iliocostalis thoracis muscles	Angles of ribs 7 to 12	Angles of ribs 1 to 6; transverse process of vertebra C7
Iliocostalis lumborum muscles	Erector spinae tendon, sacrum, iliac crest, iliolumbar ligament, sacroiliac ligament	Angles of ribs 7 to 12
Longissimus capitis muscles	Transverse processes of vertebrae T1 to T5; articular processes of vertebrae C5 to C7	Inferior border of mastoid process
Longissimus cervicis muscles	Tendons attached to transverse processes of vertebrae T1 to T5	Tendons attached to transverse processes of vertebrae C2 to C6
Longissimus thoracis muscles	Erector spinae tendon, transverse and accessory processes of lumbar vertebrae, thoracolumbar fascia	Transverse processes of all thoracic vertebrae, tubercles of inferior 10 ribs
Spinalis capitis muscles	Fibers blend with semispinalis capitis muscles (see Table 5–2)	Fibers blend with semispinalisi capitis muscles (see Table 5–2)
Spinalis cervicis muscles (inconstant)	Lower ligamentum nuchae and spine of vertebra C7	Spine of vertebra C2 (axis)
Spinalis thoracis muscles	Spines of vertebrae T11 to L2	Spines of vertebrae T1 to T8

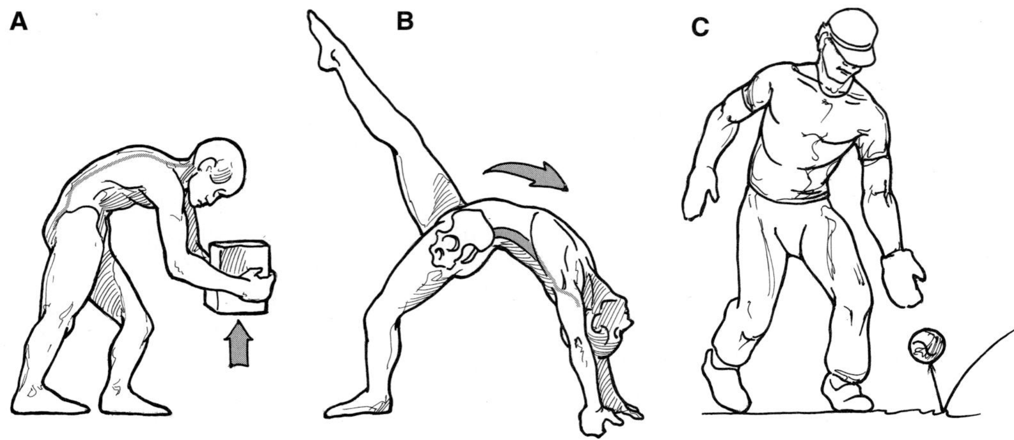

FIGURE 5–5
Movements effected by extensors of the back. **A.** Extension (improper lifting). **B.** Hyperextension. **C.** Lateral flexion. Lateral extension occurs when one returns from a position of lateral flexion.

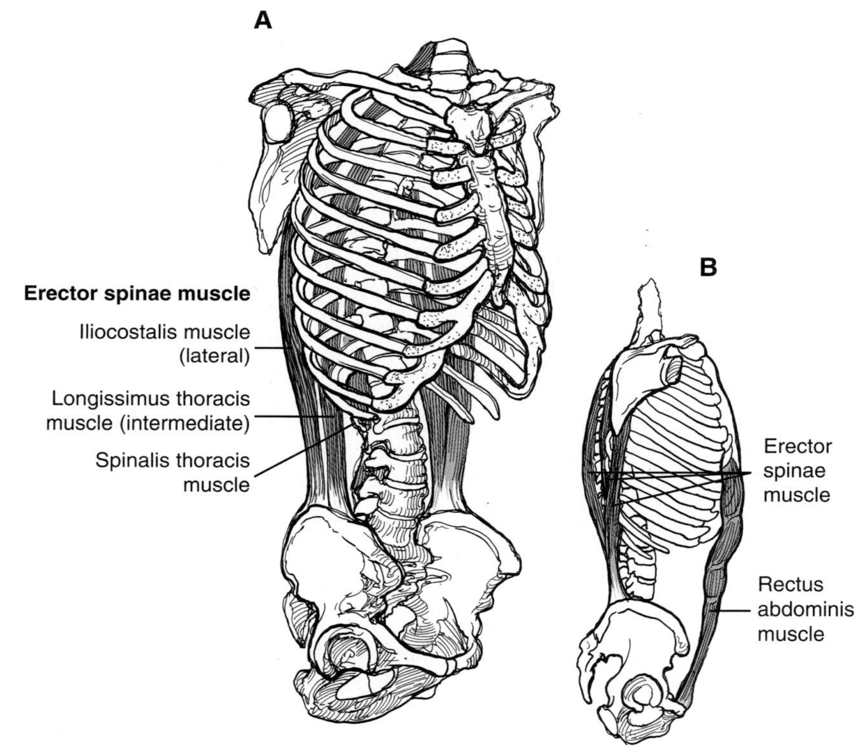

FIGURE 5–6
Synergism of erector spinae and rectus abdominis muscles. Actions of erector spinae muscles are countered by those of rectus abdominis muscles and vice versa.

muscles initiates extension of the vertebral column (Fig. 5–5*A* and *B* and see Table 5–3 for attachments of erector spinae muscles). This movement is directly countered, however, by constant contraction of the ventral rectus abdominis muscles (Fig. 5–6). Conversely, dynamic flexion of the vertebral column may be initiated by contractions of the rectus abdominis muscles, which are then countered by contractions of the erector spinae muscles. The erector spinae muscles appear, in a way, to produce dynamic movement in extension but act as static muscles during flexion of the vertebral column. Conversely, the rectus abdominis muscles flex the vertebral column against the static resistance of the erector spinae muscles. Thus these dorsal and ventral muscles intermittently maintain stability or generate movement of the axial skeleton (including the sternum and ribs) by acting as "guy wires" that tense or relax as they oppose each other's actions (Fig. 5–6*B*).

Moreover, the long extensors on opposite sides of the vertebral column play similar complementary roles during active lateral flexion of the vertebral column (see Fig. 5–5C). For example, as the trunk is laterally flexed to the right by contraction of erector spinae muscles on the right side of the vertebral column, erector spinae muscles on the left side contract to produce tension that opposes this movement (see Fig. 3–25C and D).

Short "postural" muscles also play a dynamic role in movements of the trunk

Short deep back muscles also play a dual role. Although these muscles have been described as simply maintaining the rigidity of the vertebral column to hold the body in an upright position or to keep it stable during active movements of the trunk, it is likely that the interspinous, intertransversarii, and semispinalis muscles also behave as extensors or lateral flexors of the trunk. For example, based on descriptions of attachments of intertransversarii muscles (see Table 5–1), it should not be surprising that the extension and lateral flexion produced by these short deep muscles must occur primarily in the cervical and lumbar regions. Indeed, little flexion, extension, or lateral flexion can occur in the thoracic region because of hindrance by the ribs.

The rotatores and multifidus muscles on one side of the vertebral column have been implicated in rotating the trunk to the opposite side. The rotatores muscles are best developed and possibly most active in the thoracic region, whereas the multifidus muscles are well developed throughout the cervical, thoracic, and lumbar regions (see Fig. 3–25E).

▲ Clinical Disorders of Deep Back Muscles

Back Pain

Anterior and posterior or right and left imbalances of back muscles may lead to back pain

As has been noted above, true deep back muscles behave synergistically in performing virtually all of the muscular activities of the trunk (i.e., in maintaining spinal curvatures and posture and providing stability during dynamic movements of the vertebral column). Disruption of these normal synergistic relationships resulting from imbalance in tension between the posterior and anterior musculature or between muscles on the right and left sides of the vertebral column may result in pain, postural problems, and rotational problems during standing, walking, or running. Disorders of all true deep muscles of the back may lead to **low back muscle pain.** The erector spinae muscles are more frequently involved when improper lifting has occurred (see Fig. 5–5A), whereas muscles of the transversospinal group, intertransversarii muscles, and interspinales muscles may be implicated when the patient complains of pain on standing or rotating.

Muscle Strain

A common muscle disorder leading to low back pain is **muscle strain,** which is a stretch injury to the muscle or its tendon, or both. This differs from a **sprain** in which only ligamentous tissue is stretched. The strained muscle **spasms** (contracts involuntarily), resulting in increased tension between its points of attachment.

Improper lifting, sports activities, and **trauma from automobile accidents** are common causes of back muscle strain. In addition, **obesity** and **pregnancy** tend to predispose individuals to back muscle strain because of the weight imbalance imposed by these conditions. The increased weight in the anterior region imposed by obesity and pregnancy disrupts the synergy of anterior and posterior muscles, causing posterior muscles to actively contract during activities in which they would routinely be relaxed. Patients suffering from the consequent chronic back pain (in the absence of associated orthopedic or neurologic problems) are treated conservatively. Rest; treatment with muscle relaxants, antiinflammatory agents, or analgesics; and heat or cold therapy are common remedies. Following treatment of a specific episode, patients are advised to resolve conditions that predispose them to back problems. Overweight patients are usually placed on a weight control program, instructed in proper lifting techniques ("back school"), and admonished to undertake mild exercises designed to strengthen the erector spinae and short deep back muscles.

Skeletal Disorders Resulting from Muscle Strain or Hypertrophy

Back muscle strain or hypertrophy may even lead to skeletal disorders

Muscle strain causing **bilateral spasm** of the deep back muscles tends to **flatten the lumbar curvature,** whereas **unilateral spasm** may create mild **scoliosis,** or lateral bending of the vertebral column. Muscle strain is not the only cause of this condition, however. Any **abnormal hypertrophy** of the musculature may result in abnormal bending of the vertebral column. **Bilateral hypertrophy** of muscles within a limited region of the back may result in alterations of vertebral column curvatures. This is commonly found in **swimmers,** particularly those who use the butterfly stroke. Muscles in the thoracic region hypertrophy, resulting in flattening of the thoracic and lumbar curvatures. **Adolescents** undergoing rapid growth may also experience bilateral muscle stress on the spinal column, especially in the lumbar region, as a consequence of relatively rapid growth of bone compared with muscle.

Hypertrophy of back muscles **on one side only** may occur in individuals who use the upper limb on that side for long periods of time. The resulting imbalance in tension on the vertebral column may lead to **lumbar scoliosis.**

These alterations are usually mild, but the resulting discomfort may be significant and have a profound effect on the patient's quality of life, particularly if the patient is an **adolescent** or a **young adult.**

Nerve Compression and the Spine

Muscle strains associated with orthopedic disorders may lead to nerve compression

Typically, muscle strain alone will not result in sufficient compression of the **intervertebral foramen** to squeeze the nerve root. If the vertebral arch or a portion of it is weakened, however, the added tension resulting from muscle strain and spasm often causes compression of the nerve root. An example of this is **spondylolysis,** in which a portion of the vertebral arch has fractured as a consequence of genetic predisposition, repeated stress, or both. This injury is commonly seen in **young (preadolescent) gymnasts** and in **football linemen** and is more common in **girls** than boys. Treatment frequently involves suspension of the activity aggravating the condition, stretching exercises designed to improve flexibility of the hamstring muscles (see Chapter 17), and use of a brace. In cases where this conservative treatment is unsuccessful, **posterior spinal fusion** may be performed.

Visceral Pain Referred to the Back

Visceral pain referred to the back may be mistaken for somatic back pain

Although visceral pain is more commonly referred to the abdomen and anterior thorax, it may be referred to the back (see Fig. 4–14). Stomach, gallbladder, pancreatic, and colonic pain may be referred to the upper back, whereas kidney, rectal, prostate, and uterine pain may be referred to the lower back (Fig. 5–7).

An **aortic aneurysm** frequently refers pain to the back at the same level at which the aneurysm has occurred. The patient may attribute this pain to "back problems" when the condition may be much more serious. A proper physical examination is important in determining whether back pain is caused by skeletal or muscular disorders or is referred from another site in order to make the appropriate diagnosis and design a proper course of treatment.

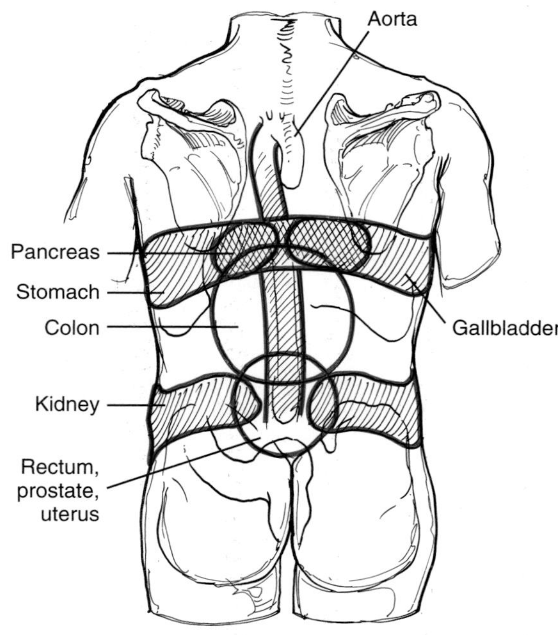

FIGURE 5–7
Pain referred to the back. Pain from thoracic, abdominal, and pelvic viscera may be referred to the back. This referred pain may be interpreted as somatic back pain.

SUBOCCIPITAL MUSCLES

Suboccipital muscles are a specialized group of "deep back muscles" of the neck

Attachments of the Suboccipital Muscles

As was discussed in Chapter 2, the suboccipital muscles are a specialized group of deep back muscles of the neck within the **suboccipital region** (Fig. 5–8). These are the **superior oblique (obliquus capitis superior), inferior oblique (obliquus capitis inferior), rectus major (rectus capitis major),** and **rectus minor (rectus capitis minor) muscles.** All of these muscles arise from epimeres and are innervated by the dorsal primary ramus of the first cervical nerve, which is sometimes called the **suboccipital nerve.**

An appreciation of the anatomic relationships of these muscles may be gained by reviewing the skeletal anatomy in this region and identifying each of these muscles one by one (Fig. 5–8).

- Once the **trapezius, splenius capitis,** and **semispinalis capitis muscles** are reflected, the **spine of vertebra C2** can be observed as the site of the superior attachment of the **semispinalis cervicis muscles** (circled 1 in Fig. 5–8 and see Table 5–2).
- This bony prominence also provides the inferior attachment site for the **rectus major muscle,** the fibers of which ascend to the **lateral part of the inferior nuchal line** at the base of the skull (circled 2 in Fig. 5–8 and see Table 5–4).
- Just above the spine of vertebra C2, the **posterior arch of vertebra C1** (circled 3 in Fig. 5–8) provides an inferior attachment site for the **rectus minor muscle** (circled 4 in Fig. 5–8), the fibers of which ascend to attach superiorly along the **medial part of the inferior nuchal line** (Fig. 5–8).
- Returning to the **spine of vertebra C2,** the medial attachment of the **inferior oblique muscle** (circled 5 in Fig. 5–8) may be observed. This muscle courses to the tip of the **transverse process of vertebra C1 (atlas)** (circled 6 in Fig. 5–8), which also provides the inferior attachment for the **superior oblique muscle** (circled 7 in Fig. 5–8).
- The superior oblique muscle is attached to the **occipital bone between the inferior and superior nuchal lines** (see Fig. 5–8).

Functions of the Suboccipital Muscles

Suboccipital muscles and other muscles of the neck perform both static and dynamic functions

Inferior oblique muscles enjoy a relatively large mechanical advantage because of the length of the transverse processes of vertebra C1 and thus play a major role in turning the face to the same side as the unilaterally contracting muscle (Fig. 5–9*A* and Table 5–4). The rectus capitis major and minor and superior oblique muscles extend the head when they contract bilaterally, but when muscles on one side contract unilaterally, they also turn the face to that side (Fig. 5–9*B*). However, these latter three pairs of suboccipital muscles are thought to behave more typically as postural muscles because they contract to counter the effect of gravity on flexion of the neck. The sternocleidomastoid muscles and other extensors of the head may possibly assist these muscles (Fig. 5–9*B* and see Chapter 24).

▲ Suboccipital Triangle

Visualizing the suboccipital region may be aided by locating a suboccipital compartment defined by a region called the suboccipital triangle

A **suboccipital triangle** can be defined on each side of the midline. The **superomedial border** of the suboccipital triangle is the rectus major muscle; the **superolateral border** is the superior oblique muscle; and the **inferior border** is the inferior oblique muscle (see Fig. 5–8). These muscles make up the **walls of a suboccipital compartment,** which (as is the case in other anatomic compartments or three-dimensional spaces such as "tunnels" and "canals") also possesses a **floor** and a **roof.**

TABLE 5–4
Suboccipital Muscle Attachments

Muscle	Inferior Attachment	Superior Attachment
Rectus capitis major muscle	Spine of vertebra C2 (axis)	Lateral part of inferior nuchal line
Rectus capitis minor muscle	Spine of vertebra C1 (atlas)	Medial part of inferior nuchal line
Obliquus capitis inferior muscle	Spine of vertebra C2	Transverse process of vertebra C1
Obliquus capitis superior muscle	Transverse process of vertebra C1	Occipital bone between inferior and superior nuchal lines

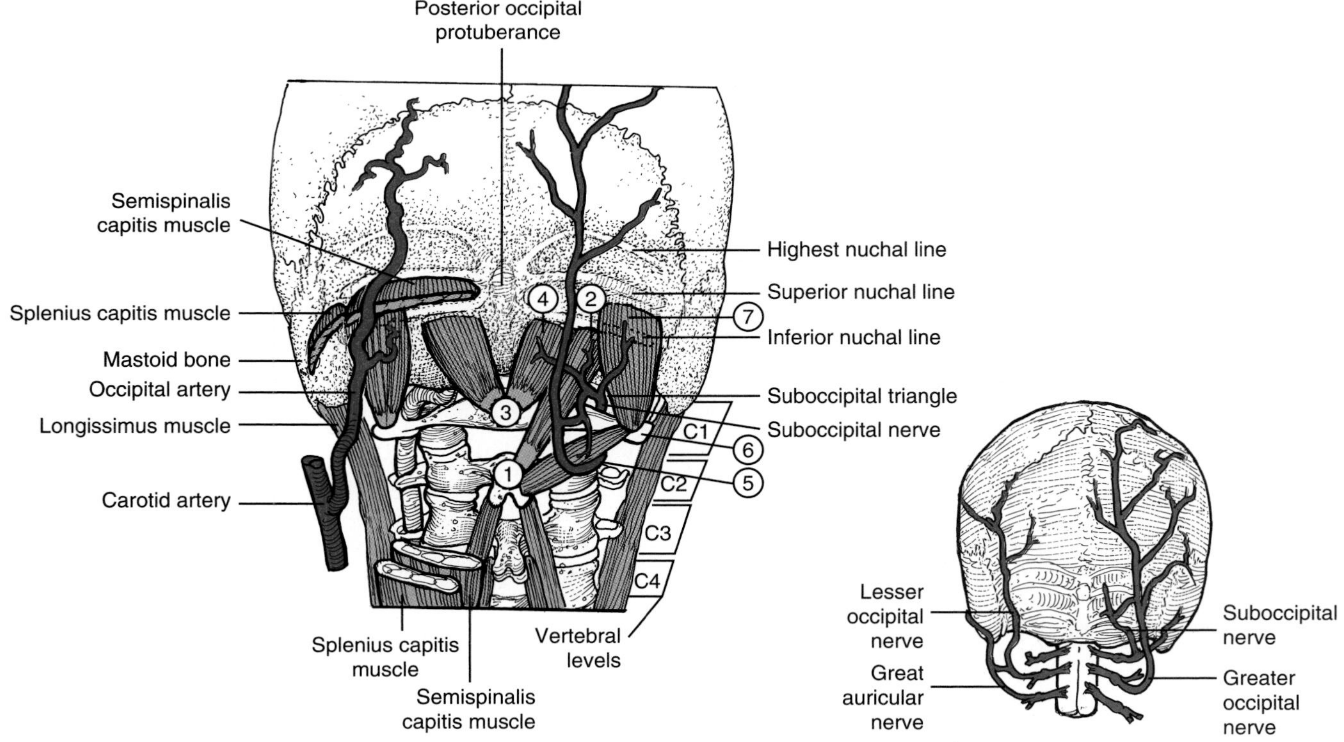

FIGURE 5–8
Suboccipital muscles. Spines of vertebrae C1 and C2 and tips of transverse processes of vertebra C1 provide palpable frames of reference for understanding organization of suboccipital muscles and associated nerves (i.e., greater occipital, suboccipital, lesser occipital, and great auricular) and arteries (i.e., vertebral and occipital). *1,* Spine of vertebra C2 (axis); *2,* rectus major muscle; *3,* posterior arch of vertebra C1; *4,* rectus minor muscle; *5,* inferior oblique muscle; *6,* transverse process of vertebra C1 (atlas); and *7,* superior oblique muscle.

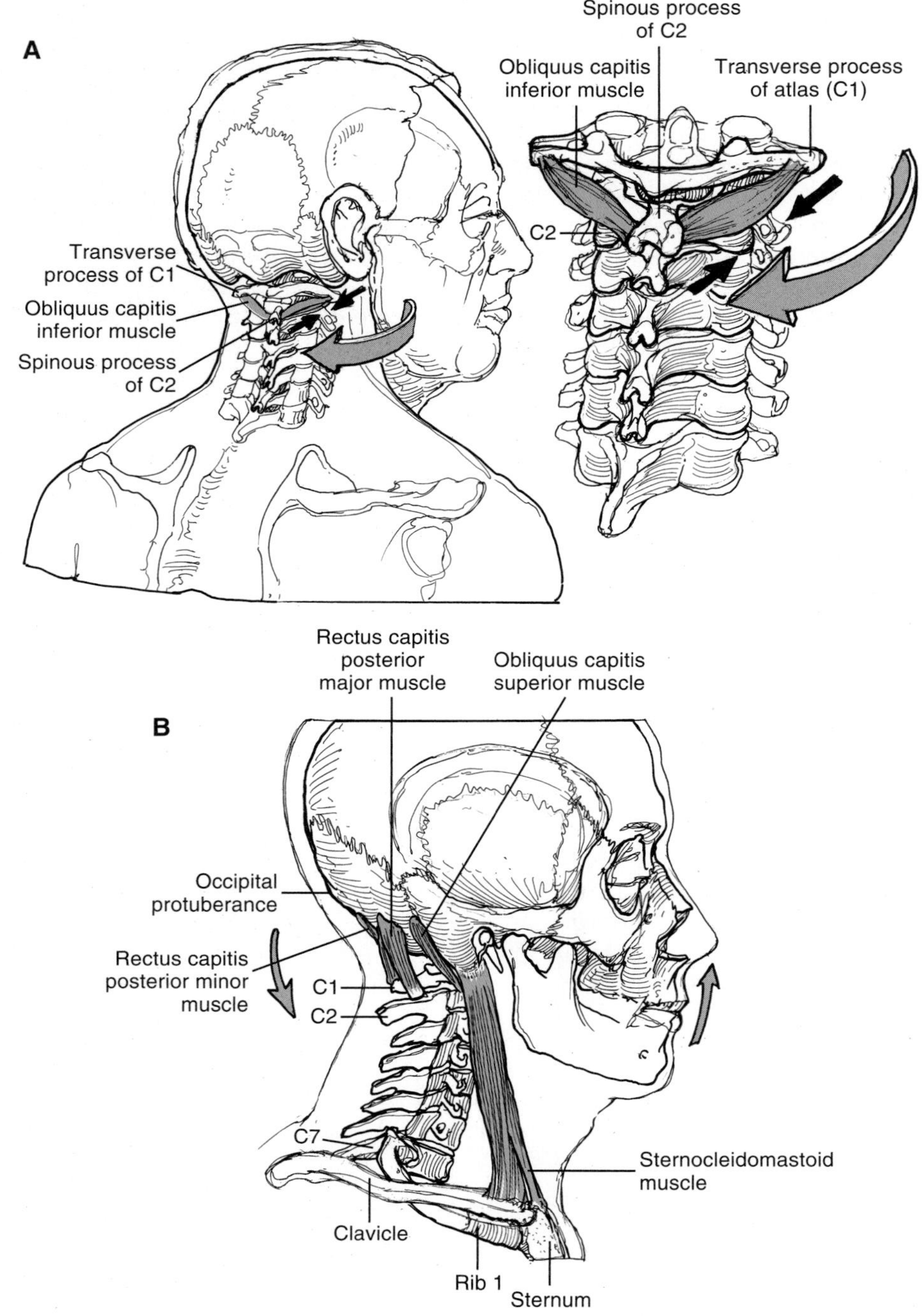

FIGURE 5–9

Actions of suboccipital muscles. **A.** Long transverse processes of vertebra C1 provide a lever for action (cervical rotation) of inferior oblique muscle. **B.** Posterior superior oblique, rectus major, and rectus minor muscles act together with anterolateral sternocleidomastoid muscles. Thus they extend or hyperextend the neck.

The roof of each suboccipital compartment is the **semispinalis capitis muscle.** The deeper, more anterior floor of each suboccipital compartment is the **posterior atlantooccipital membrane** and the **posterior arch of the atlas (C1).** The atlantooccipital membrane is a flat ligament connecting the base of the skull just posterior to the foramen magnum to the posterior arch and transverse processes of the atlas (see Fig. 5–8).

▲ Identification of Nerves and Arteries of the Suboccipital Region

Anatomic relationships of several vascular and neuronal elements of the posterior neck can be readily visualized because of their spatial relationships to regions in and around the suboccipital triangle

The **greater occipital nerve** (a branch of the dorsal ramus of spinal nerve C2) pierces the semispinalis and splenius capitis muscles to provide sensory innervation to the posterior scalp (see Fig. 5–8). Just deep to the semispinalis muscles, the greater occipital nerve emerges along the inferior border of the inferior oblique muscle (i.e., just inferior to the inferior wall of the suboccipital compartment) (see Fig. 5–8). The greater occipital nerve also provides innervation to the inferior oblique, splenius capitis, semispinalis capitis, and longissimus capitis muscles (see Table 2–1).

The **suboccipital nerve** emerges from within the suboccipital triangle (see Fig. 5–8). It contains the motor fibers of spinal nerve C1. It may combine with sensory fibers from spinal nerve C2 and then supply all of the suboccipital muscles and the semispinalis capitis muscle. Spinal nerve C1 by itself typically lacks a dorsal root ganglion and sensory fibers, unlike any other spinal nerve (see Table 2–1).

A small section of the **vertebral artery** may also be visualized deep within the suboccipital compartment, just superior to the transverse process of the atlas (vertebra C1) (see Fig. 5–8 and Chapter 2). The **occipital artery** (which is a branch of the **external carotid artery**) emerges onto the posterior scalp from a location just deep and lateral to the superior oblique muscles (see Fig. 5–8).

▲ **Nerve Compression in the Suboccipital Region**

Strains may occur in muscles of the neck, most frequently as the result of **flexion-extension (whiplash) injury.** The resultant swelling may either increase or decrease the cervical curvature and, in some cases, put direct pressure on a nerve. For example, the **greater occipital nerve** passes through the **semispinalis capitis muscle** and provides sensory innervation to the posterior half of the scalp (see Fig. 5–8). When the semispinalis muscle is swollen due to strain, it may compress the nerve where it penetrates the muscle. The patient experiences pain across the posterior aspect of the scalp, commonly describing the discomfort as a **"headache."** Nerve compressions, however, most frequently result from **entrapment.** The conventional definition of an entrapped nerve is a nerve that is compressed against firmer tissue, such as bones or ligaments.

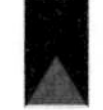

INTERMEDIATE LAYER OF BACK MUSCLES

Muscle Attachments and Functions of So-called Respiratory Muscles

The role of so-called respiratory muscles is unclear

Attachments of the **serratus posterior superior muscles** suggest that these muscles raise ribs 2 to 5, and attachments of the **serratus posterior inferior muscles** suggest that these muscles depress the lower four ribs (Fig. 5–10 and Table 5–5). Attachments of the **levatores costarum muscles** suggest that they raise all 12 pairs of ribs (see Fig. 5–1 and Table 5–1). It has been argued, therefore, that these muscles would support the **respiratory movements** that accompany **inspiration** because

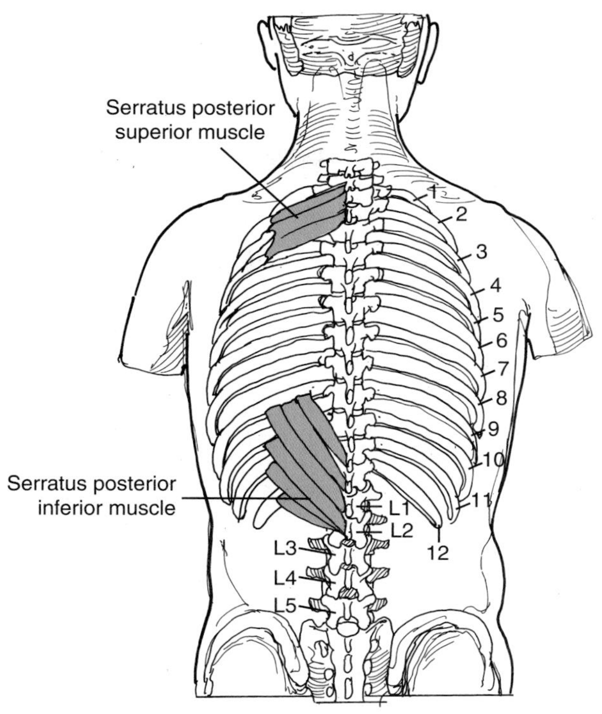

FIGURE 5–10

Attachments of superior and inferior serratus muscles. Attachments of serratus posterior superior muscles tend to implicate them in raising the upper ribs. Attachments of serratus posterior inferior muscles tend to implicate them in depressing the lower ribs.

their actions would tend to increase the volume of the thoracic cavity (see Chapter 6). The **kinesiologic** (science of muscle action) evidence available at this time is controversial, however, and it is not clear whether or not these so-called respiratory muscles play only static roles.

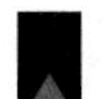

APPENDICULAR MUSCLES

Attachments of Appendicular Muscles

Appendicular muscles and associated skeletal elements migrate onto the back during early development

Anatomic and functional relationships of deep back muscles and their skeletal attachment sites, innervation, and vascularization are particularly dependent upon the coordinated segmental development of their respective precursors. On the other hand, the **migration** of muscle anlagen and their associated skeletal elements plays an equally important role in establishing anatomic relationships of the proximal upper extremity appendicular muscles to the axial skeleton of the superior trunk.

Muscles of the upper extremities arise from the mesoderm that initially migrates into the developing upper limb buds from somites C5 to T1. This mesoderm develops in close proximity to skeletal elements of the upper limb at the base of the upper limb buds between the fourth and eighth weeks of development. As precursors of proximal limb muscles and bones begin

TABLE 5–5
Serratus Posterior Muscle Attachments

Muscle	Proximal Attachment	Distal Attachment
Serratus posterior superior muscles	Spines of vertebrae C6 to T2	Angles of ribs 2 to 5
Serratus posterior inferior muscles	Spines of vertebrae T11 to L2 (with latissimus dorsi muscles)	Lower borders of ribs 9 to 12

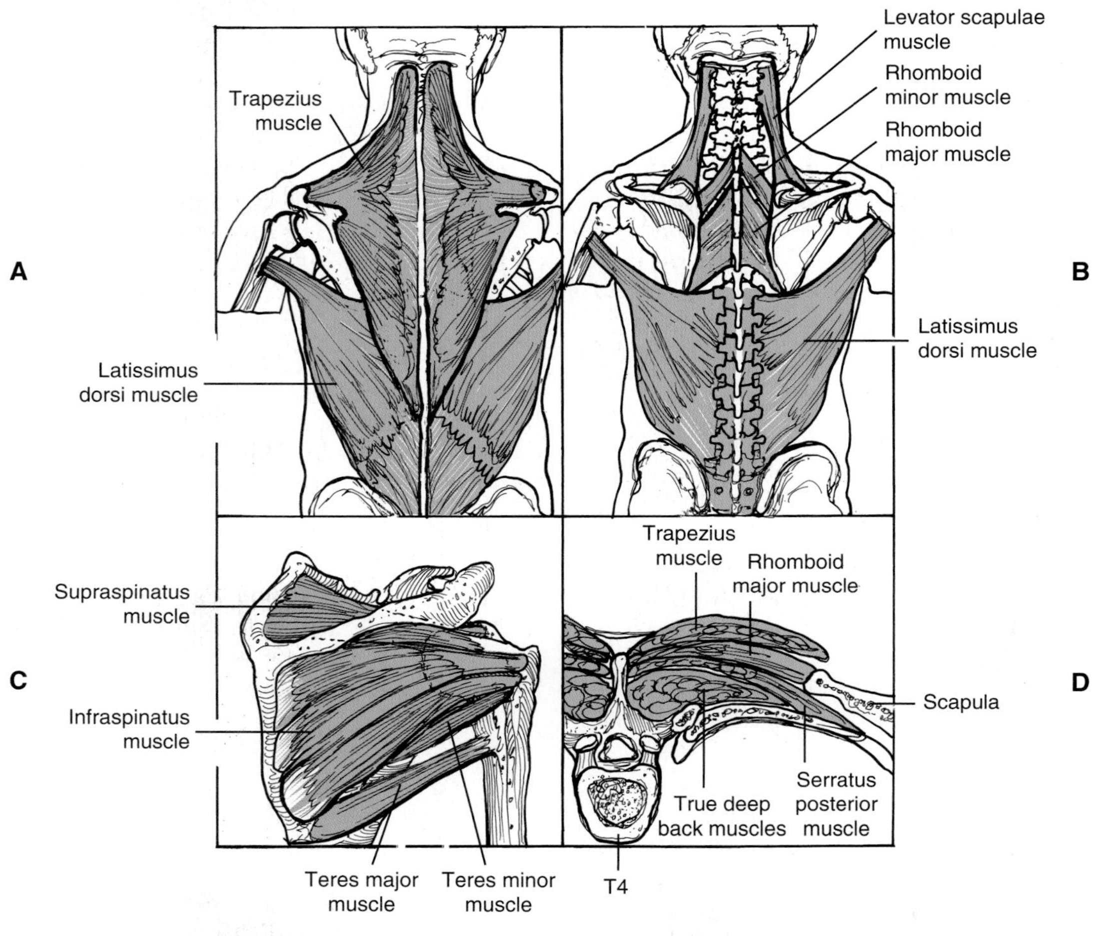

FIGURE 5–11
Attachments of appendicular muscles. Appendicular muscles of the back are primarily responsible for moving scapula, humerus, or both and for maintaining poise of shoulder. **A.** Trapezius and latissimus dorsi muscles. **B.** Levator scapulae, rhomboid major and rhomboid minor, and latissimus dorsi muscles. **C.** Supraspinatus, infraspinatus, and teres major and teres minor muscles. **D.** Cross section at vertebra T4. Appendicular muscles are most superficial of all back muscles.

to differentiate, they migrate medially, dorsally, and inferiorly over the developing deep back muscles of the posterior trunk. The nerves that innervate these muscles elongate as the muscles migrate from their sites of formation. (These nerves arise from a brachial plexus of nerves as described in Chapter 21.) Thus, even though many of the appendicular muscles of the upper extremities, including the levator scapulae, rhomboid, and latissimus dorsi muscles, become attached to the vertebral spines of the axial skeleton, these attachments are all superficial to those of the true deep back muscles and intermediate muscles of the posterior trunk.

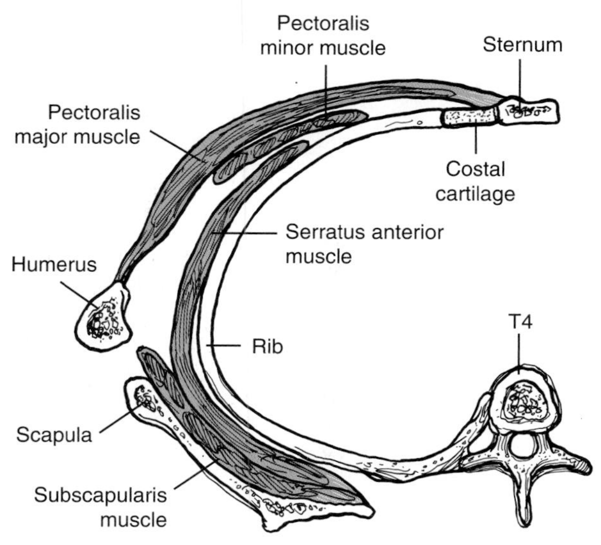

FIGURE 5–12
Attachments of serratus anterior muscle. Serratus anterior muscle holds scapula against the trunk. When its action is disrupted, as in an injury to the long thoracic nerve, the scapula is raised as a "wing scapula."

The most superficial muscle of the appendicular group, the **trapezius muscle,** is attached to the tips of the thoracic spines, the ligamentum nuchae, and the occipital bone (Fig. 5–11*A* and *D*). Its more lateral attachments include the spine of the scapula, and lateral half of the clavicle. A deeper layer of posterior appendicular muscles, associated with the scapulae, include the **levator scapulae, rhomboid major** and **minor, supraspinatus** and **infraspinatus, teres major** and **minor,** and **subscapularis muscles** (Fig. 5–11). The levator scapulae and rhomboid muscles attach the scapula to the vertebral spines at sites just deep to those of the trapezius muscle but superficial to those of the true deep back muscles (Fig. 5–11*B* and *D*). The supraspinatus, infraspinatus, teres major and minor, and subscapularis muscles all connect the humerus to the scapula and are responsible for the movement and stability of the shoulder joint (see Figs. 5–11 and 5–12 and Chapter 21). The **latissimus dorsi muscle** directly connects the humerus to the axial skeleton and other structures of the trunk (Fig. 5–11*A* and *B*). Specifically, the proximal attachments of the latissimus dorsi muscle include aponeuroses attached to the six inferior thoracic spines, all five lumbar spines, the sacral spines, and the iliac crest. The distal attachment of the latissimus dorsi muscle is the anterior surface of the upper humerus.

Of the appendicular muscles of the posterior trunk, only the **serratus anterior muscle** is directly attached to the ribs. Its attachments are to the outer surfaces and upper borders of the 9 or 10 superior ribs near their connections to the corresponding costal cartilages (Fig. 5–12 and Chapter 21). The insertion of this muscle at the medioanterior border of the scapula provides a mechanism to hold the scapula against the trunk. The **pectoralis major** and **pectoralis minor muscles** are also attached to the rib cage (including the sternal and costal cartilages) on the ventral side of the thorax (Fig. 5–12). The innervation, vascularization, and specific attachments and actions of all of the appendicular muscles of the upper extremities are described in detail in Chapters 19 to 21.

▲ Functions of Appendicular Muscles

Appendicular muscles of the back move and steady their associated skeletal elements

Appendicular muscles of the back are primarily involved in movements of the clavicle, scapula, and humerus bones of the appendicular skeleton. These muscles and their functions will be described in detail in Chapter 20, but their general functions are briefly discussed here.

It should be understood that the only bony connection of the upper extremity to the axial skeleton is at the **sternoclavicular joint.** It is, therefore, primarily the muscles associated with the clavicle, scapula, and humerus that provide the most significant attachments of the upper limbs to the body.

The delicacy of upper limb movements is achieved in much the same way as the smooth movements of the vertebral column; that is, through the contractions of opposing muscle groups.

Movements of the scapula provide a good example of this. The scapula is elevated by superior fibers of the trapezius and levator scapulae muscles working together (Fig. 5–13). The scapula is depressed by inferior fibers of the trapezius muscle acting with the serratus anterior muscles. Depending on which fibers are active, the trapezius and serratus anterior muscles also act together to protract (i.e., move toward the midline) and rotate the scapula laterally with respect to its inferior angle. The scapula can also be retracted (i.e., moved laterally) and rotated medially by the trapezius and rhomboid major and minor muscles. Finally, the trapezius muscle may act with the suboccipital muscles to extend the head when the scapula is fixed.

The trapezius muscle also behaves as a **postural muscle,** steadying the scapula and shoulder of a person during movement or when a heavy object such as a suitcase is being carried. The trapezius muscle has been described as being primarily responsible for maintaining the proper position or poise of the shoulder. However, the rhomboids, levator scapulae, and other muscles attached to the scapula may also act as postural muscles, countering dynamic movements and thus imposing control on movements of the upper extremity. A detailed discussion of actions of upper extremity muscles is provided in Chapter 20.

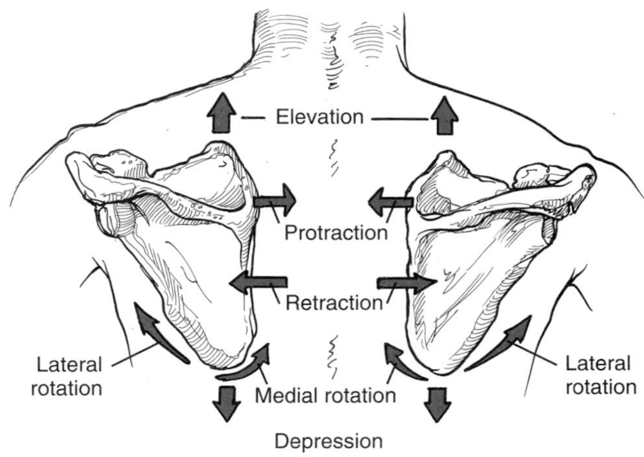

FIGURE 5–13

Movements of scapula. Scapula may be protracted (moved medially), retracted (moved laterally), elevated (moved superiorly), or depressed (moved inferiorly). Scapula may also be rotated laterally (i.e., inferior scapular angles are rotated laterally) or medially (i.e., inferior scapular angles are rotated medially).

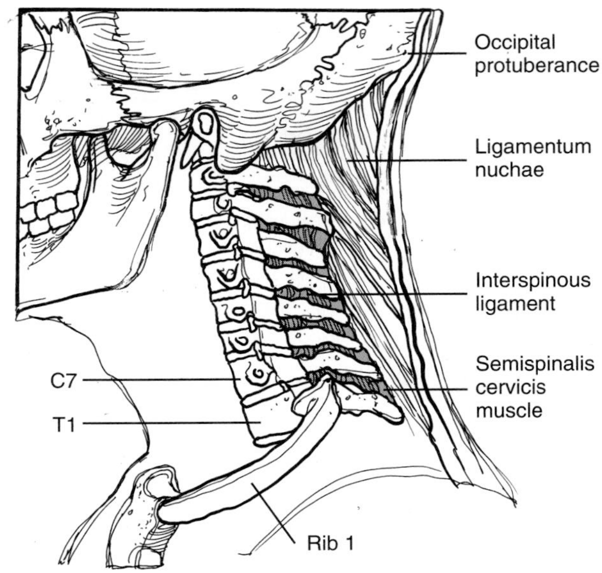

FIGURE 5–14

Ligamentum nuchae is a specialization of interspinous ligaments in the cervical region and is an attachment site for spinalis and splenius muscles in the neck.

INTEGRATION OF BACK MUSCLE ANATOMY AND ACTIONS

Connective tissue elements of the posterior trunk connect and bind together muscular and skeletal elements

As with the vertebral column, connective tissue elements play an essential role in binding together muscular elements of the back and providing attachment sites that support their integrated function. These include

- the superficial fascia (throughout the back;
- the ligamentum nuchae, a specialization of the supraspinous ligaments (in the cervical region);
- the thoracolumbar fascia, which is a specialization of the deep fascia (in the thoracic and lumbar regions); and
- a complex of tendons and ligaments in the lower back.

Superficial Fascia of the Back

Superficial fascia of the back protects underlying muscles and bones

The superficial fascia of the cervical and superior thoracic region is especially tough, thick, and fatty and is firmly connected to the overlying skin. This complex of posterior integument and hypodermis tightly and securely encloses the underlying trapezius muscle and other appendicular muscles in this region. In contrast, the loose connection between the superficial and deep fascia investing these appendicular muscles allows the scapula to move freely beneath the skin (see Fig. 5–13).

Ligamentum Nuchae

The ligamentum nuchae provides an important attachment site for muscles of the cervical region

Several specialized aponeuroses of connective tissue play a prominent role in maintaining integrity and function in the back. The ligamentum nuchae, which is the cervical extension of supraspinous ligaments, has been discussed above as a major attachment for deep back muscles of the neck such as the spinalis and splenius cervicis muscles (Fig. 5–14). These muscles are far more massive in quadrupedal animals because they play a more prominent role in holding up the head. As a consequence, the ligamentum nuchae is far better developed in quadrupeds than in upright bipedal humans.

Thoracolumbar Fascia

Thoracolumbar fascia is a specialization of deep fascia

Every muscle of the body is individually invested by deep fascia, although these investments may be fused with those of adjacent muscles. The **deep fascia of the back** is made up of dense connective tissue, which invests all of the muscles of the posterior body wall. In this region of the body, the deep fascia is well developed and plays an important role in binding together and integrating the wide array of deep back muscles in the thoracic, lumbar, and sacral regions and in separating the deep back muscles from the appendicular and serratus posterior muscles. This fascia is so well developed that it is given the specific name of **thoracolumbar fascia** (Fig. 5–15).

As the thoracolumbar fascia extends superiorly, it merges with the deep fascia, the **deep cervical fascia,** covering the deep muscles of the neck. In the thoracic region, the thoracolumbar fascia is made up of a single tough layer interposed between the serratus posterior

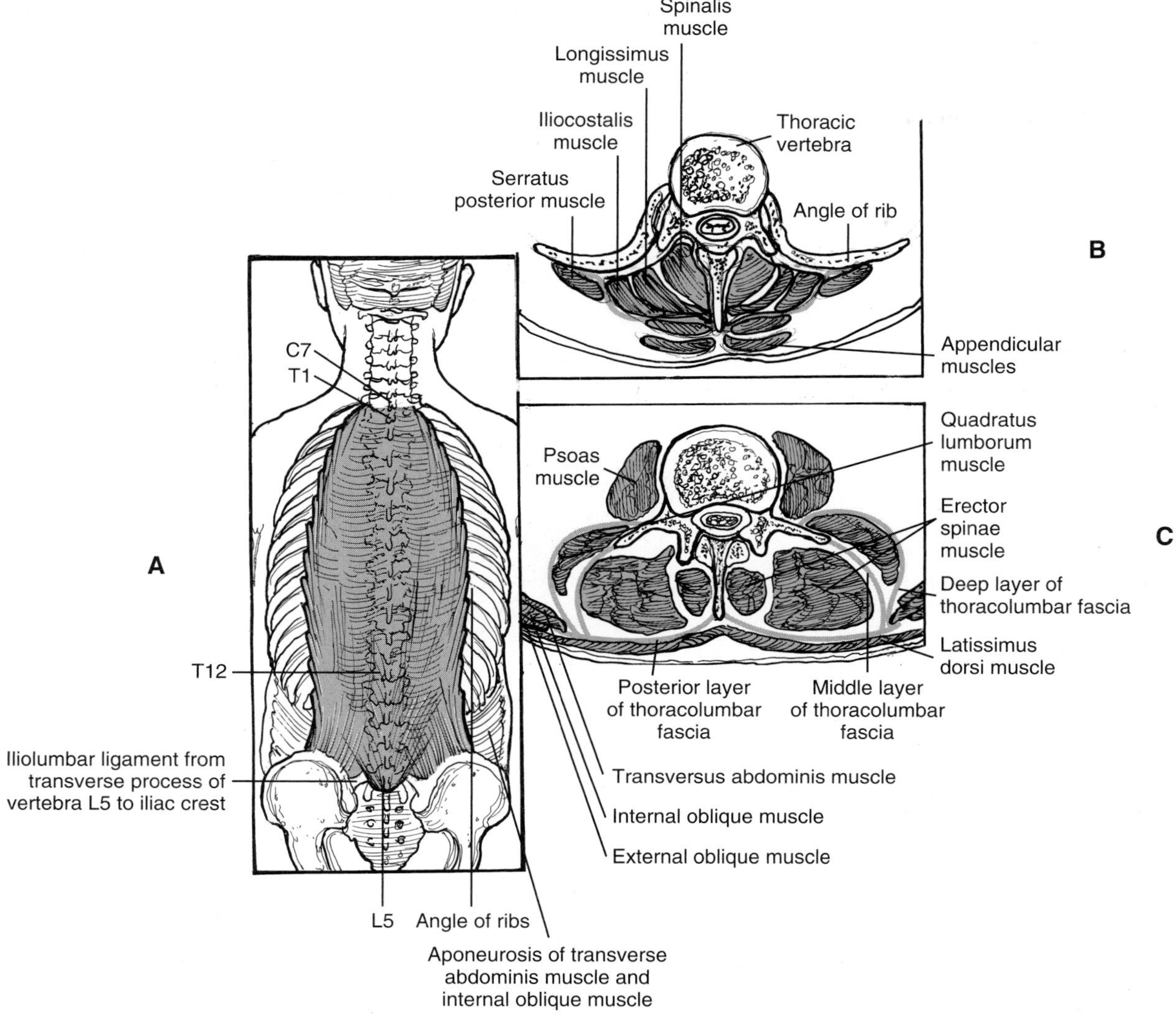

FIGURE 5–15

Thoracolumbar fascia. Deep fascia of the back is specialized to provide attachment sites for back musculature. **A.** As its name implies, fascia courses throughout thoracic and lumbar regions of the back. **B.** In the thoracic region, fascia is elaborated as a single tough membrane that provides attachment sites for erector spinae muscles and separates true deep muscles of the back from appendicular muscles. **C.** In the lumbar region, three layers of thoracolumbar fascia separate psoas muscle from quadratus lumborum muscle (deep layer), quadratus lumborum muscle from erector spinae muscle (middle layer), and quadratus lumborum muscle from latissimus dorsi muscle (posterior layer). Laterally, thoracolumbar fascia provides attachment site for transversus abdominis and internal oblique muscles of ventrolateral abdominal wall.

and erector spinae muscles (Fig. 5–15*A* and *B*) and is attached medially to all 12 thoracic vertebral spines and laterally to the angles of the ribs (Fig. 5–15*B*). It is worthwhile to note that this layer of thoracolumbar fascia separates all of the true deep back muscles from the appendicular muscles and the serratus posterior muscles. This is also relevant to the classification of the levatores costarum muscles, which are so-called respiratory muscles, as deep back muscles. They, along with other deep back muscles, are located deep to the thoracolumbar fascia. In contrast, the other respiratory muscles, the serratus posterior muscles, are superficial to the thoracolumbar fascia.

In the lumbar region, the thoracolumbar fascia is made up of three distinct, well-defined layers (Fig. 5–15*C*). The most superficial (posterior) layer separates the erector spinae muscles from the overlying appendicular latissimus dorsi muscles. This superficial layer of deep fascia is connected medially to spines of the lumbar and sacral vertebrae. A middle layer of deep fascia is attached medially to transverse processes of the lumbar vertebrae, separating the anterior surface of the erector

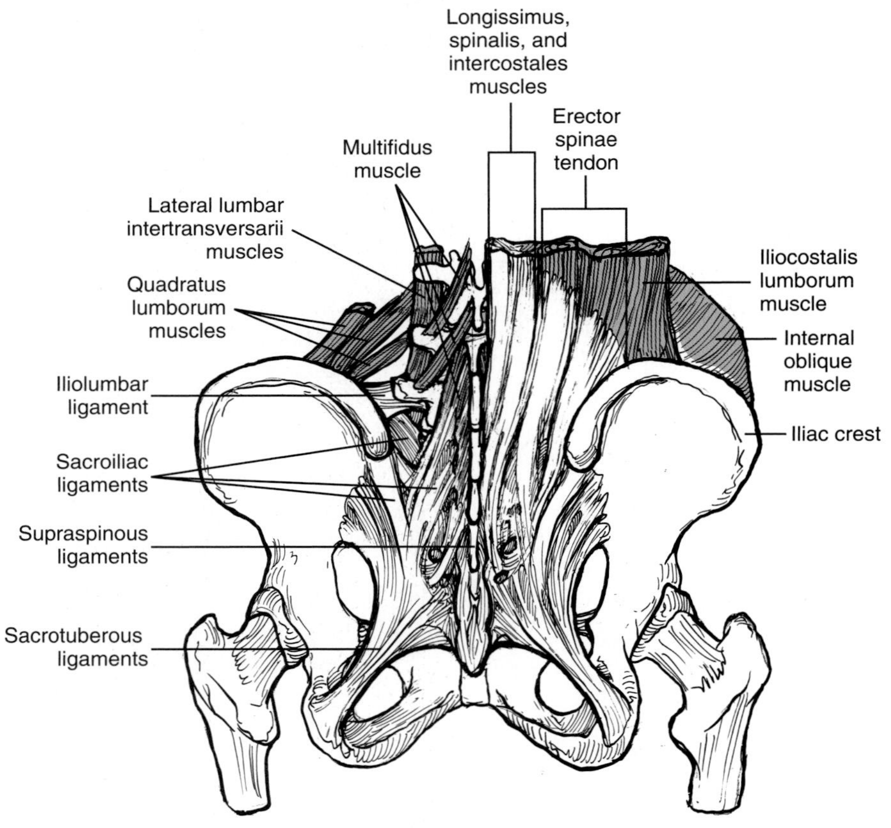

FIGURE 5–16

Connective tissues of lower back. Ligaments of pelvis and sacroiliac joint and iliolumbar ligaments provide inferior attachment sites for erector spinae and multifidus muscles.

spinae muscles from the underlying see **quadratus lumborum muscles** (Fig. 5–15*C* and see Chapter 13). The most anterior (deepest) layer of thoracolumbar fascia in this region is attached to anterior surfaces of the lumbar transverse processes and separates the quadratus lumborum muscles from the deeper **psoas muscles** (Fig. 5–15*C* and see Chapter 13).

The posterior and middle layers of thoracolumbar fascia are fused at the lateral borders of the erector spinae muscles. This combined fascia is fused with the anterior layer of thoracolumbar fascia at the lateral border of the quadratus lumborum muscles. These fused fascial layers form an **aponeurosis** (i.e., a fibrous connective tissue sheet that provides a site for muscle attachment) for the attachment of abdominal muscles, including the **transversus abdominis** and **internal oblique muscles** (Fig. 5–15*C* and see Chapter 11).

The thoracolumbar fascia is attached inferiorly to the iliolumbar ligament (see Chapter 3) and iliac crest (see Fig. 5–15 and Fig. 5–16). The fascia is a major structural component of the posterior body wall in the region of the lumbar triangle (see Chapter 2). When it is weakened at this point, it may allow the herniation (rupture or protrusion) of the underlying musculature or abdominal contents. It has also been suggested that the posterior layer of thoracolumbar fascia may function synergistically with deep back and abdominal muscles to resist flexion of the lumbar vertebral column.

▲ Connective Tissues of the Lower Back

A well-developed complex of tendons and ligaments in the lower lumbar and sacral regions provides a strong anchor for the massive muscles of the lower back

The specialized erector spinae tendon and iliolumbar and sacroiliac ligaments, along with the lower lumbar vertebrae and sacrum, provide attachment sites for the lower back muscles (see Figs. 5–4 and 5–16). Although the erector spinae tendon and iliolumbar and sacroiliac ligaments can be distinctly defined (see Chapter 14), their fibers mesh to form an integrated complex that binds together the origins of the erector spinae muscles and multifidus muscles of the transversospinal group. The fibers of thoracolumbar fascia are blended with this ligamentous and bony network, which consequently further ties together the inferior erector spinae and multifidus muscles with the more superior fasciculi of the erector spinae and transversospinal groups as well as the quadratus lumborum and psoas muscles and abdominal musculature (see discussion of thoracolumbar fascia, above).

6 The Thorax: The Thoracic Body Wall

The thorax is the region of the human trunk bounded by the 12 thoracic vertebrae, ribs, and sternum. This chapter provides an introduction to the thorax and, especially, the thoracic body wall. The structures contained within the thorax will be described briefly here as they relate to the body wall and more thoroughly in subsequent chapters. The basic organization of the thoracic cavities and viscera is described in Chapter 7. The pleural cavities and lungs are described in Chapter 8 and the superior, anterior, and middle mediastinum (including the pericardial cavity and heart) in Chapter 9. The posterior mediastinum and diaphragm are described in Chapter 10.

BOUNDARIES OF THE THORAX

Vertebrae, Ribs, and Sternum

Skeletal elements of the thorax include the 12 thoracic **vertebrae** (see Chapter 3), the 12 pairs of **ribs** and associated **costal cartilages,** and the **sternum.** These elements of the osteocartilaginous framework define the **bony boundaries** of the thoracic body wall (Fig. 6–1*A*). The **superior bony boundary** of the thoracic region is defined anteriorly by the **jugular notch** and **articulations for the clavicle** at the superior edge of the **manubrium;** laterally by the superior surfaces of the **first ribs;** and posteriorly by the superior surface of **vertebra T1.** The superior boundary defined by these bony elements is the **thoracic inlet** (Fig. 6–1*A*).

The **inferior bony boundary** of the thoracic region is defined posteriorly by the inferior surface of **vertebra T12;** posterolaterally by the tips of **ribs 11** and **12;** anterolaterally by the inferior surfaces of the **costal cartilages of ribs 7 to 10;** and in the anterior midline by the **xiphoid process** at the inferior end of the sternum (Fig. 6–1*A*). The inferomedial boundary of costal cartilages 7 to 10 is called the **infrasternal angle.** The complete inferior boundary defined by the xiphoid process, infrasternal angle, ribs 11 and 12, and vertebra T12 is called the **thoracic outlet.**

Diaphragm

The thoracic outlet provides attachment sites for a thin striated muscle sheet, the **diaphragm,** which is the most important **respiratory muscle** (see Fig. 6–1*B* to *D*). The diaphragm also defines the **inferior muscular boundary** of the thoracic region. Because the diaphragm is dome shaped and rises and falls during respiration, its level in relation to the vertebral column changes in various regions and during different phases of the respiratory cycle (see below).

CAVITIES OF THE THORAX AND THEIR CONTENTS

Thoracic cavities are devoted largely to cardiovascular and respiratory functions

The thoracic region contains three main cavities, which are derived from the **intraembryonic coelomic cavity** (see Chapter 7). These are the **definitive pericardial cavity** and **left** and **right pleural cavities** (Fig. 6–2 and see Chapter 7). The superior apices of the left and right pleural cavities extend above the thoracic inlet as well as the superior surfaces of the clavicles (Fig. 6–2*A* and Chapter 7). The definitive pericardial cavity, with its enclosed heart, is in the midline region, or **mediastinum** (from the Latin for "middle septum"). The mediastinum is a partition of tissue that also contains the **thymus gland, great vessels, trachea, lymphatic ducts,** and **esophagus** (Fig. 6–2). It is interposed between the sternum with its associated costal cartilages and the posterior thoracic vertebral column (Fig. 6–2). The left and right lungs, within the left and right pleural cavities, are located laterally on either side of the mediastinum and are enclosed by 12 thoracic ribs on each side of the thorax.

The mediastinum and the thoracic cavities and their contents are discussed in detail in Chapters 7 to 10.

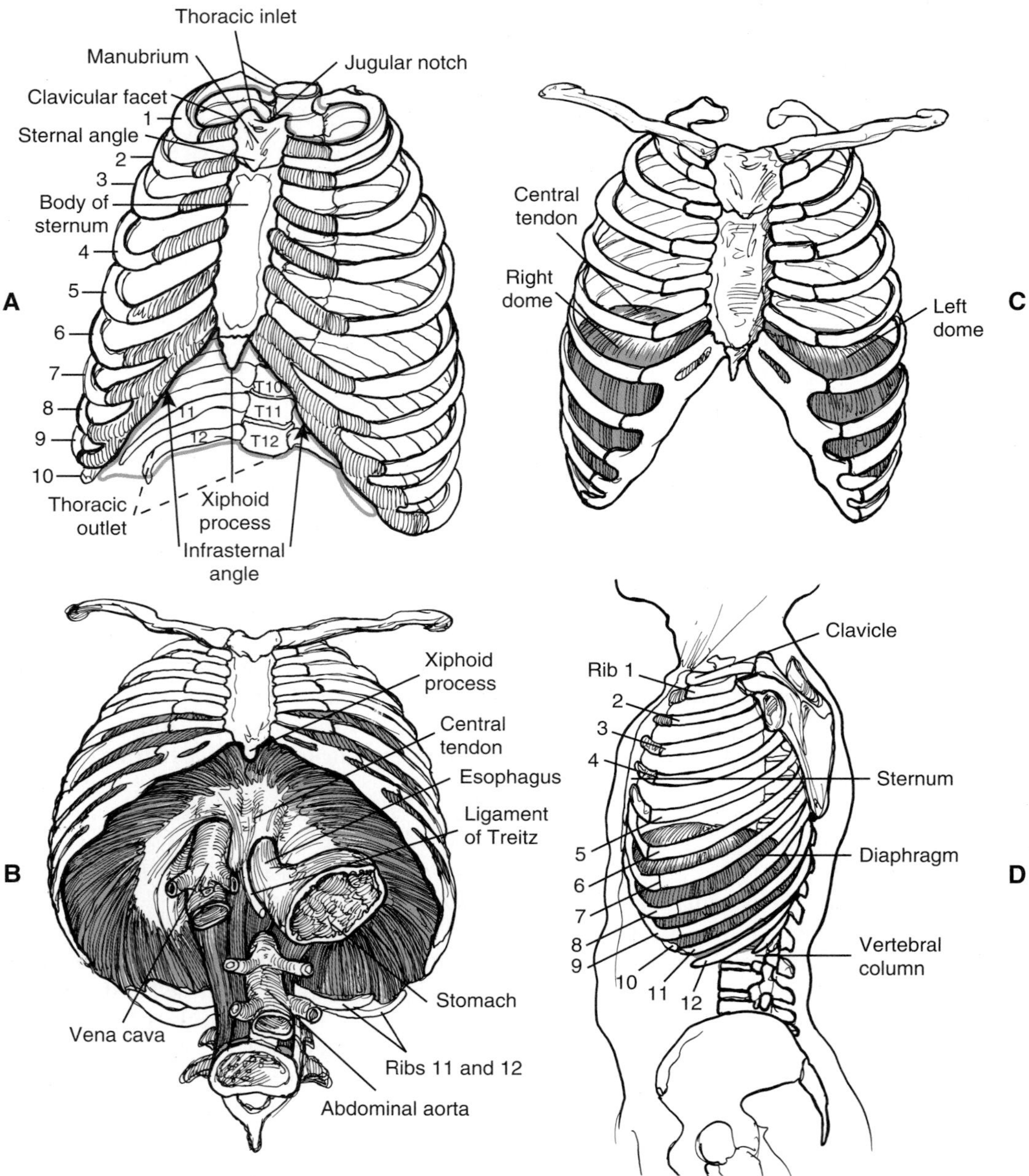

FIGURE 6–1

Bony structures and boundaries of the thoracic region. **A.** Anterior view of the rib cage, including ribs 1 to 12, the costal cartilages, and the sternum. The landmarks of the rib cage can be seen, including the thoracic inlet, thoracic outlet, and infrasternal angle. The landmarks of the sternum are also evident, including the manubrium, with its jugular (sternal) notch and clavicular facets; the connection between the manubrium and the sternal body (sternal angle); and the xiphoid process. **B.** An inferior view shows the diaphragm, which demarcates the inferior limit of the thoracic region. **C.** An anterior view of the rib cage shows the dome-shaped diaphragm. **D.** A lateral view of the rib cage shows the inferior and superior limits of the dome-shaped diaphragm.

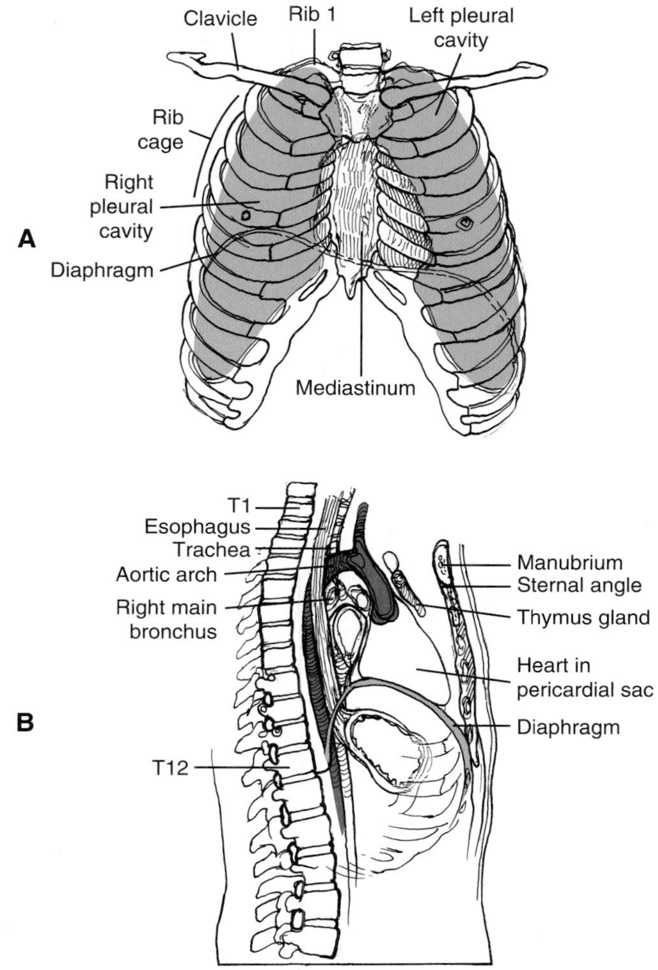

FIGURE 6–2
Organization of the thorax. **A.** The thorax contains two lateral pleural cavities containing the lungs with an interspersed medial region called the *mediastinum* (middle septum). **B.** The mediastinum contains the third major cavity of the thorax (pericardial cavity) in which the heart is situated.

Evolutionary Origins and Functions of Thoracic Structures

The thoracic body wall retains some of the most primitive elements of human vertebrate ancestors, whereas the thoracic viscera are some of the most highly specialized, highly evolved organs of the body

In contrast to the cervical region of the trunk, thoracic body wall segments are comprised of nerves, vessels, and muscles organized in simple, segmentally repeating units with little variation from one to another. This is similar to the structure of the metameric body units of lower organisms. **Metameric units** are repeating homologous segments. The ribs, which are found only in the thoracic region of humans, are descendants of bony body wall elements used for structural support in virtually all regions of the trunk in many lower animals.

In contrast, the visceral contents of the human thorax have become highly specialized over the course of evolution, mainly because of the need to adapt to life on dry land. This led to the development of the **lungs** and a more **complex blood-pumping mechanism (four-chambered heart),** which can serve both the **systemic** and **pulmonary circulations.** Most of the thorax is filled by the right and left **pleural cavities,** which contain the right and left **lungs,** and by a central region called the **mediastinum,** which includes the **pericardial cavity,** containing the **heart.**

The paradoxic juxtaposition of primitive and advanced structures in the thoracic region can perhaps be explained in the following way:

1. The ribbed, segmental, repeating units found throughout the trunk in fishes and used primarily by those swimmers for locomotion could be readily adapted to serve the more specialized function of respiration in land-dwelling mammals. In order to serve the function of respiration, the body wall must be both rigid and expandable. This allows for the development of negative pressure at inspiration. The rib cage has these fundamental attributes (see below and Chapter 7).
2. The vital lungs and heart must be protected from injury in order for humans to survive, and this protection is also afforded by the rib cage. The ribs in ancestors of humans had a protective function as well.
3. Finally, the rib cage in humans provides a relatively stable site for the attachments of appendicular muscles of the prehensile upper extremities, which are uniquely mobile tools (see below and Chapters 19 to 21).

SKELETAL FRAMEWORK OF THE THORACIC WALL

It is already evident that the thoracic skeleton almost completely encompasses and defines the region of the thorax (see Boundaries of the Thorax, above). Although the inferior boundary of the thorax (diaphragm) is not skeletal, its outline is described by the bony landmarks of the skeletal infrasternal angle and thoracic outlet.

The thoracic skeleton serves as a base for muscle attachments. Therefore, it can be used to determine the locations of muscles and structures associated with them. Knowledge of the sites of thoracic muscle attachments provides the basis for understanding muscle functions, particularly the function of respiration (see below).

Finally, the bony landmarks of the thoracic skeleton provide a means of diagnosing visceral disease. The pain of some visceral diseases may be referred to the thoracic wall. Skeletal surface landmarks reveal the location of specific thoracic dermatomes by which the pain is referred. Knowledge of thoracic surface anatomy is, therefore, critical for the health care professional.

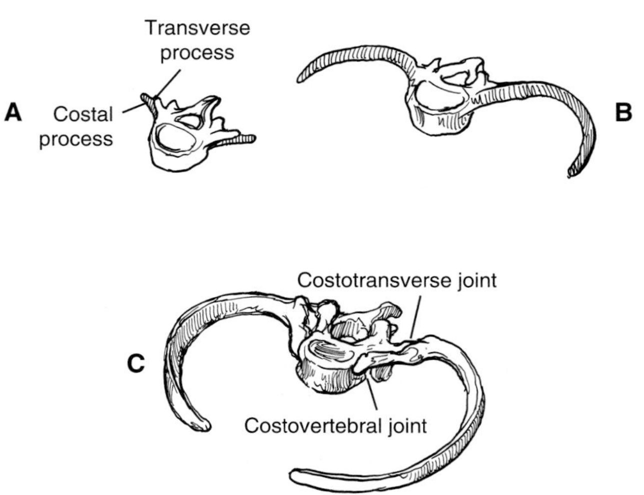

FIGURE 6–3
Development of the ribs. **A** and **B.** The ribs grow laterally and anteriorly during the early part of the sixth week as the costal processes of the thoracic vertebrae lengthen. **C.** By the end of the sixth week, costotransverse and costovertebral joints have differentiated.

Development and Anatomy of the Thoracic Vertebrae

Development of the cervical and thoracic vertebrae results in differences in the numbering of cervical and thoracic spinal nerves in relation to their associated vertebrae

The development and anatomy of the thoracic vertebrae are described in Chapters 2 and 3. The caudal and cranial parts of adjacent sclerotomes form each vertebra. Thus, the vertebrae are intersegmental structures, whereas the intervertebral discs and spinal nerves induced by each somite are segmental structures. This mode of development causes the relationship between spinal nerves and vertebrae in the cervical region to be fundamentally different than in all other regions, including the thoracic region.

Because there are eight cervical somites, eight cervical nerves are induced to sprout from the neural tube (see Fig. 2–4). The first cervical vertebra, however, is formed by the caudal part of the first cervical sclerotome. Thus, the first cervical nerve passes between the skull and vertebra C1, while the eighth cervical nerve passes between vertebra C7 and vertebra T1. Each of the

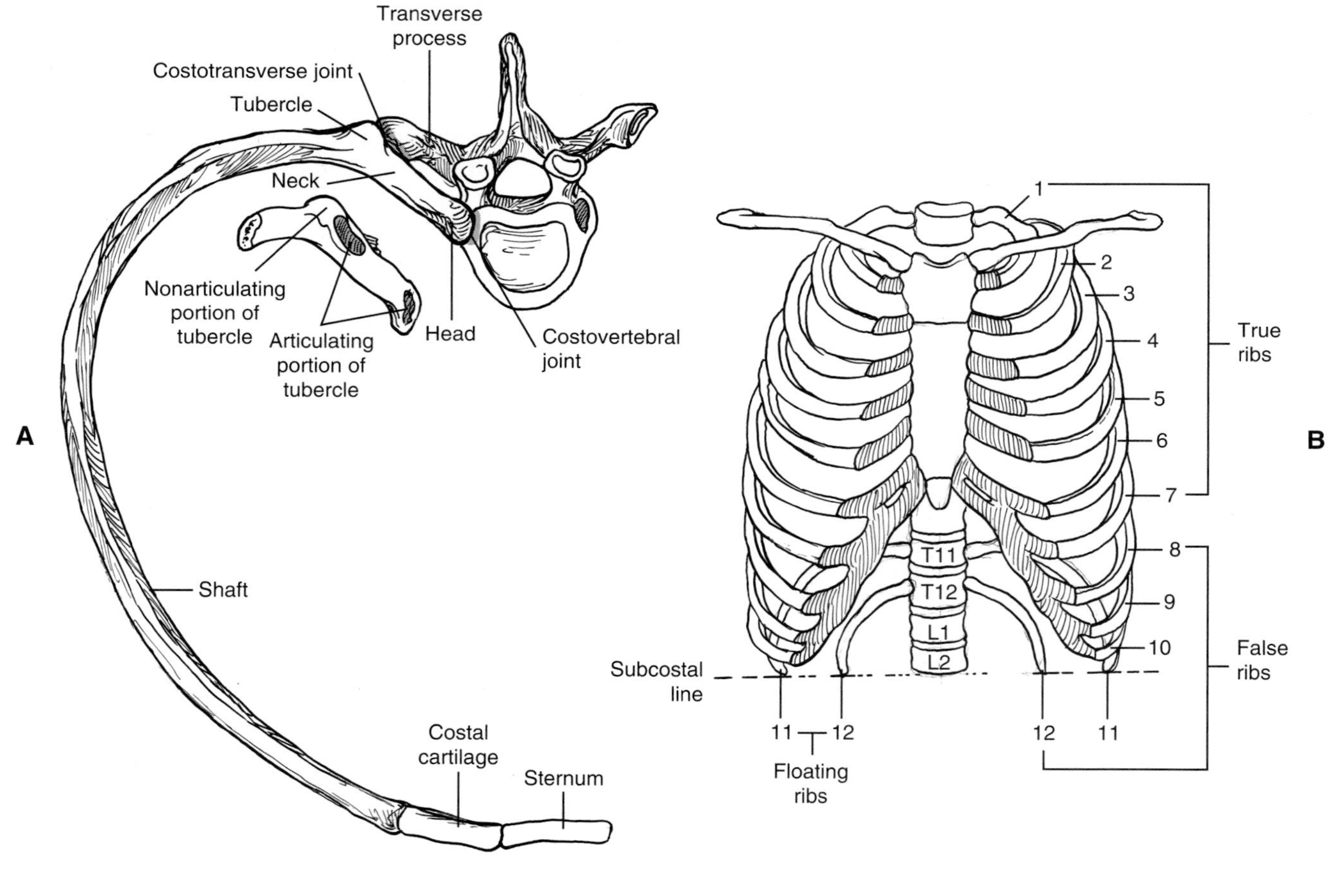

FIGURE 6–4
Structure of a differentiated true rib. **A.** A typical true rib has a head, neck, and shaft and a costal cartilage on its distal end that connects it to the sternum. (The true ribs are ribs 1 to 7 [see also Fig. 6–1]). The proximal end of the rib articulates with the vertebral bodies and transverse processes of the spine. **B.** Ribs 8 to 12 are called *false ribs* because the costal cartilages at their distal ends do not articulate directly with the sternum. Ribs 11 and 12 are also called *floating ribs* because the costal cartilages at their distal ends do not articulate with any cartilaginous or bony structure.

first seven cervical nerves exits the vertebral canal superior to the vertebra of the same number.

The first thoracic vertebra, however, is formed by the caudal part of the eighth cervical sclerotome and the cranial part of the first thoracic sclerotome. Because the first thoracic nerve is induced to form by the first thoracic somite, the first thoracic nerve exits the vertebral canal just caudal to vertebra T1 (see Fig. 2–4). Likewise, the second thoracic nerve exits just under vertebra T2, the third thoracic nerve exits just under vertebra T3, and so on, to the end of the spine.

The thoracic vertebrae are specialized with respect to their long downward-pointing spines, their vertically oriented articular processes, and their associated ribs (see Chapter 3 and Figs. 6–4*A* and 6–5). These features provide an innate rigidity to the thoracic region of the vertebral column and limit the movements of flexion, extension, lateral flexion, and lateral extension. This rigidity of the thoracic vertebral column and rib cage is essential for the function of respiration (see below).

Development and Anatomy of the Ribs and Associated Structures

Ribs, which are specialized outgrowths of thoracic vertebrae, are also components of the axial skeleton

During the embryonic period, the **costal processes** of the thoracic vertebrae appear as outgrowths of the vertebral arches. In the thoracic region, these intersegmental mesenchymal condensations rapidly elongate between the segmental myotomes to form the precartilaginous mesenchymal precursors of the **ribs** (Fig. 6–3*A*). At the same time, the slightly more dorsal transverse processes grow laterally (but to a limited extent) along the dorsal side of each costal process (Fig. 6–3*B*). Eventually, the mesenchyme between the costal and transverse processes differentiates into ligaments and associated structures of the **costotransverse joints** (from vertebrae T1 to T10) (Fig. 6–3*C*). In a similar fashion the mesenchyme between the costal processes and presumptive vertebral bodies forms all 12 pairs of **costovertebral joints** (Fig. 6–3*C*).

The mesenchymal precursors of the ribs chondrify during early fetal life. The distal ends of the ribs remain unossified as **costal cartilages,** but their midregions and proximal ends ossify within the months just prior to birth (Fig. 6–4). Ribs 1 to 10 differentiate into three distinct regions, a head, neck, and shaft (Fig. 6–4*A*), whereas ribs 11 and 12 form only a head and shaft (Fig. 6–4*B*). The **heads,** which are at the proximal ends of the ribs, articulate with vertebral bodies via **costovertebral joints** (see below). The short, flattened **necks** of ribs 1 to 10 extend distally to form dorsal processes called the **tubercles of the ribs** (Fig. 6–4*A* and see Fig. 6–5). Each **tubercle** has an articulating part, which contributes to the **costotransverse joint** (see below), and a nonarticulating part, which provides a surface for the attachment of a ligament that connects the rib to the transverse process (see Fig. 6–5). Ribs 11 and 12 have no tubercles and, thus, articulate only with vertebral bodies via costovertebral joints. All of these joints are synovial joints

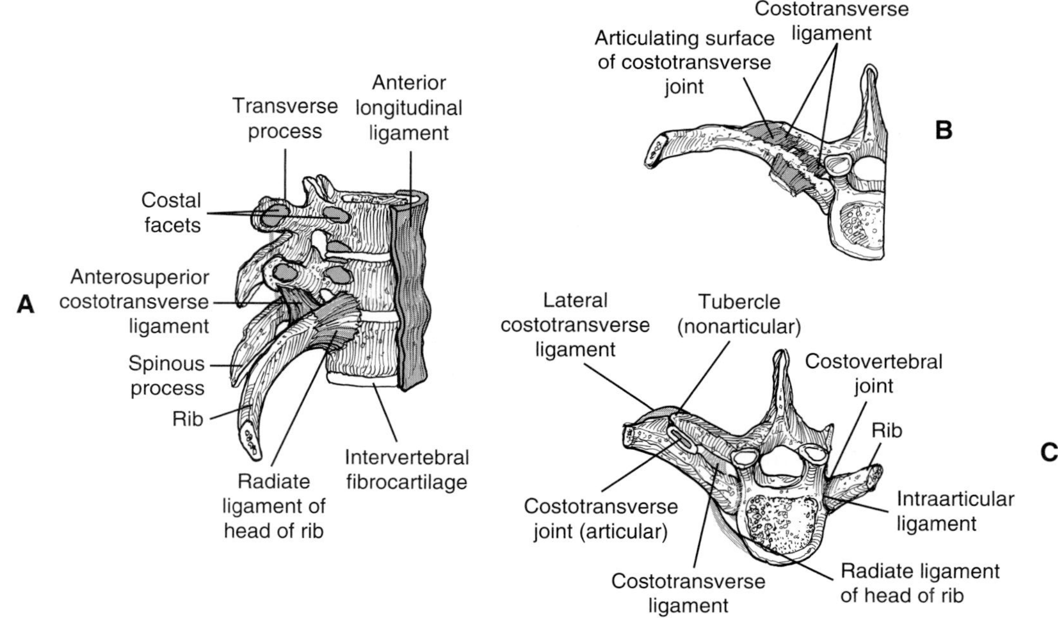

FIGURE 6–5

Structure of the costovertebral and costotransverse joints. **A.** A lateral view shows the costal facets on the transverse processes and vertebral bodies and the ligaments that strengthen the joint capsules. **B.** A superior view of the costovertebral and costotransverse joints shows the superficial ligaments of the joint capsules. **C.** A superior view of the costovertebral joint shows the intraarticular ligament. This view also shows the costotransverse joint, with the articular and nonarticular regions of the tubercle of the rib.

designed to provide a mechanism for the slight gliding movements required in respiration (see below).

The **shafts** of ribs 1 to 10 extend from the tubercle laterally and distally to the anterior end of the rib and its **costal cartilage,** which articulates with the **sternum** (Fig. 6–4*A*). Ribs 1 to 7 are distinguished from ribs 8 to 12 by their attachments to the sternum via the costal cartilages. The costal cartilages of ribs 1 to 7 are connected directly to the sternum, and these ribs are called **true ribs** (Fig. 6–4*B*). In contrast, each costal cartilage of ribs 8 to 10 is connected to the sternum via the cartilage of the rib superior to it, while the small costal cartilages of ribs 11 and 12 are not connected to the sternum or the cartilages of other ribs at all. Ribs 8 to 12 are, therefore, called **false ribs,** and ribs 11 and 12 are further characterized as **floating ribs** (Fig. 6–4*B*).

Costovertebral and Costotransverse Joints. The costovertebral and costotransverse joints are invested by fibrous capsules, which are further strengthened by specialized thickenings (Fig. 6–5). The thickenings of the fibrous capsules of the costovertebral joints include the **intraarticular ligament,** which connects the head of the rib to the connective tissue covering the adjacent intervertebral disc. The more superficial **radiate ligaments** fan out from the head of the rib to completely enclose it and firmly attach it to the bodies of the adjacent vertebrae and the connective tissue covering the adjacent intervertebral disc (Fig. 6–5).

The specialized ligaments of the costotransverse joints include the **lateral costotransverse ligament,** which courses from the tip of the transverse process to the nonarticular portion of the **tubercle** of the corresponding rib. The **superior costotransverse ligament** connects the superior aspect of each vertebral neck with the inferior surface of the adjacent transverse process (Fig. 6–5).

Specialized ligaments connecting the atlas (vertebra C1) and axis (vertebra C2) to the occipital bone of the skull are discussed in Chapter 24.

▲ Development and Anatomy of the Sternum and Associated Structures

Specialized mesenchymal condensations of the anterior thoracic wall form the sternum, which is a ventral component of the axial skeleton

As the ribs grow laterally and anteriorly, a pair of mesenchymal **sternal bars** condenses and forms within the ventral body wall (Fig. 6–6*A*). By the eighth week of development, these bars begin to chondrify into **cartilaginous sternal plates** and then fuse into a single midline structure (Fig. 6–6*B*). As the sternal plates fuse together, the superior seven pairs of ribs, which are growing and have also begun to chondrify, make contact with the lateral edges of the plates. The fused **sternal plates** later ossify to form the **sternum** through the development of several **ossification centers,** giving rise to the distinctive anatomy of the adult sternum (Fig. 6–6*C* and Fig. 6–7*A*). The definitive sternum thus consists of a superior plate of bone called the **manubrium;** four **sternebrae,** which fuse tightly together to form the **body of the sternum (mesosternum);** and an inferior **xiphoid process.** The manubrium and sternal body begin to ossify late in fetal life. The xiphoid process does not begin to ossify until a child is about 3 years of age.

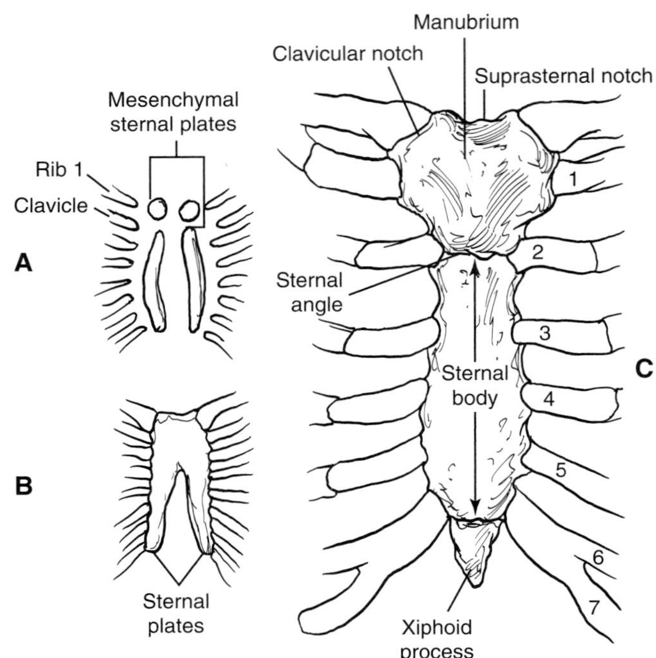

FIGURE 6–6
Development of the sternum. **A.** Two pairs of mesenchymal bars condense in the ventral body wall early in the seventh week. These are precursors of the manubrium and body of the sternum. **B.** By the end of the seventh week, the sternal plates begin to fuse, first at the cranial end and then at the caudal end, just as the distal ends of the ribs join their lateral borders. **C.** The sternal bars ossify from cartilaginous precursors between the fifth month of fetal life and the early months after birth to form the definitive sternum.

The line of fusion between the manubrium and body of the sternum is the **sternal angle,** which is useful as a bony reference point for locating underlying viscera (Figs. 6–6*C* and 6–7*A*). The superior border of the manubrium is indented at a **jugular (suprasternal) notch.** The **clavicular notches** at the superior angles of the manubrium articulate with the clavicles (Fig. 6–6*C*).

Sternocostal and Interchondral Joints

Costal cartilages at the anterior ends of the first seven ribs articulate with the sternum through fibrocartilaginous joints

The **sternocostal joints** are between the costal cartilages of ribs 2 to 7 (at the anterior ends of the ribs) and the sternum. They are generally classified as synovial joints (see Fig. 6–7). In the sternocostal joint of the first rib, the cavity that is present in the other synovial joints is absent, and a thin dense lamina of fibrocartilage is interspersed between the costal cartilage and manubrium.

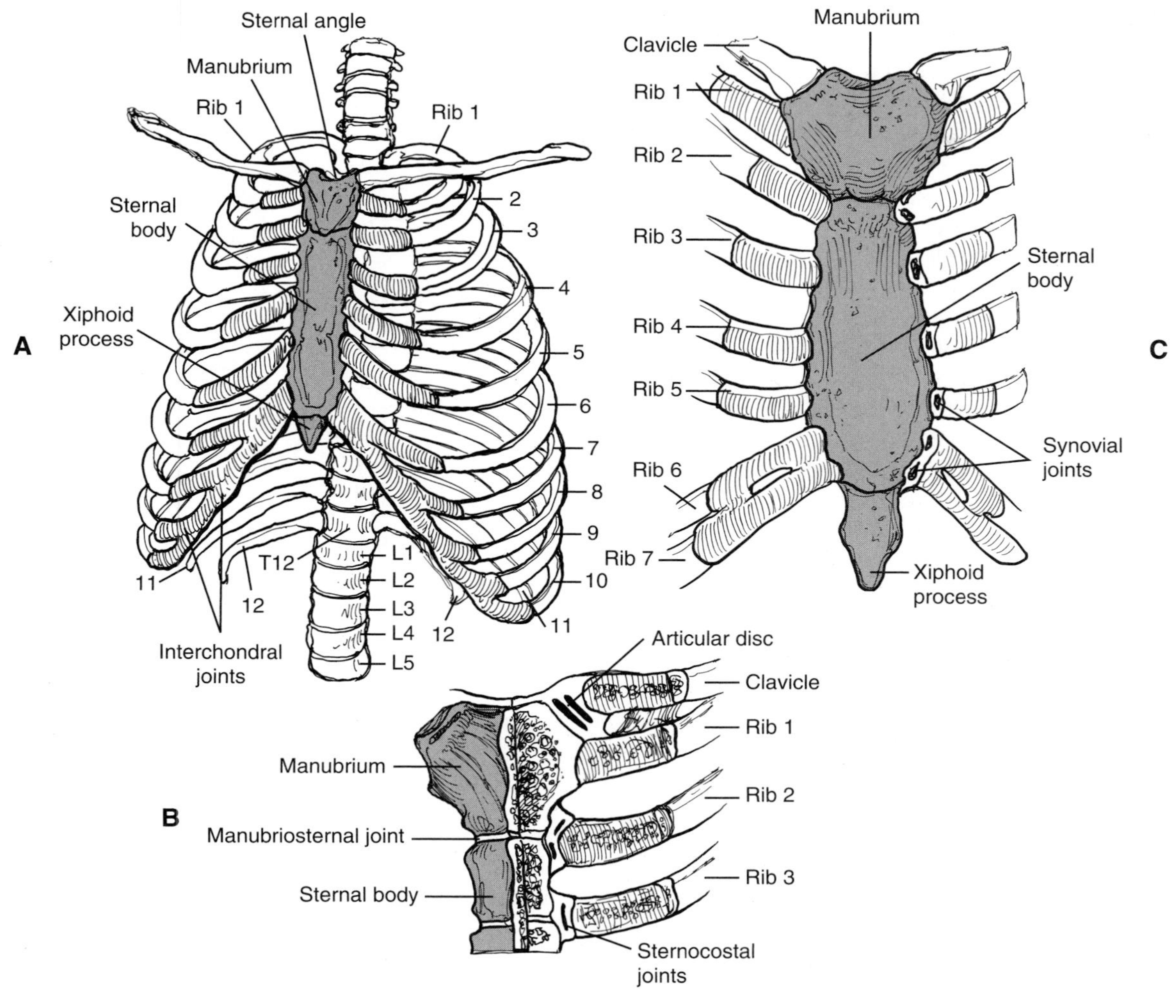

FIGURE 6–7
Joints of the sternum. **A.** Most of the costal cartilages of the sternocostal joints and interchondral joints are simple synovial joints, with the exception of the sternocostal joint of the first rib. **B.** The sternocostal joint of the first rib lacks a synovial cavity and is classified as a type of synarthrosis. **C.** The sternoclavicular joint contains an articular disc. The sternocostal joint of the second rib has two synovial cavities instead of one. The manubriosternal joint may be classified as a simple symphysis.

This joint is an unclassified variety of **synarthrosis** (see Fig. 6–7). The sternocostal joints provide the limited range of movement required for respiration. The costal cartilages of the first ribs are joined to the manubrium, while those of the second ribs are joined to the **sternal angle**, the junction of the manubrium and the sternal body. The costal cartilages of the seventh ribs join the sternum at the junction of the sternal body and xiphoid process, while those of the intervening ribs join directly with the lateral borders of the sternal body.

The costal cartilages of ribs 8 to 10 are connected by synovial **interchondral joints** to costal cartilages of the superior adjacent ribs (see Fig. 6–7*A*).

Sternoclavicular Joint

The appendicular skeleton of each upper extremity has only one small bony connection with the axial skeleton

The clavicular notches at the superior angles of the manubrium (just above the attachments of the first ribs) articulate with the appendicular skeleton of the upper extremities via the clavicles at **sternoclavicular fibrocartilaginous joints** of the synovial type (see Fig. 6–7*B*). In addition to the elements described earlier, these joints contain an intervening articular disc, which is a specialized form of the articular cartilage of the clavicle. This joint and its movements are described in greater detail in Chapter 19.

▲ Clinical Disorders of the Ribs

Cervical Ribs

In normal embryonic development, ribs form in the thoracic region only. In some embryos, however, ribs form in the cervical region, especially in association with vertebra C7. They may be rudimentary or extend from vertebra C7 to the sternum. They may become clinically significant if they interfere with vascular elements (typically the **subclavian arteries)** restricting the blood flow, or with neurologic elements (i.e., nerves within the **brachial plexus** that provide innervation to the upper extremity), disrupting motor and sensory function.

Fracture of the Ribs

Fractures of the ribs range from benign to life threatening. Fractures of one or two ribs result in sharp localized pain and tenderness. They tend not to be life threatening unless one or more of the upper three ribs are involved, in which case there are often associated injuries to underlying vascular and neural elements. Fractures of four or more ribs often result in **flail chest,** which causes hypoventilation. Patients with flail chest may also present with contusion of the underlying respiratory elements and require some form of mechanical ventilation.

Ribs fractured by traumatic forces may cause significant injury to the friable lungs within the pleural cavities or to the liver and spleen within the abdominal cavity. Puncture of the pleural cavities by broken ribs may break the seal between the pleural cavity and the outside of the body, resulting in **pneumothorax** and collapse of a lung (see Chapter 8).

▲ Clinical Disorders of the Sternum

Incomplete Fusion of Sternal Plates

The sternum is the site of a variety of congenital malformations resulting from defective fusion of cartilaginous sternal precursors. These include **pectus excavatum (sunken chest), pectus carinatum (pigeon chest),** and **sternal fissure.** All of these conditions may impair ventilation and cardiac function. Sternal fissure may have severe effects on the patient, particularly if it involves the entire sternum or inferior region of the sternum. Synthetic prostheses may be required for correction of this condition.

Injury of the Sternum

The human sternum is resistant to injury, in part, because of the elastic recoil of the ribs.

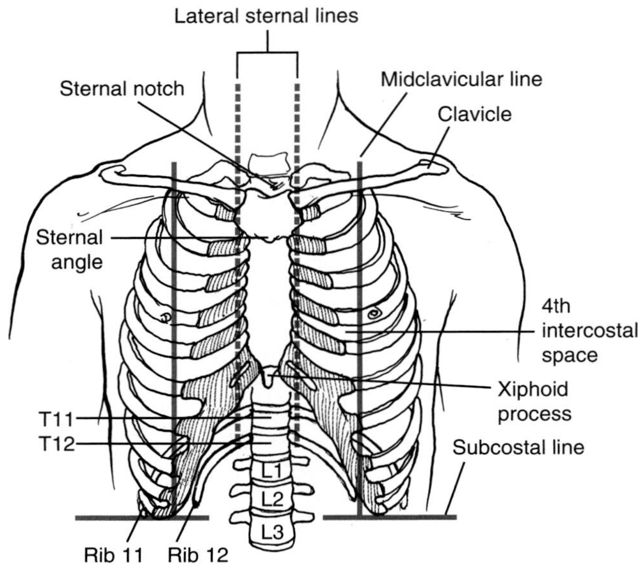

FIGURE 6–8
Landmarks of the chest. These chest landmarks are often used by physicians in the clinic to describe the location of direct somatic pain or referred visceral pain of the anterior thoracic wall.

SOFT TISSUE STRUCTURES OF THE THORACIC WALL

Surface Anatomy of the Thorax

Osteocartilaginous elements of the thoracic body wall can be used as reference points for localizing and examining internal thoracic viscera and diagnosing diseases of thoracic and abdominal organs

Learning the location of bony and cartilaginous landmarks of the anterior thoracic wall is an important objective for the student of anatomy because these landmarks are useful in visualizing the internal viscera and assessing cardiac and pulmonary function in living patients. They also serve as a set of coordinates for localizing referred pain (Fig. 6–8 and see below and Chapters 3, 5, 7, and 10) and for auscultation (see Chapter 9).

The landmarks include specialized areas of the **sternum** such as the **manubrium, body of the sternum, xiphoid process, jugular (suprasternal) notch,** and **sternal angle; ribs 1 to 12; costal cartilages** of ribs 7 to 10; **tips** and **angles** of ribs 11 and 12; **intercostal spaces,** especially the **fourth** and **fifth spaces;** and **thoracic vertebral spines,** especially of vertebrae T1 and T12 (see Fig. 2–2*A* and *B*). The **jugular notch** is at the level of vertebra T2. The **sternal angle,** just inferior to the jugular notch, is at the level of vertebra T4. This landmark is useful for locating the second rib, which is attached to the sternum at this point. The sternal angle is also in the same plane as the proximal end of the aortic arch and the bifurcation of the trachea (see Chapter 7). The **xiphoid process,** at the inferior end of the sternum, is located at the same level as vertebra T10. Imaginary lines, including lateral sternal and midclavicular lines, are also used as thoracic references (Fig. 6–8).

The student should palpate these landmarks on his or her own body. Their significance will be described at appropriate points in the discussions of structure, function, and clinical problems of the thorax throughout this and the following three chapters.

▲ Organization of the Thoracic Wall

The thoracic body wall is a stratified complex of different tissues

The **body wall of the intercostal spaces** can be thought of as a symmetrically organized **"sandwich" of**

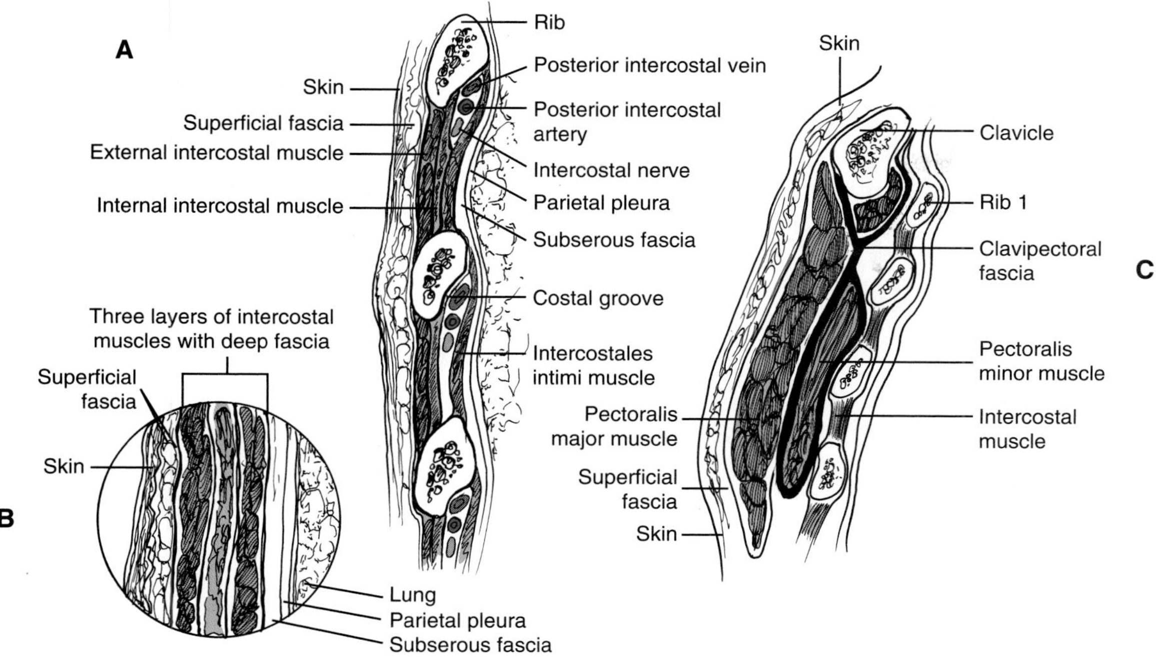

FIGURE 6–9
Elements of the thoracic wall.

tissue layers (Fig. 6–9*A* and *B*) with complementation between the outer **skin** and inner **parietal layer of serous membrane (parietal pleura);** the outer **superficial fascia** and inner **subserous fascia;** and the three layers of **intercostal muscles** with their investing deep fascia, which are positioned within the center of this stratified complex.

In some regions, however, several **appendicular muscles,** including the **pectoralis major** and **minor, subclavius, deltoid,** and **serratus anterior muscles,** have also migrated over the trunk to provide attachments of the upper extremities to the thoracic axial skeleton (Fig. 6–9*C*, Chapters 2 and 5, and below). These muscles lie deep to the integument with its superficial fascia but overlie the deep fascia investing the three layers of intercostal muscles of the thoracic wall proper.

Additional specializations of the integument of the anterior thoracic wall are the **mammary glands,** which are modified apocrine glands with associated fatty and connective tissues. Mammary glands are rudimentary in males. In females, mammary glands are well-developed to produce milk for feeding an infant in the first months of life.

The high incidence of **mammary carcinoma** in females (1 in 8) is a compelling reason for learning the structure of the breast, especially its systems of vascular and lymphatic drainage (see below).

▲ Integument of the Thorax

Thoracic integument and superficial fascia contain glands and nerve endings (within the epidermis) and blood vessels (within the dermis)

The integument of the thorax is organized generally as the integument is elsewhere in the trunk (see Fig. 2–1). A superficial **epidermis,** containing **sebaceous glands, apocrine glands, sweat glands,** and **nerve endings,** overlies the **dermis,** which contains blood vessels. The sebaceous glands secrete oil, which lubricates hair and skin. The apocrine glands, which are restricted largely to the axillary and genital regions of the trunk by the time puberty begins, become especially active at sexual maturation to produce substances that are modified by bacteria into odorous compounds (see Fig. 2–1).

The **superficial fascia (hypodermis)** of the thoracic body wall is made up of loose connective tissue containing varying amounts of fat. It is penetrated by branches of segmental nerves and vessels from deeper regions of the body wall. The sweat glands, sebaceous glands, and hair follicles penetrate the dermis and hypodermis as downgrowths of the epidermis (see Fig. 2–1).

Nerves and Vessels of the Thoracic Integument and Hypodermis

Nerves and vessels of the thoracic integument and hypodermis are organized in a segmental manner

Segmental **intercostal spinal nerves** and **intercostal arteries** and **veins** course together as neurovascu-

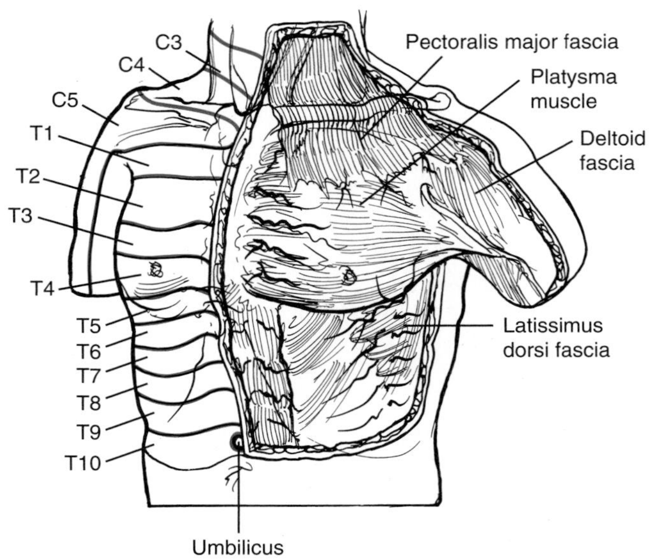

FIGURE 6–10
Segmental nerves of the anterior thoracic wall. The nipple lies within the T4 dermatome.

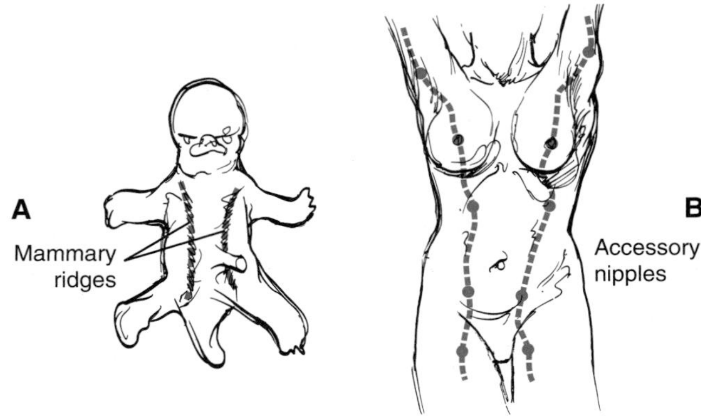

FIGURE 6–11
Development of the mammary glands. **A.** Six-week-old embryo. The mammary ridges appear as thickened lines of epidermis in the fourth week. **B.** Definitive mammary glands form in the upper thoracic region from tissue within the mammary ridge. Accessory nipples or mammary tissue may form at ectopic locations along the former mammary ridge.

lar bundles within the body wall just inferior to each rib within a **costal groove** (see Fig. 6–9*A* and below). At intervals, these vessels and nerves emit **perforating branches,** which vascularize the dermis or innervate sensory structures within the epidermis and dermis (Fig. 6–10 and see below).

▲ Mammary Glands

Embryonic Development of the Mammary Glands

Mammary glands in females are distinctive features of the anterior thoracic wall that function to support the initial postnatal growth and development of an infant

The **mammary glands,** which give mammals their name, are modified apocrine glands of the thorax. The glandular mammary tissue arises within paired epidermal thickenings **(mammary ridges)** during late embryonic and early fetal development (Fig. 6–11*A*). Mammary ridges extend from the area of the future axilla superiorly to the inguinal region inferiorly. Most of this tissue regresses, except in the thoracic region, where the paired mammary glands develop during fetal life (Fig. 6–11*B*). Paired **mammary buds** form, enlarge, and branch. Each bud forms 15–20 **lactiferous ducts,** which empty onto the skin through a **mammary pit.** Proliferation of tissue underlying the mammary pit forms a raised pigmented **papilla** called the **nipple** (Fig. 6–12*A*). Proliferation of tissue surrounding the nipple results in formation of a pigmented region containing sebaceous glands called the **areola** (Fig. 6–12*C*).

Mammary buds continue to differentiate throughout childhood and after puberty to form the **mammary glands,** which become well developed in females but are usually poorly developed in males. They function to produce milk **(lactation)** (see Function of the Female Mammary Glands below).

If, during development, mammary ridge tissue does not regress from areas other than the thorax, **supernumerary nipples (polythelia)** or **supernumerary breasts (polymastia)** may form in the axilla, abdominal region, or even the upper thigh (see Fig. 6–11*B*). Supernumerary nipples are about as common in males as in females (1% of the population). Rare cases of **congenital absence of the breast** have been reported.

The nipples of the mammary glands in males and prepubescent females are usually located at the fourth intercostal space. The nipple of the mature female breast is located at various positions, depending on the size and shape of the breast (Fig. 6–13).

The periphery of the base of each mammary gland in males and females is described by a circle. The medial margin is at the lateral boundary of the sternal body at the level of costal cartilage 4; the lateral margin is at the axilla, where the gland usually has an **axillary tail** (Fig. 6–12*A*); the superior margin is at the point where the base of the breast extends to rib 2; and the inferior margin is at rib 6 (Fig. 6–12*C*).

The deep concave surface of the breast is related to the underlying pectoralis major, serratus anterior, and external oblique muscles but is separated from them by their investments of deep fascia (Fig. 6–12*B* and *C*). In addition, **retromammary (submammary) "space"** (a zone of specialized loose connective tissue) is interposed between the base of the breast and underlying deep fascia (Fig. 6–12*B*).

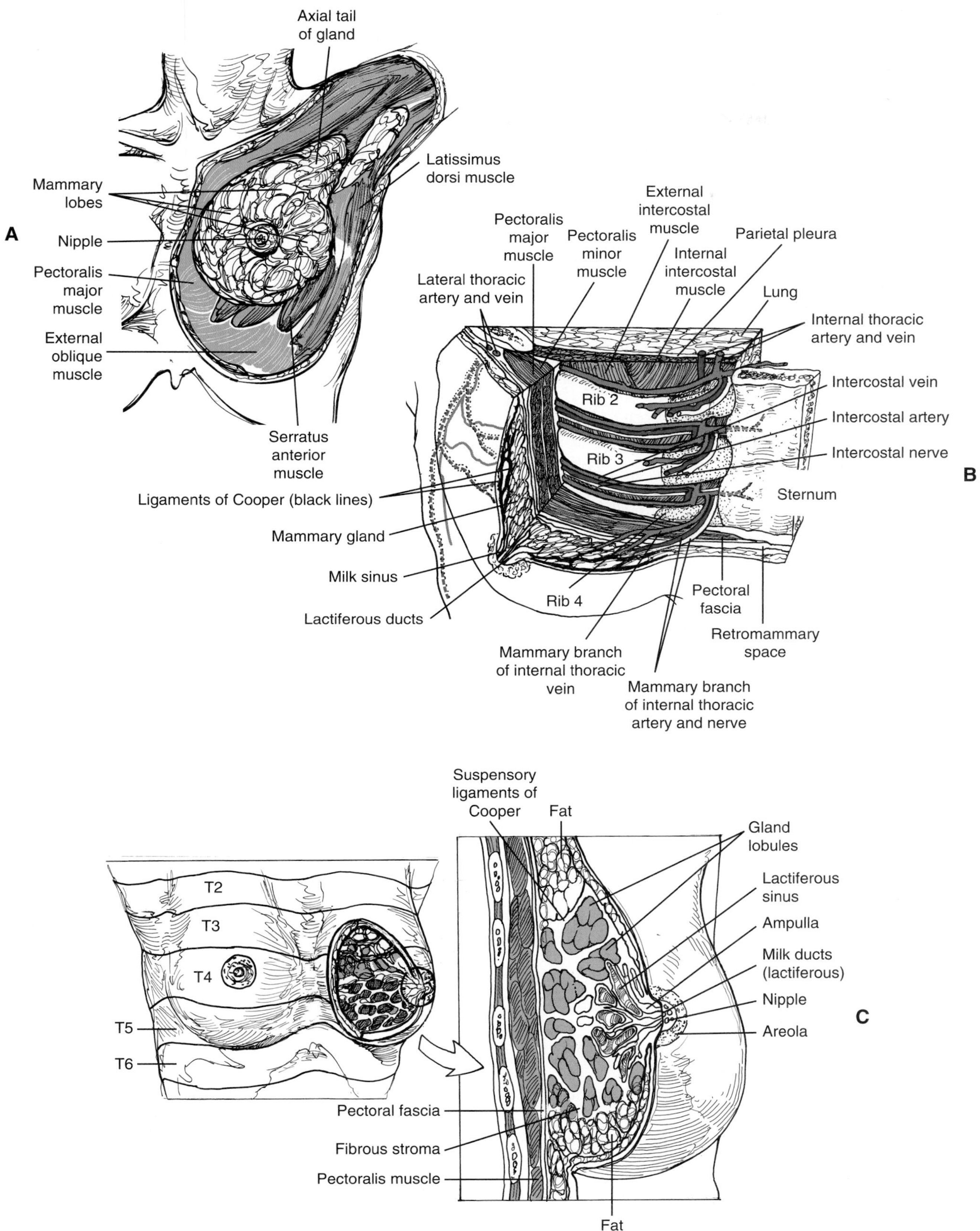

FIGURE 6–12
Structure of the female breast. **A.** Territory of breast tissue, including axillary tail. **B.** Relationship of the breast to body wall structures, including the appendicular muscles, ribs, veins, arteries, and nerves. **C.** Internal structure of the mature breast.

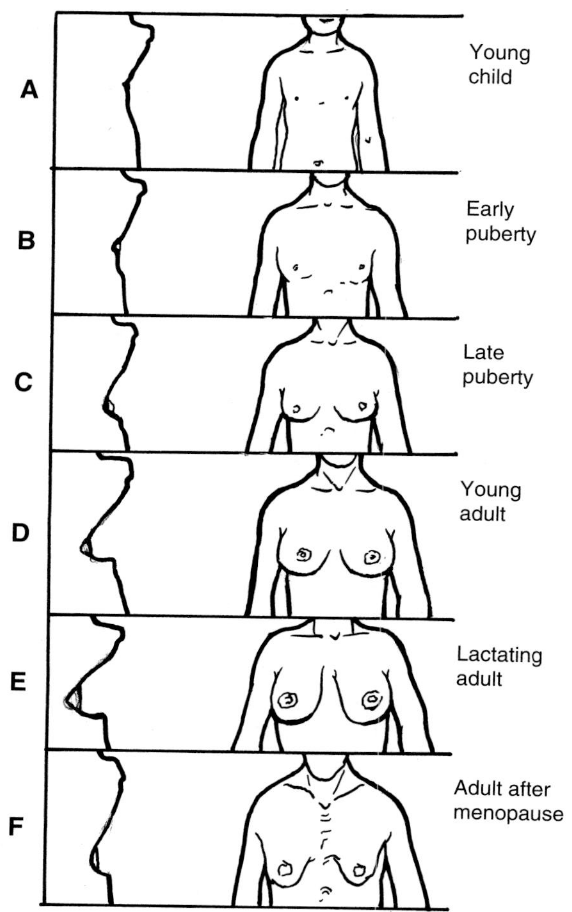

FIGURE 6–13
Changes in the breast throughout life.

Breast implants are frequently inserted just deep to this plane of loose connective tissue. Normally, the flexibility of the retromammary "space" allows some freedom of movement of the breast over the anterior thoracic wall, but fixation of the breast to the underlying musculature may occur in advanced cases of mammary carcinoma.

Physiologic Changes in the Breasts During Puberty, Pregnancy, and Menopause

Female breasts vary in size, shape, and composition at different ages and during pregnancy

The breasts of young prepubescent females and males are flattened discs characterized by a small pigmented nipple surrounded by a pigmented areola (see Fig. 6–13*A*). The poorly differentiated glandular tissue with only a moderate number of branches lies deep to the areola and nipple within the subcutaneous fascia but is not encapsulated by connective tissue.

With the onset of **puberty** in females, the breasts begin to differentiate under the influence of ovarian **estrogens** (see Fig. 6–13*B*). Once development is complete at age 16 or 17 years (see Fig. 6–13*C* and *D*), the breast of a nulliparous (never having borne children) female is comprised largely of fat. Within this fat are embedded **lactiferous glands** and **ducts,** which at this point have a greater number of branches. The blind ends of the glands form solid spherical structures, which will become **alveoli.**

A precocious onset of puberty may cause the breasts to develop prematurely, and a delayed onset may result in delayed development. The development of one breast may proceed more rapidly than the development of the other. Premature enlargement of breasts may occur in infant females in response to maternal hormones. **Gynecomastia** (breast enlargement in pubertal or early adolescent boys) may also occur as a consequence of hormonal changes usually associated with male puberty.

The fat of the breast arises from superficial fascia of the pectoral (related to the chest) region of the thorax and is organized into lobules between connective tissue septa called **suspensory ligaments (of Cooper).** These are specialized extensions of subcutaneous connective tissue and are better developed in superior regions of the gland (see Fig. 6–12*B* and *C*). These fibrous bands course between the deep fascia of the underlying musculature and dermis.

If a suspensory ligament is displaced or stretched by the growth of a **mammary tumor** (e.g., **carcinoma**), it may pull the skin at its point of attachment over to the subcutaneous fascia, causing dimpling of the skin and revealing the presence of the tumor. Mammary carcinomas usually arise from duct cells of the lactiferous epithelium.

Female breasts enlarge significantly during each **pregnancy** (see Fig. 6–13*E*). The pigmentation of nipples and areolas darkens as breasts develop the glandular apparatus required for lactation. After the infant has been weaned, the breasts decrease in size.

Following **menopause,** the lactiferous epithelium degenerates and breasts may decrease in size as fat is resorbed (see Fig. 6–13*F*).

Estrogen therapy, now often initiated following menopause, tends to prevent the typical degeneration of mammary tissue that occurs in the absence of this hormone.

Function of the Female Mammary Glands

The function of female mammary glands is regulated by ovarian and pituitary hormones

During pregnancy, increasing levels of estrogen and progesterone stimulate additional branching of the lactiferous ducts and enlargement of the alveoli. Pigmentation of the nipple and areola also increases. As the end of

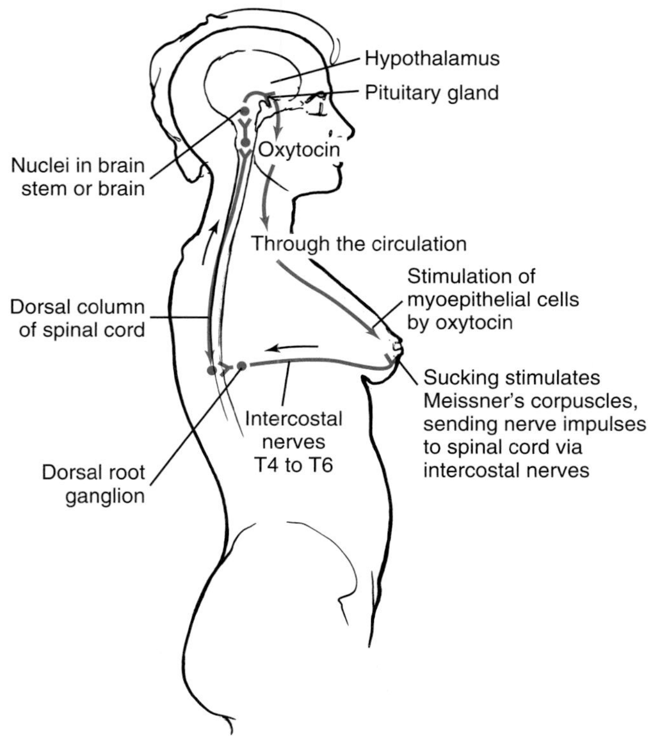

FIGURE 6–14
Neurohormonal reflex of milk expression.

gestation approaches and progesterone and estrogen levels fall, the **pituitary gland** secretes a protein hormone called **prolactin,** which stimulates secretion of a fluid called **colostrum** by the alveoli. As a consequence of alveolar enlargement and formation of colostrum, the breasts enlarge significantly. Shortly after birth, the lactiferous glands begin to produce true milk (lactation), which is elaborated through openings of the lactiferous ducts at the surface of the nipple in response to suckling by the infant (expression). Suckling stimulates sensory end-organs called **Meissner's corpuscles** and **Merkel's discs,** which are sensory fibers that end freely within the nipple and areola. This sensory stimulation causes secretion of the protein hormone **oxytocin** by the pituitary gland. Circulating oxytocin stimulates contractions of **myoepithelial cells** surrounding the lactiferous alveoli that express milk (Fig. 6–14). **Sebaceous glands** of the nipples and areolae lubricate the skin in this region.

Following birth, the mammary glands may remain enlarged and active for 5–6 months. They decrease in size when the infant is weaned, usually at about 9 months of age. The alveoli shrink and lose their lumina, the remaining milk is resorbed, and the breasts diminish in size. While the pigmentation of the nipple and areola becomes somewhat lighter, it never returns to the pale hue characteristic of nulliparous females. With each succeeding pregnancy, this cycle of mammary gland development and regression recurs.

Vascularization and Lymphatic Drainage of the Breasts

Vascularization of breasts is provided by multiple sources

Breasts are well vascularized by arteries and veins from five major sources, which penetrate the breasts around their entire circumference and at their bases. These include three branches of the **subclavian vessels** and the anterior intercostal arteries and veins (Fig. 6–15*A* and *B* and see Figs. 6–9 and 6–12*C*). Specifically, the **anterior perforating branches of the internal thoracic arteries and veins** vascularize the medial aspect of the breasts; **pectoral branches of the thoracoacromial arteries and veins** vascularize the superior aspect of the breast; and **branches of the lateral thoracic arteries and veins** vascularize the lateral aspect of the breast. In addition, vascularization of the breasts is provided by **mammary branches of anterior intercostal arteries and veins** from intercostal spaces 3 to 5, which supply and drain the base of each breast (see Fig. 6–12*B*). Some venous drainage occurs by branches of **superficial epigastric veins** (which drain inferior regions of the breasts; see Chapter 11). Branches of all of these vessels ramify into the breast tissue and anastomose with each other (Fig. 6–15*A* and see Fig. 6–12*B*). A venous anastomotic circle at the base of the nipple is called the **circulus venosus.**

Lymphatic drainage of the breasts is extensive because lymphatic channels usually follow the pattern of the many veins in this region. Lymphatic channels, like venous channels, anastomose just deep to the areola in a **subareolar plexus** (Fig. 6–15*C*). Most of the lymphatic drainage, however, is accommodated by **axillary, pectoral,** and **infraclavicular lymph nodes** associated with **superficial axillary veins,** which **parallel the cephalic vein** (Fig. 6–15*B* and *C*). These lymphatic channels may ramify extensively around the deep fascia of the pectoralis minor muscles and sternocostal heads of the pectoralis major muscles.

Alternatively, lymph may drain from the medial aspect of each breast into **parasternal lymph nodes** associated with perforating branches of the **internal thoracic veins** (Fig. 6–15*B* and *C*), from the inferior tissue of the breasts into **abdominal lymphatic ducts** associated with **superficial epigastric veins** (see Chapter 11); or **from one breast to the other.**

All of these routes are clinically significant because metastatic mammary carcinomas tend to migrate from the breasts through available lymphatic channels (see below).

Innervation of the Breasts

Breasts are well innervated to support their function

Breasts are supplied by cutaneous branches of **intercostal nerves** from spinal cord levels T4 to T6 (see Fig. 6–12*B*). The nerves contain both somatic and visceral sensory fibers, which function in the **expression** of

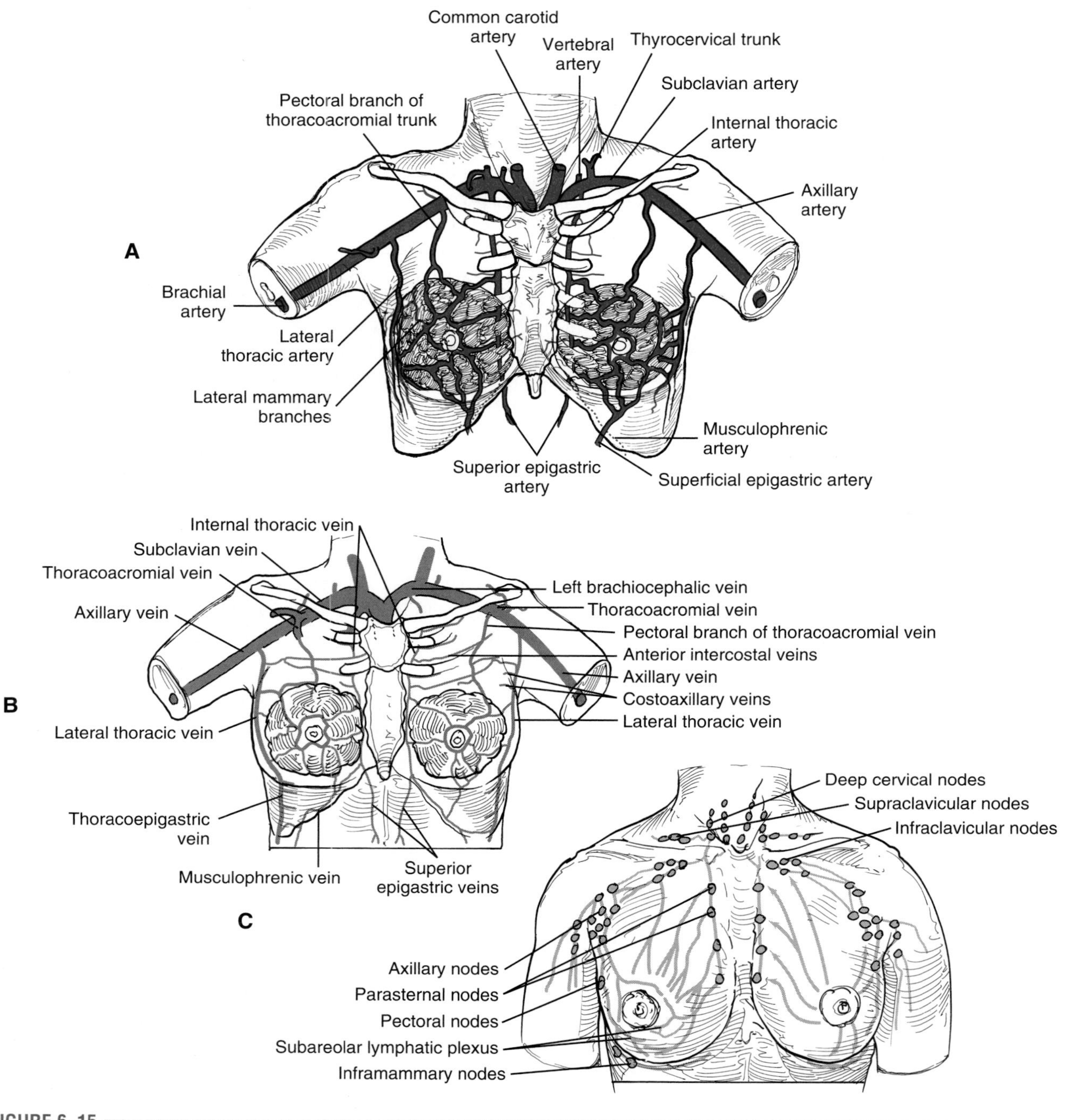

FIGURE 6–15
Breast vasculature. **A.** Arteries of the breast. **B.** Veins of the breast. **C.** Lymphatics of the breast.

milk (see Function of the Female Mammary Glands, above).

▲ Clinical Disorders of the Breasts

Clinical disorders of the breasts affect a large proportion of women

Approximately 25% of women in the United States will require medical treatment for conditions related to the breasts during their lifetimes. Although most of these conditions are resolved with appropriate treatment, some may be life threatening.

Inflammation of the Breast

The breast is subject to inflammatory conditions, which occur most commonly during lactation

Acute mastitis is an inflammatory condition occurring almost exclusively during lactation. It usually results from invasion of breast tissue by organisms that gain access through cracks or fissures in the nipples. Depending on the organism, the inflammation may be localized, forming an abscess, or more generalized, involving the entire breast. In either case, the condition is usually unilateral and is treated with antibiotic therapy.

In some cases of acute mastitis, the lactiferous ducts may become dilated, forming cysts called **galactoceles.** These may occur singly but are more commonly multiple foci. They may become infected, leading to acute mastitis with abscess formation, necrosis, and scarring. Abscesses may be surgically drained.

In unusual cases, severe pain may be experienced during periods of lactation. This results from the swelling of congenital ectopic **accessory lactiferous tissue,** which is usually found within the axilla. The tissue swells in response to hormones targeting the breast (see discussion of mammary gland development, above).

Breast Pain

Approximately 50% of women will seek treatment for breast pain during their lives

There are three common causes of breast pain, or **mastodynia** (from the Greek *mastos,* meaning breast, and *odyne,* meaning pain). The most common is **cyclic mastodynia,** which occurs just prior to the onset of menses and is experienced by most adult women. **Fibrocystic changes** (see below) are also quite common, and **referred pain** to the breast, particularly in postmenopausal women, is also common.

Benign Breast Tumors

Benign tumors of the breast are far more common than malignant tumors

Fibrocystic disease is a condition characterized by benign tumors. The lactiferous ducts become enlarged and fill with fluid. The enlargements are usually bilateral, multiple, ill-defined, and tender. Fibrocystic disease occurs most commonly in women ages 30–55 years, with increased incidence just before menopause. Treatment usually involves aspiration of fluid from the enlarged ducts.

Fibroadenomas are also benign tumors, which may occur at any time during the reproductive life of a woman. Fibroadenomas are the most common tumor in women under age 30 years. These tumors are usually small, round to discoid, freely movable, and well delineated. They are not tender. Although they are benign, they may be difficult to identify conclusively without histologic evaluation and are, therefore, usually removed surgically. Breast tissue is organized in a radial fashion, so incisions for surgery and other procedures are usually made in a radial direction. Neither fibrocystic disease nor fibroadenoma increases the risk of breast cancer.

Breast Carcinoma

Mammary carcinomas are the second leading cause of death from cancer in women

Women in the United States presently have an overall lifetime risk of 1 in 8 for mammary carcinoma. Only 20 years ago, the risk was about 1 in 20. It is not known whether the increase represents an actual change in risk or reflects the use of more sensitive diagnostic and reporting procedures, or is a combination of these two factors. Rates for different ethnic groups may differ significantly, although other factors are also important. The rate is higher in women whose mothers or sisters have had mammary carcinoma, who have never borne a child, whose first pregnancy occurs after age 30 years, whose menarche is early (before age 12 years), whose menopause is late (after age 50 years), or who are over 40 years of age. Other causative factors include exposure to ionizing radiation and dietary factors, especially a high-fat diet. Some evidence links moderate consumption of alcohol and smoking to an increased risk of mammary carcinoma. Although significant postmenopausal estrogen replacement therapy may increase the risk of breast cancer, limited moderate dosages used in controlling osteoporosis and in oral contraceptives do not seem to raise the risk.

Breast cancer may occur in males but is uncommon (about 0.6% incidence). There is an increased incidence in males with Klinefelter's syndrome or other estrogen metabolism imbalances.

Breast cancer may be diagnosed by routine self-examination or imaging techniques. Early detection and treatment of breast cancer significantly improve the likelihood of a successful outcome. **Self-examination** of the breasts is the most commonly used technique. Examination by physicians and other health professionals is common, although it is done less routinely than other screening techniques. Manual examination by the patient or health care professional does not usually detect masses less than 1 cm in diameter for which the prognosis following treatment is optimal. Other more sensitive examination techniques are now routinely available and recommended.

Thermography, sonography, and radiographic mammography are the most commonly used breast imaging techniques. Of these, the most common and standardized is **radiographic mammography (mammogram).** As the name implies, this technique is a modified x-ray examination of the breast, which is capable of detecting masses less than 1 cm in diameter. It is most often used in women over age 40 years. **Thermography** is designed to locate masses by detecting subtle differences in the temperature of tissues. The advantage of this technique is that the patient is not exposed to ionizing radiation. Unfortunately, the technique currently lacks the sensitivity to detect small masses and is not widely used. **Sonography** uses ultrasound to image the breast, but, like thermography, it lacks the sensitivity to be used as a primary screening technique.

Breast cancer therapies include surgery, irradiation, adjuvant chemotherapies, and endocrine manipulations. Surgical treatment of breast cancer was first described in 1894. The procedure, which became known as **radical mastectomy,** involved complete removal of the breast, underlying pectoralis major and minor muscles, and lymph nodes lying along the axillary vein to the region of the costoclavicular ligament (see

Chapter 21). This procedure was later modified to preserve the pectoralis muscles. Recently, more conservative techniques in which much of the breast tissue is preserved have been developed (e.g., **partial mastectomy; lumpectomy).** In this operation, the malignant growth is removed along with normal tissue immediately surrounding it. Recently, laparoscopic surgery involving introduction of a small instrument through the lactiferous ducts has been done. Whatever operation is used, axillary lymph nodes may also be removed via a separate incision and examined for metastases.

If the tumor is smaller than 2 cm in diameter, **surgery** or **radiation therapy** is usually used. Surgical removal of tumors larger than 2 cm may also be followed by radiation therapy to the breast, with particular intensity directed at the site of the tumor. Patients who have undergone surgical treatment for breast cancer are frequently given **adjuvant chemotherapy** to destroy rapidly dividing cancer cells. This is more common in **premenopausal women** with metastatic cells that have localized in some of the axillary lymph nodes, with a tumor larger than 2 cm in diameter, or for a variety of other reasons. **Hormonal therapy** with **antiestrogen compounds** is frequently used in **postmenopausal women** with mammary carcinoma because these tumors appear to be sensitive to estrogen.

Breast cancer commonly metastasizes to the skin, lungs, pleura, bone (see Fig. 3–11), liver, brain, and pericardium. The mean survival time for patients diagnosed with breast cancer that has spread to other organs is 24 months. Although no cures are presently available, chemotherapy and hormonal therapy have been moderately successful in slowing metastasis and prolonging survival rates.

MUSCULAR, VASCULAR, NEURONAL, AND CONNECTIVE TISSUE ELEMENTS OF THE THORACIC WALL

Two distinct types of muscle are located in the region of the ventrolateral thorax: segmental intercostal muscles of the body wall and appendicular muscles of the upper extremities

Three types of muscles and their associated skeletal, vascular, and neuronal elements in the back have been described:

- the deep back muscles (including the levatores costarum muscles), which are derived from epimeres;
- the appendicular muscles, which develop from migrating somitic myoblasts; and
- the intermediate layer of so-called respiratory muscles (serratus posterior muscles), which are derived from hypomeres.

Two types of muscles are associated with the ventrolateral thoracic body wall:

- the segmental muscles of the thoracic body wall proper, or **intercostal muscles,** which are derived from hypomeres; and
- the appendicular muscles related to the upper extremity **(pectoralis major, pectoralis minor, subclavius, deltoid,** and **serratus anterior muscles),** which develop from migrating somitic myoblasts.

The ventrolateral intercostal muscles of the thorax and associated appendicular muscles can be distinguished from each other by their embryonic origins, their anatomic relationships to the axial and appendicular skeletons, and the sources of their vessels and nerves.

Briefly, the **intercostal muscles of the thoracic body wall proper** are derived from hypomeres. They serve to connect adjacent ribs and function in respiration (see below). They are vascularized by intersegmental **intercostal arteries** and **veins** and innervated by thoracic **segmental spinal nerves.**

Appendicular muscles of the ventrolateral body wall arise from somitic myoblasts that migrate into the limb buds. As the muscles form, they migrate from the limb buds onto the trunk. In addition to moving and stabilizing elements of the upper extremity, these muscles assist in attaching its appendicular skeleton to the axial skeleton. They are vascularized by specific named branches of the seventh cervical intersegmental vessels (i.e., branches of the **subclavian** and **axillary arteries** and **veins**) and are innervated by named nerves that branch from the **brachial plexus** (see Chapter 21). In addition, the pectoralis major and pectoralis minor and serratus anterior muscles receive some vascularization from intersegmental (intercostal) arteries and veins (see below).

▲ Embryologic Origin and Segmental Organization of Muscles of the Thoracic Wall

The distinctive segmental organization of bony, muscular, neuronal, and vascular elements is more apparent in the thoracic body wall proper than in other regions of the trunk

As in other regions of the trunk, the thoracic myotomes split into **epimeres** and **hypomeres** (see Chapter 2). Epimeres differentiate into deep back muscles, and hypomeres give rise to anterolateral muscles of the body wall, namely, the **intercostal** and **abdominal muscles.**

Once the hypomeres of each trunk segment have formed, the hypomere on each side splits into four major parts: three anterolateral muscular sheets and one anteromedial muscular component, which is called the *rectus abdominis muscle* in the abdominal region) (see Fig. 2–3 and Chapter 11). (However, the ventral component usually does not develop within the thorax, although a thoracic rectus muscle **[sternalis muscle]** occasionally forms.) The three major ventrolateral muscle elements that usually remain in the thorax develop as a complex of **intercostal muscles** (Figs. 6–16 and 6–17 and see Table 6–1). From the most superficial to the deepest layer, they form the **external intercostal muscles (intercostales externi muscles), internal intercostal muscles (intercostales interni muscles),** and

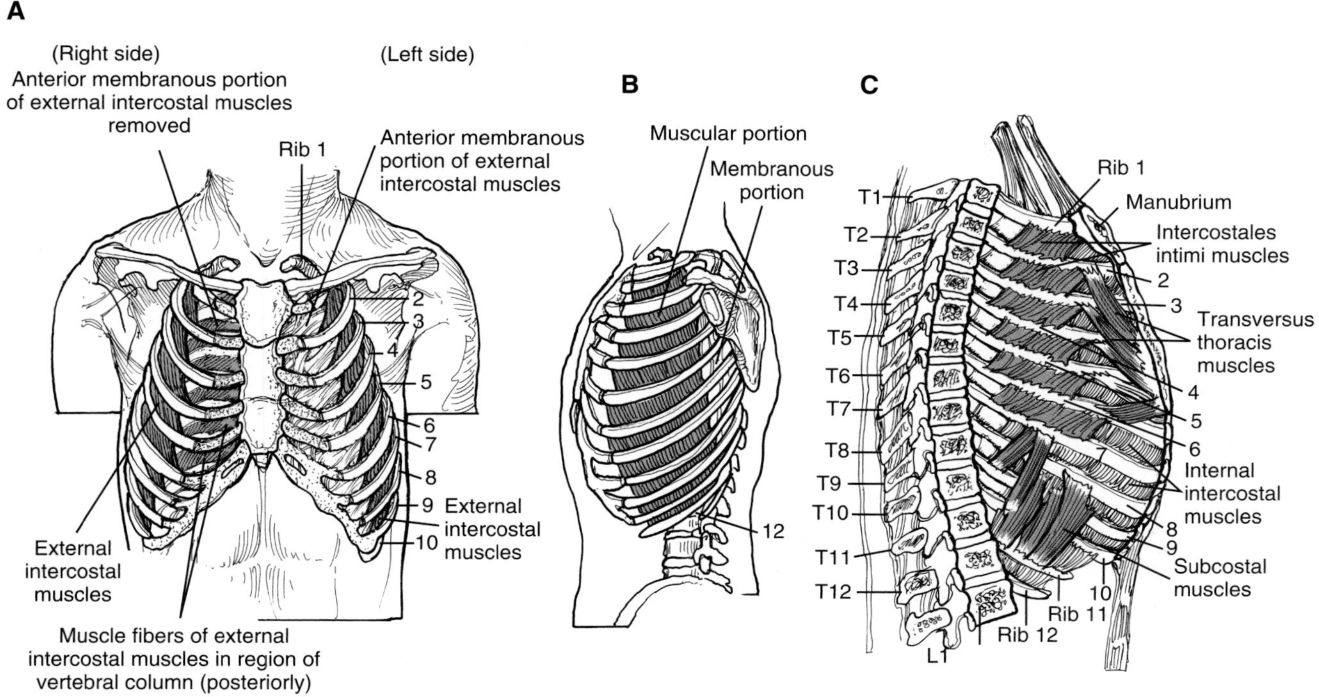

FIGURE 6–16
Intercostal muscles. **A.** The fibers of the external intercostal muscles (the most superficial layer of intercostal muscles) course inferomedially from a superolateral location. Note the anterior membranous portion of the external intercostals. **B.** Lateral view of internal intercostal muscles. (The external intercostal muscles have been removed.) Fibers of middle layer of intercostal muscles (internal intercostals) course inferolaterally from a superomedial location. Note the posterior membranous portion of the internal intercostals. **C.** Sagittal view of the innermost intercostals (the deepest layer of intercostal muscles). These muscles are confined to three regions, forming the intercostales intimi, transversus thoracis, and subcostal groups. Fibers of the intercostales intimi and subcostal groups are oriented in the same direction as fibers of the internal intercostals. Fibers of the transversus thoracis group may course obliquely or transversely.

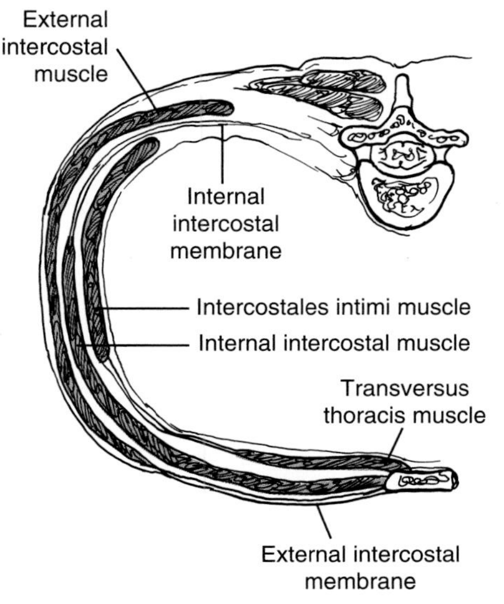

FIGURE 6–17
Section of thoracic wall showing anterior, lateral, and posterior distributions of intercostal muscles.

deepest intercostal muscles (innermost intercostal muscles) (Fig.6–16*A* to *C* and 6–17).

There are 11 pairs of external and internal intercostal muscles. These muscles lie within each intercostal space. Most of them span one segment (e.g., they connect the inferior edge of rib 1 to the superior edge of rib 2, the inferior edge of rib 2 to the superior edge of rib 3, and so on, to rib 11 [Fig. 6–16*A* and *B* and Table 6–1]). There are three subgroups of the innermost layers of intercostal muscles. These are the subcostal, transversus thoracis, and intercostales intimi muscles. The fasciculi of the transversus thoracis and subcostal muscles may span more than one segment (Fig. 6–16*C*). In all three cases, these muscles are located in restricted locations in the thoracic body wall (Fig. 6–16*C* and Table 6–1).

▲ Intercostal Muscles, Vessels, and Nerves

Intercostal Muscles

Fibers within the three layers of intercostal muscles have different orientations

Fibers of the **external intercostal muscles** course in an inferomedial direction (i.e., in the direction of one's fingers when one puts one's hands into the front pockets of one's pants) (see Fig. 6–16*A*). Fibers of the intermediate layer **(internal intercostal muscles)** are oriented at a 90-degree angle to the external intercostal muscle fibers (see Fig. 6–16*A* and *B*). Some fibers of the deepest intercostal muscles **(innermost intercostal muscles)** course horizontally (see Fig. 6–16*C*), and others course in the same direction as the internal intercostal muscle fibers (see Fig. 6–16*C*).

Some regional variations may be found in the structure and distribution of intercostal muscles

None of the three layers of the thoracic intercostal muscles is completely developed throughout the thoracic body wall. The **external intercostal muscles** are deficient near the distal ends of the ribs, represented there only by a thin **external intercostal membrane** attached to the sternum (see Figs. 6–16*A* and 6–17).

The **internal intercostal muscles** are well developed between the sternum in the region of the true ribs and costal cartilages of the false ribs until they reach the angles of the ribs. The internal intercostal muscles are deficient posterior to the angles of the ribs. They are represented in this region only by a thin intercostal membrane (see Figs. 6–16*B* and 6–17).

The **innermost intercostal muscles** can be divided into three distinct groups on the basis of location (see Fig. 6–16*C*): an anteromedial group **(transversus thoracis muscles)**, an anterolateral group **(intercostales intimi muscles)**, and a posterior group **(subcostal muscles)** (see Figs. 6–16*C* and 6–17). (All of these muscles are best developed at the middle and lower thoracic levels and are sometimes absent at higher levels. The transversus thoracis muscles attach the xiphoid process and lower thirds of the costal cartilages of ribs 3 to 6 (Table 6–1). The intercostales intimi muscles, located somewhat more laterally, each span a single intercostal space. Their fibers course in the same direction as the internal intercostal muscle fibers and are commonly confused with this more superficial layer (see Fig. 6–16*B*). The subcostal group of innermost intercostal muscles may span one or two intercostal spaces, connecting more inferior ribs in the regions of their angles (see Fig. 6–16*C*).

Intercostal Arteries

Posterior and anterior intercostal arteries provide extensive collateral circulation within the thoracic body wall

The thoracic segment of the **descending aorta** lies somewhat anterior to but slightly displaced to the left of the thoracic vertebral bodies behind a sheet of membrane called the **parietal pleura,** which lines the left **pleural cavity** (Fig. 6–18 and see Table 6–1 and Chapter 7). This major artery, which emanates from the left ventricle of the heart, distributes its well-oxygenated blood to the body wall of the trunk, the abdominopelvic organs, and the lower extremities.

TABLE 6–1
Attachments, Vascularization, and Innervation of Intrinsic Muscles of the Anterolateral Thoracic Wall: Intercostal Muscles

Muscle	Attachments	Arterial Supply and Venous Drainage	Innervation
External intercostal muscles	Lower surfaces of ribs 1 to 11 to upper surfaces of inferior adjacent ribs (ribs 2 to 12)	Posterior and anterior intercostal arteries and veins of same body segment (T1 to T11)	Intercostal nerve of same body segment (T1 to T11)
Internal intercostal muscles	Lower surfaces of ribs 1 to 11 to upper surfaces of inferior adjacent ribs (ribs 2 to 12)	Posterior and anterior intercostal arteries and veins of same body segment (T1 to T11)	Intercostal nerve of same body segment (T1 to T11)
Innermost intercostal muscles			
Transversus thoracis muscles	Xiphoid process; regions of lower sternum to deep, distal surfaces of ribs and costal cartilages 3 to 6	Mainly anterior and lateral intercostal arteries and veins of segments T3 to T6	Intercostal nerves T3 to T6
Intercostales intimi muscles	Lower surfaces of lower ribs to upper surfaces of inferior adjacent ribs	Posterior and anterior intercostal arteries and veins of inferior intercostal spaces	Lower intercostal nerves
Subcostal muscles	Lower surfaces of lower ribs to upper surfaces of inferior adjacent ribs	Posterior and anterior intercostal arteries and veins of inferior intercostal spaces	Lower intercostal nerves

Within the thoracic region, the descending aorta gives off nine pairs of **posterior intercostal arteries,** which vascularize the lowest nine intercostal spaces (i.e., intercostal spaces 3 to 11) of the thoracic body wall (Fig. 6–18 and see Table 6–1). The first two pairs are branches of the right and left **superior intercostal arteries,** which branch from the right and left **costocervical trunks** (Fig. 6–18 and see Chapter 17). The costocervical trunks are branches of the right and left subclavian arteries. A homologous **subcostal artery** lies just inferior to rib 12 (Fig. 6–18).

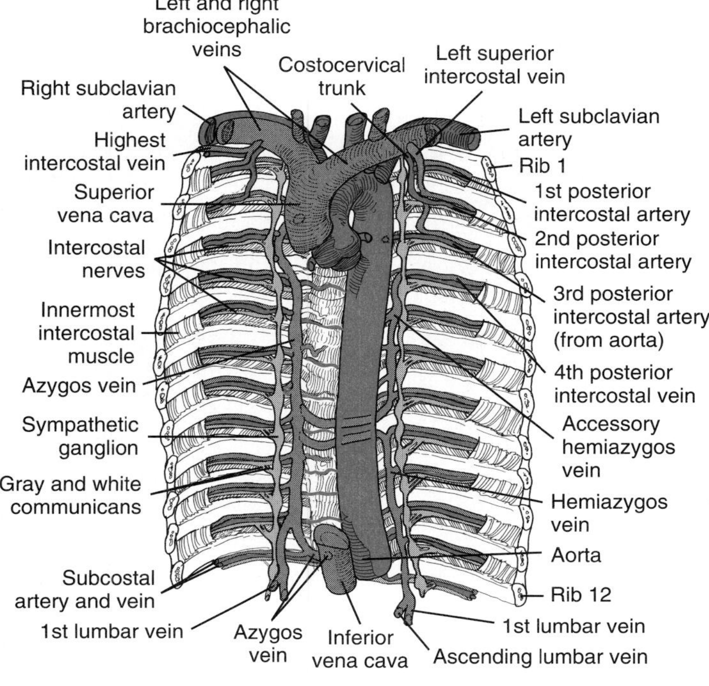

FIGURE 6–18
Anterior view of posterior thoracic wall showing the relationships of arteries, veins, and nerves.

The roots of all 12 pairs of these arteries first give off a **posterior** or **dorsal branch.** These branches supply the vertebrae, spinal cord, and deep muscles of the back (Figs. 6–18 and 6–19*A* and see Chapters 2 to 5). The main trunk of each posterior intercostal artery then gives off a small **collateral branch,** which courses along the superior border of each rib to supply the inferior region of each intercostal space. As the main trunk of each posterior intercostal artery and the subcostal artery continues on its lateral course, it enters the **costal groove,** which is located within the inferior edge of each rib. As each artery enters this protective depression, it is joined by its associated posterior intercostal vein and intercostal nerve (see below).

Each complex containing a posterior intercostal artery and vein and an intercostal nerve is covered by a sheath of connective tissue, forming a **neurovascular bundle.** The neurovascular bundles continue to course laterally and anteriorly between the innermost intercostal muscles and internal intercostal muscles within the costal grooves (Fig. 6–18 and see Fig. 6–9*A*).

Deep and superficial branches of the posterior intercostal and subcostal arteries and veins are given off at intervals to supply and drain the deeper and more superficial structures of the thoracic body wall (Fig. 6–19*A* and *B*). Likewise, the accompanying intercostal nerves

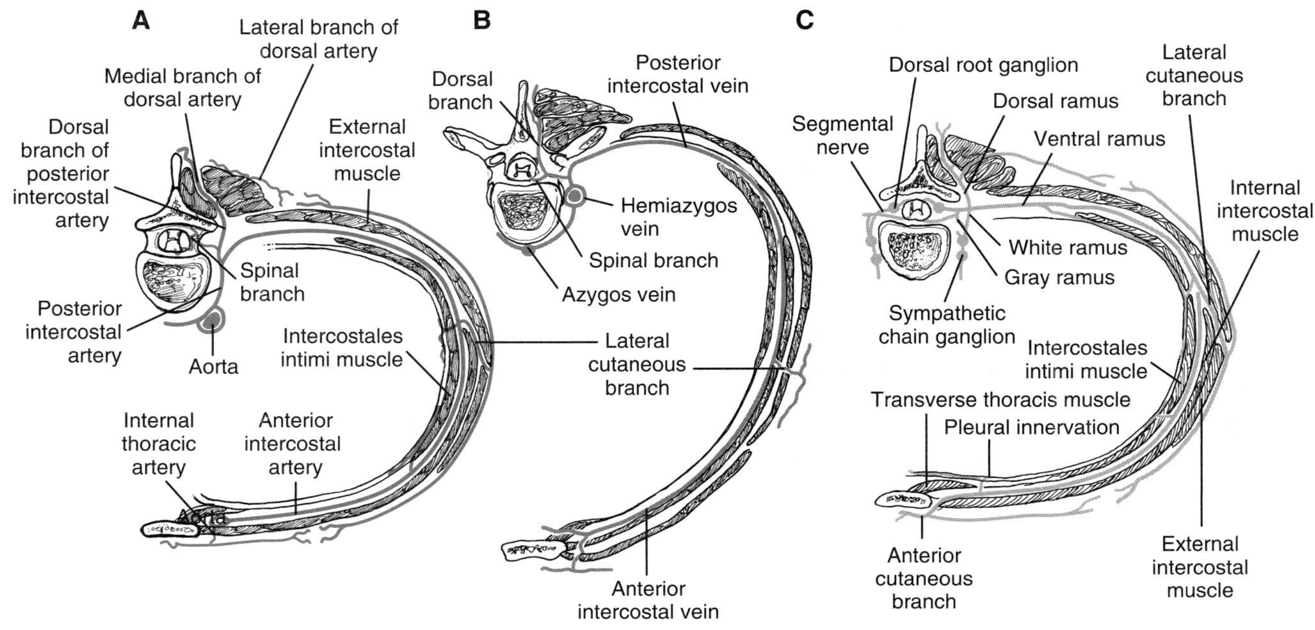

FIGURE 6–19
Transverse sections of thoracic wall showing relationship of muscle layers to the courses of arteries **(A)**, veins **(B)**, and nerves **(C)**.

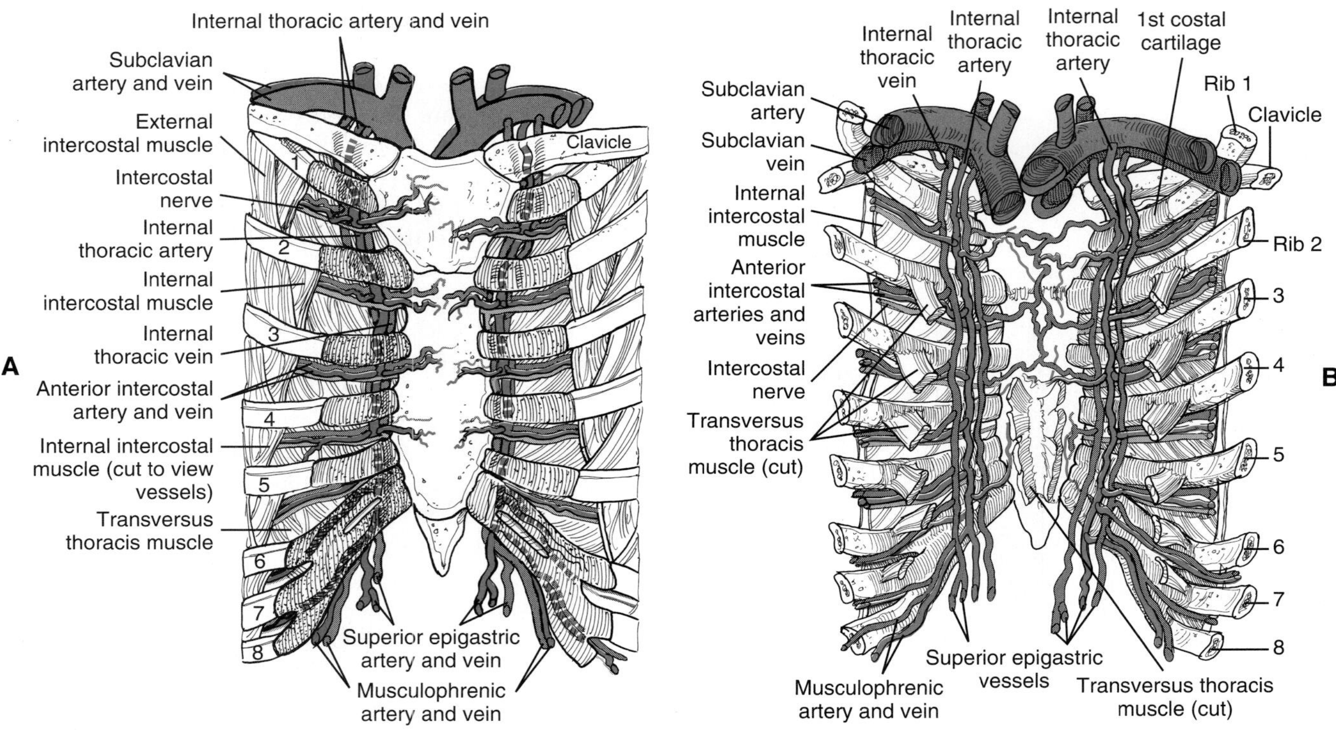

FIGURE 6–20
Anterior view **(A)** and posterior view **(B)** of anterior thoracic wall showing the relationships of arteries, veins, and nerves.

give off deep motor and sensory branches, which innervate the innermost intercostal muscles and parietal pleura, and superficial branches, which innervate the internal and external intercostal muscles and skin (Fig. 6–19*C*). The superficial branches include large major **muscular** and **lateral cutaneous branches,** which arise along the lateral thoracic wall, and **mammary branches,** which arise from the third to fifth intercostal arteries to supply the base of each mammary gland and the pectoralis major and minor muscles (Fig. 6–19 and see Fig. 6–12*B*).

Near the distal ends of the ribs, posterior intercostal arteries anastomose directly with **anterior intercostal arteries.** The anterior intercostal arteries are branches of the paired, longitudinally oriented internal thoracic arteries, which branch from subclavian arteries (Figs. 6–19 and 6–20 and see below).

The **internal thoracic arteries** course inferiorly from the subclavian arteries along the lateral edge of the sternum (Fig. 6–20). In superior regions of the thoracic wall, they course between the **parietal pleura** and internal intercostal muscles because the innermost intercostal muscle layer is usually absent in this region. Inferior to the sternocostal joint at the level of rib 3, they course between the transversus thoracis and internal intercostal muscle layers. At each intercostal space, they give off **anterior intercostal arteries** (Fig. 6–20). These anterior intercostal arteries give off **medial cutaneous** and **lateral cutaneous branches** and then course laterally, anastomosing with cutaneous branches of the posterior intercostal arteries in the region of the lateral margins of the costal cartilages (Fig. 6–19). It should be apparent that this arrangement provides a significant amount of collateral circulation for the thoracic body wall. The internal thoracic arteries also branch to form **musculophrenic arteries,** which supply the diaphragm (Fig. 6–20*A* and see Chapter 8). The internal thoracic arteries terminate as **superior epigastric arteries,** which supply the rectus abdominis muscles (Fig. 6–20 and see Chapter 9).

Intercostal Veins

Posterior intercostal veins are branches of azygos and hemiazygos veins, while anterior intercostal veins are branches of internal thoracic veins

The major venous drainage of the thoracic body wall occurs via two large longitudinal veins lying on either side of the anterior midline of the vertebral bodies: the **hemiazygos vein** on the left and the **azygos vein** on the right (see Figs. 6–18 and 6–19*B* and Chapter 10).

The blood within the hemiazygos vein drains across the midline (through **median anastomoses**) into the azygos vein, and then all of the deoxygenated blood of the thoracic body wall drains into the **superior vena cava** and **right atrium** of the heart (see Fig. 6–18). However, a **superior hemiazygos vein** may drain the upper two or three left intercostal spaces directly into the left brachiocephalic vein.

The azygos and hemiazygos veins receive branches (tributaries) called **posterior intercostal veins,** which course with posterior intercostal arteries and intercostal nerves within the costal grooves (see Fig. 6–19*B*). These veins usually anastomose with **anterior intercostal veins** in the region of the lateral boundaries of the costal cartilages as do the corresponding arteries (see Fig. 6–20). Branches of the posterior and anterior intercostal veins tend to parallel branches of the intercostal arteries, although it is not uncommon to find that **medial cutaneous veins** and laterally coursing anterior intercostal veins drain blood into two separate and distinct **internal thoracic veins.** The internal thoracic veins drain into **subclavian veins** (see Fig. 6–20).

Intercostal and Subcostal Nerves

Intercostal and subcostal nerves course with arteries and veins within the costal grooves

The **intercostal** and **subcostal nerves** that innervate muscles derived from hypomeres T1 to T12 course from the intervertebral foramina between the thoracic vertebrae and the first lumbar vertebra. They then course laterally between the innermost and internal intercostal muscle layers within the **costal groove** on the inferior edge of each rib (see Fig. 6–9*B*). They are accompanied by associated **posterior arteries** and **veins** (see Fig. 6–19*A* and *B*). Each pair of intercostal nerves gives rise to branches that innervate all three muscle layers of a given segment, the integument, and the lining of the pleural cavities, as well as terminal medial branches that innervate the skin within the ventral thoracic midline (see Fig. 6–19*C* and Chapter 7). The cutaneous branches of each dermatome tend to overlap because each segmental nerve provides some innervation to the dermatomes superior and inferior to it, as well as to its own specific segment.

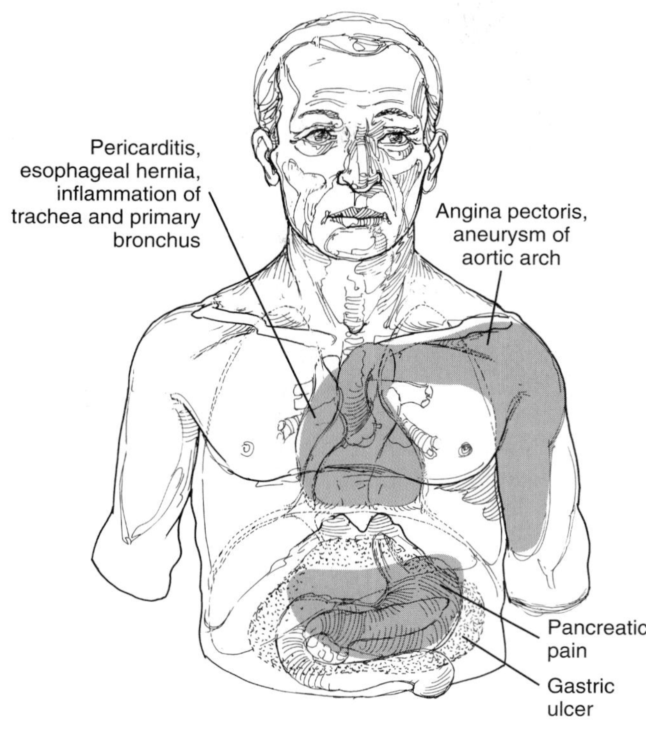

FIGURE 6–21
Visceral pain referred to the anterior thoracic wall.

Pain Referred to the Thoracic Wall

Pain referred to the thoracic body wall may be generated by diseases of thoracic and abdominal viscera

Because thoracic organs obtain their sympathetic innervation from fibers that originate at superior thoracic levels of the spinal cord, pain from thoracic viscera is referred to dermatomes of the thoracic walls. Because more than one dermatome is served by a single spinal nerve, the pain referred from visceral organs is experienced as relatively diffuse (Fig. 6–21).

Chest pain is usually pain referred from the heart, but it may also be referred from other organs within the thoracic cavity (Fig. 6–21). Pain referred from the heart is usually intense pain over the area of the sternum, spreading into the neck and sometimes into the jaw and one or both upper limbs (see Chapter 9). Aneurysm (swelling) of the aortic arch or thoracic aorta may generate a pattern of pain similar to that of cardiac pain or may refer pain to the posterior thoracic wall.

Inflammation of the trachea (tracheitis), primary bronchi (bronchitis), pericardium (pericarditis), or mediastinum (mediastinitis) frequently results in referral of pain to the central sternal region of the thorax.

Because there are no sensory nerve endings within the lung tissue or visceral pleura, inflammation or disease of these tissues does not cause pain to be referred to the thoracic wall (see Chapter 8). However, direct somatic pain of the thoracic wall may occur when inflammation of the lungs spreads to the parietal pleura, which has extensive sensory innervation. Esophageal diseases, irritations of the esophagus from gastric reflux, or hiatal hernia of the esophagus (see Chapter 10) may refer pain to the medial thorax. Pain may also be referred to the thoracic body wall from abdominal viscera innervated by the greater splanchnic nerve (Fig. 6–21 and see Chapter 11).

▲ Appendicular Muscles, Vessels, and Nerves

Appendicular Muscles

Appendicular muscles developing within limb buds of the upper extremity migrate over the anterior thoracic wall and become attached to elements of the axial skeleton

A detailed discussion of upper limb musculature may be found in Chapter 20. A brief description of the upper limb muscles associated with the ventral aspect of the thoracic region of the trunk will be given here, however, because these muscles will first be encountered in the study of the thoracic region. Precursors of all of the upper extremity muscles associated with the thoracic region migrate from the upper extremity limb buds onto the developing anterior, lateral, or posterior rib cage by the eighth week of embryonic life (see Fig. 6–9C and Chapters 2 and 5). The appendicular muscles of the anterolateral thoracic region are the **pectoralis major, pectoralis minor, subclavius, deltoid,** and **serratus anterior muscles.**

Each of the paired pectoralis major muscles usually has two heads: a **sternocostal** and a **clavicular head** (Fig. 6–22*A* and *B*). The proximal end of the sternocostal head is attached to half of the anterior surface of the sternum, to costal cartilages 1 to 6, to the anterior part of rib 6, and to the **aponeurosis of the external oblique muscle** just inferior to the xiphoid process (Table 6–2 and Fig. 6–22*A*). The proximal end of the **clavicular head** is attached to the medial (sternal) half of the clavicle (Fig. 6–22*B* and Table 6–2). The sternocostal and clavicular heads of the pectoralis major muscles are usually separated by a shallow cleft, but their more distal tendons join together to insert upon the **lateral lip of the intertubercular sulcus of the humerus bone** (Fig. 6–22*B* and Table 6–2). The base of the breast lies immediately over much of the pectoralis major muscle (see above).

Pectoralis minor muscles arise from the upper margins and anterior surfaces of ribs 3 to 5, and their distal tendons insert on the **coracoid processes** of the scapular bones (Fig. 6–22*C* and *D* and Table 6–2).

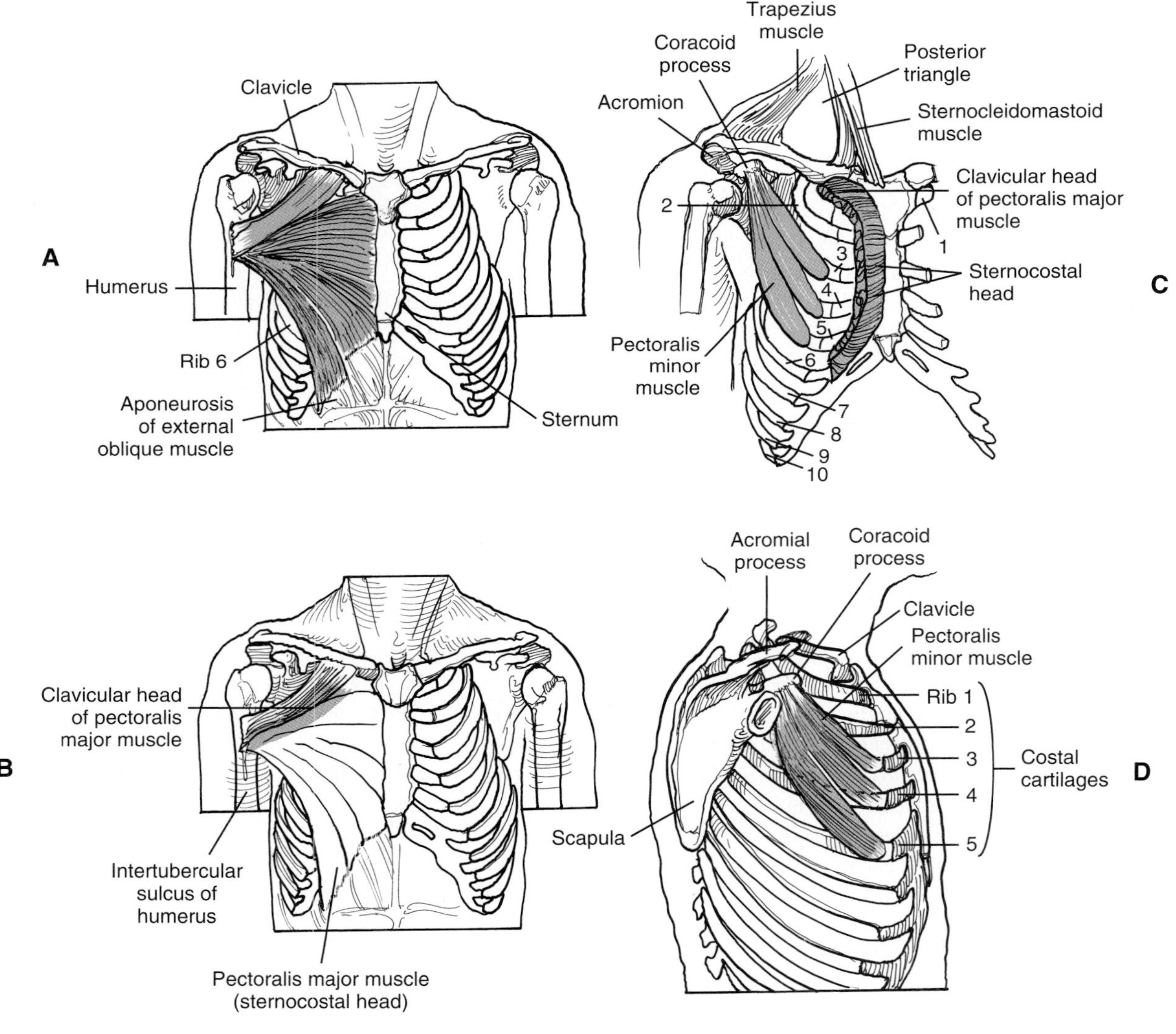

FIGURE 6–22
Appendicular muscles of the anterior thoracic wall. **A.** Sternocostal head of pectoralis major muscle. **B.** Clavicular head of pectoralis major muscle. **C.** Anterior view of pectoralis minor muscle. **D.** Lateral view of pectoralis minor muscle.

Subclavius muscles are small triangular muscles that attach the inferior surface of the middle region of the clavicle to the first ribs in the region of their junctions with the costal cartilages. Rarely, attachments of subclavius muscles to the clavicles extend laterally to the **coracoid processes** of the scapular bones (Fig. 6–22*E* and Table 6–2).

Deltoid muscles are triangular muscles that overlie the shoulder joint and several deeper muscles of the upper extremity and some of their proximal attachments to the scapula (Fig. 6–22*F* and Table 6–2 and see Chapter 17). The proximal portion of the deltoid muscle is attached to three distinct appendicular skeletal elements, including the lateral third of the clavicle, superior surface and lateral margin of the **acromial process** of the scapula, and the scapular spine.

Fibers from all regions of the muscle converge to form a distal tendon, which is attached to the **deltoid tuberosity,** a lateral protrusion in the midregion of the **humeral shaft.**

Each of the paired **serratus anterior muscles** arises from the upper edges and outer surfaces of the most superior 10 ribs, so that the collective digitations form a serrated anterior border. This broad sheet of muscle sweeps laterally and posteriorly to attach to the medial border of the scapula (Fig. 6–22*G* and *H* and Table 6–2 and see Chapter 17).

Appendicular Vessels and Nerves

Appendicular muscles of the anterior and lateral thorax are vascularized by branches of the seventh intersegmental vessels and innervated by branches of the brachial plexus

Pectoralis major muscles, like appendicular muscles of the back (see Chapter 5), are vascularized by branches that sprout from the seventh embryonic cervical intersegmental artery and vein (i.e., **pectoral** and

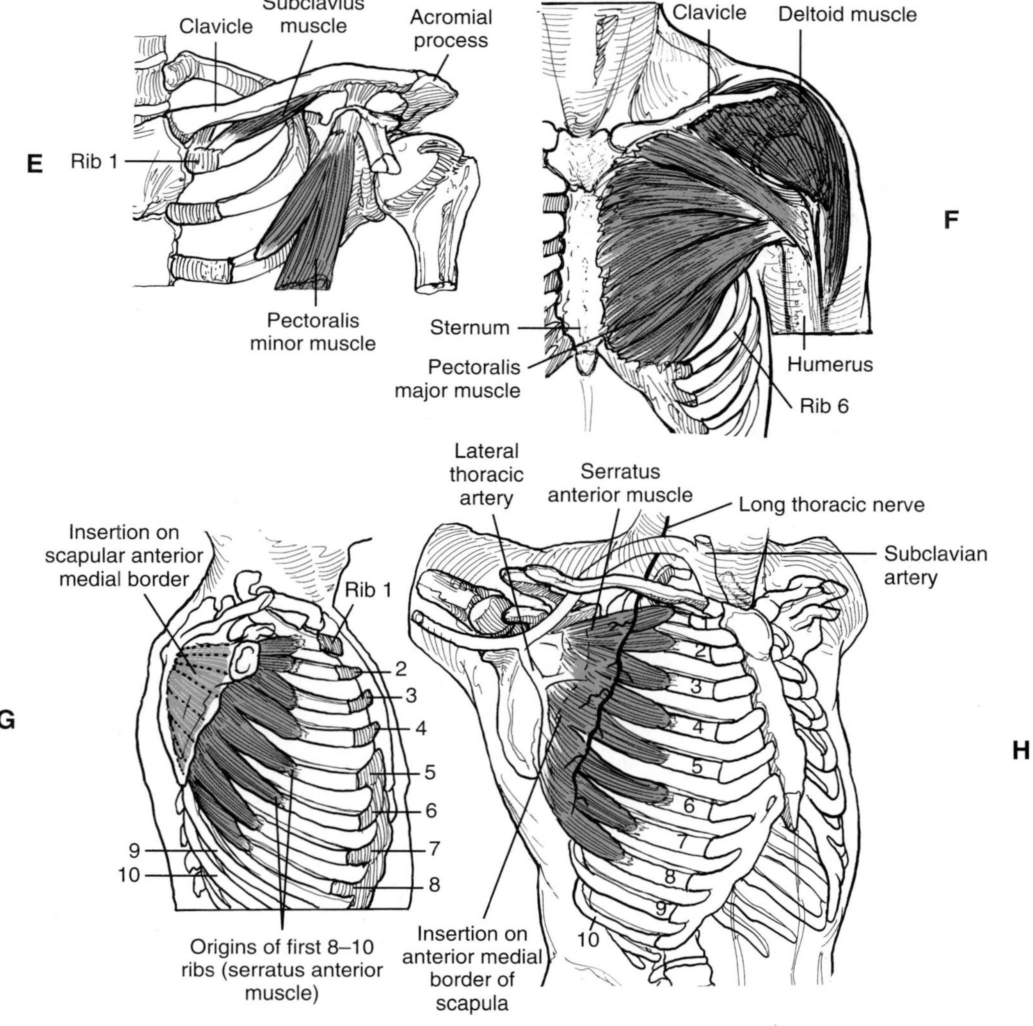

FIGURE 6–22, cont'd
E. Subclavius muscle. **F.** Deltoid and pectoralis major muscles. **G.** Lateral view of serratus anterior muscle. **H.** Anterior view of serratus anterior muscle.

TABLE 6–2
Attachments, Vascularization, and Innervation of Thoracic Appendicular Muscles

Muscle	ATTACHMENTS Proximal	Distal	Arterial Supply and Venous Drainage	Innervation
Pectoralis major muscles				
Sternocostal head	Half of sternum, costal cartilages 1 to 6, aponeurosis of external obliquus muscle	Lateral lip of intertubercular sulcus of humerus	Pectoralis and deltoid branches of thoracoacromial trunk, branches of lateral thoracic vessels, branches of intercostals and intercostal spaces 3 to 5	Medial pectoral nerve
Clavicular head	Medial half of clavicle	Lateral lip of intertubercular sulcus of humerus		Lateral pectoral nerve
Pectoralis minor muscles	Ribs 3 to 5	Coracoid process of scapula		Medial pectoral nerve
Subclavius muscles	First rib	Medial clavicle	Clavicular branch of thoracoacromial trunk	Nerve to subclavius
Deltoid muscles	Lateral third of clavicle, acromion, and spine of scapula	Deltoid tuberosity of humerus	Acromial and deltoid branches of thoracoacromial trunk	Axillary nerve
Serratus anterior muscles	Angles of superior 10 ribs	Medial border of scapula	Lateral thoracic vessels	Long thoracic nerve

deltoid branches of the **thoracoacromial trunk** and branches of the **lateral thoracic artery** and **vein**) (Fig. 6–23 and see Fig. 6–22*H*). Thus, in their definitive form, these vessels branch from **axillary vessels,** which are extensions of **subclavian arteries** and **veins** (see Table 6–2 and Chapters 20 and 21). Likewise, innervation of the pectoralis major muscle fibers is provided by branches of the brachial plexus (i.e., the **lateral pectoral nerve,** which is a branch of the **lateral cord** of the brachial plexus [clavicular head; spinal nerves C5 and C6] and **medial pectoral nerve** [sternocostal head; spinal nerves C7, C8, and T1]) (Fig. 6–23 and see Table 6–2 and Chapters 20 and 21).

Pectoralis minor muscles are vascularized by pectoral branches of the thoracoacromial trunk and innervated by the **medial pectoral nerve** (Fig. 6–23 and see Table 6–2 and Chapters 20 and 21). The apparent discrepancy between the seemingly reversed superficial locations and names of the lateral and medial pectoral nerves is explained by the fact that they are named for their origins from lateral and medial cords of the brachial plexus.

Each subclavius muscle is vascularized by the **clavicular branch** of the thoracoacromial artery and vein, which also serves the sternoclavicular joints. Each subclavius muscle is innervated by the **"nerve to the subclavius"** (spinal nerves C5 and C6), a branch of the **upper trunk** of the brachial plexus (see Table 6–2 and Chapters 20 and 21).

Deltoid muscles are vascularized by **acromial** and **deltoid branches** of the thoracoacromial trunk and innervated by the **axillary nerve** (spinal nerves C5 and C6), which is a branch of the posterior cord of the brachial plexus (Fig. 6–23 and see Table 6–2 and Chapters 20 and 21).

An obvious superficial landmark located within the groove between the deltoid and pectoralis major muscles is the **cephalic vein,** which is a superficial vein draining the upper extremity (Fig. 6–23 and see Table 6–2 and Chapter 18). This vein is so named because it "points toward" the head, but it is not involved in drainage of the head. It penetrates the body wall within the **clavipectoral fascia** (see below) and empties its blood into the axillary vein.

Serratus anterior muscles are vascularized by **lateral thoracic arteries** and **veins,** which branch from axillary arteries and veins just lateral to the thoracoacromial trunk (see Fig. 6–22*H*, Table 6–2, and Chapters 20

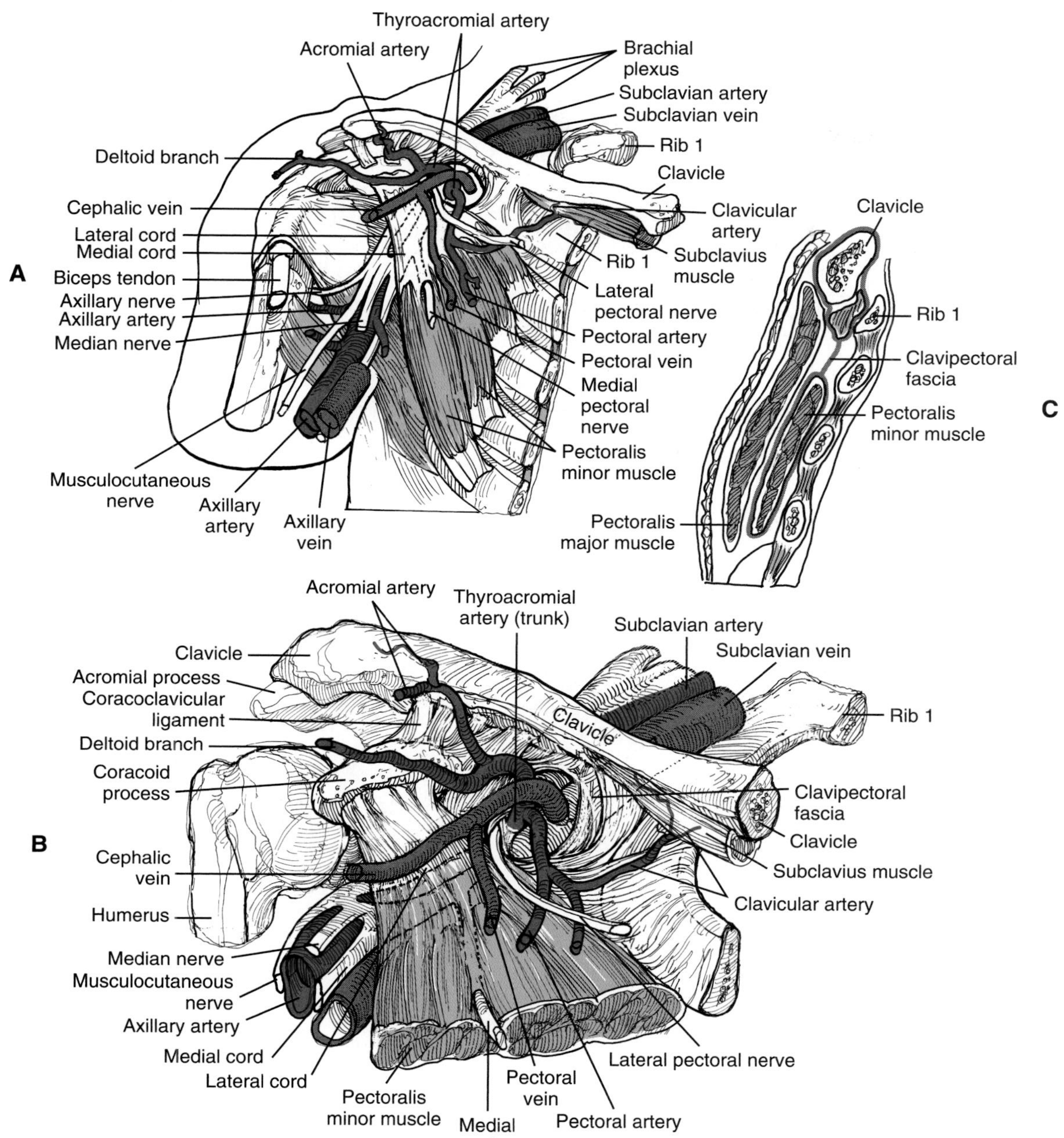

FIGURE 6–23

Clavipectoral fascia and structures that penetrate it. **A.** Structures deep to the clavipectoral fascia. **B.** Superficial structures after they have penetrated the clavipectoral fascia. **C.** Sagittal section through the clavipectoral fascia. Note that the medial pectoral nerve may be lateral to the lateral pectoral nerve at the level of the thoracic wall. These nerves are not named for their positions within the thoracic wall, but rather for their origins from the medial and lateral cords of the brachial plexus (see Chapter 21).

and 21). These muscles are innervated by **long thoracic nerves,** which are formed by a combination of branches from the **roots** of spinal nerves C5 to C7 of the brachial plexus (see Table 6–2 and Chapters 20 and 21).

▲ Clavipectoral Fascia

The clavipectoral fascia lies posterior to the clavicular part of the pectoralis major muscle. It fills the interval between the pectoralis minor and subclavius muscles and splits to invest the anterior and posterior surfaces of these muscles (see Fig. 6–23C). Superiorly, the clavipectoral fascia is attached to the inferior surface of the clavicle (on either side of the attachment of the subclavius muscle) and is continuous with the deep cervical fascia. The clavipectoral fascia is attached to the first rib medial to the attachment of the subclavius muscle, and laterally,

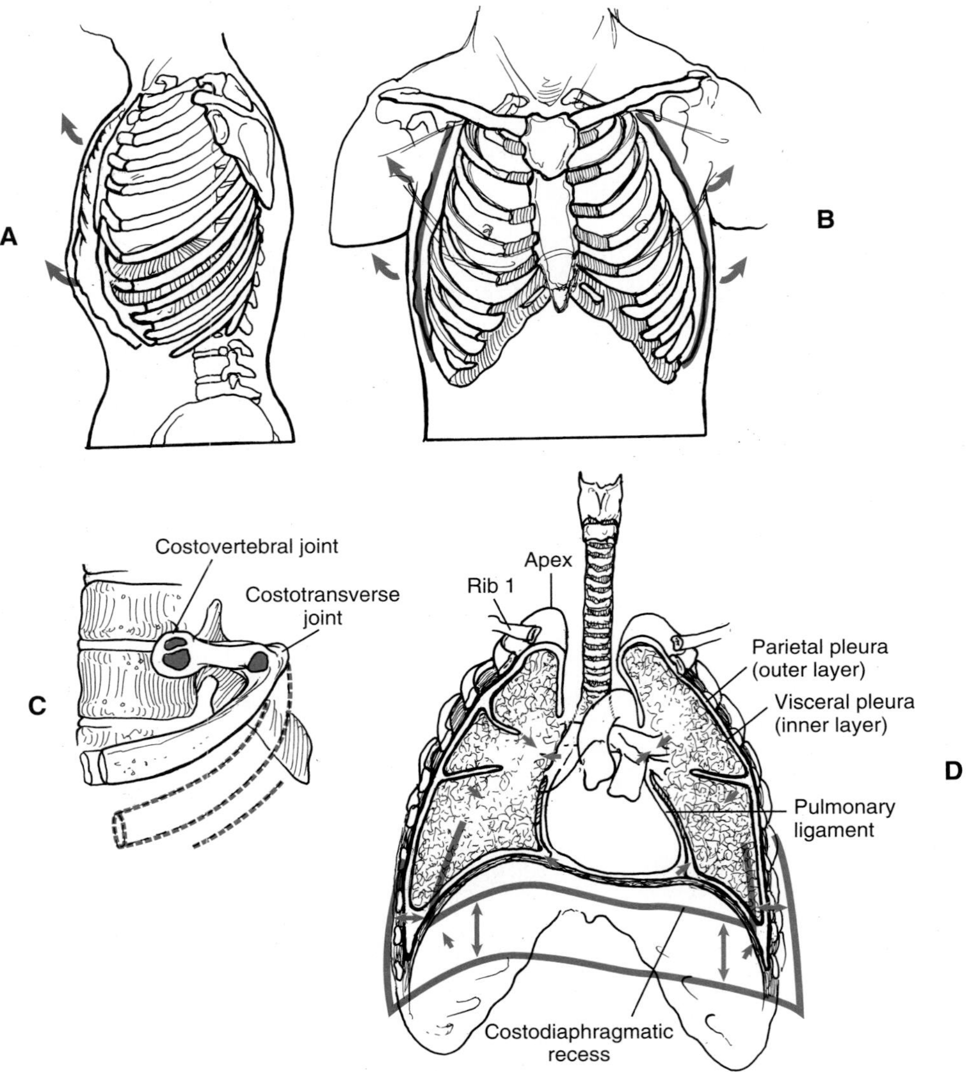

FIGURE 6–24

Movements of the thoracic wall in respiration. **A.** Anteroposterior dimensions of thoracic body wall (pump handle movement). **B.** Lateral dimensions of thoracic body wall (bucket handle movement). **C.** Superoinferior movement of diaphragm. **D.** Changes in vertical dimensions of thoracic region.

it is attached to the coracoid process and coracoclavicular ligament (see Chapter 21). Inferior to the pectoralis minor muscle, it blends with the deep fascia of the axillary (see Chapter 21) region in the back. The cephalic vein, pectoral branches of the thoracoacromial artery and vein, and lateral pectoral nerve must pierce this fascia as they course between the superficial fascia and deeper compartments of the thoracic body wall.

▲ Respiratory Function of the Thoracic Muscles and Skeleton

Movements of the thoracic wall are required for respiratory function

Respiration, or the cyclic **inspiration** and **expiration** of air between the alveoli of the lungs and the outer atmosphere, is facilitated by increases and decreases in the volume of the pleural cavities (Fig. 6–24 and see Chapter 8). An increase in volume creates negative pressure within the cavities, resulting in expansion of the pliant lungs and inspiration of air through the nose and mouth, pharynx, trachea, and bronchi. A decrease in volume results in a decrease in negative pressure, elastic recoil of the pliant lungs, and expiration of air (see Chapter 8). These fluctuations in volume may occur through increases and decreases:

- ♦ in the anteroposterior dimension of the thoracic body wall **(pump handle movement)** (Fig. 6–24*A* and *C*);
- ♦ in the lateral dimension of the thoracic body wall **(bucket handle movement)** (Fig. 6–24*B* and *D*); and

TABLE 6–3
Muscle Actions in Respiration

Function	Muscles Used	Muscle Actions
Quiet inspiration	Inferior intercostal muscles	Increase anteroposterior and lateral dimensions by raising inferior ribs and inferior part of sternum and widen infrasternal angles
	Diaphragm	Increases vertical dimension of pleural cavities; central tendon descends about 1.5 cm
Deep inspiration	All intercostal muscles	Increase anteroposterior and lateral dimensions by raising ribs 2 to 12
	Anterior and medial scalene muscles	Raise first ribs and manubrium slightly
	Diaphragm	Contracts more forcefully downward against abdominal viscera, aided by fixation of rib 12 by quadratus lumborum muscle
Forced inspiration	All intercostal muscles	Raise ribs 2 to 12
	Anterior and medial scalene, sternocleidomastoid, sternothyroid, sternohyoid muscles	Raise first ribs and manubrium
	Pectoralis major and pectoralis minor muscles	Raise superior ribs, raise ribs when scapula is fixed by trapezius, rhomboid major and rhomboid minor, and levator scapulae muscles
	Diaphragm	Contracts even more forcefully downward against abdominal viscera, again aided by fixation of rib 12 by quadratus lumborum muscle; central tendon may descend 9 to 10 cm
	Erector spinae muscles	Contract forcefully to decrease spinal curvature, thus increasing vertical dimensions of thorax
Quiet expiration	Lower intercostal muscles	Relax to lower inferior ribs and inferior part of sternum
	Diaphragm	Relaxes, diminishing vertical dimension of pleural cavities
	Abdominal muscles	Recoil elastically
Deep expiration	All intercostal muscles	Relax to lower all ribs and sternum
	Anterior and medial scalene muscles	Relax to lower manubrium
	Diaphragm	Relaxes, diminishing vertical dimensions of pleural cavities
	Abdominal muscles	Recoil elastically
Forced expiration	All intercostal muscles	Relax to lower ribs and sternum
	Anterior and medial scalene, sternocleidomastoid, sternothyroid, sternohyoid muscles	Relax to lower manubrium
	Diaphragm	Relaxes, decreasing vertical dimensions of pleural cavities
	Erector spinae muscles	Relax to decrease vertical dimensions of thorax
	Abdominal muscles	Forcefully contract, increasing intraabdominal pressure to push diaphragm upward and pull ribs medially and downward
	Latissimus dorsi muscles	Forcefully contract, increasing intraabdominal pressure to push diaphragm upward
Coughing and sneezing	Abdominal muscles, latissimus dorsi muscles	Contract forcefully against a closed glottis, resulting in build up of expiratory pressure, which is released when laryngeal muscles relax
	Scalene muscles	Prevent inferior displacement of upper ribs
Vocalization	Diaphragm	Relaxes in precise increments with aid of quadratus lumborum muscle, which fixes position of rib 12

- in the vertical dimension of the thoracic region (Fig. 6–24*D*).

Changes in the anteroposterior and lateral dimensions of the thoracic body wall associated with **quiet respiration** are primarily facilitated by contraction and relaxation of intercostal muscles and the diaphragm (Table 6–3). It should be noted, however, that the contraction of intercostal muscles during inspiration and expiration also prevents the intercostal spaces from bulging inward or outward. It is thought that the external intercostal muscles may roll the lower edges of the ribs outward, thereby helping to rotate the ribs upward at their costotransverse joints (Fig. 6–24*C*). Alterations of the vertical dimension of the thoracic region in quiet respiration are mediated by contraction and relaxation of the diaphragm. Quiet respiration supports the cyclic exchange of 500–750 ml of air. The exchange of 3–5 L of air per cycle typified by **deep** or **forced respiration** thus requires the participation of other muscles not usually classified as respiratory in function. These include the pectoralis major, pectoralis minor, and subclavius muscles; scalene muscles of the cervical region (see below and Chapter 24); erector spinae muscles (see Chapter 5); and abdominal muscles (see Chapter 10). Other respiratory movements such as coughing, sneezing, and vocalization require the use of specific subsets of muscles, which are described in Table 6–3. Further details relevant to the function of the pleural cavities and lungs in respiration are described in Chapter 8.

7 The Thoracic Cavities, Compartments, and Viscera

PARTITIONING AND DEVELOPMENT OF THE THORACIC CAVITIES

The intraembryonic coelomic cavity is partitioned into four cavities, three of which are in the thoracic region

Splitting of the lateral plate mesoderm and embryonic folding during the fourth week of development result in formation of a single **intraembryonic coelomic cavity.** This single cavity is split into four cavities: the pericardial cavity, which contains the heart; the two pleural cavities, which contain the lungs; and the peritoneal cavity, which contains much of the gastrointestinal tract and several urinary and genital organs. In some cases, these visceral organs are suspended by thin double mesothelial membranes called **mesenteries** (see Chapter 12). These organs, as well as the inner walls of the intraembryonic coelomic cavity, become lined by a continuous mesothelial membrane derived from lateral plate mesoderm.

Partitioning of the single intraembryonic coelomic cavity into four separate cavities occurs during the embryonic period. At first, the **septum transversum,** which was originally located superior to the developing brain, is translocated caudally and ventrally into the area that will become the lower thoracic region. Here, the septum transversum partially divides the intraembryonic coelomic cavity into a superior **primitive pericardial cavity** and an inferior **peritoneal cavity.** At this stage, the primitive pericardial cavity and peritoneal cavity continue to communicate through unobstructed posterior openings called **pericardioperitoneal canals** (Fig. 7–1*A*). The embryonic peritoneal cavity will become the **definitive abdominopelvic (peritoneal) cavity** (see Chapter 12).

Before further division of the primitive pericardial cavity occurs, the embryonic **lungs** begin to grow into their posterior regions from their origin at the superior end of the presumptive **esophagus.** Then additional coronal partitions called **pleuropericardial folds** grow from the lateral thoracic walls (Fig. 7–1*B* and *C*). These folds meet and fuse with each other in the midline and also fuse with mesoderm on the anterior side of the esophagus, dividing the primitive pericardial cavity into three distinct cavities: the **left pleural cavity, right pleural cavity,** and **definitive pericardial cavity.**

The anterior definitive pericardial cavity encloses the **heart,** the posterior left pleural cavity encloses the **left lung,** and the posterior right pleural cavity encloses the **right lung** (Fig. 7–1*C*). The pleuropericardial folds form the **pericardial sac** (Fig. 7–1*B* and *C* and see below).

The heart within its pericardial sac, the great vessels, thoracic esophagus, trachea, nerves, and lymphatic channels are thus enclosed within the connective tissue of a "median septum" called the **mediastinum,** which is located between the two pleural cavities (see below).

By the end of the embryonic period, a final pair of partitions, the **pleuroperitoneal membranes,** completely seals off the pericardioperitoneal canals, separating the pleural cavities from the peritoneal cavity (Fig. 7–1*D*). These membranes, along with the septum transversum and some of the esophageal and body wall mesoderm, form the definitive diaphragm (see Chapter 10).

As each of the presumptive body cavities becomes partitioned from the original intraembryonic coelomic cavity, the mesothelial membranes lining each new cavity and its enclosed viscera are given a specific name. The membrane lining the heart is the **epicardium (visceral pericardium).** The membrane lining the inner surface of the pericardial cavity is the **parietal pericardium.** The membrane lining the lungs is the **visceral pleura,** and the membrane lining the pleural cavities is the **parietal pleura.** The membrane lining the abdominopelvic viscera is the **visceral peritoneum,** and the membrane lining the abdominopelvic (peritoneal) cavity is the **parietal peritoneum.**

All of these membranes are **serous membranes** because they secrete **serous fluid,** which lubricates their surfaces and reduces friction between organs or between organs and the inner lining of the body wall. As much as 5–10 ml of serous fluid are present within each pleural cavity, and the pericardial cavity may contain 40–50 ml of serous fluid. The distribution and function of the abdominal peritoneum is discussed in Chapter 12.

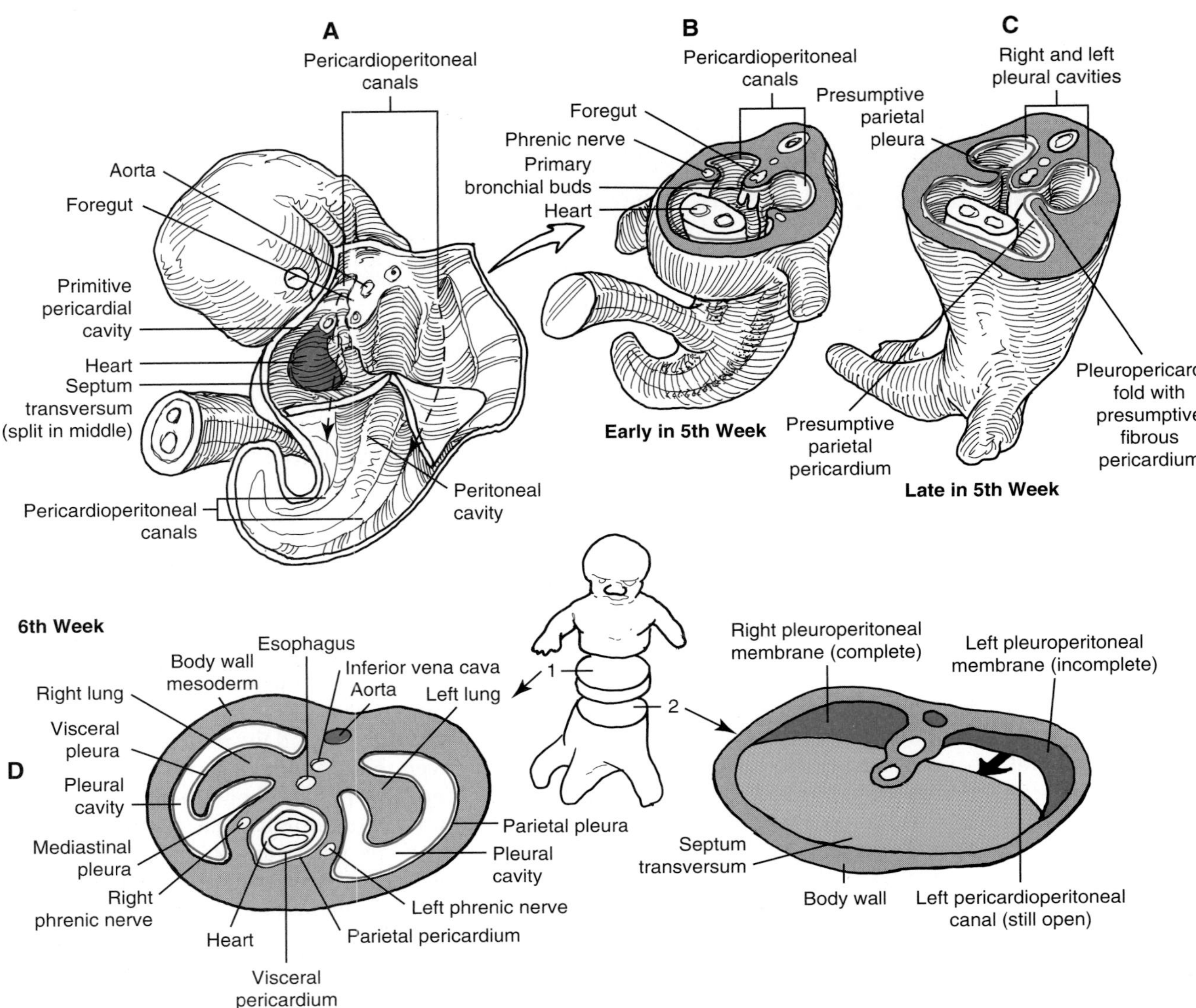

FIGURE 7–1
The intraembryonic coelom is split into four cavities. **A.** At first, the septum transversum divides the intraembryonic coelom into a superior primitive pericardial cavity and an inferior peritoneal cavity. The two cavities remain in communication, however, via posterior pericardioperitoneal canals. **B.** Coronal pleuropericardial folds grow from the lateral body wall on each side toward the midline. **C.** They divide the primitive pericardial cavity into three cavities as they meet in midline and fuse with the mesoderm around the esophagus: the left and right pleural cavities and the definitive pericardial cavity. Note that the phrenic nerves are swept into the pleuropericardial folds with associated body wall mesoderm, which becomes the fibrous pericardium. **D.** Finally, the pleuroperitoneal membranes seal off the pericardioperitoneal canals to completely separate the pleural cavities from the peritoneal cavity.

▲ Pericardial Sac

The pericardial sac has three layers

As the pleuropericardial folds grow medially from the lateral body walls, the serous membrane lining the primitive pericardial cavity is pulled out to line both sides of these evaginations (Fig. 7–1*B* and *C*). The membrane lining the anterior side becomes the parietal pericardium, while the membrane lining the posterior side becomes the parietal pleura (Fig. 7–1*D*). The body wall mesoderm incorporated within the pleuropericardial folds becomes the fibrous pericardium. In this way, the three layers of the pericardial sac are formed: the **mediastinal pleura** (outer layer); **fibrous pericardium** (middle layer); and **parietal (serous) pericardium** (inner layer) (Fig. 7–2).

The **visceral pericardium** investing the heart will be described in Chapter 9.

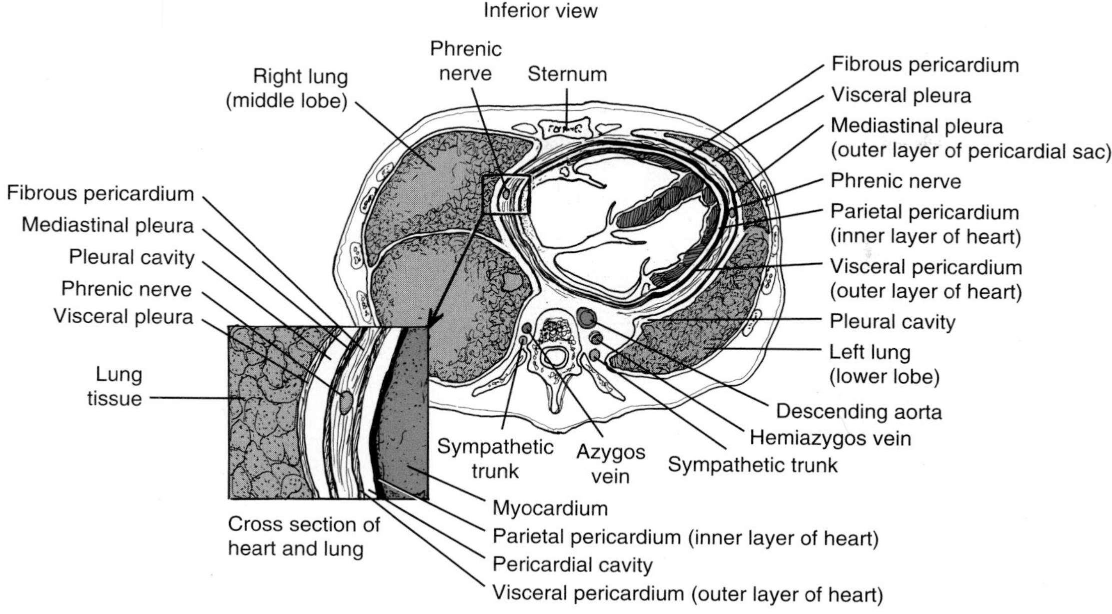

FIGURE 7–2

Inferior view of transverse section through thorax, showing relationships of pleural and pericardial cavities to the three layers of the pericardial sac. From inside to outside, the layers of the pericardial sac are the serous parietal pericardium, fibrous pericardium, and serous mediastinal pleura. Note that the phrenic nerves are embedded within the fibrous pericardium, which descends from the body wall mesoderm along with the embryonic pleuropericardial folds.

▲ Phrenic Nerves

Phrenic nerves course within the fibrous pericardium

As the presumptive diaphragm (septum transversum) descends, it becomes populated by myoblasts from cervical myotomes. These myoblasts thus become innervated by spinal nerves C3 to C5. Together, these nerves form **phrenic nerves,** which ultimately provide both motor and sensory innervation to the definitive diaphragm. During formation of the pericardial sac, the phrenic nerves evaginate inward with the pleuropericardial folds and are pulled away from their original locations within the lateral body walls (see Fig. 7–1*B* and *C*). Thus, the phrenic nerves also become situated between the parietal pericardium and mediastinal pleura, along with the fibrous pericardium and, ultimately, are positioned within the lateral walls of the **pericardial sac** (Fig. 7–2). Their pericardial branches provide sensory innervation to all three layers of the sac. The pericardiophrenic branches of internal thoracic arteries and veins provide vasculature to the pericardial sac (see Chapter 9).

▲ Mediastinum

The mediastinum lies between the two pleural cavities

The **mediastinum** lies posterior to the sternum, anterior to the vertebral column, inferior to the thoracic inlet, and superior to the diaphragm (Fig. 7–3). The mediastinum contains a variety of structures. Most of these support respiratory and cardiovascular function, while others, such as the esophagus, pass through the region to serve functions of the gastrointestinal tract. The largest single structure within the mediastinum is the **heart** within its **pericardial sac** (Fig. 7–3 and see Fig. 7–2). The mediastinum also contains the **thymus gland, great vessels, autonomic nerves, phrenic nerves, esophagus, trachea,** and **lymphatics** (Table 7–1).

Portions of the **azygos system** of veins, **descending aorta,** and **splanchnic nerves,** which lie somewhat lateral to the vertebral column, are, by convention, usually included with the contents of the mediastinum (Fig. 7–3 and see Fig. 7–2). However, the **sympathetic trunks,** which lie just posterior to the azygos vein on the right and posterior to the descending aorta on the left, will not be considered to reside within the mediastinum.

Once the fundamental organization of the mediastinum and its major visceral contents has been understood, it is easier to establish the anatomy of accessory structures. In addition, the anatomic relationships of structures within the mediastinum can be more easily seen by dividing it into four subregions.

Regions and Contents of the Mediastinum

The mediastinum is divided into major and minor subregions

There are two major subregions of the mediastinum: the **superior mediastinum** and **inferior medi-**

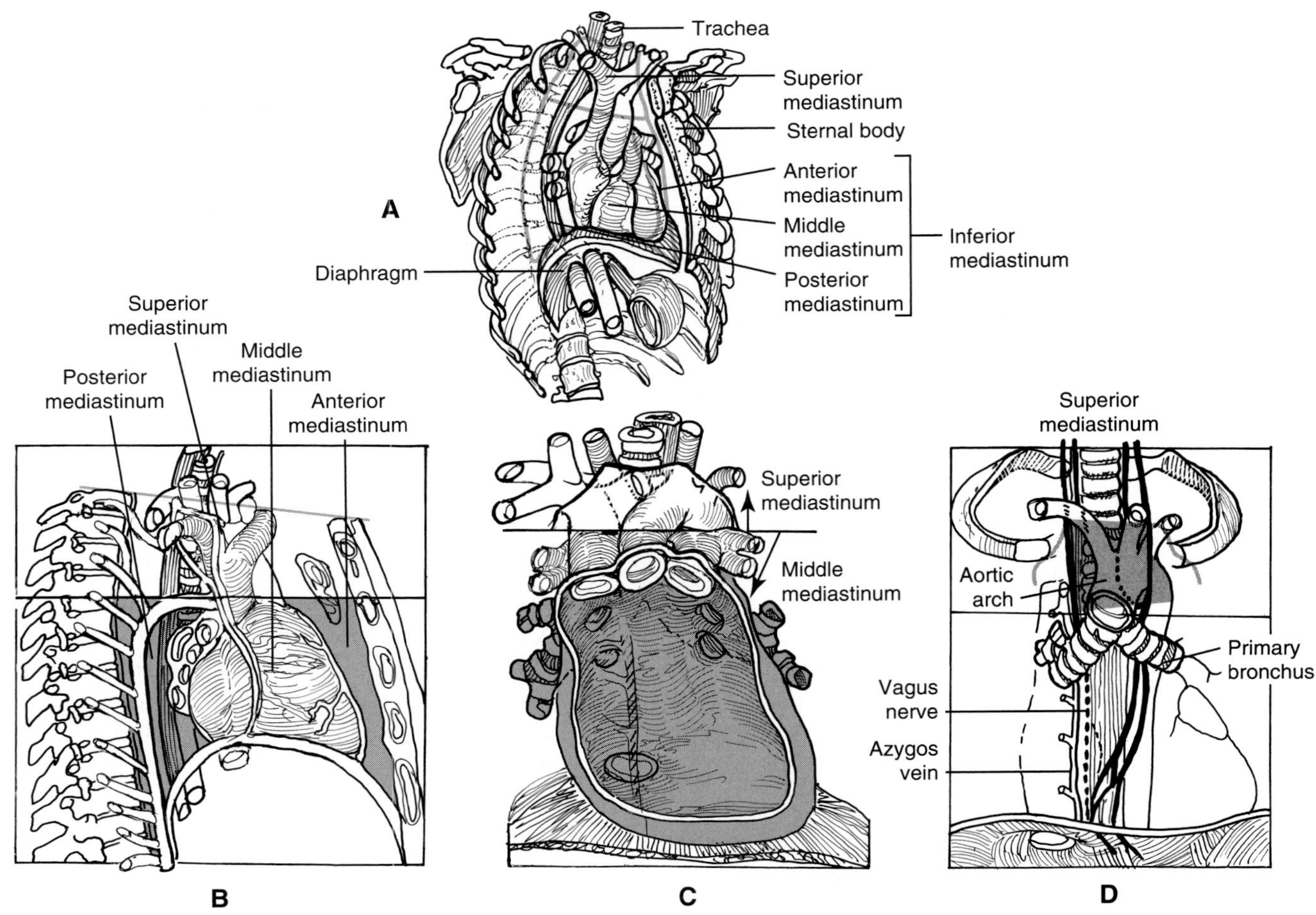

FIGURE 7–3
Organization and contents of the mediastinum.

astinum. The imaginary plane separating these two regions courses from the **sternomanubrial joint (sternal) angle** anteriorly to the inferior surface of vertebra T4 posteriorly (Fig. 7–3).

The **superior mediastinum** thus lies between the manubrium anteriorly and the superior four thoracic vertebrae posteriorly (Fig. 7–3). The superior mediastinum contains the great arteries and veins, trachea, esophagus, and associated structures (Table 7–1 and see Chapter 9). The **inferior mediastinum** lies between the body of the sternum anteriorly and the inferior eight thoracic vertebrae posteriorly (Fig. 7–3). The inferior mediastinum may, in turn, be divided into three subregions: the **anterior mediastinum,** the **middle mediastinum,** and the **posterior mediastinum** (Fig. 7–3).

The **anterior mediastinum** is a shallow compartment lying just posterior to the body of the sternum and anterior to the pericardial sac, and it contains only a few structures (Fig. 7–3*A* and *B* and Table 7–1 and see Chapter 9). The **middle mediastinum** contains mainly the **pericardial sac, heart,** and roots of the great vessels (Fig. 7–3*A* and *B* and Table 7-1 and see Chapter 9. The **posterior mediastinum** is bounded anteriorly by the bifurcation of the trachea, pulmonary vessels, and posterior wall of the pericardial cavity and posteriorly by the bodies of the inferior eight thoracic vertebrae. It mainly contains a variety of structures and organs that pass through the diaphragm into the abdominopelvic cavity (Fig. 7–3*A* and *D* and Table 7-1 and see Chapter 10).

Fig. 7–4 shows MRI scans of the normal mediastinum in a child and an adult.

PLAN FOR THE STUDY OF THORACIC STRUCTURES

The study of structures within the thorax is organized according to functional considerations as well as the usual order of dissection

Although Table 7–1 indicates that the thorax contains a diverse collection of organs with a variety of functions, closer inspection reveals that these functions may be organized into three main categories:

1. **respiratory function,**
2. **cardiovascular function,** and
3. in the case of the posterior mediastinum, the **trans-**

TABLE 7–1
Major Contents of the Superior, Anterior, Middle, and Posterior Mediastinal Compartments

Mediastinal Compartment	Contents
SUPERIOR COMPARTMENT	*Visceral organs:* Superior end of thymus gland or its remnants, trachea, superior end of esophagus
	Arteries: Aortic arch, brachiocephalic artery, left common carotid artery, left subclavian artery
	Veins: Brachiocephalic veins, left superior intercostal vein, superior half of superior vena cava
	Lymphatics: Thoracic duct and paratracheal, tracheobronchial, brachiocephalic lymph nodes
	Nerves: Vagus nerves, left recurrent laryngeal branch, cardiac branches of vagus nerves, cardiac nerves and superficial part of cardiac plexus, pulmonary nerves, phrenic nerves
INFERIOR COMPARTMENT Anterior compartment	*Visceral organs:* Inferior end of thymus gland or its remnants
	Arteries: Mediastinal branches of internal thoracic arteries
	Veins: Mediastinal branches of internal thoracic veins
	Lymphatics: Some lymph nodes
	Ligaments: Sternopericardial ligaments
Middle compartment	*Visceral organs:* Heart and pericardium, tracheal bifurcation, both main bronchi
	Arteries: Ascending aorta, pulmonary trunk, proximal parts of right and left pulmonary arteries, distal part of bronchial arteries
	Veins: Inferior half of superior vena cava, proximal part of azygos vein, right and left pulmonary veins, distal part of bronchial veins
	Lymphatics: Tracheobronchial lymph nodes
	Nerves: Deep part of cardiac plexus, pulmonary plexus, phrenic nerves within fibrous pericardium
Posterior compartment	*Visceral organs:* Esophagus
	Arteries: Descending thoracic aorta, esophageal arteries, proximal part of bronchial arteries
	Veins: Azygos and hemiazygos veins, esophageal veins, proximal part of bronchial veins
	Lymphatics: Thoracic duct, posterior mediastinal lymph nodes
	Nerves: Vagus nerves, splanchnic nerves

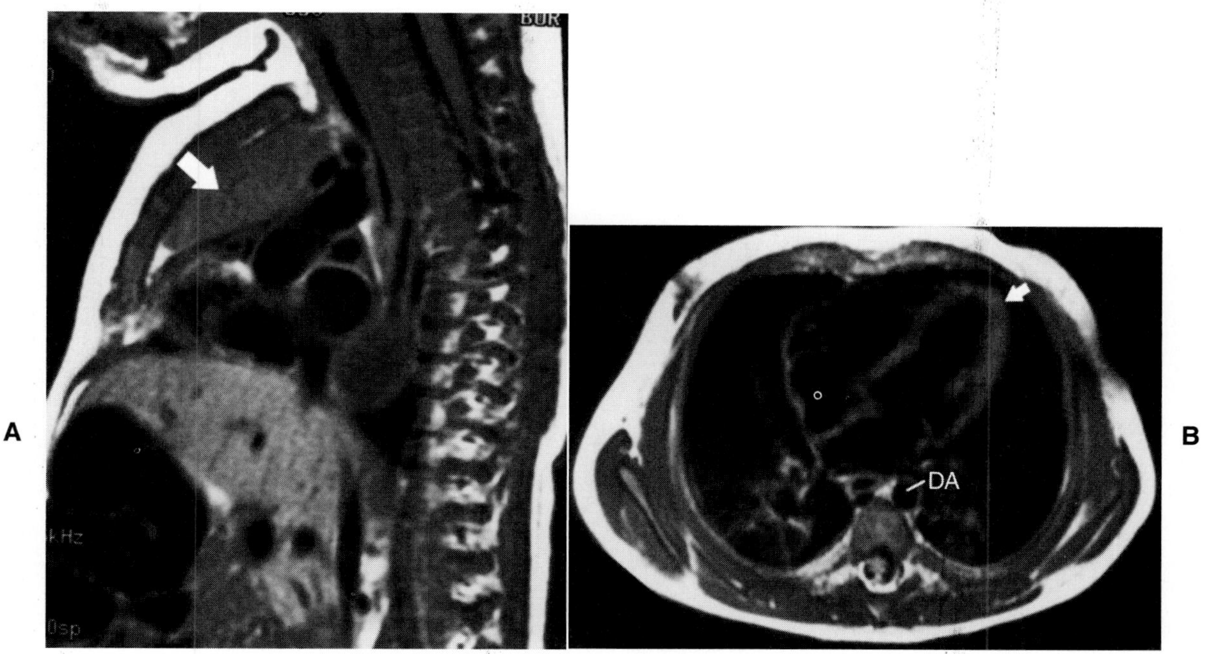

FIGURE 7–4
A. Sagittal MRI of the normal mediastinum of a juvenile. Note the large thymus gland *(arrow)* within the anterior mediastinum. **B.** Transverse MRI of the normal mediastinum. Note the apex of the heart *(arrow)* within the middle mediastinum and the thoracic segment of the descending aorta *(DA)* within the posterior mediastinum.

port of structures between the neck above and abdomen below.

For example, the pleural cavities, with their enclosed lungs, are primarily devoted to respiratory function. Therefore, Chapter 8 will focus on the pleural cavities and lungs.

In contrast, the anterior and middle compartments of the inferior mediastinum and much of the superior mediastinum are specialized for cardiovascular function. Chapter 9 will therefore describe the structure and contents of the anterior, middle, and superior mediastina together.

Finally, the posterior mediastinum and median posterior body wall contain many structures that pass through the thorax or that distribute thoracic structures to the neck or abdomen. Structures passing between the thorax and the abdomen must pierce the diaphragm. Therefore, Chapter 10 will focus on the posterior mediastinum and diaphragm.

8 The Trachea, Lungs, and Pleural Cavities

The **pulmonary airway** consists of the nasal and oral cavities, pharynx, larynx, trachea, and the left and right lungs within the left and right pleural cavities. The nasal and oral cavities, pharynx, and larynx are discussed in Chapters 22 to 24, with the head and neck. This chapter will focus on the **trachea, lungs,** and **pleural cavities.**

ANATOMY OF THE PLEURAL CAVITIES

Development of the Pleural Cavities

The pleuropericardial folds and pleuroperitoneal membranes completely separate the left and right pleural cavities from the pericardial and peritoneal cavities and from each other

When the **primitive pericardial cavity** and **presumptive abdominopelvic cavity** have become partially separated by the **septum transversum,** the **pleural cavities** begin to form. They form when the **primitive pericardial cavity** is divided by coronally oriented **pleuropericardial folds,** which grow from the lateral body wall. The **definitive pericardial cavity** is completely separated from the presumptive **left** and **right pleural cavities** by this process (see Fig. 7–1).

Subsequently, posterior canals, which allow communication between each of the pleural cavities and the peritoneal cavity, are filled in by the growth of a **pleuroperitoneal membrane,** which completely separates both of the pleural cavities from the presumptive **abdominopelvic cavity** and, indirectly, from each other. Once the growth of the pleuroperitoneal membranes is complete, each lung continues growing into its **definitive pleural cavity** (Fig. 8–1 and see Fig. 7–1).

▲ The Definitive Pleural Cavities

Once each definitive pleural cavity is formed, the cavity extends superiorly as an inverted cup-shaped recess, or **cupula,** which projects slightly above the first rib and clavicle (Fig. 8–1 and see Figs. 6–2*A*). Inferiorly, each pleural cavity is limited by the diaphragm. The diaphragm is not positioned in a truly

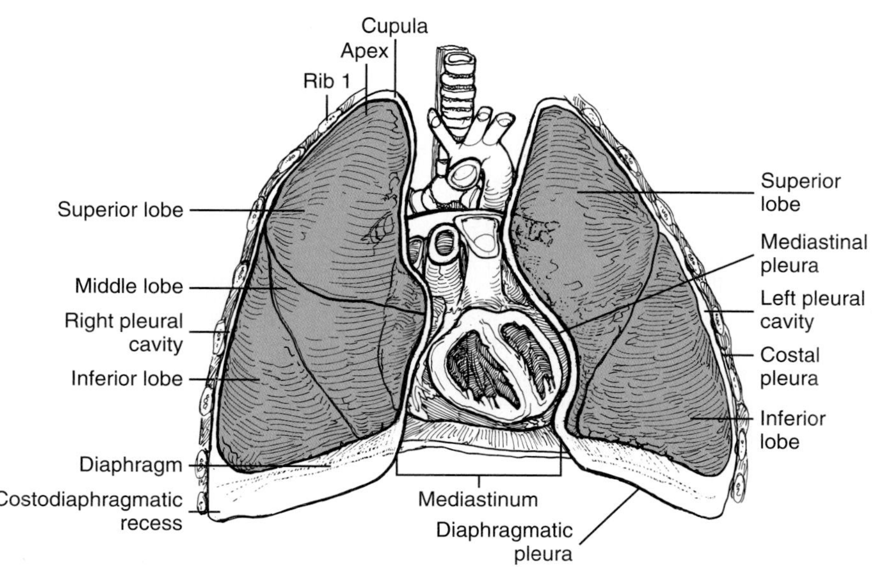

FIGURE 8–1
The right and left lungs in the right and left pleural cavities and the mediastinum (coronal section). Note the close fit between the surface of the lung and the wall of the pleural cavity. The pleural cavities are closed off from the atmosphere and are separate from each other.

horizontal plane. Its anterior edge is attached to the **xiphoid process;** its lateral edges are attached to the cartilages of ribs 7 to 10, which make up the **infrasternal angle,** and to the tips of ribs 11 and 12; and its posterior edge is attached to vertebral bodies L1 to L3 (see Figs. 6–1 and 10–9).

Deep recesses of the pleural cavities are located at the points where the mediastinum and costal cartilages meet anteriorly, the **costomediastinal recesses,** and at the **costodiaphragmatic recesses** where the diaphragm and ribs are connected inferiorly (Fig. 8–1).

▲ Function of the Pleural Cavities in Respiration

The lungs are highly elastic, but they are able to expand and contract only in response to variations in pressure within the pleural cavities. These variations result from the cyclic increase and decrease in pleural cavity volume resulting from actions of the diaphragm and respiratory muscles of the thoracic and abdominal walls (see below and Chapter 6). Each lung almost fully occupies its pleural cavity only when negative pressure is maintained within the cavity. When the pressure within a pleural cavity increases to the same level as the atmospheric pressure, as occurs in **pneumothorax,** the lung undergoes elastic recoil and becomes deflated. The lung volume is reduced to 25–35% of the volume of a fully inflated lung.

▲ Clinical Disorders

Rib Fracture and Loss of Negative Pressure in the Pleural Cavity

In order for the appropriate level of negative pressure to be maintained within the pleural cavities so that the lungs can be properly inflated, the thoracic wall must be rigid and elastic as well as airtight. If several ribs are fractured, the rigidity of the thoracic wall may be compromised, and contraction of the respiratory muscles may not be sufficient to increase the pleural cavity volume required for inflation of the lung. As a consequence, ventilation of the alveoli is reduced.

Open Pneumothorax and Tension Pneumothorax

Puncture of the thoracic wall may lead to pneumothorax

If the thoracic wall is punctured, air may enter the pleural cavity directly and cause serious disruption of respiratory function because the negative pressure needed to inflate the lung cannot be maintained **(collapsed lung)** (Fig. 8–2*A*). This condition is called **open pneumothorax.** If it is left untreated, mediastinal structures will deviate toward the affected side during inspiration, further compromising the lung's respiratory capacity. In addition, circulatory collapse within the affected lung may lead to significant diminution in the pulmonary venous return.

In some cases, air may be able to enter the punctured pleural cavity with each inspiration but may not be able to escape during expiration. The resulting increase in pressure pushes mediastinal structures toward the unaffected side, compromising respiratory efficiency of the healthy lung. This condition is called **tension pneumothorax** (Fig. 8–2*B*).

Both open pneumothorax and tension pneumothorax are life-threatening emergencies and require rapid, careful management.

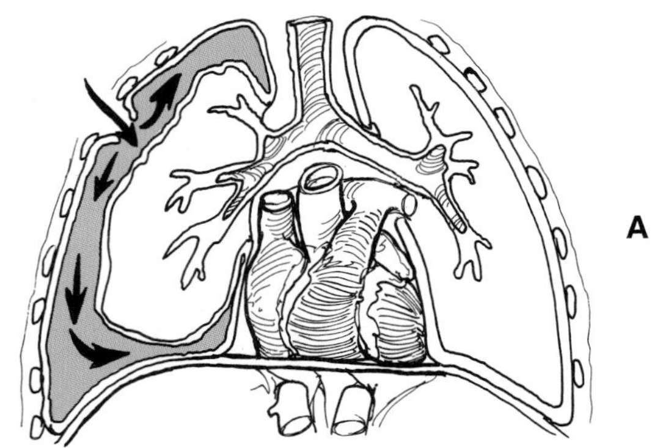

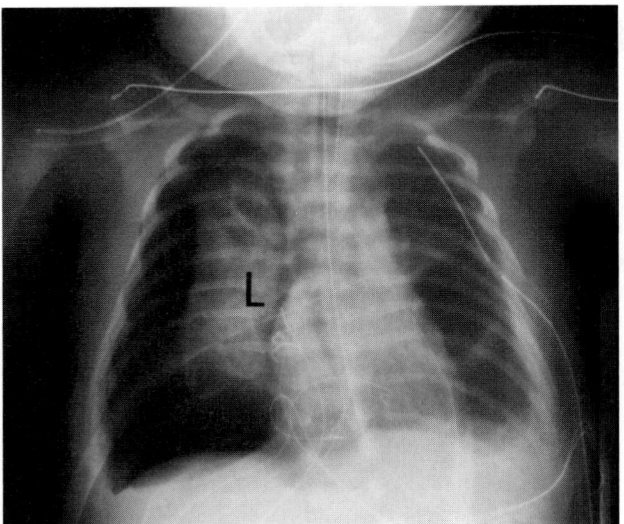

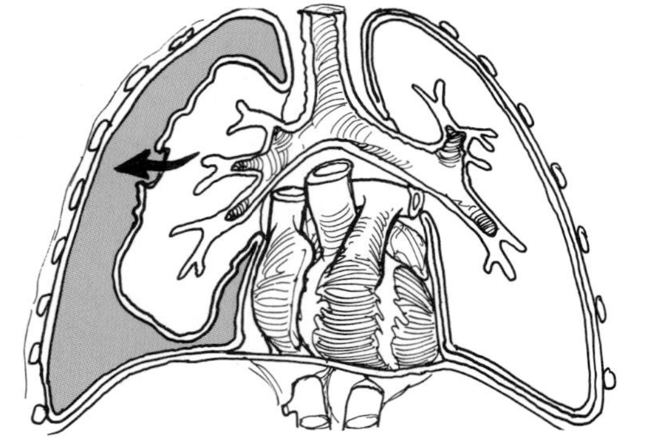

FIGURE 8–2
Pneumothorax. **A.** Open pneumothorax. **B.** X-ray of infant with tension pneumothorax. Notice deflated right lung *(L)* and air *(black area)* within the pleural cavity. The mediastinum is pushed toward the left side. **C.** Spontaneous pneumothorax.

Spontaneous Pneumothorax

Pneumothorax may occur without injury to the thoracic wall

A patient without obvious injury to the thoracic wall may complain of **dyspnea** (shortness of breath) and chest pain worsened by respiratory movements and may have some degree of **cyanosis** (bluish coloration of nail beds, gums, and lips) indicative of lung collapse. These symptoms may result from a type of spontaneous pneumothorax that occurs following "spontaneous" internal rupture of the bronchial tree and visceral pleura (typically at the site of a lung disorder such as a pulmonary cyst; see below). Such an internal injury results in direct communication between the atmosphere (via the pulmonary airway) and the pleural cavity, preventing the generation of negative pressure within the pleural cavity (Fig. 8–2*C*). The typical patient with spontaneous pneumothorax is a tall, slender male 20–40 years old who is a cigarette smoker. A wide range of individuals may suffer from this condition, however. Older patients suffering from emphysema or tumors of the lung, neonates, patients with cystic fibrosis, or adolescents may also develop spontaneous pneumothorax. Very mild cases may be asymptomatic and are usually managed by observation. More severe cases may require reinflation of the lung and removal of excess air from the pleural cavity via a tube inserted through a surgical incision in the thoracic wall. Small internal ruptures of the lung wall often close without direct treatment, although it may be necessary to suture very large ruptures or to close large cysts that have not yet ruptured.

Pleural Effusion (Serous Fluid Collection)

Collection of fluids within the pleural cavity may impair ventilation

The development of excess fluid within the pleural cavities is a **pleural effusion.** The average amount of serous fluid produced and reabsorbed by the pleura during a 24-hour period is 600–1000 ml. However, because production and reabsorption are normally balanced, only 5–10 ml of pleural fluid are present within each of the pleural cavities at any given time.

The buildup of serous fluid may result from excess production caused by hypertension related to congestive heart failure (see Chapter 9) or from increased permeability of the microvasculature caused by inflammation. Alternatively, excess serous fluid may result from decreased reabsorption, usually as a consequence of kidney failure (see Chapter 13), pneumothorax, or impaired lymphatic drainage (often resulting from blockage by tumors).

Collection of Pus, Blood, or Lymph Within the Pleural Cavity

Pus, blood, or lymph may also collect within the pleural cavities

Empyemas are effusions of purulent fluid (i.e., containing pus), which usually arise from bacterial infections of the pleural cavity. The collection of blood within the pleural cavity **(hemothorax)** may result from bleeding of pulmonary, intercostal, or internal thoracic vessel branches. Lymphatic fluid may also collect within the pleural cavities following rupture of the thoracic duct. Regardless of its source, excess fluid within the pleural space interferes with the dynamics of ventilation by decreasing the space available for lung expansion.

ANATOMY OF THE LUNGS AND TRACHEA

Development of the Lungs and Trachea

Each developing lung grows into its pleural cavity as a sprout of the embryonic gastrointestinal tract

The lungs arise from a ventral endodermal outgrowth of the **gastrointestinal tract** called the **lung bud (respiratory diverticulum)** during the fourth week of development. The location of the lung bud demarcates the more superior **pharyngeal part of the foregut** from the rest of the gastrointestinal tract (see Chapter 10). The lung bud grows into the mesoderm surrounding the esophagus (Fig. 8–3). The endoderm of the lung bud and its surrounding mesoderm give rise to all of the differentiated tissues of the pulmonary airways and parenchyma (see below).

Bronchial Tree

Initially, the endodermal lung bud forms the **trachea** (see Figs. 8–3 through 8–5). It soon bifurcates to form the right and left **primary bronchial buds,** which become **primary (main) bronchi** of the right and left lungs (Fig. 8–3). The right bud branches into three **secondary buds,** which give rise to **secondary bronchi** of the three lobes of the right lung, and the left bud branches to form secondary bronchi of the two left lung lobes (Fig. 8–3). The tertiary generation of branching establishes the pattern of the **bronchopulmonary segments** of which there are usually about 10 on each side (Figs. 8–3 and 8–4 and Table 8–1). After about 14 additional generations of branchings, the bronchial buds form **terminal bronchioles,** which branch to form **respiratory bronchioles** (Fig. 8–5). Finally, **terminal sacs** are formed by branching of the respiratory bronchioles, which become differentiated into **mature alveoli** just before birth (Fig. 8–5). Between 20 and 80 million alveoli are formed before birth, and, ultimately, in late childhood there are about 300 million alveoli.

During late fetal life, the alveoli are inflated by fluid absorbed from pulmonary tissues or by amniotic fluid that has been inspirated by the fetus. After birth, this fluid is expelled and the alveoli fill with air. The exchange of gases then occurs within the mature alveoli during each **respiratory cycle** (see above).

The complete system of bifurcating bronchial branches is the **bronchial tree.** Although the pattern of branching is largely established by inductive influences of the surrounding mesoderm on the growth of endodermal bronchial buds, the endoderm itself gives rise

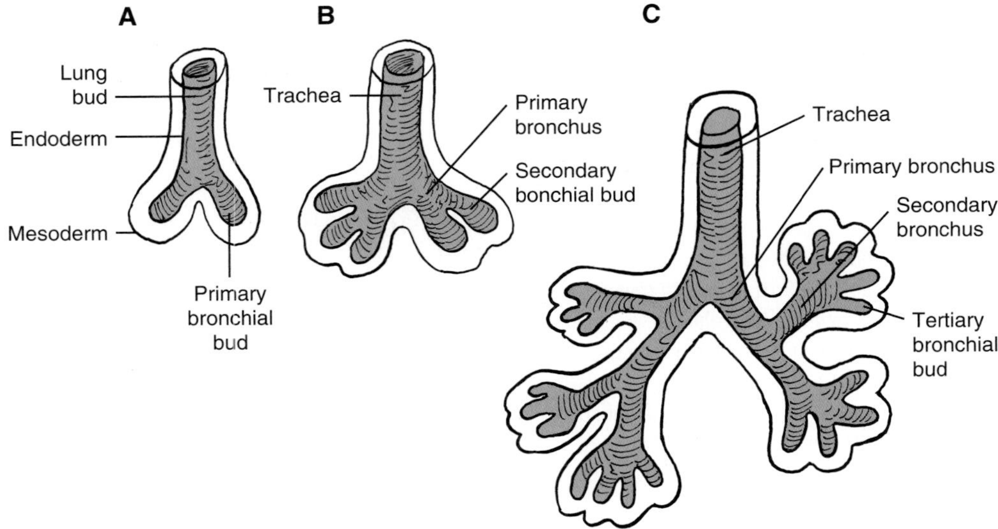

FIGURE 8–3
The lung bud sprouts from the esophagus by 25 days and bifurcates **(A)** to form the primary bronchial buds (future primary bronchi) by day 28. **B.** By 30 days, three secondary bronchial buds are produced on the right and two secondary bronchial buds are produced on the left. **C.** By 38 days, the secondary bronchial buds give rise to the tertiary bronchial buds, which become the bronchopulmonary segments.

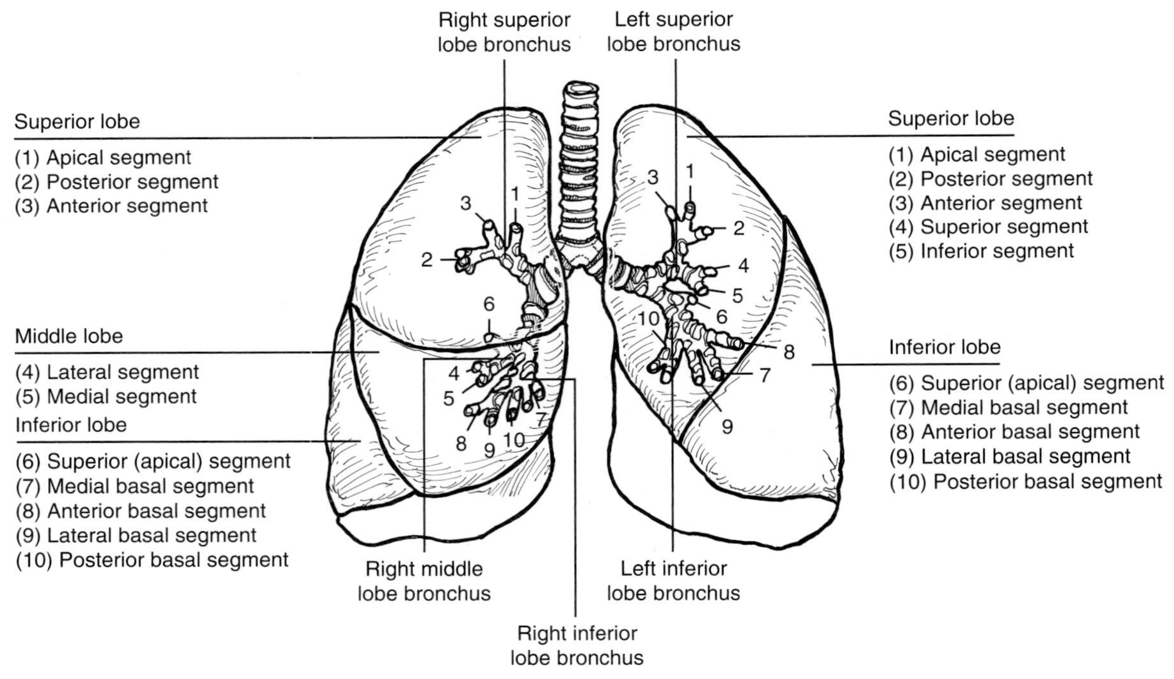

FIGURE 8–4
Bronchopulmonary segments of the right and left lungs.

only to the epithelium of the bronchial tree from the trachea to the alveoli. In contrast, the mesoderm, initially investing the lung bud, forms many structures, including the **bronchial cartilages, bronchial** and **bronchiolar smooth muscle, pulmonary** and **systemic vasculature** of the lungs, **stroma** (connective tissue) of the pulmonary parenchyma, and **visceral pleura** (serous membrane) investing each lung.

▲ The Definitive Trachea

The trachea extends from the larynx to the bifurcation of the right and left principal bronchi at the level of the sternal angle

TABLE 8–1
Naming and Numbering of the Bronchopulmonary Segments

Lobe	Right Lung	Left Lung
Superior lobe	1. Apical segment	1. Apical segment
	2. Posterior segment	2. Posterior segment
	3. Anterior segment	3. Anterior segment
		4. Superior lingular segment
		5. Inferior lingular segment
Middle lobe	4. Lateral segment	
	5. Medial segment	
Inferior lobe	6. Superior (apical) segment	6. Superior (apical) segment
	7. Medial basal segment	7. Medial basal segment
	8. Anterior basal segment	8. Anterior basal segment
	9. Lateral basal segment	9. Lateral basal segment
	10. Posterior basal segment	10. Posterior basal segment

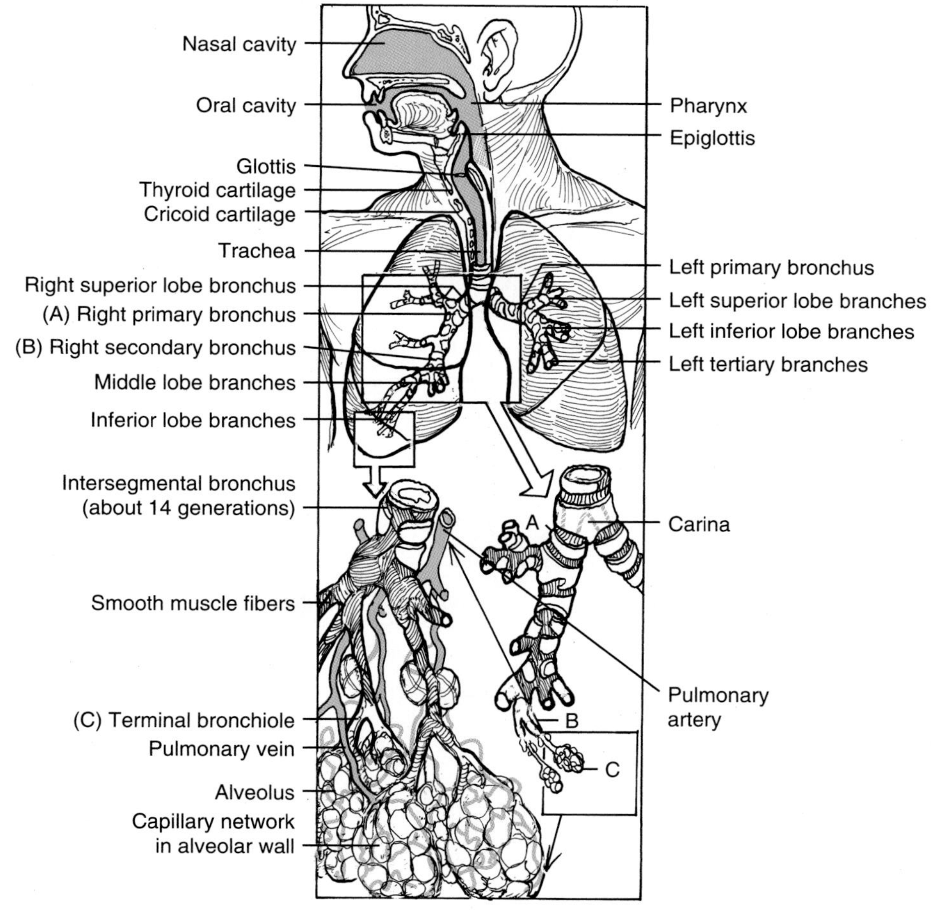

FIGURE 8–5
The bronchial tree. Once the bronchopulmonary segments are formed, about 14 additional generations of branching produce the terminal bronchioles. These branch, in turn, to form respiratory bronchioles, which branch to form the terminal sacs, which will become the alveoli. All of the bronchi are reinforced by cartilaginous rings. Bronchioles lack cartilaginous rings.

The trachea can be divided into cervical and thoracic regions. In adults, the cervical and thoracic parts of the trachea together are 10–12 cm in length.

Cervical Trachea

The **cervical part of the trachea** courses from vertebra C6 to the inferior plane of the body of vertebra C7. This section of the trachea is covered anteriorly by the integument and superficial fascia (Fig. 8–6*A*). The **isthmus of the thyroid gland** and the **sternothyroid** and **sternohyoid muscles** are sandwiched between the cervical trachea and superficial fascia (Fig. 8–6 and see Chapter 27), and the esophagus lies immediately posterior to it, separating it from the anterior surface of the

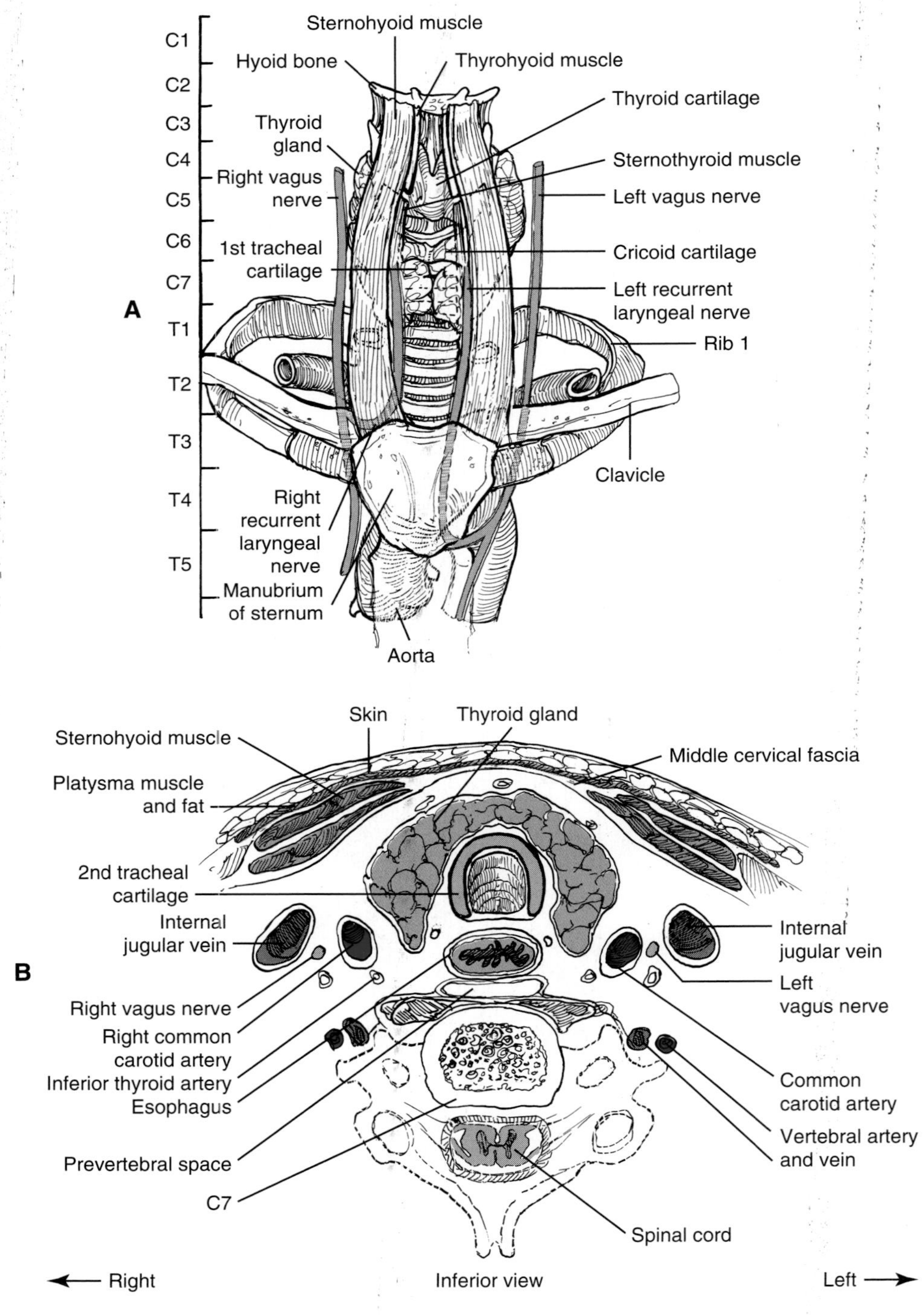

FIGURE 8–6
The cervical trachea. **A.** Frontal view of the cervical trachea at the levels of vertebrae C6 and C7. **B.** Inferior view of transverse section of the trachea at the level of vertebra C7.

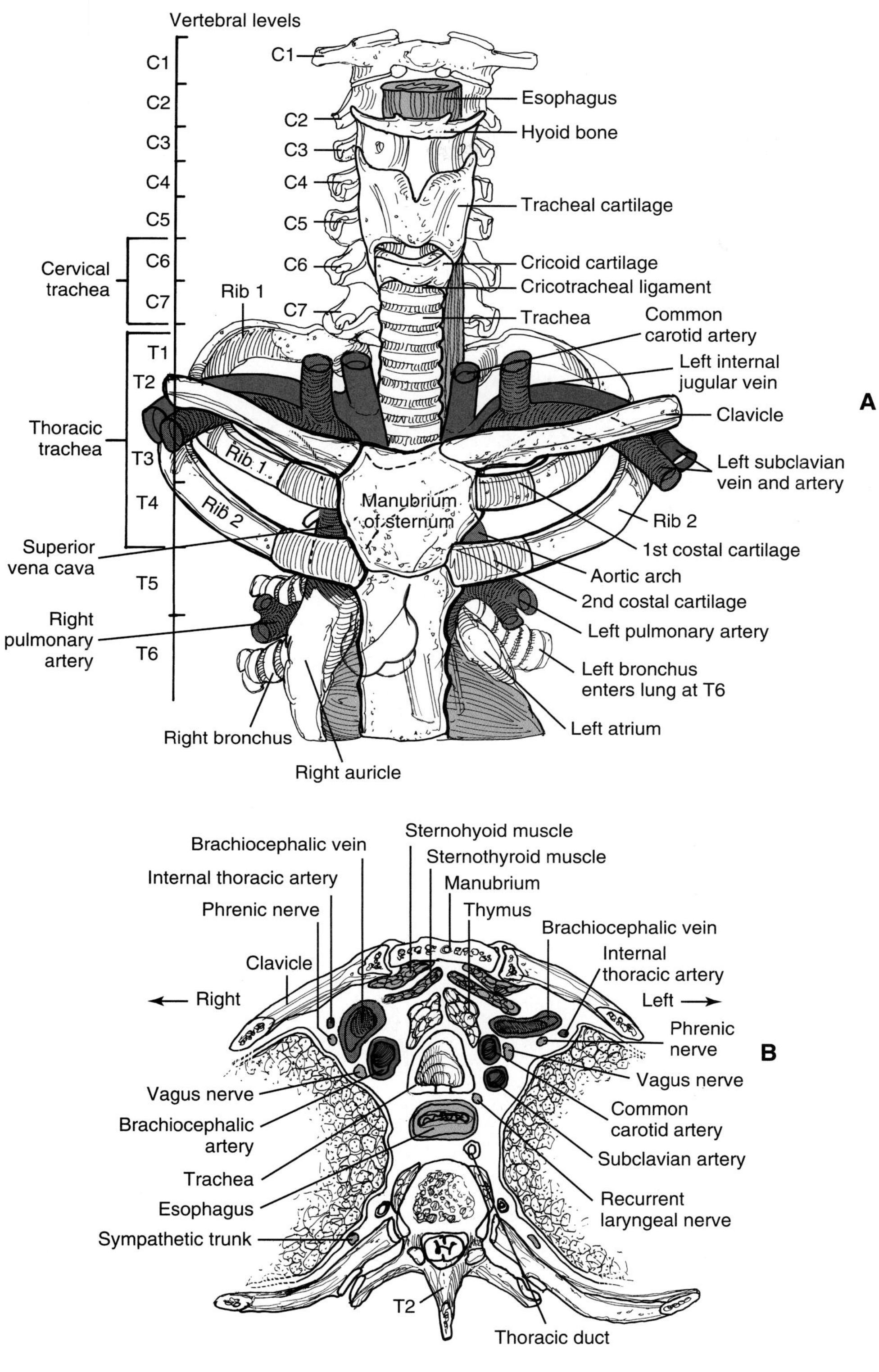

FIGURE 8–7
The thoracic trachea. **A.** Frontal view of the thoracic trachea at the levels of vertebrae T1 to T4. **B.** Inferior view of transverse section at vertebra T2.

Continued

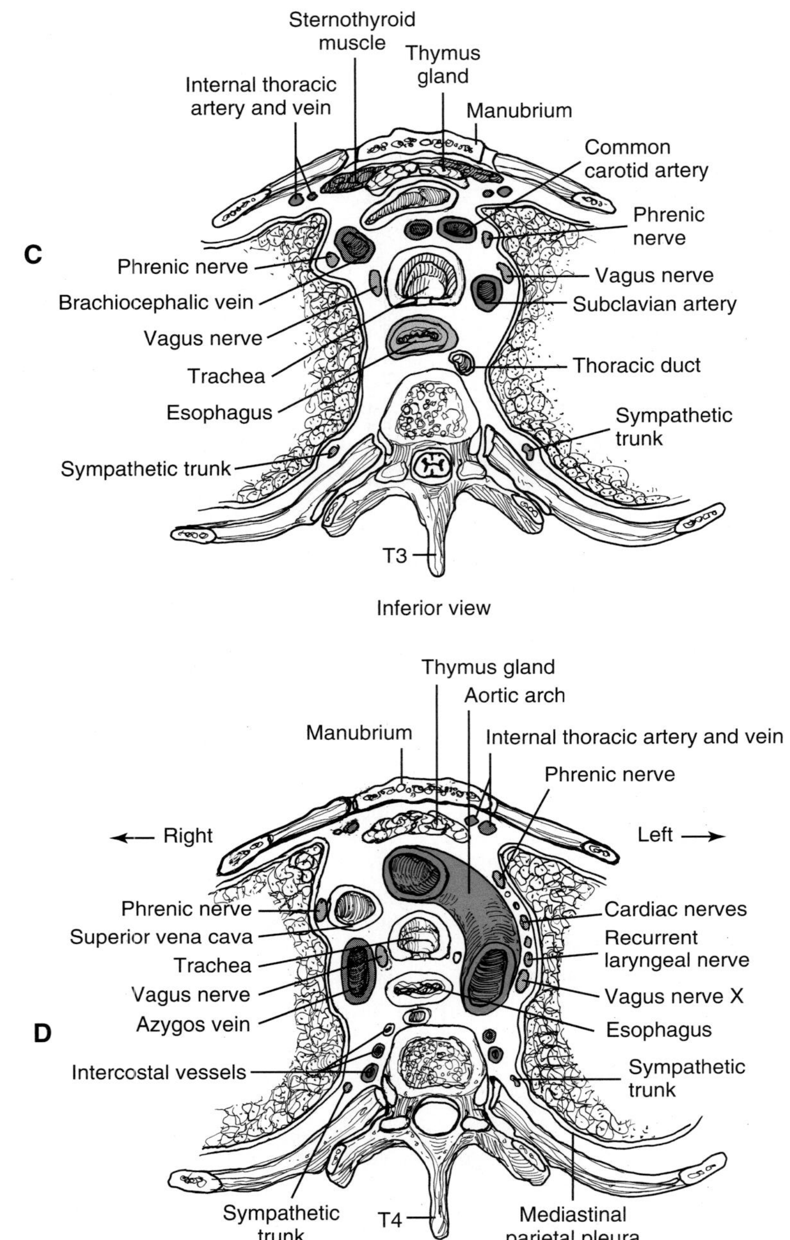

FIGURE 8–7, cont'd
C. Inferior view of transverse section at vertebra T3. **D.** Inferior view of transverse section at vertebra T4.

body of vertebra C7 (Fig. 8–6*B*). The left and right **recurrent laryngeal nerves** and lobes of the **thyroid gland** lie laterally to the cervical trachea (Fig. 8–6).

Thoracic Trachea

The **thoracic part of the trachea** lies within the **superior mediastinum,** coursing from the level of vertebra T1 to the level of the superior boundary of vertebra T5 (Fig. 8–7*A* and see Chapter 9). Its inferior end passes just posterior to the **manubrium,** the inferior attachments of the sternothyroid and sternohyoid muscles, and the vestiges of the **thymus gland** (Fig. 8–7*B*). Sandwiched between the trachea and the manubrium are parts of some of the **great vessels,** including the **left brachiocephalic vein, arch of the aorta, left carotid artery,** and **brachiocephalic artery** (Fig. 8–7*A* to *D* and see Chapter 9). The esophagus lies just posterior to the thoracic part of the trachea, which separates it from the thoracic vertebral bodies. The **superior vena cava, azygos** and **right brachiocephalic veins, right vagus**

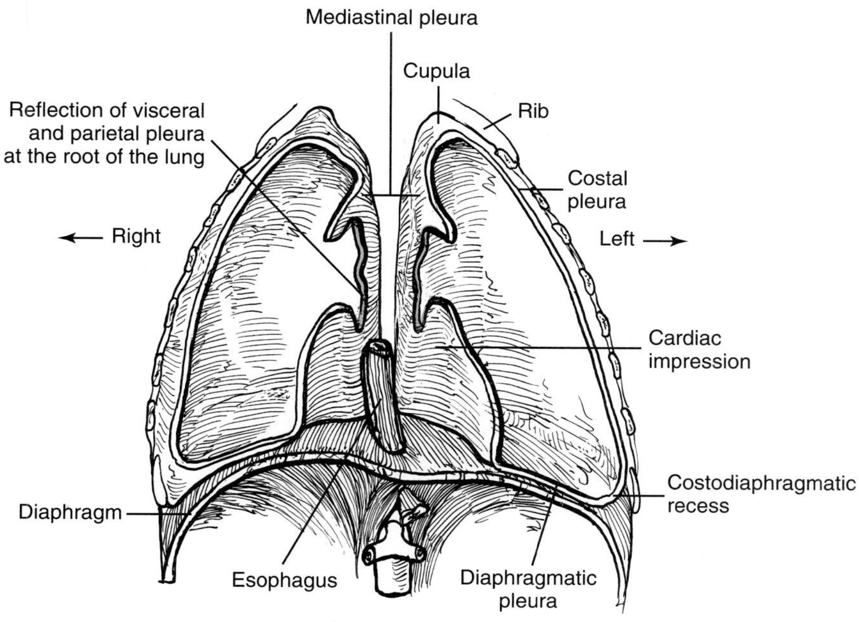

FIGURE 8–8
Parietal pleura and pleural recesses.

nerve, right recurrent laryngeal nerve, and **right sympathetic trunk** lie on the right side of the thoracic part of the trachea (Fig. 8–7). The **arch of the aorta, left common carotid** and **subclavian arteries, left vagus artery, left recurrent laryngeal nerve,** and **left sympathetic trunk** lie lateral to its left side (Fig. 8–7).

Cartilaginous "Rings" of the Trachea

Tracheal patency is maintained by 16–20 cartilaginous "rings"

The trachea is somewhat rounded anteriorly and flattened posteriorly. Its shape and patency are maintained by 16–20 incomplete cartilaginous "rings," which are shaped like horseshoes and are about 4 mm wide and 1 mm thick. These rings reinforce the anterior and lateral walls of the trachea (see Fig. 8–6*B*). The internal diameter of the trachea is less than 3 mm during the first year of life. During childhood and early adolescence, a maximum internal diameter of 9–16 mm is reached, with the measurement in millimeters corresponding roughly to the age of the child in years. Other components of the tracheal wall include connective tissue, smooth muscle, and epithelium of the tracheal lumen. These latter tissues are the only components of the posterior tracheal wall, as the tracheal cartilages are deficient in this region (see Fig. 8–6*B*).

The first tracheal cartilage is attached to the most inferior cartilage of the larynx, the **cricoid cartilage,** by a **cricotracheal ligament** (see Fig. 8–7*A*). Each tracheal cartilage is securely connected to the next by a **fibrous membrane** consisting mainly of collagen and elastin fibers. The most inferior tracheal cartilage is thicker and wider in the middle, forming a hook-shaped ridge, the **carina,** between the left and right principal bronchi (see Fig. 8–5).

Bifurcation of the Trachea

The **bifurcation of the trachea** into the left and right **principal bronchi** occurs at about the level of the **sternal angle (sternomanubrial joint),** demarcating the boundary between the superior and middle mediastina (see Figs. 7–3 and 8–7*A*). Further branching of the bronchi is described in the discussion of the lungs.

▲ The Definitive Lungs

Lung Roots and Membranes

The definitive lungs are suspended within the pleural cavities by lung roots

Each **lung root,** which consists mainly of the major bronchus and associated pulmonary vasculature, emerges from the left or right lateral wall of the mediastinum at about the level of vertebral bodies T5 to T7 posteriorly and rib 3 anteriorly (see Figs. 8–1 and 8–7*A*). Each lung is freely suspended by its root and almost fills its pleural cavity.

Each lung is completely invested by the **visceral pleura,** which is a thin, tough membrane (see below). The pleural cavities are lined by an apposed layer of **somatic (parietal) pleura** (Fig. 8–8). These are named the *costal, mediastinal,* and *diaphragmatic pleura* because they line the costal, mediastinal, and diaphragmatic surfaces of the pleural cavities (Fig. 8–8). The visceral and parietal pleura secrete a slippery serous fluid, which lubricates their surfaces (see above), allowing easy slippage of the lungs upon the inner walls of the pleural cavities during respiratory movements. The visceral and parietal pleura are continuous with each other in the region of the lung roots. A flap of pleura reflected inferiorly from each lung root is called the **pulmonary ligament** (see Figs. 8–9 and 8–11).

Shapes and Surfaces of the Lungs

The definitive lungs are cone shaped and have an apex; a base (diaphragmatic surface); mediastinal and costal surfaces; and anterior, posterior, and inferior borders

Each cone-shaped lung narrows toward its superior end into an **apex,** which extends superiorly above the anterior and lateral parts of the first rib within the superior region of the pleural cavity called the **cupula** (see Fig. 8–1). The **base** of each lung, the **diaphragmatic surface,** is concave, conforming precisely to the shape of the superior surface of the diaphragm (Fig. 8–9). Each lung has a **mediastinal (medial) surface,** which is apposed to the mediastinum, and a **costal surface,** which is apposed to the inner circumference of the entire rib cage from the

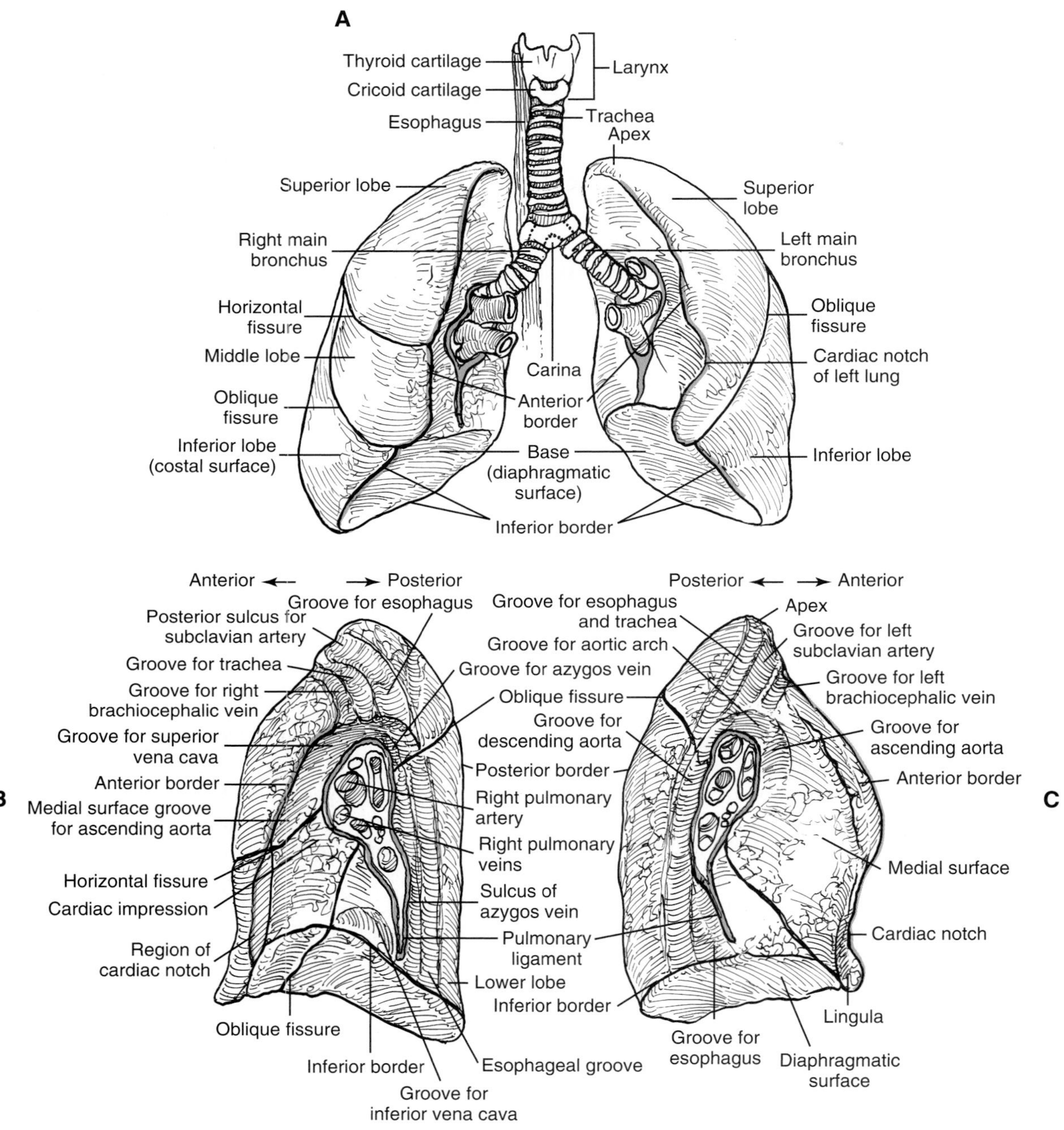

FIGURE 8–9

Surface features of the lungs. **A.** Frontal view of right and left lungs showing lobes and fissures. **B.** Medial view of right lung showing impressions of mediastinal organs. **C.** Medial view of left lung showing impressions of mediastinal organs.

heads of the ribs posteriorly to the distal ends of the ribs anteriorly. Each lung also has a sharply defined **inferior border,** an **anterior border,** and a more rounded **posterior border** (Fig. 8–9). The edge of each lung base (inferior border) extends into its costodiaphragmatic recess, and the anterior border of each lung extends into its costomediastinal recess (Fig. 8–9 and see Fig. 8–8).

The **medial surface** of each lung (Fig. 8–9) is contoured with the impressions of organs that protrude from the lateral walls of the mediastinum. For example, the medial surfaces of both lungs bear a **cardiac impression,** an impression of the heart. The cardiac impression on the right lung is primarily of the **right auricle,** a vestigial tag covering part of the anterolateral region of the **right atrium** (Fig. 8–9*B* and see Chapter 9). The cardiac impression on the left lung is primarily of the left side of the **left ventricle** and the **left auricle** (Fig. 8–9*C* and see Chapter 9). This cardiac impression of the left lung extends anteriorly, creating an indentation in the anterior border of the lung called the **cardiac notch** (Fig. 8–9*C*).

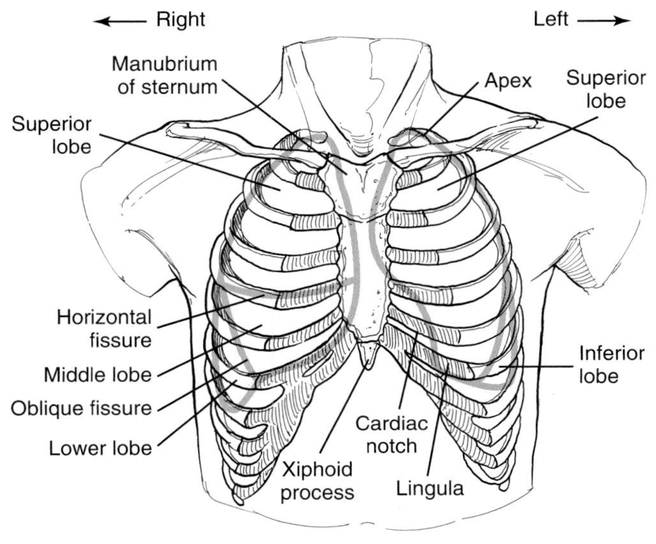

FIGURE 8–10
Projection of the lungs and their fissures onto the rib cage in quiet respiration.

The medial surface of the **left lung** bears impressions of the **arch of the aorta, descending aorta,** and **left subclavian artery** (Fig. 8–9*C*). The medial surface of the **right lung** bears impressions of the **esophagus** and arch of the **azygos vein,** which courses anteriorly to empty into the **superior vena cava** (Fig. 8–9*B*).

Other features of the medial surfaces of the lungs include the **hilum,** through which all vessels and nerves enter or depart, and **fissures** between the lung lobes. Because the **left lung** has **superior** and **inferior lobes** only, it has only a single **oblique fissure** (Fig. 8–9*C*). The **right lung,** in contrast, has **oblique** and **horizontal fissures** separating its **superior, middle,** and **inferior lobes** (Fig. 8–9*B*). The fissures of each lung are also apparent on their **costal surfaces** where they have relatively invariable spatial relationships to anterior thoracic skeletal landmarks (Fig. 8–10).

Structures That Pass Between the Mediastinum and the Lungs

Structures within each lung root enter the hilum and form branches that terminate in distal regions of the lung

The pulmonary ligament and reflected pleura covering each lung root (Fig. 8–11 and see Fig. 8–9) enclose

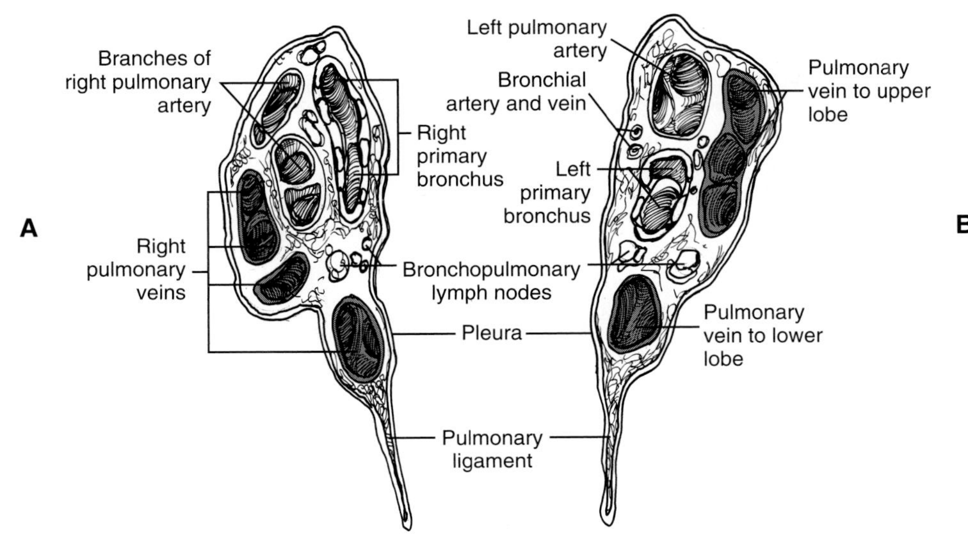

FIGURE 8–11
Lateral and medial views of the roots of the lungs and their contents. **A.** Lateral view of the right lung root. **B.** Lateral view of the left lung root.
Continued

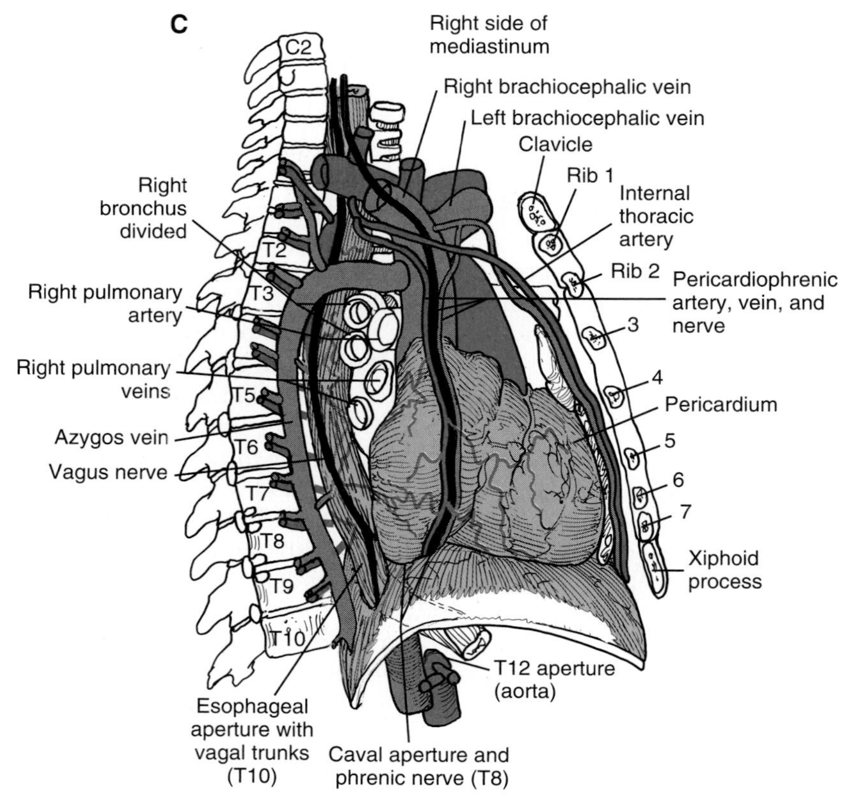

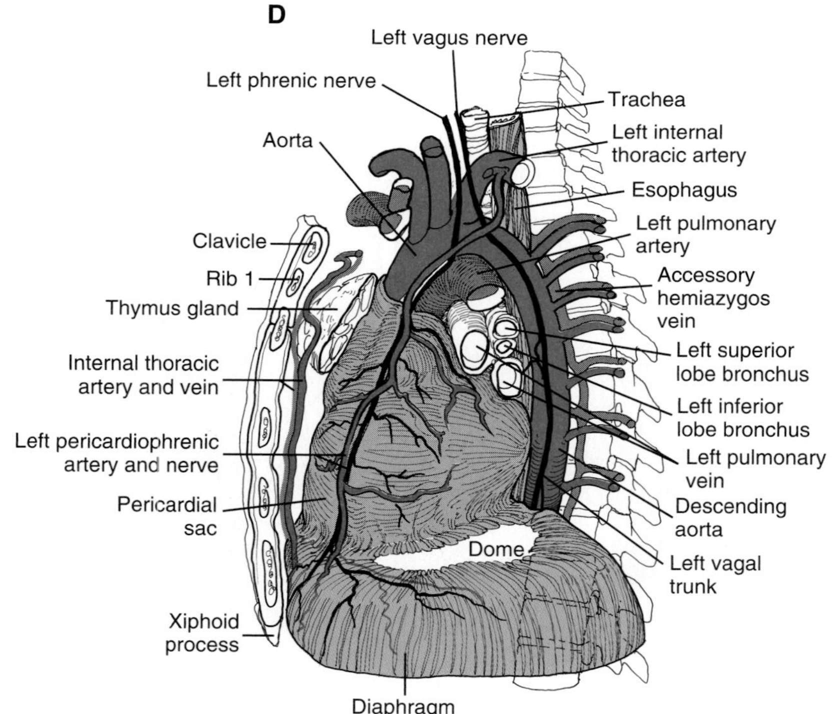

FIGURE 8–11, cont'd

C. Medial view of the right lung root and lateral wall of the mediastinum. **D.** Medial view of the left lung root and lateral wall of the mediastinum.

the supporting connective tissue and following structures that pass between the mediastinum and the lungs:

- principal bronchi,
- pulmonary arteries and veins,
- bronchial arteries and veins,
- autonomic and visceral afferent nerve fibers,
- lymphatic vessels and bronchopulmonary lymph nodes,
- connective tissue.

Structures within each lung root enter the medial surface of the lung at the hilum (Fig. 8–11 and see Fig. 8–9). Just as it enters the hilum of the right lung, the right principal bronchus gives off a **right superior lobe bronchus** (Fig. 8–11*A* and *C* and see Figs. 8–4 and 8–5). After it enters the lung, the continuation of the right principal bronchus (right intermediate bronchus) splits into a **right middle lobe bronchus** and **right inferior lobe bronchus.** The left principal bronchus branches into two secondary (lobar) bronchi, which serve the upper lobe **(left superior lobe bronchus)** and lower lobe **(left inferior lobe bronchus)** (Fig. 8–11*B* and *D* and see Figs. 8–4 and 8–5).

Primary Bronchi

Anatomic differences between the left and right primary bronchi predispose the right primary bronchus to aspiration of foreign objects

The **right principal,** or **primary, bronchus** is only about 2.5 cm in length. It enters the right lung at the level of vertebra T5 and is oriented in a somewhat vertical plane (see Figs. 8–4 and 8–5). The **left principal,** or **primary, bronchus** is about 5 cm long. It enters the lung at the level of vertebra T6 and is oriented in a more horizontal plane than the right principal bronchus. It is also smaller in diameter. As a consequence, foreign objects are more frequently aspirated into the right lung than the left lung.

Secondary Bronchi

The number of secondary bronchi branching from the left and right primary bronchi corresponds to the number of lobes in the left and right lungs

The right principal bronchus branches into three **lobar,** or **secondary, bronchi.** The first branch, the **right superior lobe bronchus,** branches from the right primary bronchus within the middle mediastinum, and the **middle** and **inferior lobe bronchi** bifurcate within the lung itself (see Figs. 8–4 and 8–5). The left principal bronchus bifurcates into two lobar bronchi after it enters the lung. These are the **left superior lobe bronchus** and **left inferior lobe bronchus** (see Figs. 8–4 and 8–5).

Tertiary Bronchi

The branches of lobar bronchi are distributed to independent functional units of the lungs called bronchopulmonary segments

Tertiary bronchi, which branch from lobar bronchi, are called **segmental bronchi** because they are distributed to the **bronchopulmonary segments,** which are subdivisions of each lung lobe (see discussion of lung development, above). Each bronchopulmonary segment is separated by a connective tissue sheath from adjacent segments. Therefore, a single segment may be surgically removed if disease is restricted to that segment only. Each bronchopulmonary segment is named and numbered for its relative position in the lung (see Fig. 8–4 and Table 8–1). There are usually 10 bronchopulmonary segments in each lung, even though the right lung has three lobes and the left two.

Terminal Bronchi, Bronchioles, and Alveoli

Approximately 11 more generations of branching produce the **terminal bronchi,** the smallest structures of the airways containing cartilaginous rings (Fig. 8–12 and see Fig. 8–5). Terminal bronchi branch into **lobular bronchioles,** which branch further into **terminal bronchioles,** which branch again into **respiratory bronchioles** (Fig. 8–12 and see Fig. 8–5). Bronchi and bronchioles are readily distinguished by two characteristics:

1. A **bronchus** is larger than 1 mm in diameter, and a **bronchiole,** which is more distal, is smaller than 1 mm in diameter.

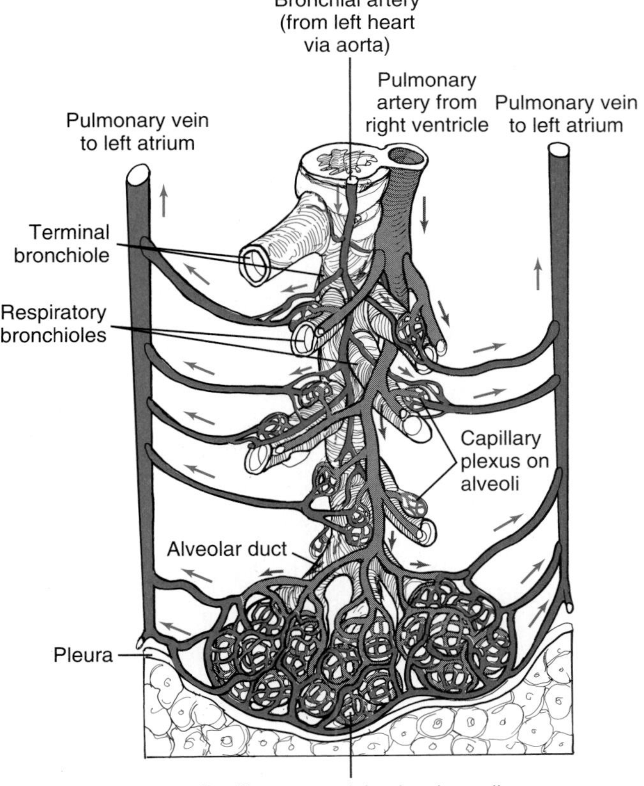

FIGURE 8–12
Pulmonary circulation within the lung.

2. Walls of the bronchi contain well-defined cartilaginous rings, but walls of the bronchioles do not (Fig. 8–12 and see Fig. 8–5).

The most distal branches of the bronchial tree, the **alveoli,** branch from respiratory bronchioles. These microscopic structures are the sites of respiratory gas exchange (Fig. 8–12 and see Fig. 8–5). It has been estimated that alveoli of the mature lungs provide as much as 900 square feet of surface area for the exchange of gases.

▲ Vasculature of the Lungs

Systemic Vasculature

The systemic vasculature serves the bronchial tree from the principal bronchi to the level of the respiratory bronchioles

The systemic circulation of the lung tissues, including parts of the bronchial tree from the principal bronchi to the respiratory bronchioles, is provided by systemic bronchial arteries and veins (Fig. 8–13). A single **right bronchial artery** usually branches from the **third posterior intercostal artery,** and two **left bronchial arteries** usually branch from the **dorsal aorta,** one near vertebra T5 and one inferior to the left principal bronchus (Fig. 8–13*A*). The two **bronchial veins** on the right branch from the **azygos vein,** and the two **bronchial veins** on the left branch from the **accessory hemiazygos vein** or from the **superior intercostal vein** (Fig. 8–13*B*). Thus, the bronchial arteries sprout from the dorsal aorta or its intercostal branches, and the bronchial veins from the azygos system of veins or their branches.

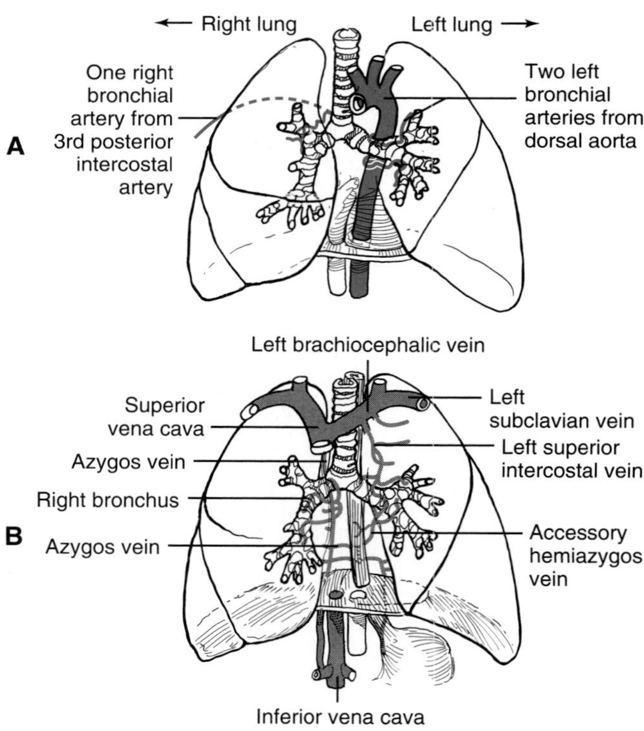

FIGURE 8–13
Vasculature of lung parenchyma and bronchi. **A.** Bronchial arteries. **B.** Bronchial veins.

During development, the presumptive bronchial arteries and veins grow into the lung buds to connect with distal networks of bronchial vessels that are developing within the mesoderm investing each lung (see Fig. 8–12). The pattern of development and branching of the bronchial arteries and veins follows the pattern of the bronchial tree. **Bronchial arteries** and **veins** usually supply and drain elements of the bronchial tree as distal as the **respiratory bronchioles** (see Fig. 8–12).

Pulmonary Vasculature

The pulmonary vasculature serves the alveoli only

The developing pulmonary vessels penetrate to the most distal regions of the lungs, but their primary functions are to carry carbon dioxide produced in the tissues to the alveoli for removal during expiration and to take up oxygen within the alveolar sacs for transport to the left atrium (see below). The roots of the **pulmonary arteries** sprout from the **fourth** and **sixth aortic arches** (see Chapter 9), and the **pulmonary veins** sprout from the left side of the **primitive atrium** of the developing heart. These sprouts anastomose with pulmonary vessels developing within the mesoderm surrounding the lung bud.

A single major pulmonary artery traverses the root of each lung to enter the hilum, and two major pulmonary veins also enter each lung (see Fig. 8–11). Although the pulmonary arteries and veins usually supply and drain the alveoli (see Fig. 8–12), anastomoses may occur between distal bronchial and pulmonary arterial branches so that some systemic bronchial blood may be returned to the left atrium of the heart directly through the pulmonary venous system (see Fig. 8–12). This may be an important consideration in lung transplantation because bronchial vessels are not usually reanastomosed in this procedure.

▲ Lymphatic Drainage of the Lungs

At the tracheobronchial nodes, lymphatic channels converge from deep and superficial regions of the lungs

Lymphatic channels draining the **lung parenchyma** accompany bronchial vessels back to the region of the hilum of each lung where they drain into **tracheobronchial lymph nodes** (Fig. 8–14). This group of nodes, from proximal to distal, includes **paratracheal nodes, superior tracheobronchial nodes, inferior tracheobronchial nodes, bronchopulmonary nodes,** and **pulmonary nodes** (Fig. 8–14).

Efferent lymphatic channels emanating from these nodes may drain into **parasternal** or **brachiocephalic nodes** or into major right or left lymphatic channels, including the **thoracic duct** (see Chapter 10). These major right and left lymphatic channels (including the thoracic duct) usually empty into the venous system at the junction of the subclavian and jugular veins on the right and left sides.

▲ Innervation of the Lungs

Autonomic Innervation

Autonomic innervation of pulmonary vessels, smooth muscle, and glands arises from the pulmonary plexus

Some of the postganglionic sympathetic fibers (see Chapter 4) that emanate from sympathetic ganglia of spinal nerves T2 to T6 as **cardiac nerves,** as well as postganglionic fibers emanating from cervical chain ganglia, course through the superior mediastinum to the region of the tracheal bifurcation. Here they join with preganglionic parasympathetic fibers from the **vagus nerve** to form a complex **pulmonary plexus** (Fig. 8–15). On the left side, this plexus includes fibers from the **left recurrent laryngeal nerve,** which is a branch of the vagus nerve.

Postganglionic sympathetic fibers and preganglionic parasympathetic fibers course from the pulmonary plexus along the pulmonary veins, arteries, and bronchi into the hilum of each lung. Here, preganglionic vagal fibers innervate small **peripheral ganglia.** From this point, postganglionic sympathetic and postganglionic parasympathetic fibers course into the lungs, branching to follow vessels and bronchioles to innervate the vascular and bronchial smooth muscle as well as mucous glands within the bronchi. These fibers also innervate vessels that terminate within the visceral pleura, but they do not innervate the visceral pleura itself.

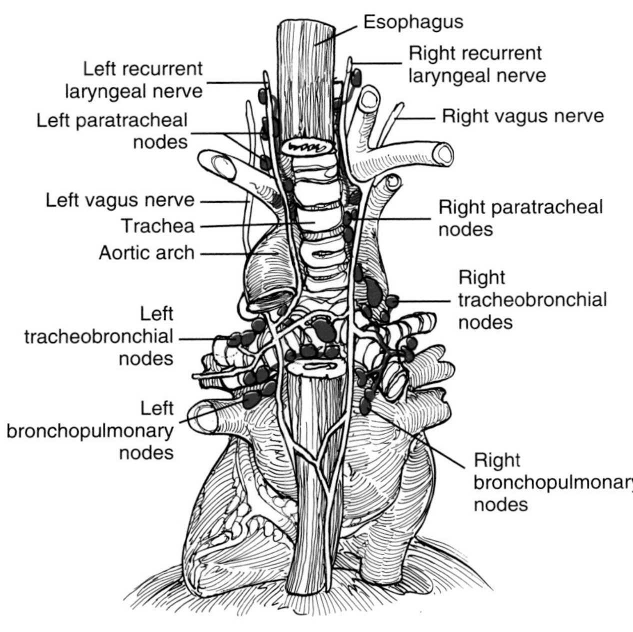

FIGURE 8–14
Tracheal and bronchial lymph nodes.

Sensory Innervation

Afferent visceral fibers that innervate a wide variety of sensory end-organs within the pulmonary mucosa and blood vessel walls carry afferent sensory impulses. These are carried mainly via visceral afferent fibers arising from neurons within sensory ganglia associated with the vagus nerve in the brainstem and afferent fibers (associated with sympathetic nerves) returning to levels T2 to T6 of the spinal cord through the dorsal root at each of these levels.

▲ Function of the Lungs: Regulation of the Respiratory Cycle

During quiet respiration, each respiratory cycle has an **inspiratory phase** that lasts about 1 second and an **expiratory phase** that lasts about 3 seconds. Inspiration of air through the nose and mouth, into the trachea and bronchi, and then into more distal regions of the bronchial tree occurs as contractions of inspiratory muscles increase the anteroposterior, lateral, and vertical dimensions of the pleural cavities (see Chapter 6 and Table 6–3). As inspiration is initiated, the pleural cavity expands and the level of pressure within the cavity is reduced, leading to reduction of pressure within the bronchial tree. During quiet inspiration, a negative pressure of −6 to −12 cm of water is generated by the action of the diaphragm. As a consequence, 500–700 ml of air passively enters the airways and there is an infe-

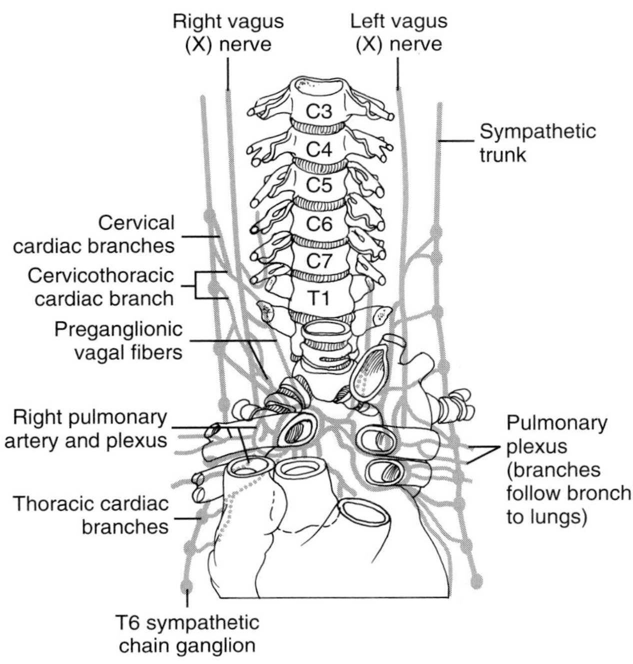

FIGURE 8–15
Parasympathetic (vagal) and sympathetic (cardiac) nerves innervation of the lung.

rior excursion of the diaphragm of approximately 1.5 cm. About 400 ml of air is delivered to the terminal alveoli, and approximately 150 ml remains within the **anatomic dead space** between the nose and terminal bronchioles. The dead space has several important functions, including humidification, warming, and filtering of air that is ultimately delivered to the alveoli. When additional respiratory muscles are recruited during forced inspiration (see below and Chapter 6), the negative pressure generated within the pleural cavities usually ranges from −12 to −18 cm of water and may even reach −40 cm of water for brief periods. Up to 4600 ml of air may be exchanged during each cycle of forced inspiration and expiration.

Neural Control of Respiration

A respiratory center within the brainstem controls the strength and rate of respiration

Three diffuse collections of neurons within the **medulla** and **pons** of the brainstem appear to regulate the respiratory cycle and are collectively called the **respiratory center.** The medulla and pons are regions of the hindbrain containing **nerve fiber tracts** and collections of neuronal cell bodies called **nuclei** that mainly relay activity between the spinal cord and higher brain centers in the cerebral cortex. A general description of the medulla and pons appears in Chapter 26.

One of the three collections of neurons of the respiratory center is called the **dorsal respiratory group,** or **inspiratory center** (Fig. 8–16). It is located in the dorsal region of the medulla and is specifically involved in the stimulation of inspiration. Another group of neurons, called the **pneumotaxic center,** is located in the superior part of the pons and regulates the duration of inspiration by inhibiting the inspiratory center. A third group of neurons is found in the ventral region of the medulla and is called the **ventral respiratory group.** This region regulates both inspiration and expiration, especially during forced respiration.

During quiet respiration, the cyclic activity of the inspiratory center usually stimulates **contraction of the inspiratory muscles** (see Table 6–3), chiefly the di-

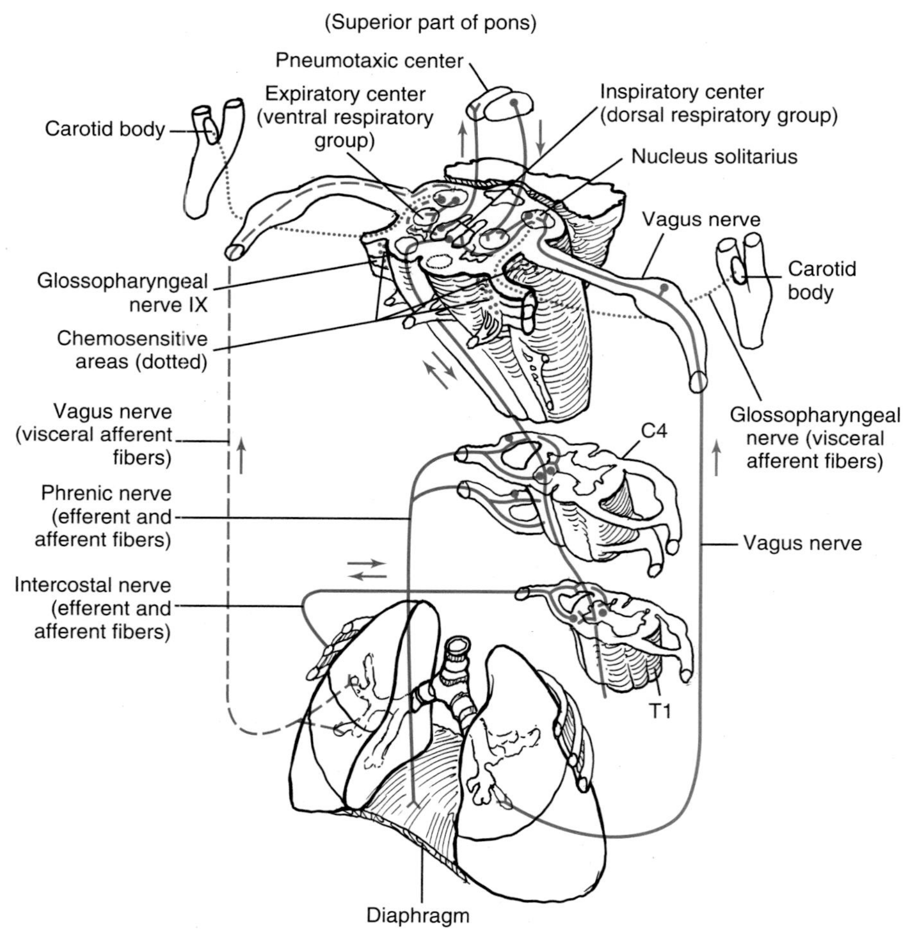

FIGURE 8–16
Reflex regulation of respiration.

aphragm (via the phrenic nerve), to induce an **inspiratory phase** of the cycle. Cessation of activity of the inspiratory center, imposed by activity of the pneumotaxic center, results in relaxation of the diaphragm and initiation of the **expiratory phase** through **passive recoil** of the thoracic wall and lungs.

The **innate rhythmic activity** of the respiratory center may be modified by stimuli from a **chemosensitive area** in the brainstem that can "measure" the concentration of hydrogen ions caused by the dissociation of carbonic acid (which occurs when carbon dioxide and water are combined) within the blood, interstitial fluid of the medulla, or cerebrospinal fluid. When the chemosensitive neurons sense that the concentration of hydrogen ions has risen, they stimulate the inspiratory center to increase the force of inspiration and to increase the rate of the respiratory cycle.

In addition, peripheral **chemosensory endings** in the great vessels and **stretch receptors** in the bronchial walls, lung parenchyma, and respiratory muscles also play important roles in the complex reflex regulation of respiration. For example, **rising carbon dioxide** or **hydrogen ion levels** in the blood stimulate specialized peripheral chemosensors in **carotid bodies** located at the junctions of internal and external carotid arteries or in **accessory carotid bodies** in the region of the aortic arch, right subclavian artery, and ligamentum arteriosum (see Chapter 9). Nervous impulses arising within these end-organs travel to the respiratory center in the brainstem via visceral afferent fibers associated with the glossopharyngeal or vagus nerves (Fig. 8–16 and see Chapter 26). Here, the activity of these sensory inputs stimulates the inspiratory center (via the nucleus solitarius), increasing the strength of inspiration and rate of the respiratory cycle (Fig. 8–16).

In addition, as the lung is **stretched** during deep inspiration, stretch receptors within the lung parenchyma are activated. Impulses are carried back to the inspiratory center via visceral afferent fibers within the vagus nerves, and this causes shortening of the inspiratory phase and increases the rate of respiration. The resistance against which the inspiratory and expiratory muscles work also varies during each sequence. However, a smooth, constant contractile force is maintained during contraction of these muscles **against different levels of resistance** through feedback between muscle spindles within the tendons of the respiratory muscles and the respiratory center. This process is called **load compensation.**

Sensory receptors within the right atrium also influence respiration by monitoring the **blood pressure** and **body temperature** (e.g., when they detect an increase in body temperature caused by fever, the respiratory rate is increased). **Conscious control of respiration** may also be influenced by higher brain centers.

Finally, in strenuous exercise, signals are transmitted from chemosensory end-organs to **ventral respiratory neurons** and the dorsal inspiratory center. Inspiratory neurons within the ventral respiratory center, along with neurons of the dorsal inspiratory center, cause the strength of the inspiratory phase and the rate of the respiratory cycle to increase. For example, in the inspiratory phase, accessory inspiratory muscles are recruited under these conditions (e.g., the scalene, pectoral, and sternocleidomastoid muscles are recruited to raise the upper ribs during the inspiratory phase) (see Table 6–2). With activation of expiratory neurons within the ventral respiratory center to initiate the expiratory phase, the internal and innermost intercostal muscles, abdominal muscles, and latissimus dorsi muscles are stimulated to actively reduce the volume of the pleural cavities (see Table 6–2).

Neural Control of the Airways in Respiration

Sympathetic and parasympathetic reflexes regulate the diameter of the airway

As respiratory muscles contract during forced inspiration, air passively enters the trachea via the nose, mouth, oral cavity, and pharynx. As incoming air increases the pressure on the walls of the airways, stretch receptors in the bronchial and bronchiolar walls are activated and send sensory impulses back to respiratory centers within the central nervous system via visceral afferent fibers associated with sympathetic pathways (within the pulmonary plexus and cardiac nerves). These signals trigger activity of the sympathetic pulmonary preganglionic neurons within the spinal cord, which transmit neural impulses back to smooth muscles of the airways via the cardiac nerves and pulmonary plexus. This results in the release of neurotransmitters called **catecholamines,** which cause the bronchial and bronchiolar smooth muscles to relax. This results in dilatation of the airways, increasing their capacity. This is the reason why the catecholamines **epinephrine** and **isoproterenol** are often administered exogenously to dilate the airways of patients who are asthmatic or suffering from allergic reactions.

As the bronchi and bronchioles stretch to their maximum diameter at the end of the inspiratory phase, stretch receptors innervated by visceral afferent fibers associated with the vagus nerve are activated. The resulting afferent signals return to respiratory centers in the brainstem to activate vagal motor neurons, which send impulses back to the airway walls via motor fibers of the vagus nerve. This results in release of the neurotransmitter **acetylcholine,** causing contraction of bronchial and bronchiolar smooth muscle. The consequent reduction in diameter of the airways prevents their overdistension and assists in expiration of air from the lungs as the striated respiratory muscles relax.

Absence of Autonomic Reflex Control in Patients Following Lung Transplantation. Elements of the complex reflex just described have been persuasively implicated in the control of respiration. It should be noted, however, that patients who have undergone lung transplantation and have no autonomic innervation of the lungs may still undertake strenuous exercise.

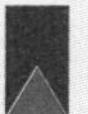

CLINICAL DISORDERS

Chronic Respiratory Disease

Respiratory airway disorders are common and costly

A significant number of individuals are affected by chronic respiratory diseases, which usually require constant medical treatment. These diseases may incapacitate an individual for varying periods or may be life threatening. Costs of treatment and lost productivity are significant.

Although respiratory diseases have diverse causes, they tend to be characterized by cough, chest pain (sharp or ill-defined), and dyspnea (shortness of breath). Ill-defined respiratory chest pain may be confused with cardiac pain (see Chapters 6 and 9).

Asthma

Asthma is the most common chronic disease of the airways

Asthma is characterized by periodic transient obstructions of the bronchioles. Obstructions may resolve spontaneously or following treatment with a catecholamine, which dilates the airways (see above). A small proportion of asthma patients dies each year as a direct consequence of inability to resolve the obstruction. The cause of asthma is unknown. Attacks are often initiated by an allergic reaction.

Chronic Obstructive Pulmonary Disease

Chronic obstructive pulmonary disease is a major cause of chronic disability and death

Chronic obstructive pulmonary disease is a general term describing a variety of pulmonary diseases characterized by reduced expiratory flow. Chronic bronchitis and emphysema are the two most common conditions associated with chronic obstructive pulmonary disease. The conditions present with similar symptoms. Typical symptoms include **barrel chest** (increased anterior or posterior dimension) and **hypertrophy of accessory respiratory muscles** (see Chapter 6).

Chronic Bronchitis. Chronic bronchitis is a cough that lasts at least 3 months a year for 2 consecutive years. It is characterized by excess mucous secretion in the larger airways. It may arise from cigarette smoking, air pollution, occupational exposure to toxic chemicals, or repeated pulmonary infection.

Emphysema. Emphysema is permanent enlargement of the alveoli accompanied by destruction of the alveolar walls. The ratio of alveolar surface area to lung volume diminishes as the alveoli fuse together and enlarge. It may result from cigarette smoking, exposure to air pollution, occupational exposure to toxic chemicals, or repeated pulmonary infection.

▲ Acute Pulmonary Disease

A variety of acute pulmonary diseases affect respiratory function

Acute Bronchitis

Acute bronchitis is a self-limiting, viral-induced inflammation of the trachea and bronchi occurring more frequently in the winter months. It may affect all ages and sexes but is more common in smokers and individuals suffering from chronic obstructive pulmonary disease or asthma. The condition is characterized by wheezing, coughing, fatigue, low-grade fever, and chest pain similar to heart pain. Bronchitis is usually self-limiting in healthy individuals.

Pneumonia

Pneumonia is a communicable acute respiratory infection of the bronchioles and alveoli (Fig. 8–17*A*). Fifteen to twenty percent of individuals affected must be hospitalized, and 10% of these die of the disease. Pneumonia arises from bacterial, viral, or fungal infections. The production of exudate results in coughing, dyspnea, sputum (sometimes bloody), chest pain, fever, and confusion.

▲ Tuberculosis

Tuberculosis is a bacterial disease communicated by prolonged exposure to individuals with an active case (see Fig. 8–17*B*). Immunocompromised and malnourished persons are at greatest risk. The incidence in the United States is rising as a consequence of the human immunodeficiency virus (HIV) epidemic and the emergence of new, more virulent strains of the tuberculosis bacteria.

Patients develop inactive tuberculosis initially. In 90–94% of cases, the disease never becomes active. Symptoms of **active tuberculosis** include weight loss, fatigue, intermittent fever, and more serious signs such as cough, production of sputum (which is frequently bloody), high fever and chills, dyspnea, pleural effusions, and chest pain (localized to the pleural cavities).

Antibiotic treatment has effectively replaced the "sanatorium," in which patients were isolated and given supportive treatment. A typical regimen of treatment includes a variety of antibiotics given over a period of several months. As has been noted, strains resistant to this strategy have begun to appear.

▲ Cystic Fibrosis

Cystic fibrosis is the most common lethal genetic disease in the United States

Mucous secretions from glands within the bronchial tree of individuals suffering from cystic fibrosis are unusually viscous and tend to block the smaller air passages. This results in **atelectasis,** the partial collapse of focal regions of lung tissue creating conditions favorable for bacterial infections and chronic bronchitis. Chronic necrotizing infection of the bronchi and bronchioles ensues, leading to permanent dilatation of the bronchioles. Successive bouts of pulmonary infection then lead to episodes of respiratory failure and death. Significant supportive strategies have been developed that have pushed the median survival age to 25 years, but there is no cure at the present time.

▲ Tumors of the Lungs and Airways

Several types of tumors may develop in the lungs and airways

A wide variety of benign and neoplastic tumors affect the lungs. The most common are malignant **bronchogenic carcinomas,** which are the leading single cause of cancer deaths in the United States. The typical patient is a male smoker between 45 and 75 years of age who has sought treatment for persistent coughing, dyspnea, or coughing up of blood. In most cases, these symptoms do not occur until the disease has progressed to an advanced stage, and the patient usually dies within 1 year. Unfortunately, rates of bronchogenic carcinoma have increased among females in recent years.

Tumors of the lung are often diagnosed through their **obstruction of** or **impingement on** adjacent structures. Tumors may obstruct blood flow within the superior vena cava, leading to cyanosis of the head and neck and even the upper limbs; an absence of venous pulsations in the neck; distension of the superficial veins of the upper thorax; and edema of the face, neck, upper limbs, and upper thoracic wall. Alternatively, lung tumors may impinge on neural elements within the thorax, such as the sympathetic trunk or cardiac plexus (see Chapter 9). In these instances, the patient may experience pain similar to that referred from the heart (see Chapters 6 and 9).

▲ Congenital Respiratory Disease of Newborn Infants

Congenital diseases of the lung compromise the respiratory function of newborn infants

Preterm infants have high rates of illness and death, chiefly because their lungs are not completely developed. Infants born before 28 weeks of gestation are especially prone to suffer from **respiratory distress syndrome** (pulmonary insufficiency accompanied by gasping and cyanosis) because the primitive alveoli have not yet formed. Infants born after 32 weeks are more likely to survive because this period is characterized by rapid differentiation of the alveoli. Nevertheless, respiratory function in these infants may be compromised because of insufficient production of **surfactant** (a mixture of phospholipids and proteins produced within the terminal airways that reduces surface tension within the alveoli). These infants may be treated with exogenous surfactant obtained from animals or from amniotic fluid, or with synthetic surfactant.

Respiratory insufficiency at birth may result from abnormal development of the bronchial tree. In some cases, the normal branching pattern is disrupted, resulting in defects as severe as **pulmonary agenesis** (total absence of a lung). Less severe anomalies of the branching process may result in defects that reduce the number of pulmonary segments or alveoli, a condition called **pulmonary hypoplasia.** More typically, pulmonary hypoplasia results from conditions that indirectly affect the growth of the lungs by reducing the size of the pleural cavities (e.g., **oligohydramnios,** or insufficiency of amniotic fluid). Reduction of the space within the pleural cavity is most commonly caused by congenital herniation of abdominal organs through a defect in the diaphragm (see Chapter 10).

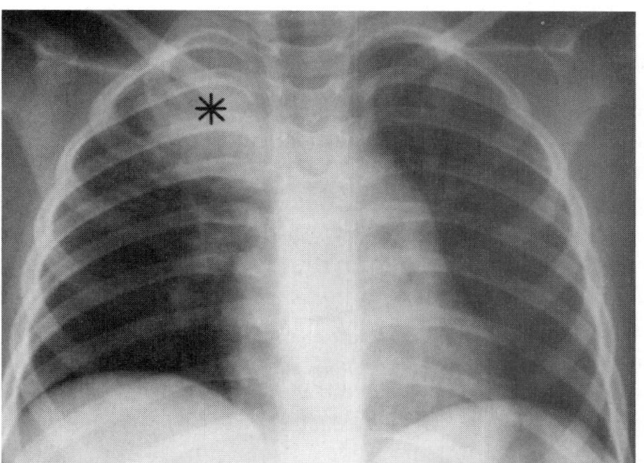

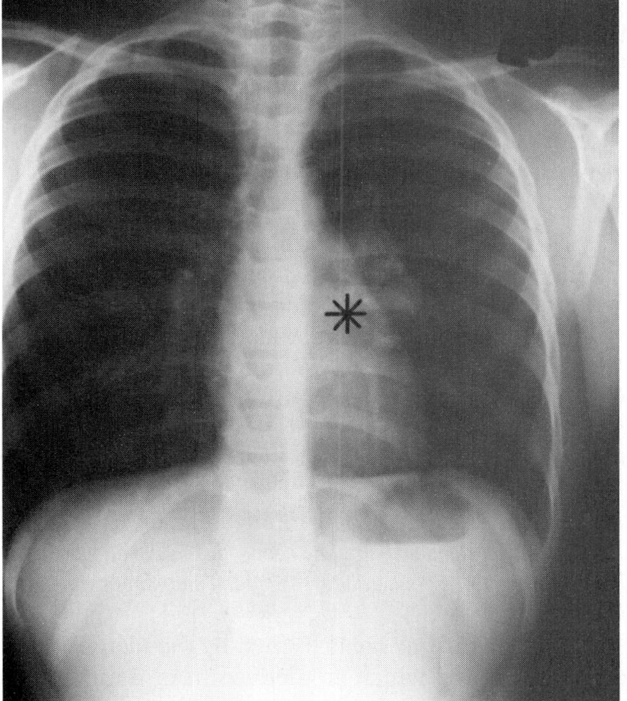

FIGURE 8–17
X-rays of infections of the lung. **A.** Pneumonia. Note the diffuse opacity in the superior lobe of the right lung *(*)*. ***B.*** Tuberculosis. Note the opaque bronchi near the root of the left lung *(*)*.

9 The Anterior, Middle, and Superior Mediastina; Cardiovascular System

Most of the structures located within the superior mediastinum and anterior and middle compartments of the inferior mediastinum serve the **cardiovascular system** (Table 9–1 and Fig. 9–1). Therefore, this chapter will focus mainly on cardiovascular anatomy, function, and disorders. Only a few structures are located within the **anterior mediastinum,** namely, the **thymus gland** or its vestiges, small vessels, and sternopericardial ligaments. The heart and its investing pericardial sac are the chief occupants of the **middle mediastinum.** Many structures within the **superior mediastinum** are accessories to the heart and lungs, including the great vessels, autonomic and somatic nervous elements, and portions of the airways. Contents of the **posterior mediastinum** are described in Chapter 10.

STRUCTURES OF THE ANTERIOR MEDIASTINUM

The anterior mediastinum is a subdivision of the inferior mediastinum lying just posterior to the sternal body and anterior to the pericardial sac

The anterior mediastinum is a shallow compartment containing only a few structures of note (Fig. 9–1 and see Fig. 9–2). These include:

- the **sternopericardial ligaments,**
- **thymus gland** or its **remnants,**
- **mediastinal branches of internal thoracic arteries** and **veins** and some **lymph nodes,** and
- **loose areolar tissue.**

Connective Tissues of the Pericardial Sac

The pericardial sac is stabilized by connective tissue attachments of its fibrous pericardium, mainly the sternopericardial ligaments

The **pericardial sac** is formed by the pleuropericardial membranes, which are derived from mesoderm of the lateral body wall (see Chapter 7). These coronal membranes at first separate the posterior pleural cavities from the definitive anterior pericardial cavity (see Fig. 7–1). However, as the roots of the pleuropericardial membranes move to a position just deep to the sternum, they form a sac that completely encircles the heart. Condensing connective tissue within the fibrous pericardium in the substernal region (anteriorly) forms strong **superior** and **inferior sternopericardial ligaments,** which provide firm attachments of the pericardial sac to the upper and lower regions of the sternal body (Fig. 9–2).

Further stability of the pericardial sac with its enclosed heart is provided by firm connections between the fibrous pericardium and central tendon of the diaphragm inferiorly (see Chapter 10) and between the fibrous pericardium and connective tissue within the walls of the great vessels superiorly.

Thymus Gland

The inferior end of the thymus gland or its remnants may also be found within the anterior mediastinum

The **thymus gland** initially develops from tissue associated with the paired third pharyngeal pouches of the embryonic pharynx from a region of the pharyngeal wall just inferior to the developing palatine tonsils (see Chapter 20). The thymic primordia, however, detach and migrate inferiorly to a location just deep to the sternum, forming the definitive thymus gland (Fig. 9–2).

The thymus gland is primarily active in childhood as a major organ of the lymphoid system. In prepubertal children, the gland grows and may ultimately weigh as much as 40 g. It may extend inferiorly to the fourth costal cartilage within the anterior mediastinum and superiorly to the level of the thyroid gland in the neck. After puberty, however, the gland typically involutes and is slowly replaced by fat. By the time an adult reaches middle age, the thymic remnant may weigh only about 10 g.

STRUCTURES OF THE MIDDLE MEDIASTINUM

Pericardial Sac and Pericardial Cavity

The pericardial sac segregates the heart from other mediastinal organs

As was described in Chapter 7, the **pericardial sac** is formed as the medial edges of the pleuropericardial folds fuse with each other *and* with mesoderm surrounding the esophagus. Then, as their lateral roots are

TABLE 9–1
Structures of the Anterior, Middle, and Superior Mediastina

STRUCTURES OF THE ANTERIOR MEDIASTINUM

- Sternopericardial ligaments
- Inferior end of thymus gland or its remnants
- Mediastinal branches of internal thoracic arteries and veins
- Lymph nodes
- Loose areolar tissue

STRUCTURES OF THE MIDDLE MEDIASTINUM

- Pericardial sac
- Pericardial cavity
- Heart
    - Right and left coronary arteries
    - Great, middle, and small cardiac veins
    - Coronary sinus
    - Right and left atria
    - Right and left ventricles
    - Cardiac skeleton
    - Pacemaker and conduction system
        - Sinoatrial node (pacemaker)
        - Atrioventricular node
        - Atrioventricular bundle
        - Ventricular plexuses of Purkinje's fibers
    - Sympathetic and parasympathetic nerves
    - Visceral afferent fibers
- Great vessels of pulmonary circulation
    - Left and right pulmonary veins
    - Pulmonary trunk
    - Proximal portions of left and right pulmonary arteries
    - Pulmonary plexus
    - Posterior portion of cardiac plexus
    - Root of left recurrent laryngeal nerve
    - Ligamentum arteriosum

STRUCTURES OF THE MIDDLE MEDIASTINUM—cont'd

- Ascending aorta
- Inferior portion of superior vena cava
- Terminal region of azygos vein
- Root of inferior vena cava
- Major channels of airways serving lungs
    - Bifurcation of trachea
    - Left and right primary bronchi

STRUCTURES OF THE SUPERIOR MEDIASTINUM

- Arch of aorta
- Arteries
    - Brachiocephalic artery
    - Root of left common carotid artery
    - Root of left subclavian artery
- Veins
    - Left and right brachiocephalic veins
    - Superior portion of superior vena cava
- Nerves
    - Vagus nerve
    - Cardiac nerves
    - Phrenic nerves
    - Left recurrent laryngeal nerves
- Airways
    - Trachea
    - Superior end of esophagus
- Superior end of thoracic duct
- Superior end of thymus gland or its remnants
- Lymph nodes
    - Peritracheal lymph nodes
    - Brachiocephalic lymph nodes
    - Tracheobronchial lymph nodes

displaced to an anterior location just deep to the sternum, the sac encloses the heart within the **definitive pericardial cavity** (Fig. 9–3).

Initially, the heart tube is straight and the entire posterior midline of the straight heart tube is suspended from the posterior wall of the pericardial sac by a dorsal mesentery consisting of reflected pericardium. Later, this mesentery ruptures so that the remaining dorsal mesentery is reflected onto the parietal pericardium of the posterior wall of the pericardial sac only in the region of the roots of the presumptive vena cavae and pulmonary veins and the aorta and pulmonary trunk. As the heart tube undergoes a looping step (bringing the precursors of the presumptive heart chambers into their definitive anatomic position [see below]), the outline of this reflected mesentery is described by an upside-down L in the region where the major veins enter the pericardial cavity (Fig. 9–4). A more superior complex of reflected pericardium is located at the roots of the aortic and pulmonary trunks (Fig. 9–4*B*). Thus, while the heart tube folds, these connections and pericardial reflections partially isolate two subregions of the pericardial cavity just posterior to the heart: the **transverse pericardial sinus** and **oblique pericardial sinus** (Fig. 9–4*B*).

Both the parietal and visceral pericardia secrete a slippery **serous fluid,** which allows the beating heart to slide easily against the inner wall of the pericardial sac. Normally, the pericardial sac contains 30–40 ml of serous fluid. As in the case of the pleural cavity, negative pressure within the pericardial cavity ensures close contact between the surface of the heart and inner lining of the pericardial sac.

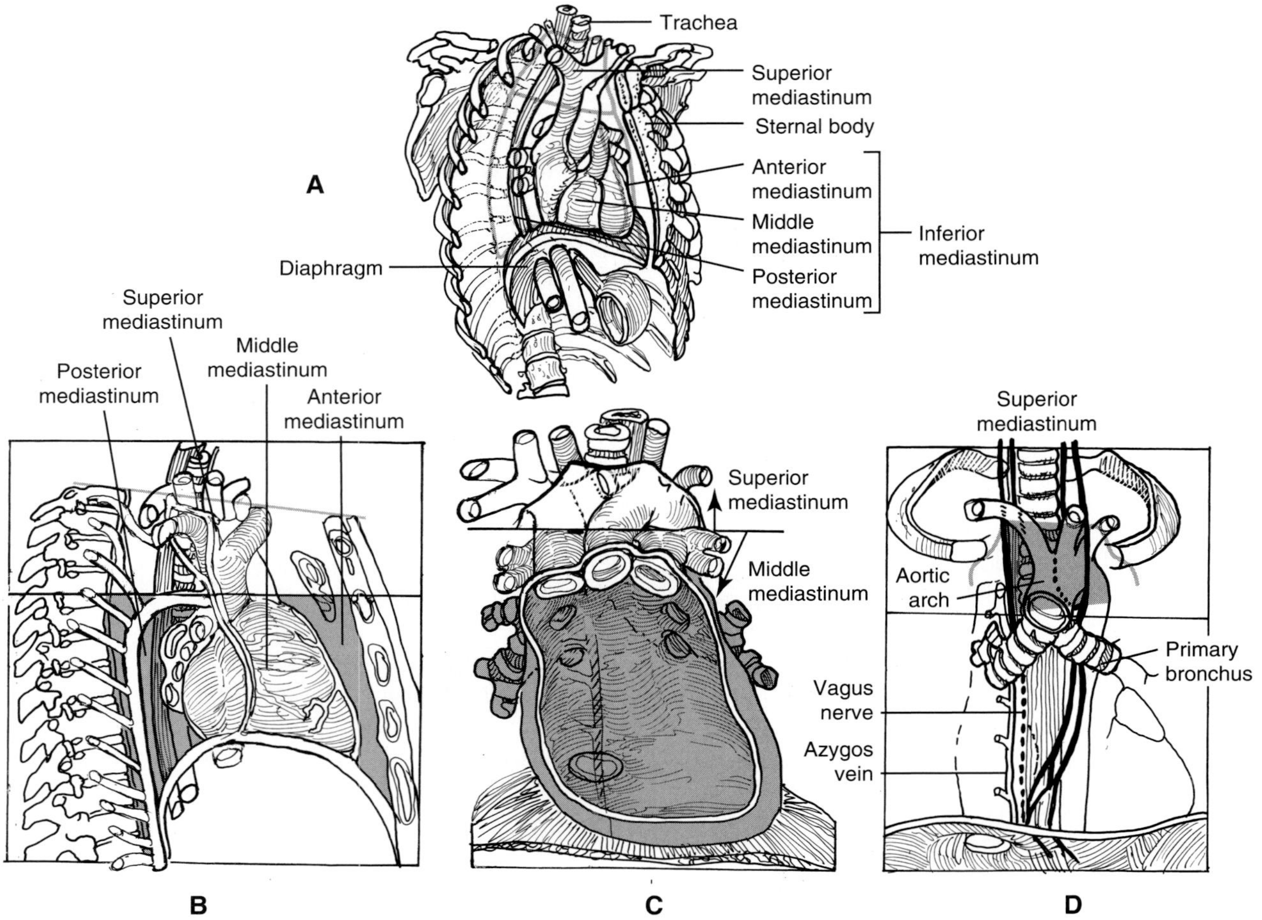

FIGURE 9–1
Regions of mediastinum.

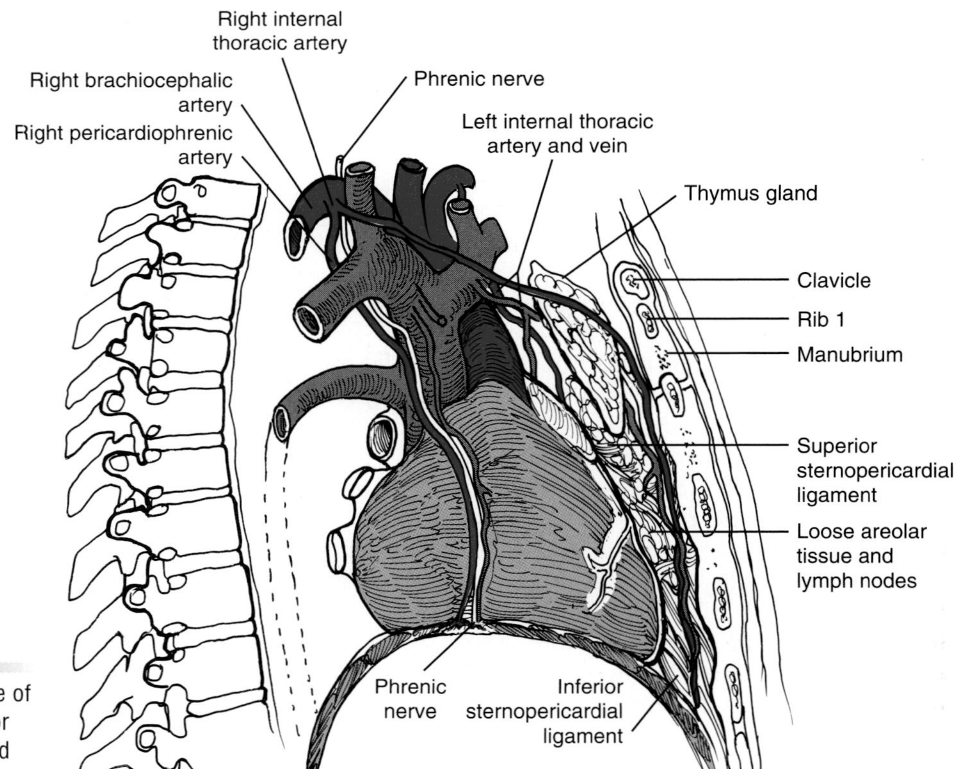

FIGURE 9–2
Medial view showing right lateral surface of the mediastinum and contents of anterior mediastinum, including the thymus gland and sternopericardial ligaments.

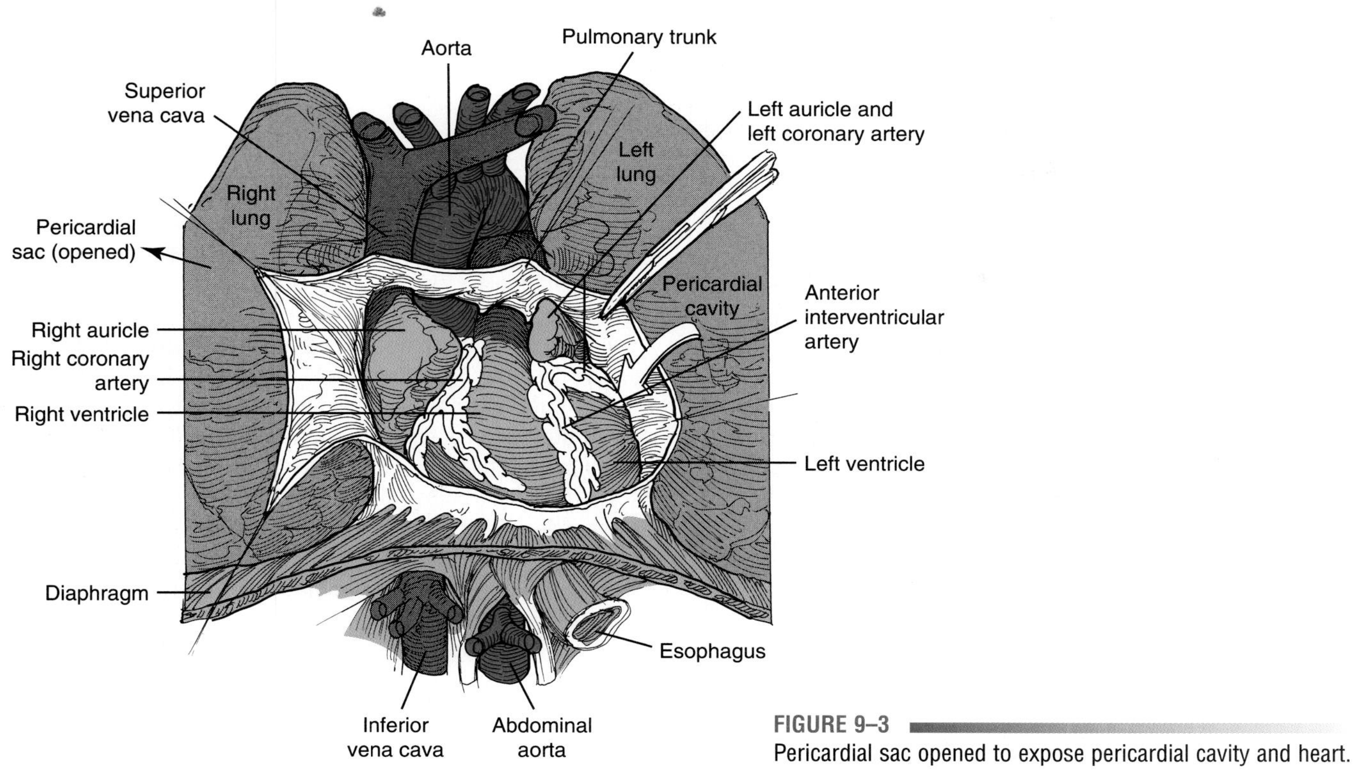

FIGURE 9–3
Pericardial sac opened to expose pericardial cavity and heart.

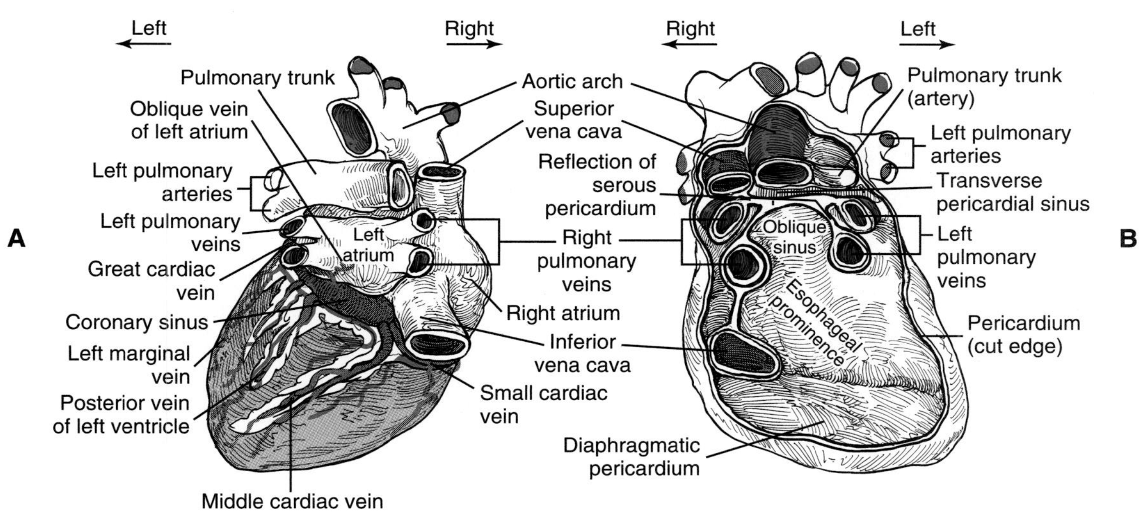

FIGURE 9–4
Heart removed from pericardial sac to reveal reflections of parietal and visceral pericardium (epicardium) and oblique and transverse pericardial sinuses. **A.** Posterior view of heart. **B.** Anterior view of heart (posterior wall of pericardial sac).

The pericardial sac is vascularized by branches of the **internal thoracic artery** and **vein** called **pericardiophrenic arteries** and **veins** (Figs. 9–2 and 9–5). As is suggested by their names, these vessels also serve the diaphragm (see Chapter 10). The pericardial sac is innervated by visceral afferent fibers associated with the **phrenic nerves,** which course within the **fibrous pericardium** (Fig. 9–5). The pericardial sac is also innervated by the vagus and cardiac nerves, including the visceral afferent fibers (see below). These visceral afferent fibers mainly innervate the parietal layer of the pericardium. The afferent fibers within the cardiac nerves carry afferent impulses to upper thoracic regions of the spinal cord (see fol-

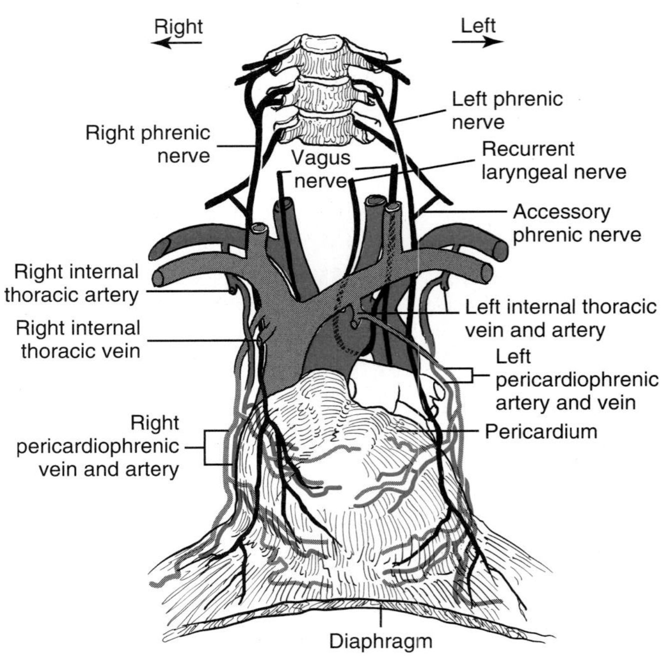

FIGURE 9–5
Innervation and blood supply to pericardial sac.

lowing discussion of referred pain from the pericardium, below).

Pericardial Disease

Pericardial disease affects the pericardial sac and has a wide range of severity

Pericarditis. Infectious agents, radiation therapy, and trauma can give rise to **acute pericarditis** (inflammation of the pericardium). This condition often results in **angina pectoris** because visceral afferents that accompany the sympathetic innervation (cardiac nerves) of the pericardium arise from dorsal root ganglia at spinal cord levels T1 to T4.

Constrictive pericarditis results in thickening of the pericardium through fibrosis and calcification (Fig. 9–6*A*). Trauma, tuberculosis or other infections, or radiation therapy can give rise to constrictive pericarditis, although, in many cases, the actual cause is not known. The pressure necessary to fill the heart during diastole is elevated, resulting in venous congestion. Constrictive pericarditis may be treated by complete removal of the pericardium.

Pericardial Effusion. Production of excess pericardial fluid (pericardial effusion) results in an increase in pres-

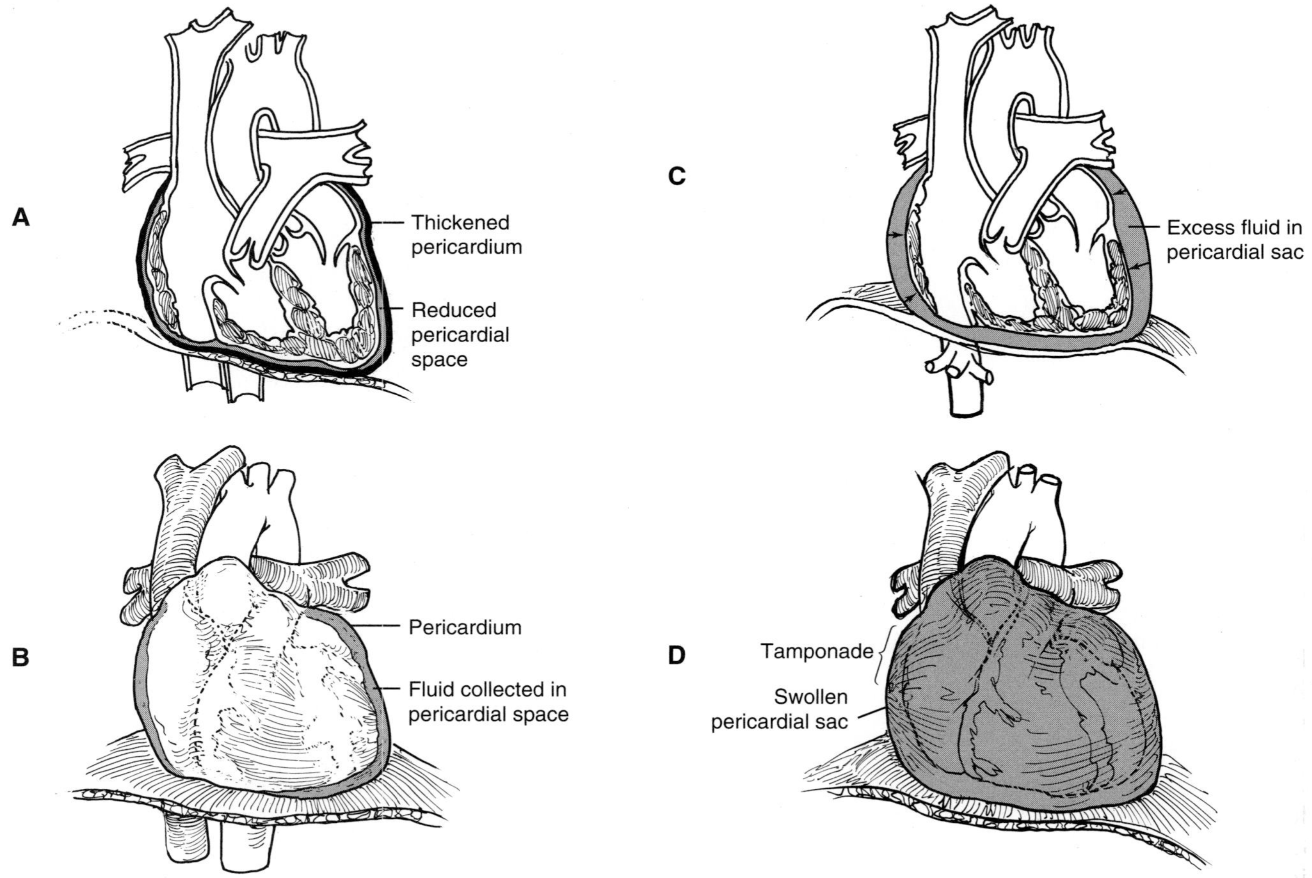

A
Thickened pericardium
Reduced pericardial space

C
Excess fluid in pericardial sac

B
Pericardium
Fluid collected in pericardial space

D
Tamponade
Swollen pericardial sac

FIGURE 9–6
Diseases of the pericardium. **A.** Constrictive pericarditis. **B.** Pericardial effusion. **C** and **D.** Cardiac tamponade.

sure within the pericardium (Fig. 9–6*B*). Slight pressure increases of 3 to 4 mm Hg do not result in symptoms, but higher pressures may interfere with refilling of the heart. **Cardiac tamponade** results when the pressure within the pericardium approaches the level of the pressure of the returning venous blood, significantly inhibiting the flow of blood into the heart during diastole (Fig. 9–6*C* and *D*). Severe cases of cardiac tamponade are life threatening. Excess fluid may be removed by passing a needle into the pericardial cavity via the fifth or sixth intercostal space near the sternum or in the region of the left costoxiphoid angle.

HEART

Development of the Heart

The heart arises from a simple longitudinal tube; definitive cardiac chambers are created by looping and septation of the primary heart tube

Initially, the longitudinal primary heart tube has symmetric left and right inflow tracts at its inferior end and symmetric left and right outflow tracts at its superior end. Soon after its formation, the tube folds asymmetrically via **cardiac looping.** This moves the presumptive cardiac chambers into their definitive positions and causes the inflow vessels to be translocated superiorly and posteriorly.

After an infant is born, all of the systemic blood in the definitive heart drains into the right atrium and all of the pulmonary blood drains into the left atrium. The inflow vessels on the left side of the heart are, therefore, remodeled to form the **oblique vein of the left atrium** and **coronary sinus,** which drain only the heart wall (see descriptions of coronary circulation and structures of the superior mediastinum, below). Inflow vessels on the right side become the **superior** and **inferior vena cavae** (see below).

The definitive atrial chambers become partially separated from each other in embryonic and fetal life by the development of two incomplete atrial septa: the **septum primum** and **septum secundum.** The thin-walled septum primum has a superior opening called the **ostium secundum,** and the septum secundum has an inferior opening called the **foramen ovale** (see Fig. 9–18*A*). During embryonic and fetal life, blood is shunted from the right atrium to the left atrium through these two foramina (see below). Blood that is shunted into the right ventricle from the right atrium, however, does not reach the pulmonary circulation because, upon ejection into the pulmonary trunk, it is shunted to the aorta through a special shunt called the **ductus arteriosus** (see Fig. 9–18*A* and Structures of the Superior Mediastinum and descriptions of heart function, below).

In the late embryonic period, at 7 to 8 weeks of life, the membranous ventricular septum spirals within the initially single outflow tract as it grows, separating the left and right ventricles and the aorta and pulmonary trunk from each other. Thus, the aorta and pulmonary trunk are twisted around each other in the definitive heart.

Shapes, Surfaces, and Borders of the Heart

Descriptions of the shape and surface anatomy of the definitive heart are useful for clinical diagnosis

The location and pattern of internal cardiac structures, such as the heart **valves** and **septa,** and external structures, such as coronary **arteries** and cardiac **veins,** can be appreciated by relating them to specific regions of the heart's surface and borders. Projection of specific **cardiac surfaces** onto bony landmarks of the body wall is also a way of localizing internal cardiac elements for several clinical procedures, including auscultation, biopsy, and cardiac imaging (Tables 9–1 and 9–2) (see below).

The heart is shaped like a slightly deformed cone, with its **base** projecting posteriorly and to the right and its **apex** pointing to the left (Fig. 9–7*A* and *B*). Other surfaces of the heart are the **anterior (sternocostal) surface, inferior (diaphragmatic) surface** (which rests upon the diaphragm), **right surface** (consisting of the rounded right lateral edge of the heart), and **left surface** (consisting mainly of the leftward-facing posterior wall of the apex) (Fig. 9–7*A* and *B*). It should be noted that the base of the heart does not lie upon the diaphragm, as does the base of each lung; rather, the **inferior surface** of the heart lies upon

TABLE 9–2
Shapes, Surfaces, and Borders of the Heart

SHAPES

- Cone-shaped structure
- Apex points to the left
- Base faces posteriorly and to the right

SURFACES

- Anterior (sternocostal) surface
- Inferior (diaphragmatic) surface (rests upon the diaphragm)
- Right surface (rounded right lateral edge of heart)
- Left surface (left-facing posterior wall of heart)

BORDERS

- Left border (left ventricle and portion of left auricle)
- Right border (right atrium)
- Inferior border (right ventricle and portion of left ventricle)
- Superior border (right and left auricles and superior portion of right ventricle)

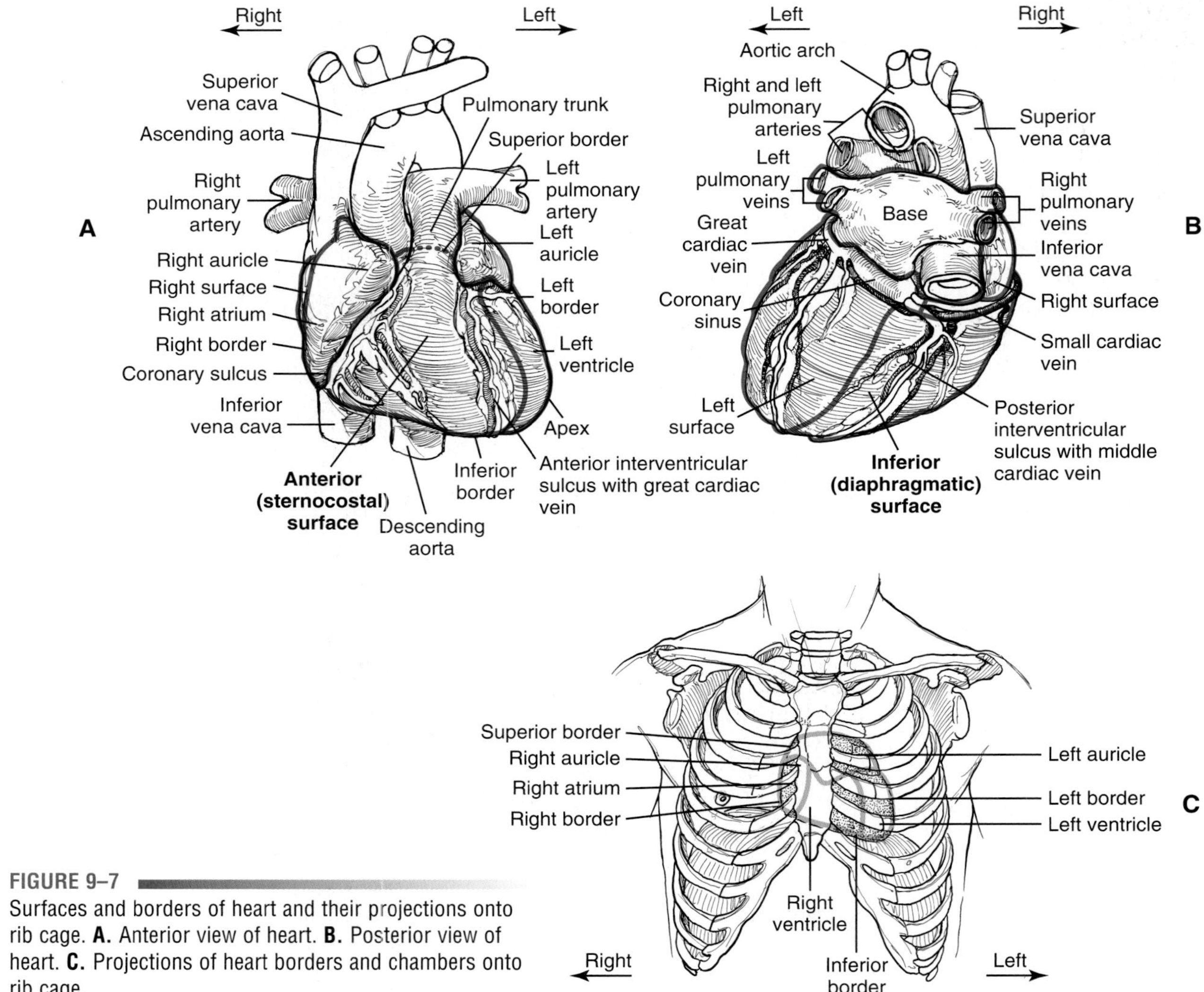

FIGURE 9–7
Surfaces and borders of heart and their projections onto rib cage. **A.** Anterior view of heart. **B.** Posterior view of heart. **C.** Projections of heart borders and chambers onto rib cage.

the diaphragm. The **base** of the heart is defined as the base of the cone with which the general shape of the heart is compared (Fig. 9–7*A* and *B*). It consists mainly of the rightward-facing posterior wall of the left atrium but includes a strip of the posterior wall of the right atrium and small portions of the superior parts of the right and left ventricles. The base of the heart is an important anatomic entity because all of the great vessels emanate from this geometrically defined region (Fig. 9–7), including, superiorly, the **pulmonary trunk, aorta,** and **superior vena cava;** posteriorly, the two **right** and two **left pulmonary veins;** and inferiorly, the **inferior vena cava.**

The **apex** of the heart consists mainly of the left ventricle and a portion of the right ventricle, but the heart's **anterior surface** includes major contributions from the walls of both ventricular chambers (Fig. 9–7). In addition, a small region of the left auricle, the right auricle, and a portion of the anterior wall of the right atrium also contribute to the anterior surface. The **right surface** of the heart consists of the right lateral wall of the right atrium (Fig. 9–7), and the **left surface** consists of the leftward-facing posterior wall of the left ventricle (Fig. 9–7). The **inferior surface** of the heart consists of the inferior walls of the right and left ventricles (Fig. 9–7).

The four borders of the heart are also useful landmarks of cardiac anatomy

The heart has four distinct borders: **left, right, inferior,** and **superior borders** (Fig. 9–7 and Table 9–2). All of these borders together define the anterior outline, or projection, of the heart on the inner surface of the rib cage (Fig. 9–7*C*). The **left border** outlines the left ventricle and a portion of the left auricle; the **right border** is defined by the right atrium; the **inferior border** is essentially defined by the right ventricle but includes part of the left ventricle; and the **superior border** is defined by both the right and left auricles and the superior part of the right ventricle (Fig. 9–7).

TABLE 9–3
Regions of the Heart, Their Sulci, and Their Typical Patterns of Vasculature

	STRUCTURES WITHIN SURFACE OR SUBREGION	
Surface or Subregion	**Wall or Sulcus**	**Vessels**
Anterior surface	Anterior wall of right auricle	
	Anterior wall of right atrium	Sinoatrial artery, right atrial arteries, anterior cardiac veins
	Anterior wall of left auricle	
	Anterior wall of left atrium	Left atrial arteries
	Coronary sulcus	Right coronary artery, small cardiac vein (on right side), left coronary artery, circumflex artery, great cardiac vein (on left side)
	Anterior wall of right ventricle	Conal branch of right coronary artery, right anterior ventricular arteries, anterior cardiac veins, right marginal artery, right marginal vein
	Anterior wall of left ventricle	Diagonal artery
	Anterior interventricular sulcus	Anterior interventricular artery, great cardiac vein
Right surface	Right wall of right atrium	
	Coronary sulcus	Right coronary artery, small cardiac vein
Base	Small posterior strip of right atrium	Superior vena cava, inferior vena cava
	Rightward-facing posterior wall of left atrium	Right and left pulmonary veins, oblique vein of left atrium
	Superior end of left ventricle	Aorta
	Superior end of right ventricle	Pulmonary trunk
Left surface	Leftward-facing posterior wall of left ventricle	Left marginal vein, posterior vein of left ventricle
	Coronary sulcus	Coronary sinus, great cardiac vein, circumflex artery, atrioventricular nodal artery
Inferior surface	Inferior wall of left ventricle	
	Inferior wall of right ventricle	
	Coronary sulcus	Coronary sinus, small cardiac vein
	Posterior interventricular sulcus	Posterior interventricular artery, middle cardiac vein

▲ Sulci

The surface of the heart contains a system of intrinsic grooves (sulci)

The **sulci** are surface indicators of intrinsic divisions between the underlying four chambers of the heart. They are also important as surface landmarks because major arteries and veins course within them (Fig. 9–7 and Table 9–3).

The **coronary (atrioventricular) sulcus** separates the atria from the ventricles and contains the main trunks of the right and left coronary arteries (Figs. 9–7 and 9–8). It encircles the heart at the level of the paired atrioventricular canals (Fig. 9–8). To appreciate the anatomy of the coronary sulcus, the student should begin to examine the anterior surface of the heart (Fig. 9–7*A*). The coronary sulcus may be observed just anterior to the root of the aorta. From this point, it descends to the right, just inferior to the **right auricle** and superior to the **right ventricle** (Figs. 9–7*A* and 9–8*A*). It then loops posteriorly around the right border onto the posteroinferior region of the right surface, just inferior to the root of the **inferior vena cava** (Figs. 9–7*B* and 9–8*B*). In a posteroinferior view of the heart (Fig. 9–7), the posterior region of the coronary sulcus is visible. At first, it ascends to the left along the border between the **right atrium** and **right ventricle** (on the inferior surface) and then along the border between the **left atrium** and **left ventricle** (on the left surface). If the heart is turned so that one can directly view the superior part of its left border, the coronary sulcus can be observed looping anteriorly around the **left auricle** onto the anterior surface (Figs. 9–7 and 9–8). Finally, if one views the anterior surface of the heart again (Fig. 9–7*A*), the coronary sulcus is apparent as it courses to the right, just anterior to the base of the **pulmonary trunk,** back to its starting point at the root of the **aorta.** The coronary sulcus, therefore, encircles the heart like the rim of a crown (Figs. 9–7 and 9–8), and this feature gives it its name.

The internal partition between the right and left atria, the **atrial** or **interatrial septum,** is demarcated by a faint surface groove on the **base of the heart.** This is the **interatrial sulcus,** which is barely perceptible between the left and right atria in posterior views of the heart (see Fig. 9–7*B*). Its position roughly corresponds to the reflection of pericardium demarcating the right superior limit of the **oblique pericardial sinus** on the right side of the heart base. Inferiorly, the interatrial sulcus intersects the coronary sulcus just to the left of the root of the inferior vena cava.

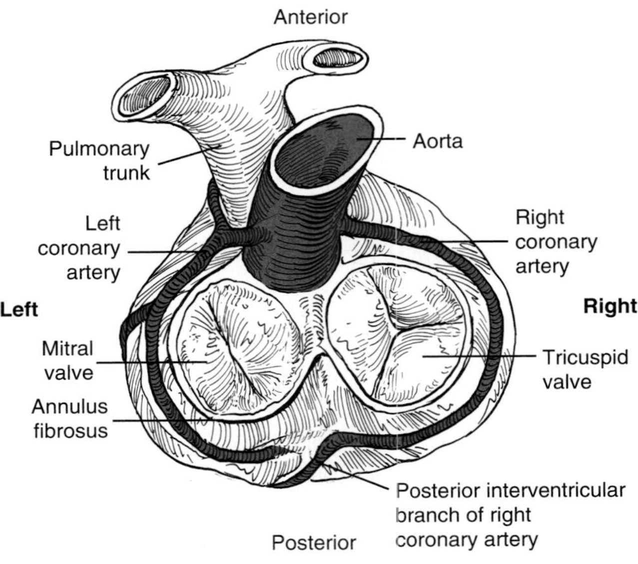

FIGURE 9–8
Superior view of heart showing right and left coronary arteries of a right dominant heart (posterior descending artery is a branch of the right coronary artery). Notice how the coronary arteries encircle the heart like a crown within the coronary sulcus.

On the anterior surface of the heart, the **anterior interventricular sulcus** demarcates the internal partition between the left and right ventricles, the **ventricular septum** (see Fig. 9–7*A*). This groove descends from the region of the **left auricle** toward the **apex** of the heart and then loops around the apex onto the **inferior surface** as the **posterior interventricular sulcus.** In posteroinferior views of the heart (see Fig. 9–7*B*), the posterior interventricular sulcus is seen to course upon the inferior surface from the **apex** to the right to intersect with the **coronary sulcus.** It should, thus, be noted that the posterior interventricular sulcus is actually located on the inferior heart surface and, for this reason, is sometimes called the **inferior interventricular sulcus.**

Arteries of the Heart

Patterns of coronary vasculature are best understood in relation to the heart's surface anatomy because sulci provide conduits for major blood vessels of the heart

In most persons, only two major **coronary arteries** emanate from the root of the aorta and course within the heart sulci to distribute their highly oxygenated blood to the heart muscle through an extensive system of arterioles and capillary beds (Fig. 9–8 and Table 9–3).

The **right coronary artery** branches from the root of the aorta just superior to the right **cusp** of the **aortic semilunar valve** (Figs. 9–8 and 9–9*A* and see below). Blood is forced into the artery from the space within the aortic lumen, which is partially enclosed by the right cusp of the aortic valve. One such partially enclosed blood-filled space is associated with each cusp (i.e., right, left, or posterior cusp) of the aortic semilunar valve; these spaces are the **aortic sinuses (of Valsalva).**

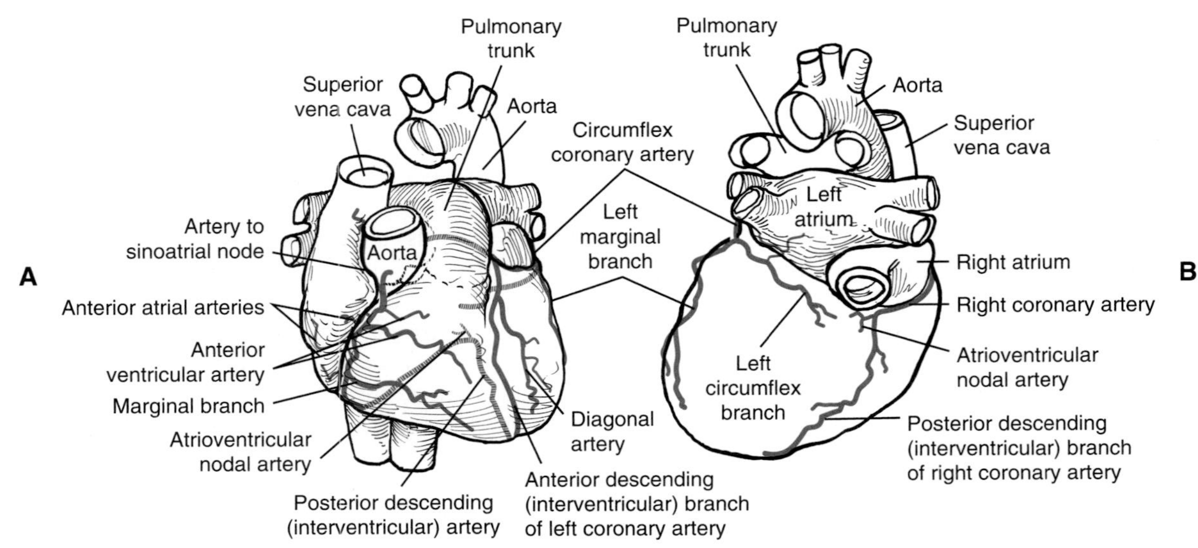

FIGURE 9–9
Coronary arteries of right-dominant heart. Anterior view **(A)** and posterior view **(B)** of heart and coronary arteries.

After emerging from the root of the aorta, the right coronary artery courses to the right and inferiorly within the coronary sulcus, between the right atrium and right ventricle (Fig. 9–9*A*). In over half of individuals, the right coronary artery almost immediately gives off a small **artery to the sinoatrial node** (Fig 9–9*A*). As the right coronary artery continues to the right within the coronary sulcus, it gives off a small **right conus artery,** which supplies the superior part of the right ventricle; one or more **anterior ventricular arteries;** and much smaller **anterior atrial arteries** (Fig. 9–9*A*). The final branch of the right coronary artery on the anterior heart surface is the **right marginal artery,** which courses inferiorly and leftward (toward the apex), just superior to the inferior border of the heart. In posteroinferior views of the heart, the right coronary artery typically courses within the coronary sulcus on the inferior surface of the heart and then turns leftward (toward the apex) to become the **posterior descending (interventricular) artery** (Fig. 9–9*B*). Just as it turns, this segment of the right coronary artery typically gives off a small, but important, **atrioventricular nodal artery.** The posterior interventricular artery continues on its leftward oblique course toward the apex within the posterior interventricular sulcus. Usually, however, the posterior interventricular artery terminates within the posterior interventricular sulcus near the apex of the heart on its inferior surface (Fig. 9–9*B*).

The **left coronary artery** branches from the root of the aorta in the region of the **left aortic sinus.** This vessel usually divides immediately (just anterior to the left auricle) into two branches: the **anterior descending (interventricular) artery** and the **circumflex artery** (Fig. 9–9*A*). The anterior descending (interventricular) artery descends from the region of the left auricle within the anterior interventricular sulcus toward the apex, giving off branches to the left and right ventricles. Among these branches, there is often a prominent one to the left ventricle called the **diagonal artery.** The anterior descending (interventricular) artery then courses around the inferior border of the heart and terminates within the posterior interventricular sulcus on the heart's inferior surface (Fig. 9–9*A* and *B*).

From the point at which it bifurcates from the anterior descending (interventricular) artery, the **circumflex artery** courses leftward, within the coronary sulcus, and quickly gives off small **left atrial branches.** Just before departing from the anterior surface of the heart, it may give off a **left marginal branch,** which supplies the left border of the heart (Fig. 9–9*B*). It then loops sharply onto the left surface of the heart, remaining within the coronary sulcus (Fig. 9–9*B*). Typically, the circumflex branch of the left coronary artery terminates within the coronary sulcus, at the point where it intersects with the posterior interventricular sulcus.

▲ Coronary Artery Disease

Coronary artery disease is a leading cause of death

The pathologic narrowing of coronary arteries (Fig. 9–10*A*), which leads to symptomatic ischemia (localized anemia resulting from obstructed blood flow), was first described in the eighteenth century. Then, as now, coronary artery disease was debilitating and led to early death. Approximately one third of United States citizens die of coronary artery disease, and yearly costs associated with its treatment are $80 to $105 billion. Although the relative number of patients diagnosed with this disease has been decreasing, the absolute number continues to rise.

Symptoms of coronary artery disease may appear late in the course of the disease. The coronary arteries are able to dilate to a much greater degree than other arteries within the body. As a result, their narrowing typically does not produce symptoms until they have been occluded by as much as 75%. Thereafter, symptoms first appear during exercise and, if untreated, become more frequent, until they are present at all times.

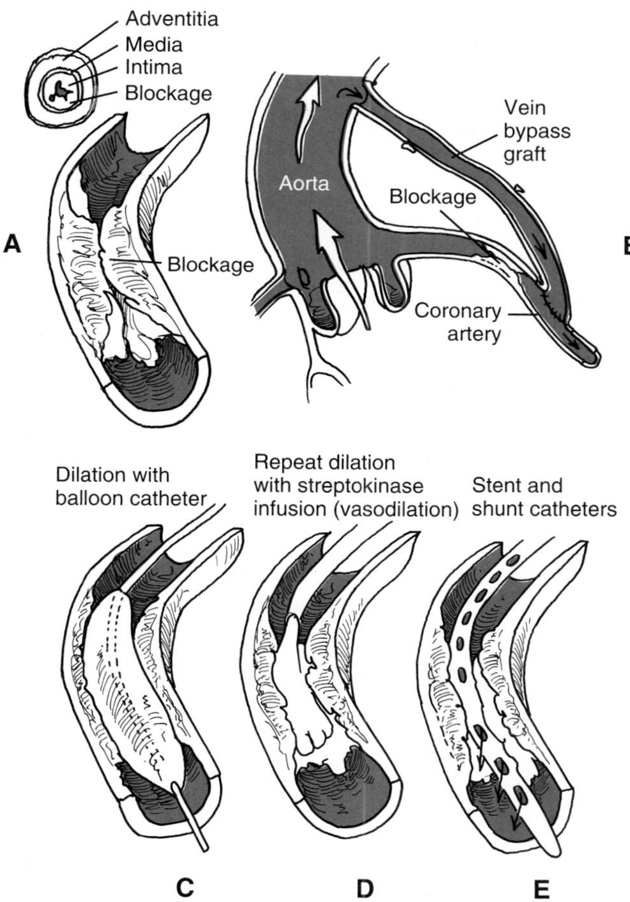

FIGURE 9–10
Coronary artery disease and its treatment. **A.** Blockage of a coronary artery by atherosclerotic plaque. **B.** Coronary bypass surgery using a vein graft. **C.** Percutaneous transluminal coronary angioplasty. **D.** Streptokinase infusion. **E.** Catheterization of the coronary artery.

The most characteristic symptom is **angina pectoris,** which is temporary discomfort within or adjacent to the chest that is aggravated by exercise or emotional stress and relieved by relaxation. Angina may be **stable** or unstable. **Unstable angina** is discomfort that is elicited more frequently by less and less stress and is a warning sign for impending **myocardial infarction** (i.e., interruption of the blood supply to a portion of the heart, which produces a macroscopic area of necrosis).

Risk factors for coronary artery disease include high serum cholesterol concentrations, elevated blood pressure, smoking, diabetes, family history of heart disease, obesity, high-fat diet, sedentary lifestyle, and personality traits such as compulsive behavior and frequent anger.

Recently, it has become apparent that females are more likely to develop significant heart disease than was previously thought, particularly after age 65 years. Females may also be at greater risk because their pattern of symptoms tends to differ significantly from that of males and, therefore, may not be recognized by the individual or the physician. Females typically do not experience the unstable angina that most male patients experience, and diagnostic tests thus frequently fail to reveal early pathologic dysfunction in females as efficiently as they do in males. As a result, coronary artery disease often progresses further prior to diagnosis in females than in males. Estrogen therapy has been effective in reducing the risk of coronary artery disease in postmenopausal women and may be used in cases where other significant risk factors exist.

Coronary artery disease can be **treated** with various techniques. Because of the clinical significance of coronary artery disease, effective management remains a focus of considerable research. One popular treatment is coronary bypass surgery, which was first successfully performed in 1962. This technique typically involves grafting a piece of saphenous vein between the root of the blocked coronary artery and a point distal to the block. Alternatively, the internal thoracic artery may be dissected from the chest wall and anastomosed with the blocked artery (Fig. 9–10*B*).

A less invasive technique for management of blockages of single vessels is **percutaneous coronary angioplasty (PTCA).** PTCA was first successfully performed in 1977 and has become a treatment of choice for single-vessel blockages. Specialized catheters equipped with an inflatable balloon and a guide are introduced into the femoral artery and advanced to the opening of the affected coronary artery. The deflated balloon is threaded into the stenotic (narrowed) vessel, so that the balloon spans the constriction. The balloon is inflated and deflated 2 to 3 times before being withdrawn (Fig. 9–10*C*). This procedure restores at least 50% of maximal flow in approximately 90% of patients.

Alternative therapies can be used to treat chronic and acute coronary artery disease. Stenotic (narrowed) coronary arteries can become suddenly occluded by a thrombus (blood clot), resulting in acute myocardial infarction (loss of blood supply to the myocardium). In order for a patient to survive these events, the blood flow must be reestablished rapidly. **Thrombolytic (thrombus-dissolving) agents** have reduced mortality rates by approximately 14%. **Streptokinase,** an agent that activates thrombus-dissolving factors in the blood, is growing in popularity because of its relatively low cost and low rate of bleeding complications (particularly stroke) and allergic reactions, the two most common side effects of thrombolytic therapy (Fig. 9–10*D*). Alternatively, noncollapsible catheters may be implanted within the occluded coronary vessel (Fig. 9–10*E*).

▲ Veins of the Heart

A system of cardiac veins returns blood from the heart walls to the right atrium

Blood is returned to the right atrium via a system of **cardiac veins** and the **coronary sinus,** which tend to lie within specific sulci of the heart (Fig. 9–11*A* and *B* and see Table 9–3). The main cardiac veins include the **great cardiac vein, middle cardiac vein,** and **small cardiac vein.** All three flow directly into the **coronary sinus** within the coronary sulcus on the **left surface** of the heart (Fig. 9-11*B*).

The **coronary sinus** is a rudiment of the embryonic left sinus venosus. During embryonic development, growth of the left horn of the sinus venosus does not keep pace with that of the right horn, and the left horn loses its connection with veins draining blood from the left side of the head and the neck and trunk and is pulled to the right. The only remnants of the left sinus horn in adults are the coronary sinus and **oblique vein of the left atrium,** which drain only the muscular wall of the heart. In the definitive heart, the coronary sinus empties all of its blood into the right atrium.

The **great cardiac vein** can be observed within the coronary sulcus connected to the left superior end of the coronary sinus (Fig. 9–11). Blood that is emptied directly from the great cardiac vein into the sinus at this point is typically collected from the walls of both ventricles in the region of the anterior interventricular sulcus and from the left border of the heart via a branch called the **left marginal vein** (Fig. 9–11 and 9–12*B*).

The **middle cardiac vein** courses from the region of the apex of the heart within the posterior (inferior) interventricular sulcus on the inferior surface of the heart. Therefore, it empties blood directly into the right inferior end of the coronary sinus (Fig. 9–11*B*).

The **small cardiac vein** also empties blood into the coronary sinus in this region (Fig. 9–11*B*). One of its tributaries may be the **right marginal vein,** which collects blood from the anterior surface of the heart, just superior to its inferior border (Fig. 9–11*A*). More typically, however, the right marginal vein empties its blood into an **anterior cardiac vein** (see Fig. 9–13*A*).

Other veins that empty into the coronary sinus include **posterior ventricular veins** (Fig. 9–11*B*) and

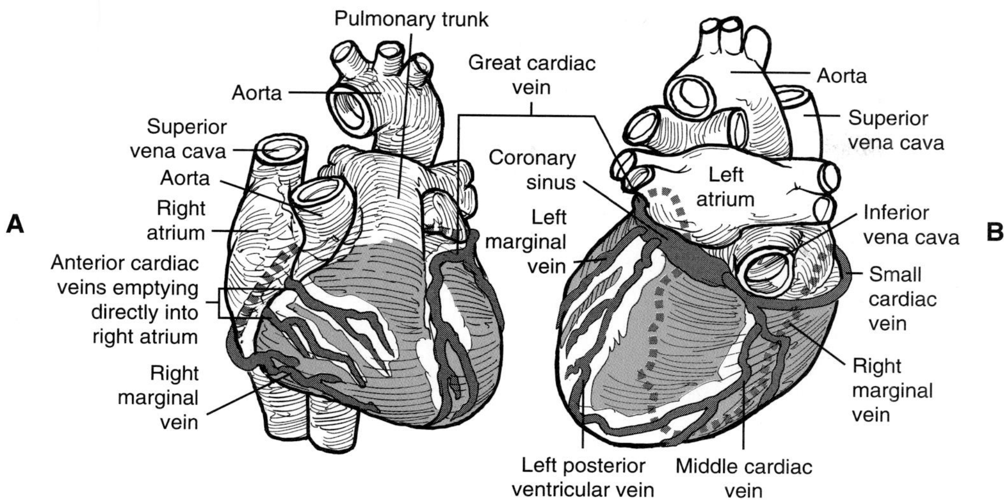

FIGURE 9–11
Cardiac veins. Anterior view **(A)** and posterior view **(B)** of the heart and venous system.

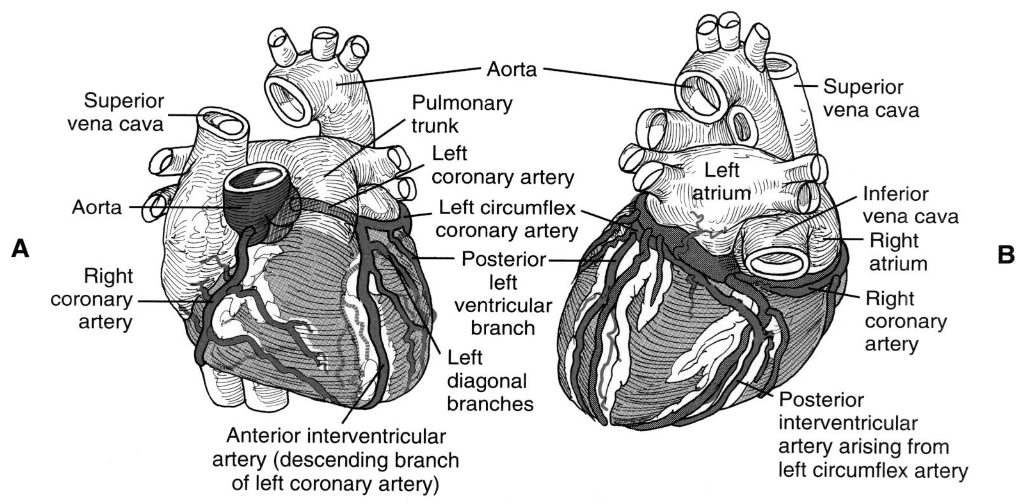

FIGURE 9–12
Coronary arteries of left dominant heart. Anterior view **(A)** and posterior view **(B)** of the heart and coronary arteries.

small veins that drain the posterior wall of the right atrium and left atrium, including the **oblique vein of the left atrium.**

In anterior views of the heart, small **anterior cardiac veins** can be seen draining the anterior wall of the right ventricle. These veins emanate from the right anterior ventricular wall and course superiorly to cross the coronary sulcus. They may pass under or over the right coronary artery (Fig. 9–11*A*). These small veins empty directly into the right atrium near the coronary sulcus.

Variability in Patterns of Cardiac Vasculature

There is extensive variability in patterns of cardiac arteries and veins

The organizational patterns of coronary arteries and cardiac veins described above are relatively common but not universal. Typical variations include independent origination of the **right conus artery** from the right aortic sinus rather than from the right coronary artery; origination of the **anterior descending (interventricular) artery** and **circumflex artery** at different points along the left aortic sinus; and origination of the **sinoatrial artery** from the circumflex artery rather than the right coronary artery. This atypical origin of the sinoatrial artery usually occurs when the posterior descending (interventricular) artery also arises from the circumflex artery instead of the right coronary artery. This latter condition is called **"left dominance"** of the coronary system in contrast to the more typical **"right dominance"** of the coronary arterial vasculature described above (Fig. 9–12).

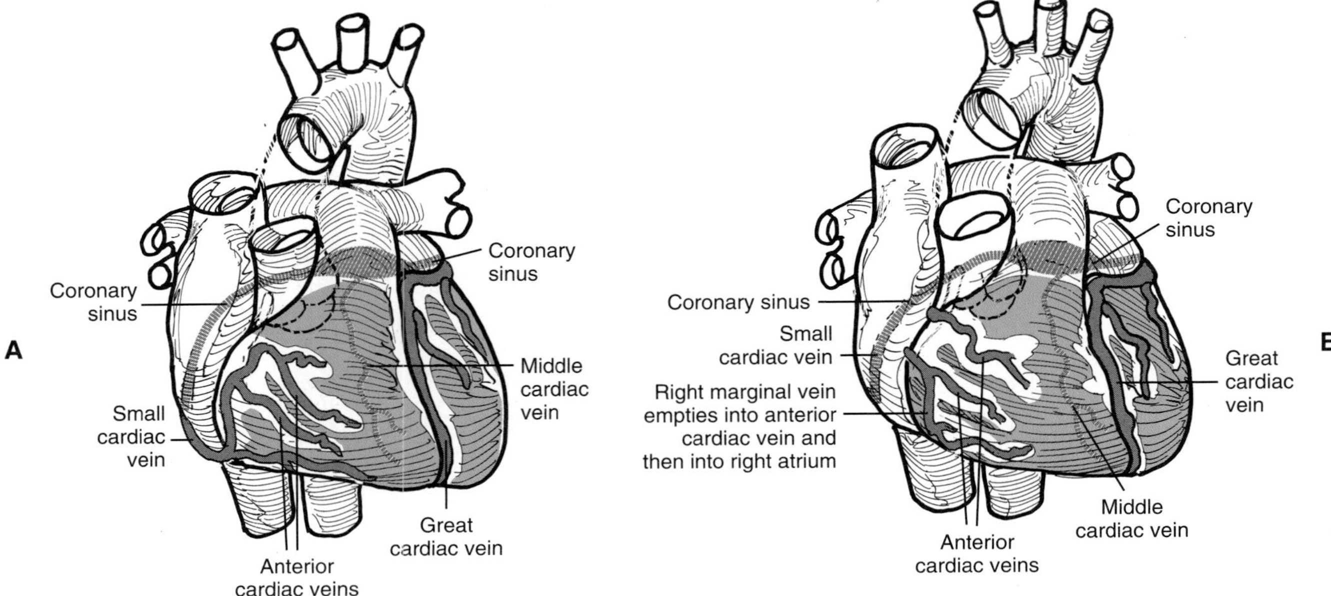

FIGURE 9–13
Variations of venous return from wall of heart. **A.** Anterior cardiac veins empty into the small cardiac vein (less typical). **B.** The right marginal vein empties into the anterior cardiac vein (common).

The most frequently described variations in the distribution of cardiac veins are connections of **anterior cardiac veins** to the small cardiac vein, which then empty into the coronary sinus or into the cardiac sinus directly (Fig. 9–13*A*). More often than not, the **right marginal vein,** which is sometimes a tributary of the **small cardiac vein** (see Fig. 9–11), empties its blood into an anterior cardiac vein instead of the coronary sinus (Fig. 9–13*B*).

▲ Disorders Caused by Abnormal Cardiac Vasculature

Infrequently, the entire coronary arterial vasculature is derived from either a single right or single left coronary artery. This condition may be asymptomatic but is often cited as the cause of sudden death in children and young adults following strenuous physical activity. Another clinically important variation is extensive development of **arteriovenous fistulas** (direct connections between coronary arteries and cardiac veins), resulting in the bypassing of capillary beds within the myocardium.

▲ Chambers of the Heart

The definitive human heart has four chambers: right and left atria and right and left ventricles

Right Atrium

Atrial chambers of the heart are thin walled and flaccid

The **right atrium** is somewhat anterior to the left atrium and extends somewhat more inferiorly (Fig. 9–14 and Table 9–4 and see Figs. 9–7*A* and 9–15). Its anterior wall largely comprises the upper right region of the **anterior surface of the heart** and all of the **right surface of the heart.** The crenated muscular pouch that extends from the superoanterior border is the **right auricle** (see Figs. 9–3, 9–7*A*, and 9–15*A*), a vestigial remnant of the embryonic atrium. The walls of the **definitive right atrium** are derived from the embryonic right sinus venosus.

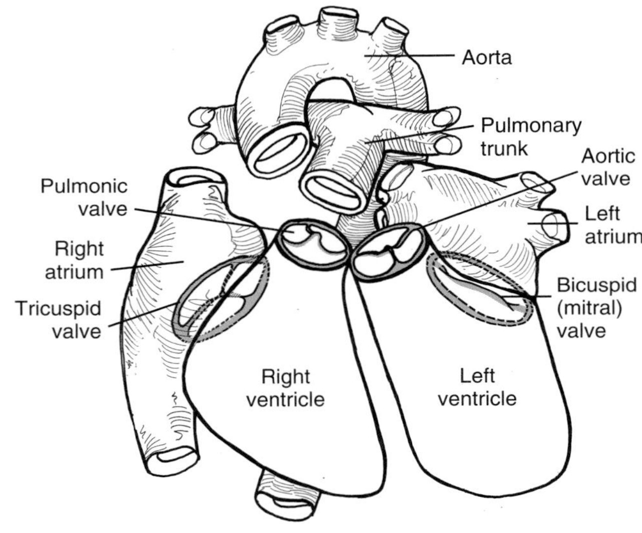

FIGURE 9–14
Exploded view of the heart showing general relationships of cardiac chambers.

Compared with the walls of the ventricular chambers, the walls of the right atrium are thin and some-

TABLE 9–4
Features of the Atria and Ventricles of the Heart

ATRIA

Left Atrium

- Left atrium is slightly larger than the right atrium.
- Walls are thin and flaccid anteriorly from left atrium.
- Musculi pectinati in left auricle are fewer and smaller than those in the right auricle.
- Right posterior wall contains openings of two right and two left pulmonary veins.
- Function is to deliver oxygenated blood from pulmonary circulation to left atrium.
- Septum primum makes up most of medioanterior wall.
- Left atrioventricular canal is smaller than the right atrioventricular canal.

Right Atrium

- Walls are thin and flaccid.
- Right auricle is crenated muscular pouch extending from the superoanterior border of the right atrium.
- Layers, from outermost to innermost, are epicardium, subepicardial fat (containing coronary vasculature), thin muscular layer, and endocardium.
- Musculi pectinati are comb-shaped muscles of the anterolateral wall, which extend into the right auricle.
- Function is to receive deoxygenated blood from superior vena cava, inferior vena cava, coronary sinus, and anterior cardiac veins.
- Sinus venarum is the smooth posterolateral portion of the atrial wall containing openings of the superior and inferior vena cavae and coronary sinus.
- Crista terminalis is the smooth-walled muscular ridge forming the boundary between the right atrium and the right auricle.
- Septum secundum is the thick muscular septum forming most of the medioposterior wall.
- Septum primum is a thin, flaccid septum located to the left of the septum secundum.
- Fossa ovalis is a distinctive depression on the septal wall (vestige of embryonic opening in septum secundum called *foramen ovale).*

Right Atrium—cont'd

- Right atrioventricular canal opens into the right ventricle from the left inferior boundary of the right atrium.

VENTRICLES

Left Ventricle

- Wall is two or three times thicker than the wall of the right ventricle.
- Trabeculae carneae are found at inflow region.
- Aortic vestibule is a smooth-walled outflow region.
- Function is to circulate oxygenated blood to the systemic circulatory system.
- Muscular interventricular septum makes up most of the right wall.
- Valves are the bicuspid (mitral) valve and the aortic semilunar valve.

Right Ventricle

- Walls are thick and muscular.
- Trabeculae carneae are roughened ridges of round or irregular muscle columns at inflow end.
- Conus arteriosus (infundibulum) is a cone-shaped chamber leading into an outflow tract (pulmonary trunk).
- Function is to circulate deoxygenated blood to pulmonary circulation of the lungs.
- Interventricular septum, having muscular and membranous portions, makes up the left wall (malformations of this septum are life threatening).
- Atrioventricular tricuspid valve prevents regurgitation of blood into the right atrium.
- Septomarginal trabecula (moderator band) is a prominent ridge of muscle connecting the muscular interventricular septum with the anterior papillary muscle.
- Valves are the tricuspid valve and the pulmonary semilunar valve.

what flaccid in the unfilled state. As is the case with all other chambers of the heart, the outer surface of the right atrium is covered by **epicardium, (visceral pericardium)** under which typically lies a layer of **subepicardial fat** within which the coronary vasculature is embedded. The thin muscular layer of the right atrium lies deep to the subepicardial fat and just superficial to the **endocardium,** which is the endothelial lining of the heart (Fig. 9–15*A*).

A view of the inner walls of the right auricle reveals parallel ridges called **musculi pectinati** (comb-shaped muscles). These muscles cover its entire inner wall as an interconnected network (Fig. 9–15*A*). The inset shows trabecular carneae in the ventricle. This is in contrast to the smooth inner walls of the definitive right atrium (Fig. 9–15*A*).

As was noted above, the right atrium may receive deoxygenated blood from several **systemic venous sources,** including the **superior vena cava, inferior vena cava, coronary sinus,** and **anterior cardiac veins.** The large openings of the inferior and superior vena cavae are readily observed within the opened atrium

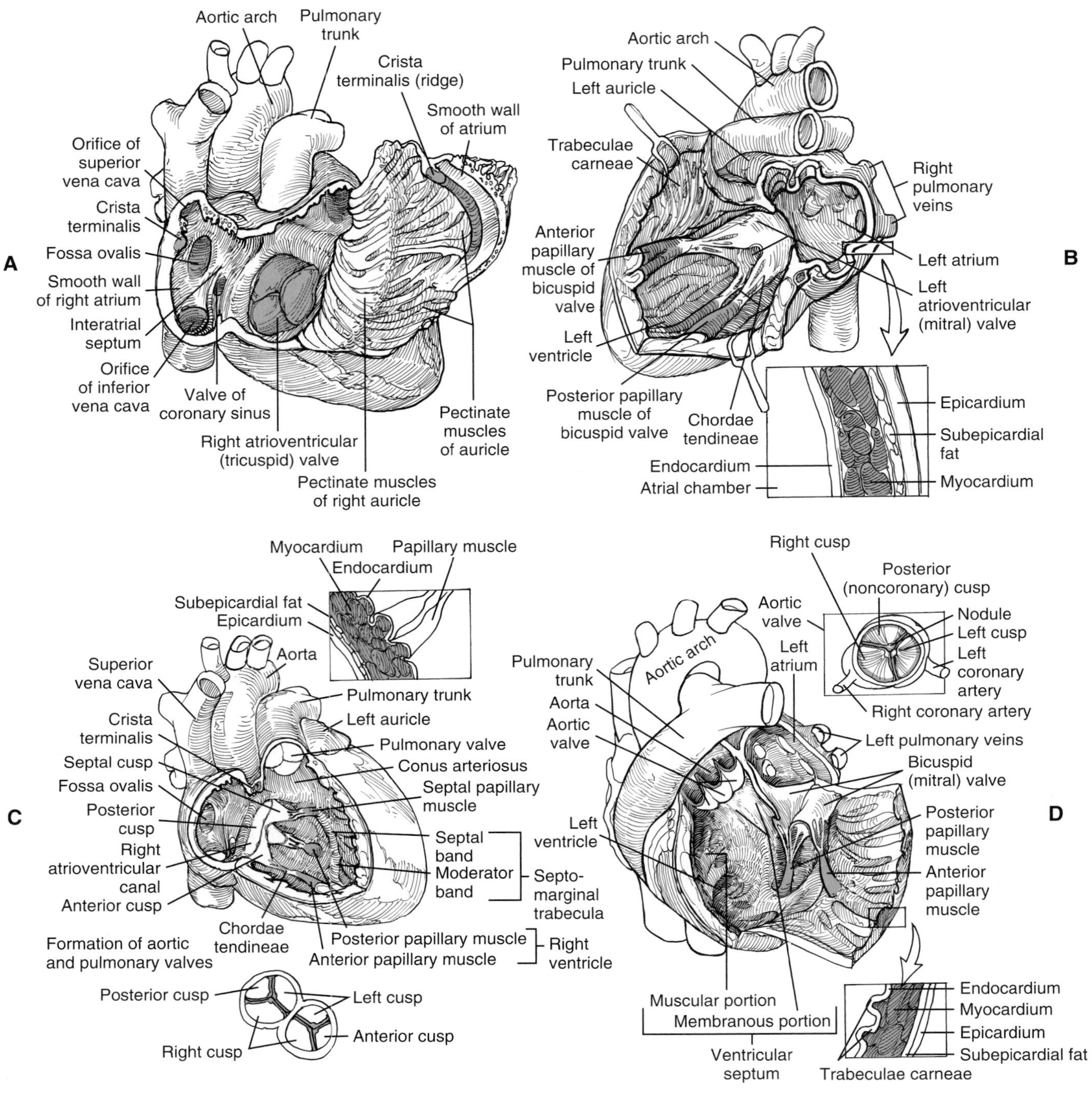

FIGURE 9–15
Interiors of the heart chambers. **A.** Medial view of the interior of the right atrium. **B.** Medial view of the interior of the left atrium. **C.** Anterior view of the interior of the right ventricle. **D.** Medial view of the interior of the left ventricle.

(Fig. 9–15*A*). They are located within a region of smooth posterolateral atrial wall called the **sinus venarum,** which is derived originally from the embryonic right sinus venosus. The more inferior orifice of the inferior vena cava is characterized by a crescent-shaped flap, which in embryonic and fetal life directs blood entering from the inferior vena cava into the left atrium via the interatrial shunt (see Function of the Heart, below).

The smaller, more medial orifice of the **coronary sinus** is also obvious within the smooth-walled sinus venarum. This opening is also partially covered by a flap, or valve, which prevents regurgitation of blood into the coronary sinus during atrial filling (Fig. 9–15*A*).

The boundary between the definitive right atrium and the right auricle is quite obvious in views of the inner wall of this chamber because it is demarcated by a prominent ridge of tissue called the **crista terminalis.** This smooth-walled muscular ridge courses from a position just superior to the orifice of the superior vena cava, inferiorly around its right edge, and laterally (to the right) to the orifice of the inferior vena cava, where it is connected to the right valve of the inferior vena cava (Fig. 9–15*A*).

The **medioposterior (septal) wall** of the right atrium is largely made up of the **septum secundum.** This thick muscular septum, along with a thin, flaccid **septum primum** located to the left of the septum secundum (thus forming the medial wall of the left atrium; see below), grows from the atrial roof during embryonic life to partially separate the right and left atria from each other. Prominent on this septal wall is a distinctive depression called the **fossa ovalis,** which is the vestige of an opening in the septum secundum called the **foramen ovale** (Fig. 9–15*A* and below).

Finally, the left inferior boundary of the right atrium is characterized by an opening into the right ventricle called the **right atrioventricular canal.** This constricted orifice is 10–12 cm in circumference and bounded by three cusps of an **atrioventricular tricuspid valve** (see Function of the Heart, below).

Left Atrium

The definitive **left atrium** is slightly larger than the right atrium and lies somewhat posterior and to the left of it (Figs. 9–7, 9–14, and 9–15*B* and Table 9–4). Its right posterior wall largely comprises the **base of the heart** and a small superior region of the **left border of the heart** (see Figs. 9–3 and 9–7). A crenated pouch, the **left auricle,** extends laterally and anteriorly from the left atrium, contributing to a small part of the **anterior surface,** the **left border,** and a small part of the **left surface of the heart** (see Figs. 9–3, 9–7, and 9–15*B*).

The left auricle, like the right auricle, is a vestige of the embryonic atrium. The definitive left atrium is formed by the intussusception of **pulmonary veins** as the primitive left atrium becomes the left auricle.

Like the walls of the definitive right atrium, the walls of the definitive left atrium are relatively thin and flaccid in the unfilled state. The inner surfaces of the left atrial walls are smooth, like most of those of the definitive right atrium (Fig. 9–15*B*). The inner walls of the left auricle are also characterized by **musculi pectinati,** although they are fewer in number and smaller than those in the right auricle.

The right posterior wall of the left atrium is distinguished by four large openings: the orifices of two **right pulmonary veins** and two **left pulmonary veins** (Fig. 9–15*B*). These vessels deliver **oxygenated** blood from the pulmonary circulation to the left atrium (see Function of the Heart, below).

The anteromedial wall of the left atrium is made up mainly of the **septum primum,** which is typically fused tightly with the more muscular septum secundum (Fig. 9–15*B*). Although the **ostium secundum** is usually not discernible in internal views of the left atrium, a depression indicating the position of the fossa ovalis on the other side of the thin septum primum may be apparent in views from the right atrium (Fig. 9–15*A*).

If one again views the left atrium from inside, one can see that its inner left inferior boundary is the site of the **left atrioventricular canal.** This constricted orifice is smaller than that of the right atrioventricular canal (7 to 9 cm in circumference) and is bounded by a **bicuspid (mitral) atrioventricular valve** (Fig. 9–15*D*). The tricuspid and bicuspid valves will be described with the ventricles (see below).

Right Ventricle

The ventricular chambers of the heart are thick walled and muscular

The **right ventricle** lies somewhat to the left of and inferior to the right atrium (see Figs. 9–3, 9–7, and 9–15*C* and Table 9–4). Its anterior wall makes up much of the **anterior surface of the heart,** from the coronary sulcus separating the right ventricle from the right atrium on the right, to the boundary defined by the anterior interventricular sulcus on the left (see Figs. 9–7 and 9–15*C*) The inferior wall of the right ventricle also forms most of the **inferior border** and some of the **inferior surface of the heart** (see Fig. 9–7).

The walls of the right ventricle are considerably thicker than those of the atria and, as a consequence, are quite inflexible in the morbid state. Much of their inner surface is studded by ridges of muscular tissue called **trabeculae carneae,** but these roughened ridges of round or irregular muscular columns are confined to the inflow end of the right ventricle in the region of the right atrioventricular canal (Fig. 9–15*C, inset*). It has been suggested that the rough-walled inflow end of the ventricle slows incoming blood during filling of the ventricle. The superior outflow region of the right ventricle is called the **conus arteriosus** or **infundibulum.** This cone-shaped chamber leads into the outflow tract of the right ventricle, or **pulmonary trunk** (Fig. 9–15*C*). The inner wall of the infundibulum is smooth walled, and this may facilitate ejection of blood into the pulmonary trunk. The function of the right ventricle is, thus, to circulate deoxygenated blood to the pulmonary circulation of the lungs.

The left wall of the right ventricle is made up of an **interventricular septum,** which is formed by two separate components: an inferior **muscular septum** and a superior **membranous septum.** The development of this septum is complex, and disruptions of its formation account for the single most life-threatening congenital abnormality in humans, **ventricular septal**

defect (about 25% of all congenital cardiac malformations) (see below).

As was noted above, the atrioventricular orifice is bounded by an **atrioventricular tricuspid valve** (Fig. 9–15*C*). This valve prevents regurgitation of blood into the right atrium as blood is ejected from the infundibulum into the pulmonary trunk. The components of this valve include an **anterior leaflet,** or **cusp,** connected by **chordae tendineae** to an **anterior papillary muscle** with its associated **septomarginal trabecula;** a **posterior leaflet,** or **cusp,** connected by **chordae tendineae** to a **posterior papillary muscle;** and a **septal leaflet,** or **cusp,** connected by **chordae tendineae** to a **septal papillary muscle.** Each valve is named for its relative position within the right ventricular chamber (Fig. 9–15*C*).

The cusps of the tricuspid valve consist of two layers of endothelium (one on each surface) with an intermediate fibrous layer. The cusps are relatively thick in the middle but quite delicate at their margins. Their bases are attached to a fibrous ring, which is part of the **cardiac skeleton** that encircles the right atrioventricular canal (see below). Margins of the cusps are attached at intervals to thin delicate cords called **chordae tendineae,** which, in turn, are connected to the papillary muscles (Fig. 9–15*C*).

The **papillary muscles** and **septomarginal trabecula** are specialized trabeculae carneae. The septomarginal trabecula is a prominent ridge of muscle connecting the muscular interventricular septum with the anterior papillary muscle (Fig. 9–15*C*). This specialized trabecula carnea contains the **right limb** of the **atrioventricular bundle,** which is part of the **conduction system** of the heart serving the right ventricle (see Function of the Heart, below). Because the septomarginal trabecula may help to prevent overdistension of the ventricle during filling, it is sometimes called the **moderator band.**

The **tricuspid valve** develops during embryonic life by sculpting of the ventricular muscular wall by apoptosis, or programmed cell death. Typically, the septal leaflet and its chordae tendineae and papillary muscle are the last structures to form. They may be absent in some individuals.

The **pulmonary semilunar valve** is located at the boundary between the outflow channel **(infundibulum; conus arteriosus)** of the right ventricle and the pulmonary trunk (Figs. 9–14 and 9–15*C*). This valve prevents backflow of blood from the pulmonary trunk into the right ventricle. The anatomy of the pulmonary valve is somewhat different from that of the tricuspid valve. The pulmonary valve is made up of three cup-shaped cusps composed of two layers of endocardium with an intermediate fibrous layer, but the marginal edges of the cusps are not stabilized by chordae tendineae and papillary muscles. Rather, their free edges are stabilized by tendinous fibers, which radiate from the attached edge of each cusp to a **nodule,** a central thickening, at its free edge. The base of each cusp is further stabilized by a fibrous ring, which is part of the cardiac skeleton (see below) and which surrounds the pulmonary trunk at the level of the valve. The **pulmonary valve,** therefore, consists of a right cusp, a left cusp, and an anterior cusp (see Fig. 9–13*C*).

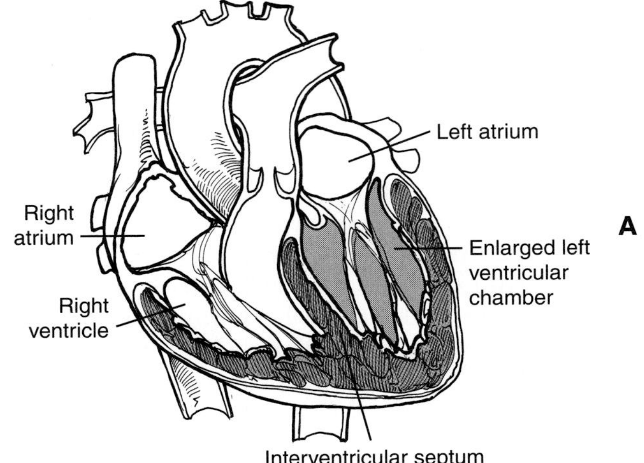

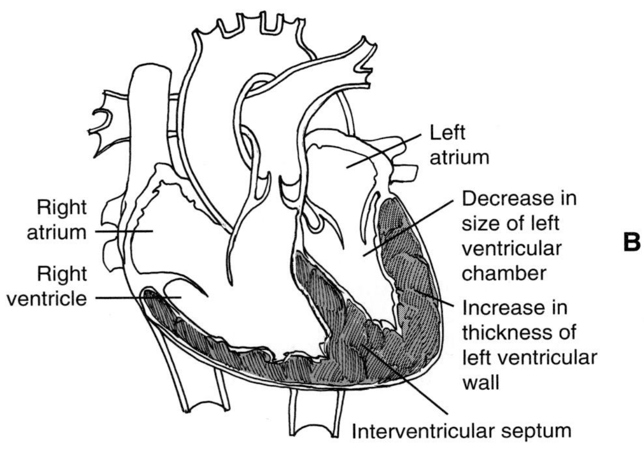

FIGURE 9–16
Cardiomyopathies. **A.** Dilated cardiomyopathy. **B.** Hypertrophic cardiomyopathy.

Left Ventricle

The **left ventricle** is conical in shape and forms most of the **apex** of the heart (see Fig. 9–3 and Table 9–4). A small portion of the left ventricle comprises a small part of the **anterior surface of the heart** just to the left of the anterior interventricular sulcus, anterior interventricular artery, and great cardiac vein (see Figs. 9–3 and 9–7*A* and *C*). The left posterior wall of the left ventricle, however, comprises most of the **left border** and **left surface of the heart** (see Fig. 9–7). The inferior wall of the left ventricle also contributes to a substantial part of the **inferior surface of the heart** (see Fig. 9–7).

The wall of the left ventricle is two to three times thicker than the wall of the right ventricle (see Fig. 9–15*C* and *D*) because the left ventricle does more work

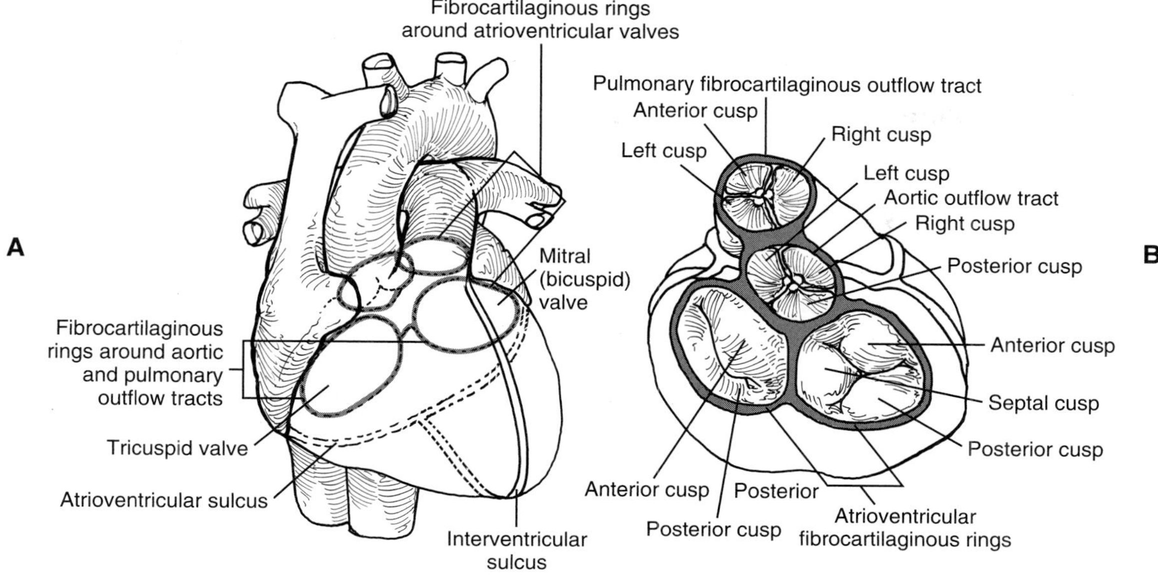

FIGURE 9–17
The cardiac skeleton, with its four fibrous rings. **A.** Anterior view of heart and cardiac skeleton. **B.** Superior view of heart and cardiac skeleton, with atria removed. This view shows ventricular contraction. The heart is in systole.

than the right ventricle. As is the case with the right ventricular wall, much of the substance of the left ventricular wall is accounted for by **trabeculae carneae.** These muscular ridges, however, are confined to the inflow region of the left ventricular chamber, presumably to slow the flow of blood received from the left atrium via the left atrioventricular canal. In contrast, the outflow region of the left ventricle, the **aortic vestibule,** is smooth walled as is the infundibulum of the right ventricle. This characteristic presumably contributes to efficient ejection of blood into the **aorta** from which blood is distributed to the head, neck, trunk, and extremities. The function of the left ventricle is, thus, to circulate oxygenated blood to the systemic circulatory system.

The right wall of the left ventricle is made up mainly of the **muscular interventricular septum** (see Fig. 9–15*D*). A small oval-shaped region just inferior to the root of the aorta can be discriminated as part of the **membranous interventricular septum** (see Fig. 9–15*D*).

The left atrioventricular canal is bounded by a **bicuspid (mitral) valve,** which prevents the regurgitation of blood into the left atrium while blood is being ejected from the left ventricle into the aorta (see Fig. 9–15*D*). This valve, like the tricuspid valve, is made up of **cusps,** or **leaflets, chordae tendineae,** and **papillary muscles.** However, as its name implies, the bicuspid valve has only two valvular units composed of a cusp, chordae tendineae, and papillary muscles: an **anterior valve** and a **posterior valve.** The term *mitral* refers to a bishop's miter, which is a hat with two vertical parts. Although the bicuspid valve does not have a septal cusp, its mode of development and its fundamental structure are identical to those of the tricuspid valve (see above). The cusps of the bicuspid valve are named for their relative positions within the left ventricular chamber (Fig. 9–17*B* and see Fig. 9–15*D*).

The **aortic semilunar valve** at the orifice between the **aortic vestibule** of the left ventricle and the root of the aorta is virtually identical in structure and composition to the pulmonary valve described above (Fig. 9–17*B* and see Fig. 9–15*D*). The bases of its cusps are also stabilized by a fibrous ring that encircles the base of the aorta at the level of the valve. Its three cusps include a right cusp, left cusp, and posterior cusp (Fig. 9–17).

▲ Disorders of Cardiac Chambers

Cardiac Hypertrophy

There are many causes of cardiac hypertrophy, one of which is valvular stenosis

If valvular stenosis develops, a higher blood pressure must be generated within the upstream chamber responsible for forcing blood through the valve. Consequent thickening of the myocardium of that chamber is likely to occur over time. Stenotic valves are frequently detected as a **murmur,** although pain similar to that associated with angina may also occur. Detection of the murmur during childhood or early adulthood suggests a congenital basis for the condition. Detection later in life is often indicative of degenerative disease. Stenosis may be so limited that no true symptoms are observed or may be severe enough to warrant surgical replacement of the valve.

Cardiomyopathy

Cardiomyopathy is a primary disease of the heart muscle

Dilated cardiomyopathy occurs when the volume of a ventricle increases without hypertrophy of the walls or septum (see Fig. 9–16*A*). A common cause is inflammation, which destroys cardiomyocytes. These myocytes do not regenerate. They are replaced by connective tissue, causing weakening of the heart wall in the region. At the present time, cardiac transplantation is the only cure for this condition.

Hypertrophic cardiomyopathy has a genetic origin. It results in thickening of the left ventricular walls to a degree that significantly diminishes the ventricular volume (see Fig. 9–16*B*). Patients with hypertrophic cardiomyopathy may remain asymptomatic until as late as 60 years of age. Sudden death is the most serious threat to these patients, particularly to younger, active patients. Such patients may have no symptoms until the terminal episode occurs, often during a period of exercise.

Restrictive cardiomyopathy is the least common of the cardiomyopathies. It is an impaired ability of the ventricle to sufficiently relax and fill during diastole.

Congestive Heart Failure

In congestive heart failure, the heart is unable to meet the circulatory needs of organs and tissues

Inability of the heart to pump adequate blood into the systemic or pulmonary circulation may develop because the contractile ability of the heart muscle becomes reduced (due to coronary artery disease or cardiomyopathy) or because an otherwise normal heart must pump against increased vascular resistance or high blood pressure within the systemic or pulmonary circulation. In all cases, the affected chambers fail to empty sufficiently during systole.

Congestive heart failure usually begins on one side of the heart but eventually tends to involve both sides. As the disease progresses, the heart chambers enlarge to increase the stroke volume and their walls thicken to increase the systolic blood pressure (see below). Any compensatory improvement achieved by these changes is temporary, in part because the heart is unable to meet the increased metabolic demands of its increasing mass. The results are death of the myocardial cells and replacement of them by connective tissue. In the absence of treatment to correct the causes of the disease, congestive heart failure is usually fatal.

Congestive heart failure may arise from a variety of causes, but patients with long-standing hypertension (high blood pressure) are among the most common to develop this disorder. The typical patient presents with dyspnea (shortness of breath), weakness, and fatigue. Management is based on treatment of the conditions that gave rise to the disease, control of factors that exacerbate the condition, and treatment of clinical manifestations of the disease.

▲ Function of the Heart

Cardiac Skeleton

The cardiac skeleton provides a solid foundation for the musculature of each cardiac chamber, so that the chambers can function independently and efficiently

The heart is composed of a complex musculature that functions dynamically and statically. For example, during initial contraction of the ventricles, **static tension** must be created momentarily to exert sufficient intraventricular pressure to close the atrioventricular valves and open the semilunar valves. **Dynamic contractions** that reduce the volume of the ventricles then eject blood into the aorta and pulmonary trunk. Moreover, the actions of the myocardium within the walls of the atria and ventricles take place in a well-regulated sequence to propel blood through the heart and into the systemic and pulmonary outflow tracts (see below).

In order for each heart chamber to serve its unique function in complement with the other chambers, the muscles within its walls must have rigid attachment sites on which they can pull without interfering with the activities of the other chambers. Anchorage for all of the chambers is provided by the **cardiac skeleton,** a system of fibrous and fibrocartilaginous bands and tendons (Fig. 9–17). The cardiac skeleton is composed mainly of four **fibrous rings** (one of which encircles each of the atrioventricular canals and pulmonary and aortic valves) and the **fibrous sheets** and **tendons** that connect the four rings (Table 9–5). In some mammals, part of the cardiac skeleton is ossified as a distinct bone, the **os cordis.**

Not only does the cardiac skeleton provide the rigid foundation required for appropriate cardiac muscle action, but also it prevents collapse or overdistension of the atrioventricular canals and pulmonary and aortic outlets. Moreover, the cardiac skeleton provides rigid attachment sites for cusps of the atrioventricular

TABLE 9–5
Structures that Assist the Heart in Functioning as a Unit

CARDIAC SKELETON
Four fibrous rings (one of which encircles each atrioventricular canal and its pulmonary and aortic valves) and fibrous sheets and tendons connecting each ring with the others, serving as firm attachment sites for heart muscles
PACEMAKER AND CONDUCTION SYSTEM
Sinoatrial node (pacemaker), atrioventricular node, atrioventricular bundle, and plexuses of Purkinje's fibers integrate functions of heart chambers
SYMPATHETIC, PARASYMPATHETIC, AND VISCERAL AFFERENT INNERVATION OF THE HEART

and semilunar valves and thus facilitates their function. The cardiac skeleton may also contribute to the inherent integrity and electrophysiologic continuity that the heart requires for proper function of its intrinsic conduction system (see below).

▲ Development of Heart Function

The heart is a single-pump system during embryonic and fetal life and is converted to a double-pump system at birth

At about 22 days of development, even before the primary heart tube has looped, the tube begins beating sluggishly, causing blood to ebb and flow within the embryonic vasculature. The heart has only a single chamber at this stage, and this primitive circulation is entirely systemic. Indeed, during the entire span of embryonic and fetal life, even after septation of the heart, the heart acts as a single-pump system, receiving oxygenated placental blood and deoxygenated blood from peripheral tissues and delivering this mixture of blood

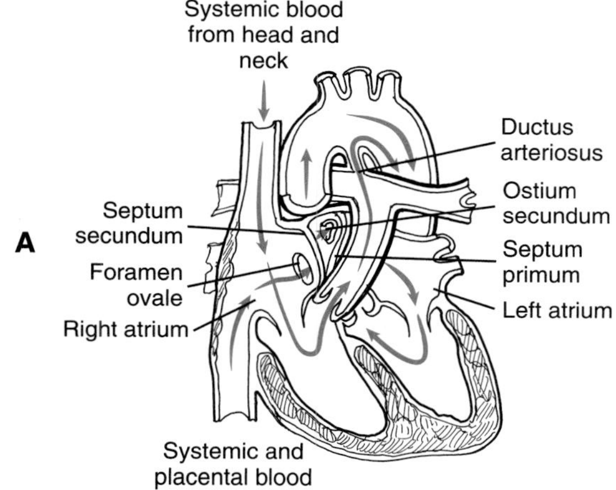

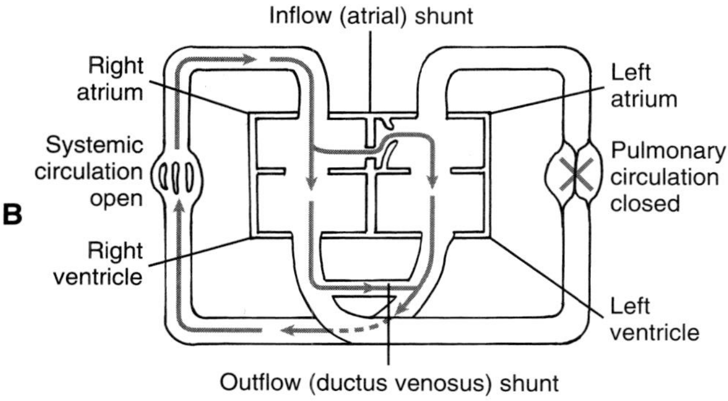

FIGURE 9–18
Flow of blood through heart before birth. **A.** Anatomic depiction. **B.** Diagrammatic depiction. At the inflow (atrial) shunt, systemic blood (mainly from the inferior vena cava) is directed to the left atrium. Systemic blood from the superior vena cava is directed to the right ventricle. At the outflow (ductus venosus) shunt, blood from the right and left heart is recombined and directed to the systemic circulation.

primarily to the systemic circulation and to the placenta. Thus, before birth, the heart receives virtually no blood from the pulmonary circulation and the single-pump function of the heart is ingeniously carried out by all four chambers. After birth, however, only two of these chambers serve the systemic vascular circuit, while the other two must serve the pulmonary circuit.

The four-chambered heart is transformed from a single pump that serves only the systemic circulation during prenatal life to a double-pump system following birth. This transformation is possible because of the presence of two shunts: a special interatrial shunt near the inflow end of the heart, the **foramen ovale** and **ostium secundum,** and another shunt connecting the outflow tracts, the **ductus arteriosus.** Prior to birth, some of the systemic blood entering the right atrium is delivered to the right ventricle (mainly blood entering the heart from the superior vena cava) and some is diverted to the left atrium via the interatrial shunt (mainly blood diverted by the valve of the inferior vena cava). In this way, all incoming systemic blood is distributed to the two atria (Fig. 9–18). However, virtually all of the blood ejected from both ventricles is subsequently recombined when blood from the right ventricle and pulmonary trunk is shunted through the ductus arteriosus to the aortic arch, where it mixes with blood from the left ventricle (Fig. 9–18).

After birth, the interatrial shunts and ductus arteriosus are rapidly closed off as the pulmonary circulation is established (Fig. 9–19). The interatrial shunt closes immediately because of increased pressure within the left atrium. Complete separation of the systemic and pulmonary circulations typically occurs about 15 hours after birth, when the ductus arteriosus closes (Fig. 9–19). Once this occurs, all of the deoxygenated systemic blood received by the right atrium flows into the right ventricle, which pumps the blood into the pulmonary trunk and then into the pulmonary circuit. After this blood is oxygenated within the **pulmonary circulation,** it is delivered to the left atrium via the pulmonary veins. All of this oxygenated blood flows into the left ventricle, which then pumps it into the **systemic circulation** (Fig. 9–19).

▲ Common Congenital Abnormalities of the Heart That Interfere With the Normal Separation of Systemic and Pulmonary Blood After Birth

Many disorders of the heart and great vessels arise during embryonic life; congenital abnormalities of the heart are the most prevalent life-threatening congenital malformation in humans

The disturbance of virtually any process related to development of the heart may lead to gross cardiac abnormalities. Many of these are clinically relevant, and a few are briefly described below. Many of these defects may be observed in the gross anatomy laboratory.

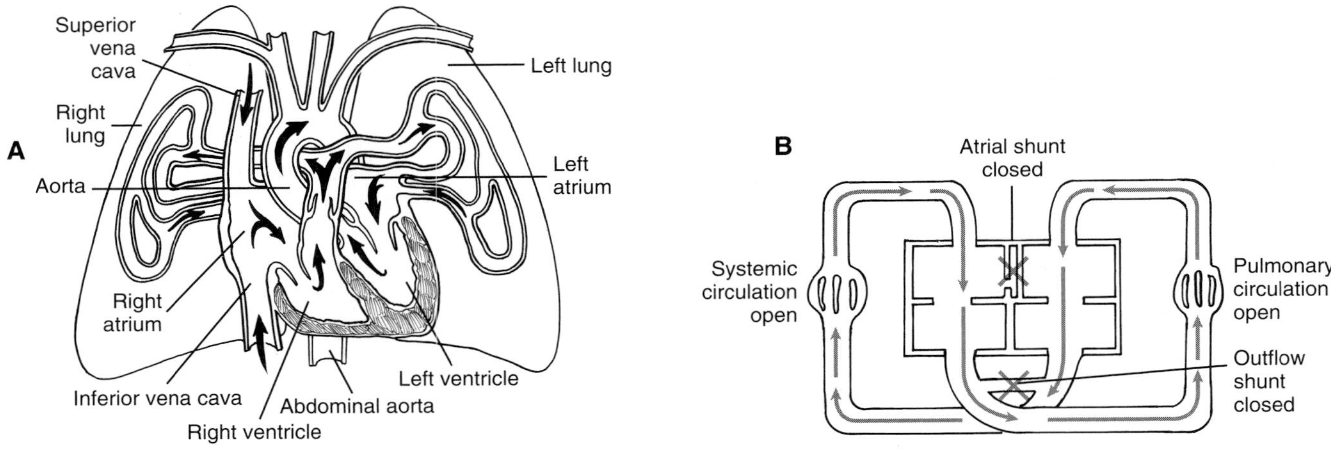

FIGURE 9–19
Flow of blood through the heart after birth. **A.** Anatomic depiction. **B.** Diagrammatic depiction.

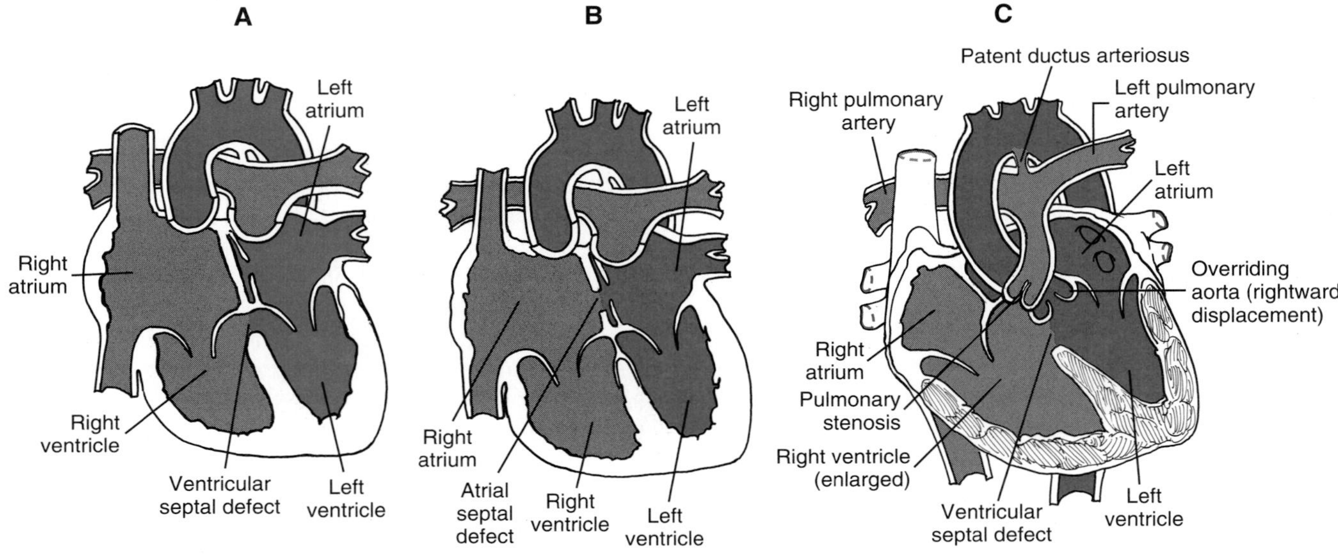

FIGURE 9–20
Congenital cardiac defects. **A.** Ventricular septal defect. **B.** Atrial septal defect. **C.** Tetralogy of Fallot. The four defects in tetralogy of Fallot are pulmonary stenosis, ventricular septal defect, overriding (rightward) displacement of the aorta, and an enlarged right ventricle.

Ventricular Septal Defect. The most common life-threatening heart defect is ventricular septal defect, which is massive shunting of blood from the left to the right ventricle and consequent **pulmonary hypertension** and enlargement of the right ventricle (Fig. 9–20*A*). Surgical correction typically restores normal pulmonary blood pressure, and the right side of the heart returns to its normal size.

Atrial Septal Defect. Atrial septal defect typically results in massive shunting of blood from the left to the right atrium, with consequent enlargement of the right ventricle (Fig. 9–20*B*). This condition may remain asymptomatic or result in cardiac failure later in life.

Tetralogy of Fallot. Tetralogy of Fallot is the most common congenital cause of **cyanosis** (a dark bluish color of the skin). Its four components include pulmonary stenosis, ventricular septal defect, rightward displacement of the aorta, and hypertrophy of the right ventricle (Fig. 9–20*C*). Patency of the ductus arteriosus also occurs in individuals afflicted with this malformation, but this abnormality is not considered one of the four anomalies of the "tetralogy."

Pacemaker and Conduction System of the Heart

A myogenic conduction system rhythmically depolarizes the heart

The functional integration of heart chamber activities is provided largely by an intrinsic pacemaker and conduction system (Fig. 9–21). Its components are modified cardiac muscle fibers rather than neurons, and

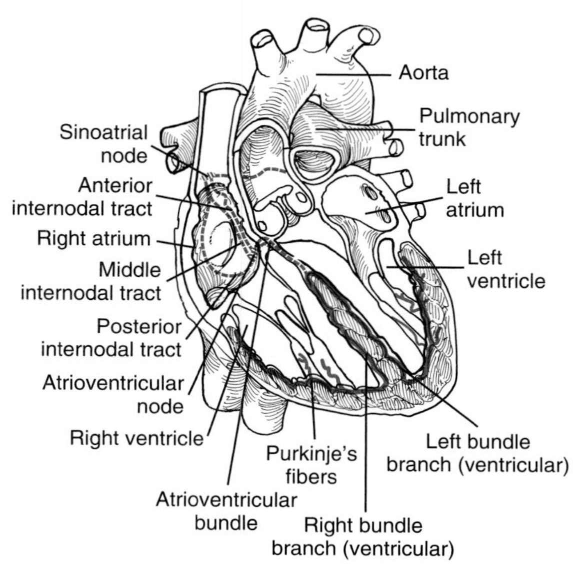

FIGURE 9–21
Conduction system of heart.

it is, therefore, considered to be **myogenic** rather than **neurogenic** in nature. Major elements of the cardiac pacemaker and conduction system include the **sinoatrial node; atrioventricular node; atrioventricular bundle,** including **right** and **left limbs;** and **ventricular plexuses of Purkinje's fibers.**

The **sinoatrial node (SAN)** is located just to the right of the orifice of the superior vena cava in the superior end of the crista terminalis of the right atrial wall (see Fig. 9–21). It is a small horseshoe-shaped concentration of modified fusiform (spindle-shaped) myocardial fibers embedded within the surrounding myocardium. It is within the SAN that each contraction and relaxation cycle of the heart is initiated, and, for this reason, it is called the **pacemaker of the heart.**

The **atrioventricular node (AVN)** is located just superior to the orifice of the coronary sinus (Fig. 9–21). Some anatomists believe that specialized myocardial fibers connect the sinoatrial node with the atrioventricular node. This theory is based upon descriptions of slightly modified atrial myocardial cells within three separate tracts called the **anterior, middle,** and **posterior internodal bundles** (Fig. 9–21). Another school of thought supports the possibility that typical myocardial cells of the entire atrial wall provide all necessary anatomic and functional connections between the SAN and AVN. According to this theory, impulses generated in the sinoatrial node spread throughout both atria via the myocardial cells and then to the atrioventricular node.

The atrioventricular node is clearly connected to ventricular muscle fibers via a recognizable specialized conduction system, the **atrioventricular bundle.** From the region of the atrioventricular node, atrioventricular bundle fibers course into the upper edge of the muscular ventricular septum, just inferior to the membranous part of the ventricular septum. Within the muscular ventricular septum, they split into the **right** and **left limbs** of the atrioventricular bundle.

The right limb (right bundle branch) courses anteriorly along the right upper edge of the muscular ventricular septum and then along the right side of the septum, into the **septomarginal trabecula,** to the base of the **anterior papillary muscle.** Other branches of the right atrioventricular bundle course within the trabeculae carneae to the bases of the posterior and septal papillary muscles. Here, each branch breaks up into a plexus of specialized myocardial cells called **Purkinje's fibers,** which ramify throughout the walls of the right ventricle.

Similarly, the left limb of the atrioventricular bundle (left bundle branch) courses upon the left side of the ventricular septum, breaking up into several branches, which are distributed to the bases of the papillary muscles through the trabeculae carneae. At these sites, the atrioventricular bundle branches break up into plexuses of Purkinje's fibers, which then ramify throughout the walls of the left ventricle.

The atrioventricular node and atrioventricular bundles are completely ensheathed by connective tissue and are, thus, insulated from the surrounding myocardium.

Sympathetic and Parasympathetic Innervation

The heart is innervated by sympathetic and parasympathetic fibers

The heart is innervated by both sympathetic and parasympathetic fibers and by visceral afferent fibers. Central neurons, which provide sympathetic innervation to the heart, are located at spinal cord levels T1 to T4 (Fig. 9–22). The preganglionic fibers that emanate from these neurons innervate peripheral neurons in chain ganglia associated with spinal nerves T1 to T4, or they ascend within the sympathetic trunk to innervate neurons within the cervical chain ganglia (Fig. 9–22). Parasympathetic innervation arises from branches of the vagus nerve (cranial nerve X). The heart is also innervated by visceral afferent fibers that arise from cervical and upper thoracic dorsal root ganglia and from sensory ganglia associated with the vagus nerve (Fig. 9–22).

The sympathetic postganglionic fibers emanating from thoracic chain ganglia that are destined to innervate the heart, along with their accompanying visceral afferent fibers, are called **cardiac nerves.** These cardiac nerves combine with postganglionic fibers issuing from cervical chain ganglia (Fig. 9–22) and with **cardiac branches** of the vagus nerve and the **left recurrent laryngeal nerve** (which is a branch of the vagus nerve) (Fig. 9–22). These vagal branches contain preganglionic parasympathetic and visceral afferent fibers. Together,

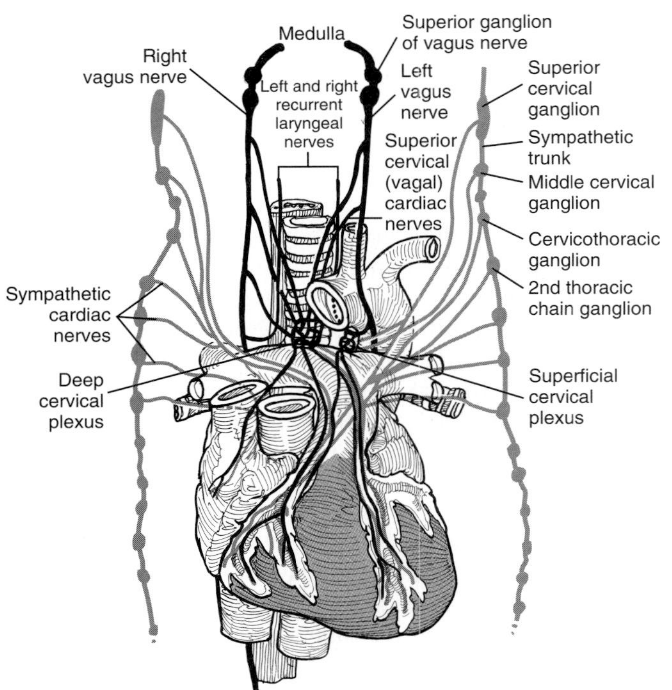

FIGURE 9–22
Parasympathetic and sympathetic innervation of the heart.

the cervical sympathetic postganglionic fibers, cardiac nerves (sympathetic nerves), and cardiac branches of the vagus and left recurrent laryngeal nerves (parasympathetic nerves) form the **superficial** and **deep cardiac plexuses.** These plexuses also contain peripheral parasympathetic ganglia, which are innervated by parasympathetic preganglionic fibers (Fig. 9–22).

Specific regions and tissues of the heart are, then, innervated by postganglionic sympathetic or parasympathetic fibers, which emanate from the cardiac plexuses. The atria and conduction system (see above) are well innervated by both sympathetic and parasympathetic fibers, while the ventricles are innervated mainly by sympathetic fibers and by fewer parasympathetic fibers. It is thought that the larger branches of the coronary arteries are innervated primarily by sympathetic fibers, while finer branches are innervated primarily by parasympathetic fibers.

Visceral afferent fibers accompanying sympathetic and parasympathetic nerves of the heart are important both clinically and functionally. Visceral afferent fibers associated with sympathetic cardiac nerves carry sensations of **pain (angina pectoris)** back to spinal cord levels T1 to T4 from regions of ischemia (i.e., local anemia resulting from obstruction of blood flow) within the heart wall. These impulses are, therefore, experienced as referred pain within the shoulder and arm (see Chapter 6). Normally, visceral afferent fibers associated with both the sympathetic cardiac nerves and the vagus nerve carry sensations back to the central nervous system that participate in reflex activity regulating the function of the heart.

TABLE 9–6
Cardiac Cycle

The cardiac cycle consists of the following:

- Systole (phase of right and left ventricular contraction)
- Diastole (phase of right and left ventricular relaxation)
- Atrial systole (atrial contraction) occurs during latter third of diastole
- Atrial diastole (atrial relaxation) occurs during systole and first two thirds of diastole

During resting state, cycle lasts about 1 second.

During strenuous exercise, cycle lasts about ⅓ second.

Autonomic Innervation of the Pericardial Sac

Branches of the cardiac plexus also innervate the pericardial sac

As was noted above, visceral afferent fibers within parasympathetic branches of the vagus nerve, branches of the sympathetic cardiac nerves, and phrenic nerves innervate the parietal layer of the **pericardial sac.** The visceral afferent fibers associated with sympathetic innervation of the pericardium typically refer pain back to spinal cord levels T1 to T4, mimicking symptoms of **angina pectoris** (see below).

Cardiac Cycle

Heart function can be defined by the cardiac cycle, which is characterized by a phase of ventricular contraction followed by a phase of ventricular relaxation

All four chambers of the definitive heart contract and relax in a sequence that propels blood through both sides of the heart and then ejects it from the left and right ventricles into the systemic and pulmonary circulations. This sequence is the **cardiac cycle.** When a person is resting, each cardiac cycle lasts about 1 second, but when a person is exercising strenuously, each cycle may last only about one third of a second (Table 9–6 and see below).

The cardiac cycle can be divided into two major phases: **systole,** the period of right and left ventricular contraction (Figs. 9–23*A* and *B* and 9–24), and **diastole,** the period of right and left ventricular relaxation (Fig. 9–23*C* and *D* and 9–24). The term *systole,* when used to describe the cardiac cycle, refers only to ventricular contraction, and the term *diastole* refers only to ventricular relaxation. It should be emphasized, however, that atrial contraction (sometimes called *atrial systole*) occurs during the latter third of diastole, and that atrial relaxation (sometimes called *atrial diastole*) occurs during systole and the first two thirds of diastole (see Fig. 9–24).

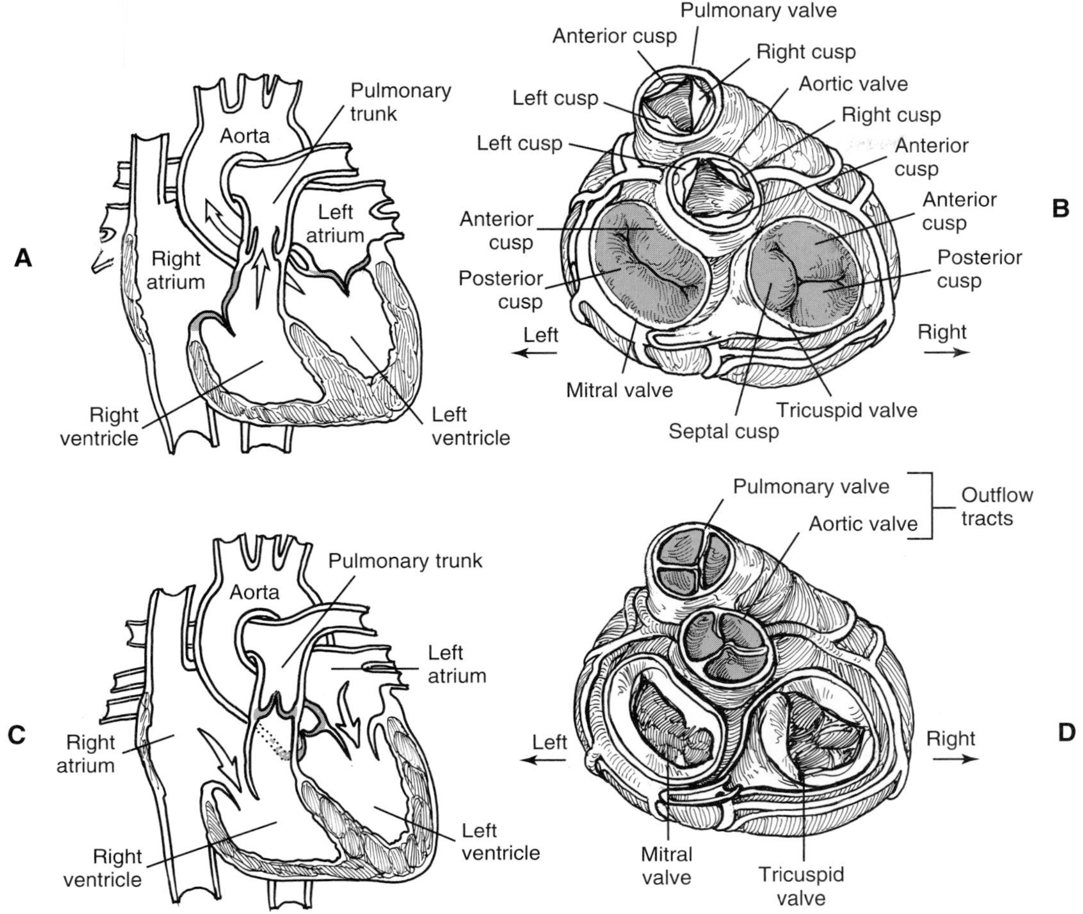

FIGURE 9–23
Disposition of heart valves in systole and diastole. **A.** Anterior view of heart valves during systole. During systole, the outflow valves are open and the mitral and tricuspid valves are closed. **B.** Superior view of the heart valves (with atria removed) during systole. **C.** Anterior view of heart valves during diastole. During diastole (ventricular dilatation), aortic and pulmonic outflow valves are closed and the mitral and tricuspid valves are open. **D.** Superior view of the heart valves (with atria removed) during diastole.

Pattern of Depolarization and Repolarization of the Heart

Specific activities of the conduction system are related to contraction and relaxation of specific heart chambers

Heart muscle cells contract when they are electrically **depolarized. Electrical repolarization** of the cardiac muscle cell membrane initiates relaxation. The pattern of depolarization and repolarization of the entire heart can be shown on an **electrocardiogram (ECG)** (Fig. 9–24 and Table 9–7). This is obtained by applying electrodes to the skin of the thorax in reference to specific bony landmarks and recording the electrical activity of the heart. The ECG may then be correlated to systole and diastole and to the status of specific valves of the heart (Fig. 9–24).

The initial wave of depolarization causing the various heart chambers to contract arises within the sinoatrial node, or pacemaker, in the region of the superior vena cava. The wave of depolarization first spreads from the sinoatrial node throughout the walls of the right and left atria, producing the initial upward deflection, or **P wave,** of the ECG (Fig. 9–24). This wave of depolarization initiates atrial contraction, which occurs during the last third of diastole (Fig. 9–24).

The wave of depolarization spreads into the AVN (possibly via the definitive internodal conduction pathways described above). However, the atrioventricular node delays the spread of depolarization into the ventricles to prevent them from contracting prematurely before maximal emptying of the atria has been completed.

From the atrioventricular node, the wave of depolarization spreads into the left and right ventricles via the atrioventricular bundle, trabeculae carneae, papillary muscles, and Purkinje's fibers and then into the ventricular walls as described above. This depolarization of the ventricles produces a slightly more complex series of deflections, called **QRS waves,** on the ECG (Fig.

A

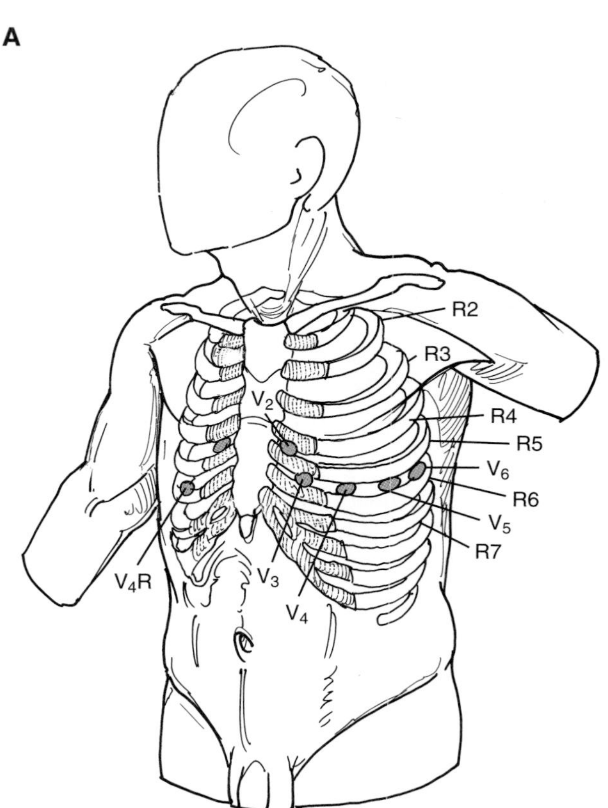

B

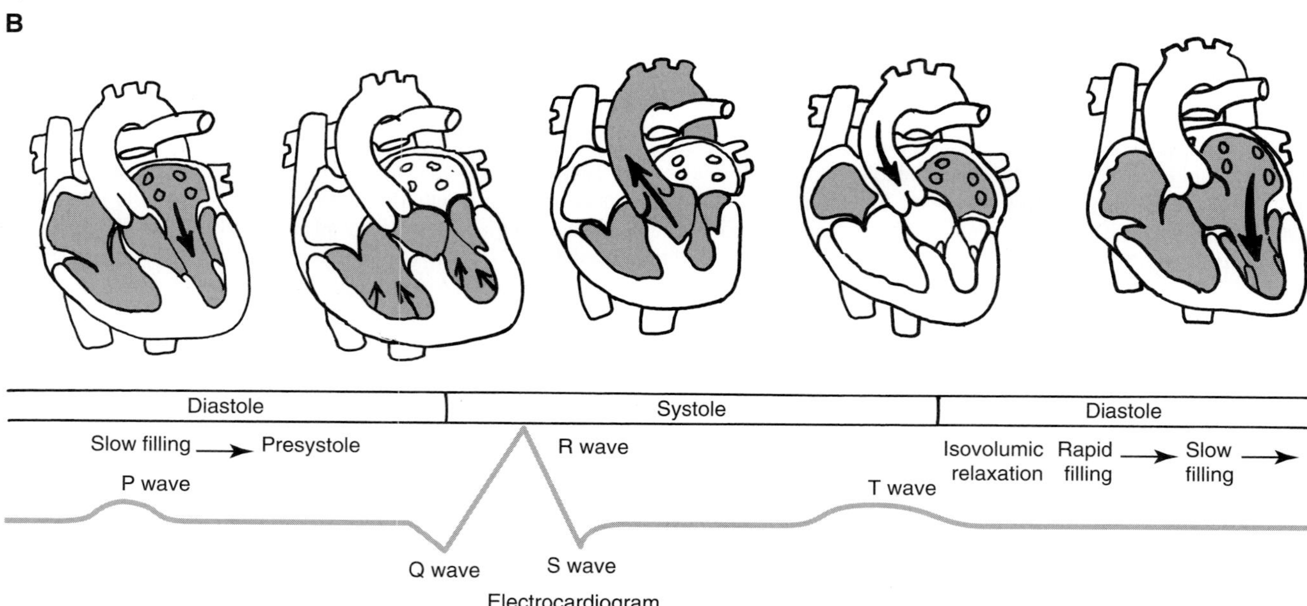

FIGURE 9–24
A. Placement of electrodes on chest for electrocardiogram (ECG).
B. ECG showing cardiac cycle.

TABLE 9–7
Waves of Depolarization and Repolarization of the Heart

Wave	Type	Action Initiated
P wave	Depolarization	Atrial contraction
QRS wave	Depolarization	Ventricular contraction
T wave	Repolarization	Ventricular relaxation

9–24). QRS waves initiate contraction of the ventricles, or the systolic phase of the cardiac cycle.

Finally, repolarization of the ventricles occurs during the last half of systole and is indicated by the **T wave** on the ECG. The T wave initiates diastole, or ventricular relaxation (Fig. 9–24). It should be noted that repolarization of the atrial walls occurs during the last part of atrial systole, but this electrical activity is obscured by the QRS waves of the ventricle.

TABLE 9–8
Important Features of Cardiac Function

STROKE VOLUME

Volume of blood ejected from ventricle during systole (about 70 ml for each ventricle in resting person)

HEART SOUNDS

- First heart sound: long, low-pitched sound heard as atrioventricular valves close at beginning of systole
- Second heart sound: sharp snap heard as semilunar valves slam shut at conclusion of systole

CLARK-STARLING'S LAW

Capacity of heart to pump out whatever volume of blood is delivered to it (within limits)

HEART RATE

- Normal resting heart rate is 60 to 70 beats per minute
- Heart rate is regulated by many factors, including ion concentrations, temperature, and autonomic activity (slowed by parasympathetic activity and increased by sympathetic activity)

Stroke Volume; Heart Sounds

Atrioventricular and semilunar valves ensure one-way propulsion of blood from the inflow end to the outflow end of each side of the heart

Blood passively enters the atria as they relax during ventricular systole and during the initial two thirds of diastole. When the semilunar valves close and the atrioventricular valves open at the beginning of diastole, blood within the atria flows passively into the ventricles. About 70% of the blood flowing into the ventricles enters them passively during the first two thirds of the diastolic phase. Only during the last one third of diastole do the atria contract to complete the filling of the ventricles.

At the initiation of systole, the atrioventricular valves close immediately as the blood pressure rises initially within the ventricles. During the entire systolic phase, the papillary muscles contract to prevent cusps of the atrioventricular valves from ballooning into the atria. Ventricular blood pressure then continues to rise during an **isometric phase** of systole. When ventricular pressure rises sufficiently (within 0.02 to 0.03 second), the semilunar valves pop open, allowing expulsion of about 60% of the blood present within the ventricles at the end of diastole. The volume of blood ejected from the ventricle during systole is the **stroke volume,** which is about 70 ml of blood for each ventricle in resting individuals (Table 9–8). At the end of systole, about 50 ml of blood remains within each ventricle. A practical appreciation of the magnitude of the ventricular stroke volume can be illustrated with a dramatic clinical example. If one assumes that the heart rate is about 70 beats per minute and the stroke volume of the left ventricle is 70 ml, then about 4900 ml of blood is pumped through the systemic circulation every minute. This volume of blood is almost exactly equivalent to the total blood volume of an average adult. One can easily imagine how quickly an acutely ruptured aneurysm of the thoracic descending aorta would cause exsanguination (loss of circulating blood) under these conditions (see Chapter 10).

The sounds of valves closing can be heard, or **auscultated,** with a **stethoscope.** Valve opening is slow and, therefore, produces no recognizable sound. However, as the atrioventricular valves close at the beginning of systole, a relatively long, low-pitched sound, the **first heart sound,** is heard. At the conclusion of systole, a sharp snap is heard as the semilunar valves slam shut, which is the **second heart sound** (see Table 9–8).

The specific sound of closure of the right and left atrioventricular valves and each semilunar valve can be separately discriminated through auscultation within the specific regions of the thorax indicated in Fig. 9–25.

Clark-Starling's Law: Heart Rate

The amount of blood pumped by the heart depends upon two major variables: the volume of blood pumped during each cardiac cycle and the frequency of the cardiac cycle

The greater the amount of blood that enters the atria, the more the atria relax and fill, and the same is true of the ventricles. The greater the amount of blood present within the ventricles, the more blood they forcefully eject into the aorta and pulmonary trunk. This capacity of the heart to pump out whatever volume of blood is delivered to it (within limits) is called **Clark-Starling's law.**

Obviously, the **heart rate** also affects the overall pumping capacity of the heart. The heart rate is regulated by a variety of factors, including ion concentra-

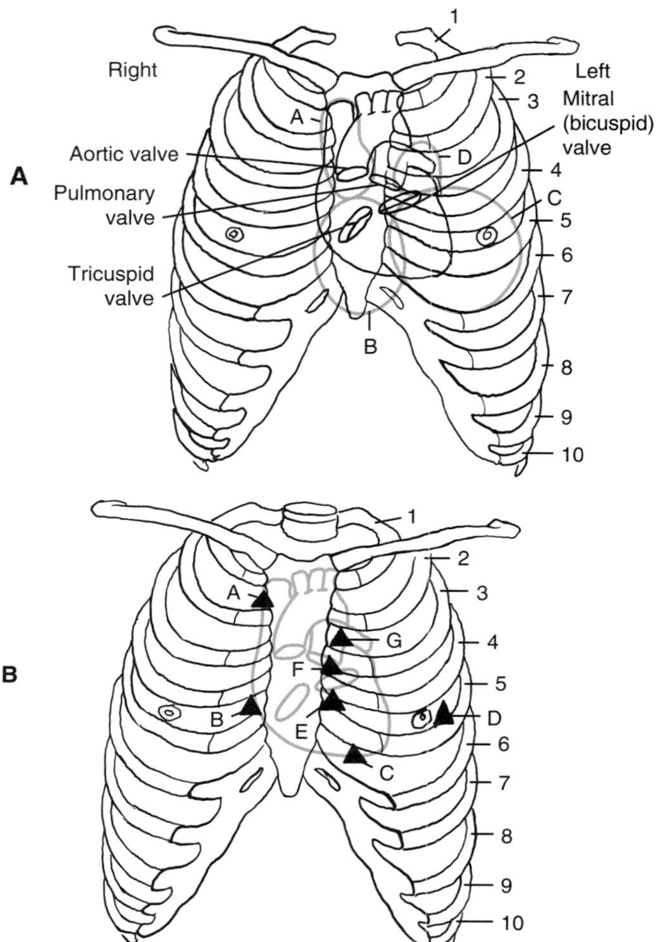

FIGURE 9–25
Auscultation of heart sounds and positions of heart valves. **A.** Areas of chest that can be auscultated to detect sounds from specific heart valves. *A*, Aortic valve; *B*, right ventricular region; *C*, left ventricular region; *D*, pulmonary valve. **B.** Relative positions of heart valves to skeletal elements of the rib cage. *A*, Aortic valve; *B*, tricuspid valve; *C*, mitral valve (apex); *D*, mitral valve (in intercostal space); *E*, mitral valve (in fourth intercostal space); *F*, aortic valve; *G*, aortic or pulmonary valve.

tions (particularly of potassium, sodium, and calcium), temperature, and autonomic innervation. Increased concentrations of potassium and sodium within the blood and lower temperatures depress the heart rate, while increased calcium concentrations and higher temperatures increase the heart rate.

Effect of Autonomic Activity on the Heart Rate

Autonomic activity, particularly of the sympathetic system, plays an active role in regulation of the heart rate and in the strength of cardiac contraction

Parasympathetic activity slows the heart rate, while sympathetic activity increases **contraction frequency.** Typically, the normal resting heart rate of 60 to 70 beats per minute is maintained under conditions of "moderate" parasympathetic activity and "slight" sympathetic control. Maximal parasympathetic stimulation accompanied by the complete inhibition of sympathetic stimulation may slow the heart rate to 20 to 30 beats per minute. On the other hand, maximal sympathetic stimulation in the absence of parasympathetic activity may increase the rate to as much as 250 beats per minute.

Sympathetic and parasympathetic activity also influences the **strength of heart contractions.** Maximum sympathetic stimulation may double the strength of contraction, while maximum parasympathetic stimulation decreases contractile strength by about 30%.

Metabolic Requirements of the Myocardium

Blood flow within the coronary vasculature is regulated primarily by metabolic requirements of the myocardium

Blood flow through the coronary circulation depends mainly upon the local metabolic activity of the heart musculature, although the autonomic system may play a minor role. The greater the activity and, hence, the lower the oxygen tension within the heart muscle, the greater the dilatation of coronary vessels and flow of blood within them. Reduced cardiac activity resulting in

TABLE 9–9
Diseases of the Heart and Pericardium
Cardiac Diseases

CARDIAC DISEASES

- Coronary artery disease
  - Angina pectoris
  - Myocardial infarction
- Cardiac hypertrophy
  - Valvular stenosis
  - Heart murmur
- Cardiomyopathy
  - Dilated cardiomyopathy
  - Hypertrophic cardiomyopathy
  - Restrictive cardiomyopathy
- Congestive heart failure
- Congenital abnormalities of the heart
  - Ventricular septal defect
  - Atrial septal defect
  - Tetralogy of Fallot

PERICARDIAL DISEASES

- Pericarditis
  - Acute pericarditis
  - Constrictive pericarditis
- Pericardial effusion
  - Cardiac tamponade

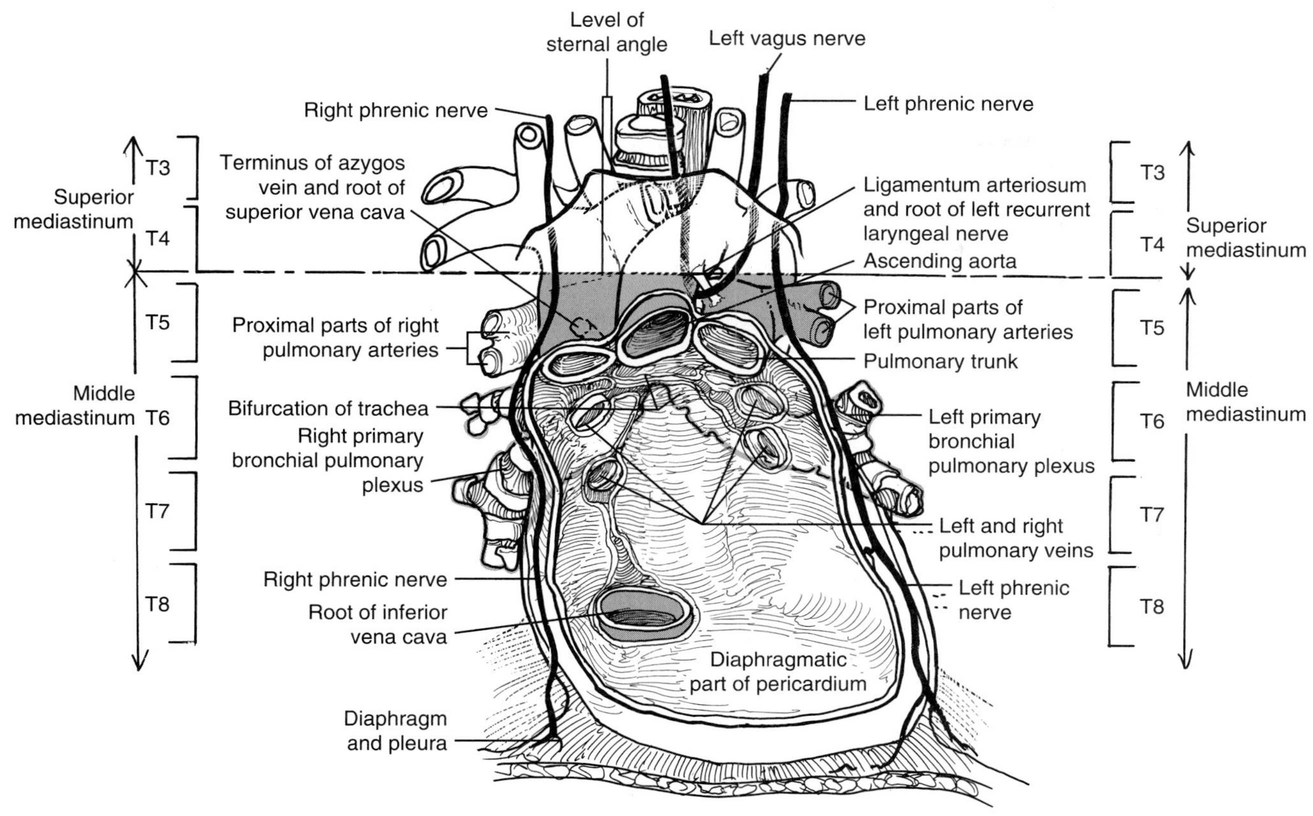

FIGURE 9–26
Other structures of the middle mediastinum.

reduction of metabolic requirements results, conversely, in coronary vessel constriction.

Table 9–9 lists diseases of the heart and pericardium.

▲ Other Structures of the Middle Mediastinum

Many of the other major structures of the middle mediastinum are components of the pulmonary system

Although the heart and pericardial sac occupy most of the space within the middle mediastinum, several other important organs are also located within this compartment (see Table 7–1). These are the roots of great vessels of the **pulmonary** and **systemic circulatory systems** and structures that make up **major channels of the airways** serving the lungs (Fig. 9–26). Included among them are

- the paired **left** and **right pulmonary veins,**
- **pulmonary trunk,**
- proximal portions of the **left** and **right pulmonary arteries,**
- **bifurcation of the trachea,**
- **left** and **right primary bronchi,**
- **pulmonary plexus,**
- **posterior part of the cardiac plexus,**
- root of the **left recurrent laryngeal nerve,**
- **ligamentum arteriosum,**
- **ascending aorta,**
- inferior portion of the **superior vena cava,**
- terminal region of the **azygos vein,** and
- root of the **inferior vena cava.**

The pulmonary veins are formed by sprouting from the left posterior wall of the embryonic atrium. This accounts for their intimate definitive relationship with the middle mediastinum. The pulmonary trunk, like the **ascending aorta,** is derived from what was originally the single outflow tract of the heart, the **truncus arteriosus.** The left sixth aortic arch forms the **ductus arteriosus.** This shunt diverts blood from the pulmonary trunk to the aorta during embryonic and fetal life but, after birth, becomes obstructed to form the **ligamentum arteriosum.** All of these vessels are intimately related to the heart and, hence, reside within the middle mediastinum.

■ STRUCTURES OF THE SUPERIOR MEDIASTINUM

The boundary between the inferior and superior mediastina is a plane intersecting the sternal angle (the site of union between the manubrium and the body of the sternum) and the intervertebral disc between vertebrae T4 and T5 (Fig. 9–27). This inferior boundary of

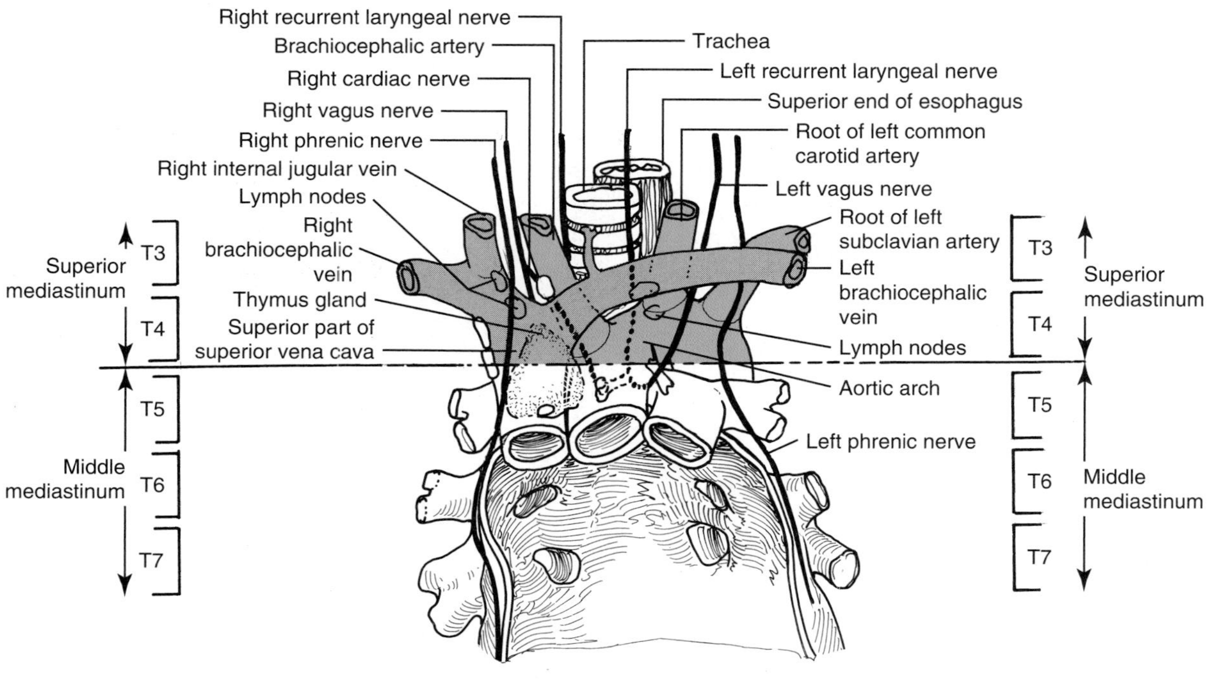

FIGURE 9–27
Structures of the superior mediastinum.

the superior mediastinum, therefore, passes just superior to the pericardial sac. The upper boundary of the superior mediastinum is a plane that intersects the superior edge of the manubrium anteriorly and the superior edge of vertebra T1 posteriorly. Many of the structures localized within this compartment, therefore, include segments of the great vessels that support the systemic circulation. Others, however, are related to gastrointestinal and respiratory functions and still others to lymphatic drainage (see Table 7–1). Thus, structures within the superior mediastinum (Fig. 9–27) include

- the **arch of the aorta;**
- **brachiocephalic artery;**
- root of the **left common carotid artery;**
- root of the **left subclavian artery;**
- **left** and **right brachiocephalic veins;**
- superior part of the **superior vena cava;**
- **vagus, cardiac, phrenic,** and **left recurrent laryngeal nerves;**
- **trachea** and superior end of the **esophagus;**
- superior end of the **thoracic duct;**
- superior end of the **thymus gland** or its remnants; and
- peritracheal, brachiocephalic, and tracheobronchial **lymph nodes** (see Chapter 8).

The development and detailed relationships of these structures will be described in Chapters 23 and 27. Continuations of the aorta, esophagus, and thoracic duct within the posterior mediastinum are described in Chapter 10.

10 The Posterior Mediastinum and Sympathetic Trunk; The Diaphragm

The **posterior mediastinum,** like other subregions of the inferior mediastinum, is located between the paired pleural cavities. It lies posterior to the pericardial sac (i.e., behind the middle mediastinum) and anterior to the vertebral bodies of T5 to T12 (Fig. 10–1). The boundary between the superior and inferior mediastina is a plane that passes through the **sternal angle** (which is the articulation of the manubrium and the body of the sternum) anteriorly and the **intervertebral disc** between **vertebrae T4** and **T5** posteriorly. Because the posterior mediastinum is a subdivision of the **inferior mediastinum,** it is located inferior to this plane but superior to the diaphragmatic attachment to vertebra L1.

Structures of primary significance within the posterior mediastinum include

- parts of the **thoracic descending aorta;**
- **roots of the posterior intercostal arteries** and their **bronchial, phrenic,** and **esophageal branches;**
- the **azygos system** and **roots of the posterior intercostal veins** and their **bronchial, phrenic,** and **esophageal branches;**
- the **esophagus;**
- the **thoracic duct;**
- the **left** and **right vagal trunks;**
- the **esophageal vagal plexus;**
- the **esophageal sympathetic nerves;** and
- the **splanchnic nerves.**

Many of these structures are located primarily within the posterior mediastinum but also extend into the **superior mediastinum** or **medioposterior walls of the pleural cavities.** For example, the superior end of the **descending thoracic aorta** of the posterior mediastinum extends into the superior mediastinum as the **arch of the aorta.** The esophagus and vagus nerves course throughout the entire thorax, specifically within the superior and posterior mediastina. The splanchnic nerves, located within the posterior mediastinum, arise from the **sympathetic trunks** within the medioposterior walls of the pleural cavities.

STRUCTURES OF THE POSTERIOR MEDIASTINUM

Thoracic Descending Aorta and Azygos Venous System

The descending aorta and the azygos venous system are closely associated with the vertebral column

Continuations of great vessels within the **superior mediastinum** serve the trunk and lower extremities after coursing within the posterior mediastinum (see Chapter 9). For example, as the arch of the aorta turns inferiorly and to the left at the level of the lower border of vertebra T4, it becomes the **thoracic descending aorta** of the posterior mediastinum. It continues along an inferior course within a longitudinal axis somewhat to the left of the midline. Its position upon the anterolateral surfaces of the thoracic vertebral bodies and intervertebral discs classifies it as a component of the posterior mediastinum.

The descending aorta gives off intersegmental branches of the inferior nine intercostal spaces (i.e., the third to eleventh **posterior intercostal arteries**). It also gives rise to the subcostal artery just inferior to the twelfth rib. The roots of these branches are, therefore, considered to reside within the posterior mediastinum (Fig. 10–2). The descending aorta also gives rise to **bronchial branches** (see Chapter 8), **esophageal** and **phrenic branches** (Fig. 10–2*A* and *B*), and minor pericardial and mediastinal arteries. The thoracic descending aorta becomes the **abdominal aorta** at the point where it penetrates the diaphragm at the level of the lower border of vertebra T12 (Fig. 10–2). Branches of this major vessel then distribute blood to the lumbar and anterior abdominal regions of the body wall (see Chapters 5, 11, and 13), intestinal viscera (see Chapter 12), pelvic organs (see Chapter 14), perineum (see Chapter 15), and lower extremities (see Chapter 18).

Blood is collected from the thoracic body wall by a longitudinal **azygos vein** on the right and the **hemiazygos** and **accessory hemiazygos veins** on the left (Figs. 10–2 and 10–3 and see Chapter 6). The hemiazygos and accessory hemiazygos veins lie upon the anterior surfaces of vertebral bodies and intervertebral discs and somewhat to the left and posterior to the descending aorta, while the azygos vein lies upon the anterior sur-

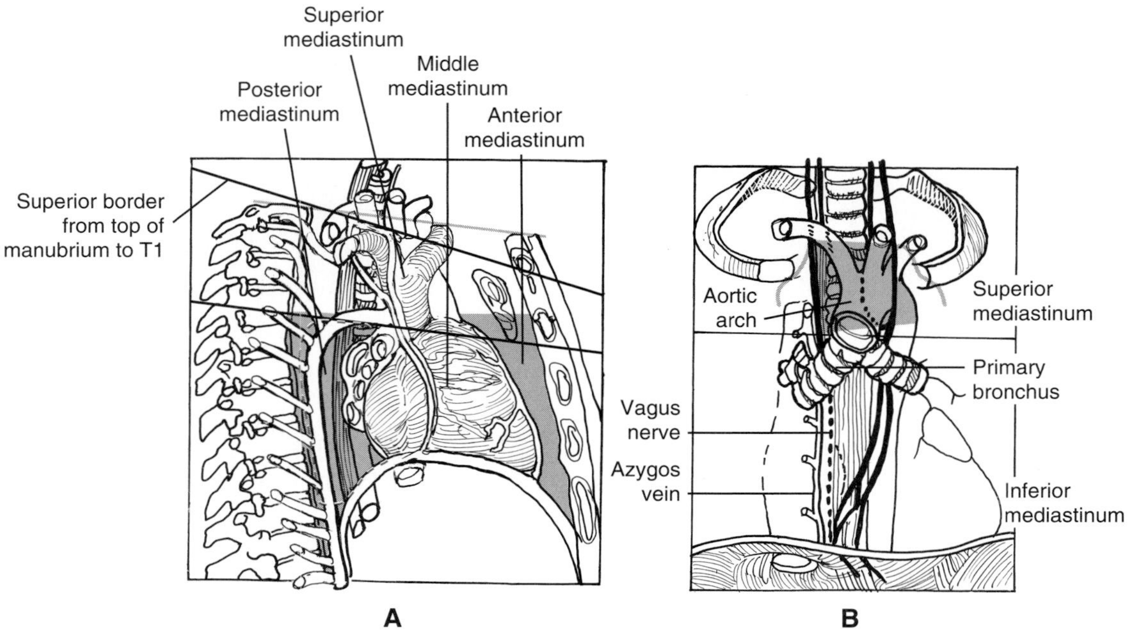

FIGURE 10–1
Regions of the mediastinum.

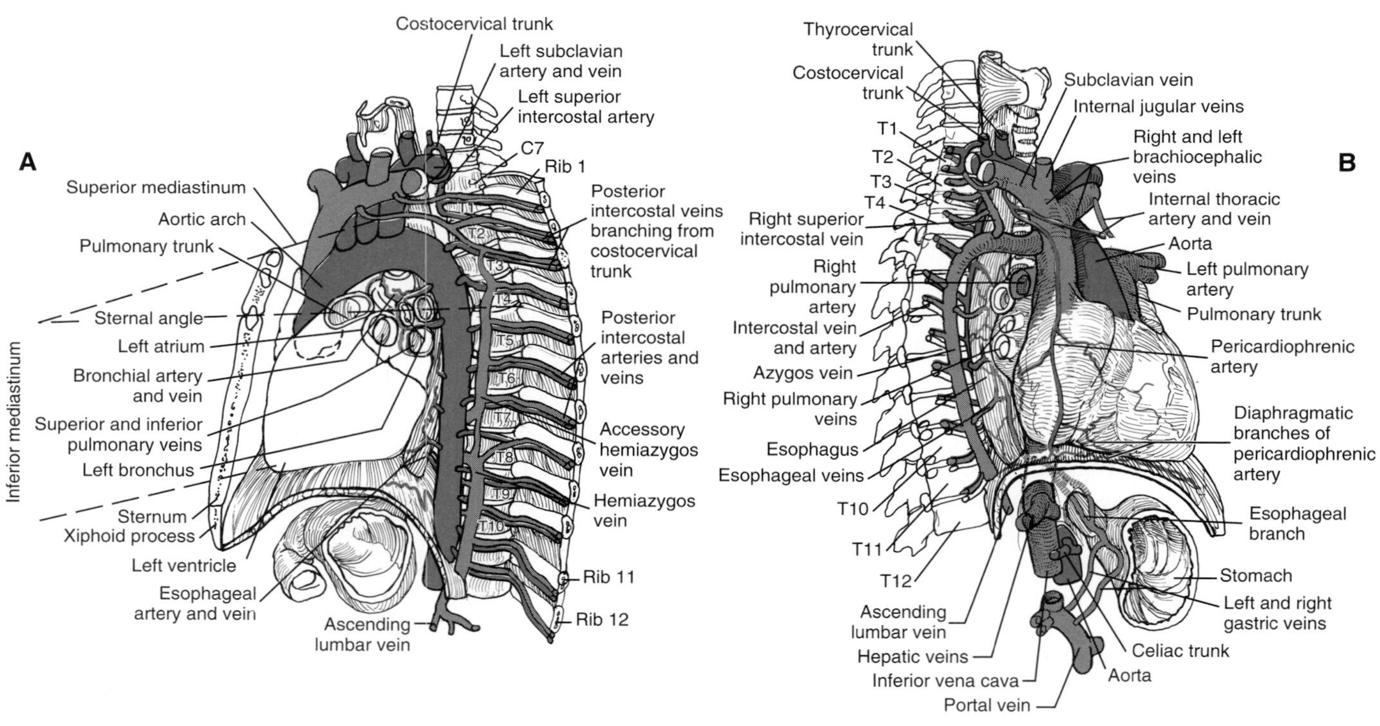

FIGURE 10–2
Medial views of structures within the posterior mediastinum from **(A)** the left side and **(B)** the right side.

face of the vertebral column just to the right of the thoracic descending aorta (Figs. 10–2 and 10–3). The median anastomoses that connect the hemiazygos, accessory hemiazygos, and azygos veins lie behind the aorta, crossing over the anterior surface of the vertebral column within the posterior mediastinum. The azygos, accessory hemiazygos, and hemiazygos veins predominantly drain the thoracic body wall via the **posterior intercostal veins,** whose roots are, therefore, considered to lie within the posterior mediastinum (Figs. 10–2 and

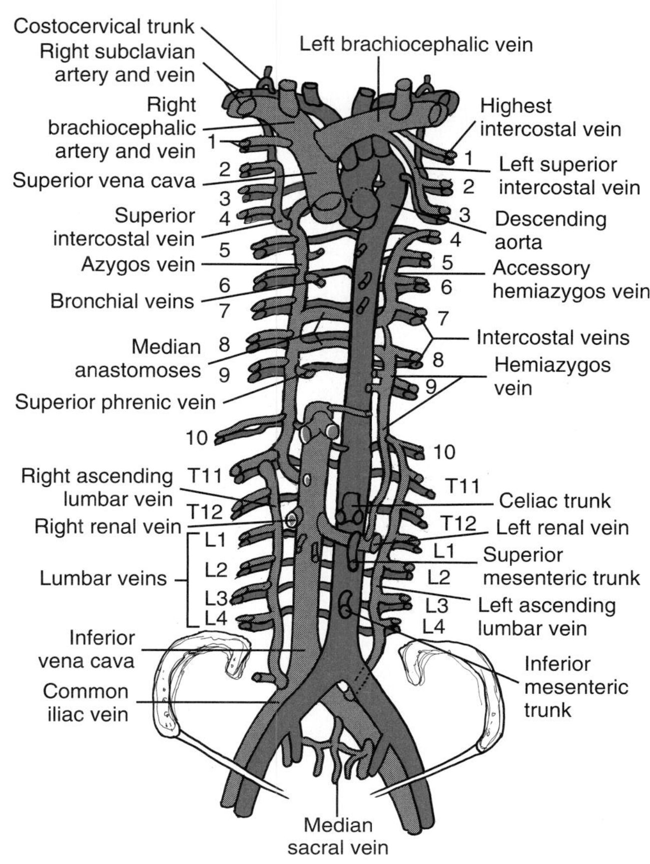

FIGURE 10–3

Arteries and veins within the posterior mediastinum, including the thoracic aorta and its branches and the azygos system and its tributaries.

10–3). The accessory superior hemiazygos veins drain the intercostal spaces above the eighth rib, while the hemiazygos vein drains the intercostal spaces below the eighth rib (Fig. 10–3). Usually, the first intercostal space is drained by a first posterior intercostal vein, which, in turn, drains into the corresponding brachiocephalic vein (Fig. 10–3).

After descending within the posterior mediastinum, the aorta gains entry into the abdominopelvic cavity via the **aortic aperture of the diaphragm** (see Apertures of the Diaphragm, below). A small ascending lumbar vein within the left side of the posterior abdominal wall pierces the diaphragm lateral to the aortic aperture to continue into the thorax as the hemiazygos vein (see Figs. 10–2 and 10–3). A small ascending lumbar vein on the right pierces the diaphragm to become the azygos vein.

Function of the Thoracic Aorta

The thoracic aorta is unusually distensible

Once the **arch of the aorta** has given off its carotid and vertebral branches to the head and neck and its subclavian branches to the upper extremities, it turns sharply and inferiorly to provide blood to the thoracic and abdominal body walls, including the spinal cord and vertebral column, diaphragm, abdominopelvic organs, and lower extremities. The only significant supplementary supply of blood to these inferior structures is via the **internal thoracic arteries,** which branch from the **subclavian arteries.** Normally, however, these latter vessels provide only a small proportion of blood to the anterior body wall, diaphragm, and superior region of the anterior abdominal wall via their terminal branches, the **superior epigastric arteries** (see Chapter 11).

Because the aorta serves as the main trunk of the systemic circulation, the fluctuation of blood pressure within it is rapid and frequent, accompanying each phase of systole and diastole of the cardiac cycle (see discussion of the cardiac cycle in Chapter 9 and Vascular Disease of the Thoracic Aorta, below). The aorta's ability to absorb and mitigate these sharp fluctuations in blood pressure is attributed to its inherent capacity to distend and contract. A consequence of this action is that the blood pressure and flow within more distal arteries and arterioles is relatively constant.

The distensibility or elasticity of the proximal aorta is ascribed to the presence of large amounts of the protein **elastin** within the **tunica media,** which is the middle layer of the aortic wall. This elasticity is slowly lost during the aging process as calcium and other deposits accumulate within this large vessel as a result of vascular disease (see below). These deposits are usually obvious in a cadaver in the gross anatomy laboratory and should be examined and palpated.

Vascular Disease of the Thoracic Aorta

Vascular disease of the aorta may be life threatening and may cause pain mimicking angina pectoris

The thoracic aorta is subject to fluctuations in blood pressure during each cardiac cycle so that during an average life span, the aorta is subjected to approximately 3 billion pulsations. Its ability to withstand these fluctuations in pressure is attributed to its inherent distensibility. If its elasticity is lost, as may occur during aging or as a consequence of vascular disease, an **aneurysm** (local dilatation of a vessel) may develop. Aneurysms may occur within any blood vessel, but aortic aneurysms are the most common and clinically significant.

Dissecting aneurysms of the thoracic aorta occur when blood penetrates the inner surface of the vessel and enlarges it by further separating or dissecting the layers (Fig. 10–4). Death results when the dissection traverses the full thickness of the arterial wall and blood escapes into the pleural, peritoneal, or pericardial cavity (see discussion of cardiac tamponade in Chapter 9). The risk of death from a dissecting aortic aneurysm is significant. About 20% to 25% of victims die within 15 minutes of the onset of symptoms, and 75% die within 1 week. Dissecting aortic aneurysms most commonly occur in males 40 to 60 years of age, who are almost always **hypertensive.** Symptoms include sudden substernal chest

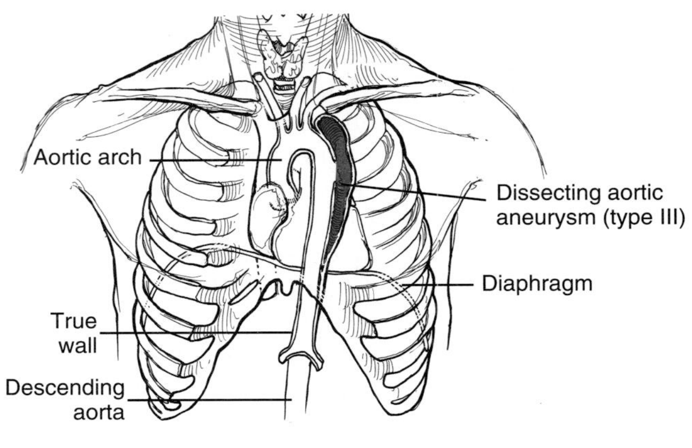

FIGURE 10–4
Dissecting aortic aneurysm.

pain that is usually so severe that the individual immediately seeks medical attention. The pain may be confined to the chest but may also extend into the back and abdomen and radiate into the neck and limbs. (See discussions of referred pain in Chapters 5, 6, and 11).

Following diagnosis, aortic aneurysms are almost always treated surgically, although some may be successfully managed with drugs designed to lower blood pressure.

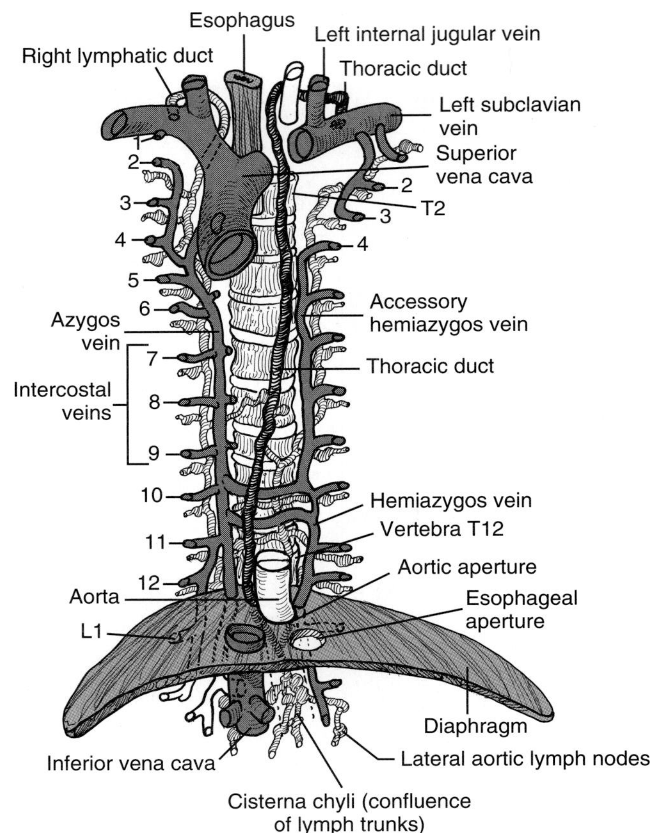

FIGURE 10–5
Lymphatic vessels within the posterior mediastinum, including the thoracic duct.

Inferior Vena Cava

The **inferior vena cava** barely gains entry into the posterior mediastinum of the thoracic compartment. The root of the inferior vena cava is connected to the right atrium of the heart at its base, just at the convergence of the right and inferior borders of the heart (see Chapter 9). Thus, this major vessel penetrates the diaphragm from the abdominopelvic cavity through a discrete **vena caval aperture** (see Apertures of the Diaphragm, below) but then terminates immediately as it opens into the right atrium of the heart.

Lymph Vessels and Thoracic Duct

Lymphatic vessels drain lymph from the abdomen and thorax into the venous system near the junction of the internal jugular and subclavian veins

The lymphatic system is **asymmetric** on the left and right sides of the body as are many other organs, including the heart, lungs, stomach, and intestines. However, the single **thoracic duct** is formed from parts of a system that was originally bilaterally symmetric. The inferior part of the duct is derived from lymphatic channels on the right side and the superior part from lymphatic channels on the left side. Thus, the inferior end is positioned at the midline or slightly to the right of the midline at the level of vertebra T10 (Fig. 10–5). After the thoracic duct gains access to the thorax (through the aortic aperture) and ascends within the posterior mediastinum, it crosses from right to left at the level of the aortic arch to drain its lymph into the venous system near the junction of the **left internal jugular** and **left subclavian veins** within the root of the neck (Fig. 10–5).

Thoracic Lymphatics on the Left Side of the Body

The **lumbar nodes** drain lymph from the abdominal wall (see Chapter 11), pelvis (see Chapter 14), perineum (see Chapter 15), and lower extremities (see Chapter 18). The **intestinal trunks** drain lymph from the stomach to the midregion of the rectum (see Chapter 14). The **descending intercostal trunks** drain the lower intercostal spaces of the thoracic wall. This confluence of lymphatic channels is sometimes characterized by a widened area called the **cisterna chyli,** but this is a rare occurrence. In most cases, once the channels converge at about the level of vertebra L2, the single **thoracic duct** ascends from the abdominal cavity into the **posterior mediastinum** via the **aortic aperture** of the diaphragm (see Apertures of the Diaphragm, below) (Fig. 10–5).

Most of the thoracic wall is also drained by the thoracic duct (Fig. 10–5), which receives tributaries from the left **upper intercostal trunks,** draining the upper intercostal spaces. The thoracic duct may also receive lymph from other sources, including the **left broncho-**

mediastinal trunks, which drain the left side of the bronchial tree and most of the heart, pericardial sac, and thoracic esophagus; **left subclavian trunk,** which drains the left upper extremity; and **left jugular trunk,** which drains the left side of the head and the neck. More typically, these latter three trunks drain separately into the venous system near the junction of the left internal jugular and left subclavian veins.

Thoracic Lymphatics on the Right Side of the Body

The thoracic lymphatic system on the right side is smaller but plays an important role in lymphatic drainage

Many structures on the right side of the thorax may drain lymph through discrete vessels into the venous system near the confluence of the right internal jugular and right subclavian veins (Fig. 10–5). Major lymphatic trunks on the right side include the **right bronchomediastinal trunk,** which drains the right side of the bronchial tree, the thoracic wall on the right side, a small part of the right side of the heart, the pericardial sac, and the esophagus; the **right subclavian trunk,** which drains the right upper extremity; and the **right jugular trunk,** which drains the right side of the head and neck.

Bicuspid valves in the regions where the lymphatic channels are connected to the venous system prevent reflux of blood into the lymphatic system.

Function of the Lymph Vessels

Lymphatic vessels are muscular structures that contain valves

Lymph is excess fluid that accumulates within **interstitial spaces** (the spaces between cells) because the **reabsorption pressure** of the venous system is lower than the **filtration pressure** of the arterial system. About one tenth of the fluid reaching the tissues from the arterial circulation is returned to the heart through the lymphatic system rather than directly through venous channels.

Lymph is squeezed into the blind-ended lymphatic ducts between endothelial cells when interstitial pressure increases as mechanical compression of tissue occurs (e.g., during muscle contraction, particularly during exercise, when lymphatic flow may be increased 10 to 30 times). Once lymph has been captured by a lymphatic vessel, distension of the vessel stimulates smooth muscle contraction within its walls, and this propels the lymph through a one-way valve into the next segment of the vessel (Fig. 10–6). This segment also expands and contracts, propelling the lymph into the next segment, and so on. Some of this segmentation may be apparent in the thoracic duct of some cadavers.

Lymph nodes, expansions of the lymphatic vessels, appear at intervals and are distributed throughout the body. As lymph passes through these structures, it is concentrated by diffusion of water into capillaries surrounding the nodes. Large organisms such as bacteria that have gained entry into the lymphatic system are destroyed by phagocytic lymphocytes, which reside within the nodes. The extensive distribution of lymph nodes

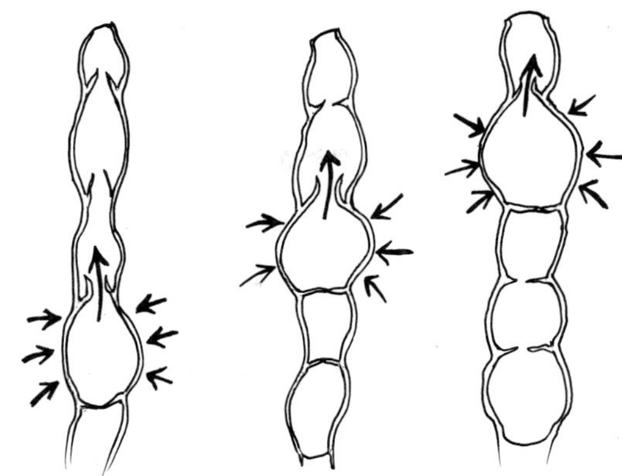

FIGURE 10–6
Lymph vessel valves and the propulsion of lymphatic fluid.

throughout the many tributaries of the lymphatic system provides a mechanism for neutralizing local infection before it spreads more widely.

Because the lymphatic circulation is a favored route for the spread of cancer cells, including cancers of the lymphoid system itself, its organization is of major pathologic significance (e.g., see the discussion of breast cancer in Chapter 6).

Edema

Edema results from inability of the lymphatic system to adequately drain interstitial fluid from the site of an injury

Edema is an increase in the relative amount of water in the extracellular compartment. It may be localized or generalized. **Localized edema** occurs when swelling results from an **inflammatory response** (e.g., an infection or allergic reaction). **Generalized edema** occurs when arterial pressure is significantly reduced and venous pressure increases, as in advanced **congestive heart failure** (see Chapter 9); when the plasma protein content is reduced, as in **cirrhosis of the liver** (see Chapter 12); in cases of **excessive sodium retention;** or in cases of **lymphatic vessel obstruction.**

In severe edema, increased hydrostatic pressure within the extracellular space results in increased filtration of fluid into the blind ends of lymphatic vessels, often resulting in abnormal dilatation. Dilatation may be so great that lymphatic valves become incompetent and are unable to drain lymphatic fluid from the affected tissues.

Edema in subcutaneous tissues or in many organs does not represent a clinically significant condition, but edema within the brain or lungs (see Chapter 8) may be life threatening.

▲ Thoracic Esophagus

The esophagus connects the pharynx, in the neck, to the stomach, in the abdominal cavity, by passing through the posterior mediastinum

The pharyngeal portion of the cervical foregut narrows to become the **esophagus** at the level of vertebra

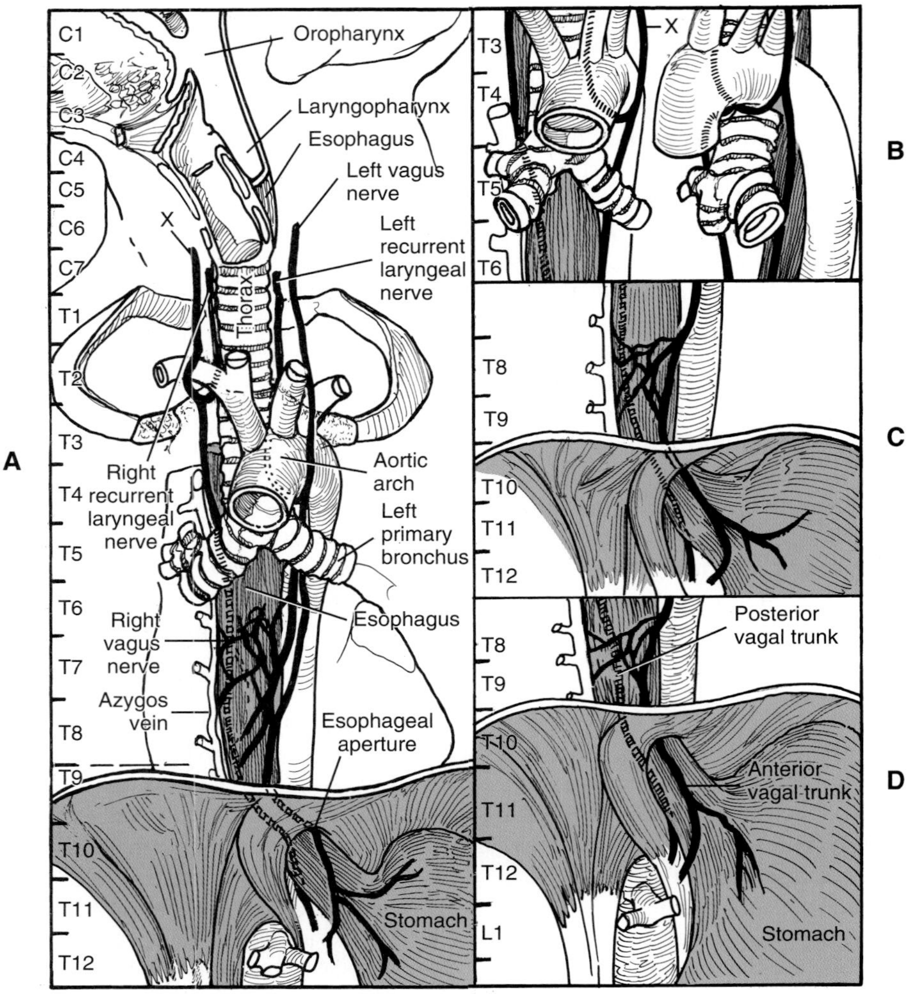

FIGURE 10–7
The esophagus within the posterior mediastinum, constriction sites of the esophagus, and innervation of the esophagus by branches of the vagus nerve (cranial nerve X).

C6 (see Chapter 26 for a discussion of the pharynx). Thus, a short cervical segment of esophagus courses anteriorly to vertebrae C6 and C7 and then enters the superior mediastinum as the **thoracic esophagus** (Fig. 10–7 and see Fig. 10–2*B*). After coursing for a short distance just anterior to vertebrae T1 to T4 and posterior to the **trachea, ascending aorta,** and **left brachiocephalic vein,** the esophagus enters the posterior mediastinum just posterior to the pericardial sac (in the middle mediastinum) (see Figs. 10–2*B* and 10–7*A* and *B* and Chapter 8). Here it lies somewhat anterior to and to the right of the **descending thoracic aorta** but posterior to the **arch of the aorta** within the superior mediastinum. The esophagus also lies anterior to the azygos system and thoracic duct throughout the length of the posterior mediastinum (see Fig. 10–2*B*).

For most of its course within the posterior mediastinum, the esophagus remains located just medial and anterior to the descending aorta. After passing through the **esophageal aperture** of the diaphragm (see below), the short **abdominal esophagus** widens into the stomach (see Fig. 10–7*A*, *C*, and *D*).

The esophagus is the narrowest part of the gastrointestinal tract and can be easily recognized within the thorax as a muscular tube with a relatively constant diameter. However, four clinically significant **constrictions** can be seen at the points

- where the esophagus originates from the pharynx,
- where it is crossed by the arch of the aorta,
- where it is crossed by the left principal bronchus, and
- where it enters its diaphragmatic aperture (see Fig. 10–7 and below).

These landmarks are important with respect to the passage of feeding tubes and instruments into the esophagus.

Vascularization of the Thoracic Esophagus

Blood is supplied to the thoracic esophagus via branches of the thoracic descending aorta, and blood is drained via the azygos system

Arteries of the thoracic esophagus are embryonic derivatives of a network of arteries that originally supplied the yolk sac of the embryo. Therefore, they belong to the same class of arteries (i.e., **celiac, superior mesenteric,** and **inferior mesenteric arteries**) that supplies the abdominopelvic part of the gastrointestinal tract (see Chapter 12).

The thoracic esophageal arteries anastomose with more superior branches of the **inferior thyroid arteries** (see Chapter 27). Inferiorly, they anastomose with **phrenic branches** of the aorta (which supply the superior surface of the diaphragm) and the **left gastric artery,** a branch of the **celiac trunk** within the abdomen (see Fig. 10–2*B*).

Blood is drained from the esophagus by **esophageal veins,** which are branches of the azygos and hemiazygos veins. These veins also anastomose with esophageal branches of the **left gastric vein,** which is a branch of the **portal vein** (see Chapter 12).

Blockage of blood flow through the liver may result in **portal hypertension** and backflow of blood from the portal system into the azygos system via this anastomosis. This may lead to **esophageal varices,** which are weakened areas of dilatation or expansion of the esophageal veins (see Chapter 12).

Innervation of the Thoracic Esophagus

Autonomic innervation of the esophagus is by the vagus nerve and by sympathetic fibers originating at spinal cord levels T2 to T5

After giving off their recurrent laryngeal branches, the vagus nerves descend onto the anterior wall of the esophagus where they break up immediately into a complex **vagal esophageal plexus** (i.e., a network of interconnecting fibers) (see Fig. 10–7). These preganglionic parasympathetic fibers innervate **enteric ganglia** (ganglia embedded within the wall of the esophagus), which, in turn, innervate smooth muscles and glands of the thoracic esophagus. Visceral afferent fibers accompany the vagal parasympathetic fibers and function in reflexes that regulate swallowing movements (see below).

The esophagus is also innervated by the **sympathetic nervous system.** These nerves are not easy to locate, however. Their preganglionic fibers originate within the intermediolateral columns of the spinal cord at levels T2 to T5. These preganglionic fibers then innervate neurons within the chain ganglia at their respective levels. Postganglionic fibers emanating from chain ganglia between vertebrae T2 and T5 collect within the **cardiac plexus** (see Chapter 9) and are distributed to the esophagus. These sympathetic fibers are accompanied by visceral afferent fibers (see below).

Function of the Thoracic Esophagus

Cranial nerve reflexes regulate peristalsis of the esophagus

The esophagus connects the pharynx to the stomach, allowing ingested food to pass to inferior regions of the gastrointestinal tract. Once a **food bolus** has been consciously moved to the back of the throat, it is propelled into the esophagus initially by **peristalsis,** a wave of contractions originating within the **pharynx.** This wave is a reflex action: The presence of food is sensed in the back of the throat; sensory impulses are conducted to the brainstem; neurons then "fire" in the "swallowing center"; motor neurons associated with **cranial nerves V, IX, X,** and **XII** are stimulated; and contraction of the pharyngeal muscles is stimulated.

Once the bolus of food is ejected into the esophagus, it is rapidly propelled into the stomach (within 5 to 8 seconds), typically with the additional support of secondary peristaltic waves generated by reflexes of visceral afferent fibers and parasympathetic motor fibers of the **vagal plexus.** (This is in contrast to the reflex actions produced when visceral afferent fibers accompanying sympathetic fibers innervating the esophagus are activated in conditions of "fight and flight," which inhibit the peristaltic activity stimulated by the vagus.) In disorders of the esophagus, these visceral afferent fibers may carry referred pain, mimicking angina pectoris, to the upper thoracic body wall (see below).

Esophageal Disorders

Conditions affecting the esophagus may result in symptoms that mimic those of angina pectoris

Dysphagia is difficulty in swallowing. It is commonly associated with disorders of the upper esophageal sphincter or muscles of the pharynx. This condition may refer pain to the region of the suprasternal notch or substernal region, mimicking **angina pectoris.**

Reflux of gastric contents into the esophagus, known as **gastroesophageal reflux,** irritates the lining of the esophagus, resulting in referral of pain to the xiphoid area (dermatome T7), which mimics **angina pectoris** and is typically described as **"heartburn."** The pain usually worsens when the patient bends over or lies down and may be accompanied by vomiting, whereas true angina pectoris is usually relieved by lying down.

Inability of the esophagus to effectively transport a bolus of ingested material to the stomach frequently results in **esophageal colic,** crushing substernal pain that may radiate to the back, neck, and arms. This pain may range in intensity from mild to overwhelming and may last only 5 to 10 seconds or as long as several hours. Differentiation between this condition and **angina pectoris** may not be possible based on clinical examination and history alone. In some cases, esophageal colic, like angina pectoris, may be related to exercise and may respond to treatment with nitroglycerin (which dilates the blood vessels).

Esophageal varices are dilated esophageal veins resulting from an increase in blood pressure within the portal system **(portal hypertension)** (see Chapter 12). This is an insidious condition that does not produce pain but is initially indicated by vomiting of blood. As a result, bleeding varices can be catastrophic, with a mortality rate as high as 60%. Control of bleeding, restoration of blood volume, and decreasing portal venous pressure are the primary treatment objectives.

▲ Sympathetic Nerve Trunk

The sympathetic trunk and thoracic chain ganglia technically lie within the posteromedial walls of the pleural cavities and not within the posterior mediastinum

In this description, the **dorsal** and **ventral spinal nerve roots, sympathetic trunk, chain ganglia,** and roots of the **splanchnic nerves** are considered to lie posterior to the posterior mediastinum. They lie upon the lateral walls of thoracic vertebral bodies and intervertebral discs but are not considered to lie "within" the pleural cavities because they are completely invested by parietal pleura (Fig. 10–8).

The left and right **sympathetic trunks** course the entire length of the thoracic vertebral column. Each trunk extends superiorly to the level of the second intervertebral disc (between vertebrae C2 and C3) and inferiorly to the level of the coccyx, where the left and right trunks unite to form a single median ganglion **(ganglion impar)** (see Chapter 12).

Elements of the sympathetic trunks and associated structures are described in detail in Chapter 4, and elements of the sympathetic system present within the thorax are illustrated in Figure 10–8. Briefly, the trunks are primarily made up of sympathetic preganglionic fibers that originate from neuronal cell bodies within intermediolateral columns at spinal cord levels T1 to L2, exit the spinal cord through the ventral rami, enter spinal nerves T1 to L2, and exit each spinal nerve via a white ramus communicans to enter the chain ganglion at the same level. These fibers then take one of several routes:

1. they synapse with a peripheral neuron within this chain ganglion;
2. they pass superiorly through the sympathetic trunk to synapse with a peripheral neuron within a chain ganglion at another level;
3. they pass inferiorly through the sympathetic trunk to synapse with a peripheral neuron within a chain ganglion at an inferior level; or
4. they pass directly out from chain ganglia T5 to L2, forming **splanchnic nerves** that innervate the **prevertebra,** or **preaortic, ganglia** of the abdominopelvic cavity (see Chapter 12).

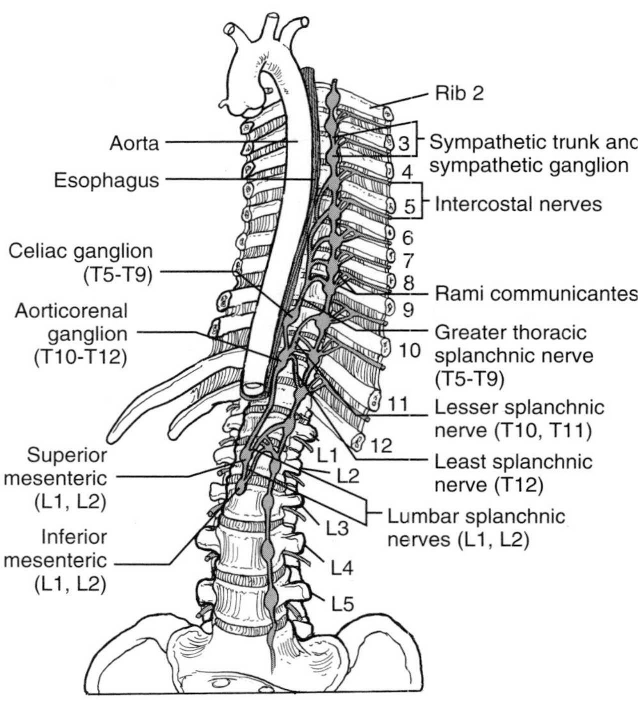

FIGURE 10–8
The sympathetic trunk does not lie within the posterior mediastinum, but the splanchnic nerves do.

▲ Splanchnic Nerves

Three pairs of **splanchnic nerves** arise within the thorax, and one pair arises within the abdominopelvic cavity. The preganglionic sympathetic splanchnic nerve fibers exiting the chain ganglia associated with spinal cord levels T5 to T9 course anteroinferiorly and combine to form the **greater splanchnic nerve,** which, because of its more ventral location, is considered to lie within the posterior mediastinum (see Fig. 10–8). The **lesser splanchnic nerve** is made up of preganglionic fibers emanating from chain ganglia associated with spinal cord levels T10 and T11, and the **least splanchnic nerve** is formed by fibers issuing from the chain ganglion at spinal cord level T12 (see Fig. 10–8). The lesser and least splanchnic nerves are also classified as structures within the posterior mediastinum. A fourth pair of splanchnic nerves, the **lumbar splanchnic nerves,** is formed by preganglionic sympathetic fibers that emanate from chain ganglia within the abdominal cavity associated with spinal cord levels L1 and L2.

Because the greater, lesser, and least splanchnic nerves originate within the thorax, they gain entrance into the abdominal cavity by piercing the musculature of the **diaphragmatic crura** (see Apertures of the Diaphragm, below). After passing into the abdomen, these preganglionic sympathetic fibers innervate neurons within the **celiac, superior mesenteric, aorticorenal,** and **inferior mesenteric ganglia** (see Chapter 12).

THE DIAPHRAGM

The diaphragm is a composite structure that separates the pleural and peritoneal cavities

The anteromedial part of the diaphragm originates from a large block of mesodermal tissue called the **septum transversum,** which forms at the most cranial edge of the embryo early in development prior to embryonic folding (see Chapter 7). As the embryo folds, the septum transversum is translocated caudally to form the bulk of the diaphragm. As the septum transversum travels through the cervical region, it picks up myoblasts from cervical somites, which are innervated by ventral rami of spinal nerves C3 to C5. These fibers combine to form the paired **phrenic nerves.**

Translocation of the septum transversum does not result in complete sealing off of the superior **primitive pericardial cavity** from the inferior **peritoneal cavity** (see Chapter 7). Bilateral openings called **pericardioperitoneal canals** remain at the conclusion of the folding process. However, soon after the definitive pericardial cavity and left and right pleural cavities are formed, specialized membranes, the **pleuroperitoneal membranes,** grow across the pericardioperitoneal canals to completely segregate the peritoneal cavity from both pleural cavities (see Chapters 7 to 9).

The myoblasts within the septum transversum migrate into the pleuroperitoneal membranes and to the periphery of the septum transversum, dragging the phrenic nerves with them to form the posterolateral and anterior **muscular regions of the diaphragm.** The central part of the former septum transversum remains relatively devoid of muscle to form the **central tendon of the diaphragm,** which supports the heart and middle mediastinum on a central flattened plateau (Fig. 10–9*A*).

Other embryonic precursors also contribute to the formation of the diaphragm. These include some of the mesoderm surrounding the esophagus, which forms the **right** and **left crura** of the diaphragm. These structures provide solid posterior attachments of the diaphragm to the vertebral column, specifically to vertebral bodies L1 to L3 on the right and L1 and L2 on the left (Fig. 10–9*B*). The crura, however, are also innervated by the phrenic nerves. Finally, the outer rim of the diaphragm arises from body wall mesoderm in the regions where the diaphragm is attached to the body wall. This peripheral region is provided with innervation by spinal nerves T7 to T12 (Fig. 10–9).

Attachments of the Diaphragm

The diaphragm is securely connected to the inferior thoracic aperture

Anteriorly, the **sternal part of the diaphragm** is typically attached to the posterior surface of the **xiphoid process** by two muscular slips (Fig. 10–9). The **costal part of the diaphragm** is connected to the inner surfaces of the costal cartilages of ribs 7 to 10 and the distal ends of ribs 11 and 12, while the **lumbar part of the diaphragm** is attached to the **lateral** and **medial arcuate ligaments** (Fig. 10–9*B*). The lateral arcuate ligaments are bands of fascia that arch over the anterior surfaces of the **quadratus lumborum muscles** (see Chapter 13) from the transverse process of vertebra L1 to the tip of rib 12 (Fig. 10–9). The **medial arcuate ligaments** are tendinous bands that arch over the **psoas muscles** (see Chapter 13) from the body of vertebra L2 to the anterior surface of the transverse process of vertebra L1 (Fig. 10–9*B*).

Apertures of the Diaphragm

Apertures of the diaphragm permit structures to pass between the thoracic and abdominopelvic cavities

The locations of the diaphragmatic apertures can most easily be remembered by realizing that the diaphragm inclines inferiorly from anterior to posterior (see Fig. 10–9*B*) and by noting the anteroposterior relationships of relevant structures that penetrate the diaphragm (Fig. 10–9*A* and Table 10–1). For example, the **inferior vena cava** penetrates the diaphragm somewhat anteriorly and to the right of the midline within the region of the central tendon, gaining access to the middle mediastinum to connect with the right atrium of the heart. Thus, the **vena caval aperture** is located at the level of **vertebra T8** (Fig. 10–9). The **right phrenic nerve,** which courses within the right lateral wall of the pericardial sac in the middle mediastinum, may also gain access to the inferior surface of the diaphragm via

TABLE 10–1
Apertures of the Diaphragm

Aperture	Vertebral Level
Vena caval aperture	T8
Inferior vena cava	
Right phrenic nerve	
Left phrenic nerve aperture	T8
Esophageal aperture	T10
Esophagus	
Left and right vagal trunks	
Aortic aperture	T12
Descending aorta	
Azygos and hemiazygos veins	
Thoracic duct	
Aperture of greater splanchnic nerve	
Aperture of lesser splanchnic nerve	
Apertures of musculophrenic branches of internal thoracic artery	

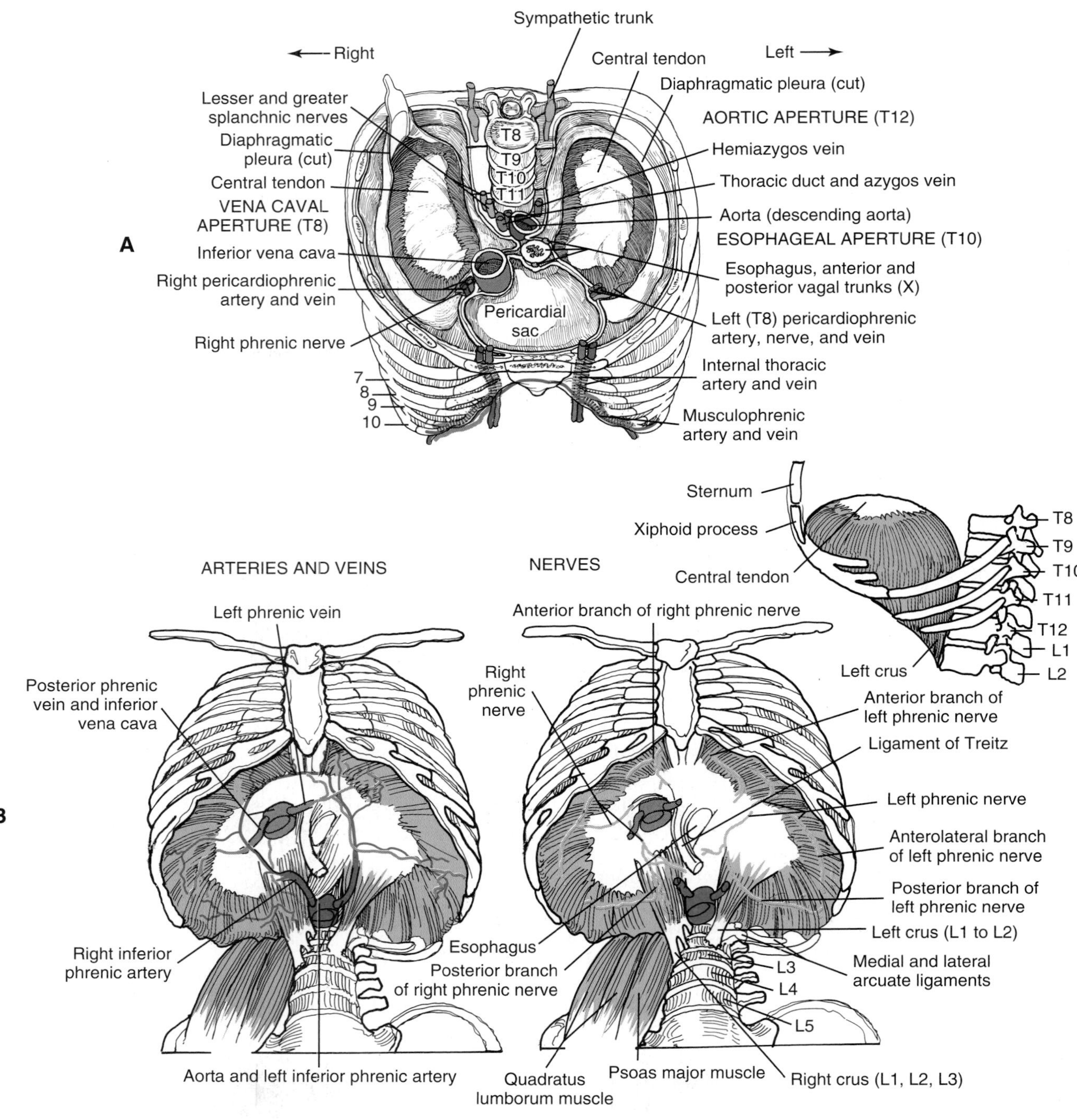

FIGURE 10–9

A. Apertures of the diaphragm. **B.** Inferior view of the diaphragm showing arteries and veins in the left view and nerves in the right view.

this vena caval aperture. The **left phrenic nerve,** after exiting the left lateral wall of the pericardial sac, penetrates a muscular region of the diaphragm at the level of vertebra T8 but to the left of the midline and slightly anterior to the vena caval orifice via its own specific aperture (Fig. 10–9*B* and see Fig. 10–10*B*).

The thoracic **esophagus** is positioned somewhat more posteriorly to the inferior vena cava within the anterior part of the posterior mediastinum and so gains access to the abdominal cavity via the **esophageal aperture** at the level of **vertebra T10** (Fig. 10–9*A* and *B*). The **left** and **right vagal trunks,** which adhere closely to the esophagus, are also transmitted to the abdominopelvic cavity via this esophageal hiatus.

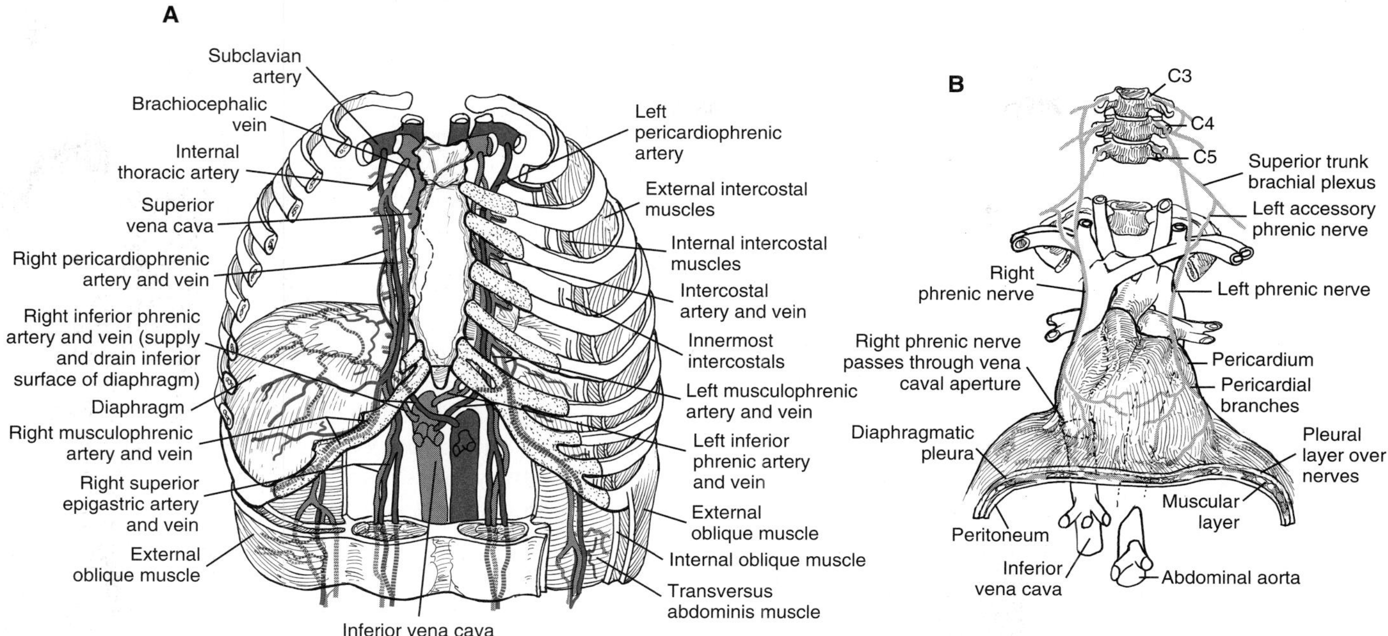

FIGURE 10–10
Vascularization and innervation of the diaphragm. **A.** Superior and inferior phrenic arteries and veins of the diaphragm. **B.** Innervation of the diaphragm by the phrenic nerves.

The **descending aorta** lies directly upon the anterior longitudinal ligament of the vertebral column in the posterior region of the posterior mediastinum and so penetrates the diaphragm via the **aortic aperture** at the level of **vertebra T12** (see Fig. 10–9*A* and *B*). This aperture is formed by interdigitating fibers **(median arcuate ligament)** of the left and right **diaphragmatic crura** (Fig. 10–9*B*). The aorta is, therefore, usually described as passing **posterior** to the diaphragm. The **azygos** and **hemiazygos veins** and **thoracic duct,** which lie close to the aorta, also pass between the thoracic and abdominopelvic cavities via this aortic aperture (Fig. 10–9*A*). The anatomy of the aortic aperture prevents these major vascular channels from becoming constricted during the inspiratory phase of respiration.

The **greater** and **lesser splanchnic nerves** gain access to the abdominal cavity via two small apertures within each of the **crura,** and **musculophrenic branches** of the internal thoracic artery penetrate the diaphragm through small apertures near its connection with the costal cartilages of ribs 7 to 9 (Fig. 10–9*A* and see below).

▲ Vasculature of the Diaphragm

Multiple arteries and veins serve the diaphragm

The diaphragm is supplied with blood mainly by branches of the **internal thoracic artery** and **descending aorta** (Fig. 10–10*A*). The internal thoracic artery gives rise to pericardiophrenic (see Chapter 9) and musculophrenic arteries. After supplying the pericardium, the pericardiophrenic arteries join the phrenic nerves to supply the **central region of the diaphragm** (Fig. 10–10). The diaphragmatic branches of the pericardiophrenic vessels also anastomose with the musculophrenic branches of the internal thoracic arteries, which penetrate the diaphragm near its attachments to costal cartilages 7 to 9, providing blood to the **anterior border of the diaphragm** and some of the musculature of the anterior abdominal wall (Fig. 10–10*A*).

The descending aorta provides small branches, the **superior phrenic arteries,** that vascularize the **superior surface of the diaphragm.** After the descending aorta passes into the abdominopelvic cavity, it gives off **inferior phrenic branches,** which vascularize the **inferior surface of the diaphragm** (Fig. 10–10*A*). The inferior phrenic branches anastomose with other arteries in their vicinity, including the tenth and eleventh intercostal arteries and musculophrenic arteries.

Venous drainage of the diaphragm typically occurs via vessels that accompany the arteries just listed. However, the **right inferior phrenic vein** usually empties into the **inferior vena cava,** and the **left inferior phrenic vein** empties into the **left renal vein** (see Chapter 13).

▲ Innervation of the Diaphragm

Innervation of the diaphragm occurs mainly via the phrenic nerves

Innervation of the diaphragm must be discussed in relation to the origin of specific regions of this respiratory muscle. While spinal nerves contribute to innervation of the periphery of the diaphragm (see above), innervation occurs primarily via the specialized phrenic nerves, which originate at spinal cord levels C3 to C5 (Table 10–2 and see Fig. 10–10*B*). Contributions from the fourth cervical nerve are the major components of the phrenic nerves. These nerves are sufficiently important to the function of the diaphragm that injury to either of their main trunks or any of their branches results in cessation of contractions to the area of the diaphragm supplied and, ultimately, to atrophy of the area. It should be noted, however, that **accessory phrenic nerves** may be present in some individuals. These nerves may be derived from spinal nerves C4, C5, or C6 and descend into the thorax independently of the **phrenic nerves,** remaining anatomically distinct to the level of the first rib or even below the root of the lung. Respiration in these individuals may not be so completely compromised when traumatic injury occurs to the phrenic nerves only.

At the level of the diaphragm, the phrenic nerves give off sensory branches that innervate the parietal pleura above and parietal peritoneum below; these membranes enclose the musculature of the diaphragm. Each nerve then typically splits into three major branches, which tend to course within or just inferior to the musculature of the diaphragm (see Fig. 10–10*B*). These branches include an **anterior** or **sternal branch, anterolateral branch,** and **posterior branch.** These main diaphragmatic branches of the phrenic nerves carry both motor and sensory fibers. It is essential to avoid injury to these nerves during surgery involving the diaphragm.

Respiratory function of the diaphragm is discussed in Chapters 6 and 8.

TABLE 10–2
Innervation of the Diaphragm

Region of Diaphragm	Origin of Region	Innervation of Region
Central tendon of diaphragm	Septum transversum	Phrenic nerves from C3 to C5 (motor and sensory)
Muscular regions		
Posterolateral pleuroperitoneal membranes	Myoblasts from septum transversum	Phrenic nerves from C3 to C5 (motor and sensory)
Periphery	Body wall mesoderm	Spinal nerves from T7 to T12 (sensory)
Crura	Esophageal mesoderm	Phrenic nerves from C3 to C5 (motor and sensory)

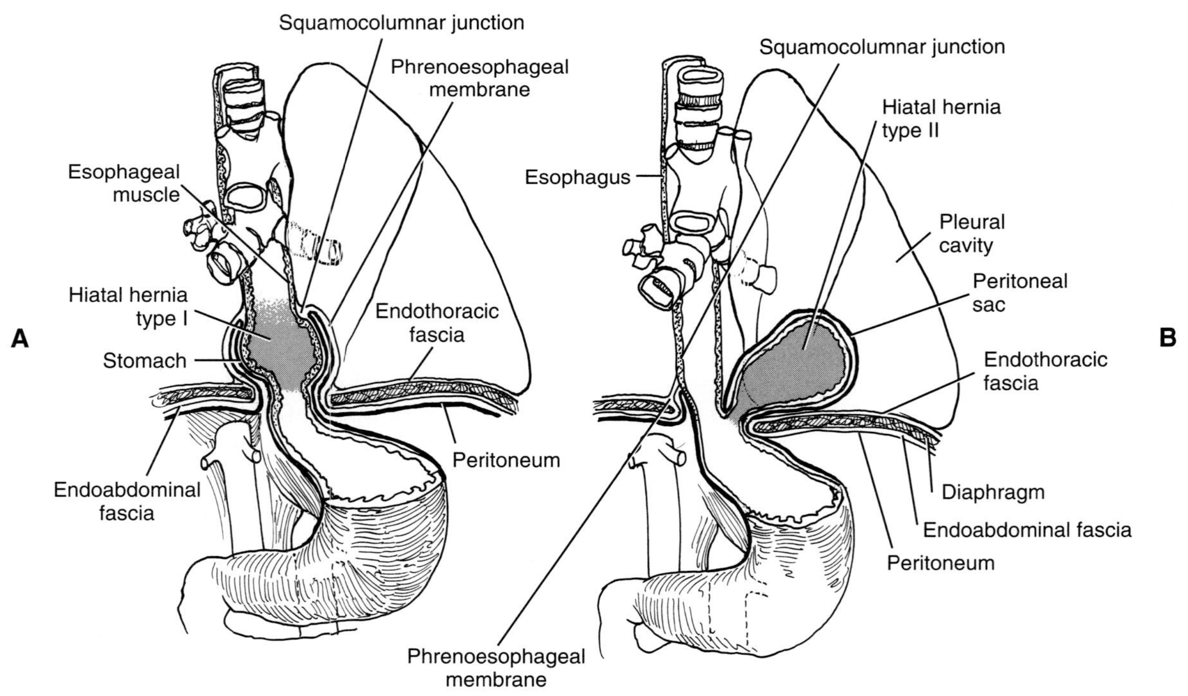

FIGURE 10–11
Hiatal hernias of the esophagus. **A.** Type I. **B.** Type II.

Clinical Disorders of the Diaphragm

Disorders of the diaphragm may affect respiratory or gastrointestinal function

Congenital Diaphragmatic Hernias. Congenital diaphragmatic hernia is a significant cause of **pulmonary hypoplasia** in infants. It is most often caused by failure of the left **pleuroperitoneal membrane** to fully close off the left **pericardioperitoneal canal** (see above and Chapter 7). As a consequence, developing abdominal organs may herniate through the opening during fetal life to occupy the pleural cavity, restricting growth of the lung on the affected side. Infants with this condition may suffer from life-threatening **pulmonary insufficiency.**

Hiatal Hernias in Adults. One type of hiatal hernia of the diaphragm in adults occurs when the connective tissue that anchors the esophagus within its hiatus is weakened, allowing the esophagus to slide superiorly (Fig. 10–11*A*). This condition may result in chronic esophageal reflux of stomach contents, causing substernal pain that mimics **angina pectoris** and damage to the epithelial lining of the esophagus.

A much more serious and insidious type of hiatal hernia in adults occurs when the esophagus itself remains anchored in place within its hiatus while the **stomach herniates into the thorax** via expansion of the weakened esophageal hiatus (Fig. 10–11*B*). Much of the stomach may herniate into the thorax before symptoms are noticed, but, eventually, these patients may complain of shortness of breath, difficulty in swallowing, vomiting, and a feeling of fullness after eating small meals. In severe cases, the herniated stomach may twist upon itself, restricting its blood supply (see Chapter 12). This represents a life-threatening condition that requires prompt surgical repair.

11 Introduction to the Abdomen: Structures of the Anterolateral Abdominal Wall

INTRODUCTION TO THE ABDOMEN

The **abdomen** is the region of the trunk located between the **thorax** and the **pelvis.** It includes the anterolateral walls of the trunk, the deep regions of the posterior wall of the trunk (see Chapter 13), and the abdominal cavity and viscera within the abdominal cavity. Chapters 11 through 13 focus upon the abdominal region. It should be noted, however, that the abdominal and pelvic cavities are contiguous, forming the **abdominopelvic (peritoneal) cavity.** Moreover, some visceral organs or systems are located partly in the abdominal cavity and partly in the pelvic cavity. It is, therefore, necessary to consider some aspects of the abdomen (especially the viscera) within the larger context of the abdominopelvic cavity.

The **abdominopelvic cavity** contains most of the **gastrointestinal tract,** including the **abdominal esophagus, stomach,** and **small** and **large intestines** (see Fig. 11–2 and Chapter 12). It also contains the **spleen,** which is an organ of the immune system, and accessory digestive organs, such as the **liver, gallbladder,** and **pancreas** and their ducts. **Urinary organs** in the abdominopelvic cavity include the **kidneys** and **ureters.** The ureters course from the abdominal cavity to the pelvic cavity. Most of the **bladder** is located within the anterior wall of the abdominopelvic cavity. The **suprarenal glands** are located at the superior poles of the kidneys (see Chapter 13). **Genital organs** such as the **ovaries, oviducts,** and **uterus** in females and **spermatic ducts (vasa deferentia)** in males are located within inferior regions of the abdominopelvic cavity (see Chapter 14). A detailed discussion of the abdominopelvic cavity and its viscera is found in Chapter 12.

Embryonic Development of the Abdominopelvic Cavity

The abdominopelvic cavity, like all of the body cavities, develops from the intraembryonic coelomic cavity. The first division of the coelomic cavity by the **septum transversum** creates a superior primitive **pericardial cavity** and an inferior **peritoneal cavity.** The **peritoneal cavity** gives rise to the **definitive abdominopelvic (peritoneal) cavity,** which is bounded superiorly by the diaphragm and inferiorly by a group of muscles called the **pelvic diaphragm** (see Chapter 14). Two subcavities of the abdominopelvic cavity are the **abdominal cavity** and **pelvic cavity.** The abdominal cavity and pelvic cavity can be separated by an imaginary plane defined by the **pelvic brim** of the pelvic bone (Fig. 11–1 and see Fig. 14–2).

Boundaries of the Abdominal Cavity

The posterior longitudinal boundary of the abdominal cavity is defined by the lumbar vertebrae and their intervertebral discs (Fig. 11–1 and see Chapter 13). Anteriorly, the superior boundary is demarcated by the **xiphoid process** and **infrasternal angle** (defined by the costal cartilages of ribs 6 to 10, the tips of ribs 11 and 12, and the inferior border of rib 12). Posteriorly, the superior boundary is demarcated by the intervertebral disc between vertebrae T12 and L1 (Fig. 11–1). The superior boundary of the abdominal cavity rises and falls with the dome of the diaphragm (Figs. 11–1 and 11–2 and see Chapter 10). As has been noted, the inferior boundary of the abdominal cavity is described by the **pelvic brim,** which may be palpated only in the region of the pubic symphysis and pubic crest anteriorly. Other prominent landmarks of the pelvis in this region that are easily palpated include the **pubic tubercles, inguinal ligaments, anterior superior iliac spines (ASIS),** and **iliac crests** and **tubercles** (Figs. 11–1 and 11–2).

Regions of the Abdominal Wall

Conventional descriptions of abdominal surface anatomy are useful in determining the location of somatic pain of the body wall and referred pain from abdominal and pelvic viscera

In order to identify the location of direct somatic or referred visceral pain in the abdominal wall, it is useful to divide the abdominal wall into four or nine regions by drawing imaginary lines between bony landmarks (Fig. 11–2). The anterior abdominal wall can be divided into **four regions** by drawing a longitudinal line at the midline and the **transumbilical line**—a transverse line through the umbilicus. This divides it into **upper right, upper left, lower right,** and **lower left quadrants** (Fig. 11–2*A*). The anterior abdominal wall can be divided into **nine regions** by drawing two longitudinal **mid-**

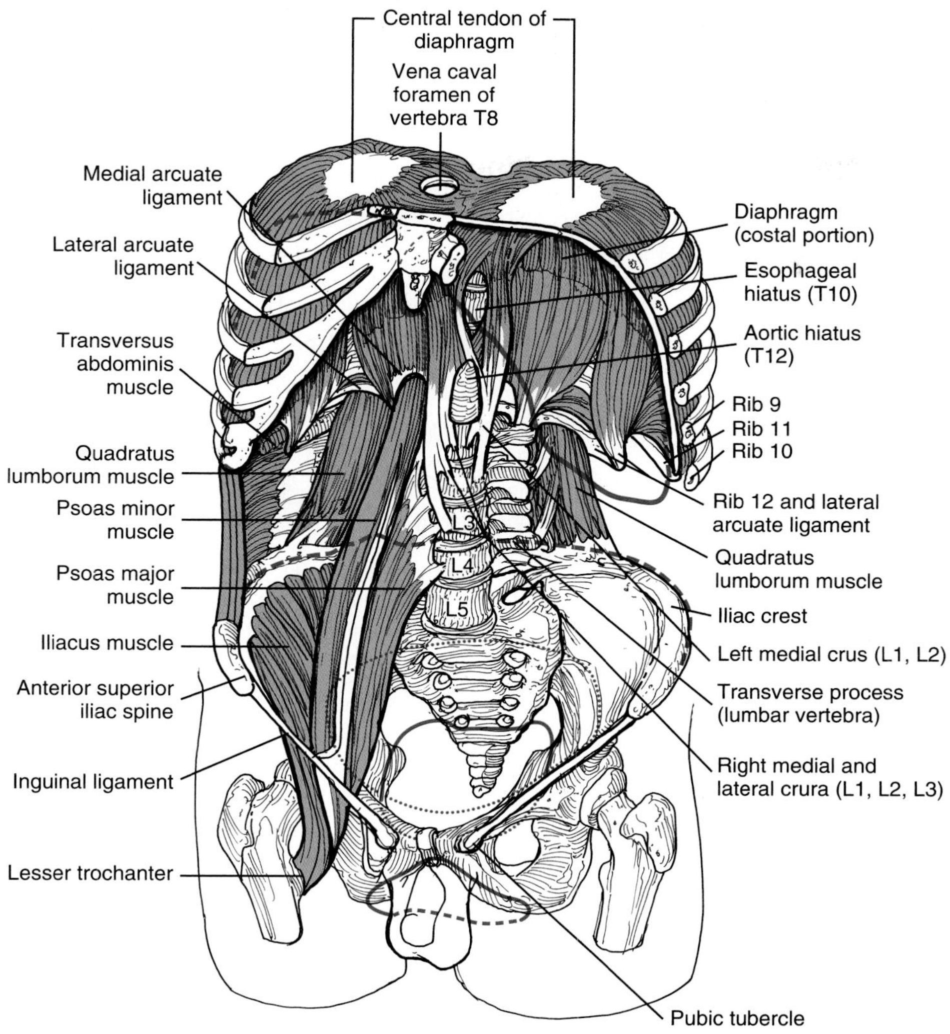

FIGURE 11–1

Boundaries of the abdomen and the abdominal cavity. The abdomen is the part of the trunk between the thorax and the pelvis, excluding the back. The abdominal cavity is bounded superiorly by the diaphragm and inferiorly by an imaginary plane drawn through the pelvic brim of the pelvic bone. The posterior boundary includes the lumbar vertebrae and the psoas and quadratus lumborum muscles. The anterolateral boundary of the abdomen is defined by the external oblique, internal oblique, transversus abdominis, and rectus abdominis muscles. The true pelvic cavity is continuous with the abdominal cavity and is located inferior to the plane defined by the pelvic brim. The false pelvis is the inferior part of the abdominal cavity within the regions of the iliac fossae.

clavicular (midinguinal) lines, a superior **subcostal line,** and an inferior **intertubercular,** or **interspinous, line.** These lines divide the anterior abdominal wall into the **left hypochondriac, epigastric, right hypochondriac, left lateral (lumbar), umbilical, right lateral (lumbar), left iliac (inguinal), hypogastric (pubic),** and **right iliac (inguinal) regions** (see Fig. 11–2*B*). It is also useful to draw a **spinoumbilical line** on the anterior abdominal wall to describe the relative location of the appendix. Typically, the appendix is located at a point between the lower one third and upper two thirds of the spinoumbilical line. This is called **McBurney's point** (see Fig. 11–2*B*).

Abdominal Wall Pain

The location of referred pain within specific dermatomes of the anterior abdominal wall can be used as a diagnostic tool

Referred pain originates in the abdominal or pelvic viscera but is felt in the abdominal wall (see Chapters 4, 9, 10, 12, and 15). This type of pain is usually diffuse because it is referred to several contiguous dermatomes. This may be in contrast to **direct somatic pain of the anterolateral abdominal wall,** which tends to be sharp and localized to the area of trauma, irritation, or injury. Referred pain may be referred from the **stomach, pancreas, gallbladder, biliary ducts, small** or **large intestine,** or **appendix** (Fig. 11–3). Irritation caused by ulceration, inflammation, or stretching of a viscus

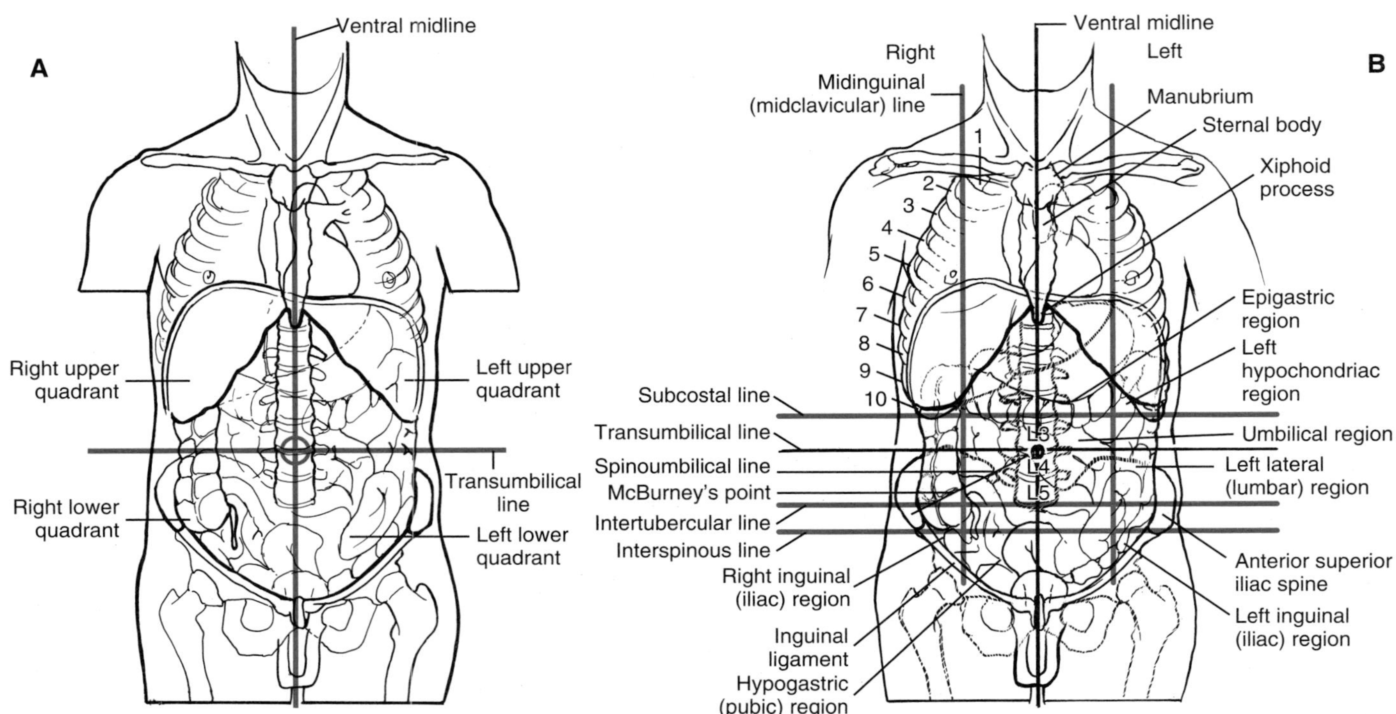

FIGURE 11–2
Mapping the anterior abdominal wall for diagnostic purposes. **A.** The anterior abdominal wall can be divided into four regions by a vertical midline and a horizontal transumbilical line. These four regions are the right upper quadrant, left upper quadrant, right lower quadrant, and left lower quadrant. **B.** The anterior abdominal wall can be divided into nine regions by two vertical midclavicular (midinguinal) lines, a transverse subcostal line, and a transverse intertubercular line. Alternatively, a transverse interspinous line can be substituted for the intertubercular line. These nine regions are the right hypochondriac, epigastric, and left hypochondriac regions; the left lateral (lumbar), umbilical, and right lateral (lumbar) regions; and the right inguinal (iliac), hypogastric (pubic), and left inguinal (iliac) regions. A line drawn from the anterior superior iliac spine (ASIS) of the pelvis to the umbilicus is called the *spinoumbilical line.* McBurney's point is a point dividing the lower one third of this line from the upper two thirds. McBurney's point designates the typical location of the appendix.

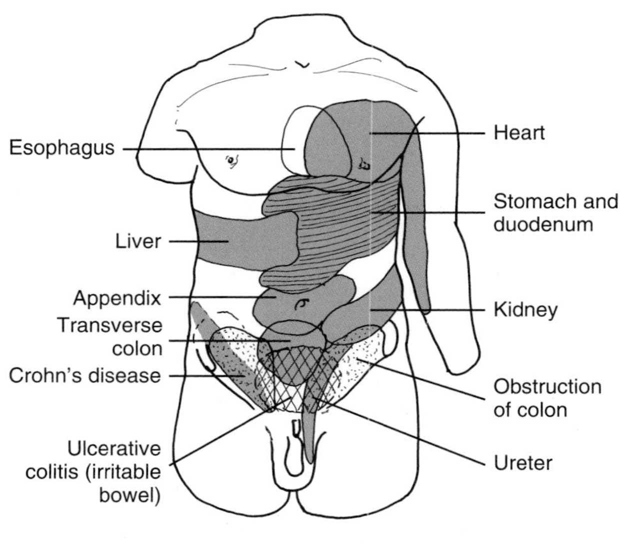

FIGURE 11–3
Visceral pain from abdominal and pelvic organs is referred to dermatomes of the anterolateral abdominal wall. Specific areas to which the pain of inflammation, stretching, or ulceration of various organs is referred are shown.

is a common cause of referred pain. It may also result from irritation of the **visceral peritoneum** by blood or other body fluids. A "map" of the abdominal wall can be used to pinpoint the location of the pain for diagnostic purposes. The location of that pain may be described with the **four-quadrant** or **nine-region methods** (see Figs. 11–2 and 11–3).

Other Disorders of the Anterolateral Abdominal Wall

The four-quadrant or nine-region system may be used to describe other disorders of the anterolateral abdominal wall

Disorders of the abdominal wall may be revealed by anatomic alterations of structures within the wall itself. The presence of **enlarged lymph nodes** within the abdominal wall may be symptomatic of intra-abdominal cancer. Areas of discoloration around the umbilicus **(Grey Turner's sign)** indicate that **retroperitoneal hemorrhage** (i.e., hemorrhage between the peritoneum and abdominal wall) has occurred. **Caput medusa,** in which the veins within the superficial fascia become dilated in the region of the umbilicus, results from blockage of the portal system and consequent portal hypertension (see below and Chapter 12).

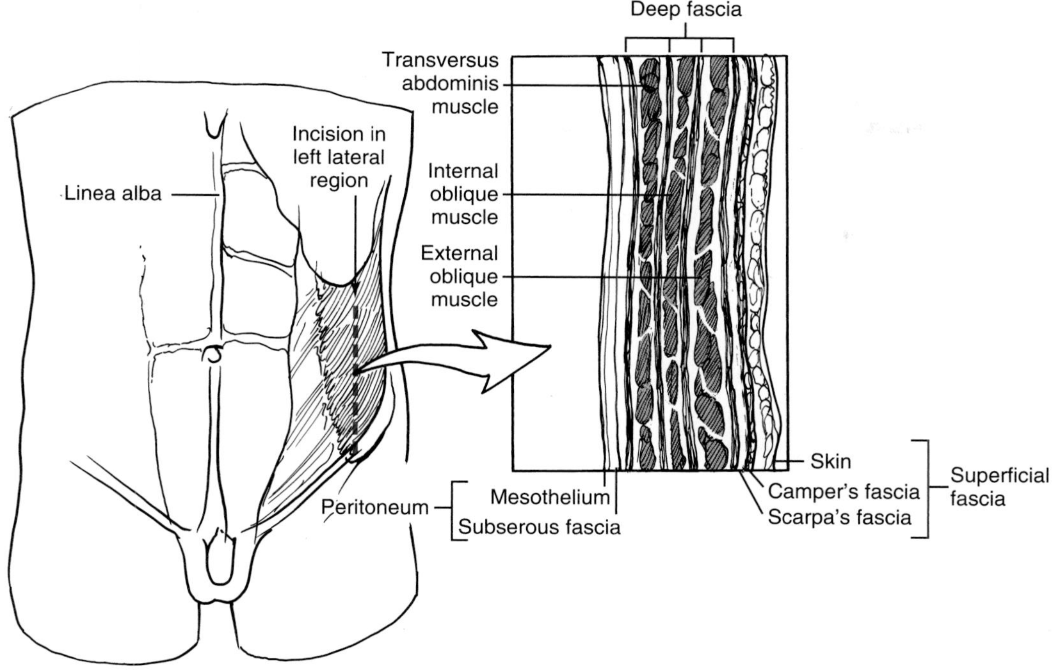

FIGURE 11–4
Layers of the abdominal wall are easily remembered because they are symmetrically organized. From superficial to deep, the layers include the integument, superficial fascia, three layers of muscle (each of which is invested by deep fascia), subserous fascia, and peritoneum.

LAYERS OF THE ABDOMINAL WALL

The skin on the outside of the abdomen and the mesothelium lining the abdominal cavity enclose three intermediate layers of muscle and associated fascia

As in the thoracic wall (see Chapter 6), the layers in most regions of the abdominal wall are organized symmetrically (Fig. 11–4). From superficial to deep, these layers are the **integument (skin), superficial fascia (hypodermis,** or **subcutaneous fat), deep fascia, external oblique muscle, deep fascia, internal oblique muscle, deep fascia, transversus abdominis muscle, deep fascia,** and **peritoneal membrane (peritoneum),** which has a layer of more superficial **subserous fascia** and a deeper layer of **mesothelium.** In the specialized regions of the rectus sheaths and inguinal canals, the arrangement of these layers has been modified (see below).

Integument of the Abdomen

Integument of the abdomen contains specialized integumentary organs

The abdominal integument has a superficial layer of epidermis and a deep layer of dermis (see Fig. 2–1). The epidermis contains sensory nerve endings and end organs of the spinal nerves, which sense pain, temperature, and touch (see below). The dermis contains blood vessels, which exchange nutrients and wastes and regulate the temperature of the body. Hair, sebaceous glands, and sweat glands are present in the epidermis and grow downward into the dermis (see Fig. 2–1). The abdominal region does not have specialized apocrine glands such as those located in the areola of the breast (see Chapter 6).

Superficial Fascia

Superficial fascia (hypodermis) lies just deep to the dermis

In the abdominal wall, as in the back and thorax, the superficial fascia (hypodermis) lies just deep to the dermis. This is a layer of loose connective tissue (Figs. 11–4 and 11–5). In the abdominal wall, two layers of this tissue can be easily identified. These are the thick **fatty outer layer (Camper's fascia)** and thin **membranous inner layer (Scarpa's fascia).** The outer layer, which is a major fat depot, is easy to appreciate as a definitive entity at dissection, especially in older males. This layer may become thickened with age, even if it is transplanted with its associated integument to another region of the body (e.g., the dorsal surface of the hand), as was done in reconstructive surgery. The superficial fascia continues into the labium majus and perineum of females and into the perineum and scrotum of males (see Chapter 15). In these regions in both sexes, it is known as **Colles' fascia** (Fig. 11–5). In the scrotal wall of the male, however, the superficial fascia contains nonstriated muscle and is called the **tunica dartos** or **dartos muscle** (Fig. 11–5). The tunica dartos contracts to pull the testes closer to the body wall in cold temperatures.

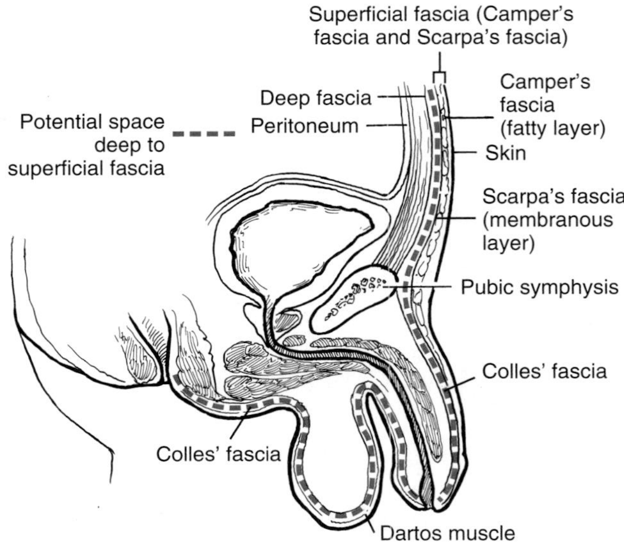

FIGURE 11–5
The superficial fascia (hypodermis) consists of a superficial fatty layer (Camper's fascia) and a deeper membranous layer (Scarpa's fascia). The layers adhere tightly to each other. These two layers continue into the perineum, where they are collectively called *Colles' fascia.* The superficial fascia of the scrotal wall contains smooth muscle fibers and is called the *tunica dartos (dartos muscle).*

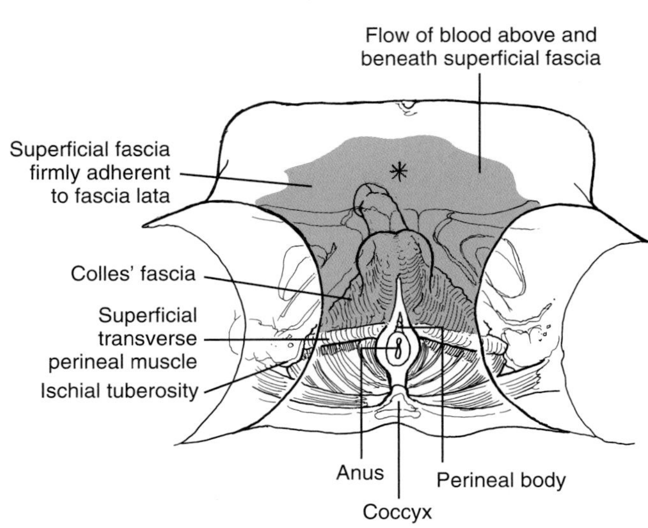

FIGURE 11–6
The membranous layer of superficial fascia is only loosely connected to the underlying deep fascia, except along a line between the ischial tuberosities (in the region of the superficial transverse perineal muscles) and at the boundaries of the thighs. Following accidents to the perineum, blood or urine may be released into the space just deep to the superficial fascia. The blood or urine cannot enter the thighs but may seep upward, into the abdominal region.

Scarpa's fascia is difficult to appreciate at dissection because it tends to be so closely adherent to the overlying layer of Camper's fascia (Fig. 11–5). Because Scarpa's fascia is not firmly bound to the underlying deep fascia covering the external oblique muscle, however, a space may develop between these layers, resulting from seepage of blood or urine following injury to the urethra or perineal vessels (Figs. 11–5 and 11–6). Scarpa's fascia and Colles' fascia, however, are firmly fused to the underlying deep fascia at the boundary between the abdomen and the thigh, at the boundary between the perineum and the thigh, and along a strip of deep fascia connecting the **ischial tuberosities of the pelvic bone.** This fusion prevents blood and urine from seeping into the thigh and anal triangle of the perineum (Fig. 11–6 and see Chapter 15).

▲ Muscles of the Abdominal Wall

The three layers of abdominal wall muscles are homologous to muscles of the thoracic wall, but there is also a fourth segment of muscle in the abdominal wall (and sometimes a fifth)

The reader will recall that the trunk musculature develops from the segmental somites, which split into myotomes, sclerotomes, and dermatomes during the fourth week of development (see Chapters 3 and 5). At first, each myotome splits into an **epimere** and a **hypomere.** Each epimere is innervated by a **dorsal primary ramus** of a spinal nerve, and each hypomere is innervated by a **ventral primary ramus** of a spinal nerve. True deep back muscles are derived from epimeres and are, therefore, innervated by dorsal primary rami. Intercostal muscles of the thoracic region are derived from hypomeres and are innervated by ventral primary rami (Fig. 11–7).

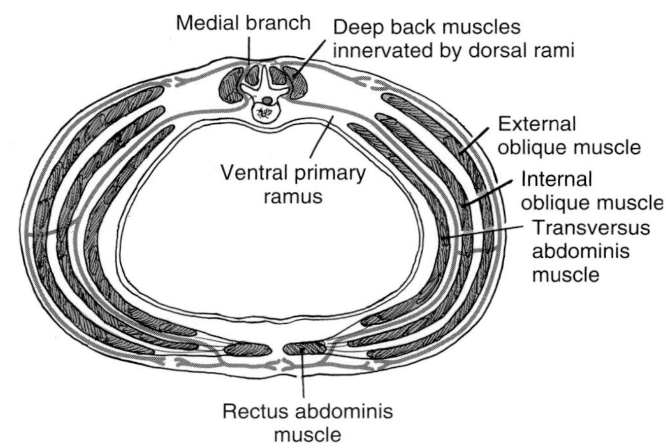

FIGURE 11–7
Innervation of muscles that have descended from hypomeres.

Like the intercostal muscles, the **abdominal muscles** are derived from pairs of **hypomeres.** In the case of the abdominal muscles, however, each hypomere splits into four parts rather than three (Figs. 11–7 and 11–8).

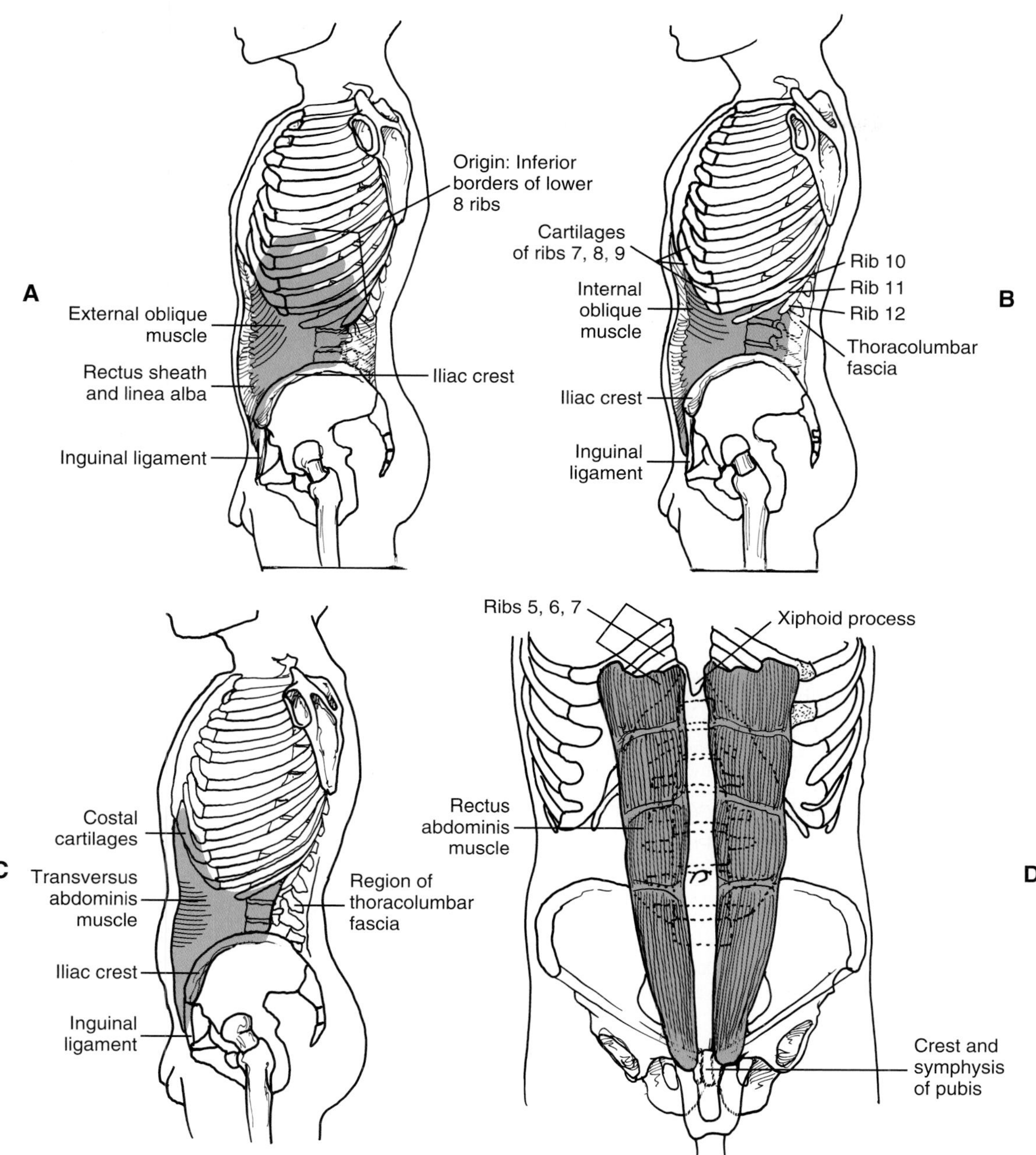

FIGURE 11–8

Muscles of the anterolateral abdominal wall. **A.** The external oblique muscles arise from the outer surfaces and lower borders of the most inferior eight ribs. The distal tendon inserts upon the xiphoid process, linea alba, and pubic symphysis; the pubic tubercle; and the anterior half of the iliac crest of the pelvis bone. Fibers of the external oblique muscle are directed inferomedially. The inferior border of the external oblique muscle forms the inguinal ligament, which connects the pubic tubercle and the anterior superior iliac spine (ASIS). **B.** The internal oblique muscles arise from the thoracolumbar fascia, the anterior two thirds of the iliac crests, and the lateral two thirds of the inguinal ligament. These muscles insert upon the pubic crest, pubic symphysis, and linea alba. The fibers of the internal oblique muscles are directed at right angles to those of the external oblique muscles. **C.** The transversus abdominis muscles arise from the costal cartilages of ribs 7 to 10; from ribs 11 and 12; and from the thoracolumbar fascia, the anterior two thirds of the iliac crest, and the lateral one third of the inguinal ligament. Their most inferomedial fibers blend with those of the internal oblique muscles to form the conjoined tendons. The conjoined tendons insert upon the pubic crest and pubic symphysis. Fibers of the transversus abdominis muscles course horizontally. **D.** The rectus columns are attached inferiorly to the pubic crest and pubic symphysis and superiorly to the xiphoid process and costal cartilages of ribs 5 to 7. They are marked by tendinous intersections that reveal the regions of fusion between adjacent hypomeres. Each of the rectus columns is enclosed within a specialized rectus sheath formed by the aponeuroses of the external oblique, internal oblique, and transversus abdominis muscles (see Fig. 11–15).

Three of these parts correspond to the precursors that give rise to the external, internal, and innermost intercostal muscles of the thoracic region. In the abdominal wall, these are the **external oblique, internal oblique,** and **transversus abdominis muscles** (Figs. 11–7 and 11–8 and see Fig. 2–3). The fourth segment gives rise to the **rectus abdominis muscles (rectus columns),** which flank the abdominal ventral midline (Figs. 11–7, 11–8*D*, and 11–9). A fifth pair of muscles, the **pyramidalis muscles,** is sometimes present also (Fig. 11–9). The origins and insertions of these muscles are described in Table 11–1.

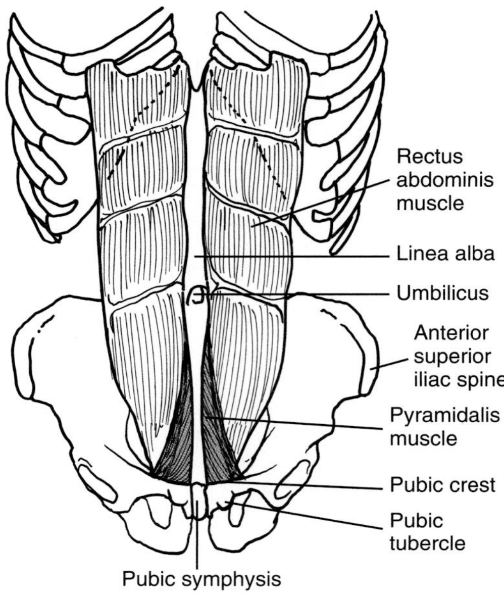

FIGURE 11–9
The pyramidalis muscles. These inconstant muscles arise from the pubic crest and pubic symphysis to insert upon the inferior end of the linea alba.

External Oblique Muscles

The external oblique muscles are the most superficial of the abdominal wall muscles

As with the external intercostal muscles, the fibers of the external oblique muscles course obliquely from a lateral superior region of the abdomen to more inferior medial regions (i.e., in the same direction that the fingers are pointing when the hands are in the front pockets) (see Fig. 11–8*A*). The superolateral attachments (often referred to as *origins*) of these paired muscle sheets are from the outer surfaces and lower borders of the most inferior eight ribs (Table 11–1). However, muscle fibers of the external oblique muscles are confined to the superolateral regions of the anterolateral body wall. They rarely descend further than the level of a line drawn between the anterior superior iliac spine (ASIS) and the umbilicus (a spinoumbilical line). At this point, muscle fibers give way to a strong tendinous **aponeurosis,** which is an expanded fibrous sheet of tendon. The medial and inferior terminations of this aponeurosis are the insertions of the external oblique muscle (see Fig. 11–8*A*).

Thus, the medial insertion of the external oblique muscle is a ventral midline tendon formed by fusion of the paired external oblique, internal oblique, and transversus abdominis muscle tendons. This is the **linea alba,** which is characterized as a tendinous **raphe** (i.e., the line of union of two contiguous bilaterally symmetric structures). It courses from the **xiphoid process** superiorly to the **pubic symphysis** inferiorly (see Figs. 11–8*A* and 11–9). The most inferior border of the external oblique muscle is a thickened tendon called the **inguinal ligament.** This tough band of tendon extends from the **pubic tubercle** to the **ASIS** of the iliac bone. It is folded under and inward slightly, forming a shallow trough deep to the inferior edge of the external oblique aponeurosis (see Figs. 11–8*A* and 11–19). The most pos-

TABLE 11–1
Origins and Insertions of Abdominal Muscles

Muscle	Origins	Insertions
External oblique	Outer surfaces and lower borders of ribs 5 to 12	Anterior half of iliac crest, anterior superior iliac spine, pubic tubercle, pubic crest, pubic symphysis, linea alba, xiphoid process
Internal oblique	Thoracolumbar fascia, anterior two thirds of iliac crest, lateral two thirds of inguinal ligament	Pubic crest, pubic symphysis, linea alba, costal cartilages of ribs 7 to 9, inferior borders of ribs 11 and 12
Transversus abdominis	Costal cartilages of ribs 7 to 10, inferior surfaces of ribs 11 and 12, thoracolumbar fascia, anterior two thirds of iliac crest, lateral one third of inguinal ligament	Xiphoid process, linea alba, pubic symphysis, pubic crest
Rectus abdominis	Pubic symphysis, pubic crest	Costal cartilages of ribs 5 to 7, xiphoid process
Pyramidalis	Pubic symphysis, pubic crest	Linea alba to point halfway between pubic symphysis and umbilicus

terior region of the external oblique muscle, which arises from ribs 11 and 12, is inserted onto the anterior half of the **iliac crest** (see Fig. 11–8 and Table 11–1).

Internal Oblique Muscles

Internal oblique muscles lie deep to the external oblique muscles

The internal oblique muscles are thinner than the external oblique muscles, and their fibers course at an angle approximately 90 degrees from the direction of the external oblique muscle fibers. The internal oblique muscles arise from the anterior edge of the **thoracolumbar fascia,** the anterior two thirds of the **iliac crests,** and the lateral two thirds of the **inguinal ligament** (see Figs. 5–15 and 11–8*B* and Table 11–1). Fibers of the internal oblique muscles arising from the most medial regions of their attachments to the inguinal ligaments arch over the **spermatic cord** in males or **round ligament of the uterus** in females to blend with deeper fibers of the transversus abdominis muscles, forming the **conjoined tendon (falx inguinalis)** (see Fig. 11–19*C* to *E*). The fibers of the conjoined tendon insert upon the **pubic crest** and **pubic symphysis** (see Table 11–1). Internal oblique fibers arising from the more lateral regions of the inguinal ligament and most regions of the iliac crest insert along the ventral midline within the **linea alba** and superiorly upon the cartilages of ribs 7 to 9. The internal oblique fibers arising from the most posterior regions of the iliac crest insert onto the inferior borders of ribs 10 to 12 (see Fig. 11–8*B* and Table 11–1).

The **cremaster muscle** is a specialized region of the internal oblique muscle that invests the spermatic cord in males. This muscle will be described in the discussion of the **inguinal canal,** below (see Figs. 11–16, 11–17, and 11–22).

Transversus Abdominis Muscles

The deepest layer of anterolateral abdominal muscles is the transversus abdominis muscles

The transversus abdominis muscles are named for the direction of their fibers, which course horizontally (see Fig. 11–8C). The origins of these muscles include the lateral one-third of the inguinal ligament, anterior two-thirds of the iliac crest, thoracolumbar fascia, ribs 11 and 12, and costal cartilages of ribs 7 to 10 (see Fig. 11–8C and Table 11–1).

As was noted above, the most inferomedial fibers of the transversus abdominis muscle intermingle with fibers of the internal oblique muscle to form the **conjoined tendon,** which inserts on the **pubic crest** and **pubic symphysis** (see Fig. 11–19*C* to *E*). All of the remaining fibers of the transversus abdominis muscle insert upon the entire length of the linea alba, from the pubic symphysis to the xiphoid process (see Fig. 11–8*C* and Table 11–1).

Rectus Abdominis Muscles

The fourth group of muscles in the abdominal region is the paired rectus abdominis muscles

The rectus abdominis muscles are attached inferiorly to the pubic crest and pubic symphysis and superiorly to the costal cartilages of ribs 5 to 7, in the vicinity of the xiphoid process (see Fig. 11–8*D* and Table 11–1). The rectus abdominis muscles are usually marked by three (and sometimes as many as five) horizontal bands of connective tissue called **tendinous intersections.** These bands develop at the points where muscle precursors of adjacent myotomes have fused to form the rectus muscles. The bands are also fused to the inner aspect of the overlying tendon of the **rectus sheath,** which is a specialized tendinous structure enclosing each of the rectus columns. The sheath is formed by tendons of the external oblique, internal oblique, and transversus abdominis muscles (see below).

Pyramidalis Muscles

A fifth pair of small triangular-shaped muscles is sometimes found within the inferior region of the anterior abdominal wall

The small paired pyramidalis muscles may be attached inferiorly to the pubic symphysis and pubic crest and superiorly to the linea alba at a point about halfway between the pubic crest and the umbilicus (see Fig. 11–9 and Table 11–1). The pyramidalis muscles tense the linea alba and, like the rectus abdominis muscles, are enclosed within the rectus sheath (see below).

▲ Function of Abdominal Wall Muscles

Anterolateral abdominal muscles may function dynamically or to maintain tension

The most obvious function of the abdominal musculature is to create the **tonus** that is required to keep the abdominal viscera in place when a person is standing or sitting. The internal oblique muscle is especially active in this process, and it is possibly the most important function accomplished by the transversus abdominis muscle. Static contraction of the rectus abdominis muscle also maintains posture of the trunk by preventing hyperextension of the vertebral column caused by gravitational forces or contraction of the erector spinae muscles (see Chapter 5).

Anterolateral abdominal muscles are also used in active movements of the trunk, notably **flexion** and **rotation.** Dynamic contraction of the rectus abdominis muscles against the forces of gravity or against the resistance of the erector spinae muscles of the back results in **flexion** of the vertebral column (see Chapter 5). Contraction of the external oblique and internal oblique muscles on both sides of the anterolateral abdominal wall may aid in this movement. Usually, however, one of the oblique muscles on only one side of the trunk contracts during twisting or rotational movements. In this regard, the external oblique and internal oblique muscles have opposite effects. For example, when a person is in a standing or sitting position with the pelvis fixed, contraction of the external oblique muscle on one side of the body rotates that side of the trunk anteriorly (Fig. 11–10*A*). Contraction of the internal oblique muscle on the same side pulls the opposite side of the body in an anterior direction (Fig. 11–10*B*). Thus, rotational movements of the trunk are facilitated by the coordinated contractions of an external oblique muscle on one side and an internal oblique muscle on the other side (Fig. 11–10*C* and *D*). The innervation of and functions of anterolateral abdominal muscles are summarized in Table 11–4.

Expulsion of Feces, Urine, and Vomitus; Childbirth

When the rib cage and pelvis are fixed, contraction of the anterolateral abdominal muscles increases the pressure within the abdominal cavity and aids in the expulsion of air or substances from thoracic and abdominopelvic organs

When the diaphragm is relaxed, contraction of the anterolateral abdominal muscles aids in forced expiration, coughing, and sneezing (see Chapter 6). The in-

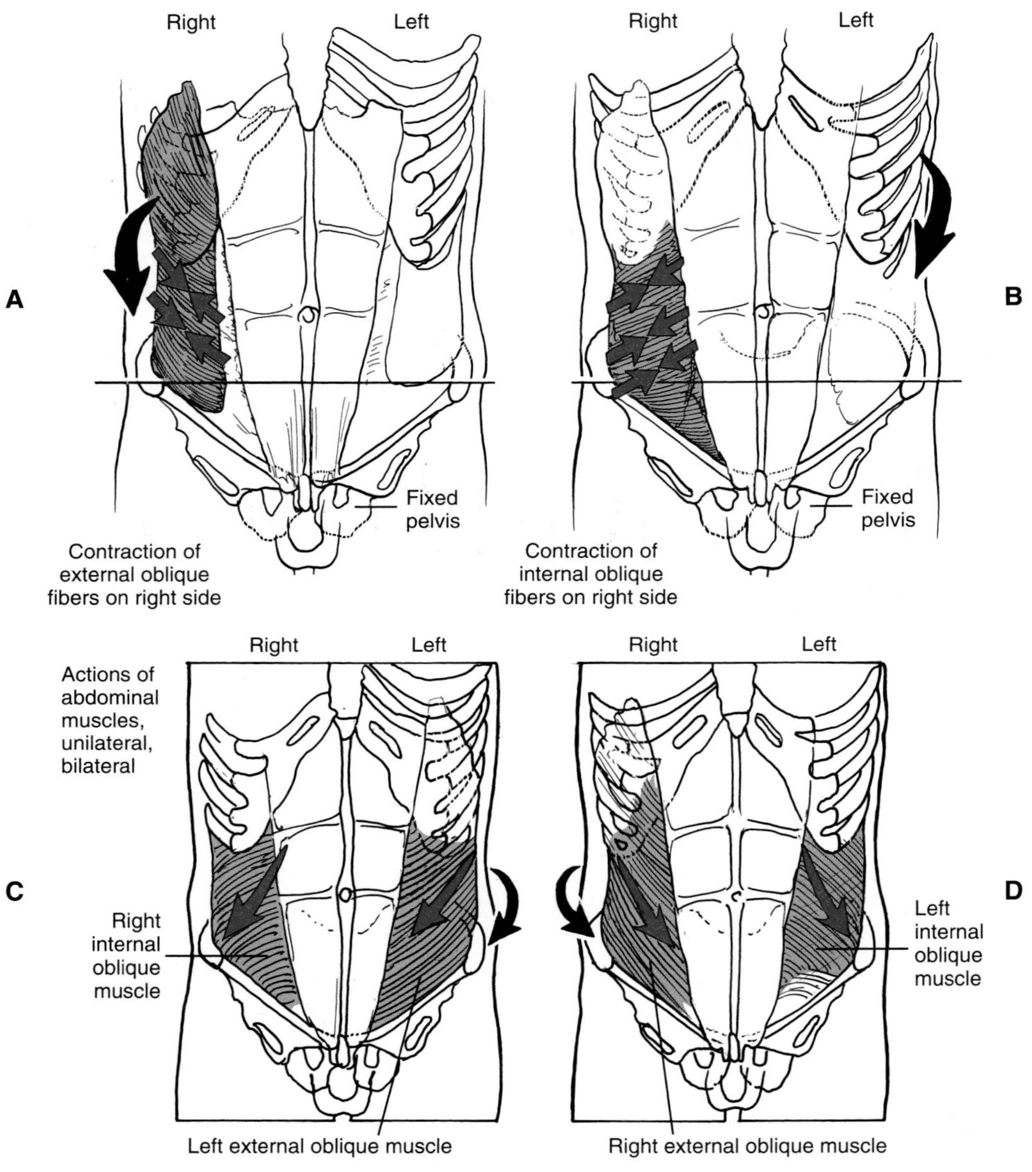

FIGURE 11–10
Rotational movements affected by the external oblique and internal oblique muscles. **A.** With the pelvis fixed, independent contraction of the external oblique muscle on one side rotates that side of the trunk anteriorly. **B.** With the pelvis fixed, independent contraction of the internal oblique muscle on one side rotates the opposite side of the trunk anteriorly. **C** and **D.** Simultaneous contractions of the external oblique and internal oblique muscles on opposite sides coordinately rotate the trunk.

crease in intra-abdominal pressure forces the diaphragm to move upward suddenly, causing a rapid reduction in the volume of the pleural cavities. When the diaphragm is fixed, however, contraction of the abdominal muscles results in an increase in intra-abdominal pressure, causing a reduction in the volume of the gastrointestinal tract, bladder, or uterus. Thus, the processes of vomiting, defecation, micturition, and childbirth may be regulated to some degree by voluntary contractions of the anterolateral abdominal muscles and diaphragm. This is the basis for the panting and pushing regimens used to regulate the progress of childbirth (see Chapter 14). Although the rectus abdominis muscles play no direct role in these functions, the increase in intra-abdominal pressure created by contraction of the external oblique, internal oblique, and transversus abdominis muscles is mediated, in part, by imposition of increased tension on the rectus sheath and linea alba.

Protection of Abdominal Viscera

The most fragile abdominal viscera are protected by the ribs and vertebral column, while other organs are protected by an abdominal reflex

Of the abdominal viscera, the **liver, pancreas, spleen,** and **kidneys** (see Chapter 12) are the most injury-prone, or **friable** (from the Latin, meaning to crumble or to be brittle), organs of the abdominal cavity. They are located within the most superior reaches of the cavity, either within the dome of the diaphragm or adjacent to the vertebral column. They are, therefore, surrounded and protected by the lower ribs or adjacent massive lumbar vertebrae (Fig. 11–11). The kidneys and suprarenal glands are also protected by a thick investment of extraperitoneal fat elaborated just deep to the transversalis fascia (see Chapter 13).

The gastrointestinal tract (see Chapter 12) is highly mobile and deformable and does not require the protection that the ribs afford more vulnerable organs, such as the heart and lungs in the thorax and the friable abdominal organs just mentioned. Indeed, the deformability of the gastrointestinal tract is functionally advantageous (see above and Chapter 12). However, because the zone of abdominal muscle just deep to each dermatome is innervated by motor and sensory branches of the same spinal nerve (see Fig. 11–14), reflex activity allows abdominal muscles to contract rapidly in response to a blow to the abdominal wall, affording some protection to the underlying intestines.

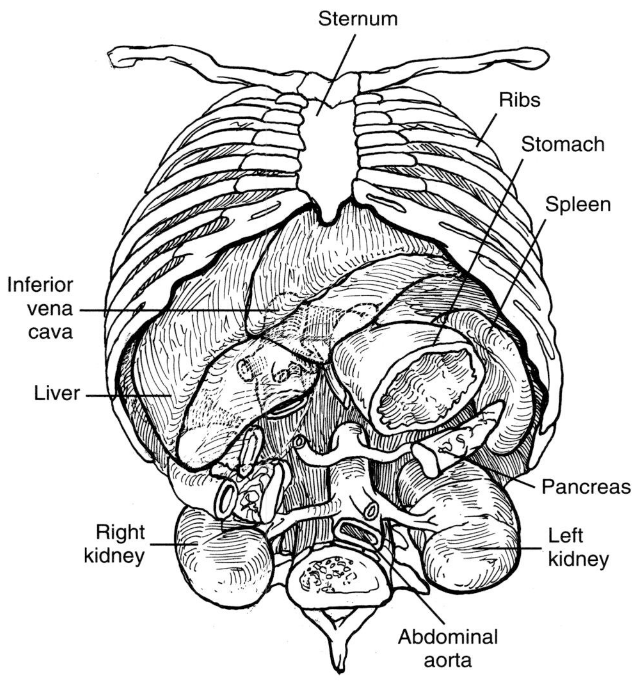

FIGURE 11–11
The rib cage and lumbar vertebral column protect the friable organs of the abdominal cavity, including the liver, spleen, and kidneys. Superior view from under the diaphragm.

▲ Transversalis Fascia

Transversalis fascia underlies the transversus abdominis muscle and is continuous with other layers of deep fascia within the anterolateral abdominal wall

As in the skeletal muscles in the back and thorax, a thin layer of deep fascia invests each of the muscles of the anterolateral abdominal wall (Fig. 11–12). Like the thoracolumbar fascia of the back (see Chapter 5), all of the deep fascia surrounding the muscles of the anterolateral abdominal wall is contiguous. The deepest layer

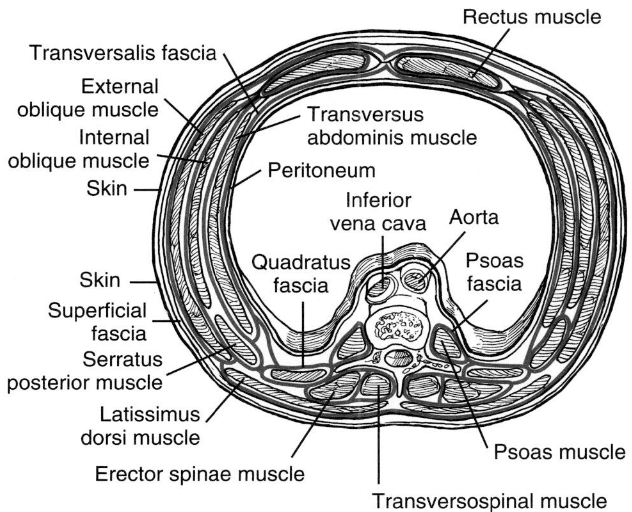

FIGURE 11–12
Deep fascia invests all of the musculature of the body wall. A specific region of this deep fascia is named for the muscle it encloses. Note the transversalis fascia (enclosing the transversus abdominis muscle), the quadratus fascia (enclosing the quadratus lumborum muscle), and the psoas fascia (enclosing the psoas muscle).

of fascia, which invests the deep side of the transversus abdominis muscle, is known as the *transversalis fascia* (Fig. 11–12). Part of the reason for this specific designation is that, in its definitive condition, the transversalis fascia can be identified as a distinct entity in at least two regions of the wall (i.e., it makes up the floor of the **inguinal canal** and gives rise to the **internal spermatic fascia**) (see Fig. 11–16). In addition, the transversalis fascia and peritoneum are the only layers separating the lower ends of the rectus muscles from the peritoneal cavity in a region where posterior walls of the **rectus sheaths** are deficient (see below).

The transversalis fascia is, thus, continuous with the deepest layer of deep fascia in all regions of the abdominal and pelvic walls. However, each region of this layer of deep fascia is named for the specific muscle it invests. For example, in the region where the deepest layer of deep fascia invests the inner surface of the quadratus lumborum muscle, it is called **quadratus fascia,** and in the region where it invests the psoas muscle, it is called **psoas fascia** (Fig. 11–12). This naming convention is somewhat analogous to the convention used in naming the different regions of the parietal pleura (see Chapter 8).

Peritoneum

The peritoneum is a membrane with two layers consisting of mesothelium and subserous fascia

The **peritoneum (peritoneal membrane)** has two layers: a deep layer of **mesothelium** lining the abdominopelvic cavity and an adjacent superficial layer of **subserous fascia** just deep to the transversalis fascia (see Fig. 11–4). The subserous fascia is usually quite thin, but in some regions of the body wall it is elaborated to form thicker supportive ligaments (e.g., the **uterine ligaments** within the pelvic floor in females) or extensive fatty deposits (e.g., those surrounding the kidney in the posterior abdominal wall). Usually, this layer of fascia serves another important function by providing a medium through which **retroperitoneal structures** may course from one area of the abdominopelvic wall to another (see Chapter 12). A simple example is the abdominal segment of the descending aorta, which courses within subserous fascia of the posterior body wall. Likewise, the ureters course within the plane of subserous fascia from the kidneys in a superior region of the abdominal cavity to the posterior wall of the bladder within the pelvic cavity. The subserous fascia transports the **inferior epigastric** and **deep circumflex iliac vessels,** which ascend within this plane from their origins at the distal ends of the **external iliac vessels.** The subserous fascia also serves as a "thoroughfare" for the physical transportation of the testes during embryonic and fetal life as they move from an inferior thoracic level through the inguinal canals and into the **scrotal swellings** (see Fig. 11–17).

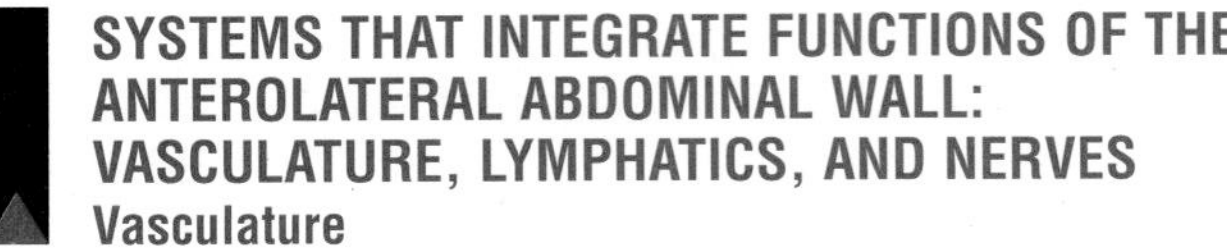

SYSTEMS THAT INTEGRATE FUNCTIONS OF THE ANTEROLATERAL ABDOMINAL WALL: VASCULATURE, LYMPHATICS, AND NERVES

Vasculature

Lumbar Vessels

The abdominal **dermatomes** of the body wall are segmental regions, each of which is innervated by a specific spinal nerve (see below and Chapter 4). Each successive dermatome is also vascularized by sequentially organized **intercostal** or **lumbar arteries** that accompany the nerves. These arteries branch from the **descending aorta** (Fig. 11–13*A* and *C* and see Chapter 6). Each abdominal dermatome is also drained by successive **intercostal veins** that branch from the **azygos vein** (on the right) and **hemiazygos vein** (on the left) and by **lumbar veins** that branch from the **inferior vena cava** (Fig. 11–13*B* and *C* and see Chapter 6). The specific segmental vessels involved in the supply and drainage of the anterolateral abdominal wall are the distal portions of **intercostal vessels** at T7 to T11, subcostal vessels at T12, and lumbar vessels at L1. The region of the xiphoid process is vascularized by T7 intercostal vessels and the umbilicus by T10 intercostal arteries and veins. The pubic (hypogastric) region is vascularized by L1 arteries and veins. The vascular fields of lumbar vessels L2 to L4 are restricted to more posterior regions of the trunk (Fig. 11–13*A* and *B*). The origin and usual course of intercostal vessels within the thoracic region are described in Chapter 6.

All four pairs of lumbar arteries originate from the aorta (Fig. 11–13*A*). The lumbar veins arise from the inferior vena cava (Fig. 11–13*B*). Both the arteries and veins then course laterally, posterior to the sympathetic trunks (Fig. 11–13*C*). They first give off dorsal branches, which supply the spinal cord (spinal radicular branches) and deep muscles and skin of the posterior lumbar region (Fig. 11–13*C*). The main trunks of these vessels pass posteriorly to the psoas muscle and lumbar plexus and then course posteriorly (at L1, L2, or L3) or anteriorly (at L4) to the quadratus lumborum muscle. They pierce the posterior aponeurosis of the transversus abdominis muscle and course in a lateral direction within the body wall between the innermost layer of muscles (i.e., transversus abdominis muscles) and middle layer of muscles (i.e., internal oblique muscles) (Fig. 11–13*C*). Deep branches supply and drain the body wall muscles and peritoneum, and superficial branches supply and drain the integument and superficial fascia.

Inferior Epigastric and Deep Circumflex Iliac Vessels

The peritoneum of the abdominal body wall is also served by branches of external iliac arteries and veins

Longitudinal branches of arteries and veins emanate from the distal regions of the **external iliac arteries** and **veins** to supply and drain the peritoneum of the anterolateral abdominal wall (see Fig. 11–13*D* and *E*).

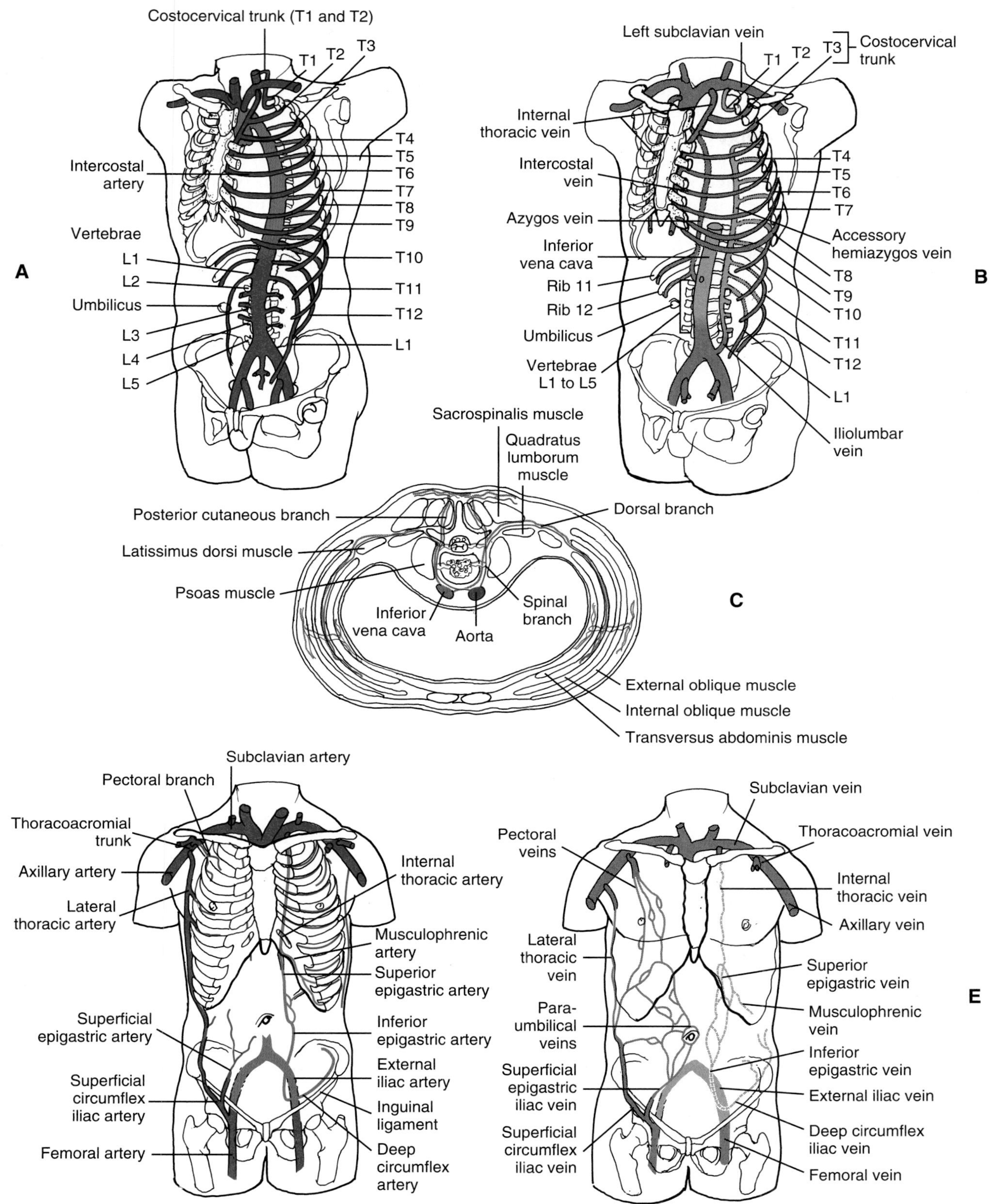

FIGURE 11–13

Vasculature of the abdominal region. **A.** The arterial supply to the more posterior regions of the abdominal wall includes several inferior intersegmental intercostal arteries and lumbar arteries. **B.** The distribution of intersegmental veins in the abdominal regions parallels that of the intersegmental arteries. **C.** Intersegmental arteries and veins pass posterior to the psoas muscle and then posterior to the quadratus lumborum muscle (at the levels of vertebrae L1, L2, and L3) or anterior to the quadratus lumborum muscle (at the level of vertebra L4). Intersegmental arteries and veins then course between the internal oblique and transversus abdominis muscles. **D.** The distribution of the superficial epigastric and circumflex iliac arteries and veins within the superficial fascia and the distribution of the inferior epigastric and deep circumflex iliac arteries within the subserous fascia of the anterolateral abdominal wall. **E.** The distribution of superficial epigastric and circumflex iliac veins within the superficial fascia and of inferior epigastric and deep circumflex iliac veins within the subserous fascia of the anterolateral abdominal wall.

These arteries and veins each have two major branches, the more medial **inferior epigastric arteries** and **veins** and the more lateral **deep circumflex iliac arteries** and **veins.** These vessels ascend through the abdominal subserous fascia, eventually anastomosing with terminal branches of the **internal thoracic vessels** (**superior epigastric** and **musculophrenic arteries** and **veins**) (see Fig. 11–13*D* and *E*). The deep circumflex iliac vessels also anastomose with branches of intercostal and lumbar arteries and veins.

The inferior epigastric arteries and veins also serve the rectus abdominis muscles by coursing superiorly within the subserous fascia from the point at which they originate from the external iliac vessels. By penetrating the transversalis fascia, they enter the rectus columns within the rectus sheath (see Fig. 11–15*D* and *E*).

In the region of the umbilicus, some branches of the inferior epigastric veins course into the abdominal cavity along the rudiment of the embryologic left umbilical vein (i.e., **ligamentum teres hepatica,** or **round ligament of the liver**). Here, the inferior epigastric branches anastomose with branches of portal veins within the abdominal cavity (see Chapter 12).

Superficial Epigastric and Superficial Circumflex Iliac Vessels

Superficial fascia of the abdominal body wall is served by branches of femoral arteries and veins

As the external iliac arteries and veins course inferiorly deep to the inguinal ligament into the thighs, they become the **femoral arteries** and **veins.** Two major branches emanate almost immediately from the proximal ends of these femoral vessels and rise superficially to course back over the inguinal ligament and up into the superficial fascia of the anterolateral abdominal wall. These vessels are the **superficial epigastric arteries** and **veins** and **superficial circumflex iliac arteries** and **veins** (see Fig. 11–13*D* and *E*). These superficial vessels and their branches parallel closely the inferior epigastric and deep circumflex iliac vessels and their branches that course within the subserous fascia.

Branches of the superficial circumflex iliac arteries and veins anastomose with superior branches of the lateral thoracic arteries and veins (see Fig. 11–13*D* and *E*). The superficial epigastric arteries usually terminate within the inferior abdominal wall (see Fig. 11–13*D*). The more extensive superficial epigastric veins, however, anastomose with pectoral, clavicular, and deltoid branches of the thoracoacromial trunk (see Fig. 11–13*E*).

Paraumbilical Veins

The paraumbilical veins are superficial epigastric venous branches that make up an extensive complex radiating from the region of the umbilicus (see Fig. 11–13*E*). These veins are clinically important because they anastomose with the deeper inferior epigastric veins, which, in turn, anastomose with portal veins draining the round ligament of the liver. This allows blood to flow from portal to systemic vessels in certain pathologic conditions (see Chapter 12).

Function of Abdominal Wall Vasculature

A pivotal function of vessels of the trunk, particularly those of the dermis, is the regulation of body temperature. In colder conditions, sympathetic activity causes constriction of peripheral vessels to prevent heat loss. In warmer conditions, sympathetic vasoconstrictor activity and dilatation of the cutaneous vessels ceases, resulting in an increased rate of heat loss. Release of the hormone **bradykinin** also plays an important role in the vasodilatation of body wall vessels.

▲ Lymphatics

Lymphatic drainage of the anterior abdominal wall occurs via lymphatic vessels that accompany superficial and deep arteries within the superficial and subserous fascia (see Fig. 11–13*D*). However, lymph fluid flows in a direction opposite to that of arterial blood, that is, downward into external iliac nodes and then lumbar nodes or upward into nodes associated with internal thoracic arteries.

▲ Nerves

Thoracic Nerves

Thoracic spinal nerves (see Chapter 4) of the abdominal integument are distributed segmentally in a craniocaudal sequence from spinal nerves T6 and T7 (in the region of the xiphoid process) to spinal nerve T12 (within the inguinal and pubic regions) (Fig. 11–14*A*). The tenth thoracic nerve is located at the level of the umbilicus. The horizontal "belt" of innervation of each spinal nerve within the abdominal wall is called a **dermatome** (see Fig. 2–7 and 11–14*A*). All of these nerves course within the wall between the innermost layer of muscles (i.e., transversus abdominis muscles) and middle layer of muscles (i.e., internal oblique muscles), along with blood vessels (Fig. 11–14*B*), in a manner similar to that described in the thoracic region (see Chapters 4 and 6).

Lumbar Nerves (Iliohypogastric, Ilioinguinal, and Genitofemoral Nerves)

Nerves that branch from the **lumbar plexus** also innervate structures within the anterior abdominal wall (see Chapter 13). Two of these are branches of spinal nerve L1, namely, the more superior **iliohypogastric nerve** and more inferior **ilioinguinal nerve.** Another branch is the **genitofemoral nerve,** which includes fibers from spinal nerves L1 and L2 (see Figs. 11–14*A* and 11–24 and Chapter 13). The iliohypogastric nerve innervates the anterior abdominal wall just superior to the pubic crest, while the ilioinguinal nerve supplies the medial thigh and proximal region of the external genitalia in males and females (see Fig. 11–14*A* and below).

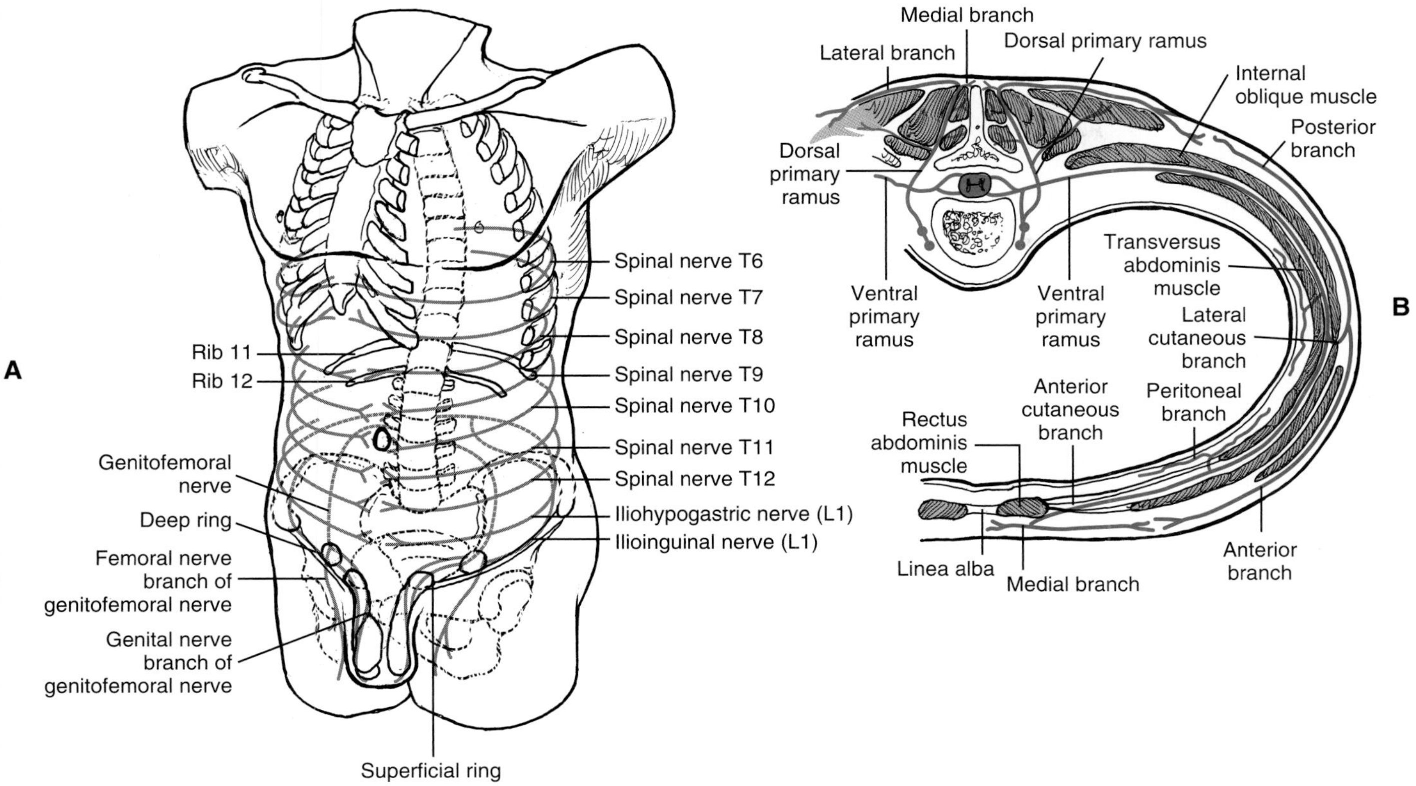

FIGURE 11–14
Spinal nerves of the anterolateral abdominal wall. **A.** Skin, muscles, and parietal peritoneum of the anterolateral abdominal wall are innervated by ventral rami of spinal nerves T7 to L1 and by the genitofemoral nerve, which branches from the lumbar plexus (see Chapter 13). Spinal nerve T7 innervates the body wall in the region of the xiphoid process. Spinal nerve T10 innervates the body wall in the region of the umbilicus. Spinal nerve L1 branches to form the iliohypogastric and ilioinguinal nerves, which innervate the lowest dermatomes of the anterior abdominal wall. The genital branch of the genitofemoral nerve innervates the cremaster muscle, a specialization of the internal oblique muscle (see Fig. 11–24). **B.** Ventral rami that innervate the anterolateral abdominal wall course between the internal oblique and transversus abdominis muscles.

The point along its length at which spinal nerve L1 splits to form the iliohypogastric and ilioinguinal nerves may vary significantly from one individual to another (see Chapter 13).

The **genitofemoral nerve** is best known for its innervation of a specialized region of the internal oblique muscle, namely, the **cremaster muscle (cremasteric fascia) of the spermatic cord.** It also innervates a small region of the medial thigh (see Fig. 11–14A and 11–24). The genitofemoral nerve is made up of motor, sensory, and sympathetic fibers arising from spinal nerves L1 and L2 (see Chapter 13).

Motor, Sensory, and Sympathetic Functions of Abdominal Segmental Nerves. All of the spinal nerves within the abdominal wall contain motor components, which innervate the contractile mechanism of the underlying muscles, and sensory components, which innervate sensory end organs in the integument and muscles as well as sensory receptors within the peritoneum lining the abdominal cavity. The motor fibers of each spinal nerve innervate the same region of the body wall as the corresponding sensory fibers (see Fig. 11–14 and Table 11–4). Because the sensory territories of adjacent spinal nerves overlap, however, damage to one spinal nerve does not result in a complete deficit of sensory innervation to its dermatome.

Spinal nerves of the anterolateral abdominal wall also contain **sympathetic fibers,** which innervate a variety of structures within the integument, including the arrector pili muscles of hair follicles, myoepithelial cells of sweat glands, and smooth muscles in the walls of blood vessels. None of the nerves to the trunk or extremities contain parasympathetic fibers (see Chapter 4).

SPECIALIZED STRUCTURES OF THE ANTEROLATERAL ABDOMINAL WALL

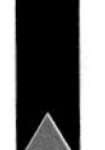

Rectus Sheaths

Tendons of abdominal muscles symmetrically invest the rectus columns above the interspinous line but cover only the outer surface of each rectus column inferior to the interspinous line

Rectus sheaths invest and enclose the paired rectus columns on each side of the ventral midline (Fig. 11–15). The sheaths are formed by fusion of the tendi-

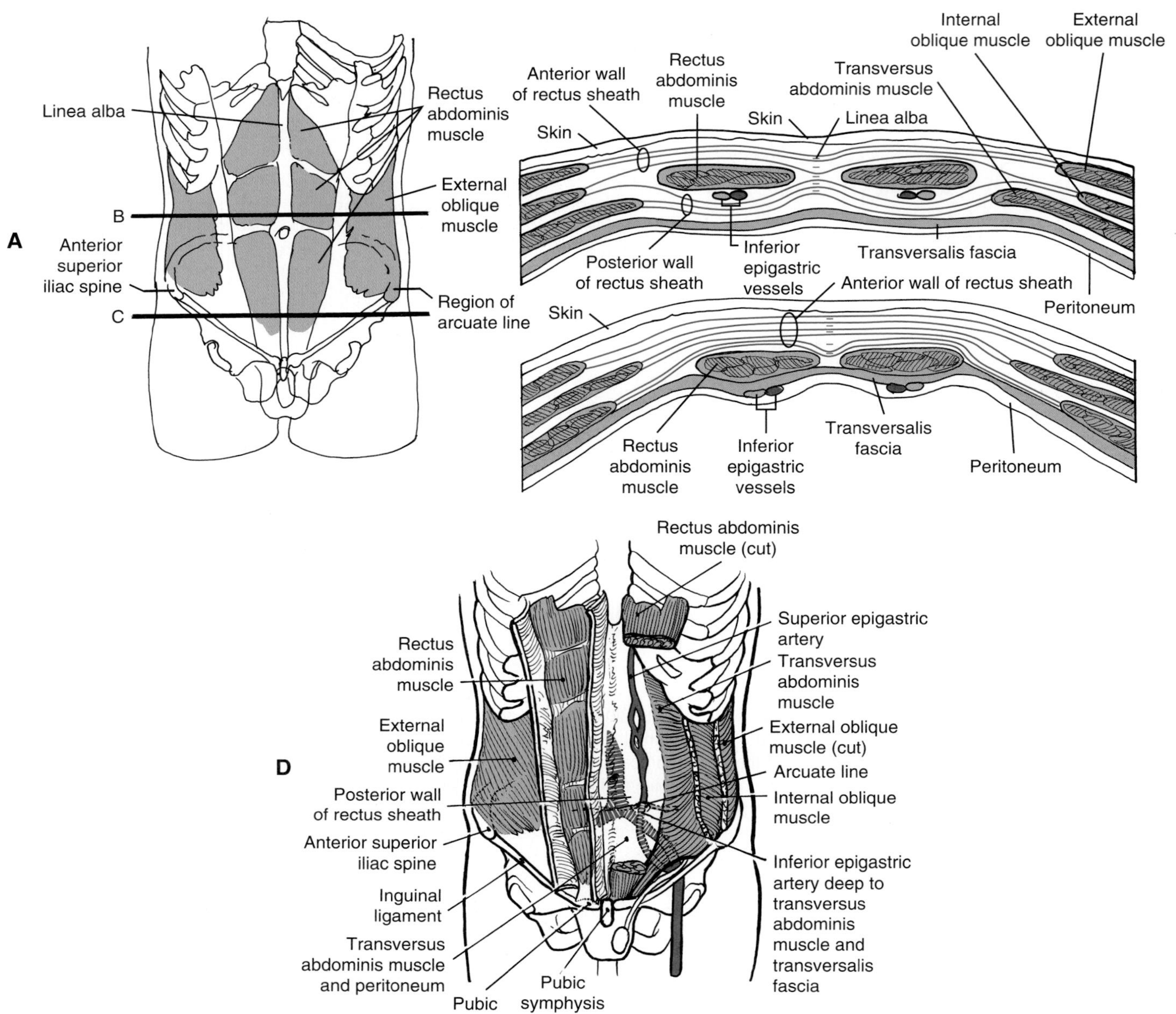

FIGURE 11–15

The rectus sheath. **A.** Anterior view of anterior abdominal wall. Each rectus column is enclosed within a rectus sheath, which is a specialization of the aponeuroses of the external oblique, internal oblique, and transversus abdominis muscles. The composition of the anterior and posterior walls of the rectus sheath is different above and below the interspinous line. **B.** Transverse section of the rectus sheaths and columns superior to the interspinous line. Superior to the interspinous line (Fig. 11–15*A*), the anterior and posterior walls of the rectus sheaths are symmetric. The anterior wall is comprised of both laminae of the external oblique muscle and the superficial lamina of the internal oblique muscle. The posterior wall of each sheath in this region is comprised of both laminae of the transversus abdominis muscle and the deep lamina of the internal oblique muscle. **C.** Transverse section of rectus sheaths and columns inferior to the interspinous lines. Inferior to the interspinous line (Fig. 11–15*A*), both laminae of all three muscles comprise the anterior wall of the rectus sheath. In this region, there is no posterior wall of the sheath. The only structures of the abdominal wall deep to the rectus muscles inferior to the interspinous line are the transversalis fascia and the peritoneum (consisting of subserous fascia and mesothelium). **D.** Anterior view of rectus sheaths. The anterior wall of the rectus sheath on the right has been reflected to show the enclosed rectus abdominis muscle. The anterior wall of the rectus column and the rectus abdominis muscle on the left have been removed to expose the anterior surface of the posterior wall of the rectus sheath. The lower boundary of the posterior wall of the sheath is at the level of the interspinous line. It can be recognized because the posterior wall of the sheath superior to this boundary is opaque. This inferior boundary is called the *arcuate line.* It marks the level at which the inferior epigastric vessels pierce the transverse fascia to enter the rectus sheath. These vessels anastomose with superior epigastric vessels posterior to the rectus abdominis muscles.

nous aponeuroses of the external oblique, internal oblique, and transversus abdominis muscles. Each of these tendons has a superficial and a deep lamina (Fig. 11–15*B* and *C*). Between the xiphoid process and the interspinous line, the **anterior wall of the rectus sheath** is formed by fusion of both laminae of the external oblique tendon and the superficial lamina of the internal oblique tendon (Fig. 11–15*B*). Between the xiphoid process and the interspinous line, the **posterior wall of the rectus sheath** is formed by fusion of the deep lamina of the internal oblique tendon with both laminae of the transversus abdominis tendon (Fig. 11–15*B*).

Inferior to the interspinous line, all laminae of the external oblique, internal oblique, and transversus abdominis tendons on each flank fuse and pass anteriorly to the rectus columns on either side of the midline. (The **flank,** or **latus,** is the side of the body between the pelvis and the ribs.) Thus, none of these tendons course deep to the rectus columns in this region. As a consequence, the inferior half of the anterior wall of the rectus sheath is well developed but the posterior wall is wholly deficient (Fig. 11–15*C* and *D*). Therefore, the only barriers between the posterior surface of the rectus column and the abdominal cavity inferior to the interspinous line are thin layers of **transversalis fascia** and **peritoneum** (Fig. 11–15*C* and *D*). These membranes are not technically considered to constitute any part of the rectus sheath, either above or below the interspinous line. The composition of different regions of the anterior and posterior walls of the rectus sheath is shown in Table 11–2.

In some individuals, the inferior boundary of the posterior wall of the rectus sheath may be sharply defined. Since the transversalis fascia and peritoneum may be more translucent than the tendinous superior posterior wall, the lower edge of the posterior wall of the rectus sheath can be seen as an **arcuate (arc-shaped) line** in these cases (Fig. 11–15*D* and see Fig. 11–18*B*). In other individuals, the arcuate line may be more diffuse and difficult to discriminate because the transfer of internal oblique and transversus abdominis tendons from the posterior wall to the anterior wall at the interspinous line may be more gradual.

Linea Alba

The rectus sheaths on each side of the abdomen are joined in the ventral midline by a tendinous aponeurosis

From the xiphoid process to the pubic symphysis, tendons of the external oblique, internal oblique, and transversus abdominis muscles converge from each side of the anterior abdominal wall to fuse into a tough midline **aponeurosis** called the **linea alba** (from the Latin, meaning *white line*) (Fig. 11–15*A* to *C*). The only deficiency in this aponeurosis is in the region of the umbilicus.

Surgical Incisions Along the Linea Alba. Making surgical incisions along the linea alba is advantageous because there is little damage to blood vessels and spinal nerves, which terminate just lateral to it. It is disadvantageous because incisions heal slowly in this region.

Umbilical Hernias

Umbilical hernias are congenital defects that result from failure of the umbilical ring to close properly

Umbilical hernias are more common in black infants than in white infants. These hernias usually resolve spontaneously. Nonetheless, surgical intervention may be indicated if the herniated mass is greater than 1 cm in diameter by the time the child is 2 years of age.

Conditions that lead to chronic elevations in intra-abdominal pressure (e.g., pregnancy, the presence of ascites, and obesity) may result in umbilical hernias in adults. Elimination of the pressure usually resolves the hernia, although surgical repair is still occasionally necessary. Umbilical hernias seldom result in strangulation of viscera. Abdominal trauma may cause the hernia to rupture, however, resulting in a life-threatening emergency situation.

TABLE 11–2
Components of Anterior and Posterior Walls of the Rectus Sheaths

Region	Components
ANTERIOR WALL OF SHEATH	
Superior to costal margin	Both laminae of external oblique tendons
Between xiphoid process and interspinous line	Both laminae of external oblique tendons; anterior lamina of internal oblique tendon
Between interspinous line and pubic crest	Both laminae of external oblique, internal oblique, and transversus abdominis tendons
POSTERIOR WALL OF SHEATH	
Superior to costal margin	No posterior wall, rectus rests on costal cartilage
Between xiphoid process and interspinous line	Posterior lamina of internal oblique tendon; both laminae of transversus abdominis tendons
Between interspinous line and pubic crest	No posterior wall, bordered only by transversalis fascia and peritoneum

Midline Epigastric Hernias

Midline epigastric herniation may result from weakness of the linea alba

The abdominal wall (i.e., muscle, fascia, and peritoneum) may protrude between the rectus abdominis muscles, resulting in **diastasis recti.** This common condition, affecting approximately 5% of the population, usually requires no treatment other than observation.

Inferior Epigastric Vessels

Inferior epigastric vessels must pierce the transversalis fascia to gain entry into the rectus sheaths

Inferior epigastric vessels branch from external iliac arteries and veins within the subserous fascia just deep to the transversalis fascia (see Figs. 11–15*D* and 11–18*B*). They course superiorly through the subserous fascia, and, in the region of the arcuate line, they pierce the transversalis fascia to gain entry into the rectus sheath in order to supply the rectus abdominis muscles. Within the posterior wall of the rectus column, the **inferior epigastric arteries** and **veins** anastomose with **superior epigastric arteries** and **veins** and **musculophrenic arteries** and **veins** (see Fig. 11–14*D*).

▲ Inguinal Canal

Embryonic Development of the Inguinal Canal and Spermatic Fascia

Inguinal canals develop at the beginning of fetal life within the anterior abdominal walls of males and females

Inguinal canals are present in both sexes. They serve as passageways for the spermatic cords in males and for the round ligaments of the uterus in females.

The inguinal canal begins to develop in the presumptive inferior abdominal wall during the eighth week of embryonic life. The **processus vaginalis,** which is a diverticulum of the peritoneum, pushes out three layers of the abdominal wall in succession to form a multilayered socklike pouch that eventually lines the inguinal canal and invests the spermatic cord in males. In both males and females, the processus vaginalis first pushes out the **transversalis fascia** in a medial direction just lateral to the midinguinal line (Fig. 11–16*A* and *B*). The deficiency produced in the transversalis fascia thus becomes the **deep inguinal ring.** The processus vaginalis then passes through a large hiatus in the transversus abdominis muscle and pushes out the **internal oblique muscle** just medial to the deep inguinal ring (Fig. 11–16*C*). Finally, in a region of the abdomen just lateral to the pubic tubercles, the processus vaginalis pushes out the **external oblique muscle** (Fig. 11–16*D*). The deficiency created in this muscle layer becomes the **superficial inguinal ring** (Fig. 11–16*D* and *E*). Therefore, as evagination progresses, the processus vaginalis becomes invested by three muscle layers. From inside to outside, these are the **internal, cremasteric,** and **external spermatic fascia.** The processus vaginalis continues to evaginate in an inferior direction into the **labioscrotal swellings** (Fig. 11–16*D* and *E*).

Male and Female Gonads in Relation to the Developing Inguinal Canal

The male and female gonads initially develop within the posterior body wall in the lower thoracic and superior lumbar regions. As the gonads form, they become attached to the superior end of the **gubernaculum,** a tough ligamentous cord that condenses within the subserous fascia. The gubernaculum is attached below to fascia between the incipient external oblique and internal oblique muscles in the region of the **labioscrotal swellings** (Fig. 11–17 and see Chapter 16). These labioscrotal swellings form the **labia majora** in females and the **scrotum** in males. Eventually, the processus vaginalis, invested by all three layers of spermatic fascia, and the inferior part of the gubernaculum extend into the inferior poles of the presumptive scrotum or labia majora (see Figs. 11–16*D* and *E* and 11–17).

Descent of the Male Gonad Through the Inguinal Canal

The male gonad is pulled into the developing scrotum as the gubernaculum shortens during fetal life

The male gonad **(testis)** is pulled into the developing scrotum by the gubernaculum, which becomes shorter during the third month of embryonic life. This results, in part, from effects of the male hormone testosterone. The gonad is pulled along within the plane of the peritoneal subserous fascia in the posterior body wall. It does not leave this plane at any time during its descent into the scrotum (see Fig. 11–17).

The **testicular arteries** and **veins,** which at first vascularize the developing gonads at about the level of vertebra T10, lengthen as the testes are pulled in an inferior direction. The **sympathetic** and **parasympathetic nerves** that accompany the arteries also lengthen to accommodate the translocation of the testes. In addition, the superior ends of the developing **spermatic ducts** are pulled inferiorly. By the end of the third month, the gubernaculum has pulled the gonad down to the region of the presumptive deep inguinal ring. The gonad, however, is still connected to blood vessels, autonomic nerves, and the spermatic duct, which trail behind it. Between the seventh and ninth months, the gubernaculum becomes even shorter, pulling the testes through the deep inguinal ring into the inguinal canals and then the scrotum (see Fig. 11–17*B*).

Origin of Spermatic Fascia

Spermatic fascia are formed by the socklike evaginations of the anterior abdominal wall that are pushed outward by the processus vaginalis during creation of the inguinal canal

As the processus vaginalis and its associated subserous fascia become invested by the three layers of the

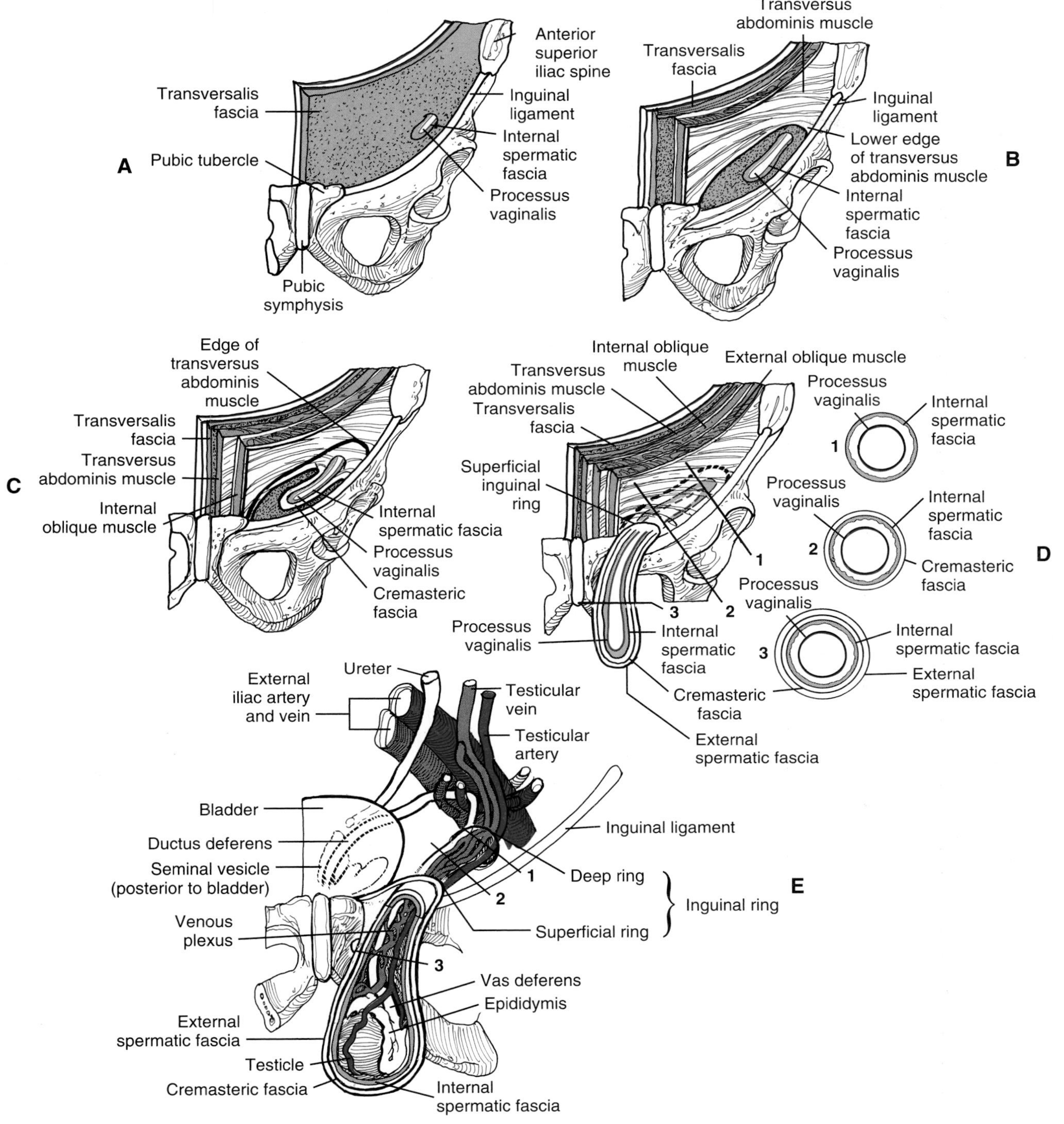

FIGURE 11–16

Formation of the inguinal canal in males and females and the presumptive spermatic fascia. The following illustrations use "artistic license," since they depict the behavior of the processus vaginalis during embryonic and fetal life within the context of the definitive structure of the anterior abdominal wall and pelvis. **A.** An evagination of the peritoneum called the *processus vaginalis* pushes a socklike extension of transversalis fascia anteriorly and medially to form the presumptive internal spermatic fascia. This is at the level of the presumptive deep ring of the inguinal canal. **B.** The processus vaginalis-internal spermatic fascia complex passes through a large hiatus in the transversus abdominis muscle, which, as a consequence, does not contribute to the formation of the spermatic fascia. **C.** The processus vaginalis-internal spermatic fascia complex continues to evaginate medially and inferiorly and pushes out a thin socklike extension of the internal oblique muscle. This evagination of the internal oblique muscle forms the presumptive cremasteric fascia. **D.** The processus vaginalis-internal spermatic fascia-cremasteric fascia complex evaginates medially and inferiorly to push out a socklike extension of the external oblique muscle, which forms the presumptive external spermatic fascia. Note that a section through the presumptive inguinal canal at *(1)* includes only the processus vaginalis and internal spermatic fascia. A section at *(2)* includes the processus vaginalis, internal spermatic fascia, and cremasteric fascia. A section at *(3),* outside the inguinal canal, includes the processus vaginalis, internal spermatic fascia, cremasteric fascia, and external spermatic fascia.

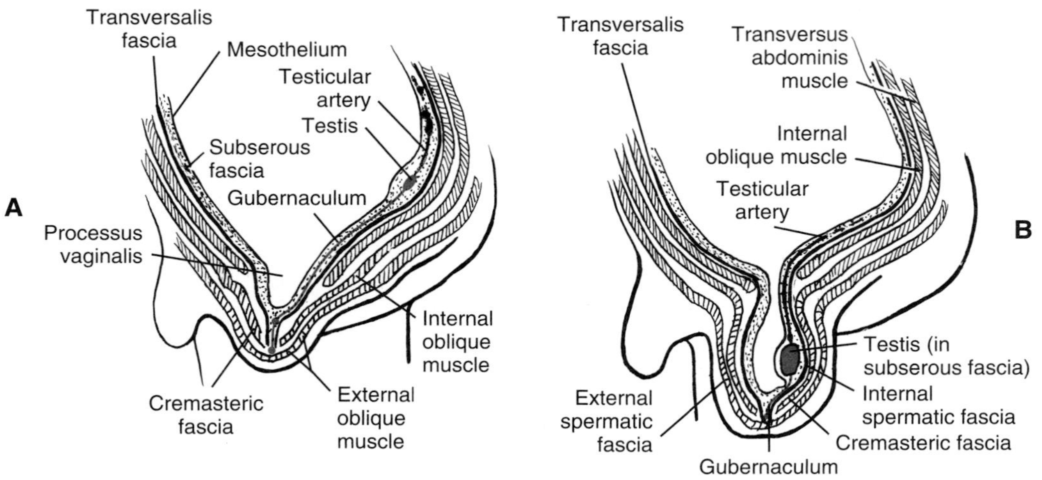

FIGURE 11–17
Descent of the testes in males. **A.** Testes form within the subserous fascia of the posterior abdominal wall between the fourth and eighth weeks of development. Their inferior poles become connected to the labioscrotal swelling by a ligamentous cord called the *gubernaculum.* **B.** The gubernaculum shortens to pull the testes to the vicinity of the deep ring between the seventh and twelfth weeks and then into the scrotum between the seventh and ninth months of gestation. The testes do not leave the plane of the subserous fascia at any time during the descent, even after they enter the inguinal canal and the scrotum.

anterior abdominal wall during its evagination into the labioscrotal swellings, the testes, vessels, and nerves trailing behind them also become invested by these three layers. The layers form the definitive **spermatic fascia** of the gonads and **spermatic cord** (see Figs. 11–16, 11–17*B*, and 11–22). These layers and their precursors, from deep to superficial, are the **internal spermatic fascia (transversalis fascia), cremasteric fascia (internal oblique muscle),** and **external spermatic fascia (external oblique muscle).** Not all regions of the definitive spermatic cord are invested by all three layers of spermatic fascia, however (see Figs. 11–16, 11–17*B*, and 11–22).

Cryptorchism

Failure of the testes to descend results in cryptorchism

In a small percentage of full-term male infants, one or both testes do not completely descend into the scrotum. Failure of the testes to descend may result from defects in androgen production. The descent may be arrested at any point along the normal route of translocation from the posterior body wall to the inguinal canal, but it is usually arrested at the level of the inguinal canal. Undescended testes do not produce viable sperm. Complete descent of the **cryptorchid testis** may occur spontaneously within the first 2 years of life. If this does not occur, surgical manipulation may be attempted. If surgical intervention is not successful, the undescended testis is usually removed in order to decrease the possibility of **testicular cancer.**

Testicular Torsion

Laxity of the tunica vaginalis or rupture of the gubernaculum may result in testicular torsion

If the testis is not anchored within the scrotal sac, it may be pulled superiorly by the action of the cremaster muscle, resulting in testicular torsion. Testicular torsion may be caused by traumatic injury to the scrotum or may occur spontaneously. Symptoms of testicular torsion include rapid onset of scrotal pain, scrotal swelling, nausea, vomiting, and fever. These symptoms may mimic those of **epididymitis** (inflammation of the epididymis). However, epididymitis may also be associated with inflammation of the prostate gland and the presence of pus in the urine. In testicular torsion, the testis may be located within the superior region of the scrotum, near the superficial inguinal ring, and may adopt a horizontal orientation.

Severe torsion, resulting in compromise of the blood supply and significant reduction in blood flow, is an emergency condition requiring repair within a few hours of the onset of symptoms. Repair is accomplished by surgical anchoring of the testis within the scrotum.

Inguinal Triangle

The region of the definitive inguinal canal can be defined by surface features and specializations of the anterior abdominal wall

In adults the inguinal canal can be identified by locating structures that form the **inguinal triangle.** The inguinal triangle is a region bounded by the lateral border of the rectus abdominis muscle (medially), the inguinal ligament (inferiorly), and the inferior epigastric vessels (superolaterally) (Fig. 11–18). The deep inguinal ring is located just lateral to the inferolateral apex of the inguinal triangle (and just lateral to the site of origin of the inferior epigastric vessels). Thus, the spermatic cord

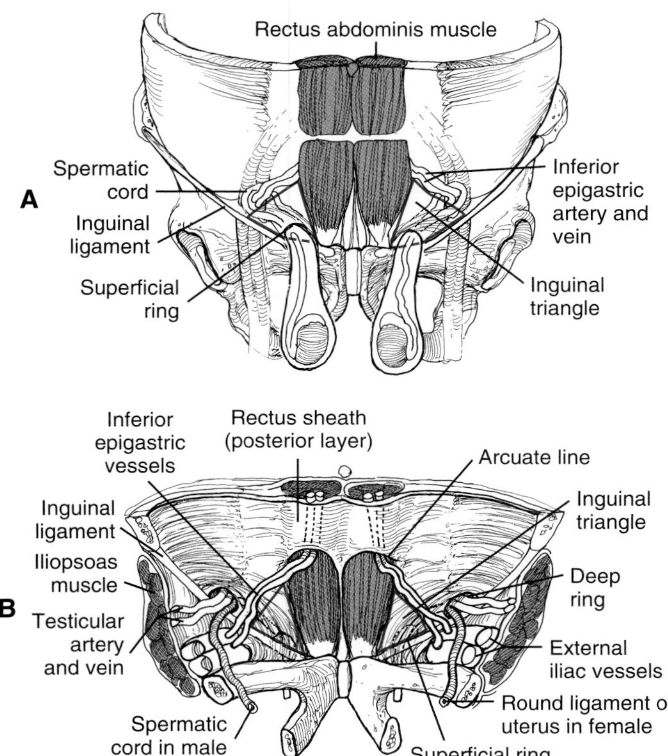

FIGURE 11–18
The left and right inguinal triangles. **A.** Anterior view. **B.** Posterior view. Each inguinal triangle is bounded inferiorly by the inguinal ligament, medially by the lateral edge of the rectus abdominis muscle, and superolaterally by the inferior epigastric vessels.

in males and the round ligament of the uterus in females loop around the inferior epigastric vessels as they enter the deep inguinal ring (Fig. 11–18).

Definitive Relationships of the Inguinal Canal to Its Contents

The definitive inguinal canal has anterior and posterior walls, a floor, and a roof

Like the suboccipital compartment (see Chapter 5), the inguinal canal has a structure that can be compared to a house, with anterior and posterior walls, a floor, and a roof. In the case of the inguinal canal, the terms *wall, roof,* and *floor* refer to structures that surround the spermatic cord and its investments of spermatic fascia. Perhaps it can also be said that the inguinal canal has a *back door* (the deep ring) and a *front door* (the superficial ring). The clearest description of the inguinal canal begins at its most posterior region and moves in an anterior or superficial direction (Fig. 11–19 and Table 11–3). Most of the **posterior wall** is made up of **transversalis fascia** only (Fig. 11–19*A*). Just posterior to the superficial inguinal ring, however, the posterior wall of the inguinal canal is also strengthened by the **conjoined tendon (falx inguinalis),** which is formed by fusion of arching fibers of the transversus abdominis and internal oblique muscles (Fig. 11–19*C* to *E*).

The exceedingly narrow **roof** of the inguinal canal is formed by **superior arching fibers of the transversus abdominis** and **internal oblique muscles** and, therefore, is no deeper (in its anterior-posterior axis) than the combined thickness of these two thin muscles (Fig. 11–19).

Most of the **anterior wall** of the inguinal canal is made up of the **external oblique muscle** (Fig. 11–19*D* and *E*). However, a small portion of the **internal oblique muscle** covers the anterior side of the most lateral part of the inguinal canal in the region of the deep inguinal ring (compare parts *A* and *B* of Fig. 11–19).

The **floor** of the inguinal canal is made up solely of the **inguinal ligament,** which is the thickened tendinous lower edge of the external oblique muscle (Fig. 11–19). The inguinal ligament is attached medially to the **pubic tubercle** and laterally to the **ASIS.** The transversalis fascia is connected to the entire length of the inguinal ligament, while the transversus abdominis and internal oblique muscles are attached only in medial and lateral regions of the ligament (Table 11–3) (see also descriptions of these muscle attachments, above).

▲ Definitive Inguinal Canal and Associated Structures in Males (Including Contents of Spermatic Cord)

Tunica Vaginalis

During the first year of life in males, the proximal neck of the processus vaginalis disintegrates, leaving the tunica vaginalis, a small distal remnant, wrapped around each testis in the scrotum

The disintegration of the proximal neck of the processus vaginalis (between the superior pole of the testis and deep inguinal ring) normally occurs during the first year of postnatal life (Fig. 11–20*A* and *B*). The **tunica vaginalis,** which is a remnant of the most distal end of the processus vaginalis, remains intact just anterior to the testis. This double-walled structure (which was an evagination of the peritoneum) wraps itself around the sides and posterior wall of the testis, enveloping most of the gonad, except for the regions of its attachment to the spermatic cord and gubernaculum (Fig. 11–20*C*). Like the testis and the part of the spermatic cord within the scrotum, the tunica vaginalis is enclosed within the three layers of spermatic fascia (Fig. 11–20*B* and *C*).

Testicular Hydrocele

Injuries or infection of the tunica vaginalis may result in testicular hydrocele

As is the case in the peritoneal cavity, the inner lining of the tunica vaginalis is comprised of mesothelium, a membrane that can secrete serous fluid. Normally, however, the

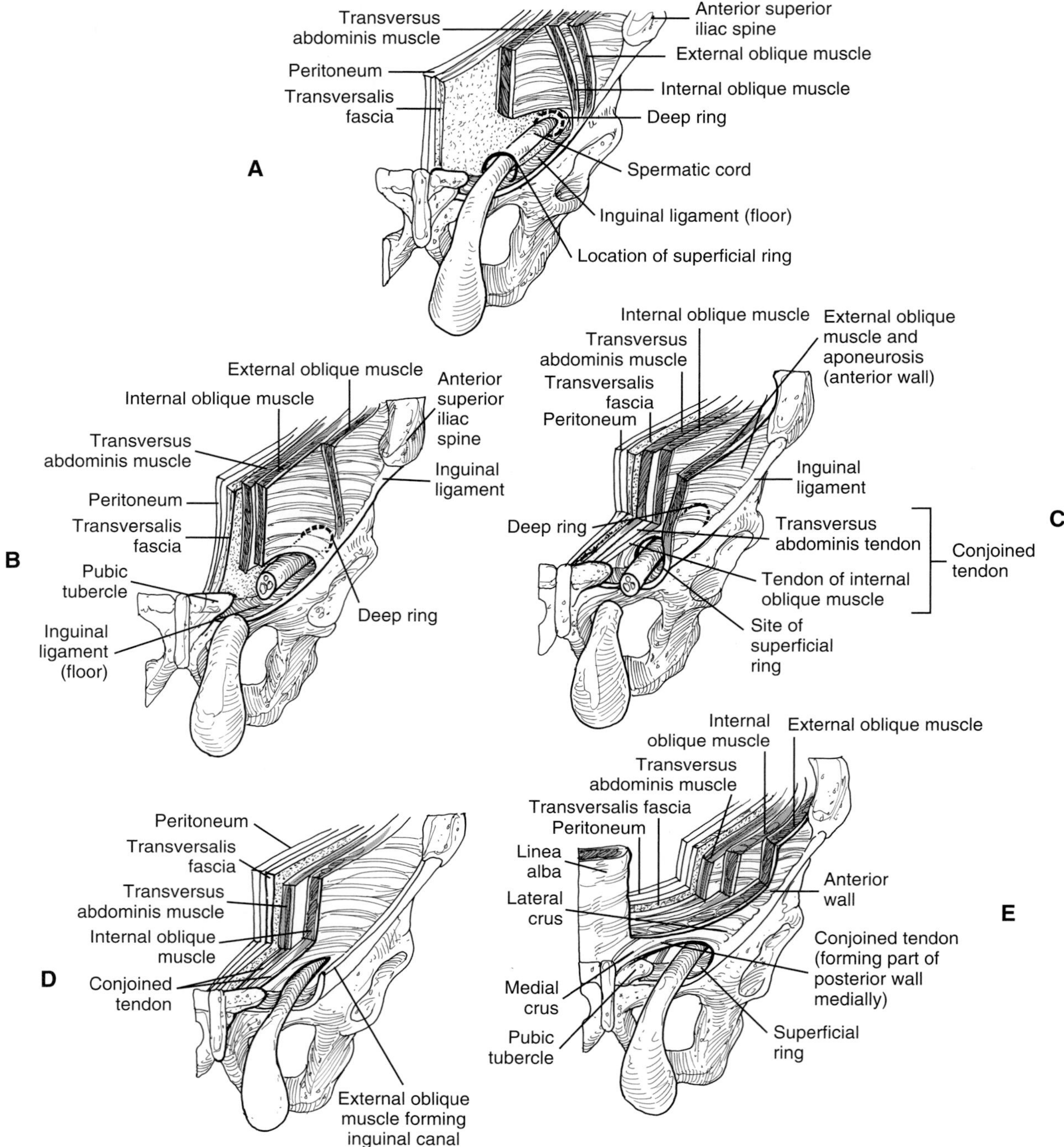

FIGURE 11–19

Anterior view of the definitive inguinal canal in males, from deep to superficial. **A.** The floor of the inguinal canal is formed by the inguinal ligament. Most of the posterior wall of the inguinal canal consists of the transversalis fascia. The deep ring of the inguinal canal represents the initial evagination of the transversalis fascia. **B.** A small part of the anterior wall of the inguinal canal (laterally) is formed by the internal oblique muscle. Arching fibers of the internal oblique and transversus abdominis muscles form the roof of the inguinal canal. **C** to **E.** The external oblique muscle forms most of the anterior wall of the inguinal canal. The fused medial regions of the internal oblique and transversus abdominis muscles (conjoined tendon) form some of the posterior wall of the inguinal canal (deep to the superficial ring). The superficial ring represents the region of external oblique muscle initially pushed out by the processus vaginalis.

TABLE 11–3
Components of the Walls, Roof, and Floor of the Inguinal Canals

Posterior Wall	Anterior Wall	Roof	Floor
Transversalis fascia	External oblique muscle	Arch of transversus abdominis muscle	Inguinal ligament
Conjoined tendon (medial)	Internal oblique muscle (lateral)	Arch of internal oblique muscle	

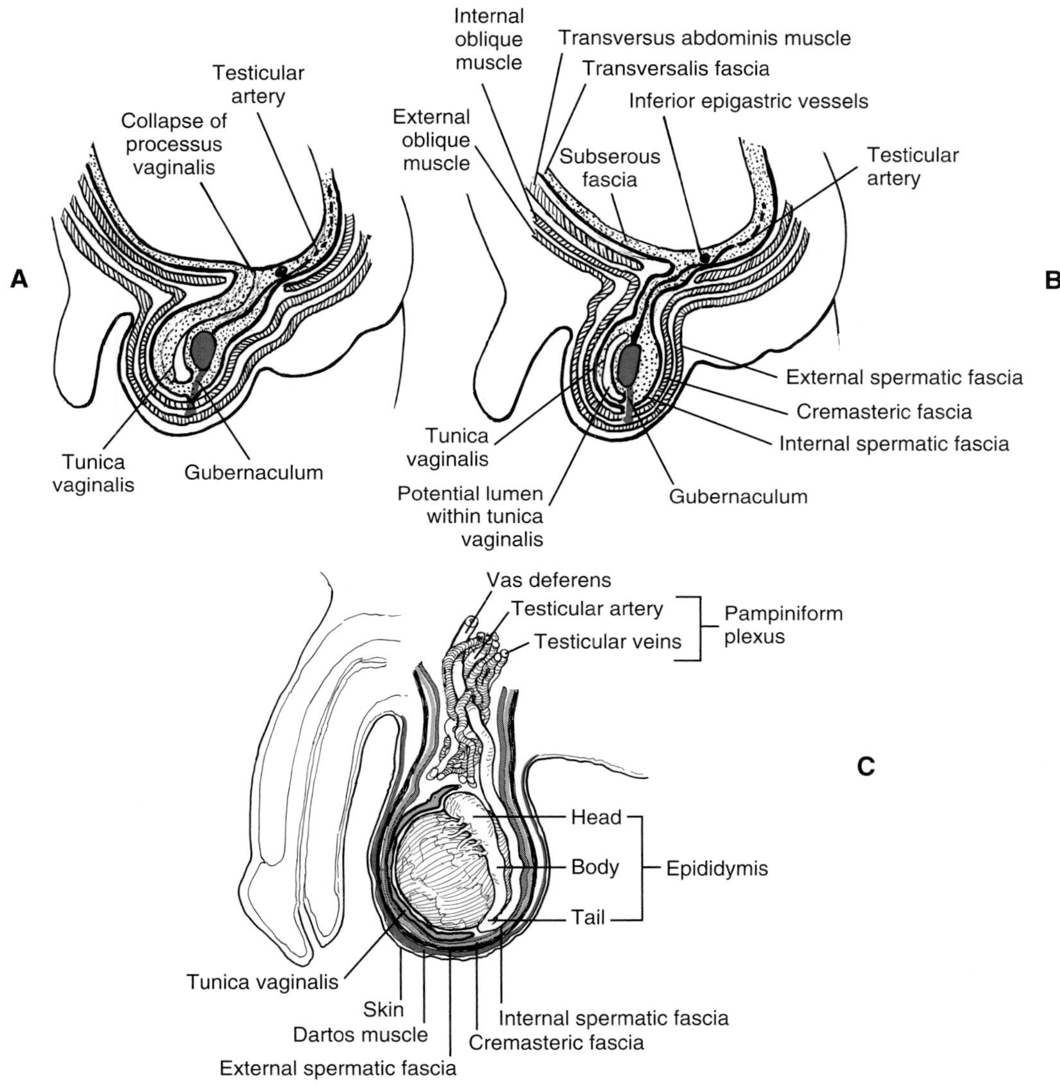

FIGURE 11–20

A and **B.** The superior regions of the processus vaginalis are obliterated during the first postnatal year, leaving a remnant of peritoneum anterior to the testis called the *tunica vaginalis.* During the descent of the testis, the testicular artery and vein, lymphatics, sympathetic nerves, and vas deferens are pulled into the inguinal canal to form the spermatic cord. **C.** The tunica vaginalis is a rudiment of the processus vaginalis. It is wrapped around the anterior surface of the testis. Because the tunica vaginalis is formed by the processus vaginalis, a former outpouching of the peritoneum, the potential space within this flattened sac may fill with serous fluid if it is injured.

tunica vaginalis contains little fluid and its cavity is difficult to define. Nonetheless, following trauma or the onset of infection, the inner lining of the tunica vaginalis may secrete excessive amounts of serous fluid, resulting in its swelling and the formation of a **vaginal hydrocele** (Fig. 11–21*A*). In some cases, the superior part of the processus vaginalis may not be obliterated, allowing direct communication between the cavity within the processus vaginalis and the peritoneal cavity (see discussion of indirect inguinal hernias, below). Peritoneal fluid may, thus, collect within the processus vaginalis, resulting in development of a **congenital hydrocele** (Fig. 11–21*B*). Occasionally, the processus vaginalis may be obliterated only in the region of the deep inguinal ring and an **infantile hydrocele** may extend into the inguinal canal (Fig. 11–21*C*). In cases where the processus is obliterated both in the region of the deep ring and superior to the epididymis, an **encysted hydrocele of the cord** may develop within the region of the processus between these two points (Fig. 11–21*D*).

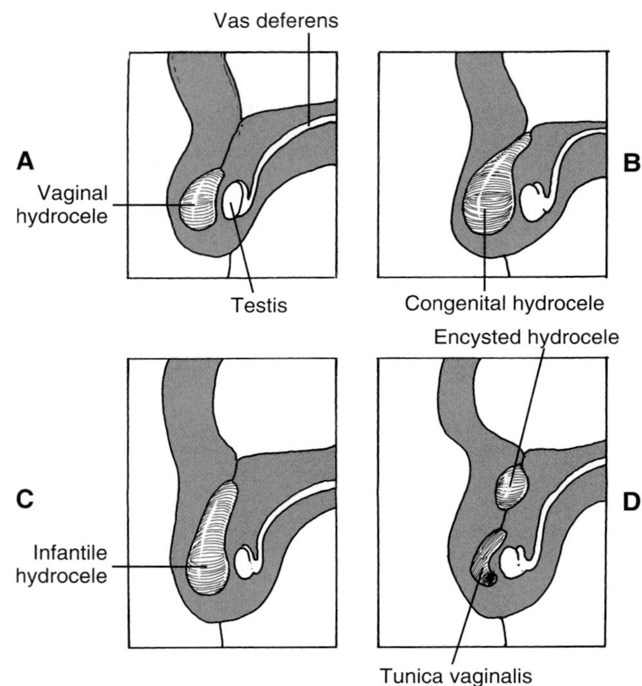

FIGURE 11–21
Hydroceles in males. **A.** Vaginal hydrocele. **B.** Congenital hydrocele. **C.** Infantile hydrocele. **D.** Encysted hydrocele.

Spermatic Cord

The spermatic cord is a complex of vessels, nerves, ducts, and accessory structures, which is formed when the testis enters the deep ring of the inguinal canal

The spermatic cord is made up of the **testicular artery** and **vein, sympathetic fibers** from the **aorticorenal ganglion** (at spinal nerves T10 and T11), **afferent visceral fibers, parasympathetic fibers** from the **pelvic splanchnic nerves, vas deferens (spermatic duct), deferent artery** and **vein, cremasteric artery,** and **lymphatic vessels** (Fig. 11–22 and see Figs. 11–16 and 11–18). These structures converge to form the spermatic cord as the testis, its trailing vessels, and the vas deferens enter the deep inguinal ring and pass through the narrow space of the inguinal canal. Thus, the spermatic cord lengthens as the gonad moves through the canal. The cremasteric artery and vein are associated with the cremasteric muscle (fascia) and are, therefore, superficial to the internal spermatic fascia. In addition, the ilioinguinal nerve does not reside within the spermatic cord (Fig. 11–22*B*). As the spermatic cord follows the gonad through the subserous fascia of the processus vaginalis into the deep ring, it is further covered by internal spermatic fascia. In more medial regions of the canal, it is further covered by the cremasteric fascia. The spermatic cord becomes covered by the external spermatic fascia only after it exits the inguinal canal through the superficial ring (Fig. 11–22 and see Fig. 11–16*D* and *E*).

Testicular Vessels

Testicular arteries branch from anterolateral aspects of the abdominal aorta about midway between the points where the superior and inferior mesenteric arteries arise (see Chapter 13). The testicular arteries descend anterior to the ureters and enter the inguinal canals through the deep inguinal rings. These arteries give off small branches to many structures along their course (e.g., to the renal fat, ureters, and cremaster muscle [see Chapter 13]), but their main trunks supply the testes (see Fig. 11–22).

Testicular veins branch from the **inferior vena cava** (on the right) and the **renal vein** (on the left) (see Chapter 13). These vessels accompany testicular arteries into the scrotum to drain blood from the testes. Within the abdomen, however, they usually split into two parallel veins, and then, within the inguinal canal, into four veins. Within the scrotum, the four veins ramify into numerous tributaries, which together make up the **pampiniform plexus** (see Fig. 11–22). This plexus invests the testicular artery, cooling the incoming blood.

As an individual ages, **varicoceles** develop within the veins of the pampiniform plexus. Because venous pressure is typically higher in the left testicular vein, varicoceles of the left pampiniform plexus tend to enlarge more rapidly. As a consequence, the left side of the scrotal sac extends more inferiorly in older men. Testicular varicoceles may also result from obstructions to venous drainage caused by pressure from the overlying descending colon or by tumors that obstruct the drainage of testicular blood.

Testicular Nerves

Sympathetic fibers to the testis arise from the aorticorenal ganglia, which are innervated by preganglionic fibers from spinal nerves T10 and T11. These nerves are

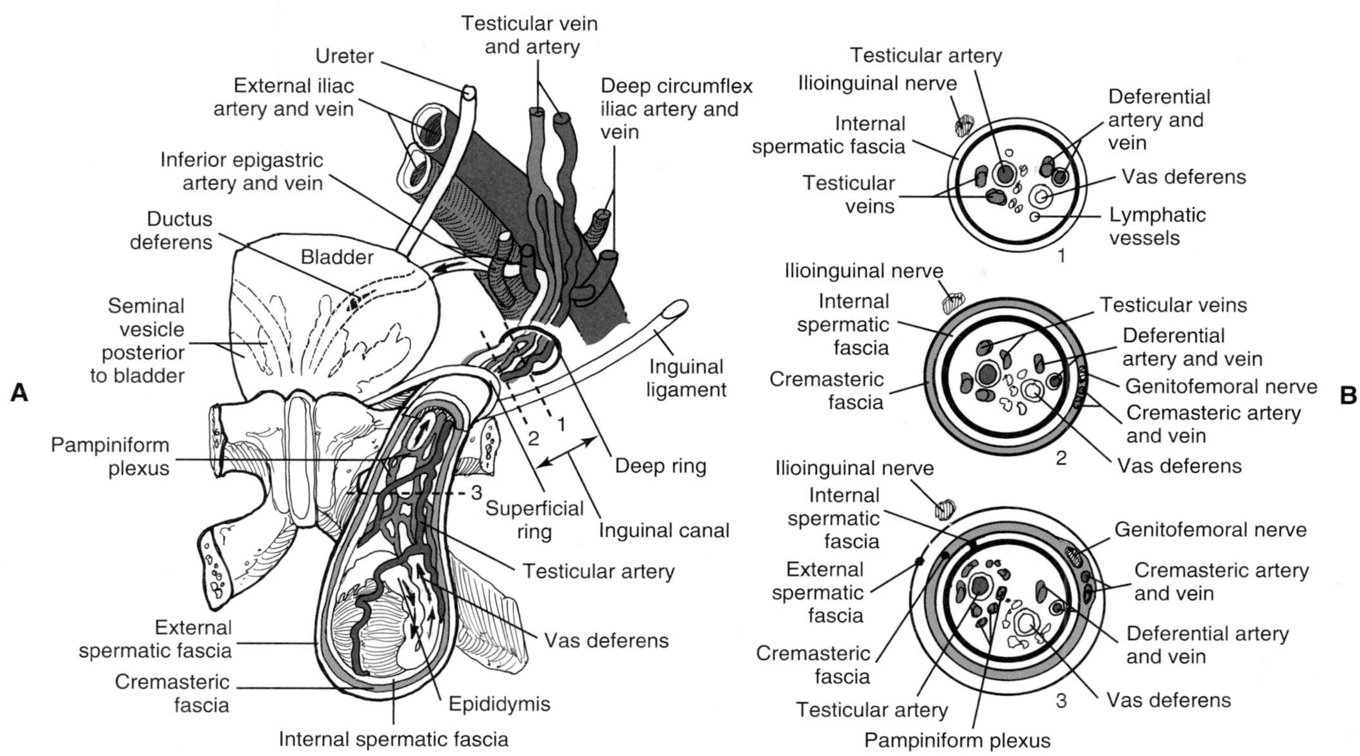

FIGURE 11–22
The definitive spermatic cord. **A.** Anterior view of the spermatic cord. **B.** Cross sections of the spermatic cord at points 1, 2, and 3 in part A from the anteroposterior view. The definitive spermatic cord contains the testicular artery and veins (pampiniform plexus), sympathetic fibers from the aorticorenal ganglion (about at the level of T10 and T11), afferent visceral fibers, parasympathetic fibers from pelvic splanchnic nerves, the vas deferens, the deferential artery and vein, the cremasteric artery, and lymphatic vessels. The ilioinguinal nerve is outside the spermatic cord but within the inguinal canal. The cremasteric vessels are embedded within the cremasteric fascia. Note the disposition of the spermatic fascia in three different regions of the cord.

accompanied by **visceral afferent fibers,** which carry sensory impulses back to the levels of spinal nerves T10 and T11. **Parasympathetic innervation** of the testes is provided by the **pelvic splanchnic nerves** (S2 to S4) (Fig. 11–22). The functions of these autonomic nerves are described in Chapter 15.

Spermatic Duct (Vas Deferens)

The vas deferens is a remnant of an embryonic urinary duct (mesonephric duct) (see Fig. 11–22). This duct completely disappears in females. In males, the inferior end of the spermatic duct becomes attached to the **prostatic utricle,** which is a slightly expanded region of the **prostatic urethra** located just inferior to the bladder (Fig. 11–23 and see Chapter 15). The superior end of the duct is attached to the developing testis, and its lumen becomes continuous with the lumina of the efferent ductules and, ultimately, with the lumina of the **seminiferous tubules.** As the testis descends during fetal life, the superior end of the vas deferens is pulled in an inferior direction into the inguinal canal and then into the scrotum.

The **function of the spermatic duct** is to transport spermatozoa from the testis into the prostatic urethra

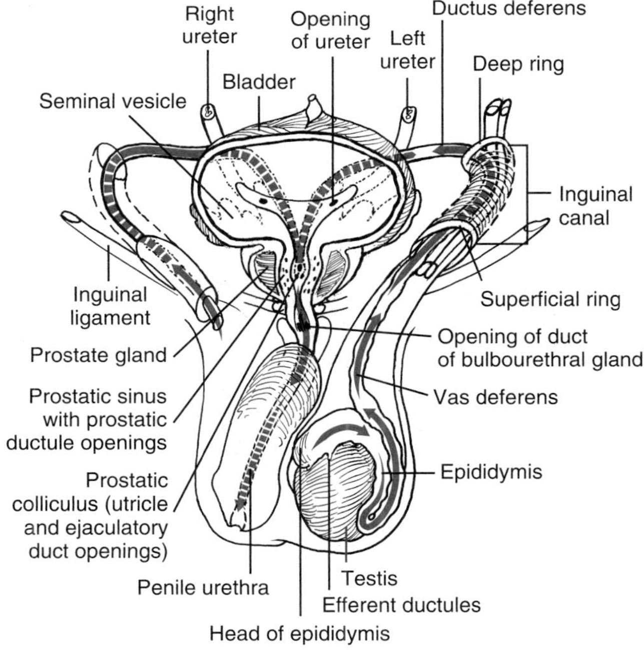

FIGURE 11–23
Route of sperm and seminal fluid from the testes and accessory glands to the penile urethra.

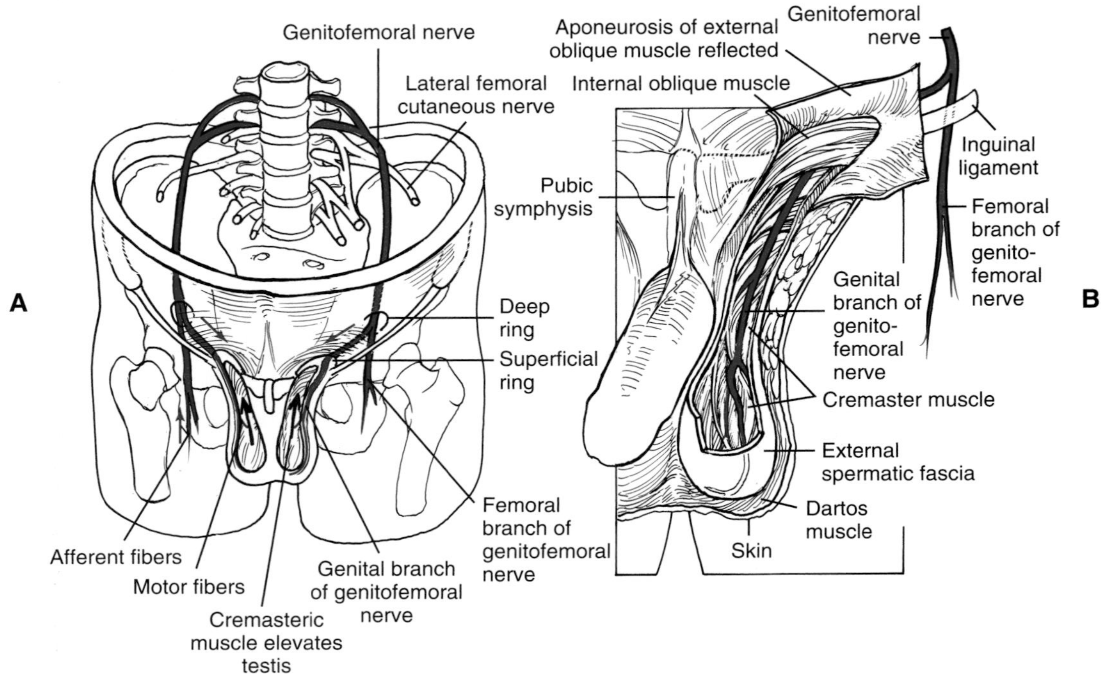

FIGURE 11–24 Innervation of the cremaster muscles and the cremasteric reflex. **A.** Stimulation of the femoral branch of the genitofemoral nerve in the medial thigh results in raising of the testicle through motor fibers within the genital branch of the genitofemoral nerve. Innervation is by the genital branch of the genitofemoral nerve. **B.** The genital branch of the genitofemoral nerve innervates the cremasteric fascia of the spermatic cord.

during ejaculation. The spermatozoa are formed in seminiferous tubules of the testis. During ejaculation, they move through efferent ductules, into the lumen of the vas deferens, and out of the scrotum; through the superficial ring into the inguinal canal; then in a superolateral direction through the inguinal canal; through the deep inguinal ring; and onto the inner surface of the abdominal wall. They are then transported in an inferior direction along the inner surface of the anterior pelvic wall, into the prostatic utricle of the prostatic urethra, and into the penile urethra (Fig. 11–23).

The neural control of the vas deferens and the function of accessory glands are described in detail in Chapter 15. The vas deferens is vascularized by **deferential arteries** and **veins,** which branch from **superior vesicle arteries** and **veins** (see Fig. 11–22 and Chapter 13).

Cremaster Muscles

Specialized muscles of the anterolateral abdominal wall raise the testes in males

The **cremaster muscles** constitute the middle layer of the spermatic fascia. This muscular layer suspends the spermatic cord from the layer of internal oblique muscle from which the cremaster muscle was created (Fig. 11–24). Contraction of the cremaster muscles causes the testes to move superiorly, closer to the perineum and inferior abdominal wall. This protects the testes from trauma and also protects them from exposure to cold temperatures. The cremaster muscles are striated. They are innervated by somatic motor fibers associated with the **genital branch of the genitofemoral nerve.** However, these muscles usually contract in a reflexive, involuntary manner **(cremasteric reflex)** in response to cold temperatures. They typically operate in concert with the **dartos muscles,** which are made up of smooth (nonstriated) muscles innervated by sympathetic (visceral motor) fibers of several nerves (Table 11–4). The cremasteric reflex may be initiated by stimulation of sensory fibers of the **femoral branch of the genitofemoral nerve,** within the superomedial thigh (Fig. 11–24). Thus, the cremasteric reflex is tested by stroking the medial thigh in a physical examination.

Other Structures of the Inguinal Canal in Males

A small **cremasteric artery** and **vein** vascularize the cremaster muscle within the wall of the spermatic cord.

Lymphatic vessels of the testis accompany testicular arteries back to **lateral aortic lymph nodes** (see Fig. 11–22*B*). Lymph is drained from the vas deferens back to **external iliac lymph nodes** (see Chapter 13).

The segmental innervation of the anterolateral abdominal wall by intercostal nerves at T7 to T11, subcostal nerves at T12, and lumbar nerves (iliohypogastric and ilioinguinal nerves) at L1 is described above. These nerves

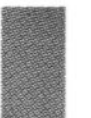

TABLE 11–4
Specific Innervation of and Actions of Anterolateral Body Wall Muscles

Muscle	Innervation of Muscle*	Specific Actions of Muscle
External oblique	Intercostal nerves T6 to T11; subcostal nerve T12	Pulls anterior wall of abdomen to opposite side and aids in flexion of vertebral column
Internal oblique	Intercostal nerves T6 to T11; subcostal nerves T12 and L1	Pulls anterior wall of abdomen to same side and aids in flexion of vertebral column
Cremaster	Genital branch of genitofemoral nerve (L1, L2, branch of lumbar plexus)	Pulls testis up toward superficial inguinal ring
Transversus abdominis	Intercostal nerves T6 to T11; subcostal nerves T12 and L1	Provides tonus of abdominal wall so that it retains abdominal viscera
Rectus abdominis	Intercostal nerves T6 to T11	Is active in flexion when resistance must be overcome; opposes action of erector spinae muscles
Pyramidalis	Subcostal nerve T12	Tenses linea alba for no known reason
Dartos	Only sympathetic and sensory fibers of genital branch of genitofemoral nerve (L1, L2); ilioinguinal nerve (L1); posterior femoral cutaneous branch of sacral plexus (S1 to S3); posterior scrotal branch (S4) of perineal nerve	Pulls testis closer to body wall

*Nerves contain motor, sensory, and sympathetic fibers unless otherwise noted. Sympathetic fibers are mainly vasoconstrictive or provide motor innervation to dartos muscles.

course from their points of origin in the posterior wall to the anterior abdominal wall between the transversus abdominis and internal oblique muscles. As the ilioinguinal nerve enters the inguinal canal, it comes to lie just superior to the spermatic cord in males, between the transversalis fascia and external oblique muscle in the region where the transversus abdominis and internal oblique muscles are absent (see Fig. 11–22*B*). The nerve exits the inguinal canal with the spermatic cord to provide sensory and sympathetic fibers to the superomedial region of the thigh and skin at the root of the penis.

Definitive Inguinal Canal and Associated Structures in Females

The definitive inguinal canal in females contains the round ligament of the uterus and the ilioinguinal nerve

In females, the processus vaginalis pushes three layers of the anterior body wall outward in a medial direction to form an inguinal canal that is just like that of the male in every respect. A **gubernacular ligament** also forms within the subserous fascia between the gonads (ovaries) and labioscrotal swellings. In the **absence of high titers of testosterone,** the gubernaculum does not become shortened as it does in males but grows at the same pace as the rest of the body. Nonetheless, the ovary is pulled inferiorly by the gubernaculum because the uterus develops by fusion of the paired **paramesonephric ducts,** each of which is connected to the gubernaculum on one side of the body. As the paramesonephric ducts fuse together, the round ligament of the uterus and gubernacular ligament are pulled into the **broad ligament of the uterus** (see Chapter 14). Thus, in the definitive condition, the gubernaculum courses from the former inferior pole of the ovary through the subserous fascia of the broad ligament to the wall of the uterus, and through the subserous fascia of the broad ligament and the anterior pelvic wall; through the deep ring into the inguinal canal; through the canal in a medial direction; out through the superficial inguinal ring; and into the labium majus (Fig. 11–25). The section of the former gubernaculum that extends from the labium majus to the lateral wall of the uterus is the **round ligament of the uterus.** The remaining section, which extends from the lateral wall of the uterus to the ovary, is the **ovarian ligament.** The combined length of the round ligament of the uterus and ovarian ligament is 15 to 20 cm. The ligament is usually somewhat flattened. At its widest point, it is 2 to 4 mm in diameter. It splays into several branches as it courses from the superficial inguinal ring into the superficial fascia of the labium majus.

As in males, the inguinal canal in females contains a portion of the **ilioinguinal nerve,** which escapes through the superficial inguinal ring to innervate the superior region of the labium majus and the **mons pubis,** which is the skin lying immediately superior to the labium majus.

Inguinal Hernias. **Indirect congenital inguinal hernias** develop when the proximal end of the processus vaginalis fails to degenerate during an infant's first year of life. As a consequence, organs of the abdominal cavity may herniate

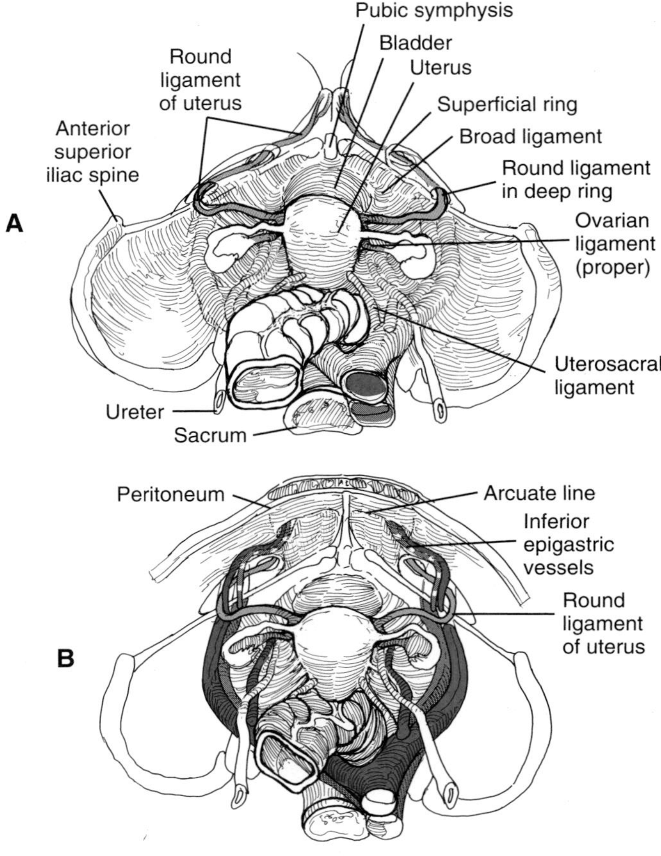

FIGURE 11–25
In females, the round ligament of the uterus and the ovarian ligament descend from the gubernaculum. **A** and **B** show the course of each of these ligaments.

into the patent lumen of the processus via the deep inguinal ring. They may then move through the inguinal canal to extrude through the superficial inguinal ring and into the scrotum in males or labia majora in females. Thus, even though these hernias may ultimately evaginate through the superficial inguinal ring, their route to this location is **indirect** because they first evaginate through the deep inguinal ring just *lateral* to the inguinal triangle (Fig. 11–26). These hernias are most often diagnosed in younger males or females.

Direct acquired inguinal hernias push through the weakened conjoined tendon to evaginate **directly** through the superficial inguinal ring *within* the inguinal triangle (Fig. 11–26). Direct inguinal hernias usually result from weakening of the abdominal muscles in persons over 40 years of age. However, direct inguinal hernias occasionally occur in younger individuals as a result of congenital failure of the anterior abdominal muscles to properly align with and "shutter" the inguinal canal.

Inguinal hernias are common. They represent approximately 75% of all abdominal hernias. Of them, 86% of them occur in males of all ages. The incidence is approximately 15 in 1000 individuals. About two thirds of inguinal hernias are indirect and one third are direct.

Fortunately, inguinal hernias are readily repairable. Surgical repair of indirect inguinal hernias in both sexes involves removal of the processus vaginalis. In females, transection of the round ligament of the uterus may also be needed. The abdominal wall must be strengthened in the region of the inguinal canal, especially in the region of the superficial inguinal ring in direct hernias and the deep inguinal ring in indirect hernias. This may be accomplished by inserting a synthetic patch or by tightening the transversalis fascia or external ab-

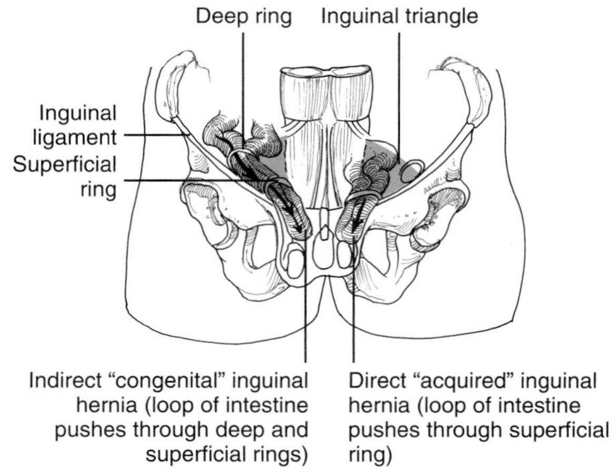

FIGURE 11–26
Anterior view of direct inguinal hernias (left side) and indirect inguinal hernias (right side). Notice that although herniation of the colon appears in the region of the superficial ring in both cases, the indirect hernia enters the processus vaginalis at the deep ring (lateral to the inguinal triangle) while the direct hernia pushes through a weakened conjoined tendon in the region of the superficial ring (within the inguinal triangle).

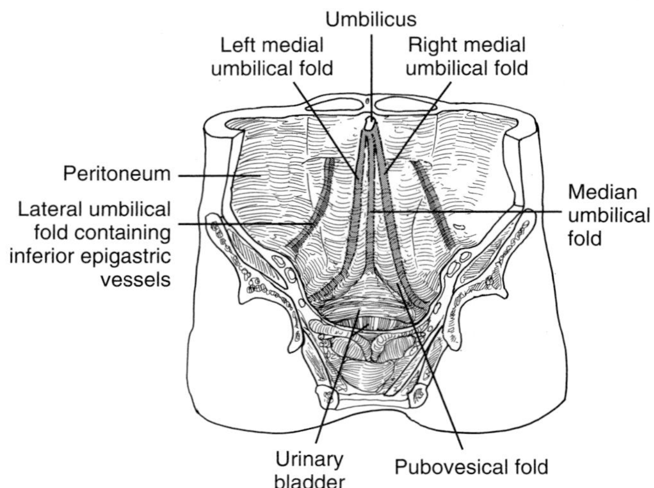

FIGURE 11–27
Posterior view of anterior abdominal wall showing the umbilical folds. The lateral umbilical folds are formed by obliterated umbilical arteries. The medial umbilical folds are formed by the inferior epigastric arteries and veins. The median umbilical fold is a remnant of the embryologic allantois called the *urachus*.

dominal oblique aponeurosis with sutures. Since 1990, more than half of inguinal hernia repairs have been done on an outpatient basis, frequently with **laparoscopic techniques.**

Inguinal hernias, like other hernias, may be life threatening if the protruding section of omentum or intestine becomes strangulated, leading to compromise of the blood supply. Unless surgical repair is done immediately, necrosis may develop and may lead to death. Clinical signs of a strangulated hernia include vomiting and severe abdominal pain lasting several hours. These symptoms are similar to and often confused with those of bowel obstruction (see Chapter 12).

▲ Umbilical Folds

Specialized umbilical folds are created by structures that course within the subserous fascia of the anterior abdominal wall

Once the anterior abdominal wall is reflected, five distinct folds of peritoneum may be observed coursing from inferior regions toward the umbilicus. These are the **paired lateral umbilical folds, paired medial umbilical folds,** and midline **median umbilical fold.**

The **lateral umbilical folds** contain the inferior epigastric vessels, which constitute the lateral boundary of the inguinal triangle. These are functional vessels that serve the anterior abdominal wall and rectus abdominis muscles. They arise just medial to the deep inguinal ring, and course superiorly to the arcuate line of the rectus sheath (Fig. 11–27 and see Figs. 11–15*D* and 11–18*B*).

The **medial umbilical folds** contain the obliterated **umbilical arteries,** which were the terminal branches of the anterior division of the **internal iliac arteries** (see Chapter 14). These arteries have become scarified ligaments and may be easily identified as extensions of the **superior vesicle arteries,** which course along the lateral surfaces of the bladder and onto the anterior abdominal wall to terminate at the umbilicus (Fig. 11–27).

The **median umbilical fold** contains the **urachus,** which is a remnant of the **allantois,** an embryologic structure that extends superiorly from the superior pole of the bladder. Like the remnants of the umbilical arteries, the urachus appears as a ligament that terminates in the region of the umbilicus (Fig. 11–27).

Umbilical hernias were previously described.

12 The Abdominal Cavity and Abdominal Viscera

The **abdominopelvic (peritoneal) cavity** is bounded by the diaphragm, anterolateral and posterior abdominal walls, and pelvic diaphragm (Fig. 12–1 and see Chapter 14). It contains the **gastrointestinal tract (alimentary canal)**, from the abdominal esophagus to the rectum, and glandular organs that arise from it, including the **liver, gallbladder, pancreas,** and **appendix.** Other important organs within the abdominopelvic cavity are the **spleen, suprarenal glands,** and organs of the **urogenital system,** including the kidneys, ureters, uterus, oviducts, ovaries, vas deferens, and bladder. The boundary between the abdominal cavity and the pelvic cavity is a plane that transects the pelvic brim (Fig. 12–1 and see below).

ANATOMY OF THE ABDOMINOPELVIC CAVITY

Boundaries of the Abdominopelvic Cavity

The sternum, ribs, vertebrae, pelvis, and several muscles are landmarks that demarcate the boundaries of the abdominopelvic cavity

The **abdominopelvic cavity** develops from the intraembryonic coelomic cavity (see Chapter 6). It is separated from the definitive superior pericardial cavity and left and right pleural cavities by the **septum transversum** and pleuroperitoneal membranes (see Figs. 7–1, 10–9, and 12–1*A*). The membranes and septum transversum form the dome-shaped diaphragm, which is the superior boundary of the definitive peritoneal cavity. The central part of the diaphragm reaches different levels during different phases of the respiratory cycle (see Chapter 8). However, its peripheral connections to the body wall are fixed at the xiphoid process anteriorly, at the infrasternal angle, upon ribs 11 and 12 laterally, and at vertebra L1 posteriorly (see Fig. 12–1*A*).

The **inferior boundary** of the definitive peritoneal cavity is a complex of muscles within the floor of the pelvis called the **pelvic diaphragm** (see Fig. 12–1*B* and Chapter 14). The pelvic diaphragm includes the **levator ani muscle** (pubococcygeus and iliococcygeus muscles) and a posterior part of the coccygeus muscle complex (sometimes called the **ischiococcygeus muscle**). These muscles also form the superior boundary of the **perineum,** which is the most inferior compartment of the trunk. The perineum contains outlets for the gastrointestinal and urinary tracts (see Chapter 15).

The **posterior boundary** of the definitive abdominopelvic cavity includes the five lumbar vertebrae, five fused sacral vertebrae, and muscles associated with these regions of the vertebral column (see Fig. 12–1*A*). Muscles associated with the lumbar region are the psoas and quadratus lumborum muscles (see Fig. 12–1*A*). Muscles associated with the superior sacral region (within the false pelvis, or iliac fossa) include the psoas and iliacus muscles. Muscles that form the posterior boundary of the peritoneal cavity in the inferior sacral region (true pelvis) include the piriformis muscle and upper borders of the coccygeus muscles (see Chapter 14).

The **anterolateral boundary** of the definitive peritoneal cavity is primarily defined by muscles (and their aponeuroses) of the anterior abdominal wall. These are the external oblique, internal oblique, transversus abdominis, rectus abdominis, and pyramidalis muscles (see Chapter 11). The anterolateral muscle boundaries within the true pelvis (just inferior to the pubic crest) include the obturator internus muscles, anterior slips of the pubococcygeus muscles, and lateral tendons of the iliococcygeus muscles (see Chapter 14).

Boundary Between the Abdominal Cavity and the Pelvic Cavity

A plane at the level of the pelvic brim divides the definitive peritoneal cavity into a superior abdominal cavity and an inferior pelvic cavity

The pelvic bone is described in detail in Chapter 14, but several of its features will be discussed here as a way of relating the peritoneal organs to prominent landmarks associated with this bony framework. By convention, the definitive peritoneal cavity is divided into two contiguous, openly communicating regions: the superior abdominal cavity and inferior pelvic cavity. The boundary between the two regions is a plane that intersects the **sacral promontory** posteriorly, **anterior rim of the ala of the sacrum** posterolaterally, **arcuate line of the ilium** laterally, **pecten pubis (pectineal line)**

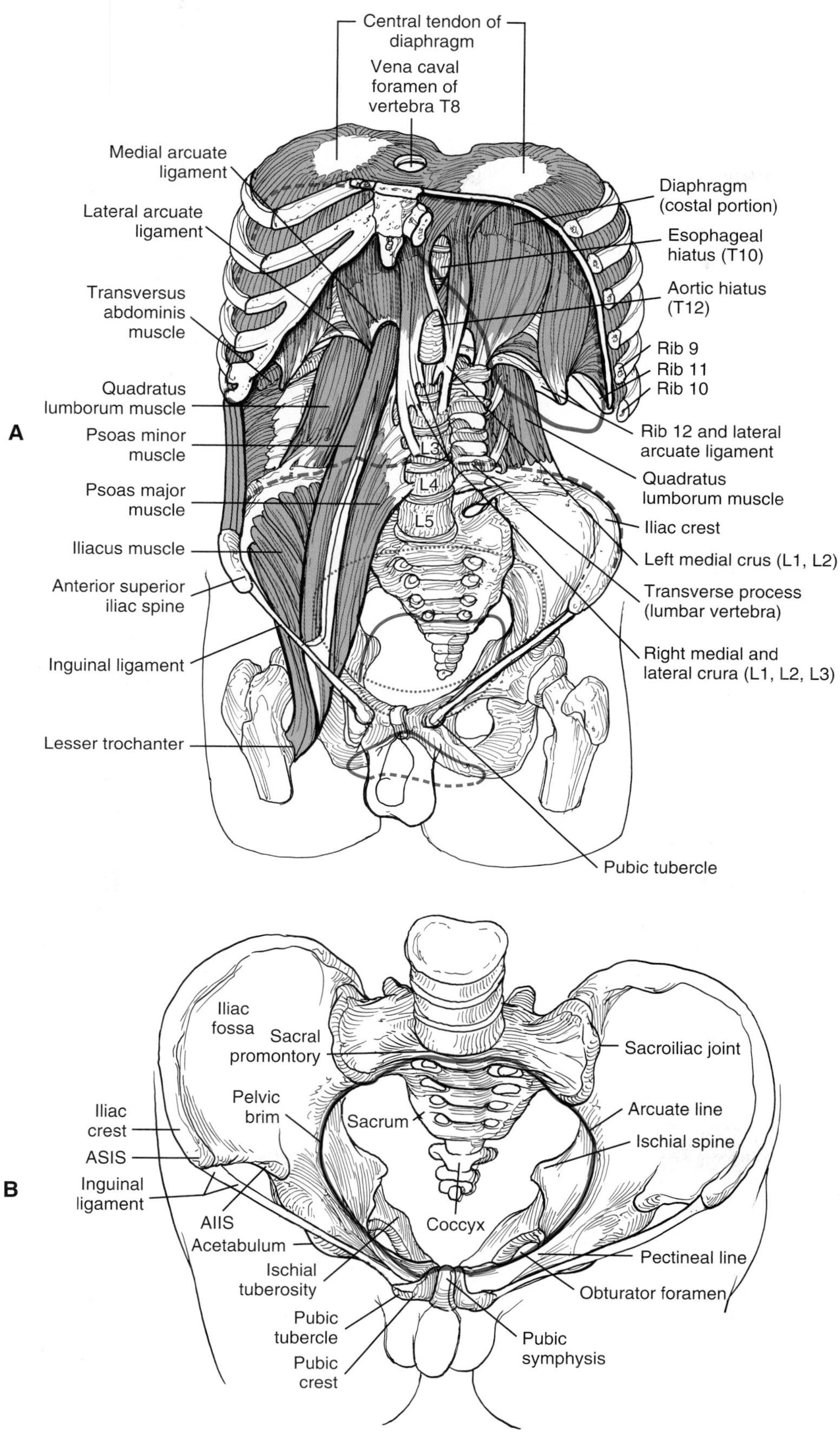

FIGURE 12–1

Boundaries of the abdominopelvic cavity. **A.** The abdominopelvic cavity is bounded superiorly by the diaphragm and its bony attachments; inferiorly by the pelvic diaphragm; posteriorly by the lumbar vertebrae, psoas, and quadratus lumborum muscles above and sacrum and piriformis muscles below; and anterolaterally by the abdominal musculature above and pelvis and obturator internus muscles below. **B.** The boundary between the abdominal cavity and pelvic cavity is the imaginary plane at the level of the pelvic brim (pelvic inlet). *ASIS,* Anterior superior iliac spine; *AIIS,* anterior inferior iliac spine.

anterolaterally, and **pubic crest** anteriorly (see Fig. 12–1). This ring of bone intersected by the imaginary plane is the **pelvic brim.** The opening between the abdominal and pelvic cavities at the level of the pelvic brim is the **pelvic inlet** (see Fig. 12–1 and Chapter 14).

A subsection of the pelvic brim is the **linea terminalis.** The linea terminalis includes the **pubic crest, pecten pubis (pectineal line),** and **arcuate line of the ilium.** It does not include the ala of the sacrum or the sacral promontory. A subsection of the linea terminalis is the **iliopectineal line,** which consists of the pecten pubis and arcuate line of the ilium only (see Fig. 12–1*B*).

The extensions of iliac bones that flare superiorly from the pelvic brim are **iliac crests,** and the concavities they create are **iliac fossae** (see Fig. 12–1*A*). The iliac fossae and the space between them are part of the abdominal cavity because they are superior to the pelvic brim. However, this inferior region of the abdominal cavity is called the **false (major) pelvis,** while the cavity inferior to the pelvic brim is called the **true (minor, obstetric) pelvis** (see Fig. 12–1*B*).

Peritoneal Membranes

Peritoneal membranes play a critical role in organization of the abdominopelvic cavity and its viscera

The peritoneal membrane lining the peritoneal cavity is the **parietal peritoneum,** and the peritoneal membrane investing the visceral organs is the **visceral peritoneum** (Fig. 12–2*A*). The parietal peritoneum completely lines the inner wall of the abdominopelvic cavity in males (Fig. 12–2B). This membrane is also reflected into the abdominopelvic cavity to form the **mesenteries,** which suspend some of the viscera and contribute to the visceral peritoneum investing them (Fig. 12–2*A* and see Fig. 12–3*A*). The parietal and visceral peritoneum form a continuous membrane, in some regions via the mesenteries. This is similar to the parietal pleura, which is a continuous lining of the pleural cavity and the reflected visceral pleura investing the lung. In females, the peritoneum is perforated at the openings of the paired oviducts (Fig. 12–2*C*). These apertures allow an oocyte to enter the mouth (ostium) of the oviduct, so that it may be fertilized and eventually reach the uterine cavity.

If it were possible to surgically remove the abdominopelvic peritoneum as an intact structure in its natural configuration, including the parietal and visceral peritoneum and mesenteries, it would be a closed sac with invaginations conforming precisely to the outlines of the abdominopelvic cavity and the abdominopelvic viscera (Fig. 12–2*B* and *C*).

Intraperitoneal, Retroperitoneal, and Secondarily Retroperitoneal Relationships

The abdominopelvic organs are of three types based on their relationships to the body wall and peritoneum. Organs such as the stomach, jejunum, ileum, and transverse colon are suspended by mesenteries from the body wall of the peritoneal cavity and are **intraperitoneal organs** (Fig. 12–2*A*). Organs embedded within the body wall behind the peritoneal membrane are **retroperitoneal organs** (Fig. 12–2*A*). These organs may be located in any region of the body wall, including the anterior region (e.g., the urachus), lateral region (e.g., the deep circumflex iliac vessels), or posterior region (e.g., the kidneys). A third group of structures appears to be retroperitoneal organs but are not because they developed in a different way than the true retroperitoneal organs. During early development, these organs were sus-

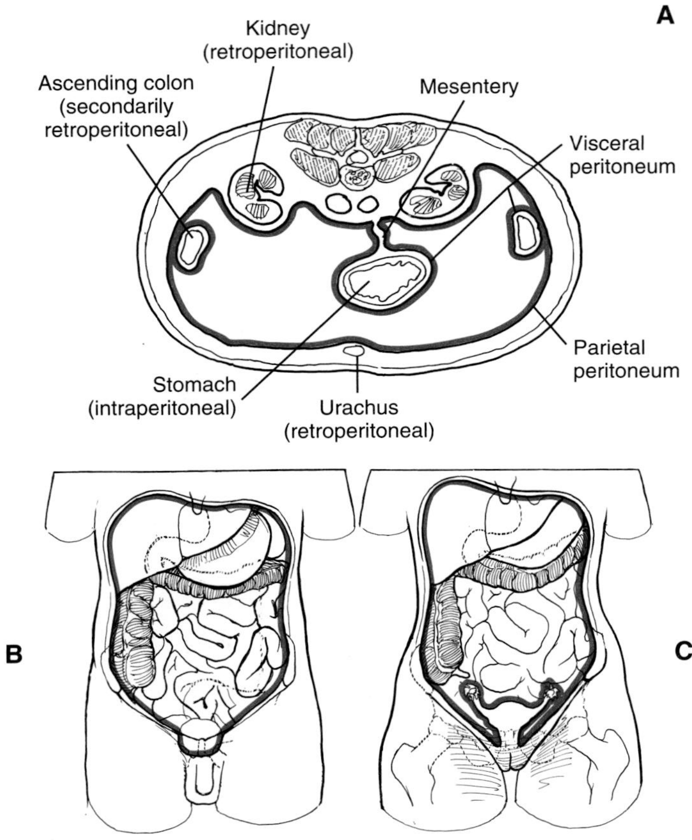

FIGURE 12–2
Relationships of the peritoneum to the abdominal wall and the viscera. **A.** Transverse section of the abdomen. Peritoneum covering the deep surface of the body wall is parietal peritoneum. Peritoneum investing the viscera is visceral peritoneum. Abdominopelvic organs that are suspended by a mesentery are intraperitoneal. Abdominopelvic organs embedded in the body wall but covered on their deep surfaces by peritoneum are retroperitoneal. Organs that appear to be embedded in the body wall but were suspended by the mesentery during embryonic life are secondarily retroperitoneal. **B.** Frontal view of the male abdominopelvic cavity. The peritoneum completely lines the abdominopelvic cavity in males. **C.** Frontal view of the female abdominopelvic cavity. In females, the peritoneum is punctured by openings at the mouths of the oviducts.

pended by the mesentery as intraperitoneal organs, but they became fused to the body wall when their mesenteries collapsed. These organs, including the duodenum, pancreas, and ascending colon and descending colon, are **secondarily retroperitoneal organs** (Fig. 12–2*A*). They may be easily separated from the body wall during surgery or dissection.

Functions of the Abdominopelvic Peritoneum

The peritoneal lining of the abdominopelvic cavity is a selectively permeable barrier; fluids, solutes, and cells may pass across the peritoneum

The **mesothelium** lining the peritoneal cavity and abdominopelvic organs can be compared to the endothelial lining of blood vessels. It is a selective barrier that allows water and solutes to cross it in both directions between the peritoneal cavity and the interstitial spaces of enclosed tissues. Wandering macrophages and lymphocytes can also cross the peritoneal membrane. Macrophages engulf debris within the peritoneal cavity and migrate to the spleen or lymph nodes, purifying the peritoneal fluid. Lymphocytes in the peritoneal fluid function in the immunologic defense of the peritoneal cavity.

Serous fluid within the peritoneal cavity is a dialysate of blood and tissue fluids containing electrolytes and proteins. Its composition may be altered in certain pathologic conditions, and, therefore, its analysis is useful in the diagnosis of some diseases. Water or drugs **injected into the peritoneal cavity** easily cross the mesothelium and enter the circulatory system. When kidney disease or dysfunction occurs, the dialysis of blood wastes may be achieved by rinsing the peritoneal cavity with large volumes of fluid.

A fundamental function of serous fluid is to lubricate the surfaces of gastrointestinal organs as they slide against one another and against the inner lining of the body wall during the contractile movements of **peristalsis** (see below).

▲ Recesses and Spaces of the Abdominal Cavity

Landmarks within the peritoneal cavity include several recesses and subregions of varying significance

Several inconstant **peritoneal recesses** have been identified in the regions of the duodenojejunal junction, ileocecal junction, and root of the sigmoid colon and its attachment to the posterior body wall. All of these recesses form between small folds of the peritoneum where the visceral structure (i.e., the jejunum, ileum, cecum, or sigmoid colon) abuts an adjacent organ or the body wall.

Of greater clinical significance are the spaces within the peritoneal cavity that isolate infected peritoneal fluid or provide a conduit for the flow of infected fluid to other regions of the cavity. Spaces that may isolate infected fluid include the supracolic space, which lies between the transverse colon and diaphragm above it (Fig. 12–3*A* and *B*), and infracolic space, which lies posterior and inferior to the transverse colon and to the right and left of the transverse mesocolon (Fig. 12–3*C*). Spaces that may serve as conduits for infected fluid include the four paracolic gutters, which lie just lateral and medial to the ascending colon and descending colon and the hepatorenal recess (Fig. 12–3*C*). In patients who are supine, infections may travel superiorly within the right lateral paracolic gutter into the hepatorenal recess and then into the lesser sac of the peritoneal cavity posterior to the stomach (Fig. 12–3*A* and see the discussion of mesenteries of the stomach and greater and lesser peritoneal sacs, below). In patients who are in the sitting position, infections may travel inferiorly into the inferior pouches (fossae) of the pelvic cavity. The inferior fossae of the pelvic cavity include the rectovesical pouch in males, rectouterine and vesicouterine pouches in females, and left and right pararectal fossae in both sexes. The pararectal fossae are the most inferior excursions of the parietal peritoneum in the pelvic cavity (Fig. 12–3*A* and see Chapter 14).

■ ANATOMY OF THE GASTROINTESTINAL TRACT AND ACCESSORY ORGANS

Most of the abdominopelvic viscera are parts of the gastrointestinal tract

The abdominal gastrointestinal tract is conventionally divided into three regions based on the organization of the three different arteries that serve it. These are the **abdominal foregut, midgut,** and **hindgut** (Fig. 12–4*A*). Each of these regions is also drained by specific portal vessels and innervated by different branches of the sympathetic nervous system. Thus, this three-part division of the abdominal gastrointestinal tract is essential for understanding its function and making clinical diagnoses based on descriptions of referred pain (see below).

▲ Organization of the Gastrointestinal Tract on the Basis of Vasculature

Vascular fields of the three embryonic vitelline arteries demarcate the abdominal foregut, midgut, and hindgut

By the fourth week of development, the vitelline system of arteries consists of the multiple ventral branches of the dorsal aorta, which are an extensive network of vessels supplying the embryonic yolk sac. As the yolk sac decreases in importance and size during the second month of development, this peritoneal vitelline network is reduced to three major ventral branches of the dorsal aorta, which provide blood to three sequential regions of the abdominopelvic gastrointestinal tract and its associated organs. These three vessels are the **celiac artery,** which supplies the abdominal foregut; **superior mesenteric artery,** which supplies the midgut; and **inferior mesenteric artery,** which supplies the

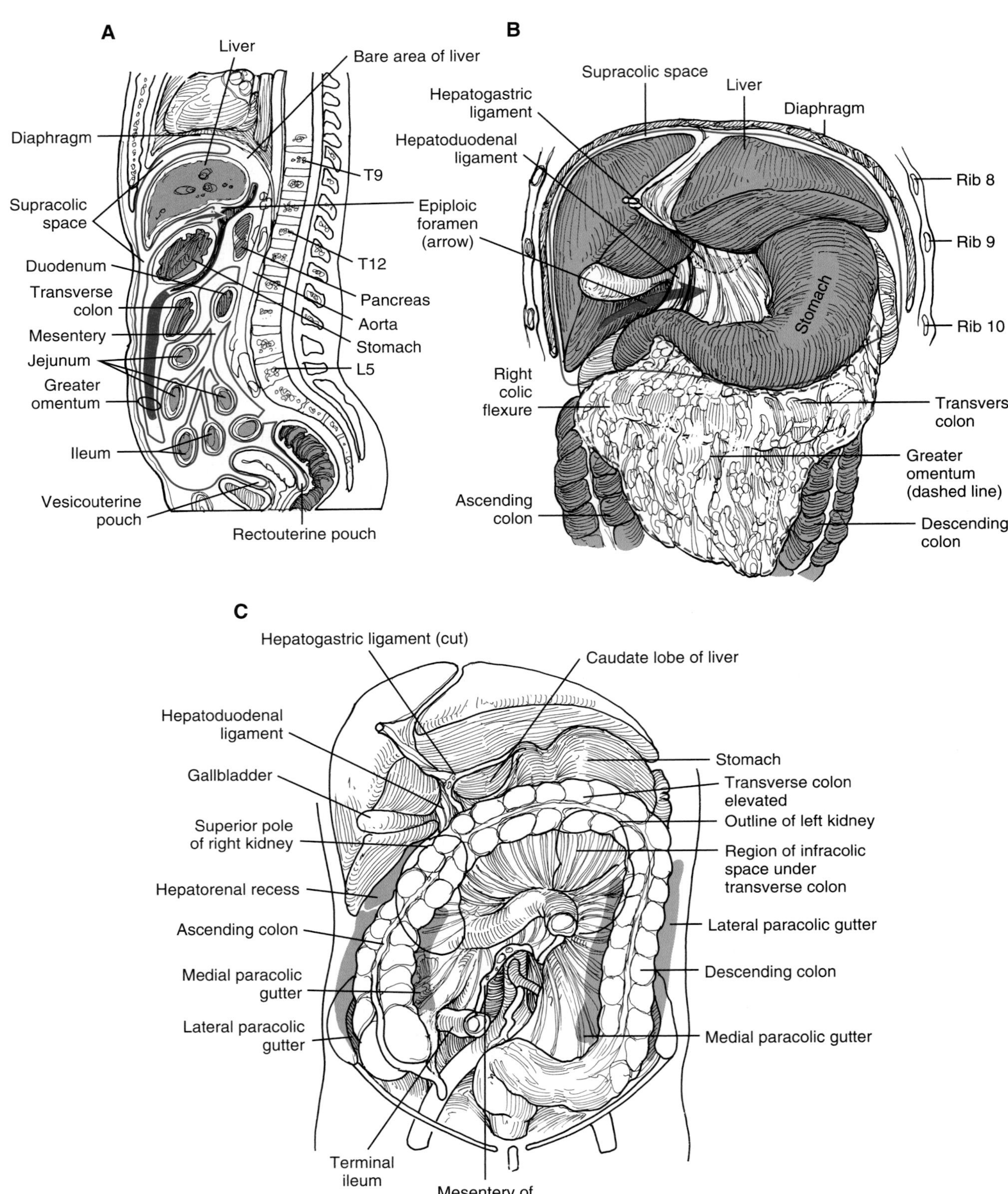

FIGURE 12–3

Recesses and spaces of the abdominopelvic cavity. **A.** This midsagittal section shows the supracolic space of the greater sac of the peritoneal cavity and the lesser sac of the peritoneal cavity. **B.** Frontal view of the abdominal cavity shows the region of the supracolic space and the epiploic foramen of Winslow, which allows communication between the greater and lesser sacs. **C.** This frontal view of the abdominal cavity shows the infracolic space, hepatorenal recess, and lateral and medial paracolic gutters. Note how infections could travel from the right lateral paracolic gutter to the hepatorenal recess, under the hepatoduodenal ligament, through the epiploic foramen of Winslow, and into the lesser sac.

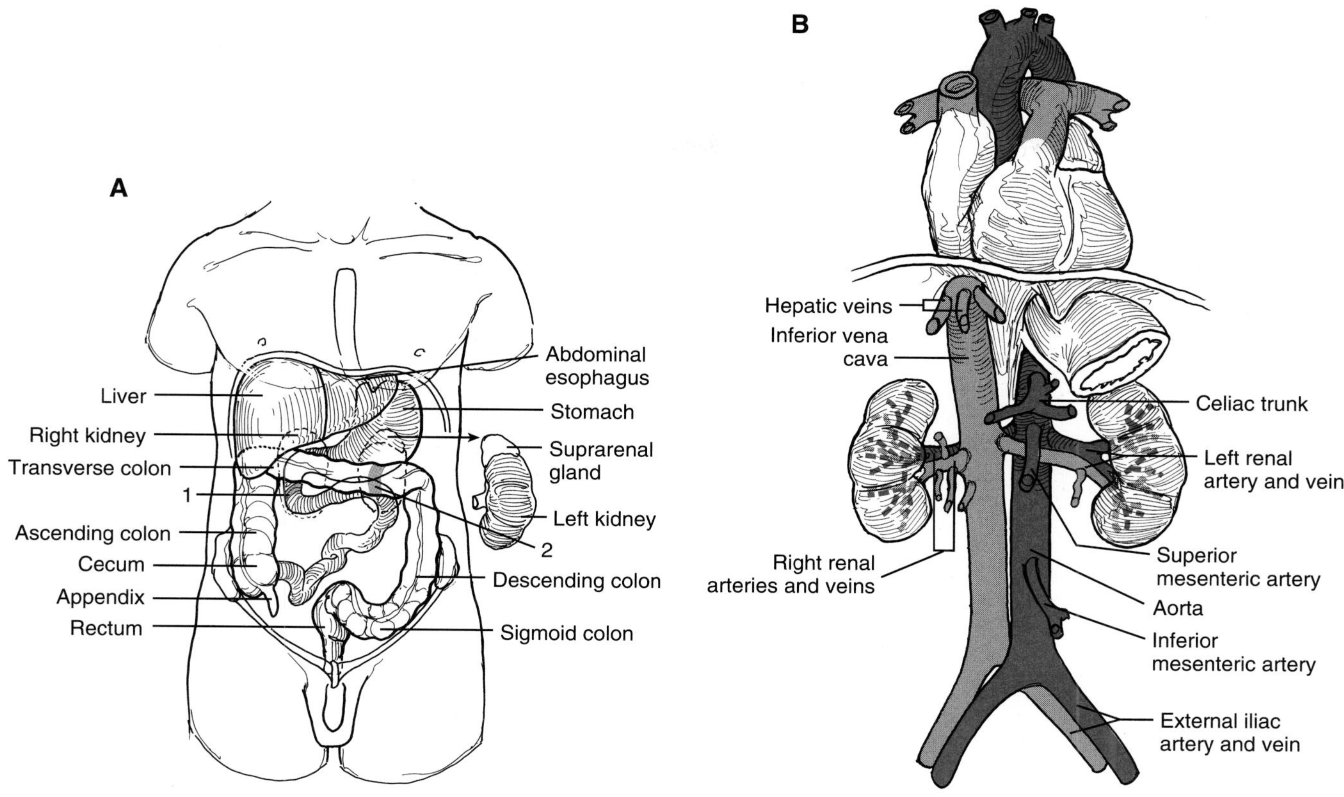

FIGURE 12–4
Organization of the abdominal gastrointestinal tract on the basis of vasculature. **A.** The abdominal part of the gastrointestinal tract is composed of the abdominal foregut (vascularized by branches of the celiac trunk), the midgut (vascularized by branches of the superior mesenteric artery), and the hindgut (vascularized by branches of the inferior mesenteric artery). *1,* Boundary between the foregut and midgut; *2,* boundary between the midgut and hindgut. **B.** The roots of the celiac, superior mesenteric, and inferior mesenteric arteries branch from the ventral surface of the abdominal aorta.

hindgut (Fig. 12–4*B*). These vessels and their branches are described in detail below.

In its definitive state, the **abdominal foregut** courses from a small superior section of the **abdominal esophagus** to the **stomach** and **superior part of the duodenum** (Figs. 12–4*A* and 12–5). The **midgut** includes the **inferior part of the duodenum,** the **jejunum** and **ileum,** the **ascending colon,** and the **proximal two thirds of the transverse colon** (Fig. 12–4*A* and see Fig. 12–15). The **hindgut** consists of the **distal one-third of the transverse colon, descending colon, sigmoid colon,** and **rectum** (Fig. 12–4*A* and see Fig. 12–19). Gastrointestinal segments characterizing each region are listed in Table 12–1.

ANATOMY OF THE ABDOMINAL FOREGUT

The foregut includes the pharynx, thoracic esophagus, abdominal esophagus, stomach, about half of the duodenum, and several accessory gastrointestinal glands

The most superior part of the foregut includes the pharynx and the thoracic segment of the esophagus. Parts of the **pharyngeal foregut (pharynx)** are located within the head, cervical region, and upper part of the thoracic region. The superior limit of the pharynx is the **oral isthmus,** between the **palatoglossal folds,** and its inferior limit is its junction with the **thoracic esophagus** (see Fig. 12–5*A* and Chapter 26). The **abdominal foregut** consists of the abdominal esophagus, stomach, and approximately one-half of the duodenum (see Fig. 12–5*B*). It is associated with several accessory gastrointestinal glands. The abdominal foregut is vascularized entirely by branches of the celiac artery (see Figs. 12–4*B* and 12–22).

▲ Abdominal Esophagus

The abdominal esophagus is a short intraperitoneal extension of the thoracic esophagus

The retroperitoneal segment of the **thoracic esophagus** pierces the diaphragm via the **esophageal hiatus** at the level of vertebra T10 (see Fig. 12–5 and Chapter 13). The **vagal trunks** accompany the esophagus into the abdominal cavity through this hiatus (see Fig. 12–5*B*). Immediately after entering the abdominal cavity, the esophagus becomes suspended by mesentery and is an **intraperitoneal organ** (see Fig. 12–5).

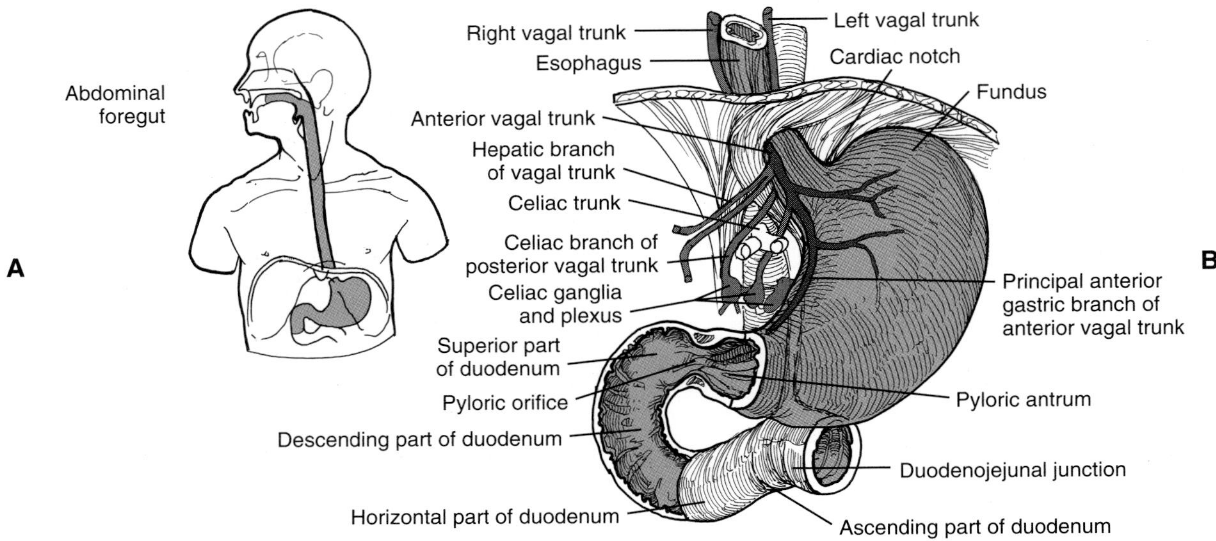

FIGURE 12–5

The foregut. **A.** The thoracic part of the foregut includes the pharynx and thoracic segment of the esophagus. **B.** The abdominal part of the foregut includes the abdominal segment of the esophagus, the stomach, and the superior half of the duodenum.

TABLE 12–1
Structures of the Foregut, Midgut, and Hindgut

Region of Gastrointestinal Tract	Arterial Vasculature	Definitive Organs
Foregut	Celiac trunk	Abdominal esophagus, stomach, superior half of duodenum
Midgut	Superior mesenteric artery	Inferior half of duodenum, jejunum, ileum, ascending colon with cecum and appendix, right two thirds of transverse colon
Hindgut	Inferior mesenteric artery	Left one third of transverse colon, descending colon, sigmoid colon, rectum

During development, this short section of suspended abdominal esophagus twists to allow the stomach to rotate on its longitudinal axis. The **left** and **right vagal trunks** originally associated with the lower part of the thoracic esophagus rotate to become the **posterior** and **anterior vagal trunks** of the abdominal esophagus and stomach (see Fig. 12–5*B* and Chapter 10).

Function of the Abdominal Esophagus

The abdominal esophagus delivers food to the stomach and prevents its reflux

Once a bolus of food is swallowed, it is transported along the entire length of the thoracic esophagus in 5 to 8 seconds (see Chapter 10). It is propelled by **peristalsis,** during which waves of esophageal contraction are followed by waves of relaxation. These coordinated peristaltic movements are regulated by parasympathetic vagal fibers and their accompanying afferent fibers. Activity of the sympathetic nervous system inhibits peristalsis of the thoracic esophagus.

Once the bolus of food has been delivered to the abdominal esophagus, it is temporarily prevented from entering the stomach. However, the presence of a structurally defined **gastroesophageal (inferior esophageal) sphincter** has not been demonstrated. Apparently, increased tonus of the cardiac orifice (see below) may regulate the entry of food into the stomach and also prevent regurgitation of gastric contents into the esophagus. This gastroesophageal "sphincter" is thought to be controlled by vagal reflex activity.

▲ Stomach

Development of the Stomach

The stomach (gaster) is a pouchlike expansion of the gastrointestinal tract

The definitive stomach is an expanded region of the foregut that is displaced to the left side of the superior abdominal cavity (Fig. 12–6). This results from differential expansion and rotation of the presumptive stomach. Between the fourth and sixth weeks of embry-

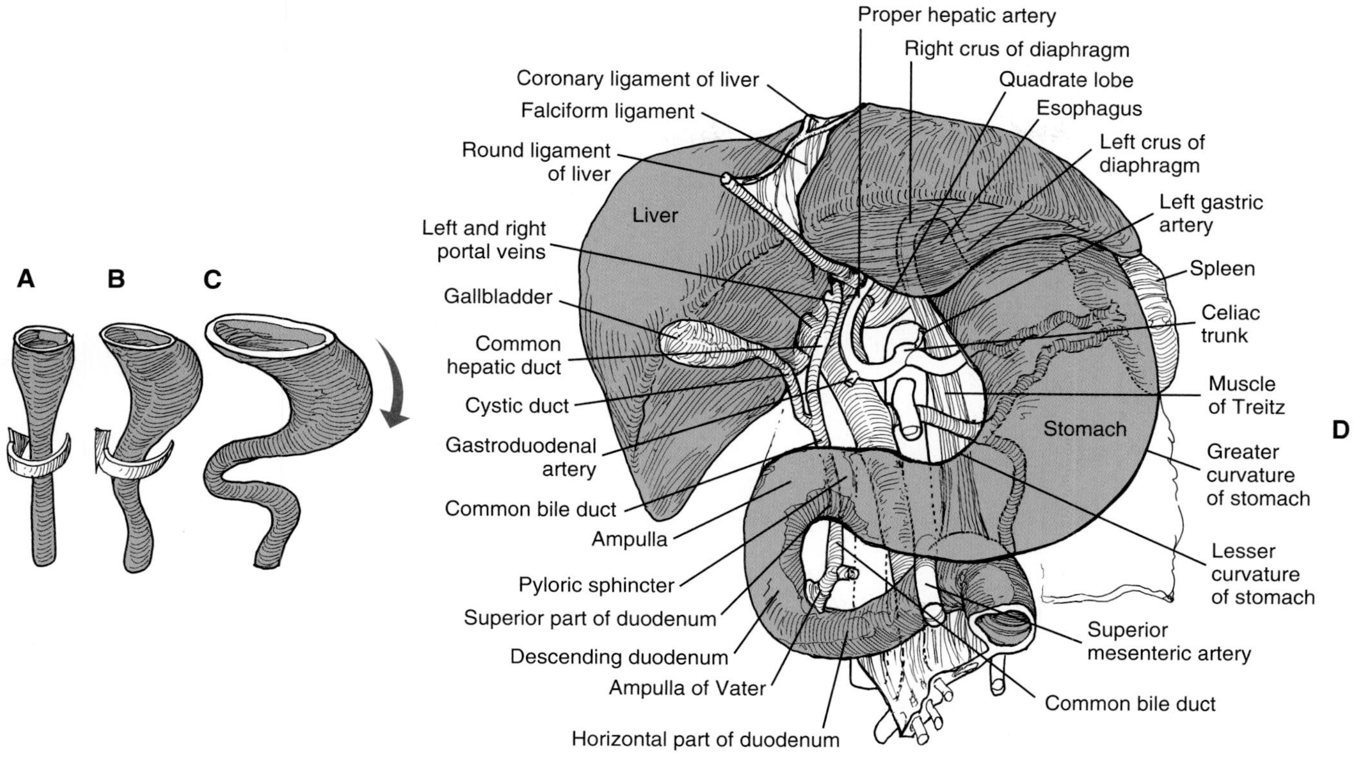

FIGURE 12–6
Expansion and rotation of the stomach between the fourth and sixth weeks of embryonic development. **A.** In the fourth week, the foregut in the region of the presumptive stomach begins to expand in its posterior region. **B.** During the fourth week, the presumptive stomach rotates clockwise along its longitudinal axis (when viewed from above). **C.** Continued clockwise rotation of the presumptive stomach displaces its posterior side to the left and its anterior side to the right. **D.** The former posterior side of the stomach becomes the greater curvature, and the former anterior side becomes the lesser curvature.

onic development, the gut tube in the region of the presumptive stomach expands, mostly at the posterior wall (Fig. 12–6). As this expansion occurs, the developing stomach and duodenum rotate 90 degrees clockwise along a longitudinal axis when viewed from above (Fig. 12–6*C* and *D*). This causes the posterior region of the stomach to turn leftward, and this convex region becomes the **greater curvature of the stomach** (Fig. 12–6*C* and *D*). The anterior wall of the gut tube becomes the right border of the stomach, which assumes a concave shape, and this is the **lesser curvature of the stomach** (Fig. 12–6*C*). The stomach then rotates again 90 degrees clockwise along a dorsoventral axis. This displaces the greater curvature in an inferior direction and the lesser curvature in a somewhat superior direction (Fig. 12–6*D*).

The constricted opening to the stomach from the abdominal esophagus is the **cardiac orifice** (Fig. 12–7*C*). The sharp angle formed by the esophagus and greater curvature of the left side of the stomach at the level of the cardiac orifice is the **cardiac notch (incisure).** The expanded part of the former posterior wall of the stomach that extends superiorly above a horizontal line drawn through the apex of the cardiac notch is the **fundus.** Most of the remainder of the stomach is the **body of the stomach,** and the narrowed inferior region is the **pyloric antrum.** The constricted opening at the lower end of the stomach that marks the boundary of the stomach with the superior part of the duodenum is the **pyloric orifice.** A superficial circular groove at the level of the pyloric orifice marks the location of the muscular **pylorus (pyloric sphincter)** within the stomach wall (Fig. 12–7*A* and *C*).

Stomach Wall

Tissues of the stomach wall are organized into discrete layers

In most areas of the stomach wall, the layers are organized in the same way as those in the rest of the gastrointestinal tract (see Fig. 12–7*B*). The outermost, **serosal layer** is made up of visceral peritoneum of the stomach (see Fig. 12–7*B*). Just deep to this is the **subserosal connective tissue,** which is loosely connected to the **external muscular layer (muscularis externa).** In the stomach, the muscularis externa has three layers of smooth muscle fibers, unlike in other regions of the gastrointestinal tract where there are only two layers (see

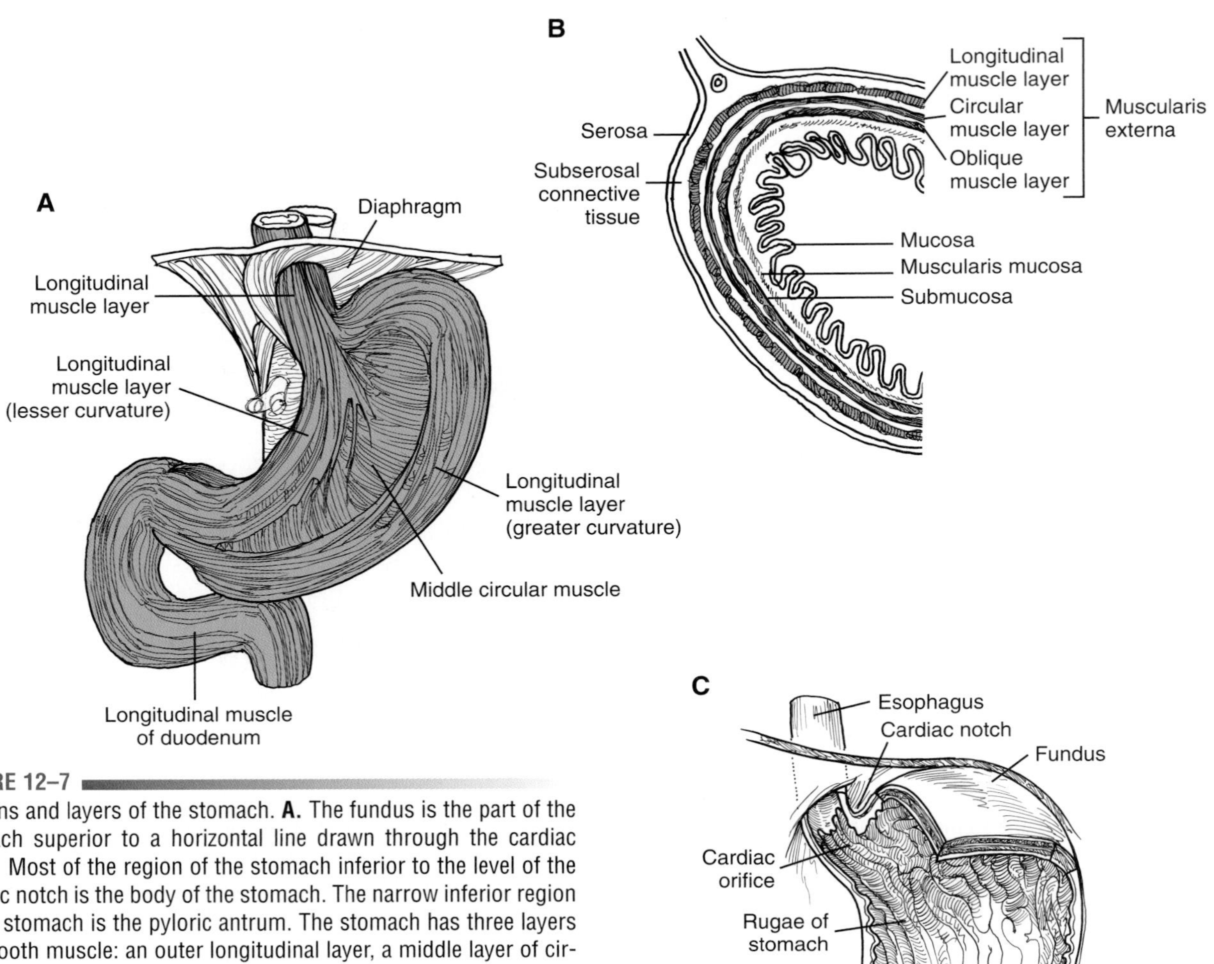

FIGURE 12–7
Regions and layers of the stomach. **A.** The fundus is the part of the stomach superior to a horizontal line drawn through the cardiac notch. Most of the region of the stomach inferior to the level of the cardiac notch is the body of the stomach. The narrow inferior region of the stomach is the pyloric antrum. The stomach has three layers of smooth muscle: an outer longitudinal layer, a middle layer of circular muscle, and a deep layer of oblique muscle fibers. These are collectively called the *muscularis externa.* **B.** A transverse section of the stomach reveals several layers of the stomach wall. From superficial to deep, they are an outer serosal layer, a deeper layer of subserosal connective tissue, the muscularis externa, a submucosal layer of loose connective tissue, and a deep layer of gastric mucosa. The gastric mucosa contains circular and longitudinal layers of smooth muscle, which are collectively called the *muscularis mucosa.* **C.** During contraction of the stomach, the mucosa is pushed into folds called *rugae.*

Fig. 12–7*A*). In the stomach, the most superficial layer of the muscularis externa is oriented along the longitudinal axis of the stomach. These **longitudinal muscle fibers** are present in two distinct regions of the stomach (see Fig. 12–7*A*). Both groups of fibers are continuous with the longitudinal muscle fibers of the esophagus and radiate into the stomach wall from the region of the cardiac orifice (see Fig. 12–7*A*). These bands of muscle split to form the longitudinal muscle bands of the lesser and greater curvatures. In both cases, these bands of fibers course rightward toward the pylorus, where they recombine (see Fig. 12–7*A*). Some of these fibers are continuous with longitudinal fibers of the duodenum, and others interdigitate with fibers of the pyloric sphincter. A uniform layer of **circular muscle fibers** is located just deep to the longitudinal muscle layer. The deepest layer of muscle fibers of the muscularis externa is comprised of **oblique muscle fibers** and is peculiar to the stomach wall (see Fig. 12–7*A* and *B*). These oblique fibers emanate from the region of the cardiac orifice, spread over the body of the stomach, and mesh with the circular muscle fibers in the region of the greater curvature.

A **submucosal layer** of loose connective tissue is located deep to the muscularis externa. Deep to the submucosa is the **gastric mucosa,** which lines the lumen of the stomach (see Fig. 12–7*B*). The gastric mucosa is a thick inner layer of the stomach made up of a columnar **mucous epithelium** interspersed with **digestive glands.**

The gastric mucosa also contains an inner circular layer and an outer longitudinal layer of smooth muscle **(muscularis mucosa)** (see Fig. 12–7*B*). When the stomach contracts during **peristaltic activity** (see below), the relatively thick uniform layer of mucous epithelium becomes organized into irregular folds called **rugae** (see Fig. 12–7*C*).

Function of the Stomach

The stomach converts the food bolus into chyme and propels it into the duodenum

Before a person has swallowed a single bite of food, vagal impulses may be initiated by the smell or taste of food or even the sight or thought of food. These **vagal impulses** stimulate the release of hydrochloric acid, pepsinogen (an inactive precursor of pepsin), and mucin (a protective gastric mucus) into the stomach lumen. The release of pepsinogen may also be mediated by the action of **gastrin,** which is a **gastric hormone** that is released from G cells of the pyloric antrum in response to vagal impulses. Gastrin circulates through the blood stream to pepsinogen-producing cells, which are the parietal cells of the body and fundus of the stomach. The secreted fluid containing pepsinogen, hydrochloric acid, and mucin is called **gastric juice.** Gastric juice is present in the stomach just prior to the delivery of food to its lumen. In addition to gastrin, the stomach also secretes a substance called **somatostatin,** which inhibits gastrin secretion. Many other hormones are secreted by segments of the intestinal tract (see below).

Upon its release into the gastric lumen, pepsinogen is converted into a mixture of activated proteases. The hydrochloric acid lowers the pH to a value conducive to protease activity, and the mucin protects the lining of the stomach from the corrosive action of the hydrochloric acid. The amount of gastric juice secreted in a single day is usually 2 to 3 L. A small amount of slightly alkaline fluid is secreted between meals. The largest amount of highly acidic gastric juice (pH 1) is secreted at the time when food is ingested.

The empty stomach is a contracted, collapsed muscular tube that passively expands as food enters its lumen. Upon entering the stomach, the food bolus lies in the region of the lesser curvature of the stomach. As additional food enters, food in the region of the lesser curvature is displaced toward the pyloric antrum, where it is mixed with gastric juice. The presence of food within the pyloric antrum results in the stretching of smooth muscles in its walls, stimulating **local reflex waves** of contraction that mix the food with gastric juice. This mixture of food and gastric juice is **chyme.** Small amounts of chyme are intermittently released into the duodenum by coordinated peristaltic contractions of the pyloric antrum and the **vagal-mediated relaxation** of the **pyloric sphincter.** Small mushy foods rich in carbohydrate may pass through the stomach quickly, whereas fatty foods that have been poorly chewed may remain in the stomach for several hours prior to their release into the duodenum.

As experience will testify, retrograde emptying of the stomach may occur on occasion. The protective **reflex of vomiting** is a function of some of the primary and accessory respiratory muscles (see Chapters 6 and 8). Infections such as gastroenteritis type A may result in nausea accompanied by sweating, secretion of salivary fluids, and slow respiratory movements. Following a particularly deep inspiration, the opening to the larynx closes. The inferior gastroesophageal sphincter (see above) and superior esophageal sphincter (see Chapter 24) open in coordination with the sudden contraction of abdominal muscles and the diaphragm, and the stomach contents are ejected out through the mouth. This **complex reflex of autonomic and somatic activity** is regulated by centers in the brain stem.

Mesenteries of the Stomach

The definitive stomach is an intraperitoneal organ that is suspended by a unique ventral mesentery and a dorsal mesentery

The definitive stomach is suspended from the posterior body wall by a **dorsal mesentery (dorsal mesogastrium),** as is much of the rest of the abdominal gastrointestinal tract. Unlike other regions of the gut tube, however, the stomach has another mesentery by which it is suspended from the ventral body wall (Fig. 12–8).

The **ventral mesentery** is formed by the thinning of the inferior region of the septum transversum. The reader may recall that the superior part of the septum transversum forms part of the diaphragm (see Chapters 7 and 10).

Soon after the formation of the ventral mesentery, a **hepatic diverticulum** sprouts from the anterior wall of the duodenum and grows into the ventral mesentery (Fig. 12–8*A* and *B*). The hepatic diverticulum penetrates between the two mesothelial membranes of the mesentery within the apposed layers of subserous fascia. As the liver expands, it separates the two peritoneal membranes. They come to invest the surfaces of the liver and provide the liver with its **visceral peritoneum** (Fig. 12–8*A* and *B*). Ultimately, the superior pole of the liver makes contact with the inferior surface of the developing diaphragm. At this point, the liver splits the membranes completely apart, and liver tissue comes into direct contact with diaphragmatic mesoderm, creating an oblong region at the upper surface of the liver called the **bare area of the liver** (Fig. 12–8*C*).

The bare area of the liver is entirely surrounded by a ring of peritoneum, which is reflected from the surface of the liver onto the inferior surface of the diaphragm (Figs 12–8*C* and 12–9). This reflected peritoneum surrounds the superior pole of the liver like a crown and is, therefore, called the **coronary ligament** (Fig. 12–9*A* and

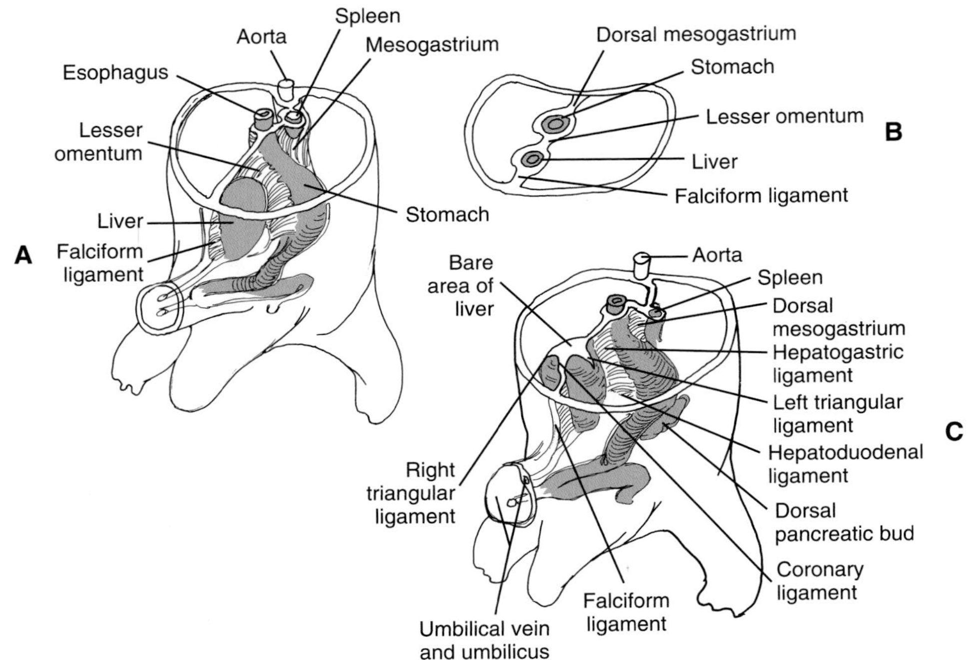

FIGURE 12–8

Ventral mesentery. **A.** The stomach is an intraperitoneal organ suspended by a dorsal mesentery and a ventral mesentery. The ventral mesentery is a specialization of the inferior part of the septum transversum. **B.** The liver grows into the ventral mesentery, splitting its two layers, which then invest the liver as its visceral peritoneum. **C.** As the liver continues to grow, it continues to split the ventral mesentery apart to make contact with the inferior surface of the diaphragm. This part of the liver is the bare area of the liver. The ventral mesentery remaining just anterior to the liver becomes the falciform ligament. The lower edge of the falciform ligament contains the former left umbilical vein, which in the definitive condition becomes a fibrous vestige called the *round ligament of the liver (ligamentum teres hepatis).* The ventral mesentery remaining between the liver and the stomach is the lesser omentum. The lesser omentum includes the hepatogastric and hepatoduodenal ligaments.

B). The far left and far right apices of the coronary ligament at the points where it sharply reverses its course, are the **left triangular** and **right triangular ligaments** (Figs. 12–8*C* and 12–9).

Even after the growth and expansion of the liver is complete, two regions of the ventral mesentery remain as mesenteric membranes. The membrane just anterior to the liver is the **falciform ligament,** and the membrane connecting the liver and stomach is the **lesser omentum** (Figs. 12–8*A* and 12–10). Both of these membranes are thin and fragile. Their lower free edges define the lower limit of the ventral mesentery and are landmarks for important anatomic structures. For example, the lower edge of the falciform ligament contains the former **left umbilical vein** (Fig. 12–10), which, in the definitive condition, becomes a fibrous vestige called the **round ligament of the liver (ligamentum teres hepatis).** This structure can be easily palpated in cadavers. Although the round ligament of the liver is not a functional structure, its significant mass is drained by both systemic and portal veins. These vessels provide continuity between the portal and systemic circulation and are a conduit for the portal-systemic shunting of blood that occurs when the portal system in the liver becomes blocked (see Fig. 12–29).

The lower free edge of the lesser omentum contains several functional vessels, ducts, and nerves. Because it connects the superior region of the duodenum with the liver, it is called the **hepatoduodenal ligament** (Fig. 12–10). The rest of the lesser omentum connects the liver with the lesser curvature of the stomach and is called the **hepatogastric ligament** (Fig. 12–10).

It must be stressed that these two ligaments of the lesser omentum, as well as other mesenteries that are referred to as ligaments, are not ligaments in the classic sense. Each of these "ligaments" is merely a distinct region of mesentery connecting the two structures for which it is named. Derivatives of the ventral mesentery are summarized in Box 12–1.

Additionally, the **hepatoduodenal ligament** is a landmark for several ducts, vessels, and nerves (Fig. 12–10). The course of the common bile duct and associated structures is somewhat complicated by the rotation of the stomach, duodenum, and ventral bud of the pancreas. For the most part, however, their locations are clearly defined by the hepatoduodenal lig-

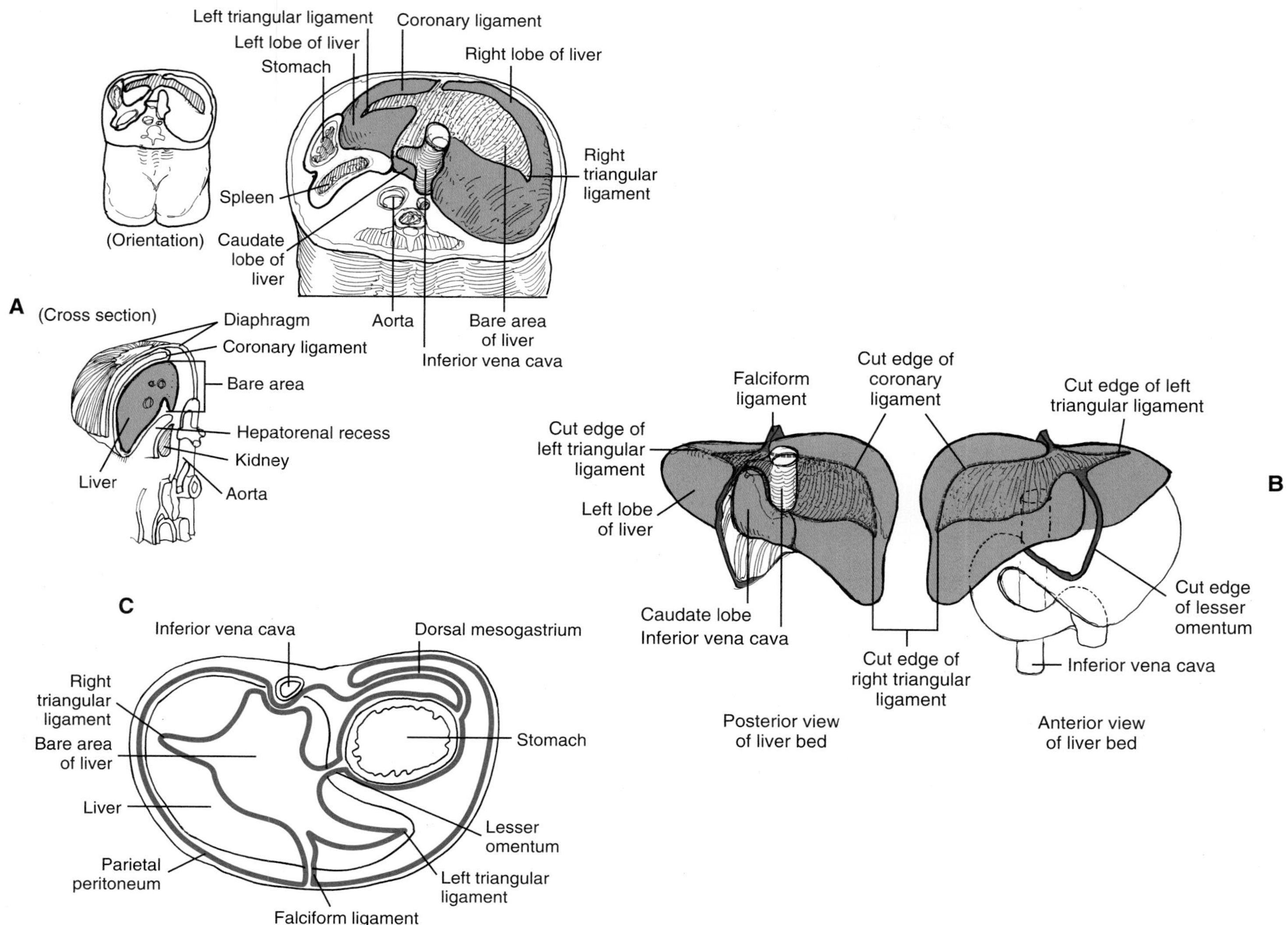

FIGURE 12–9
The bare area of the liver. **A.** The coronary ligament encircles the dome of the liver like a crown. Its sharp deviation on the right is the right triangular ligament, and its sharp deviation on the left is the left triangular ligament. The sagittal section in the inset shows the coronary ligament as a short reflection of visceral peritoneum of the liver onto the inferior surface of the diaphragm. **B.** The coronary ligament has been cut around its entire periphery to remove the liver (in the figure on the left) from the body cavity (in the figure on the right). The liver has then been flipped over to show its posterior surface. The shaded area in the figure on the left is the bare area, which is surrounded by the cut edge of the coronary ligament. The shaded area on the right is the region that the bare area of the liver apposed in the bed of the liver. **C.** This section of the trunk shows the continuity of the anterior parietal peritoneum; falciform, coronal, and hepatogastric ligaments; visceral peritoneum of the stomach; dorsal mesogastrium; and posterior parietal peritoneum.

ament at the lower free edge of the lesser omentum. The student can easily palpate the common bile duct within this ligament in a cadaver, as well as the cystic duct, common hepatic duct, hepatic artery and some of its branches, portal vein, lymphatic vessels, and vagal and sympathetic fibers (Box 12–2 and Fig. 12–10 and the discussion of the liver and porta hepatis below).

As the stomach undergoes two clockwise rotations, it remains suspended by its dorsal mesentery, which greatly expands, producing an extensive leftward-facing fold called the **greater omentum** (Fig. 12–11). After the first rotation is complete, this fold of dorsal mesentery becomes suspended from the former posterior wall of the stomach, which is now the greater curvature (Fig. 12–11*B* and *C*). After the second rotation of the stomach about its dorsoventral axis, the greater omentum faces somewhat inferiorly (Figs. 12–11*C* and 12–12*A, B,* and *D*). As in the case of the lesser omentum, certain subregions of the greater omentum are characterized as

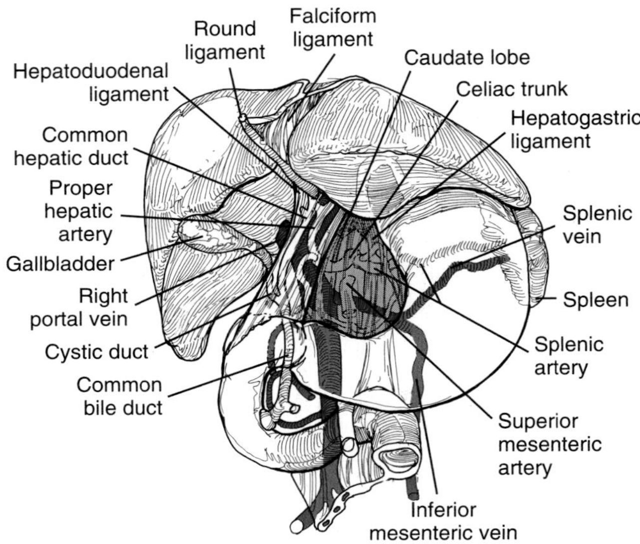

FIGURE 12–10
Contents of the hepatoduodenal ligament. The hepatoduodenal ligament (i.e., the lower free edge of the lesser omentum) contains the hepatic artery proper and its left and right branches, cystic artery, common hepatic duct, cystic duct, common bile duct, and right and left portal veins. Lymphatic vessels and hepatic lymph nodes that drain the liver are associated with the proper hepatic artery and common bile duct. These vessels tend to drain into celiac nodes associated with the aorta. The hepatoduodenal ligament also contains preganglionic parasympathetic fibers of the vagus nerve and postganglionic sympathetic fibers from the celiac ganglia (see below). Afferent fibers are associated with vagal and sympathetic nerves. All of these structures thus lie in a plane just anterior to the epiploic foramen of Winslow.

BOX 12–1

DEFINITIVE DERIVATIVES OF THE VENTRAL MESENTERY (INFERIOR PART OF SEPTUM TRANSVERSUM)

- Falciform ligament
- Visceral peritoneum of liver
- Coronary ligament
  - Left triangular ligament
  - Right triangular ligament
- Lesser omentum
  - Gastrohepatic ligament
  - Gastroduodenal ligament

mesenteric ligaments. The region between the stomach and the spleen is the **gastrosplenic ligament,** and the region connecting the spleen and the kidney is the **lienorenal (splenorenal) ligament** (Fig. 12–12C). The definitive greater omentum is primarily a storage depot for fat.

BOX 12–2

STRUCTURES WITHIN THE HEPATODUODENAL LIGAMENT

- Hepatic artery proper
  - Right hepatic artery
  - Cystic artery
  - Left hepatic artery
- Portal vein
  - Right portal vein
  - Left portal vein
- Common bile duct
  - Cystic duct
  - Common hepatic duct
  - Right hepatic duct
  - Left hepatic duct
- Descending lymphatic vessels
- Postganglionic sympathetic fibers from celiac ganglia
- Preganglionic parasympathetic vagal fibers
- Afferent fibers associated with parasympathetic and sympathetic nerves

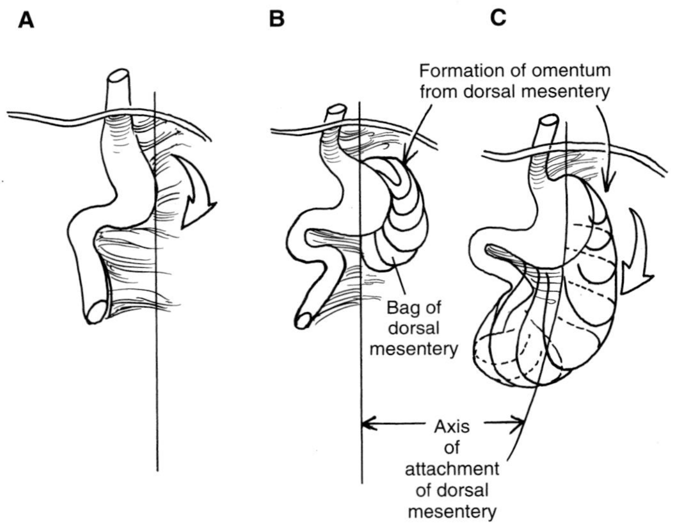

FIGURE 12–11
Formation of the greater omentum. The greater omentum is an outpouching of the dorsal mesogastrium (dorsal mesentery of the stomach).

▲ Greater and Lesser Sacs of the Peritoneal Cavity

The greater and lesser omenta, with the liver, stomach, and duodenum, segregate the greater and lesser sacs of the peritoneal cavity

When the C-shaped duodenum rotates slightly, between the fourth and sixth weeks of embryonic devel-

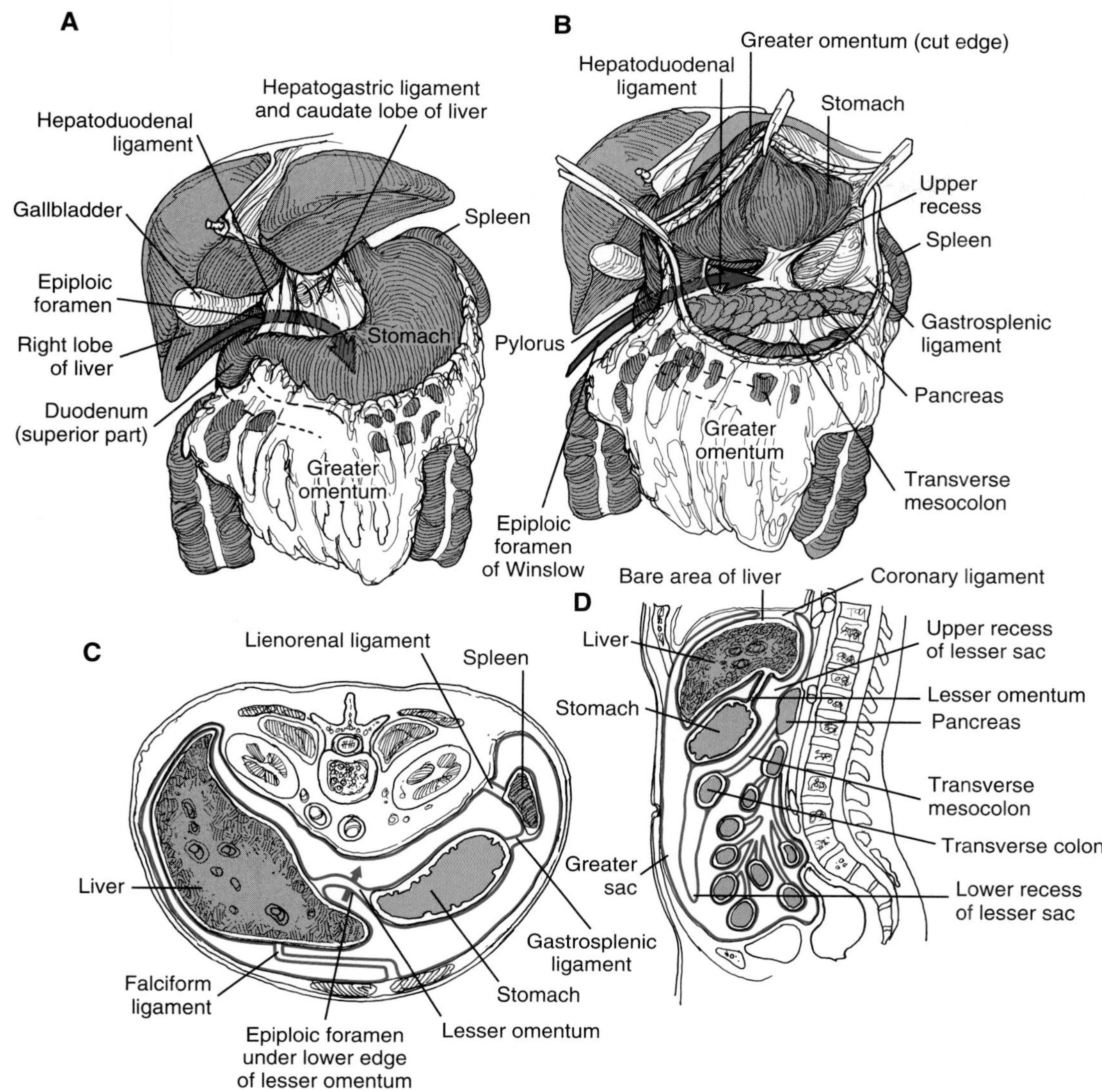

FIGURE 12–12

The definitive mesenteries of the stomach. **A.** The lesser omentum is a thin membrane connecting the stomach to the liver. Rotation of the stomach produces an enclosed space behind the stomach and lesser omentum (lesser sac of the peritoneal cavity), which communicates with the rest of the peritoneal cavity (greater sac of the peritoneal cavity) through the epiploic foramen of Winslow *(arrow).* The greater omentum is suspended from the former posterior wall of the stomach. **B.** The lesser sac of the peritoneal cavity may be entered by cutting the greater omentum from the greater curvature of the stomach (see also Fig. 12–12*D*). Elevation of the stomach then reveals the pancreas in the posterior wall of the lesser sac. **C.** Transverse section through the liver, stomach, spleen, and associated mesenteries. The region of dorsal mesentery between the stomach and spleen is the gastrosplenic ligament. The region of dorsal mesentery between the spleen and kidney is the lienorenal (splenorenal) ligament. **D.** Midsagittal section showing continuity between the upper recess of the lesser sac (behind the stomach) and the lower recess of the lesser sac (within the greater omentum).

opment, its former right surface becomes fixed to the posterior body wall just inferior to the stomach. The clockwise rotation of the stomach along the longitudinal axis (with respect to a superior view) displaces the liver to the right. The liver, however, remains suspended within its ventral mesentery (except in the region of the bare area) but is firmly pressed against the right superior posterior abdominal wall and diaphragm. This placement restricts communication between the more inferior and anterior regions of the abdominopelvic cavity and the space that has been created just posterior to the stomach by fixation of the duodenum to the posterior abdominal wall (see Fig. 12–12). This space is continuous with the cavity in the expanded dorsal mesogastrium or greater omentum **(omental bursa)** (see Fig. 12–12*D*). The entrapped space behind the stomach and within the greater omentum is the **lesser sac of the peritoneal cavity.** The remainder of the peritoneal cavity anterior and inferior to the stomach is the **greater sac of the peritoneal cavity** (see Fig. 12–12*D*). The most direct communication between these regions is a small passageway inferior and posterior to the lower free edge of the lesser omentum or hepatoduodenal ligament, which is called the **epiploic foramen of Winslow** (see Fig. 12–12*A* to *C*).

The lesser sac may be divided into two regions: the **upper (superior) recess** and **lower (inferior) recess.** The superior recess is the region of the lesser sac posterior to the lesser omentum and stomach, and the inferior recess is the cavity within the sac formed by the greater omentum (see Fig. 12–12*D*). However, the inferior recess is usually obliterated as the walls of the omental bursa fuse with each other during fetal development (see Fig. 12–3*A*).

Infection or Tumors within the Lesser and Greater Sacs. Although the lesser and greater sacs of the peritoneal cavity are, for the most part, segregated from each other, infectious organisms or tumor cells may enter the lesser sac from the greater sac via the right lateral paracolic gutter, hepatoduodenal recess, and epiploic foramen of Winslow (see Fig. 12–3*C*). This is especially true if the patient is in a supine position. The presence and entrapment of infection or cancer cells within the superior recess of the lesser sac may endanger vital organs of the thoracic cavity just on the other side of the diaphragm.

▲ Spleen

The spleen develops from a condensation of mesoderm within the greater omentum

Unlike the liver, gallbladder, and pancreas, the spleen has no endodermal components and arises independently of the gastrointestinal tract from mesoderm of the dorsal mesogastrium. Thus, in its definitive form, the spleen is a compact friable organ suspended within the dorsal mesentery of the stomach **(mesogastrium)** in the left hypochondriac region of the peritoneal cavity between the fundus of the stomach and diaphragm (Fig. 12–13*A*). It is directly connected to the stomach by the **gastrosplenic ligament** and to the posterior body wall and left kidney by the **lienorenal ligament** (Fig. 12–13*A*).

Although it is separated by peritoneal recesses from surrounding organs and structures, the convex posterolateral surface of the spleen lies against the diaphragm

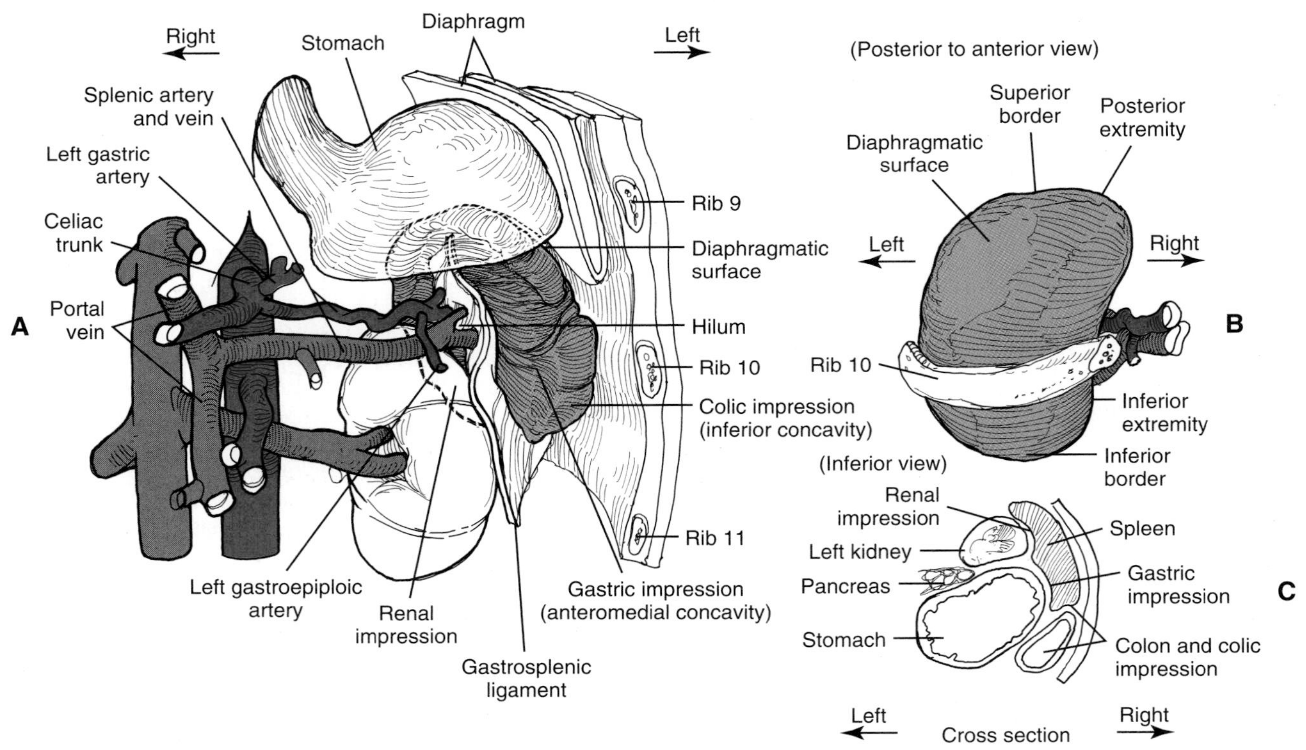

FIGURE 12–13
The spleen. **A.** The spleen is protected by the tenth rib under the dome of the diaphragm in the left superior region of the peritoneal cavity. The hilum on the medial side of the spleen is a site of entrance and egress of splenic arteries and veins. A gastric impression is located anterior to the hilum, and a renal impression is located just medial and posterior to the hilum. An inferior concavity is the colic impression. **B.** Posterior view of the spleen shows its relationship to the tenth rib and the diaphragm (diaphragmatic surface). **C.** Transverse section of the spleen shows its relationship to the kidney, stomach, and colon.

in the plane of rib 10 (Fig. 12–13*B* and *C*). The posteromedial concavity of the spleen is formed by the kidney **(renal impression)** (Fig. 12–13*C*), and the inferior concavity is formed by the left flexure of the transverse colon **(colic impression).** The anteromedial surface of the spleen is shaped by the stomach **(gastric impression)** (Fig. 12–13*C*). This impression contains a fissure, the **hilum of the spleen,** through which vessels and nerves enter and exit the spleen (Fig. 12–13*A*). The spleen also has **superior** and **inferior borders** and **anterior** and **posterior extremities** (Fig. 12–13*B*).

In adults, the spleen may weigh 100 to 300 g. Its size and weight vary according to the nutritional or health status of an individual (see below). The spleen lies so high within the dome of the diaphragm that it is well protected from traumatic injury, unless ribs 10 to 12 are fractured. In normal individuals, the spleen is not palpable. Occasionally, small nodules of splenic tissue called *accessory spleens* may be present nearby within the dorsal mesogastrium.

The spleen is an important organ of the reticuloendothelial system, which functions to filter and cleanse the blood and serve the immune system. It contains macrophages, which remove debris, dying blood cells, and bacteria from blood. It is also a site of hematopoiesis. It produces most blood cell types in the fetus and especially manufactures macrophages and lymphocytes in adults when it mounts an immune response. The spleen is a site of erythrocyte storage, and most of its weight is due to the blood that is present within it.

The functions of the spleen and its friability predispose it to serious injury following the fracture of surrounding ribs. However, surgical removal of the spleen may have little long-term effect on health. This suggests that functions of the spleen may be readily appropriated by other organs of the reticuloendothelial system such as lymph nodes and bone marrow. On the other hand, it has been documented that small accessory spleens may hypertrophy significantly following splenectomy.

▲ Duodenum

The duodenum is a short, superior, secondarily retroperitoneal segment of the small intestine

The most superior segment of the small intestine is the **duodenum,** which begins just to the right of the pyloric constriction (Fig. 12–14*A* and *B*). This short segment of the gastrointestinal tract assumes its definitive orientation during embryonic development. Like the stomach, it rotates 90 degrees along a longitudinal axis (when viewed from the front). The left side of the embryonic duodenum becomes the anterior surface of the definitive duodenum; the right side turns so that it faces in a posterior direction as the duodenum becomes secondarily fixed to the posterior body wall; the anterior surface is displaced to the right; and the posterior surface is displaced to the left (Fig. 12–14). Thus, as the duodenum rotates, it becomes a **secondarily retroperitoneal organ,** except for its most superior and inferior regions, which remain intraperitoneal (Fig. 12–14). The definitive C-shaped **duodenum** is about 10 inches in length.

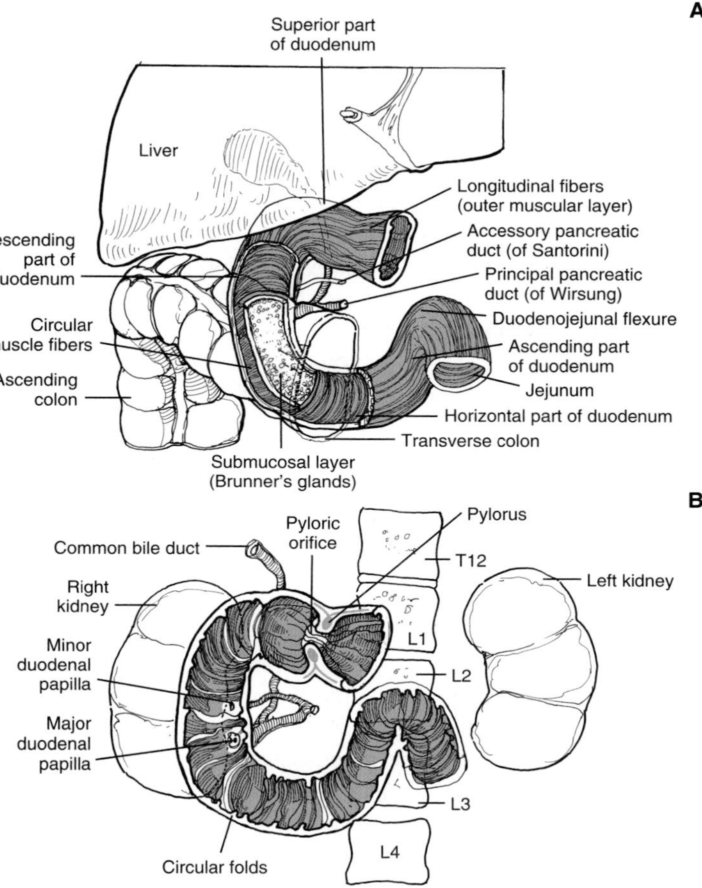

FIGURE 12–14

A. The duodenum consists of four parts: the superior, descending, horizontal, and ascending parts. The duodenum is invested by a serosal layer (visceral peritoneum) and a deeper subserosal layer of deep connective tissue. Deep to the subserosal layer is the muscularis externa, which is composed of uniform layers of longitudinal and circular muscle. **B.** Numerous duodenal glands of Brunner are embedded within a deeper submucosal layer containing longitudinal and circular smooth muscle of the muscularis mucosa. Finally, a mucosal layer is thrown into folds. The mucosal layer (including these folds) contains both circular and longitudinal layers of smooth muscle called the *muscularis mucosa.* The major pancreatic duct and common bile duct enter the duodenum at the major papilla. An accessory pancreatic duct may enter the duodenum at a minor papilla. The descending part of the duodenum overlies the right kidney. The duodenojejunal junction is located in the midline at the level of the second and third lumbar vertebrae.

As the duodenum rotates, it bends into the shape of a C in such a way that its superior end courses rightward from the pyloric sphincter. It then turns to course inferiorly as a descending segment. It turns again from right to left as a horizontal segment just under the stomach. Finally, the most inferior end of the duodenum turns superiorly just before it ends at the duodenojejunal junction. Thus, the definitive duodenum has four segments: the **superior (first), descending (second), horizontal (third),** and **short ascending (fourth) segments** (Fig. 12–14). The most superior expanded region of the **first part** of the duodenum **(ampulla)** is suspended by the gastroduodenal ligament and a short segment of dorsal mesentery and is, therefore, an intraperitoneal segment. The secondarily retroperitoneal **second part** is characterized by its connection to the **common bile duct** at an outpouching called the **ampulla of Vater** (Fig. 12–14*B* and see below). The **third part** is a secondarily retroperitoneal horizontal region (Fig. 12–14). The **fourth part** is an intraperitoneal segment, which is suspended by a short mesentery called the **suspensory muscle of the duodenum** or **muscle ("ligament") of Treitz** (Fig. 12–14 and see Fig. 12–6 and Chapter 13). This peritoneal "ligament" originates from the right crus of the diaphragm. It contains both striated and smooth muscle fibers. Contraction of its fibers in the region of the duodenojejunal junction may constrict the gastrointestinal tract at this point, creating a partial sphincter between the lower end of the duodenum and superior end of the jejunum.

Wall of the Duodenum

The wall of the duodenum contains the same fundamental series of layers that are present in the stomach (see below). A thin serosal layer (visceral peritoneum of the duodenum) is the most superficial layer. It directly overlies a thin subserosal layer of loose connective tissue. A uniform layer of longitudinal muscle and then a uniform layer of circular muscle lie just deep to the subserosal layer **(muscularis externa)** (Fig. 12–14*A*). Numerous **duodenal glands (of Brunner)** are embedded within the deeper submucosal layer. Their ducts pierce the longitudinal and circular layers of the **muscularis mucosa,** which lies just deep to the submucosa. The smooth muscle of the muscularis mucosa extends into circular mucosal folds that line the innermost surface of the duodenum (Fig. 12–14*B*).

Digestive Glands of the Duodenum

The **liver, gallbladder,** and **pancreas** and their **ducts** are sprouts of the presumptive duodenum. They all form between the fourth and seventh weeks of embryonic development.

The endodermal **liver bud (hepatic diverticulum)** sprouts from the presumptive duodenum and grows directly into the ventral mesentery, forming the **liver primordium** and its **hepatic ducts** (common hepatic duct and left and right hepatic ducts) and **bile canaliculi** (see Fig. 12–8*A* and *B*). The hepatic diverticulum forms the four lobes of the **liver:** the **right, left, quadrate,** and **caudate lobes** (Fig. 12–15). More detailed descriptions of the anatomy and function of the liver are also presented below in the discussion of the portal vasculature.

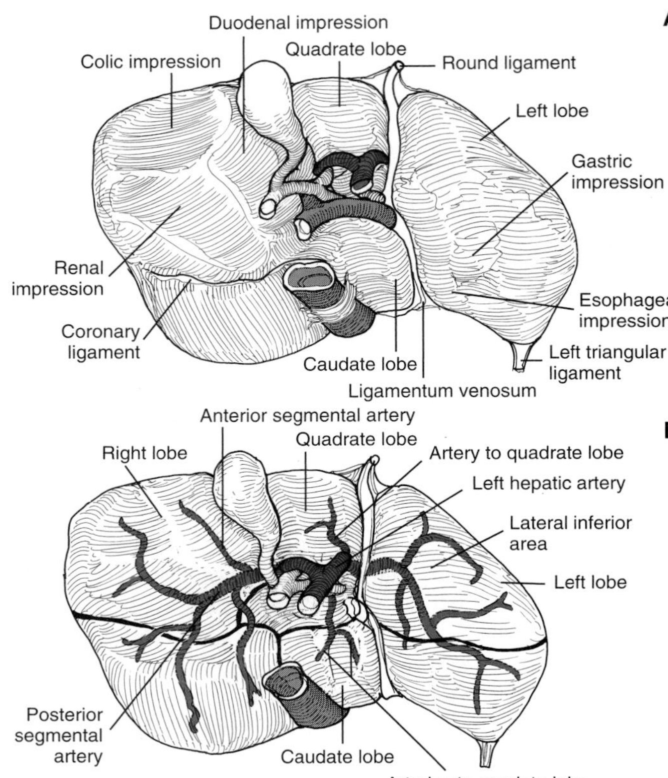

FIGURE 12–15
Lobes and porta hepatis of the liver. **A.** The porta hepatis is a transverse fissure in the inferior surface of the liver through which enter the left and right portal veins, left and right hepatic arteries, and left and right hepatic ducts. All of these elements (portal veins, hepatic arteries, and hepatic ducts) branch together within the substance of the liver to form bundles containing all three elements. These bundles are thus called *hepatic triads.* **B.** The distribution of branches of the right and left hepatic arteries is similar to that of the right and left branches of the portal vein and hepatic duct. The right branches serve the right lobe, and the left branches serve the left, quadrate, and caudate lobes.

All of the structures coursing within the hepatoduodenal ligament (see Fig. 12–10) enter the liver through a breach or fissure **(hilum)** of its inferior surface called the **porta hepatis** (Fig. 12–15). The right hepatic artery and right branch of the portal vein enter the right liver lobe, and the left hepatic artery and left branch of the portal vein provide branches to the left, quadrate, and caudate lobes (Fig. 12–15 and see Fig. 12–27). Likewise, the **right hepatic duct** is formed by the convergence of the bile canaliculi of the right hepatic lobe, and the **left hepatic duct** is formed by the convergence of the bile canaliculi from the left,

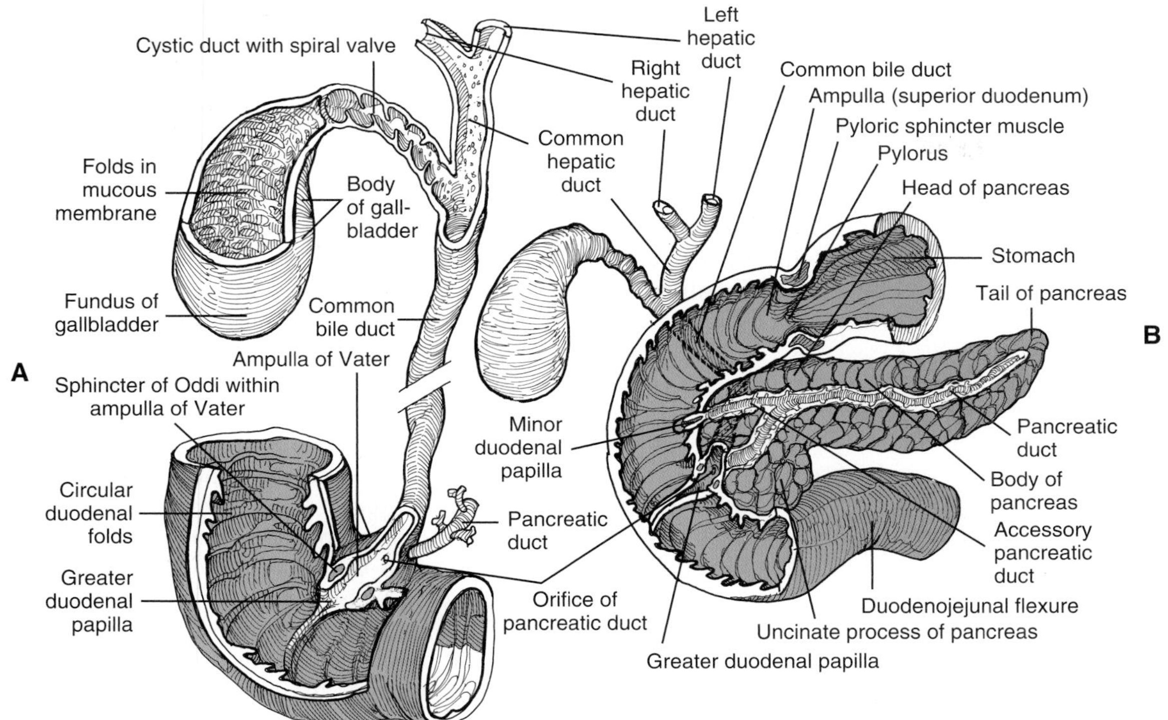

FIGURE 12–16
The gallbladder and pancreas and their ducts. **A.** The left hepatic duct drains bile from the left, quadrate, and caudate lobes of the liver, and the right hepatic duct drains the right lobe. The left and right hepatic ducts join to form the common hepatic duct, which joins with the cystic duct to form the common bile duct. Bile may circulate to the gallbladder for storage and concentration or to the common bile duct for delivery to the lumen of the duodenum through the major duodenal papilla (of Vater). The common bile duct is joined by the major pancreatic duct at the major duodenal papilla. Movement of bile into and out of the gallbladder is regulated by a spiral valve in the cystic duct. Emptying of bile into the duodenum through the major papilla is regulated by the smooth muscle sphincter of Oddi. **B.** The pancreas may also be drained by an accessory pancreatic duct through a minor duodenal papilla. The greater duodenal papilla marks the division between the foregut and midgut.

quadrate, and caudate hepatic lobes. **Descending lymphatic branches** from the interior of the liver exit the liver via the porta hepatis to drain into the hepatic lymph nodes. Postganglionic branches of the **sympathetic nerves** arising from celiac ganglia and preganglionic branches of **parasympathetic vagal branches** (see below) follow the course of the blood vessels and ducts into the liver (see below). Structures of the gastroduodenal ligament are summarized in Box 12–2.

The **cystic diverticulum** sprouts from the presumptive duodenum just inferior to the liver bud, grows into the ventral mesentery, and forms the **gallbladder** and its **cystic duct.** As cells proliferate near the roots of the hepatic and cystic ducts, the **common bile duct** forms, elongates, and ultimately carries the root of the cystic duct about 8 mm distally to its definitive junction with the **common hepatic duct** (Fig. 12–16).

The proximal end of the common bile duct, at its attachment to the duodenum, is demarcated by an expansion called the **ampulla of Vater (greater duodenal papilla)** (Fig. 12–16). It is sometimes called the **hepatopancreatic papilla** because the main duct of the pancreas usually joins the common bile duct just distal to it. The walls of the greater duodenal papilla contain a muscle called the **sphincter of Oddi,** which regulates the secretion of bile and pancreatic enzymes into the duodenum (Fig. 12–16*A*).

The **pancreas** arises from two separate evaginations of the duodenum. One develops just inferior to the cystic bud **(ventral pancreatic bud),** and the other develops from the opposite side of the duodenum **(dorsal pancreatic bud).** The duct of the ventral pancreatic bud becomes connected to the root of the developing common bile duct (Fig. 12–16*B*). As the stomach and duodenum rotate, the ventral pancreatic bud (along with the root of the common bile duct) rotates clockwise along a longitudinal axis (as viewed from above), moves posteriorly around the duodenum, and joins with the dorsal pancreatic bud. The dorsal bud forms the **head, body,** and **tail of the pancreas,** while the ventral bud gives rise to the hook-shaped **uncinate process** (Fig. 12–16*B*). The duct systems of the dorsal and ventral pancreatic buds fuse, and the original direct connection between the dorsal bud duct system and duodenum usually disappears. Secretions of the dorsal bud (i.e., the head, body, and tail of the pancreas) then drain into the ventral bud duct system and, finally, into the common bile duct at the ampulla of Vater and duodenum. Thus, the duct of the ventral bud becomes the **main pancreatic duct.** In some cases, the duct of the dorsal bud does not disappear and becomes the **accessory pancreatic duct.** This duct drains into a small expansion called the **minor duodenal papilla** (Fig. 12–16*B*).

Function of the Duodenum and Associated Digestive Glands

The duodenum further processes chyme via actions of pancreatic enzymes and bile

The liver produces 600 to 800 ml of **bile** each day. It drains into the bile canaliculi, left and right bile ducts, and common hepatic duct. It may then flow into the duodenum via the common bile duct. However, because the common bile duct is constricted at the **sphincter of Oddi,** much of the bile is diverted from the hepatic duct into the cystic duct and then into the gallbladder where it is concentrated and stored during periods when digestion is not occurring. When food is ingested and initially processed by the stomach, the interaction of chyme with the mucosal lining of the duodenum causes the mucosa to produce and secrete the hormone **cholecystokinin.** This hormone circulates through the blood stream, stimulating **contractions of the smooth muscle layers of the gallbladder** and **cystic duct** and causing the **spiral valve** to dilate. Concentrated bile is thus forced back through the cystic duct and into the common bile duct. In addition, the increased pressure within the gallbladder results in relaxation of the sphincter of Oddi, which is mediated by **vagal reflex activity.** This allows concentrated bile to be released into the duodenal lumen.

The actions of cholecystokinin and the **vagus nerve** also stimulate the secretion of **pancreatic juice** and its release into the duodenal lumen through the main and accessory pancreatic ducts. The pancreatic juice contains enzymes that split carbohydrates (α-amylase), proteins (trypsin, chymotrypsin, and carboxypeptidases), and fats (lipases, phospholipases, and esterases). The pancreas also secretes bicarbonate, which increases the pH of contents of the duodenal lumen to 7 or 8. This pH is more favorable for the actions of these enzymes. Approximately 2 L of pancreatic juice are secreted each day.

The presence of chyme within the duodenal lumen results in secretion of several other hormones, including **somatostatin,** which inhibits the secretion of **gastrin.** The duodenum also secretes the hormone **secretin,** which inhibits the secretion of hydrochloric acid by the stomach. This function is aided by secretion of another hormone called **gastric inhibitory peptide.** Secretion of the hormone **vasoactive peptide** stimulates an increase in intestinal blood flow, while secretion of the hormone **motilin** stimulates increased contractile activity by the stomach and intestines.

ANATOMY OF THE MIDGUT

The midgut contains the inferior half of the duodenum, jejunum and ileum, ascending colon, and about two-thirds of the transverse colon

The **greater papilla** marks the boundary between the foregut and the midgut (see Fig. 12–16). As has been discussed above, the liver, gallbladder, and pancreas produce or process secretions that are expressed into the duodenum at the point where their ducts converge with the **common bile duct,** about halfway down the definitive left border of the descending duodenum (see Fig. 12–16). This connection of the common bile duct to the duodenum at the major papilla roughly marks the boundary between the foregut and the midgut because it occurs approximately at the interface of the vascular fields of the celiac and superior mesenteric arteries that serve these two sections of the gastrointestinal tract (Fig. 12–17).

Thus, the definitive midgut is composed of the segment of gastrointestinal tract from the ampulla of Vater to a point just medial to the left colic flexure. Its entire territory is vascularized by branches of the **superior mesenteric artery** (Fig. 12–17 and see Figs. 12–4*B* and 12–23).

Development of the Midgut

Two rotations of the embryonic midgut produce the definitive jejunum, ileum, and large intestine

During embryonic development, the midgut grows more rapidly than the abdominal cavity. This causes the elongating **primary intestinal loop** to herniate anteriorly through the umbilical ring. As it herniates, it rotates 90 degrees counterclockwise about a dorsoventral axis (as viewed from the front). Several weeks later, it is retracted, and during this process, it rotates another 180 degrees counterclockwise. Consequently, the developing cecum becomes fixed to the right posterior abdominal wall just inferior to the liver and then descends to the lower lumbar region on the right side. A segment of the large intestine between the cecum and the hepatic flexure becomes secondarily fixed as the ascending colon (see Fig. 12–20). Secondary fixation of part of the hindgut on the left side of the posterior abdominal wall produces the descending colon (see discussion of the hindgut, below). Of the midgut segments involved in the rotation of the primary intestinal loop, the jejunum, ileum, and superior (right) two thirds of the transverse

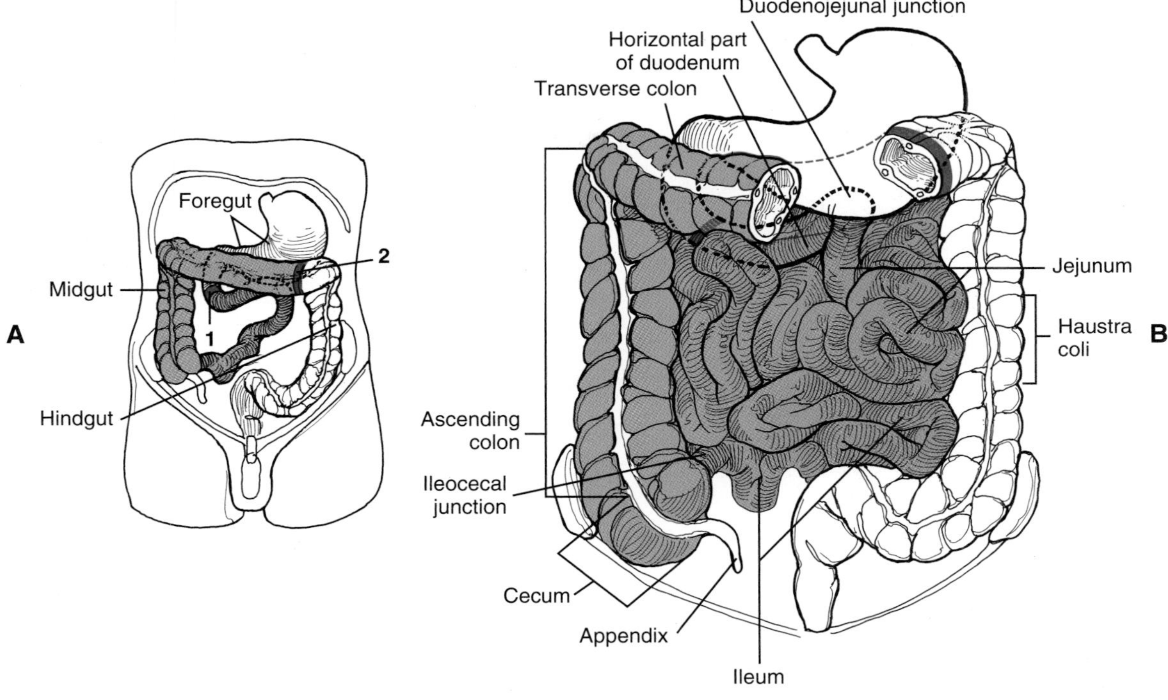

FIGURE 12–17
The midgut. The midgut begins about halfway along the duodenum in the region of the major papilla and ends at the boundary between the middle and left lateral thirds of the transverse colon. Therefore, the midgut includes the inferior half of the duodenum, jejunum, ileum, ascending colon, and right and middle thirds of the transverse colon. *1,* Boundary between the foregut and midgut; *2,* boundary between the midgut and hindgut.

colon remain suspended by mesentery and are intraperitoneal organs (Fig. 12–18*A* and see Fig. 12–19*C*).

▲ Jejunum and Ileum

The 20-foot length of the definitive jejunum and ileum is folded along a line of mesentery running from the terminus of the duodenum (duodenojejunal flexure) to the ileocecal junction

The jejunum and ileum are intraperitoneal organs that extend from the **duodenojejunal flexure** to the **ileocecal junction.** The combined jejunal and ileal segments are about 20 feet in length. They are suspended by a fan-shaped mesentery that allows relatively free movement of all regions (see Fig. 12–18*A*).

The mesentery also prevents these segments from twisting about themselves (volvulus). Such twisting results in intestinal obstruction or compromise of intestinal vasculature.

In the laboratory, the student should confirm this relationship between the intraperitoneal segment of the small intestine and its mesenteric attachment to the posterior body wall. This can be done by grasping the upper part of the jejunum with the fingertips of both hands and then alternately sliding them along the intestine toward the ileocecal junction.

This technique may be used by the surgeon to examine the mesentery for tumors such as metastatic tumors of ovarian carcinoma.

At the ileocecal junction, the **ileocecal orifice** is constricted by an **ileocecal valve** (see Fig. 12–18*B* and *C*). This valve may be shaped like a papilla with radial folds or like a mouth with upper and lower lips (see Fig. 12–18*B* and *C*). The valve is covered with mucous membrane and contains both circular and longitudinal muscle fibers, which allow it to close (see Fig. 12–18).

Boundary between the Jejunum and the Ileum

The inferior end of the jejunum and superior end of the ileum are not demarcated by a definitive boundary

There is no anatomic feature that clearly defines the border between the jejunum and the ileum. The conventional distinction is that the **jejunum** is the upper two fifths of the jejunoileal segment and the **ileum** is the lower three fifths. However, the superior part of the jejunum has several features that distinguish it from the

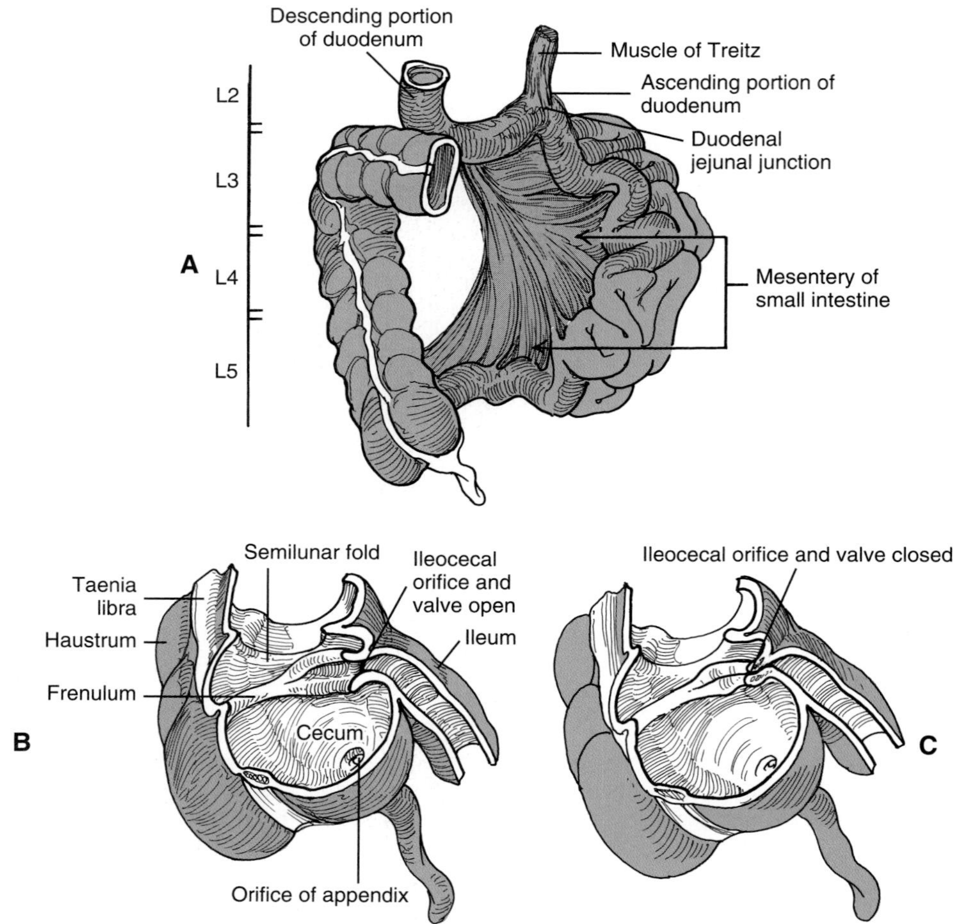

FIGURE 12–18

A. The jejunum and ileum, together, are about 20 feet long. They are suspended by a dorsal mesentery. The superior end of the jejunum begins at the terminus of the ascending part of the duodenum. The ileum terminates at the ileocecal junction. **B** and **C.** The passage of chyme from the ileum to the cecum is regulated by an ileocecal valve.

most inferior regions of the ileum, but these differences occur only gradually along the course of the small intestine.

Distinguishing Characteristics of the Jejunal and Ileal Walls

The upper part of the jejunum and lower part of the ileum are distinctively different

Most areas of the walls of the small intestine, including the walls of the jejunum and ileum, have an outer serosal layer, a muscularis externa consisting of uniform layers of longitudinal and circular muscle fibers, a deeper layer of submucosal connective tissue, and a mucosal layer lining the lumen. The mucosal layer contains columnar epithelial cells interspersed with simple tubular **intestinal glands (crypts).** As in other regions of the gastrointestinal tract, the mucosa has an inner layer of circular muscle and outer layer of longitudinal smooth muscle **(muscularis mucosa).**

The diameter of the superior part of the jejunum is slightly more than 1.5 inches, and the diameter of the ileum is slightly less than 1.5 inches. This difference may be attributed, in part, to the presence of numerous large **mucosal folds (plicae circulares)** in the upper part of the jejunum (Fig. 12–19*A*). The mucosal folds of the lower part of the ileum are small and infrequent or may be absent altogether (Fig. 12–19*B*). The upper part of the jejunum contains **solitary lymphatic follicles** but does not have the **aggregated lymphatic follicles** called **Peyer's patches** that are present in the lower part of the jejunum and the ileum (Fig. 12–19). In the lower part of the jejunum, Peyer's patches are only about 1 inch in diameter and round, whereas in the lower part of the ileum they are up to 4 inches in diameter and ovoid (Fig. 12–19*B*). In all regions where they are present, the aggregated lymphatic follicles are most numerous within the wall of the intestine opposite its attachment by the mesentery.

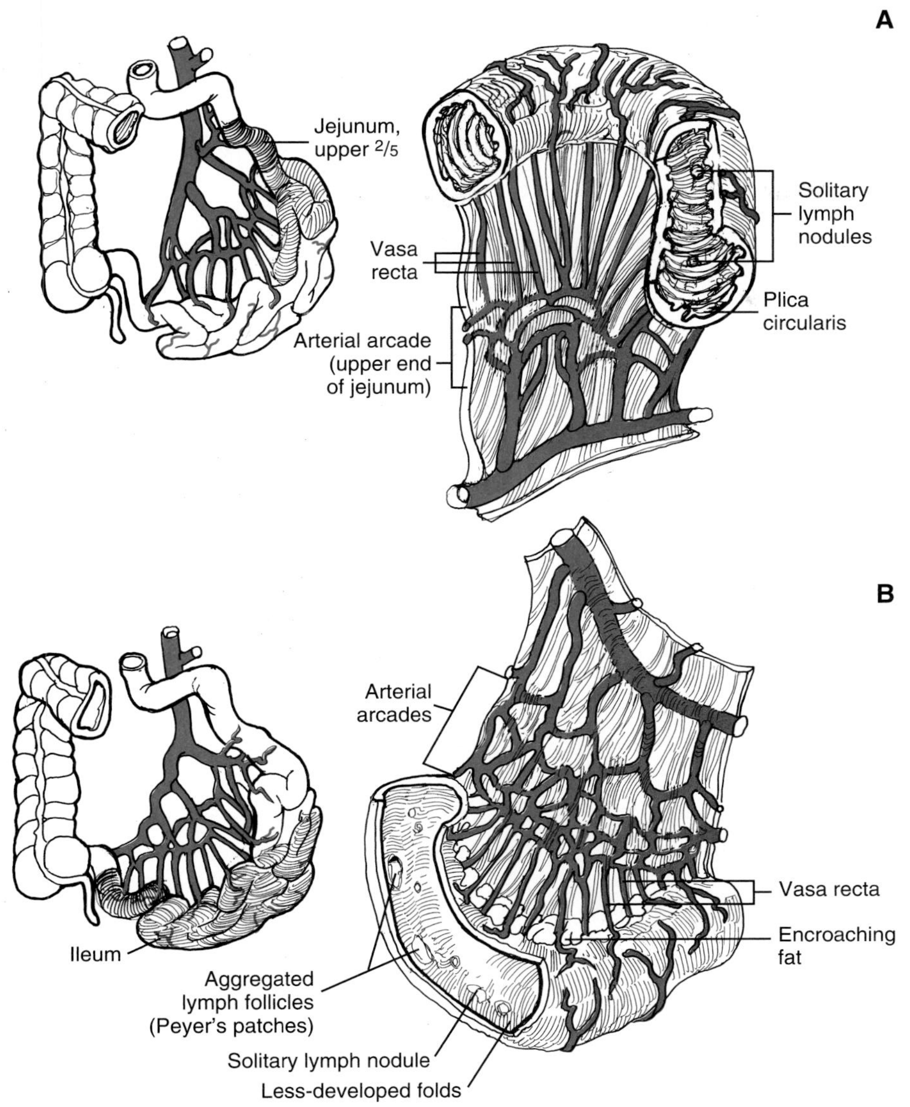

FIGURE 12–19

Comparing anatomic features of the jejunum and ileum. The jejunum **(A)** is slightly larger than the ileum, **(B),** in part because of the presence of mucosal folds (plicae circulares), which are absent in the lower end of the ileum. The lower end of the ileum contains large aggregated lymphatic follicles in its antimesenteric wall (Peyer's patches), which are absent from the jejunum. The mesentery of the jejunum is distinguished by relatively simple arterial arcades and long vasa recta, while the lower end of the ileum has more complex arterial arcades, short vasa recta, and encroaching fat adjacent to the intestine.

Distinguishing Characteristics of the Jejunal and Ileal Mesenteries

Branches of the **superior mesenteric artery** supply the midgut. These branches course within suspensory mesenteries of the small intestine (as do veins draining intraperitoneal segments of the gastrointestinal tract). At the base of the mesentery, **jejunal** and **ileal branches** of the superior mesenteric artery form a series of arches **(arterial arcades)** (Fig. 12–9). Long straight arteries called **vasa recta** emanate from the arcades to vascularize the intestinal wall usually in such a way that alternate vasa recta vascularize opposite sides of the wall (Fig. 12–9). Although the arterial vasculature is much more extensive in the upper part of the jejunum (imparting a pinkish cast in living individuals), the arterial arcades are usually more complex and the vasa recta shorter in the lower part of the ileum (Fig. 12–19).

One additional difference between the jejunum and ileum is the amount of fat deposited within the mesentery adjacent to the intestine (Fig. 12–19). This **encroaching fat** is more extensive in inferior regions of the ileum than in superior regions of the jejunum.

Table 12–2 summarizes the differences between the upper jejunum and the lower ileum.

Function of the Jejunum and the Ileum

Absorption of nutrients occurs in the small intestine

Most of the amino acids, polypeptides, oligosaccharides, and fatty acids produced by the actions of pepsin and hydrochloric acid in the stomach and by the actions of bile and pancreatic juice in the duodenum are absorbed by the mucosal lining of the duodenum, jejunum, and ileum as the substances are mixed together and propelled along these segments. Most of the 10 L of water that enter the duodenum each day (either

TABLE 12–2
Comparison of Anatomic Characteristics of Jejunum and Ileum

Anatomic Characteristic	Upper Part of Jejunum	Lower Part of Ileum
Diameter	1.6 inches	1.4 inches
Walls	Thicker	Thinner
Plicae circulares	Larger, more numerous	Smaller, infrequent
Peyer's patches	Few, small, round	Many, large, ovoid
Arterial supply	Greater	Lesser
Arterial arcades	Fewer, less extensive	Many, more extensive
Vasa recta	Longer, less numerous	Shorter, more numerous
Encroaching fat	Absent or infrequent	Extensive

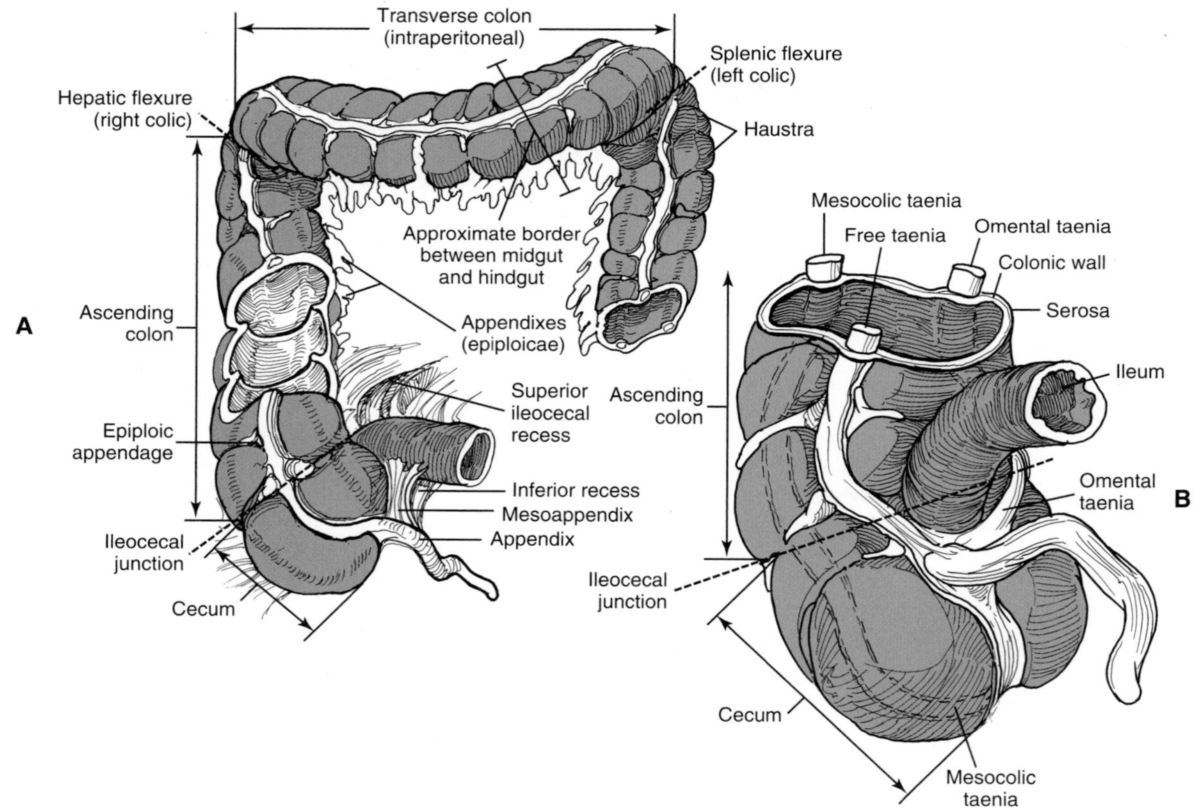

FIGURE 12–20
Ascending colon, cecum, appendix, and transverse colon. **A.** The ascending colon is a 10- to 15-inch segment, which is fixed to the right posterior abdominal wall just inferior to the liver. Its superior boundary with the transverse colon is at a sharp bend called the *hepatic (right colic) flexure.* Its inferior boundary is the ileocecal junction. The cecum is an expanded pouch at the inferior end of the ascending colon. The appendix is a lymphoid appendage of the cecum. The ascending colon is secondarily retroperitoneal and the appendix and cecum are intraperitoneal. The longitudinal muscle of the colon is segregated into three bands called *taeniae coli.* ***B.*** The taeniae coli converge at the apex of the root of the appendix.

through direct ingestion or through secretion of gastric and intestinal fluids) is also absorbed in the upper part of the small intestine.

The absorption and propulsion of chyme within the small intestine are facilitated by several distinct movements and mechanisms. **Reflexive myogenic feedback mechanisms** initiated by the presence of chyme within the small intestine result in **pendular** or **sleevelike movements** of longitudinal muscles of the intestines around the enclosed bolus of chyme. In addition, **intrinsic reflexive neurogenic feedback mechanisms** regulate the **rhythmic segmental contractions** of the circular muscle that result in further mixing of chyme. **Intrinsic neurogenic mechanisms** also regulate **peristaltic movements** of circular muscle that propel chyme along the length of the small intestine. Finally, **vagal reflexes** regulate **pistonlike movements of the intestinal villi** that facilitate the mixing of chyme at the inner surface of the intestinal lumen. It usually takes 4 to 8 hours for chyme to traverse the entire length of the small intestine.

▲ Ascending Colon, Cecum, and Appendix

The midgut continues as the ascending colon of the large intestine

The rotations of the primary intestinal loop of the midgut result in fixation of the presumptive **ascending colon** onto the right posterior peritoneal wall, just inferior to the liver (Fig. 12–20*A* and see Fig. 12–17). This segment is 10 to 15 inches in length. It begins at the ileocecal junction, where it courses from the upper sacral to upper lumbar levels just inferior to the liver. At this point, the colon bends sharply to the left at the **right colic (hepatic) flexure** and becomes the **transverse colon** (Fig. 12–20*A* and see Fig. 12–17).

Most of the ascending colon is a secondarily retroperitoneal organ. However, the **cecum** is suspended by a short mesentery, as is the **vermiform** (worm-shaped) **appendix,** which extends from the cecum's inferior apex (Fig. 12–20*A*). Both of these structures are classified as intraperitoneal structures of the midgut. The appendix is not often immediately apparent in a patient or a cadaver. In two thirds of individu-

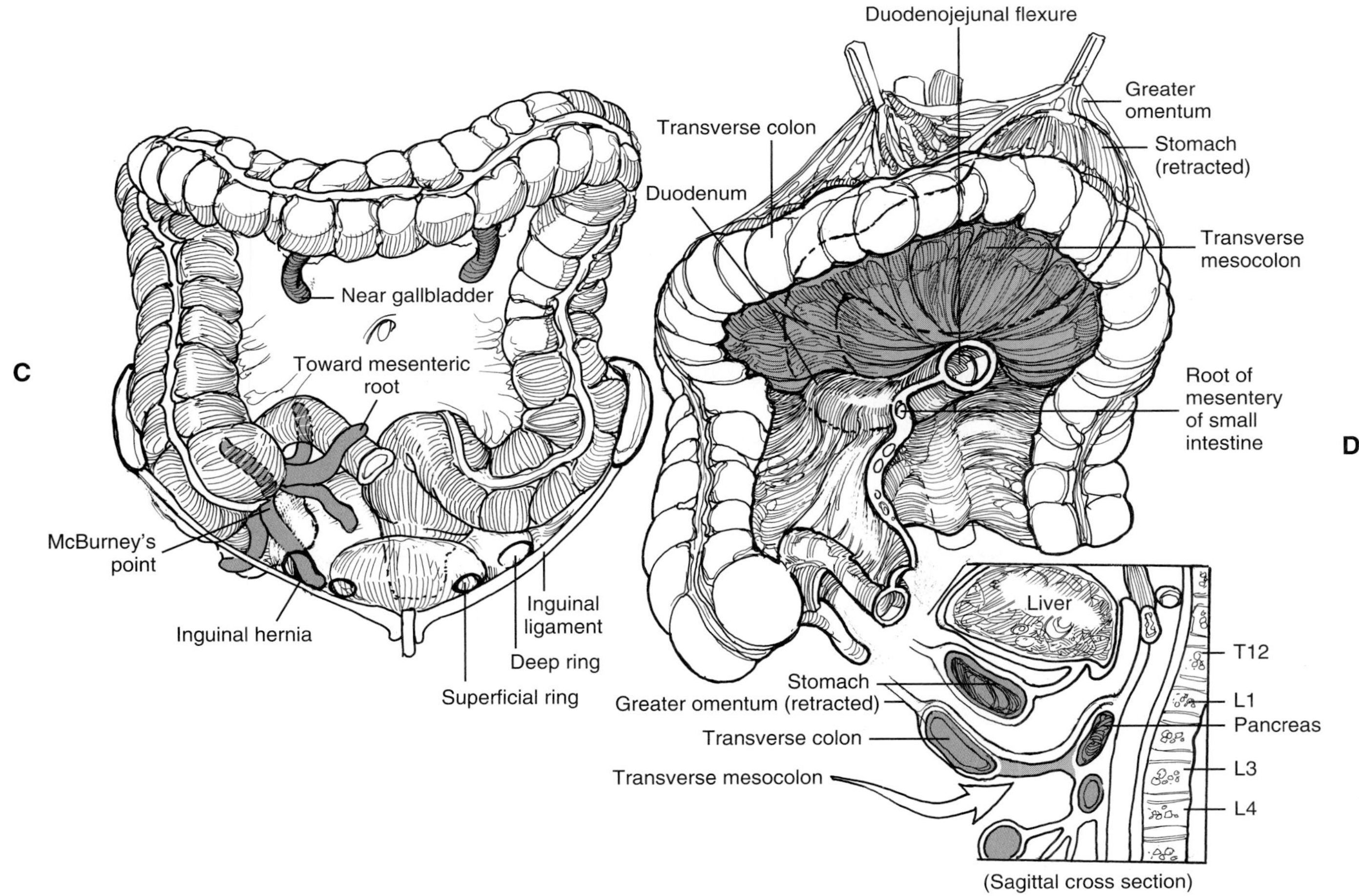

FIGURE 12–20, cont'd
C. The location of the appendix is variable. **D.** The transverse colon is intraperitoneal. The transverse colon begins at the right colic (hepatic) flexure, while its boundary with the descending colon is at the left colic (splenic) flexure.

als, the appendix is retrocecal, apparently because of the inferior displacement of the cecum relative to the posterior body wall during embryonic development (Fig. 12–20*C*). In the remaining individuals, the appendix may be visible as it dangles from the inferior end of the cecum. It is usually disposed along the longitudinal axis of the body but is occasionally deflected to the left or right. Rarely, it is displaced to aberrant locations with the rest of the large intestine as a consequence of rotational abnormalities (Fig. 12–20*C* and see below).

Because the appendix is an appendage of the cecum, it has a diminutive central lumen (see Fig. 12–18*B* and *C*), and its fundamental substructure is similar to that of the ascending colon. However, its lymphoid tissue, which is made up of **lymphoid masses,** is much more extensively developed than that of the remainder of the intestine.

▲ Muscles of the Large Intestinal Wall

A characteristic that distinguishes all parts of the large intestine (except the rectum) from the small intestine is the way in which its longitudinal muscles are organized. The outer layer of longitudinal muscle of the duodenum, jejunum, and ileum is uniformly distributed within their walls as is the inner layer of circular muscle. In the large intestine, the circular muscle is also distributed relatively uniformly throughout its walls. The longitudinal muscle, however, is thickened into three concentrated longitudinal bands called the **taeniae coli** (see Fig. 12–20*A*). These bands are clearly visible through the thin serosal layer of the large intestine. Their presence causes the walls to form pouch-like **sacculations (haustra)** (see Fig. 12–20*A*). The three bands of taeniae coli converge at the base of the cecum and at the root of the appendix. Thus, if the appendix cannot be easily located in a cadaver (or a patient), it can be found by following the taeniae coli to their point of convergence at the base of the cecum. The taeniae coli and their sacculations, the larger bore and diameter of the large intestine, and the presence of small fatty mesenteric diverticulas **(appendices epiploicae,** or **fatty tags)** distinguish the large intestine from the small intestine (Table 12–3 and see Fig. 12–20*A*).

Function of the Large Intestine

Passage of chyme into the lower end of the ascending colon is regulated by activity of the ileocecal valve

Small amounts of chyme intermittently pass from the ileum into the large intestine through opening and closing of the **ileocecal valve** (see Fig. 12–18*B* and *C*). The aperture of the valve is usually closed because of constant tonus imposed by **sympathetic stimulation** of its smooth muscle fibers. The opening of the ileocecal valve and the passage of chyme from the ileum to the ascending colon is mainly the consequence of peristaltic activity of the ileum initiated by the ingestion of food **(gastroileal reflex).**

Once chyme has entered the large intestine, it is propelled through the ascending, transverse, descending, and sigmoid colons by **slow** and **large peristaltic waves.** The slow peristaltic waves caused by circular muscle contraction are propagated over relatively short distances and serve, in large part, to mix the chyme, facilitating extraction of most of the remaining water. Large peristaltic waves are propagated along the entire length of the large intestine to propel chyme into the rectum in preparation for **defecation** (see Chapter 15). Slow and large peristaltic waves are regulated by stimulatory action of the **parasympathetic nervous system** (in part by the **vagus nerve** and in part by **pelvic splanchnic nerves** at levels S2 to S4) and by inhibitory action of **sympathetic fibers** from the **superior mesenteric, intermesenteric,** and **inferior mesenteric plexuses** (see above).

▲ Transverse Colon

The right two thirds of the transverse colon is the terminal segment of the midgut

The colon bends sharply just inferior to the liver as the ascending colon becomes the **transverse colon** (see Fig. 12–20). This is the **right colic (hepatic) flexure.** Another obvious indication of the transition between the transverse and ascending colon is the relationship of each of these segments to the posterior body wall. The ascending colon is a secondarily retroperitoneal organ, while the transverse colon is suspended by a mesentery **(transverse mesocolon)** and is an intraperitoneal organ (see Fig. 12–20). Other than this, there are no signifi-

TABLE 12–3
Anatomic Characteristics of the Small and Large Intestines

Characteristic	Small Intestine	Large Intestine
Diameter	Small	Large
Longitudinal muscle	Uniformly distributed	Organized as taeniae coli
Sacculations (haustra)	Absent	Present
Appendices epiploicae	Absent	Present

cant differences between the ascending and transverse colon. The transverse colon is about 20 inches long.

Anomalies of Midgut Rotation

Anomalies of midgut rotation may result in significant clinical symptoms. The embryonic midgut may rotate only partially, or its rotation may be reversed or uncoordinated. These anomalies may lead to volvulus, which is the twisting of the intestine around a single point, or to abnormal fixation of intestinal segments by the mesenteries to the posterior abdominal wall. Volvulus may result in obstruction of the gastrointestinal tract or constriction of blood vessels and compromise of the gastrointestinal blood supply in the affected region. The infant may be unable to pass meconium, which is the contents of the gastrointestinal tract in the fetus, or may have gastrointestinal bleeding, bowel sepsis (putrefaction), and failure to thrive. Although rotational anomalies such as these are usually diagnosed in infancy or early childhood, they may remain clinically silent until adulthood.

Meckel's Diverticulum

Meckel's diverticulum is a congenital disorder that may have symptoms similar to those produced by rotational anomalies. Meckel's diverticulum is an enlarged remnant of the yolk sac and vitelline duct, which, for unknown reasons, grows to keep pace with the body. It is usually attached to the ileum about 100 cm superior to the ileocecal valve. Other regions of the bowel may wrap around the diverticulum, resulting in obstruction of the bowel or compromise of the blood supply and sepsis. In such cases, the individual may have gastrointestinal bleeding and a sequence of umbilical and lower right quadrant pain mimicking that of appendicitis (see below).

Intestinal Stenosis or Atresia

Intestinal stenosis or atresia may result from abnormal canalization of the gastrointestinal tract in the second month of development. The gut tube is initially hollow, but the endodermal lining proliferates during the early part of the second month to completely fill the gut lumen, which is then recanalized during the last part of the second month. In some cases, canalization is incomplete or abnormal, resulting in focal duplications, narrowing, or complete obstruction of the lumen. The infant may not be able to pass meconium, may have bowel sepsis, and may fail to thrive.

ORGANIZATION OF THE HINDGUT

The hindgut includes the left one third of the transverse colon and the descending colon, sigmoid colon, and rectum

The midgut ends and the **hindgut** begins just to the right of the **splenic (left colic) flexure,** at the junction between the medial and left lateral segments of the transverse colon (Fig. 12–21*A*). Although no apparent anatomic landmark can be discerned in this region, it is agreed by convention that this is the point of interface between vascular fields of the **superior** and **inferior mesenteric arteries** (see Fig. 12–24 and discussion of the arterial vasculature below). After bending sharply just inferior to the spleen, the colon continues inferiorly for about 10 inches as the **descending colon** (Fig. 12–21*A* and *B* and see Fig. 12–20).

When the midgut is retracted into the abdominal cavity following its rotation (see above), the presumptive descending colon, like the ascending colon, becomes secondarily fixed to the posterior body wall as a secondarily retroperitoneal organ.

Sigmoid Colon

The hindgut continues as the highly mobile segment of **sigmoid colon,** which is intraperitoneal. It connects the descending colon to the superior end of the **rectum,** which is retroperitoneal, at about the level of vertebra S3 within the pelvic cavity (Fig. 12–21*B* and *C*). The sigmoid colon is about 15 inches in length.

Rectum

Division of the terminal region of the hindgut, or cloaca, results in formation of the rectum and urinary bladder

At the end of the first month of development, the hindgut terminates in a large expansion called the **cloaca** (see Fig. 15–1). During the next few weeks, its anterior and posterior regions are separated by a mesodermal **urorectal septum.** This results in formation of the **bladder** and **urethra** anteriorly and **rectum** posteriorly. The bladder and urethra become completely separated from the rest of the gastrointestinal tract. The rectum becomes the most inferior, terminal segment of the hindgut (see Chapter 15).

The rectum is never suspended by mesentery and, therefore, is a retroperitoneal organ. It is embedded within the posterior body wall just anterior to vertebrae S3, S4, and S5 and the coccygeal vertebrae (see Fig. 12–21*C*). The rectum is connected to the anterior wall of the sacrum by loose connective tissue that also encloses blood vessels and nerves (see below). It is about 5 inches long. Its diameter is approximately the same as that of the sigmoid colon except at a slightly expanded inferior region called the **rectal ampulla** (see Chapter 15). The anterior and lateral surfaces of the upper two thirds of the rectum have a serosal layer, but only the anterior surface of the lower one third is invested by peritoneum. The subserosal layer of connective tissue is not unlike that of other regions of the gastrointestinal tract, but the longitudinal muscle layer deep to it has a unique organization. Just above the junction between the sigmoid colon and rectum, the taeniae coli widen to form anterior and posterior longitudinal bands within the rectal wall. These course throughout the full length of the rectum. The circular muscle is uniformly distributed throughout most of the rectal wall but is thicker at the terminus of the rectum (i.e., the boundary of the rectum and **anal canal**) (see Fig. 12–21*D*). This thickened region of circular muscle is the **internal anal sphincter** (see Chapter 15).

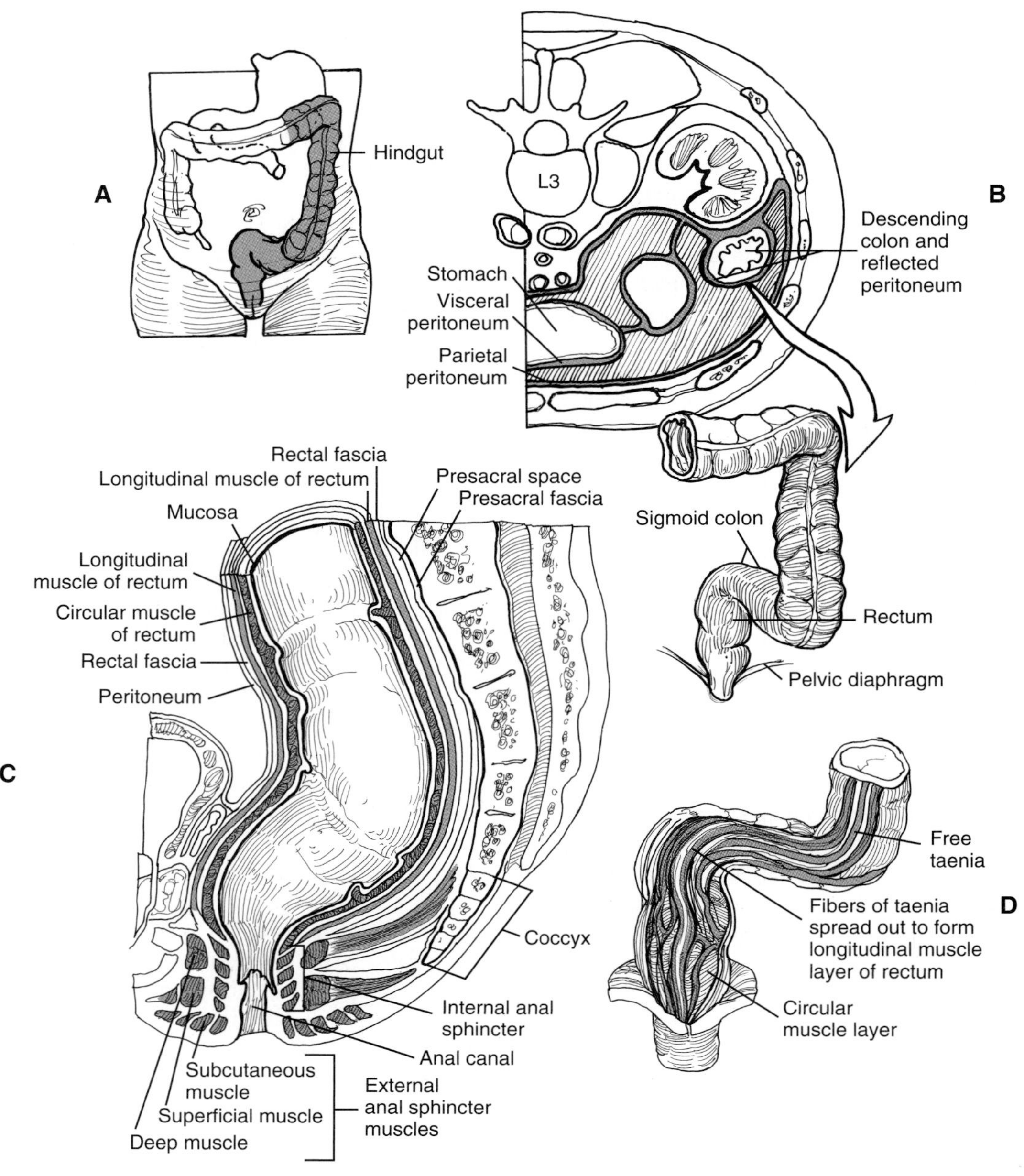

FIGURE 12–21
A. The hindgut includes the left one third of the transverse colon, the descending and sigmoid colons, and the rectum. The transverse and sigmoid colons are intraperitoneal, the descending colon is secondarily retroperitoneal, and the rectum is retroperitoneal (**B** and **C**). **C.** The uniformly distributed circular muscle of the rectum is thickened at the junction between the rectum and anal canal, forming an internal anal sphincter. Striated muscle that develops with the anal canal is organized as an external anal sphincter. **D.** The taeniae coli of the sigmoid colon splay out and widen to form anterior and posterior bands of longitudinal muscle in the wall of the rectum. (See Fig. 15–5.)

Anal Canal

The lowest segment of the gastrointestinal tract, the **anal canal,** arises from an ectodermal invagination called the **anal pit.** Striated musculature that develops with the anal pit is organized as an external anal sphincter (see Fig. 12–21C). Its vascularization and innervation are different than that of the rectum, which constitutes the upper two thirds of the **anorectal canal.**

ANATOMY OF OTHER ORGANS WITHIN THE ABDOMINOPELVIC CAVITY

The abdominopelvic cavity contains several urogenital organs

Organs of the abdominopelvic cavity, other than the gastrointestinal organs, are mainly organs of the **urogenital system.** Some of these are located within the posterior abdominal wall, such as the **kidneys** and superior regions of the **ureters.** The **suprarenal gland,** which is an endocrine organ, is located at the superior pole of the kidney (see Chapter 13).

The **pelvic cavity** contains the **ovary** and **uterus** in females and parts of the **vas deferens (spermatic duct)** and **seminal vesicles** in males. It also contains the **bladder** and lower part of the **ureters** in both sexes (see Chapter 14). Other urogenital organs, including the **prostate** and **bulbourethral glands** in males, **greater** and **lesser vestibular glands** in females, and **urethra** and **external genitalia** in both sexes, are located within an inferior compartment of the trunk called the **perineum** (see Chapter 15).

SYSTEMS THAT INTEGRATE FUNCTIONS OF THE GASTROINTESTINAL TRACT

Arteries of the Gastrointestinal Tract

The distribution of branches of the celiac, superior mesenteric, and inferior mesenteric arteries is used to define the foregut, midgut, and hindgut.

Celiac Artery and Its Branches

The **celiac trunk** is an extremely short vessel. It is difficult to locate during dissection because it is completely invested with nerve fibers and connective tissue. The definitive celiac trunk emanates from the ventral surface of the aorta at about the level of **vertebra T12** and immediately splits into three major branches: the **left gastric artery, common hepatic artery,** and **splenic artery.** The typical pattern of celiac arterial distribution is shown in Fig. 12–22*A*.

The **left gastric artery** courses superiorly and leftward from the celiac trunk within the lesser omentum. Its gastric and esophageal branches supply blood to the region of the esophagogastric junction (Fig. 12–22*A*). **Esophageal branches** supply the abdominal esophagus, and **gastric branches** supply the lesser curvature of the stomach where they anastomose with branches of the right gastric artery (see below).

The **common hepatic artery** is a large branch of the celiac trunk that courses rightward and anteriorly to the membrane of the lesser omentum (Fig. 12–22*A*). It courses rightward within the omentum, passing anteriorly toward the large portal vein. Occasionally, the common hepatic artery gives off a small **right gastric branch** that supplies the lower part of the lesser curvature of the stomach and anastomoses with the left gastric artery within the lesser curvature (see above). More typically, the common hepatic artery courses from the celiac trunk and then, just ventral to the portal vein and slightly to its left, it bifurcates into a **hepatic artery proper** and **gastroduodenal artery** (Fig. 12–22*A*). The hepatic artery proper rises superiorly within the hepatoduodenal ligament alongside (and usually anterior to) the portal vein and bile duct (see Figs. 12–6*D* and 12–10). It usually gives off a **right gastric artery** before bifurcating into **right** and **left hepatic arteries** (Fig. 12–22*A*). The left hepatic artery enters the porta hepatis of the liver to supply the left, quadrate, and caudate lobes, and the right hepatic artery supplies the right lobe only (see Figs. 12–15 and 12–26*A*). The right hepatic artery usually gives rise to a **cystic artery** that serves the **gallbladder** (Fig. 12–22*A*).

The other major branch of the common hepatic artery, the **gastroduodenal artery,** courses inferiorly posterior to the duodenum and to the left of the common bile duct (Fig. 12–22*A*). At the level of the inferior border of the superior part of the duodenum, it bifurcates into a **right gastroepiploic artery** and **superior pancreaticoduodenal artery** (Fig. 12–22*A*).

The right gastroepiploic artery courses leftward through the substance of the upper border of the greater omentum and gives off **gastric branches** serving the stomach and **epiploic branches** serving the omentum (Fig. 12–22*A*). It anastomoses with the left gastroepiploic artery, which is a branch of the splenic artery.

The **superior pancreaticoduodenal artery** usually branches into **anterior** and **posterior pancreaticoduodenal arteries.** Both the anterior and posterior branches split into **pancreatic** and **duodenal branches.** The pancreatic branches supply blood to the head of the pancreas (Fig. 12–22*B*). The duodenal branches serve the duodenum and common bile duct (Fig. 12–22*A* and *B*). The posterior pancreaticoduodenal artery also frequently arises independently from the gastroduodenal artery. In all cases, the superior pancreaticoduodenal branches anastomose with branches of the inferior pancreaticoduodenal artery, which is a branch of the superior mesenteric artery (Fig. 12–22*B*).

The **gastroduodenal artery** may also give rise to an inconstant **supraduodenal artery,** which supplies blood to the lower surface of the superior part of the duodenum, to the greater omentum, and even to the stomach (Fig. 12–22*A*).

Usually, the final (third) branch of the celiac trunk is the **splenic artery.** This is a large, contorted vessel that branches from the left side of the celiac trunk and courses leftward just adjacent to or sometimes within the substance of the superior margin of the pancreas (Fig. 12–22*A*). It gives rise to many small pancreatic branches, the dorsal (superior) pancreatic artery, large (great) pancreatic artery, caudal pancreatic artery, short gastric arteries, and left gastroepiploic artery, and it finally terminates in several splenic branches (Fig. 12–22*B*).

The **dorsal pancreatic artery** courses posteriorly to the pancreas and splits into right and left branches. The **right branches** anastomose with pancreaticoduodenal branches and assist in supplying blood to the head and uncinate process of the pancreas (Fig. 12–22*B*). The **left branches** course toward the tail of the pancreas, anastomosing with the **great** and **caudal pancreatic arteries** to serve the body and tail of the pancreas (Fig. 12–22*A* and *B*).

Five to seven **short gastric arteries** ascend from the splenic artery (or sometimes from the left gastroepiploic

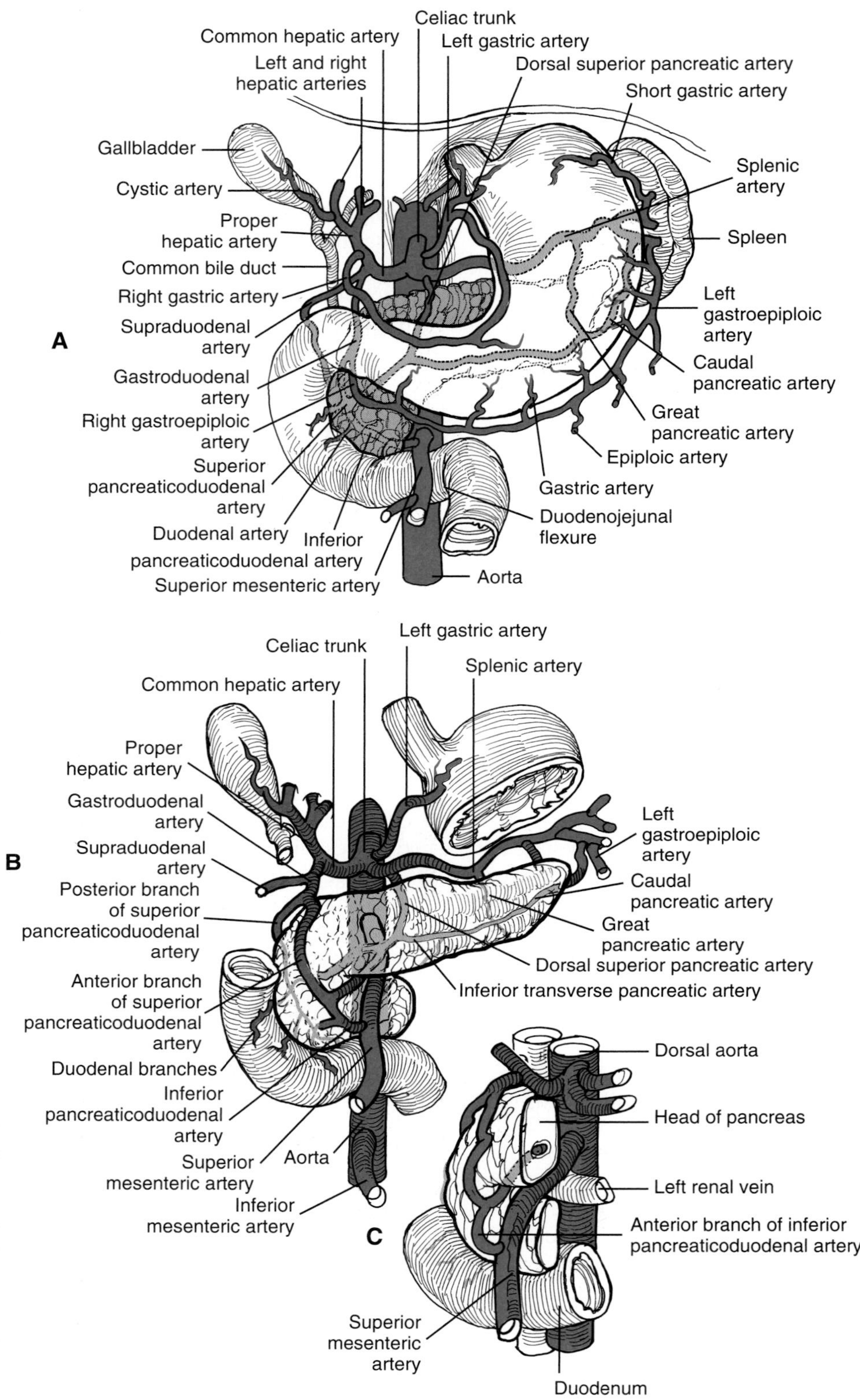

FIGURE 12–22

A. The three major branches of the celiac trunk are the left gastric artery, common hepatic artery, and splenic artery. Their branches vascularize the abdominal esophagus, stomach, superior part of the duodenum, half of the descending part of the duodenum, liver, gallbladder, pancreas, spleen, greater omentum, and lesser omentum. **B.** The pancreas receives arterial branches from the superior pancreaticoduodenal branch of the gastroduodenal artery, splenic artery, and inferior pancreaticoduodenal branch of the superior mesenteric artery. All of these have branches that anastomose within the substance of the pancreas. **C.** Left lateral view of pancreatic arteries.

artery) to supply the fundus of the stomach. Some of these may anastomose with branches of the left gastric artery (Fig. 12–22*A*).

Just before it terminates in numerous **splenic branches,** the splenic artery gives rise to a **left gastroepiploic artery** (Fig. 12–22). This vessel courses rightward, back along the greater curvature of the stomach within the greater omentum at its junction with the stomach. Like the right gastroepiploic artery, it gives off numerous **gastric** and **epiploic branches.** It then anastomoses with the right gastroepiploic artery (Fig. 12–22).

The terminal **splenic branches** course within the lienorenal ligament to enter the spleen through a fissure in its right surface called the **hilum of the spleen** (Fig. 12–22*A* and see Fig. 12–13*A*).

Superior Mesenteric Artery and Its Branches

Branches of the superior mesenteric artery supply the midgut

The large superior mesenteric artery branches from the ventral surface of the dorsal aorta at the level of **vertebra L1,** just half an inch inferior to the celiac trunk (Fig. 12–23 and see Fig. 12-22). It passes anteriorly to the left renal vein and pierces the pancreas, passing behind the body and anterior to its uncinate process. It then passes over the horizontal (third) part of the duodenum and enters the mesentery of the midgut (Fig. 12–23 and see Fig. 12–22). It usually gives rise to an inferior pancreaticoduodenal artery (see Fig. 12–22), numerous jejunal and ileal branches, an ileocolic artery, and right and middle colic arteries (Fig. 12–23). The typical pattern of superior mesenteric arterial distribution is shown in Fig. 12–23.

The **inferior pancreaticoduodenal artery** is the first branch of the superior mesenteric artery. It usually arises at the level of the upper border of the third part of the duodenum (Fig. 12–23 and see Fig. 12–22). Like the superior pancreaticoduodenal artery, it bifurcates into anterior and posterior branches, which anastomose with anterior and posterior branches of the superior pancreaticoduodenal artery (see above). The duodenal branches supply the duodenum, and the pancreatic branches supply the head of the pancreas and its uncinate process (see Fig. 12–22).

Numerous **jejunal** and **ileal branches** arise from the left surface of the superior mesenteric artery and course leftward between layers of the jejunal and ileal mesenteries to form the arterial arcades and vasa recta of the small intestine (Fig. 12–23 and see Fig. 12–19).

The **middle colic, right colic,** and **ileocolic arteries** branch from superior to inferior from the right surface of the superior mesenteric artery, each coursing rightward within the midgut mesentery to supply the remaining segments of the midgut.

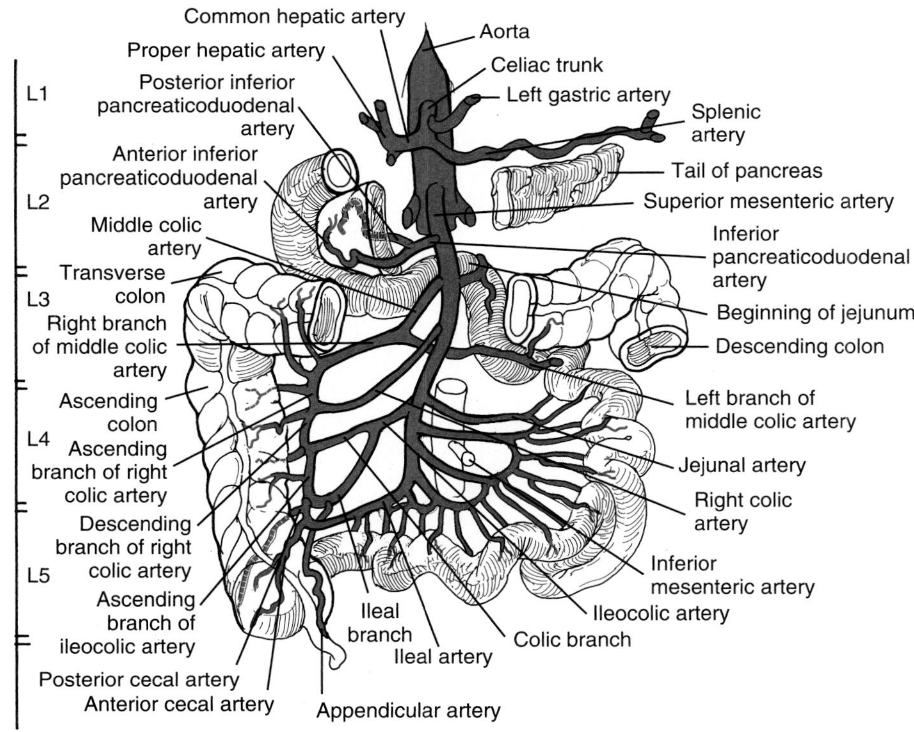

FIGURE 12–23

Major branches of the superior mesenteric artery include jejunal and ileal branches, an ileocolic branch, a right colic artery, and a middle colic artery.

The most inferior of these arteries, the **ileocolic artery,** supplies the ileocolic (ileocecal) junction. It gives rise to **ileal branches,** an **appendicular branch, anterior** and **posterior cecal branches,** and an **ascending colic branch** (Fig. 12–23).

The **right colic artery** arises from the superior mesenteric artery and passes rightward within the mesentery to supply the ascending colon (Fig. 12–23). As it approaches the wall of the colon, it splits into a descending branch and an ascending branch, each of which provide several terminal branches to the wall of the ascending colon (Fig. 12–23). The descending branch of the right colic artery courses inferiorly to anastomose with the ascending colic branch of the ileocolic artery. The ascending branch of the right colic artery anastomoses with the right branch of the middle colic artery (Fig. 12–23). Anastomoses of these terminal branches with each other and with similar terminal branches of the inferior mesenteric artery form an arterial ring shaped like an inverted U adjacent to the mesenteric surface of the ascending, transverse, and descending colons. This is sometimes called the **marginal artery** (Fig. 12–24).

The **middle colic artery** usually arises from the right surface of the superior mesenteric artery just inferior to the lower border of the uncinate process of the pancreas (Fig. 12–23). It courses within the mesentery of the transverse colon (transverse mesocolon) and then bifurcates into **right** and **left branches** (Fig. 12–23). These branches give off several short terminal branches, which supply the wall of the transverse colon. The continuation of the right branch anastomoses with the ascending branch of the right colic artery. The left branch anastomoses with terminal branches of the left colic artery, which is a branch of the inferior mesenteric artery, contributing to the horizontal segment of the marginal artery (Figs. 12–23 and 12–24).

Inferior Mesenteric Artery and Its Branches

Branches of the inferior mesenteric artery supply the hindgut

The third and final ventral splanchnic arterial trunk of the dorsal aorta is the **inferior mesenteric artery** (see Fig. 12–24). It gives rise to a **left colic artery, sigmoidal arteries,** and **superior rectal arteries,** which supply hindgut derivatives of the gastrointestinal tract. This most inferior branch of the dorsal aorta arises at the level of **vertebra L3,** about an inch above the bifurcation of the dorsal aorta into the right and left common iliac arteries. The typical pattern of inferior mesenteric arterial distribution is shown in Fig. 12–24.

The **left colic branch** of the inferior mesenteric artery is a retroperitoneal structure. It does not course

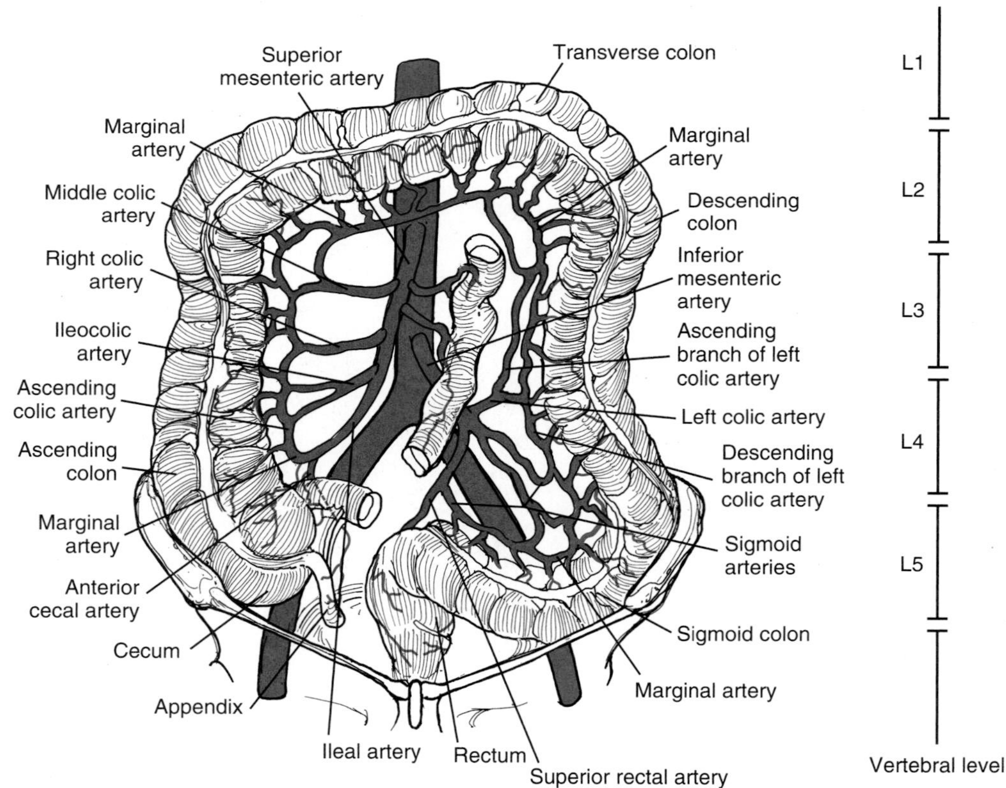

FIGURE 12–24
Major branches of the inferior mesenteric artery include the left colic artery, sigmoidal arteries, and a superior rectal artery. Terminal branches of these arteries, along with terminal branches of the middle colic, right colic, and ileocolic arteries, form an anastomosis around the entire inner border of the colon called the *marginal artery.*

within a freely suspended mesentery as do branches of the superior mesenteric artery. It passes along the posterior body wall upward and leftward from its origin on the anterior surfaces of the aorta and the left psoas and quadratus lumborum muscles and then bifurcates into **descending** and **ascending branches** (see Fig. 12–24). These branches give rise to short terminal branches, which supply the walls of the left third of the transverse colon and entire descending colon. The ascending branch anastomoses with the left branch of the middle colic artery, and the descending branch anastomoses with an adjacent sigmoidal artery to form this descending left side of the marginal artery (see Fig. 12–24).

The inferior mesenteric artery gives rise to two or three **sigmoidal branches,** which course within the mesentery that suspends the sigmoid colon to supply this intraperitoneal segment of the hindgut (see Fig. 12–24). Terminal regions of these branches may anastomose to contribute to the marginal artery.

Although the rectum is a retroperitoneal organ, the root of the most inferior branch of the inferior mesenteric artery, the **superior rectal artery,** first courses inferiorly within the mesentery of the sigmoid colon, often just to the right of the root of the most inferior sigmoidal artery (see Fig. 12–24). At about the level of vertebra S3, the superior rectal artery usually bifurcates into branches that become retroperitoneal structures as they course along the lateral surfaces of the rectum. These arteries give rise to numerous terminal branches, which supply muscular and mucosal layers of the most superior third of the rectal wall. These branches also anastomose with branches of the **middle rectal arteries** (branches of the internal iliac arteries) and **inferior rectal arteries** (branches of the internal pudendal arteries) (see Chapters 14 and 15).

Common Variations of the Arterial Supply to the Abdominal Foregut

The pattern of gastrointestinal arteries may vary dramatically from one individual to another

Although the branching patterns of the celiac, superior mesenteric, and inferior mesenteric arteries described above are common, the scheme of vascularization may vary enormously in different individuals. This fact is obviously of great clinical importance to surgeons, especially when resection of parts of the esophagus, stomach, or bowel is necessary.

The gastrointestinal vasculature develops from intricate networks of vitelline arteries and veins, which supply and drain the yolk sac of the embryo. These networks become less complex as a few vessels become larger and more dominant and others become smaller or disappear. This mechanism underlies the development of most of the other systems of vasculature as well, and for this reason, patterns of arterial and venous distribution are among the most variable in the human body.

Dramatic **variations in celiac trunk branches** may occur (Fig. 12–25). For example, the proper hepatic arteries may originate from the superior mesenteric artery (Fig. 12–25*A*). The gastroduodenal artery may branch directly from the superior mesenteric artery (Fig. 12–25*B*), right hepatic artery (Fig. 12–25*C*), or right gastric artery (Fig. 12–25*D*). There may be two gastroduodenal arteries instead of one, or this vessel may be completely absent. The cystic artery usually originates from the right hepatic artery, but it may also arise from the common hepatic or left hepatic artery. The right gastric artery usually branches from the proper hepatic artery, but it may, instead, branch directly from the common hepatic artery.

Variations of the superior mesenteric artery may also occur. For example, the inferior pancreaticoduodenal artery may originate from a superior jejunal artery. The ileocolic, right colic, or middle colic branch may share common origins from the superior mesenteric artery. In some persons, the ileocolic and right colic branches originate together from the superior mesenteric artery, and in others, the right colic and middle colic branches share a common root.

Function of the Collateral Arterial Circulation of the Gastrointestinal Tract

Collateral circulation in the gastrointestinal tract is extensive

It is obvious that the arterial supply to the gastrointestinal tract is extensive and functionally interconnected. If, for example, the common hepatic arterial branch of the celiac trunk were to become obstructed proximal to its bifurcation into the gastroduodenal and proper hepatic arteries, the liver would probably not become necrotic because blood could be delivered to the proper hepatic artery via the left and right gastric arteries or the splenic, left gastroepiploic, right gastroepiploic, and gastroduodenal arteries. If the superior pancreaticoduodenal artery were ligated or became obstructed, blood could reach the head and body of the pancreas through the splenic artery, dorsal pancreatic artery and its right branch, or superior mesenteric artery and its inferior pancreaticoduodenal branch. The collateral circulation of the ascending, transverse, descending, and sigmoid colons via the "marginal" artery has been described above.

> The multiple arteries supplying blood to the large intestine must be considered when vessels are ligated prior to surgical resection of intestinal segments.

▲ Veins of the Gastrointestinal Tract: The Hepatic Portal System

Blood delivered to the gastrointestinal tract is drained by a hepatic portal system of veins

Blood draining from the gastrointestinal tract must be filtered and processed by the liver, primarily for the purpose of extracting nutrients and water absorbed by

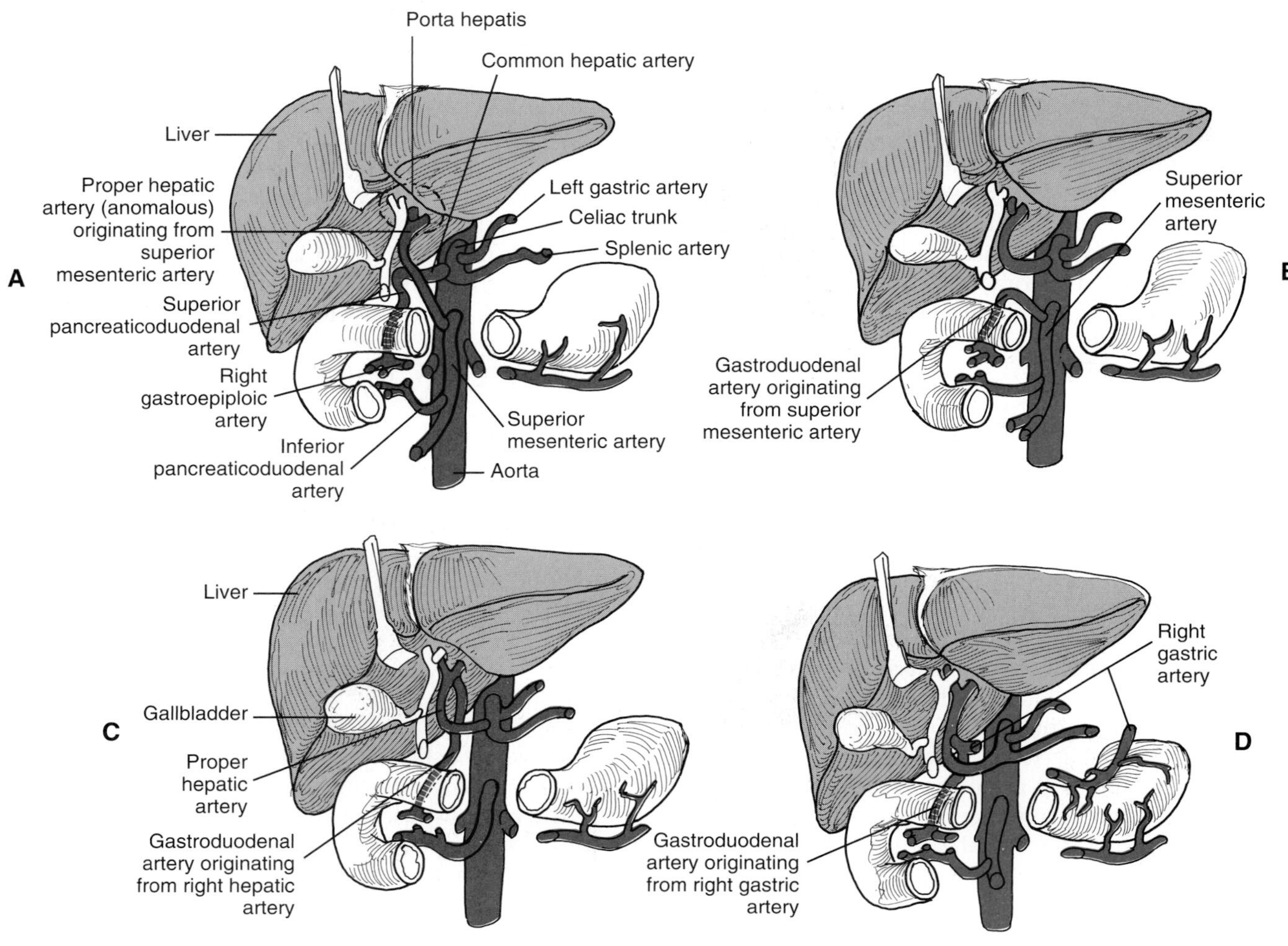

FIGURE 12–25

Common variations of the arterial supply to the abdominal foregut. **A.** The proper hepatic artery may arise from the superior mesenteric artery. The gastroduodenal artery may arise from the superior mesenteric artery, **(B)**, the right hepatic artery, **(C)**, or the right gastric artery, **(D)**.

the intestinal epithelium (see below). All of the veins draining the gastrointestinal tract converge toward the porta hepatis and merge into a single large **hepatic portal vein** (Fig. 12–26 and see Fig. 12–28).

The organization of portal veins is similar to that of the arteries that supply the gastrointestinal tract, with a few notable exceptions. It is similar in that separate groups of vessels drain the abdominal foregut, midgut, and hindgut of the gastrointestinal tract. Vessels draining the midgut converge to form the superior mesenteric venous trunk, while vessels draining the hindgut converge to form the inferior mesenteric venous trunk. Branches draining the foregut, however, empty individually into the hepatic portal vein or upper part of the superior mesenteric venous trunk (Fig. 12–26).

Left and Right Gastric Veins

The abdominal esophagus and upper part of the lesser curvature of the stomach are drained by the **left gastric vein.** This vein empties directly into the portal vein at its right side, just superior to the upper border of the pancreas (see Fig. 12–26). A **right gastric vein,** which drains the same field of the lower region of the lesser curvature that is supplied by its arterial counterpart, empties separately into the portal vein, just inferior to the left gastric vein. Like the left and right gastric arteries, the left and right gastric veins anastomose in the region of the lesser curvature of the stomach (see Fig. 12–26). A **supraduodenal vein** and **superior pancreaticoduodenal vein** also empty directly into the portal vein (Fig. 12–26).

Splenic and Gastroepiploic Veins

The **splenic vein** drains directly into the portal vein just inferior to its connection to the right gastric vein behind the body of the pancreas (see Fig. 12–26). Its drainage fields are similar to the fields supplied by the splenic artery. It collects blood from the spleen via **splenic branches,** from the fundus and body of the stomach via **short gastric veins,** from the pancreas by

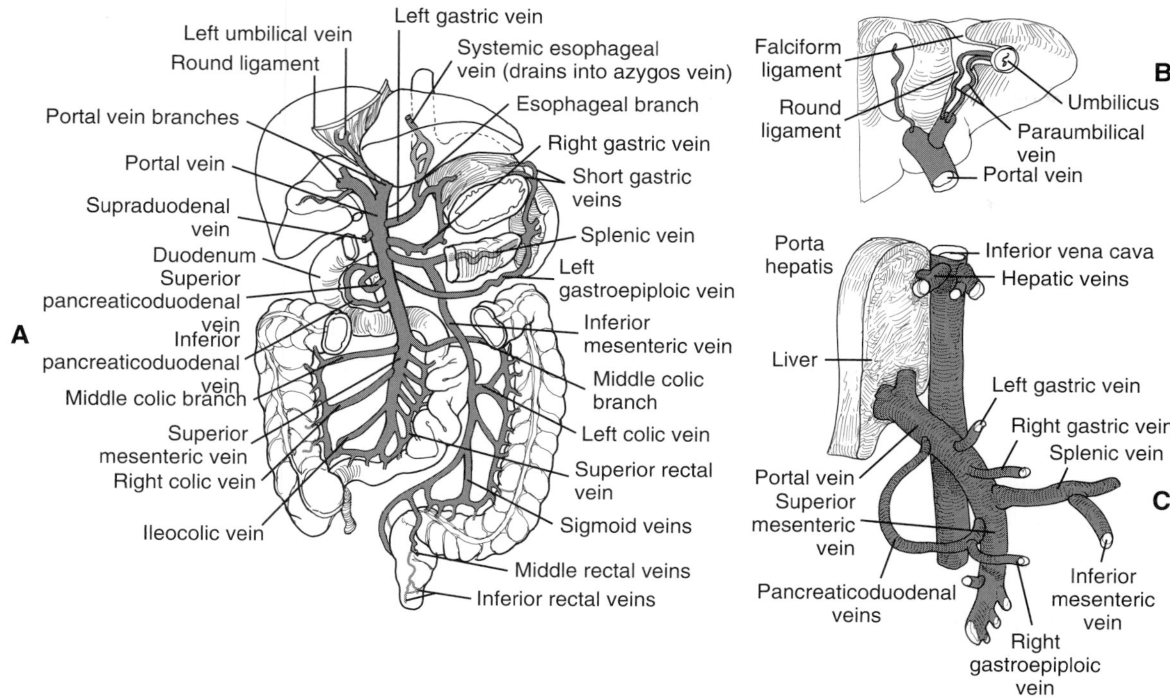

FIGURE 12–26

The hepatic portal system. Much of the foregut is drained by individual tributaries of the hepatic portal vein (see also inset). The midgut is drained by a superior mesenteric vein, which is continuous with the hepatic portal vein. Drainage of the hindgut is by an inferior mesenteric vein, which empties into the splenic vein, superior mesenteric vein, or the junction of the splenic and superior mesenteric veins. The ligamentum teres hepatica is drained by small veins, which commonly empty into the left portal vein *(inset).*

various **pancreatic branches,** and from much of the left part of the greater curvature of the stomach and greater omentum via a **left gastroepiploic vein** (see Fig. 12–26). The **right gastroepiploic vein** anastomoses with the left gastroepiploic vein in the region of the greater curvature of the stomach and drains directly into the portal vein or upper part of the superior mesenteric vein (see Fig. 12–26).

Cystic Vein

Because the portal system is designed to deliver blood to the liver from the gastrointestinal tract, there is no common hepatic or hepatic proper vein corresponding to those branches of the arterial system. The **cystic vein** must, therefore, empty directly into the hepatic portal vein or its right branch (see Fig. 12–26). A small vein draining the obliterated left umbilical vein **(ligamentum teres hepatis,** or **round ligament of the liver)** also drains directly into the hepatic portal system (see Fig. 12–26).

Superior Mesenteric Vein

Venous branches draining the midgut are similar in distribution and organization to branches of the superior mesenteric artery. These branches merge into a single **superior mesenteric vein,** which is continuous with and empties directly into the hepatic portal vein. Branches of the superior mesenteric vein include **jejunal, ileal, ileocolic, right colic,** and **middle colic branches** (see Fig. 12–26). An **inferior pancreaticoduodenal vein** may empty directly into the portal vein or right gastroepiploic vein.

Inferior Mesenteric Vein

Venous branches draining the hindgut are also similar in distribution and organization to their arterial counterparts. The **inferior mesenteric vein** collects blood from its tributaries, which include the **left colic vein, sigmoidal veins,** and **superior rectal veins** (see Fig. 12–26).

Veins of the Liver

Portal blood enters the liver via right and left branches of the hepatic portal vein and is distributed to specific lobes and areas of the liver

The four lobes of the liver are a large **right lobe,** smaller **left lobe,** smaller anterior inferior **quadrate lobe,** and posterior inferior **caudate lobe,** which is the smallest lobe (Fig. 12–27 and see Fig. 12–15). The indentation produced by the **ligamentum teres hepatis** (former left umbilical vein) and **ligamentum arteriosum** (former **ductus venosus**) appears to segregate the left lobe from the other three lobes. However, the functional division of the liver is based upon the distribution of branches of the left and right portal veins, hepatic arteries, and hepatic ducts. Right branches serve the right lobe only, and left branches serve the left, quadrate, and caudate lobes (Fig. 12–27).

Mixing of hepatic arterial blood with portal blood in the liver sinusoids and drainage of this blood into the systemic circulation via **hepatic veins** and the **inferior vena cava** are described below (see Fig. 12–28).

Function of the Liver and Portal System

The liver filters nutrient-laden blood from the gastrointestinal tract through a special portal system of veins

Blood flow to the gastrointestinal tract may be minimal during periods of "fight and flight," when digestive processes are less important than muscular work. Constriction of gastrointestinal vessels under these conditions is mainly controlled by activity of **splanchnic nerves** of the **sympathetic system.** During periods of "peace and relaxation," the **absence of sympathetic activity** results in dilatation of gastrointestinal vessels. This causes blood flow to the stomach and intestines to be maximal during digestion of a large meal. Blood delivered to the gastrointestinal tract by celiac, superior mesenteric, and inferior mesenteric arteries enters capillaries of the intestinal villi, where it picks up amino acids, fats, and sugars absorbed by the intestinal mucosa. This nutrient-laden blood is transported to the liver through branches of the **portal veins** (Fig. 12–28*A* and see Fig. 12–27*B*).

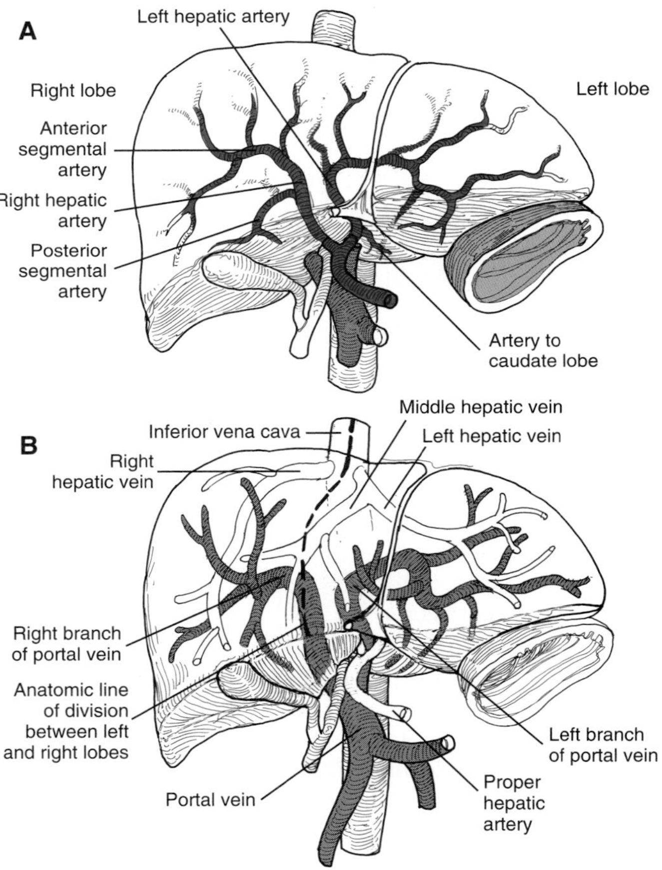

FIGURE 12–27
Functional right and left sides of the liver. **A.** The right hepatic artery supplies only the right lobe. The left hepatic artery supplies the left, quadrate, and caudate lobes. **B.** Blood from the right hepatic portal vein drains into the right lobe, whereas blood from the left hepatic portal vein drains into the left, quadrate, and caudate lobes.

Portal tributaries converge to form the hepatic portal vein, which is joined by the proper hepatic artery and common bile duct within the gastroduodenal ligament. At the level of the cystic duct, the portal vein, proper hepatic artery, and common hepatic duct enter the porta hepatis (see Fig. 12–15). All three of these structures branch together as they course to their destinations within the liver. These three elements constitute a **hepatic triad** (Fig. 12–28*C* and see Fig. 12–15*A*).

> Blood within the portal vein that has been derived from the superior mesenteric vein mixes minimally with blood that has been derived from splenic and inferior mesenteric veins. This fact may be helpful in determining the general location of a primary tumor of the gastrointestinal tract that has metastasized to the liver. The preferential seeding of metastases within the right or left liver lobes reflects the pattern of blood flow that has carried them (see Fig. 12–27*B*).

The ultimate destinations of the hepatic triads are the numerous **hepatic lobules,** which constitute the smallest functional subunits of the liver (Fig. 12–28*C*). Hepatic lobules are cylindrically shaped aggregates of hepatocytes about 1 mm in diameter. The portal triads (usually about three per lobule) are located at the periphery of each cylinder (Fig. 12–28*C*). Blood from portal veins drains directly into the radially organized liver sinusoids within the lobules. Oxygenated blood from hepatic arterioles is mixed with this sinusoidal blood. Once the blood is processed, it drains into a **central vein** within the lobule. This central vein drains the blood into **hepatic veins** and, ultimately, back into the **inferior vena cava** (Fig. 12–28*A* and *C*).

Bile, which is manufactured by hepatocytes, is collected within bile canaliculi between liver cells. Canaliculi merge to form hepatic ducts within each portal triad. Bile drains from these smaller tributaries into larger ducts and then into the right and left hepatic ducts and common hepatic duct. Bile may be concentrated within the gallbladder after transport through the cystic duct or may be directly transported to the duodenum via the common bile duct (see discussion of the function of the gallbladder, above).

Obstruction of the Hepatic Vasculature

Obstruction of the hepatic vasculature may result in backflow of blood within the hepatic portal system; hepatitis and chronic alcoholism are common causes of liver cirrhosis

Infections of the liver, chronic consumption of alcohol, and liver cancer may result in the replacement of liver cells by fibrous connective tissue (cirrhosis) or by multiple tumor foci, causing obstruction of portal blood flow within the liver. Portal blood draining from gastrointestinal organs is not able to empty into the inferior vena cava through the hepatic veins and must find an alternate pathway to the systemic circulation. With the resulting increase in portal pressure (portal hypertension), portal blood may flow backward and then into the systemic circulation at several sites of portal-systemic anastomosis (Fig. 12–29). The portal vessels have no valves, and retrograde flow of blood is therefore possible. Also, the increased portal pressure causes expansion or enlargement of the vessels (varicoceles, or varices) in these anastomotic regions.

The most clinically relevant regions of portal-systemic anastomosis are the portal and systemic esophageal branches at the inferior end of the esophagus, portal superior rectal

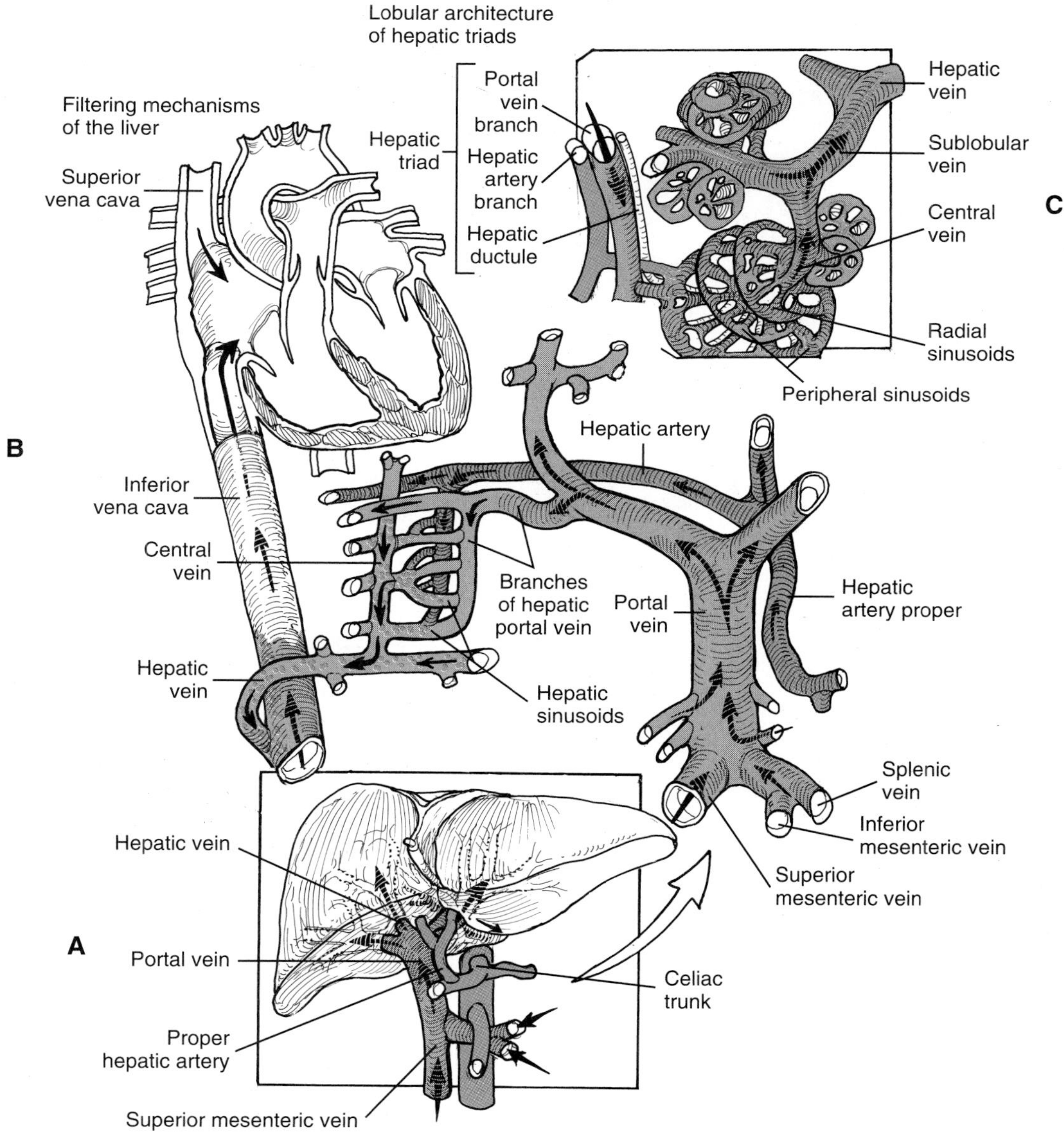

FIGURE 12–28
Filtration of portal blood by the liver. **A.** Portal blood draining the gastrointestinal tract (within the portal veins) and oxygenated hepatic arterial blood (within the hepatic arteries) enters the liver through the porta hepatis. **B.** Portal and arterial blood mixes together in the liver sinusoids, which converge to form central veins. Central veins, in turn, drain into sublobular veins. Sublobular veins converge to form hepatic veins, which empty the processed hepatic blood into the inferior vena cava at the posterior surface of the liver. **C.** The liver sinusoids are organized as peripheral and radial sinusoids.

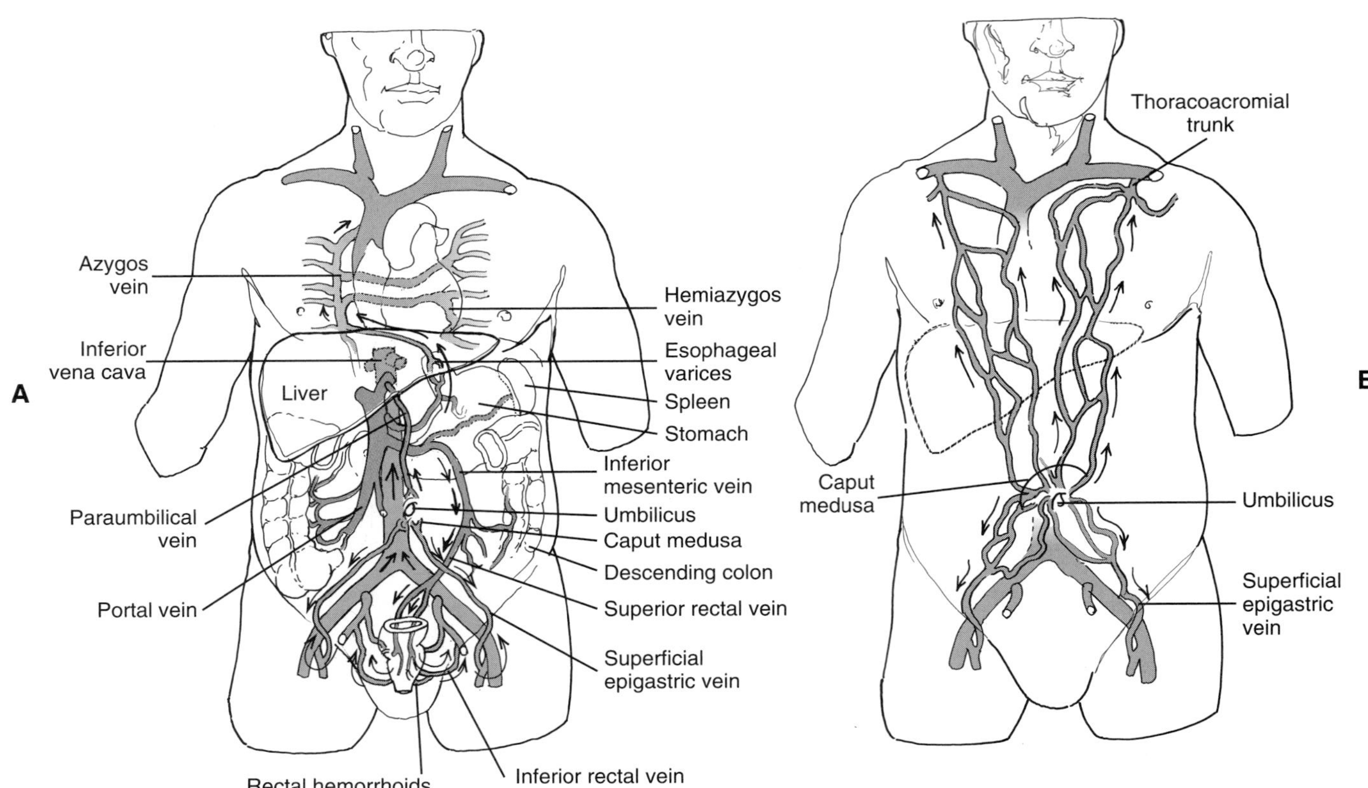

FIGURE 12–29
Obstruction of portal return. In cases of liver cirrhosis or other obstructions of the portal system, portal blood may flow backward through portal vessels and into the systemic circulation via enlarged portosystemic anastomoses. These include anastomoses between (1) superior rectal veins (branch of the portal inferior mesenteric vein) and the inferior rectal vein within the rectal mucosa, (2) portal and systemic veins that drain the round ligament of the liver, and (3) portal esophageal branches of the left gastric vein and systemic esophageal branches of the azygos system.

(hemorrhoidal) veins and systemic inferior rectal (hemorrhoidal) veins within the mucosa of the anorectal canal, and portal and systemic parumbilical veins draining the round ligament of the liver (Fig. 12–29 and see Fig. 12–26).

Serious consequences of liver cirrhosis are sometimes manifested by the development of varicoceles at the inferior end of the esophagus (Fig. 12–29). These may rupture and bleed, frequently resulting in death. Chronic alcoholism may cause backflow of portal blood into paraumbilical veins within the subserous fascia (superior and inferior epigastric veins) or superficial fascia (superficial epigastric veins), or both, of the anterior abdominal wall (Fig. 12–29). Enlargement of superficial epigastric veins within the anterior abdominal wall may be evident as snakelike radiations in the region of the umbilicus (caput medusae).

A more common manifestation of increased portal pressure is the development of and occasional bleeding of hemorrhoids, which are enlarged areas of inferior hemorrhoidal veins within the mucosa of the anal canal (Fig. 12–29). Constriction of portal vessels may be caused by pressure of the fetus in pregnant women or by excess abdominal fat in obese persons. Hemorrhoids are also common in individuals who sit for long periods of time (e.g., truck drivers, medical students, and professors of anatomy). Although it is typically not life threatening, chronic bleeding of hemorrhoids may result in a lowered hematocrit (reduced numbers of red blood cells) and loss of energy and should be treated.

Other less clinically relevant regions of portal-systemic anastomosis are at the interface between the ascending and descending colons and the posterior body wall, in the region of the bare area of the liver, and between branches of renal and inferior mesenteric veins.

▲ Lymphatic Drainage of the Gastrointestinal Tract

Lymph is drained from the gastrointestinal tract via aortic lymphatic vessels and nodes

Lymphatic vessels and associated lymph nodes draining the gastrointestinal tract from the abdominal esophagus to the upper third of the anorectal canal usually follow the course of the arterial channels that supply these organs (Fig. 12–30 and see Fig. 13–11). The liver, spleen, and stomach are drained by lymphatic vessels that terminate within **preaortic nodes** associated with the celiac trunk. Lymph that drains from the duodenum and from the rest of the midgut

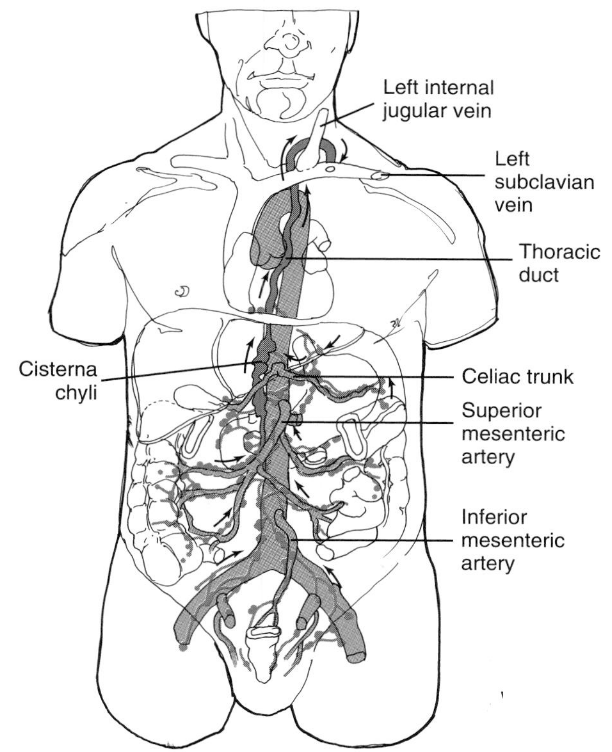

FIGURE 12–30
Lymphatic drainage of abdominopelvic organs. Abdominopelvic organs are drained by lymphatic vessels and nodes that accompany the arterial vasculature of the abdominopelvic cavity. Thus, lymph from abdominopelvic organs eventually drains back into vessels and nodes associated with the aorta (preaortic nodes) and then into the cisterna chyli, into the thoracic duct, and into the systemic circulation in the region of the junction of the left jugular and left subclavian veins.

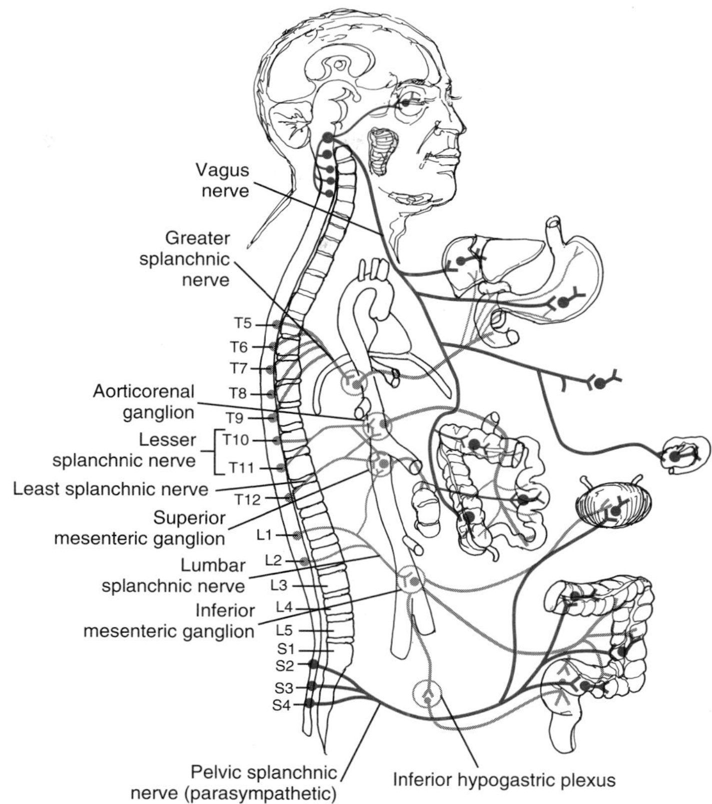

FIGURE 12–31
Autonomic innervation of abdominopelvic organs. Sympathetic innervation of the gastrointestinal tract is provided by the greater splanchnic nerves (to the foregut), lesser and least splanchnic nerves (to the midgut), and lumbar splanchnic nerves (to the hindgut). Parasympathetic innervation of the gastrointestinal tract is provided by the vagus nerves (to the foregut and midgut) and by the pelvic splanchnic nerves (to the hindgut). Visceral afferent fibers accompany all sympathetic and parasympathetic pathways.

passes through lymphatic vessels and preaortic nodes, which converge upon the root of the superior mesenteric artery. Lymph that drains from the hindgut flows to preaortic nodes associated with the inferior mesenteric artery. All of these preaortic nodes drain into the **cisterna chyli,** which drains lymph into the **thoracic duct** (see Chapter 10). The thoracic duct delivers lymph to the circulatory system near the junction of the left jugular and subclavian veins. Glands and organs located lateral to the aorta, such as the kidneys and suprarenal glands, drain into **lateral aortic lymph nodes,** which also drain into the cisterna chyli and thoracic duct.

▲ Innervation of the Abdomen and Abdominal Organs

Autonomic Innervation of the Gastrointestinal Tract

Autonomic innervation of the gastrointestinal tract follows the pattern established by the distribution of aortic arterial branches

The pattern of autonomic innervation of the gastrointestinal tract is most easily understood in relation to the embryologic subdivisions of the gut, namely, the **foregut, midgut,** and **hindgut.** In general, **preganglionic sympathetic fibers** within the greater splanchnic nerve innervate the **prevertebral (preaortic) ganglia** associated with the celiac trunk; preganglionic fibers of the lesser splanchnic nerve innervate the aorticorenal ganglia (and superior mesenteric ganglia); preganglionic fibers of the least splanchnic nerve innervate the superior mesenteric ganglia (and aorticorenal ganglia); and preganglionic fibers of the lumbar splanchnic nerves mainly innervate the inferior mesenteric ganglia (Fig. 12–31). **Sympathetic postganglionic fibers** emanating from these ganglia follow arterial branches of these major arterial trunks to innervate the gastrointestinal viscera served by their respective branches (Fig. 12–31 and see below). **Preganglionic parasympathetic innervation** is supplied to the gastrointestinal tract by the **vagus nerve** and parasympathetic **pelvic splanchnic nerves** originating with intermediolateral cell columns at levels S2, S3, and S4 of the spinal cord (Fig. 12–31). Preganglionic fibers of the vagus nerves innervate small, scattered ganglia embedded within the walls of foregut and midgut abdominopelvic viscera. Preganglionic fibers of pelvic splanchnic nerves innervate small ganglia embedded within the walls of hindgut viscera (Fig. 12–31). Chapter 4 has a more general discussion of the autonomic nervous system and its function.

Sympathetic Innervation of the Gastrointestinal Tract

Sympathetic innervation of the gut is mediated by variable and interacting splanchnic nerves, ganglia, and plexuses

The preceding introduction to the pattern of sympathetic innervation of prevertebral ganglia is somewhat simplified. Ganglia may not be discrete but may be broken into small structures that are dispersed throughout larger nerve networks called **plexuses.** Alternatively, some of the ganglia may be fused with neighboring ganglia or may be innervated by preganglionic fibers from more than one splanchnic nerve. Thus, significant variation in the pattern of autonomic innervation may occur.

However, prevertebral **celiac ganglia** are relatively large, discrete masses that can easily be observed by students in the laboratory (Fig. 12–32 and see Fig. 12–31). The ganglia have the diameter of a penny or nickel. They are located on either side of the celiac trunk between it and the superior pole of the kidney. Each ganglion lies just anterior to the diaphragmatic crura and is innervated by a visible **greater splanchnic nerve** just after it perforates the diaphragmatic crus. Postganglionic fibers that emanate from these ganglia mainly follow branches of the celiac trunk to innervate organs of the foregut, although they may be mixed with vagal nerve autonomic fibers within **plexuses** that innervate organs of the foregut and superior peritoneal cavity. These include the hepatic and left gastric plexuses (see Figs. 12–28 and 12–29).

Prevertebral **superior mesenteric ganglia** are often inferior extensions of celiac ganglia but, as is suggested by their name, are located closer to the superior mesenteric arteries (see Fig. 12–31). These ganglia also receive preganglionic fibers from the **lesser** and **least splanchnic nerves** and distribute postganglionic sympathetic fibers to the midgut.

Prevertebral **aorticorenal ganglia** are also inferior extensions of celiac ganglia and are innervated by preganglionic sympathetic fibers of the **lesser** and **least splanchnic nerves** (see Fig. 12–31). These ganglia may be difficult to find in the laboratory because their location varies considerably in relation to the root of the renal artery. Postganglionic fibers that emanate from these ganglia first pass through a secondary plexus called the

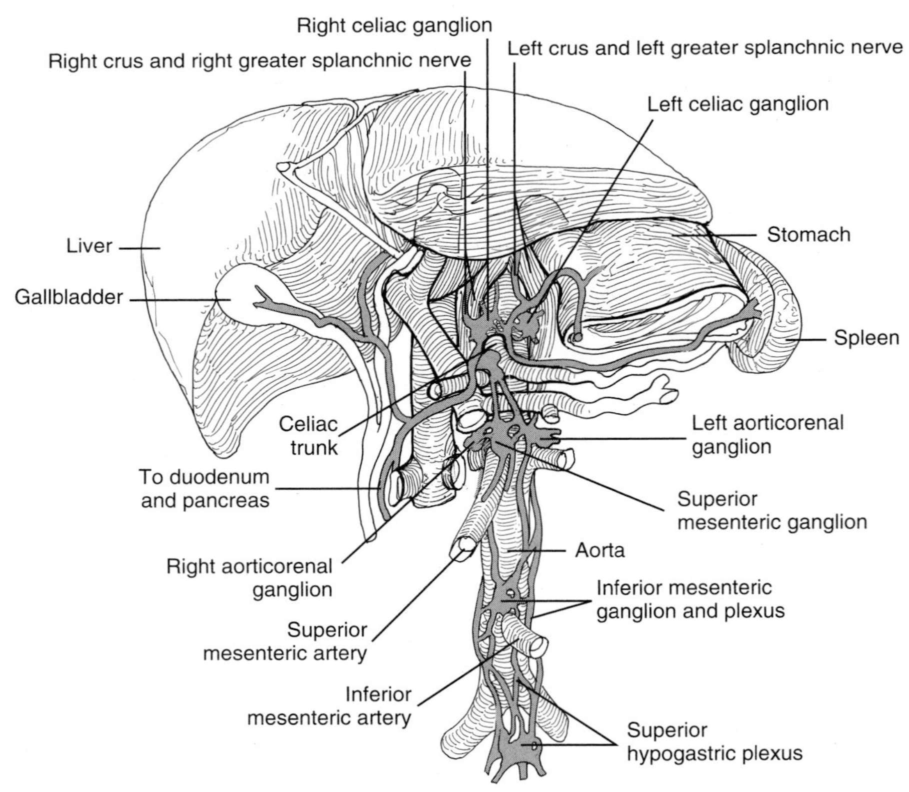

FIGURE 12–32
Preaortic ganglia and plexuses of the abdominopelvic cavity.

renal plexus, which also contains ganglia innervated by preganglionic fibers from the **least splanchnic nerve** and superior branches of the **lumbar splanchnic nerves** (see Fig. 12–31). Postganglionic sympathetic fibers that emanate from the renal plexus innervate the kidneys, ureter, and ovaries or testes.

In addition to the renal plexus, the **lumbar splanchnic nerves** innervate ganglia located within an **abdominal aortic (intermesenteric) plexus, inferior mesenteric ganglia** (which are small or difficult to visualize) associated with the inferior mesenteric artery, and **superior** and **inferior hypogastric plexuses.** Innervation of ganglia in these plexuses may also include small **lumbar splanchnic nerves,** which emanate from chain ganglia at spinal nerves L3, L4, and L5. Additional innervation may be supplied by small **sacral splanchnic nerves** arising from chain ganglia at spinal nerves S1 to S4. However, the preganglionic fibers in these small lumbar and sacral splanchnic nerves descend within the sympathetic trunk from cell bodies located at spinal cord levels L1 and L2.

The **intermesenteric plexus** distributes postganglionic fibers to the testicular or ovarian plexuses and to the lumbar segment of the **inferior vena cava.** Postganglionic fibers that emanate from the **inferior mesenteric ganglia** innervate derivatives of the hindgut (see Fig. 12–31). Postganglionic fibers emanating from the **superior** and **inferior hypogastric plexuses** provide sympathetic innervation to the hindgut and also innervate a variety of **pelvic** and **perineal organs** (see Fig. 13–12 and Chapters 14 and 15).

Parasympathetic Innervation of the Abdominal Viscera

The vagus nerve is assisted in its parasympathetic innervation of abdominopelvic viscera by the pelvic splanchnic nerves

Parasympathetic innervation of the abdominal viscera roughly corresponds to the organization just described. Small scattered ganglia within the walls of the foregut, midgut, kidneys, and adrenal glands are innervated mainly by **preganglionic parasympathetic fibers** of the vagus nerve, while ganglia within walls of the hindgut and organs of the pelvis are innervated by **preganglionic parasympathetic fibers** of the pelvic splanchnic nerves (see Fig. 12–31). The pelvic splanchnic nerves originate from levels S2 to S4 of the spinal cord. Parasympathetic ganglia within the walls of organs innervated by preganglionic parasympathetic fibers from the vagus nerve and pelvic splanchnic nerves emit short **postganglionic parasympathetic fibers** that innervate end organs, including glands and smooth muscle fibers.

Autonomic Afferent Fibers of the Abdominal Viscera

Autonomic afferent fibers accompany motor fibers of abdominopelvic sympathetic and parasympathetic nerves

General visceral afferent fibers carry sensations from abdominopelvic viscera back to the central nervous system via the same nerves that carry the autonomic (visceral efferent) fibers described above. In fact, sensory fibers make up the bulk of the vagus nerve. They also constitute a significant portion of the pelvic splanchnic nerves and the sympathetic splanchnic nerves of the abdominopelvic cavity.

The basic function of sensory fibers that accompany the sympathetic and parasympathetic nerves in the abdominopelvic cavity is **visceral reflex actions** that regulate the **peristaltic contractions** and **glandular secretions** of the gastrointestinal tract (see below). For the most part, these fibers innervate stretch receptors and chemoreceptors, which initiate reflexes that usually do not reach the level of consciousness. Nevertheless, it must be emphasized that most autonomic reflexes are not completely autonomous. Most visceral reflexes of abdominopelvic organs are initiated or modified by somatic sensations and, in addition, may be consciously manipulated by higher centers of the central nervous system (see below and Chapter 15).

In addition to the general visceral afferent fibers that regulate peristalsis and digestion through their innervation of stretch receptors and chemoreceptors within organs of the peritoneal cavity, many of the general visceral afferent fibers within the walls of these structures conduct sensations of pain. These fibers may carry sensations of visceral pain directly back to the central nervous system where they are usually perceived as dull and diffuse. Although direct visceral pain cannot be stimulated by simple cutting or crushing of viscera, it may be initiated by excessive stretching of smooth muscle or by certain pathologic conditions. Sensations from these fibers may also stimulate associated somatic pathways within the spinal cord, causing the sensation of referred pain. Referred pain is perceived as tenderness of or pain in the segment of the body wall innervated by spinal nerves that originate at the same spinal cord level to which the general visceral afferent fiber carries its impulses (see below). Thus, visceral pain or referred pain is initially mediated by general visceral afferent fibers that accompany sympathetic nerves of the abdominopelvic cavity. Exceptions to this pattern are noted below.

The Role of Intrinsic Reflexes in the Function of the Gastrointestinal Tract

Myenteric and submucous plexuses mediate, coordinate, and initiate the peristaltic, secretory, and absorptive activities of the gastrointestinal tract

In addition to the activity mediated by sympathetic or parasympathetic input, the functions of some regions of the gastrointestinal tract require the action of local **intrinsic reflexes.** This local activity, as well as all of the autonomic activity in various segments of the gastrointestinal tract, is mediated and coordinated by two complex networks of nerves and their fibers located within the walls of the abdominopelvic gastrointestinal tract. The most extensive of these plexuses is located between muscle layers of the gastric and intestinal walls and is called the **myenteric (Auerbach's) plexus.** A less complex secondary plexus is located within submucosal connective tissue of the gut and is called the **submucous (Meissner's) plexus.** These plexuses together contain as many as 100 million neuronal cell bodies. Recent evidence supports the idea that these gastrointestinal plexuses are capable of significant intrinsic activity and, in addition, may have far greater influence over higher centers of the central nervous system than was previously suspected.

Abdominal Pain: Referred Pain

Most abdominal pain in adults is associated with disorders of the gastrointestinal system

Pain from abdominal organs is usually referred to regions of the anterior body wall, which are illustrated in Fig. 12–33 and listed in Table 12–4 (see also Fig. 12–31 and Chapter 11). Impulses are carried back to the spinal cord by afferent sensory fibers at the same level from which the sympathetic innervation of the organ arises. Referred pain usually occurs when visceral organs have become stretched as a consequence of obstruction or inflammation resulting from bacterial or viral infection. Referred pain may be sharp if it is referred to a single dermatome or diffuse if it is referred to several dermatomes.

Peptic Ulcer

Perforation of a peptic ulcer is most common in males age 30 to 40 years

Peptic ulcer disease in adult males is usually localized in the duodenum rather than the stomach. The initial visceral pain is sharp, sudden, and severe and usually localized to the epigastric region. Diffuse referred pain may be felt within the entire abdominal wall and frequently in the region of the shoulders as well, especially the left shoulder (Table 12–4 and see Fig. 12–33). With complete perforation of the duodenal wall, gastric juice or chyme may drain from the duodenal lumen into the right and left paracolic gutters of the peritoneal cavity. Somatic pain resulting from consequent irritation of the parietal peritoneum may mimic the localized pain of acute appendicitis as the sensory endings of somatic afferent nerves within the dermatome are stimulated (see below). Fever and abdominal distention may accompany this condition.

Treatment of a perforated ulcer in young, healthy patients may involve patching the opening with a piece of omentum. In older, infirm patients who would suffer significant risk from surgery, antibiotics and fluid replacement may be used.

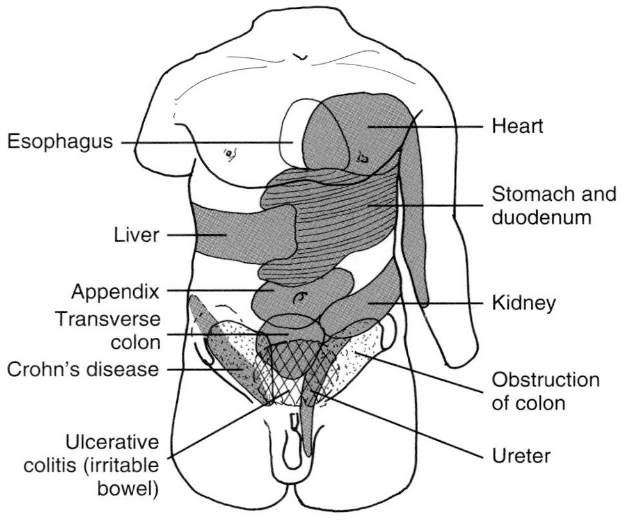

FIGURE 12–33
Referred pain. Pain from abdominopelvic organs is referred to specific dermatomes of the anterolateral and posterior body walls.

Biliary Disorders

Disorders of the biliary system are common causes of abdominal pain in obese female patients

Expression of bile from the gallbladder and bile ducts may be blocked by gallstones in the cystic duct or common bile duct, leading to infection and inflammation of the gallbladder. Although the condition may occur in males, it is most common in females 30 to 60 years old who have previously been pregnant and who suffer from digestive difficulties. These patients are commonly characterized by the four f's (female, forties, fecund, flatulent).

Referred biliary pain is initially localized in the right upper quadrant and frequently accompanied by nausea and vomiting (see Fig. 12–33 and Table 12–4). These symptoms occur most often at night or several hours after ingestion of a large meal, although it is not uncommon for pain to occur in the absence of eating. With simple obstruction of the bile duct (chronic cholecystitis), the pain may subside after several hours but then recur intermittently, sometimes over the course of several years. If the biliary tract becomes infected, the pain may not subside. This indicates progression to acute cholecystitis. In this case, referred pain may become generalized within the abdominal wall, along the right and left costal margins, and to the back (see Fig. 12–33 and Table 12–4).

Significant advances have been made in the diagnosis and surgical treatment of cholecystitis in recent years, including improvements in diagnostic imaging and laparoscopic surgical techniques.

Pancreatitis

Chronic and acute pancreatitis may result from obstruction of the pancreatic ducts, most commonly in individuals 30 to 50 years old who suffer from chronic alcoholism

Chronic pancreatitis may be silent or associated with rapid onset of constant, severe epigastric pain that radiates along the costal margins directly to the back. This is described as a piercing or knifelike pain. The pain may last a few hours to a few days (see Fig. 12–33 and Table 12–4). Although the localization of the pain resulting from pancreatitis may mimic that of peptic ulcer or biliary obstruction, the duration of episodes tends to be longer, especially when chronic pancreatitis progresses to acute pancreatitis.

In acute pancreatitis, which is characterized by autolysis (autodigestion) of pancreatic cells by their own enzymes, the duration of painful episodes often lasts even longer, from a day to a week. Patients may lose weight, be unable to digest fats, and develop diabetes mellitus because of destruction of the insulin-producing islet cells of the pancreas. Symptoms of acute pancreatitis may be exacerbated by a variety of conditions, including chronic use of alcohol, genetic predisposition to the disorder, trauma, pregnancy, infection, vascular disorders, peptic ulcer, or cystic fibrosis (see Chapter 8).

Both the chronic and acute forms of pancreatitis are suggested by the presence of pancreatic enzymes in the plasma and urine. Ultrasonography, CT scanning, or MRI may be useful in diagnosis. Treatment focuses primarily on the relief of pain resulting from distention of the pancreatic ducts. Surgical procedures include enlargement of the ampulla of Vater or main pancreatic duct and, in extreme cases, removal of the affected region of the pancreas. Nonsurgical procedures may focus on treating infection, controlling alcohol intake, or replacing pancreatic enzymes. The mortality rate from mild cases of acute pancreatitis is low, but for the more severe forms of the disease, it approaches 100%.

Appendicitis

Acute appendicitis commonly occurs in individuals age 5 to 30 years

Occlusion of the lumen of the appendix is the initiating event in the development of acute appendicitis. Pressure within the appendix increases, inhibiting venous return and arterial blood flow and resulting in necrosis and eventual perforation of the organ. Bacteria then invade the organ wall, contributing to the inflammation.

At first, patients usually complain of pain in the epigastric and umbilical regions, as in pancreatitis and peptic ulcer (see Fig. 12–33 and Table 12–4). This referred epigastric pain is the result of stretching of the appendix and conduction of impulses to spinal cord levels T10 and T11 through afferent fibers that accompany the lesser splanchnic nerve (see Fig. 12–31). In later stages, direct somatic pain is most often localized to the right lower quadrant because the perforated appendix irritates the peritoneum in this region. Direct somatic pain may result from irritation of the peritoneal lining of the body wall and conduction of impulses through the somatic sensory fibers of the spinal nerves. This pain is often caused by the entry of blood, gastric contents, pancreatic juice, urine, and bile into the peritoneal space. Intense acute peritoneal pain may cause spasm of the associated muscles of the abdominal wall. If the appendix is located within the pelvis, somatic pain associated with later stages of the disease may be localized to the lower left quadrant (see Table 12–4). If the appendix is located in a retrocecal position, pain may be localized to the right thigh or testicle. Nausea, loss of appetite, and vomiting frequently occur during episodes of appendicitis.

Ultrasound and CT scanning are useful in diagnosing acute appendicitis. Treatment almost always involves surgical removal of the inflamed appendix followed by use of antibiotics.

Intestinal Obstruction

Intestinal obstruction may result in abdominal pain

The intestine may become blocked by a mechanical obstruction or because of paralysis of the intestinal muscles. Mechanical obstruction may be the consequence of congenital disease (see above) or tumors developing within or outside of the gastrointestinal tract. Gases and fluids accumulate proximal to the obstruction, and this may trigger vomiting, dehydration, and electrolyte imbalance. Obstruction may also result in compromise of the vasculature, leading to necrosis of the affected segment.

Obstructions of the small intestine are more common in children and adolescents and are often the consequence of congenital disease. These conditions tend to cause pain in the umbilical region. Obstruction of the colon is frequently the result of a carcinoma or benign tumor and most often occurs in

TABLE 12–4
Disorders Causing Referred Pain in the Abdominal Viscera

Disorder	Region of Referred or Direct Pain
Peptic ulcer	Referred pain to entire abdominal wall
Biliary obstruction	Referred pain at first in upper right quadrant and then along right and left costal margins of back
Pancreatitis	Referred pain in epigastric regions radiating along costal margins to back
Acute appendicitis	Referred pain in epigastric and umbilical regions followed by direct pain from irritation of parietal perineum in region where appendix is located (see Fig. 12–18)
Obstruction of small intestine	Referred pain in epigastric and umbilical regions
Obstruction of colon	Referred pain in lower left quadrant
Crohn's disease	Referred pain in lower right quadrant
Ulcerative colitis	Referred pain in lower abdominal wall
Irritable bowel syndrome	Referred pain in lower abdominal wall

individuals over age 50 years. In this case, pain is more often experienced in the lower left quadrant (see Fig. 12–33 and Table 12–4).

Patients suffering from colon cancer do not necessarily experience the pain associated with intestinal obstruction. This may result in delayed diagnosis and spread of the disease to other organs, with high rates of mortality. Colon cancer accounts for 15% of all cancer deaths in the United States. Treatment of colon cancer involves surgical removal of the tumor and associated segment of colon.

Infections

Infectious disorders can result in diarrhea and consequent abdominal pain

Diarrhea is abnormally frequent defecation of liquid or semiliquid stool and is a common cause of abdominal pain. Diarrhea resulting from infectious organisms commonly occurs if individuals are living in overcrowded conditions and hygiene and sanitation are substandard or if food is improperly prepared or stored. If left untreated, diarrhea may result in severe dehydration and electrolyte imbalance and may be life threatening for young children, elderly people, or individuals whose health has been compromised by other disorders. The abdominal pain associated with infectious diarrhea may mimic that of appendicitis, obstructive bowel disease, or cholecystitis and may result in misdiagnosis of these conditions.

Dysentery is a more severe form of diarrhea characterized by watery stools frequently mixed with blood and mucus.

Noninfectious Disorders

Acute abdominal pain may result from a variety of noninfectious anatomic or physiologic disorders

Crohn's disease and ulcerative colitis present with symptoms of acute abdominal pain, diarrhea, fever, and weight loss. Patients suffering from Crohn's disease, which is a form of regional enteritis characterized by inflammation and deep patchy ulcers, tend to complain of pain in the lower right quadrant because the terminal ileum, cecum, and proximal portion of the ascending colon are most commonly affected (see Fig. 12–33 and Table 12–4). Ulcerative colitis, which is characterized by chronic inflammation and ulceration, tends to affect the rectum initially and then spreads proximally throughout the large intestine, referring pain to the lower abdominal wall (see Table 12–4). Most patients suffering from Crohn's disease or ulcerative colitis can be treated with medication. Surgical removal of the inflamed portion of the gastrointestinal tract is an option if obstruction occurs or if medical treatment is ineffective.

Irritable bowel syndrome is a common cause of abdominal pain. It may be the reason for up to 50% of visits to gastroenterologists. Patients usually present with poorly localized cramping pain in the lower abdomen, often associated with morning diarrhea or episodic diarrhea and bouts of constipation (see Fig. 12–33 and Table 12–4).

13 The Posterior Body Wall and Associated Structures

ORGANIZATION AND LANDMARKS OF THE POSTERIOR ABDOMINAL WALL

Superior, Inferior, and Lateral Boundaries

Bony landmarks of the posterior abdominal wall include the twelfth pair of ribs, lumbar vertebral bodies, sacral promontory, and iliac bones of the pelvis

With the gastrointestinal tract removed, the territory of the posterior abdominal wall can be defined by prominent, easily visualized, bony landmarks. These include the **twelfth pair of ribs, sacral promontory,** and flared **iliac bones** of the pelvis (Fig. 13–1). Soft tissue structures within this region are commonly defined by their spatial relationships to these bony landmarks.

The landmarks are also useful in diagnosing referred pain, giving injections, and performing surgery.

The **superior boundary** of the posterior body wall is defined by the **twelfth pair of ribs.** The distal end of rib 12, like that of rib 11, fails to make a cartilaginous connection with the sternum. Nonetheless, rib 12 serves as a firm anchor for the posterior region of the diaphragm and for the psoas and quadratus lumborum muscles of the posterior abdominal wall (Fig. 13–1 and see Fig. 13–2*B*).

The five massive **lumbar vertebral bodies** and their **intervertebral discs** are prominent **midline features** of the posterior abdominal wall. However, the most superior three vertebrae and their articulating discs are partially obscured by muscular slips of the diaphragm called **diaphragmatic crura** (Fig. 13–1 and see Fig. 10–9). The **right crus** extends from the tendinous anterior and right and left lateral boundaries of the esophageal hiatus superiorly and from the right anterolateral walls of vertebral bodies L1 to L3 inferiorly. The superior attachment of the **left crus** is to the central tendon just to the left of the esophageal hiatus, while its inferior attachment is to the left anterolateral walls of vertebrae L1 and L2 (Fig. 13–1 and see Fig. 10–9). Vertebral bodies L1 to L5 are also largely obscured by the abdominal aorta and inferior vena cava.

The lumbar segment of the vertebral column curves anteriorly **(lumbar lordosis)** from vertebrae L1 to L5 to meet the S1 segment of the sacrum. This superior segment of the sacrum projects anteriorly at the level of the pelvic brim and is called the **sacral promontory** (Fig. 13–1). The sacral promontory and the posterolateral regions of the right and left **arcuate lines** of the pelvic brim define the **inferior boundary of the posterior abdominal wall** (Fig. 13–1). The flared iliac bones extend superiorly from the arcuate lines of the right and left ilia to form the concavities of the **iliac fossae.** These concavities thus constitute the inferior region of the posterior abdominal wall and also define the posterior region of the **false pelvis** (Fig. 13–1 and see Chapter 12). The most superior boundaries of the iliac fossae are the prominent **iliac crests,** which can be easily palpated in living patients (Fig. 13–1 and see Chapter 14).

Muscular Boundaries

Several muscles also form boundaries of the posterior abdominal wall

The **lateral boundaries of the posterior abdominal wall** are defined by the lateral edges of the right and left **quadratus lumborum muscles.** These muscles are attached superiorly to the medial regions of each of the twelfth ribs, but the attachments are obscured by arching fibers of the diaphragm and an associated ligament called the **lateral arcuate ligament** (Fig. 13–1 and see Fig. 10–9). The quadratus lumborum muscles are attached inferiorly to the iliac crests (Fig. 13–1 and see Figs. 13–2*B* and 13–11). The lateral regions of these muscles are attached to the aponeuroses of the transversus abdominis muscles (Fig. 13–1 and see Figs. 13–2*B* and 13–11).

The **psoas major muscles** lie just between the vertebral column and the medial edges of the flanking quadratus lumborum muscles (Fig. 13–1 and see Fig. 13–11). Superior slips of these powerful **flexors of the thigh** are attached to the medial regions of the vertebral body of T12 and the vertebral bodies and transverse processes of all five lumbar vertebrae. Their most superior attachments are obscured by arching fibers of the diaphragm and an associated ligament called the **medial arcuate ligament** (see Figs. 10–9, 13–1, and 13–11). Each psoas muscle joins inferiorly with the **ili-**

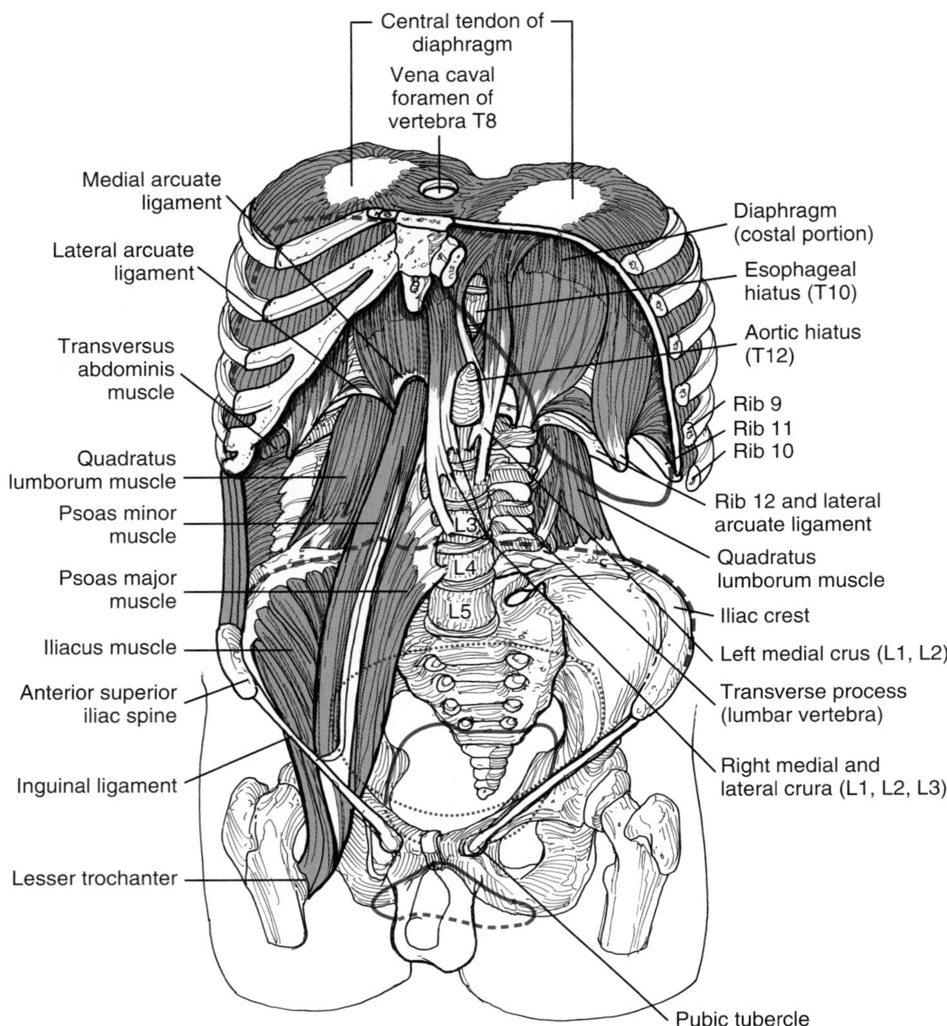

FIGURE 13–1

Skeletal and muscular elements of the posterior abdominal wall. Skeletal elements of the posterior body wall include vertebrae L1 to L5 and their intervertebral discs, the anterior surface of the sacrum, and the wings (alae) of the ilium bone on both sides of the vertebral column. The tip of floating rib 11 and most of floating rib 12 are also visible in the superior region of the posterior abdominal wall. The psoas major muscles lie adjacent to the vertebral column. A psoas minor muscle is present in 50% of individuals. The quadratus lumborum muscles are lateral to the psoas complex. Posterior fibers of the transversus abdominis muscles lie in the most lateral regions of the posterior abdominal wall (see Fig. 11–1).

acus muscle—a sheet of fibers that fills the iliac fossa (Fig. 13–1). Together, the psoas and iliacus muscles form a tendon, which extends over the anterior region of the pelvic brim but under the inguinal ligament to attach to the **lesser trochanter of the femur** (Fig. 13–1 and see Fig. 17–7). In about half of individuals, a separate slip of muscle called the **psoas minor muscle** may be observed on the anterior surface of the psoas major muscle. Its superior attachment is to the vertebral bodies of T12 and L1 and the intervening disc. Its inferior attachment is to the lateral region of the pelvic brim. The psoas and iliacus muscles are discussed in detail as muscles of the lower extremity in Chapter 17.

ORGANS AND TISSUES OF THE POSTERIOR ABDOMINAL WALL

Kidneys and Ureters

All of the organs, vessels, and nerves discussed in this chapter are **retroperitoneal structures.** They are all embedded within the subserous fascia and are visible behind a thin membrane of mesothelium that lines the posterior wall of the abdominal cavity. The definitive kidneys are retroperitoneal organs of the urinary system. During the fifth week of embryologic development, they arise from the intermediate mesoderm within the sacral region as the **metanephroi.** Between the sixth and twelfth weeks, the definitive kidneys ascend to the level

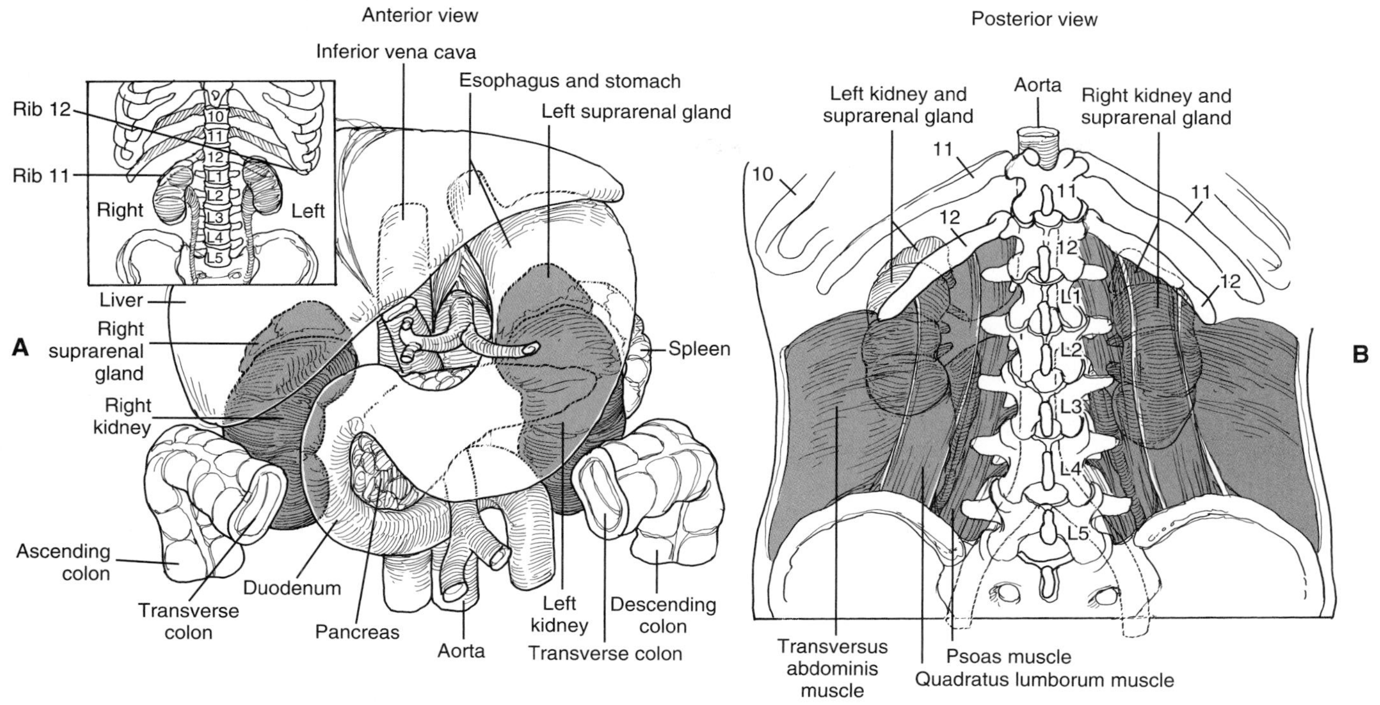

FIGURE 13–2
Relationships of organs of the posterior abdominal wall to skeletal and muscular landmarks.

of vertebrae L1 and L2. The ureters, which originally sprouted from the embryonic mesonephric ducts (see below), become implanted within the posterior wall of the bladder and elongate as the kidneys ascend. This definitive urinary system may become functional as early as the tenth week of embryonic life.

In some persons, a kidney may not ascend and so remains within the pelvis as a pelvic kidney. In others, the inferior poles of both kidneys may fuse during ascent to form a horseshoe kidney, which is caught by the inferior mesenteric artery. Kidneys may rarely ascend into the thorax through an open pericardioperitoneal canal (see Chapter 10).

In its definitive location, the right kidney is typically somewhat inferior to the left kidney, presumably because of the inferior projection of the liver on the right side (Fig. 13–2*A*). The "mapping" of structures onto the posterior surfaces of the kidneys reveals that the left kidney is closely associated with rib 11 at its superior pole, while the right kidney typically rises no higher than the lower posterior edge of the diaphragm (Fig. 13–2*B*). Other structures related to the posterior walls of both kidneys include the twelfth pair of ribs, aponeuroses of the transversus abdominis muscles, and the quadratus lumborum and psoas major muscles (Fig. 13–2*B*). Although the arrangement just described is typical, it is not universal. The relative positions of the right and left kidneys may be reversed.

The medial surface of each bean-shaped kidney is concave and contains a depression called the **hilus** (see Fig. 13–4). Arteries and veins enter and leave via the hilus. The hilus also contains the expanded renal pelvis of the collecting system of the kidney.

Fascia of the Kidneys

The fragile kidneys are protected by the eleventh and twelfth pairs of ribs and by the massive lumbar vertebral column (Fig. 13–2*B*). The kidneys are also embedded within several layers of protective fat and connective tissue, most of which differentiate from the **subserous fascia** (Fig. 13–3 and Table 13–1). The kidneys are tightly invested by a tough **fibrous capsule,** which is a derivative of the intermediate mesoderm of the developing kidney (Table 13–1 and see below). A thick specialized layer of subserous fascia, the **perirenal fat,** surrounds the fibrous capsule. This 1- to 2-inch layer of fat is further invested by a layer of connective tissue called the **renal fascia,** another specialization of the subserous fascia (Fig. 13–3). This connective tissue investment covers the kidney somewhat like an inverted sock. It has definitive **anterior** and **posterior layers,** which are fused together at the superior pole and lateral edges of the kidneys. However, the anterior and posterior layers of renal fascia do not fuse together around the medial side of each kidney. The anterior layers end blindly just anterior to the psoas muscles, while medial excursions of each posterior layer of renal fascia extend

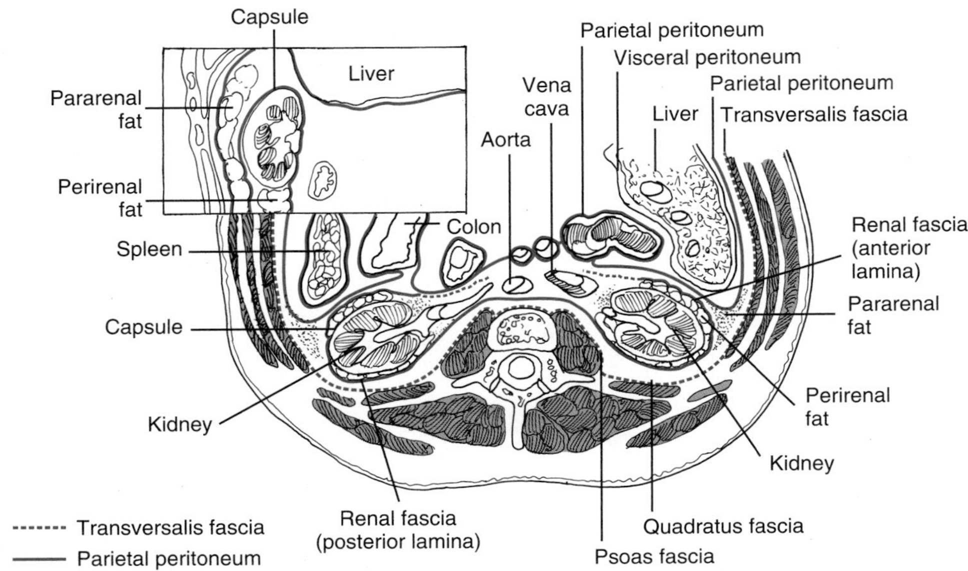

FIGURE 13–3
Specializations of subserous fascia around the kidney and their relationships to the kidney capsule and the posterior abdominal wall. Note that the renal fascia does not completely enclose the kidney and its perirenal fat in the medial and inferior regions of the kidney.

TABLE 13–1
Tissues that Cover the Kidneys From Deep to Superficial

Layer	Embryonic Origin	Region
Fibrous capsule	Intermediate mesoderm (metanephros)	All but medial
Perirenal fat	Lateral plate mesoderm (subserous fascia)	All
Renal fascia	Lateral plate mesoderm (subserous fascia)	All but medial and inferior
Pararenal fat	Lateral plate mesoderm (subserous fascia)	All but medial
Deep fascia	Lateral plate mesoderm (body wall)	All but anterior
Mesothelium	Lateral plate mesoderm (parietal lining)	Anterior

across the midline to fuse with each other (Fig. 13–3). The anterior and posterior layers of renal fascia also fail to fuse with each other inferior to the kidney (Fig. 13–3, *inset*). Another specialized type of subserous fascia, the **pararenal fat,** invests the perirenal fascia. In a lateral direction, the pararenal fat abuts the deep layer of the **fascia transversalis** and its medial continuation, the deep layers of investing fascia of the quadratus lumborum muscles **(quadratus fascia)** and psoas muscles **(psoas fascia)** (Fig. 13–3). Anterior and medial to the kidney, the pararenal fat lies adjacent to the mesothelial membrane of the peritoneum (Fig. 13–3).

Development of the Renal Units and Collecting System of the Kidneys

Development of the definitive cellular architecture of the kidneys begins when an evagination of the **mesonephric duct** called the **ureteric bud** grows into the intermediate mesoderm of the sacral region in the fifth week. This region of the intermediate mesoderm is called the **metanephric blastema.** Signals from the ureteric bud induce the formation of renal vesicles within the metanephric blastema. These vesicles form **nephric units,** which consist of the **Bowman's capsule, proximal convoluted tubule, loop of Henle,** and **distal convoluted tubule** (Fig. 13–4). In turn, signals from the metanephric blastema induce branching of the ureteric bud, which forms the **collecting system** of the kidney. The complete collecting system of each kidney includes the **collecting ducts, minor** and **major calyces, renal pelvis,** and **ureter** (Fig. 13–4). Initially, the branching ureteric bud induces formation of a lobular kidney with an uneven surface marked by numerous sulci. Normally, the sulci fill in to produce

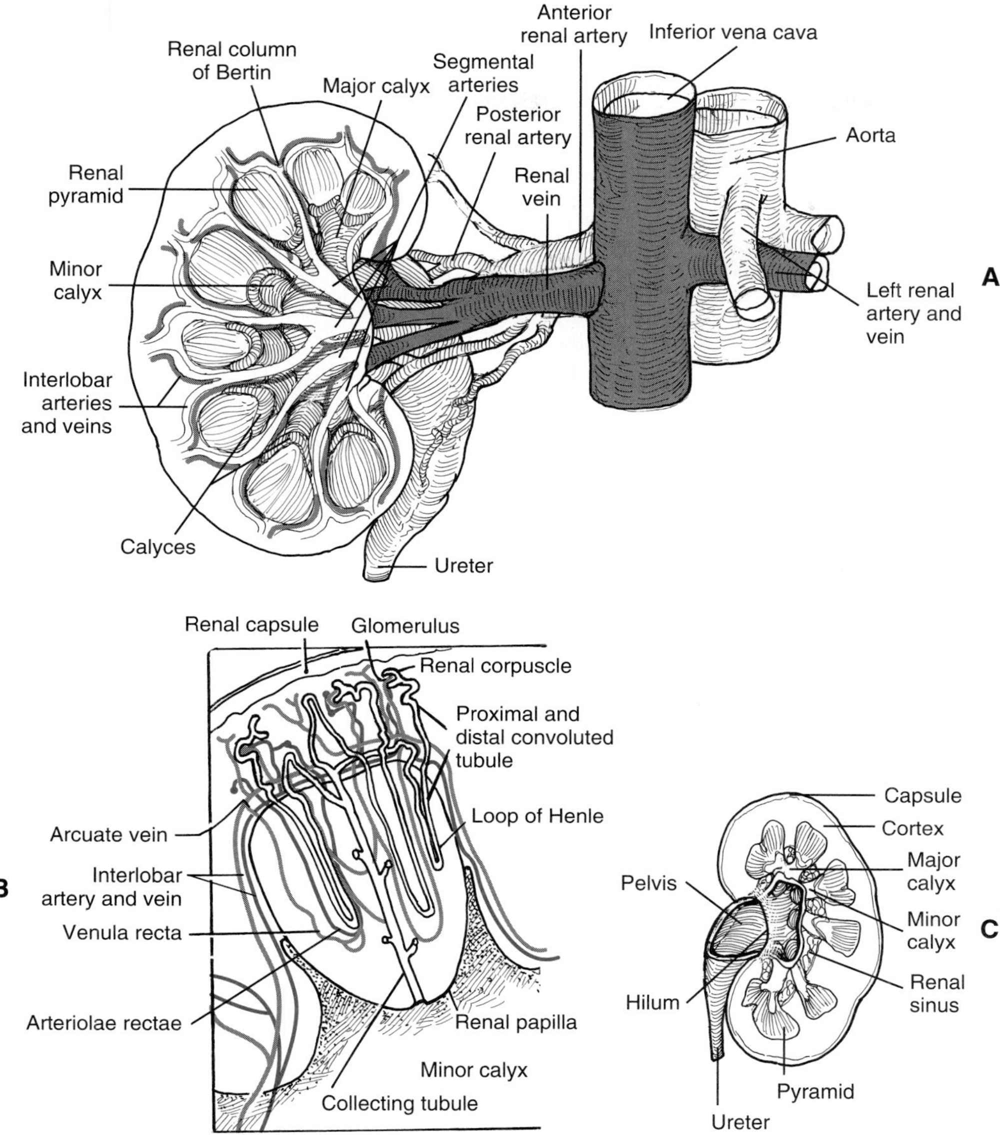

FIGURE 13–4
Architecture of the kidney. The renal cortex and columns of Bertin within the renal medulla contain the renal corpuscles (Bowman's capsules and glomeruli) and proximal and distal convoluted tubules. The collecting ducts of the kidney are located in the renal pyramids of the medulla, along with the straight arteries and veins and the loops of Henle. The collecting ducts converge at a renal papilla at the apex of a minor calyx. Several minor calyces empty into a major calyx. The major calyces empty into the renal pelvis, which, in turn, narrows to form the ureter.

the typical smooth surface of the definitive kidney. Occasionally, however, the definitive kidney retains its fetal lobulation.

A coronal section of the kidney reveals that the collecting tubules are confined to the prominent medullary **pyramids** of the kidney (Fig. 13–4). The apex of each pyramid forms a **renal papilla,** and one to three of these protrude into an expanded region of the collecting system called a **minor calyx** (Fig. 13–4C). Several minor calyces converge upon each **major calyx,** and two to four major calyces converge upon a large expansion called the **renal pelvis.** The renal pelvis narrows medially to form the **ureter** (Fig. 13–4C).

Microscopic analysis of the kidney reveals that the Bowman's capsules and proximal and distal convoluted tubules are located within the **cortical region** of the kidney and in the deeper **renal columns (of Bertin),** which lie between the pyramids. In addition to the collecting tubules, the pyramids contain the **loop of Henle, vasa recta** (straight arterioles), and **venulae recta** (straight venules) (Fig. 13–4*B*).

Ureters

The ureters are retroperitoneal organs embedded within the subserous fascia of the posterior body wall. They course inferiorly from the region of the hilus of the

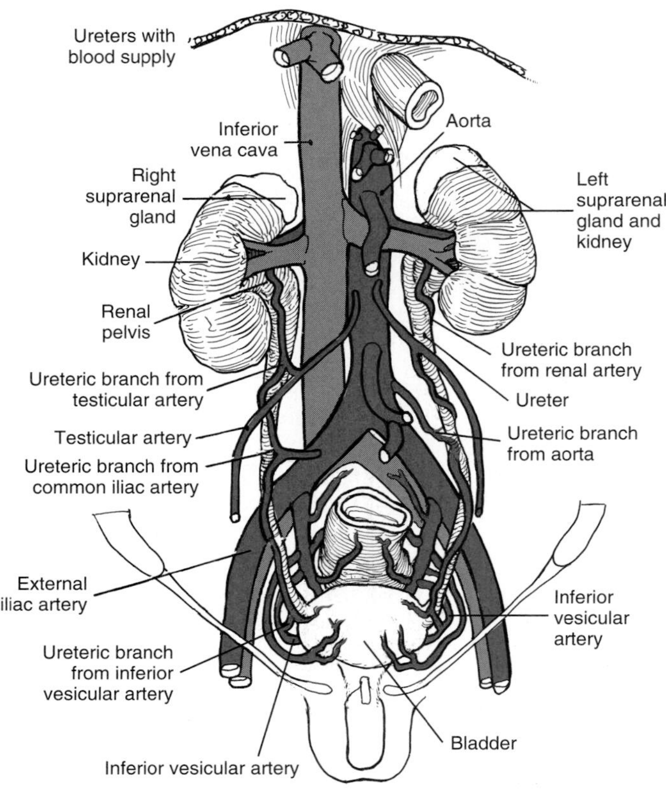

FIGURE 13–5
The ureters course from the renal pelvis of the kidney to the posterior wall of the bladder. The arterial supply is from branches of the gonadal arteries, the aorta, and the common iliac arteries.

kidney, lying posterior to the gonadal arteries and veins but anterior to the external iliac arteries and veins. The ureters course over the posterolateral edges of the pelvic brim into the pelvis and then anteriorly within the lateral pelvic wall to the posterolateral walls of the bladder (Fig. 13–5). The bladder is described in greater detail in Chapters 14 and 15.

Function of the Kidneys

The kidneys maintain the balance of sodium and water and the pH of the plasma; they also excrete toxic wastes

Initially, the kidneys produce **primary urine** by the filtration of arterial blood through the glomeruli into Bowman's capsules. The primary urine is modified by water or solutes, or both, which are reabsorbed into the vasa recta via more distal segments of the nephron and the collecting system. The urine passes through the minor and major calyces, renal pelvis, and ureter to the bladder. The kidneys eliminate wastes and maintain the osmotic homeostasis of blood via feedback mechanisms, which adjust the amounts of water and solutes eliminated in the urine according to the amounts taken in during ingestion.

The glomeruli restrict the transport of blood cells and molecules larger than 5 to 6 kDa (typically proteins) into the Bowman's capsules but freely allow the transport of water, small metabolites, and ions. The primary urine is, therefore, referred to as an **ultrafiltrate of blood.** This ultrafiltrate is modified by processes of secretion and reabsorption as it passes through more distal tubules of the nephrons and the collecting tubules on its way to the ureters and bladder. The reabsorption of sodium is primarily regulated by the mineralocorticoid hormone **aldosterone,** which is produced by the cortex of the suprarenal gland. Water is passively reabsorbed with sodium from the lumen of the **proximal tubules.** In the region of the **distal tubules** and **collecting ducts,** however, water reabsorption is actively regulated by **antidiuretic hormone,** which is produced by the pituitary gland.

As urine passes through the nephron and collecting system, it is concentrated by countercurrent mechanisms, which use the parallel arrangement of descending and ascending limbs of Henle, collecting ducts, and vasa recta within the pyramids of the **renal medulla.**

The homeostasis of other ions such as potassium and calcium is also regulated by the kidneys. Potassium excretion is directly related to sodium reabsorption in the proximal tubule and loop of Henle, but adjustments in relative proportions of plasma and urine potassium may occur within the distal tubules.

Calcium homeostasis is specifically regulated in all regions by calcitonin, which stimulates excretion, and by parathormone, which stimulates reabsorption. Both hormones are produced by the parathyroid glands.

Glucose is filtered into the Bowman's capsule without restriction, but nearly 100% of it is actively reabsorbed, mainly by the proximal tubules in conjunction with active sodium reabsorption. This occurs even in persons in whom the glucose concentration in the blood may be relatively high. However, once the blood glucose concentration approaches a threshold of approximately 2 g/L (renal threshold), glucose is excreted in the urine. In individuals lacking active insulin-secreting β-cells (e.g., patients with insulin-dependent diabetes mellitus), blood glucose levels more often exceed the renal threshold and glucose is more frequently excreted in the urine, producing the classic "sweet" urine of diabetics.

Proteins are too large to be filtered into the Bowman's capsules in healthy individuals, but amino acids freely pass through the glomerulus to become part of the primary urine. However, specific active transporters cause nearly all of the amino acids to be reabsorbed into the vasa recta as urine flows through the proximal tubules, loop of Henle, and distal tubules. Urea, an end product of protein metabolism, is filtered without restriction into the Bowman's capsules, but only about 50% of it typically remains in the final urine following its passive reabsorption and secretion by more distal segments of the nephron.

Secretion of Hormones by the Kidneys

The kidneys also secrete hormones

The kidneys secrete protein hormones, including erythropoietin and renin. **Erythropoietin** stimulates the production of red blood cells in blood-producing organs such as the marrow. **Renin** plays a key role in regulation of the liver factor **angiotensinogen.** Circulating angiotensinogen is eventually converted to angiotensin II and III (in part by the action of renin). **Angiotensin II** and **III** regulate vascular tone and stimulate secretion of the hormone **aldosterone** by the suprarenal cortex, stimulating the reabsorption of sodium and water within the proximal tubules (see above). The secretion of renin and its release by the kidney are stimulated by sodium deficiency or low blood pressure. The release of renin is also stimulated by **sympathetic excitation,** a mechanism that may affect the retention of plasma sodium and water following injury and blood loss.

Disorders of Kidney Function

Kidney function may be impaired by exogenous or endogenous conditions

As is evident from the discussion above, normal kidney function is possible only when a profuse renal blood flow maintains a certain level of hydrostatic pressure within the glomerular capillaries. Underperfusion, leading to renal dysfunction, can result from a reduction in the overall circulating blood volume (trauma and bleeding) caused by renal artery disease or vasoconstriction. These conditions commonly occur in response to kidney transplantation or as a side effect of some drugs.

Diseases of nephric tissue may also lead to renal failure. In acute nephrotic syndrome, the glomerular filtration apparatus leaks excessively, allowing unrestricted filtration of large protein molecules into the urine. Unfortunately, these conditions do not typically have overt symptoms.

Kidney Stones

Kidney stones cause severe pain with clearly diagnosable characteristics

Kidney stones (calculi) typically form when excess calcium, phosphate, or oxalate precipitates in the urine. These inorganic kidney stones may result from hyperparathyroidism, which leads to excess calcium and phosphate excretion. Alternatively, organic kidney stones may develop as a consequence of defective reabsorption of amino acids such as cysteine (cystinuria). Up to 5% of individuals develop inorganic renal calculi within their lifetimes, and most (80%) have more than one episode of calculus-related pain. At first, the calculi develop within the major or minor calyces or the renal pelvis as microscopic structures, which grow by aggregation. The patient typically has no symptoms until a calculus grows larger and enters the ureter. If the calculus is large enough, it may become stuck or impacted at various points along the ureter, most commonly in constricted regions at (1) the junction of the renal pelvis and ureter, (2) the point at which the ureter enters the true pelvis at the pelvic brim, or (3) the junction of the ureter and urinary bladder. If referred pain is produced as a consequence of impaction in each of these regions, the pain moves along the body wall from dermatome to dermatome as the calculus becomes stuck at each point (see Fig. 12–33). At first, severe pain is experienced in the flank near the costovertebral angle within dermatomes related to the lesser or least splanchnic nerves (spinal cord levels T10, T11, and T12). As the calculus becomes stuck in the ureter at the pelvic brim or at the junction of the ureter and bladder, pain may be felt in the groin (in males, in the penis and testis, and in females, in the labium majus). This occurs because the sensation of pain is experienced within dermatomes related to the lumbar splanchnic nerves (spinal cord levels L1 and L2). Pain may also be felt within the anterior region of the thigh that is innervated by the genitofemoral nerve. Consequent motor reflexes may stimulate contraction of the cremaster muscle, raising the testis in males. If impaction or swelling of the ureter has occurred, the pain may persist for hours to days following passage of the stone. However, in most cases, passage of the stone relieves the pain. Secondary effects of renal calculi include infection resulting in fever and dysuria (painful urination). Treatment consists of drinking large volumes (2–3 L/d) of fluids that do not contain the high concentrations of calcium that are found in milk or oxalate. Large stones settling in the bladder may be surgically removed or pulverized by ultrasound.

Ectopic or Bifid Ureters

Ectopic or bifid ureters may result in chronic infection of the urinary tract

In some embryos, the ureteric bud bifurcates before it reaches the metanephric blastema during the fourth and fifth weeks of development, forming a bifid (Y-shaped) ureter. One branch may end blindly. Most of the kidney is usually drained by the lower branch. Even though the two branches are derived from the same ureteric bud, their contractions may not be synchronous and urine may reflux from one branch to the other, resulting in stagnation of urine and infection. The condition may be alleviated by surgical removal of the less functional branch along with the small region of the kidney that it drains.

More than one ureteric bud may branch from the mesonephric duct during the fifth week so that two ureters are formed. The normal ureter tends to drain the larger inferior pole of the kidney, opening into the bladder in a normal location. The ectopic ureter usually drains a diminutive superior pole of the kidney, opening into an inferior ectopic location. In males, drainage may occur within the pelvic urethra, usually at a point superior to the urethral sphincter (suprasphincteric location). In females, the ectopic ureter usually drains below the urethral sphincter (extrasphincteric location) into the vestibule of the vagina or the vagina, resulting in chronic "wetting." The ectopic ureter and upper pole of the kidney may be surgically removed to alleviate the problem. In males, surgery may also be required to alleviate chronic infection in an ectopic ureter.

Kidney Transplantation

Kidney transplantation is now commonplace in many parts of the world

The first kidney transplantation was attempted in 1902. The operation was not successful, however, until the significance of histocompatibility was appreciated in the 1950s and immunosuppressive drugs were developed in the late 1970s. Donor kidneys are typically implanted within the iliac fossa. The donor renal artery is anastomosed to the external or internal iliac artery, and the renal vein is anastomosed to the external iliac vein. The ureter of the donor kidney is grafted to the wall of the bladder.

▲ Suprarenal (Adrenal) Glands

Suprarenal (adrenal) glands are retroperitoneal compound endocrine organs

The **adrenal (suprarenal) glands** cover the superior pole of each kidney like a cap (Fig. 13–6). The glands are invested by a tough capsule with septal extensions, which penetrate its cortex. These septa contain the arteries that supply the glands (see below). Each gland has a diminutive hilus, which transmits the adrenal vein. The hilus of the left gland is on its medial surface, and the hilus of the right gland is on its anterior surface. The adrenal glands are embedded within the **perirenal fat** and are invested by the **renal fascia** in the same way as the kidneys. They are, therefore, retroperitoneal organs. The medial surface of the pyramidal right adrenal gland is closely related to the inferior vena cava; the superolateral surface is related to the liver; and the posterior surface is related to the diaphragm. The anterior surface of the crescentic left adrenal gland is related to the stomach and pancreas, while the posterior surface is related to the diaphragm.

Each adrenal gland is a composite of two endocrine glands (i.e., ductless glands that secrete hormones directly into the systemic circulation). These glands are the **cortex,** which synthesizes steroid hormones (i.e., corticosteroids and sex hormones), and the **medulla,** which produces catecholamines (Fig. 13–6). The cortex arises through differentiation of the mesothelial lining of the posterior body wall during the sixth week. The medulla is produced by invading neural crest cells. At birth, the adrenal glands are one-third as large as the kidneys. In adults, however, they are only one-thirtieth as large as the kidneys because of the growth of the kidneys and the acute regression of the thick fetal cortex of the adrenal glands following birth. In the definitive adrenal gland, the cortex is about 90% of the gland's total volume, and the medulla is about 10% of the gland's total volume. The distinction between the adrenal cortex and the medulla is typically difficult to appreciate in the laboratory. However, a coronal section may reveal a contrast between a dull yellow cortex and a much smaller central gray medulla (Fig. 13–6).

Function of the Suprarenal (Adrenal) Glands

Suprarenal (adrenal) glands perform multiple functions

Each **suprarenal gland** has an outer **cortex,** which surrounds a central **medulla.** The cortex has three zones, which produce three different steroid hormones. The outermost zone produces **glucocorticoid hormones;** the middle zone, **mineralocorticoid hormones;** and the innermost zone, **sex hormones.** The adrenal medulla produces the catecholamine hormones **adrenalin** and **noradrenalin.**

Glucocorticoids are largely responsible for the regulation of glucose metabolism (including the formation of glucose from protein, amino acids, and fat) and for the conversion of glucose to glycogen. Glucocorticoids also regulate and coordinate many of the body's re-

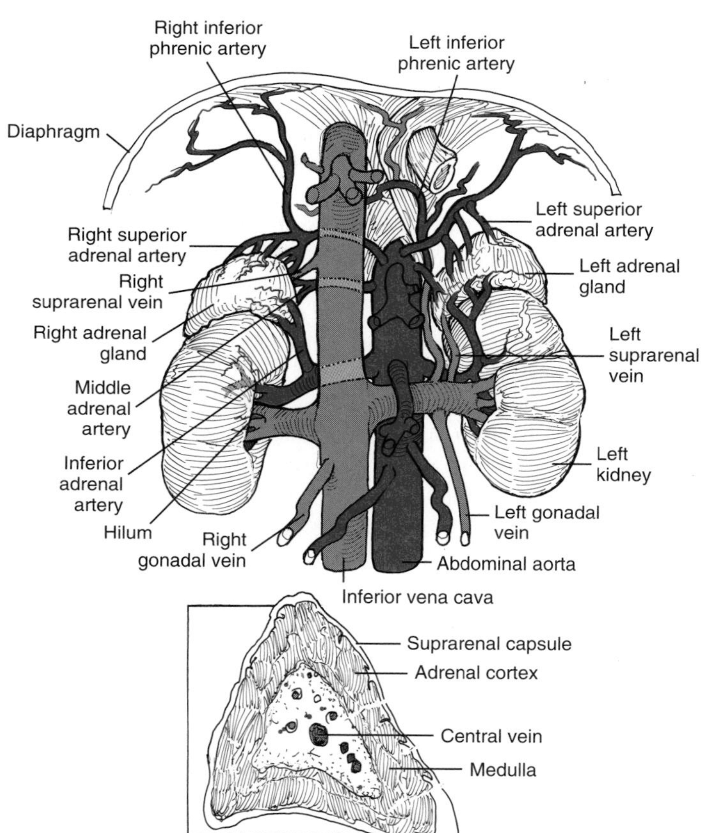

FIGURE 13–6
The suprarenal (adrenal) glands. The suprarenal glands are compound endocrine organs, which consist of a cortex and a medulla. The cortex (derived from lateral plate mesoderm) secretes steroid hormones. The medulla (derived from neural crest cells) secretes catecholamines. The arterial supply to the suprarenal gland is from branches of the aorta, branches of the renal arteries, and branches of the inferior phrenic arteries.

sponses to infection by inhibiting inflammation and suppressing the immune system. **Mineralocorticoids,** such as aldosterone, play an active role in regulating sodium and water reabsorption as well as potassium secretion by the kidneys. **Sex hormones** produced within the adrenal cortex of males and females are of greatest significance in specific pathologic states such as female pseudohermaphroditism or precocious puberty. Secretion of **adrenalin** and **noradrenalin** by the adrenal medulla typically occurs in a state of "fight or flight" during activation of the sympathetic nervous system. Therefore, as would be expected (see Chapter 4), these hormones increase the blood pressure and heartbeat, dilate the bronchi, inhibit gastrointestinal motility, and stimulate the breakdown of glycogen.

Disorders of the Adrenal Glands

Pathologic disorders of the adrenal glands may lead to hormone hyposecretion or hypersecretion

Addison's disease is characterized by hyposecretion of adrenal steroid hormones. This usually results from the destruction of adrenocortical cells. Patients with this condition experience weakness and fatigue, weight loss and anorexia (diminished appetite), hyperpigmentation (frequently misdiagnosed as "suntan"), hypotension (low blood pressure), gastrointestinal upsets (e.g., nausea, vomiting, diarrhea), a craving for salt, and dizziness. Addison's disease tends to develop slowly and insidiously. It is difficult to make the diagnosis before as many as 90% of the cells of the adrenal cortex have been destroyed.

Cushing's disease is characterized by hypersecretion of glucocorticoids. As is the case with Addison's disease, Cushing's disease develops quite slowly. Symptoms include muscle weakness and obesity, particularly in the abdomen and face. The breakdown of connective tissue results in red or purple indentations in the skin of the abdomen. The most common cause is hypersecretion of adrenocorticotropic hormone (ACTH) by the pituitary gland (either directly or as a result of increased secretion of ACTH-releasing factor by the hypothalamus). Another cause is a tumor of the adrenal cortex. Such tumors may also cause hypersecretion of sex hormones, resulting in precocious puberty in children.

▲ Lumbar Plexus

The prominent lumbar plexus can be defined in relationship to bony and muscular landmarks of the posterior abdominal wall

The **lumbar plexus** is formed by interconnecting fibers of the **ventral rami** of spinal nerves T12 to L5 (Fig. 13–7). Although this nerve plexus is a prominent feature of the posterior abdominal wall and contains nerves that innervate the wall's quadratus lumborum, psoas, and iliacus muscles, its function is more significantly related to the anterolateral abdominal wall (see Chapter 11) and lower extremities (see Chapters 16 to 18). On the other hand, the dorsal rami of the thoracic and lumbar spinal nerves, which contribute to the lumbar plexus, innervate the true deep muscles of the back (see Chapter 5). The **sacral plexus** is formed by sacral nerves (see Chapter 14). These nerves course from the pelvic cavity to innervate structures within the perineum, gluteal region, and lower extremity (see Chapters 14 to 18). A small **coccygeal plexus** is composed of interconnecting sacral and coccygeal nerves, which have minor functions in the perineum (see Chapters 14 and 15). The composition of the lumbar plexus is described in Table 13–2.

The general structure and organization of the lumbar plexus are sometimes difficult to appreciate because they may differ from one individual to another. This may be problematic in the dissection laboratory. However, individual variations may be revealed by the following approach.

Although the **subcostal nerve** is not a formal component of the lumbar plexus, it should be identified first to avoid confusing it with the more inferior nerves of the plexus proper. The subcostal nerve is closely related to the inferior edge of rib 12, a landmark that is easily palpated in cadavers or living patients (Fig. 13–7). Identification of spinal nerve L1 is problematic because it may split into the iliohypogastric and ilioinguinal nerves at varying points along its course (Fig. 13–7). The genitofemoral nerve may also be difficult to identify because it splits into its genital and femoral branches at different points along its course. It is, therefore, most useful to next define the lateral femoral cutaneous nerve, which has consistent unique, definitive characteristics. The **lateral femoral cutaneous nerve** emerges from beneath the lateral border of the psoas muscle, courses across the inferior region of the posterior abdominal wall and iliac fossa, and escapes the abdomen by coursing under the inguinal ligament just anterior to the anterior superior iliac spine onto the superior part of the lateral thigh (Fig. 13–7). To appreciate the course of this nerve in the laboratory, one should free it as it passes under the inguinal ligament and onto the lateral thigh.

If two nerves are present between the subcostal nerve and the lateral femoral cutaneous nerve, they are probably the **iliohypogastric** and **ilioinguinal nerves,** which have branched within the substance of the psoas muscle (Fig. 13–7). If only a single nerve is observed, it may be the **ventral ramus of spinal nerve L1,** which has not yet split into its iliohypogastric and ilioinguinal branches. In some cases, the ventral ramus of spinal nerve L1 may split into its iliohypogastric and ilioinguinal branches in plain view on the posterior abdominal wall (Fig. 13–7). Alternatively, it may split only after it has disappeared into the space between the opaque fibers of the transversus abdominis muscle and the internal oblique muscle within the lateral body wall

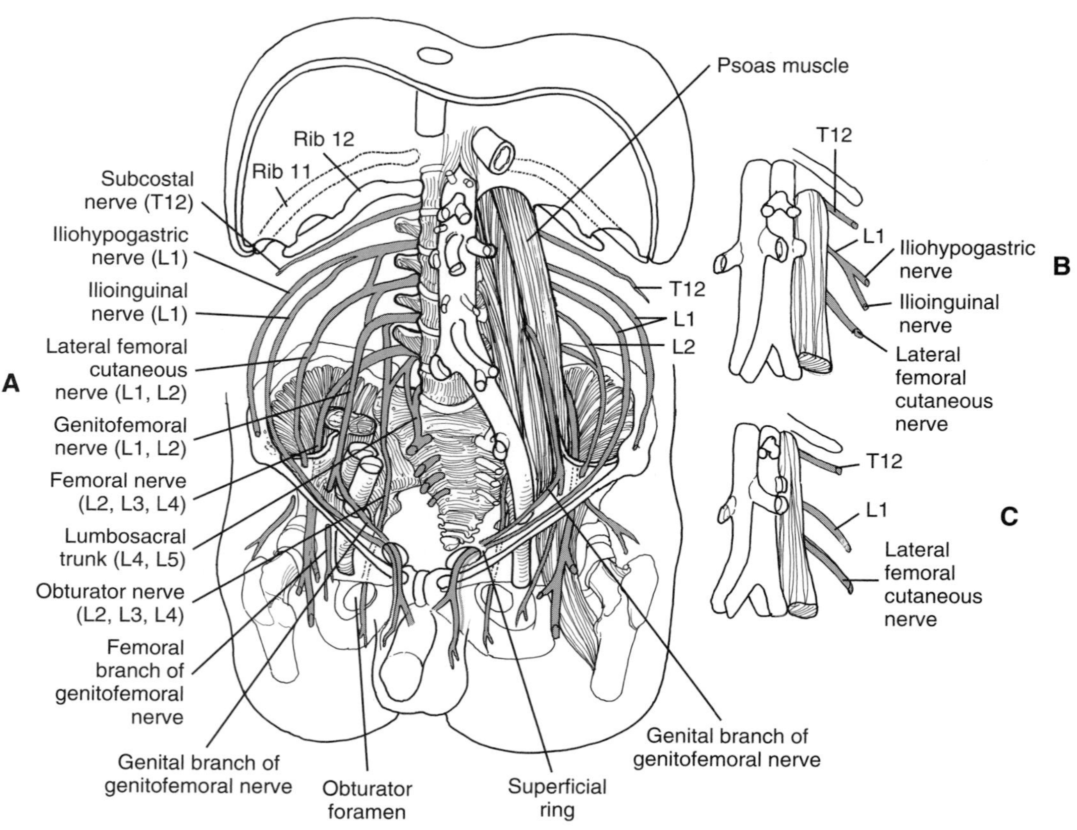

FIGURE 13–7

The lumbar plexus. Ventral rami from spinal nerves L1 to L5 interconnect to form a plexus that contributes mainly to the innervation of the lower extremity (see Chapter 18). The pattern of nerves depends to some extent upon the points at which the iliohypogastric and ilioinguinal nerves branch from spinal nerve L1 (variations shown in **B** and **C**) and the points at which the femoral and genital branches of the genitofemoral nerve (L1, L2) divide into its femoral and genital branches. The sacral and coccygeal plexuses of the pelvic cavity are described in Chapter 14.

TABLE 13–2
Nerves of the Lumbar Plexus

Nerve	Origin	Field of Innervation
Nerves to quadratus lumborum muscle	T12, L1, L2, L3	Quadratus lumborum muscle
Iliohypogastric nerve	L1	Iliac and hypogastric regions of anterior abdominal wall; its lateral cutaneous branch innervates skin of gluteal region
Ilioinguinal nerve	L1	Inferior iliac and hypogastric regions of anterior abdominal wall and skin of anterior labium majus or scrotum and medial thigh
Genitofemoral nerve	L1, L2	Genital branch: cremaster muscle, skin of scrotum, skin of labium majus and medial thigh Femoral branch: skin of anterior thigh
Lateral femoral cutaneous nerve	L2, L3	Lateral skin of thigh
Nerves to psoas and iliacus muscles	L2, L3, L4	Psoas and iliacus muscles (see Chapters 16 and 17)
Femoral nerve	L2, L3, L4	Anterior compartment of thigh (see Chapters 16 and 17); nerves to psoas and iliacus may accompany femoral nerve
Obturator nerve	L2, L3, L4	Medial compartment of thigh (see Chapters 16 and 17)
Accessory obturator nerve	L3, L4	Medial compartment of thigh (see Chapters 16 and 17)
Lumbosacral trunk nerve	L4, L5	Posterior thigh, lateral and anterior leg, dorsum of foot (Chapters 16 and 17)

(Fig. 13–7). In some cases, the ilioinguinal, iliohypogastric, or lateral femoral cutaneous nerve may be so small that it may be completely missed in laboratory dissection.

The **genitofemoral nerve** may also branch within the substance of the psoas muscle or more inferiorly, just adjacent to the anterior abdominal wall or at any point between. By identifying the lateral femoral cutaneous nerve first, the student can avoid confusing it with the **genital branch of the genitofemoral nerve,** which may lie upon the lateral wall of the psoas muscle. The genital branch may also be defined by its entry through the deep ring into the inguinal canal. The **femoral branch of the genitofemoral nerve** may be identified as it passes under the inguinal ligament to provide sensory innervation to the most superior part of the anterior thigh (Fig. 13–7). (The **thigh** is the part of the lower extremity above the knee [see Chapter 16].)

The **femoral nerve** is a large nerve lying close to the lateral side of the psoas muscle and coursing under the midregion of the inguinal ligament to enter the anterior compartment of the thigh (Fig. 13–7). In contrast, the **obturator nerve** courses deep to the psoas muscle along its posteromedial surface and cannot be easily viewed without reflecting the psoas muscle laterally. This nerve exits the pelvis via the **obturator canal** into the medial compartment of the thigh (Fig. 13–7 and Chapter 18). An **accessory obturator nerve** may also be present but is formed only from fibers of spinal nerves L3 and L4 (Fig. 13–7). It follows the same course as the obturator nerve and also enters the medial compartment of the thigh.

Finally, fibers from the ventral rami of spinal nerves L4 and L5 join together to form a large but well-hidden **lumbosacral trunk.** This massive nerve is closely associated with the vertebral column, where, in the region of the alar process of the sacrum, it joins with fibers from the ventral rami of spinal nerves S1, S2, and S3 to form nerves of the gluteal region, posterior thigh, and leg (Fig. 13–7). These fibers exit the pelvis via the **greater sciatic foramen** of the pelvis (see Chapter 15).

SYSTEMS THAT INTEGRATE STRUCTURES OF THE POSTERIOR ABDOMINAL WALL: VASCULATURE, LYMPHATICS, AND NERVES

Arteries of the Posterior Abdominal Wall

The arterial vasculature supplies the body wall and glandular and gastrointestinal viscera.

Abdominal Aorta

The abdominal aorta has three major kinds of branches and several other miscellaneous branches

The abdominal aorta lies somewhat to the right on the anterior surface of the vertebral column (see Figs. 13–1 and 13–7). It is visible superiorly at the level of the twelfth thoracic vertebral body as it enters the abdomen through the **aortic hiatus** (see Figs. 13–1 and 10–9). It courses to the level of the intervertebral disc between vertebrae L4 and L5 where it bifurcates into the **common iliac arteries** (Fig. 13–8 and see Fig. 13–5). Along this course, the abdominal aorta emits (1) the paired posterolateral **lumbar arteries,** (2) the paired lateral **glandular arteries,** (3) the three ventral **vitelline branches,** which supply the gastrointestinal tract, and (4) several **miscellaneous branches,** such as the inferior phrenic and ureteric arteries (Table 13–3 and Fig. 13–8 and see Fig. 13–9).

Posterolateral Branches of the Abdominal Aorta

Paired posterolateral branches supply the body wall and spine

As in the case of the thoracic aorta, the abdominal segment of the descending aorta emits paired posterolateral branches that vascularize the body wall, vertebral column, and spinal cord. The paired intersegmental arteries emitted at the level of vertebra L1 mimic the organization and distribution of the more superior intercostal arteries. This pair of **lumbar arteries** vascularize dermatome L1 from the back to the lateral abdominal wall (see Fig. 13–8). Their branches also vascularize the vertebral column and inferior end of the spinal cord. Indeed, an anterior radicular branch of the first left lumbar artery may provide most of the blood to the lower two thirds of the spinal cord. This artery is called the **major anterior radicular artery** or the **artery of Adamkiewicz.** In other persons, however, the major anterior radicular artery may branch from a lower posterior intercostal artery. More inferior lumbar arteries **(arteries L2 to L4)** also vascularize structures of the back, including the deep back muscles, integument, and vertebral column (see Fig. 13–8). It should be recalled from Chapter 11 that most of the anterolateral abdominal wall is vascularized by **intercostal arteries** from vertebrae T7 to T12. Because the dorsal aorta splits into the **common iliac arteries** at the intervertebral disc between vertebral bodies L4 and L5, the last lumbar artery just inferior to vertebra L5 may branch from a diminutive midline extension of the dorsal aorta, the **median sacral artery,** rather than from the aorta itself (see Fig. 13–8 and below). More often, however, artery L5 branches from the **iliolumbar branch** of the **external iliac artery** (Fig. 13–9 and see Chapter 14).

Lateral Glandular Branches of the Abdominal Aorta

Paired lateral aortic branches vascularize paired abdominal glands

The dorsal aorta emits several pairs of lateral **glandular branches,** including the **renal arteries, middle suprarenal arteries,** and **gonadal (ovarian** or **testicular) arteries.**

The **renal arteries** are usually a single pair of large lateral vessels that branch from the abdominal aorta at the level of vertebral body L1 (see Figs. 13–8 and 13–9). As the kidneys ascend during development (see above), they are vascularized by successively higher branches of

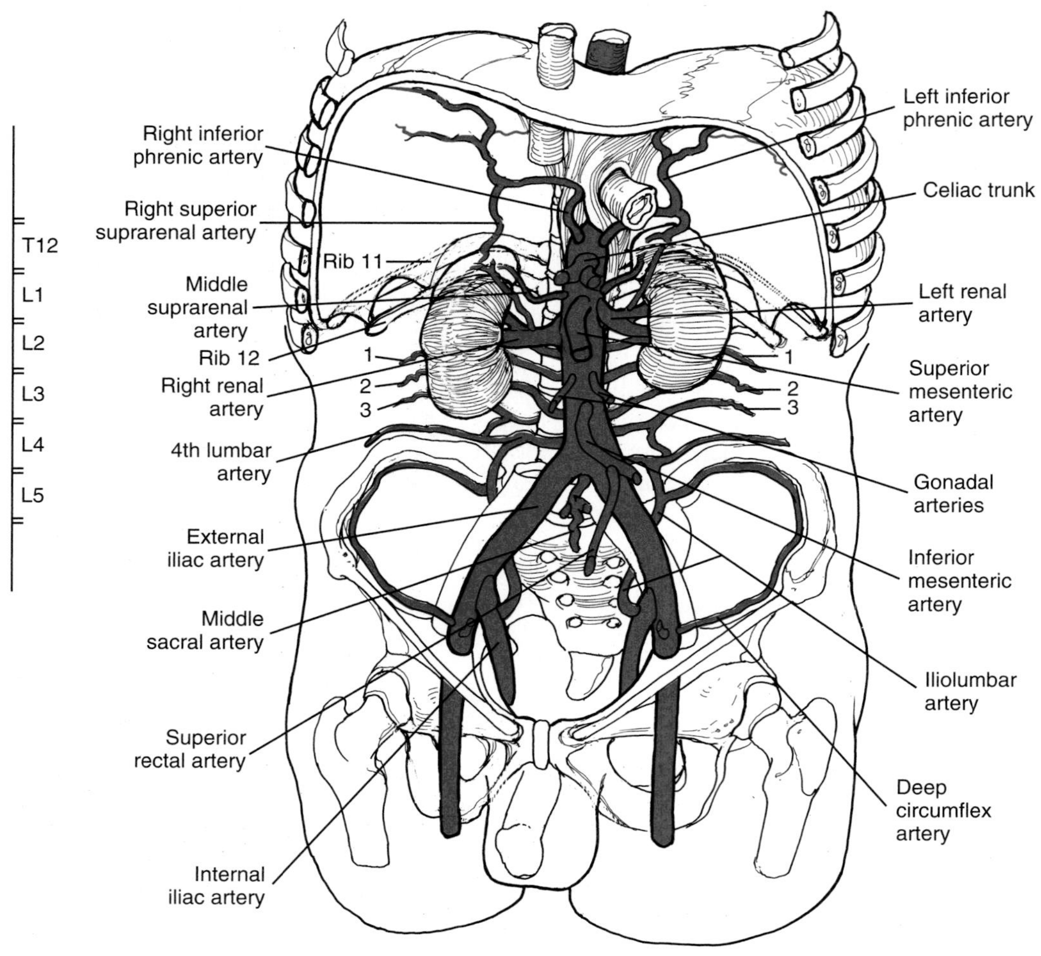

FIGURE 13–8

Arteries of the posterior abdominal wall. The aorta lies slightly to the left of the midline before it bifurcates into the left and right common iliac arteries. The aorta gives off posterolateral branches to the body wall (lumbar arteries), lateral branches to glands (renal, suprarenal, and gonadal arteries), and ventral branches to the gastrointestinal tract (celiac, superior mesenteric, and inferior mesenteric arteries). Other smaller arterial branches of the aorta supply the diaphragm, ureters, and posterior wall of the rectum.

the dorsal aorta. In some persons, however, inferior branches may not degenerate, and so these branches may form additional **accessory renal arteries.** The right renal artery usually courses posterior to the inferior vena cava, but some accessory renal arteries may pass anterior to the inferior vena cava. The renal arteries also produce **adrenal branches,** which vascularize the inferior pole of each suprarenal gland (see Figs. 13–6 and 13–9). The adrenal glands are also vascularized by branches of the aorta and the inferior phrenic arteries (see Figs. 13–6*A* and 13–8 and below).

The **gonadal arteries** branch from the abdominal aorta at the level of vertebra L2 or L3 (see Fig. 13–8). The level may vary in different individuals and from one side to the other in the same individual. Typically, the right gonadal artery branches at a more inferior level than the left. These arteries were originally branches of the descending aorta at the level of vertebra T10 during initial formation of the gonads at this level in the posterior abdominal wall. However, the roots of the gonadal arteries slowly descend to a midlumbar level during development. In addition, as the gonads descend during embryonic and fetal life, the gonadal arteries also elongate, following the ovaries into the broad ligaments of the uterus or the testes into the scrotum (see Chapter 15).

Ventral Vitelline Branches of the Abdominal Aorta

Three ventral vitelline branches vascularize the abdominal gut

The third major category of arterial branches of the abdominal aorta is the ventral derivatives of the vitelline arteries, which vascularize the gastrointestinal tract. These unpaired arteries, which branch directly from the anterior surface of the aorta, include the **celiac, superior mesenteric,** and **inferior mesenteric arteries** (see Figs. 13–8 and 13–9). These vessels and their branches are described in detail in Chapter 12.

TABLE 13–3
Branches of the Abdominal Aorta

Type	Name	Level of Origin	Vascular Field
INTERSEGMENTAL	L1	L1 vertebral body	Entire L1 dermatome, vertebral column, spinal column, back muscles and skin
	L2 to L4	L2 to L4 vertebral bodies	Vertebral column, back muscles and skin of L2 to L3 dermatomes
GLANDULAR	Suprarenal	T12 to L1 disc	Suprarenal glands
	Renal	L1 vertebral body	Kidneys (suprarenal glands)
	Accessory renal	L1 to L2 vertebral bodies	Lower poles of kidneys
	Gonadal	L2 to L3 vertebral bodies	Testes in males, ovaries in female
VITELLINE	Celiac	T12 vertebral body	Foregut
	Superior mesenteric	L1 vertebral body	Midgut
	Inferior mesenteric	L3 vertebral body	Hindgut
MISCELLANEOUS	Inferior phrenic	T12 vertebral body	Inferior surface of diaphragm (suprarenal glands)
	Ureteric	L4 vertebral body	Midregion of ureter
	Common iliacs	L4 to L5 disc	Pelvis and lower extremities
	Median sacral	L4 to L5 disc	Muscles and skin of lower back, posterior wall of rectum

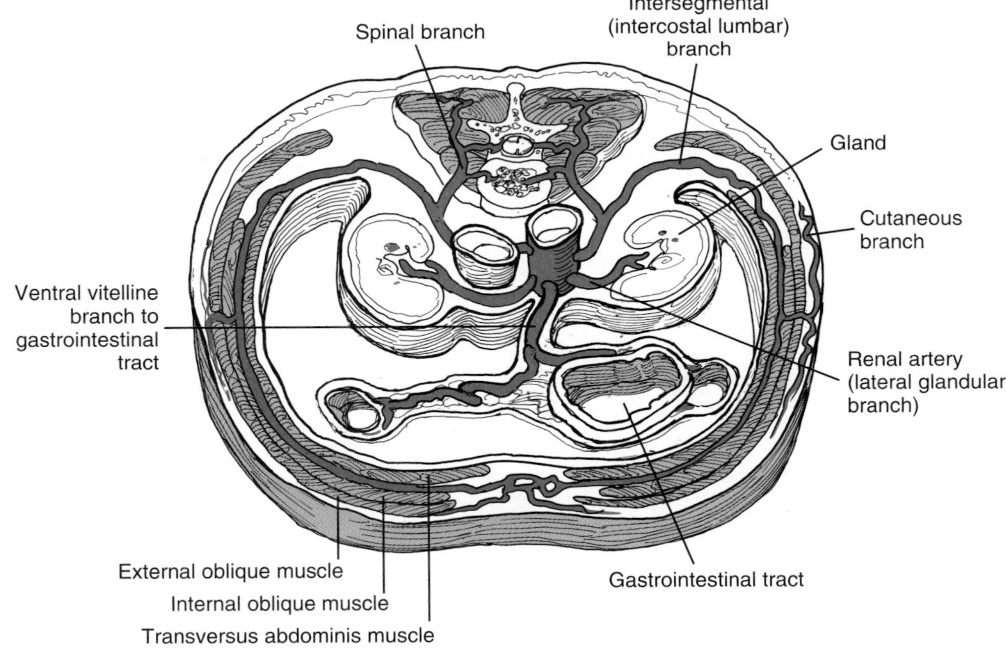

FIGURE 13–9
Generalized scheme showing the posterolateral, lateral, and ventral branches of the aorta.

Smaller Branches of the Aorta

Miscellaneous arteries of the aorta vascularize the diaphragm, adrenal glands, ureter, and posterior wall of the rectum

The aorta may emit several smaller branches that do not belong to any of the three major categories of branches described above. Small right and left **inferior phrenic arteries** may emerge from the ventral wall of the aorta just adjacent to and superior to the celiac trunk (see Figs. 13–6 and 13–8). These paired arteries supply the inferior surface of the diaphragm. As has been noted, they also produce multiple superior **adrenal branches,** which supply the medial surfaces of the right and left suprarenal glands. The branches penetrate the substance of each gland via fibrous septa, which extend from the capsule that covers the surface of each gland (see Figs. 13–6*A* and 13–8).

Small **ureteric branches** of the aorta may contribute to the vascularization of the ureters (see Fig. 13–5). The ureters also receive blood via small branches of the renal, gonadal, common iliac, and inferior vesicle arteries (see Fig. 13–5).

Finally, a small **median sacral artery** extends inferiorly from the bifurcation of the aorta into the **common iliac arteries** at the level of vertebral body L4 (see Fig. 13–8). This diminutive midline artery may give off a single pair of small lumbar branches and branches that anastomose with the **iliolumbar branches** of the **internal iliac arteries** (see Chapter 14) at the level of vertebra L5. The median sacral artery may also anastomose with the **lateral sacral arteries** (see Chapter 14). It extends to the coccyx, giving off small branches to the posterior wall of the rectum.

▲ Veins of the Posterior Body Wall

Systemic tributaries of the inferior vena cava drain the body wall and glandular viscera. Drainage of the gastrointestinal tract by the portal system is described in Chapter 12.

Abdominal Inferior Vena Cava

The abdominal segment of the inferior vena cava (and its branches) closely parallels the abdominal aorta, except that it lacks tributaries from most of the gut

The abdominal inferior vena cava is a large retroperitoneal vessel that lies on the left anterolateral surface of the vertebral column (Fig. 13–10). It originates inferiorly at the convergence of the **common iliac veins** at the level of the disc between vertebrae L4 and L5. It exits the abdominal cavity superiorly through the **vena caval aperture** at the level of vertebra T8 (see Chapter 10). The abdominal inferior vena cava is devoid of tributaries that parallel those of the celiac, superior mesenteric, and inferior mesenteric arterial

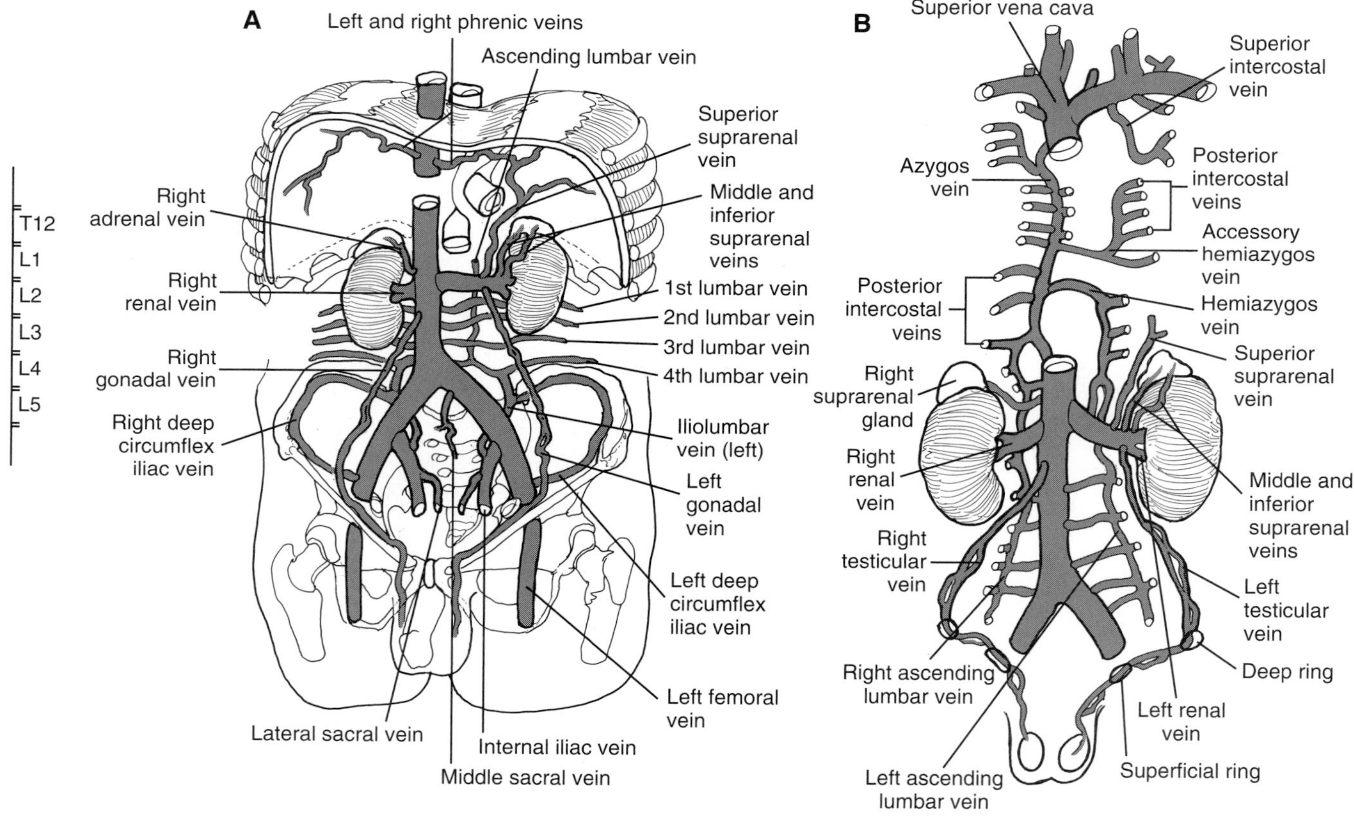

FIGURE 13–10
Veins of the posterior abdominal wall. **A.** The inferior vena cava lies somewhat to the right of the midline. Its branches include posterolateral branches (lumbar veins), which drain the body wall, and glandular branches, which drain the suprarenal glands, kidneys, and gonads. Its smaller branches drain the diaphragm and ureters. **B.** The diminutive left and right ascending lumbar veins anastomose with lumbar branches of the inferior vena cava and drain into the azygos system in the thorax. These vessels may provide collateral circulation when the inferior vena cava is obstructed. There are no venous correlates of the ventral aortic branches to the gastrointestinal tract because the stomach and intestines are drained by a special portal system of veins (see Chapter 12).

branches of the aorta. Instead, blood returning to the heart from the foregut, midgut, and hindgut is filtered through the liver via a specialized **portal system of veins** (see Chapter 12). However, the inferior vena cava does receive the paired posterolateral **lumbar veins** and the **lateral renal, suprarenal, right gonadal,** and **inferior phrenic veins** (Fig. 13–10). It also drains blood from the pelvis, perineum, and lower extremities (see Chapters 14 to 18).

Posterolateral Veins of the Body Wall

Paired posterolateral veins drain the posterolateral musculature of the lower body wall

Four pairs of lumbar tributaries of the inferior vena cava **(lumbar veins L1 to L4)** drain the posterior body wall from the level of vertebral bodies L1 to L4. The veins of L1 also drain anterolateral regions of the first dermatome in the manner of the intercostal veins. In addition, all of the lumbar veins anastomose freely with one another and with the deep circumflex iliac veins within the subserous fascia of the abdominal wall (see Chapter 11). The lumbar veins on the left are typically longer than those on the right because they must cross over the vertebral column (posterior to the aorta) to drain into the inferior vena cava (see Fig. 13–10*A*). A diminutive **median sacral vein** may accompany the median sacral artery. It typically drains into the left common iliac vein but may also drain into the junction of the **common iliac veins.** The common iliac veins branch at the same level as the common iliac arteries, but this bifurcation is skewed slightly to the right (see Fig. 13–10*A*).

The systemic veins in the lumbar region originally develop from the bilaterally symmetric subcardinal and supracardinal veins. The subcardinal and supracardinal veins on the left side eventually regress, whereas those on the right side enlarge to form the inferior vena cava. Thus, the inferior vena cava must accommodate the drainage of most of the blood from both sides of the trunk and both lower extremities back to the heart. However, a small longitudinal vein does typically remain on the left side. This left **ascending lumbar vein** usually anastomoses with segmental lumbar veins at every level (see Fig. 13–10*A* and *B*). It may also directly drain vein L1 or L2, or both, if they do not cross over to the right side to join the inferior vena cava. The left ascending lumbar vein is typically continuous with the **hemiazygos vein** within the left side of the thorax. Thus, its blood ultimately circulates to the right side into the azygos vein and superior vena cava, providing a collateral circuit for blood draining from the lower trunk or lower extremities if the inferior vena cava becomes blocked (see Fig. 13–10*B*). Anastomoses between lumbar veins on the right (lateral to the inferior vena cava) may also form a diminutive right ascending lumbar vein (see Fig. 13–10*B*). This vein may anastomose with the inferior vena cava or azygos vein, or both.

Glandular Veins

Paired glandular branches drain the adrenal glands, kidneys, and gonads

The right and left **renal veins** both empty into the inferior vena cava at about the level of vertebral body L2 (see Fig. 13–10). Since the inferior vena cava lies on the right side of the vertebral column, the left renal vein is longer, typically crossing over the abdominal aorta but just under the root of the superior mesenteric artery to reach the other side (see Fig. 13–6).

The **right suprarenal vein** issues from the medial side of the right suprarenal gland to empty directly into the inferior vena cava. The **left suprarenal vein** issues from the inferior pole of the left suprarenal gland to empty directly into the left renal vein (see Figs. 13–6 and 13–10*B*).

Similarly, the **right gonadal vein** empties directly into the inferior vena cava at about the lower second or upper third lumber level, while the **left gonadal vein** empties directly into the left renal vein (see Figs. 13–6 and 13–10). The consequent restriction of backflow on the left side results in more rapid but gradual expansion and development of varices of the left pampiniform plexus throughout life (see Chapter 11).

The organization of the right and left **inferior phrenic veins** is also somewhat different. The right inferior phrenic vein drains directly into the inferior vena cava, while one branch of the left inferior phrenic vein may drain directly into the inferior vena cava and the other into the left renal vein. Moreover, these latter two veins typically anastomose with each other (see Fig. 13–10*A*).

▲ Lymphatic System of the Posterior Abdominal Wall

The lymphatic system of the posterior abdominal wall is associated with the abdominal aorta

Organs of the posterior abdominal wall, pelvis (see Chapter 14), perineum (see Chapter 15), and lower extremities (see Chapters 16 to 18) drain into a plexus of lymphatic vessels and lymph nodes associated with the abdominal aorta as tributaries from each of these regions converge near the bifurcation of the aorta into the common iliac arteries (Fig. 13–11). At their superior extremities, the abdominal lymph ducts consolidate at about the level of vertebra L2 to form the **cisterna chyli,** an expansion of the **thoracic duct** (see Chapter 10). The cisterna chyli may course from the lower boundary of vertebra L2 to the lower boundary of vertebra T12, just to the right of and posterior to the aorta (Fig. 13–11 and see Chapter 10). The thoracic duct traverses the diaphragm via the aortic hiatus (at vertebral level T12) and ascends to the junction of the left subclavian and common jugular veins to return lymph to the systemic circulation (Fig. 13–11).

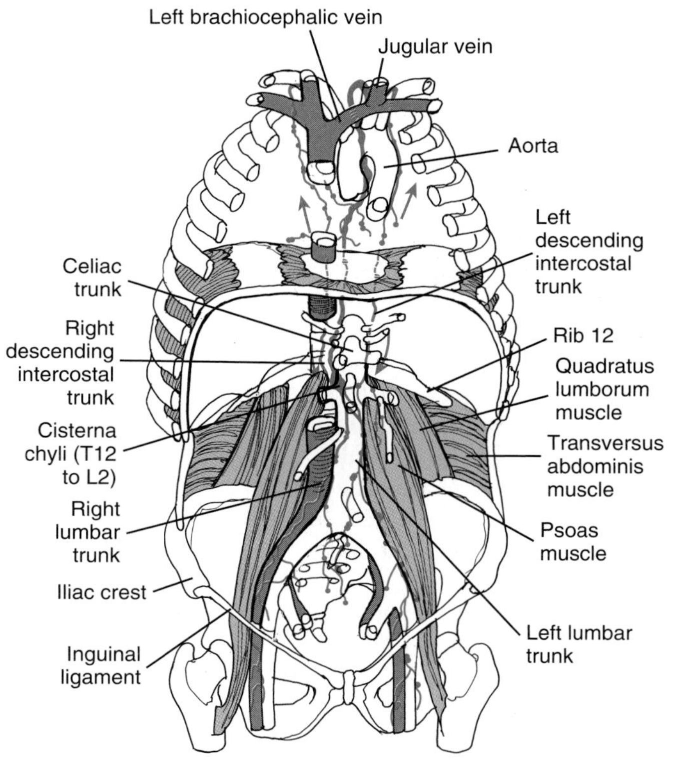

FIGURE 13–11
Organs of the posterior abdominal wall are drained by lymphatic vessels that follow the arteries that supply the organs. These lymphatic vessels sometimes converge to form an expansion at the level of vertebra L2 called the *cisterna chyli,* which continues into the thorax as the thoracic duct.

Disorders of Vascularization of the Posterior Abdominal Wall

Vascular elements of the posterior abdominal wall are subject to pathologic disorders

Although a dissecting aneurysm of the thoracic aorta may have catastrophic consequences (see Chapter 9), aneurysms of the abdominal aorta are more common, particularly those occurring just inferior to the renal arteries. They occur most commonly in males over age 60 years (the male to female ratio is 6:1) and typically result from atherosclerosis. Pain from the enlarging aneurysm is referred to the lower back (via the lumbar splanchnic innervation of the dorsal aorta) and becomes increasingly severe as the aneurysm reaches the point of bursting. In contrast to thoracic aortic aneurysms, which are not palpable, abdominal aortic aneurysms may be diagnosed by palpation, although ultrasound is now commonly used to confirm and identify the presence and location of these structures. Diseased regions of the abdominal aorta and common iliac arteries may be replaced by synthetic prostheses before an aneurysm bursts.

Obstruction of the inferior vena cava most often occurs inferior to the kidneys because of extension of deep venous thromboses from a lower limb (see Chapter 18) into the pelvis or abdomen. Typically, collateral circulation via the azygos and hemiazygos veins resolves the problem without treatment (see Fig. 13–10*B*).

Obstructions that impede the renal arterial blood flow are serious because they may result in underperfusion of the kidneys and consequent hematuria, proteinuria, and renal failure (see discussion of renal function above). Obstructions may also impede drainage of the hepatic veins, resulting in portal hypertension, ascites, and hepatic failure (see Chapter 12). These obstructions typically result from renal carcinoma or hypertrophy of the liver (hepatomegaly). Treatment may include drugs to dissolve the renal thromboses, irradiation or chemotherapy to relieve renal carcinoma, renal or hepatic transplantation, or introduction of a shunt to dilate the inferior vena cava in the region of the obstruction.

Autonomic Innervation of the Posterior Abdominal Wall Viscera

Sympathetic and parasympathetic fibers located within the posterior body wall innervate abdominal and pelvic viscera.

Sympathetic Nerves

Several elements of the sympathetic nervous system are located within the posterior abdominal wall

The most prominent nerves of the posterior abdominal wall are the somatic nerves of the lumbar plexus, described above. However, several significant elements of the autonomic nervous system are also located in this region. The continuations of the **sympathetic trunks** course within the subserous fascia along the lateral walls of the lumbar vertebral bodies. These lumbar segments gain access to the abdomen by traversing the diaphragm from the thorax via the medial **lumbocostal arch** just medial to each psoas muscle (Fig. 13–12). As in the thorax, the lumbar segment of each of the sympathetic trunks is associated with **sympathetic chain ganglia.** Typically, about four pairs of these can be identified (Fig. 13–12).

A pair of **lumbar splanchnic nerves** are also formed by preganglionic fibers that emanate from sympathetic ganglia L1 and L2 (Fig. 13–12 and see Chapters 4 and 12). The lumbar splanchnic nerves innervate cell bodies within the diffuse **inferior mesenteric ganglia.** The postganglionic fibers emitted from these cell bodies innervate the territory of the inferior mesenteric artery—namely, the hindgut.

Diminutive lower **lumbar** and **sacral splanchnic nerves** may also emanate from lower lumbar and sacral chain ganglia. The preganglionic sympathetic fibers contained within these nerves, however, originate from neurons within upper lumbar levels of the spinal cord. They innervate neurons within the hypogastric plexus, which, in turn, innervate pelvic viscera along with sym-

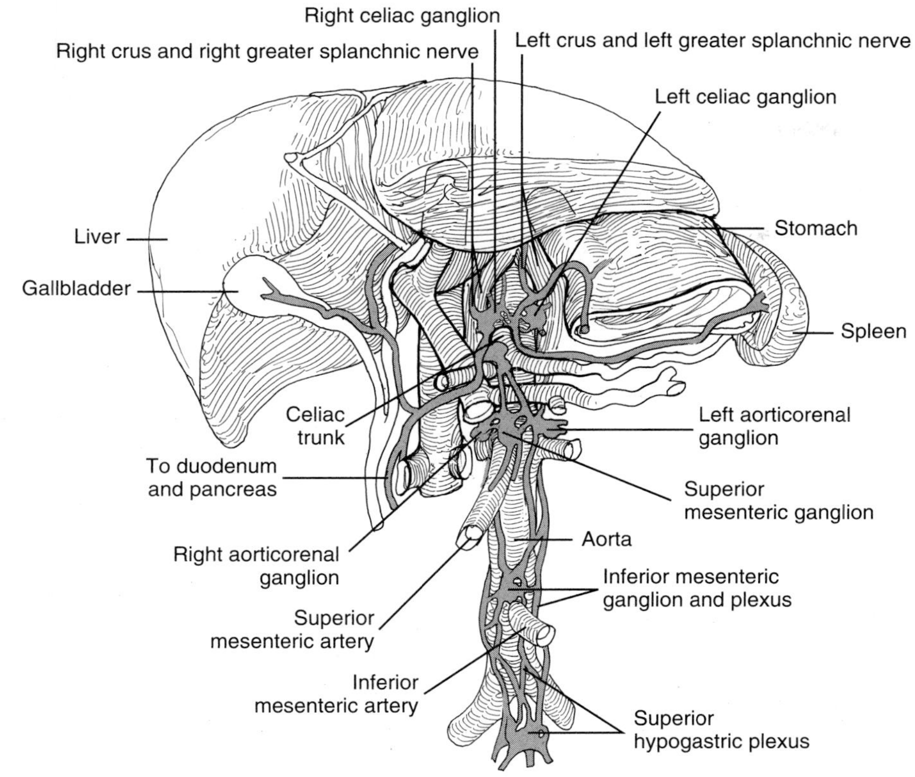

FIGURE 13–12
Autonomic structures of the posterior abdominal wall. Large celiac ganglia are associated with the celiac trunk, while aorticorenal and superior and inferior mesenteric ganglia are more diffuse. The dispersed neurons of the inferior mesenteric ganglia are intermixed with parasympathetic pelvic splanchnic nerves to form an inferior mesenteric plexus. The kidneys and arteries of the cortex and medulla and medullary cells of the suprarenal glands are innervated by postganglionic fibers from the aorticorenal ganglion, which may receive preganglionic fibers from neurons at spinal levels between vertebrae T10 and L1. Parasympathetic innervation of the kidneys is from the pelvic splanchnic nerves (spinal nerves S2 to S4). Because the gonads first developed at the lower thoracic and upper lumbar levels, they are innervated by sympathetic postganglionic fibers of neurons that receive their innervation from spinal nerves T10 to L1.

pathetic postganglionic fibers from inferior mesenteric ganglia (Fig. 13–12 and see Chapter 12).

Parasympathetic Nerves of the Posterior Abdominal Wall

Both cranial and pelvic elements of the parasympathetic nervous system are present in the posterior abdomen

The anterior and posterior vagus trunks enter the abdomen via the **esophageal hiatus** and follow the gastrointestinal tract to the termination of the midgut, giving off **gastric** and **intestinal branches** along their courses (see Fig. 13–12 and Chapter 12). These parasympathetic nerves are not, therefore, embedded within the subserous fascia of the posterior abdominal wall at any point. Parasympathetic fibers within the **pelvic splanchnic nerves** arising from sacral spinal cord origins innervate the abdominal viscera as far superior as the transverse colon in the region of the left colic flexure (see Chapter 12), kidneys, and ureters. However, the major function of the pelvic splanchnic nerves is to provide parasympathetic innervation to the pelvic viscera (see Chapter 14).

Anatomic Plexuses of the Posterior Abdominal Wall

Many autonomic nerve fibers in the posterior abdomen are distributed to the pelvic and perineal organs through the

- **testicular** or **ovarian plexus,**
- **abdominal aortic (intermesenteric) plexus,** and
- **superior** and **inferior hypogastric plexuses.**

These plexuses are located within the extraperitoneal connective tissue of the posterior abdominal and pelvic walls. The plexuses contain preganglionic fibers from the lesser (T10 and T11), least (T12), and lumbar (L1 and L2) splanchnic nerves and preganglionic parasympathetic fibers from the vagus or pelvic splanchnic nerves, or both. The scattered sympathetic ganglia contained within these plexuses are innervated in a superior to inferior order by preganglionic fibers from spinal nerves T10 to L2. The organization, contents, and functions of the superior and inferior hypogastric plexuses are discussed in Chapters 14 and 15.

14 The Pelvic Cavity, Pelvic Bone, and Pelvic Viscera

The **pelvis** is a compartment of the trunk located just inferior to the abdomen. It encloses the **pelvic cavity,** which contains the **pelvic viscera,** most of which serve functions of the urogenital and lower gastrointestinal tracts. The pelvis is bounded

- inferiorly by the **perineum,**
- superiorly by a transverse plane at the level of the pelvic brim,
- posterolaterally by the **gluteal region,** and
- anterolaterally by the **thigh.**

Thus, most of the **pelvic compartment** is enclosed by muscles and integument of the superior part of the lower extremity. It is also bounded by

- a small inverted medial triangle of integument covering the sacrococcygeal region posteriorly and
- a small region anterior to the pubic symphysis.

The embryonic origin of the pelvic cavity is described in Chapter 11. The pelvic cavity is created from the most inferior recess of the peritoneal cavity, which arises from the original intraembryonic coelom and, thus, is in continuity with the abdominal cavity. Indeed, the inferior part of the abdominal cavity, enclosed by the iliac fossae, is typically called the **false (greater) pelvis.** This false pelvis is superior to the level of the pelvic brim (Fig. 14–1). The **true (lesser) pelvis,** or **pelvic cavity,** lies just inferior to the pelvic brim. The posterior boundary of the pelvic cavity is the sacrum, and the lateral, anterior, and inferior boundaries are defined by the **pelvic diaphragm,** a composite muscle that includes the coccygeus, iliococcygeus, and pubococcygeus muscles. The lateral and anterior iliococcygeus and pubococcygeus muscles function in the conscious regulation of defecation and are together called the **levator ani muscle** (see Fig. 14–9).

The pelvic cavity is enclosed within and protected by a bony encasement called the **pelvic (innominate) bone** (Fig. 14–2). This bone can be used as a frame of reference for the anatomic relationships of the trunk, perineum, and lower limbs, so it will be described first. Its bony landmarks also serve as useful practical guides in diagnosis and treatment (see below).

PELVIC BONE

The pelvic bone is an important framework for understanding the anatomy of the pelvis

The **pelvic bone (os coxae)** is made up of three pairs of bones, namely, the **pubic bones** (anteriorly), **iliac bones** (superolaterally), and **ischial bones** (inferolaterally) (Fig. 14–2). During embryonic and fetal development, these six bones each arise from distinct ossification centers. By adulthood, however, each of the three-bone units on each side of the pelvis becomes tightly fused into a single bone. Nonetheless, some distortion of the bony pelvis is possible, especially in females during childbirth. This results from the slight flexibility of the synovial **sacroiliac joints** and **sacroiliac** and **vertebropelvic ligaments,** which bind the pelvis to the sacrum and vertebral column posteriorly (see Fig. 14–3), and of the **symphysis pubis** (syndesmosis of the pubic bones), which binds the two halves of the pelvis together anteriorly (Fig. 14–2*A* and *C*). Generally, however, these bilateral assemblies function together and with the sacrum to protect the enclosed vital organs and to serve as a foundation for the vertebral column and lower extremities. This **appendicular** pelvic bone is, thus, a stable connector between the sacrum of the axial skeleton and the movable femur of the lower extremity, supporting upright posture for sitting and bipedal locomotion.

The connection between the pelvis and femur is the synovial **hip joint,** which consists of a deep socket, the **acetabulum,** that encloses the proximal ball of the femur (Fig. 14–2*E*). The three fused bones on each side of the pelvis (the ilium, ischium, and pubis) contribute to the acetabulum (the ilium superiorly, the pubis inferiorly and ventrally, and the ischium inferiorly and dorsally).

Iliac Bones

Iliac bones support the flanks

The iliac bones have two extremities: an **upper extremity,** consisting of flared superior wings of bone, and a **lower extremity.** The upper extremity is topped by an expanded **iliac crest** anteriorly and a widened **iliac tuberosity** posteriorly (Fig. 14–2*E* and *F*). The lower extremity contributes to the superior region of the acetabulum (see below).

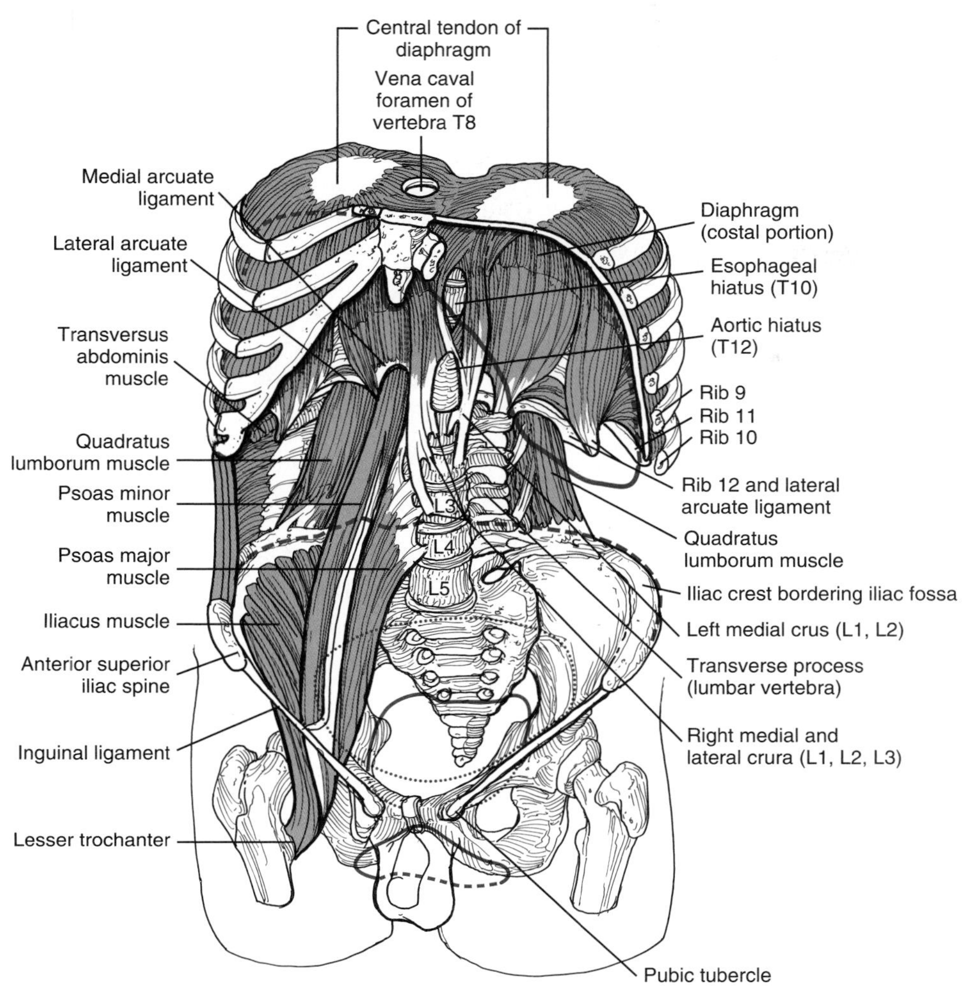

FIGURE 14–1
Boundaries of the pelvic cavity. The true pelvis is the region of the abdominopelvic cavity below a plane defined by the pelvic brim. The pelvic cavity is bounded posteriorly by the sacrum. The lateral, anterior, and inferior boundaries are defined by the muscular pelvic diaphragm. Thus, the pelvic cavity is encased by the sacrum and the bony pelvis, which is formed by the left and right ossa coxae. Each os coxae is formed by the fusion of three bones: the pubic bone, iliac bone, and ischial bone.

The **upper extremity** of the iliac bone has three surfaces: an **iliac fossa,** a **sacropelvic surface,** and a **gluteal surface.** The **iliac fossa** is the medial concave surface of the iliac bone. It contains the iliacus muscle and a middle segment of the psoas muscle (Figs. 14–1 and 14–2 and see Chapter 13). The inferomedial surface of the iliac bone is the **sacropelvic surface.** This region of the ilium includes the medial aspect of the **iliac tuberosity** and an **auricular** (ear-shaped) **surface,** which articulates with the lateral alar process of the sacrum. The sacropelvic surface of the iliac tuberosity provides an attachment site for the **sacroiliac ligaments,** ligaments that bind the ilium to the sacrum, and to the **iliolumbar ligaments** (the lumbar vertebrae). The sacropelvic surface of the lower extremity of the iliac bone also provides an attachment site for the **obturator internus muscle.** The third surface of the ilium is the posterolateral **gluteal surface** (Fig. 14–2). It is a roughened surface that serves as an attachment site for the gluteal muscles that move and stabilize the femur.

The **specialized processes** of the iliac bones, in addition to the iliac crest and iliac tuberosity mentioned above, include the **anterior superior iliac spine (ASIS)** to which the **inguinal ligament** is attached; the **anterior inferior iliac spine (AIIS),** which is the site of the superior attachment of the **rectus femoris muscle;** the **posterior superior iliac spine (PSIS),** which provides a superior attachment for the **gluteus maximus muscle;** and the **posterior inferior iliac spine (PIIS),** which provides an attachment site for the **piriformis muscle.** The **iliac crest** provides attachment sites for the **external oblique, internal oblique,** and **transversus abdominis muscles** of the anterolateral body wall and the **quadratus lumborum muscles** of the posterior body wall. The iliac tuberosities

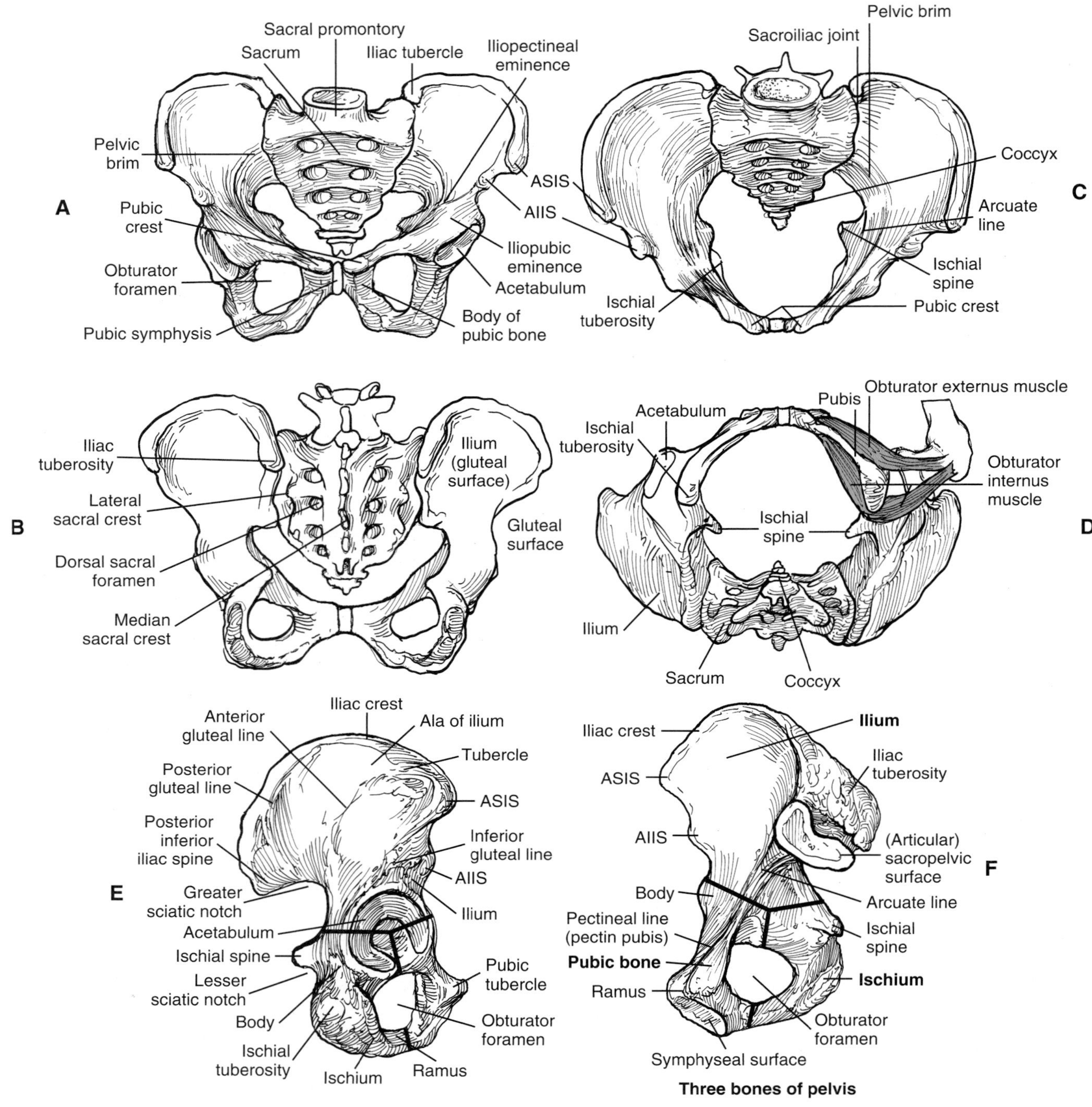

FIGURE 14–2
Anatomy of the pelvic bones. **A.** Anterior view. **B.** Posterior view. **C.** Superior view. **D.** Inferior view. **E.** Lateral view. **F.** Medial view.

provide attachment sites for the lateral fibers of the **erector spinae muscles.** The iliac contribution to the pelvic brim is the **arcuate line of the ilium** (Fig. 14–2*C*).

▲ Pubic Bones

Pubic bones make up the inferoventral region of the pelvis

Each of the paired **pubic bones** has three parts: a **body, superior ramus,** and **inferior ramus.** The pubic bones participate in the formation of the acetabulum and form the superoventral and inferodorsal margins of the **obturator foramen**—the anterior aperture of the pelvis (see Fig. 14–2*A* and below).

The body of each pubic bone has three surfaces: a **ventral, dorsal,** and **medial (symphysial) surface.** The **ventral surfaces** face inferolaterally and provide attachment sites for the **obturator externus muscle** and muscles of the medial (adductor) compartment of the thigh. The **dorsal surfaces** are apposed to the urinary bladder, which is located within the anterior wall of the pelvis. This bony surface also provides attachment sites for the **pubococcygeus** components of the **levator ani muscles** and **obturator internus muscles.** The **medial surfaces** form the **pubic symphysis,** as described above (see Figs. 14–2 and 14–9).

The **superior ramus** of the pubic bone is joined to the ilium within the acetabulum superiorly, and the **inferior ramus** is joined to the **ramus of the ischium** inferiorly. The **ventral surfaces** of the superior and inferior rami (with the pubic body) are directed somewhat inferiorly and laterally and serve as attachment sites for the **obturator externus muscle** and muscles of the medial (adductor) compartment of the thigh. The **dorsal surfaces** of the superior and inferior rami are apposed to the pelvic cavity and bladder and also provide an attachment site for the **obturator internus muscle** (see Fig. 14–2 and Chapters 11 and 17).

The **specialized processes** of the body of the pubic bone include the **pubic crest,** which is a rounded superomedial prominence that provides sites for the attachments of the external oblique, internal oblique, transversus abdominis, pyramidalis, and rectus abdominis muscles. The anterolateral projections on either side of each pubic crest are the **pubic tubercles,** which provide attachment sites for the **inguinal ligaments.** The superior ramus has a specialized attachment site for the **pectineus muscle** called the **pectineal line (pecten pubis).** The upper boundary of this **pectineal surface** is, thus, defined by the pecten pubis, which continues laterally and posteriorly to merge with the **arcuate line** of the iliac bone. The pubic crest, pecten pubis, and arcuate line of the ilium form the **linea terminalis.** This ridge plus the **sacral promontory** form the **pelvic brim.** The pecten pubis also provides attachment sites for several important ligaments in this region. The **conjoint** and **lacunar ligaments** are attached at its medial end and the **pectineal ligament** at its lateral end (see Fig. 11–19 and Chapters 11 and 17).

▲ Ischial Bones

Ischial bones make up the inferodorsal region of the pelvic bone

Each ischium consists of a **body** and **ramus.** The upper part of the ischial body joins the lower extremity of the ilium and the lateral end of the superior ramus of the pubic bone to form the acetabulum. The ischial body also forms the rough inferior expansion called the **ischial tuberosity** and contributes to the superior and posterior boundaries of the **obturator foramen.** The **ischial ramus** courses anteriorly and superiorly to fuse with the inferior ramus of the pubic bone, contributing to the inferior border of the obturator foramen (see Fig. 14–2).

The **ischial body** has three surfaces: the **femoral surface, dorsal surface,** and **pelvic surface.** The **femoral surface** is directed laterally and inferiorly toward the lateral part of the thigh and contains part of the acetabulum. It provides attachment sites for the hamstring muscles of the posterior compartment of the thigh. The **dorsal surface** is directed posteriorly and upward and includes the posterior part of the outer wall of the acetabulum, which is contiguous with the gluteal surface of the ilium. The **pelvic surface** is directed toward the pelvic cavity and also makes up part of the lateral boundary of the **ischiorectal fossa** (see Fig. 14–2 and Chapters 15 and 17).

The **ventral** and **dorsal surfaces** of the **ischial ramus** are contiguous with the ventral and dorsal surfaces of the inferior ramus of the pubic bone. The ischial ramus provides sites for attachments of muscles of the medial (adductor) compartment of the thigh. The smooth posterior surface of the ramus apposes the pelvic cavity.

Specialized structures of the ischium include the **lesser sciatic notch,** which is an indentation formed by the posterior border of the body of the ischium and the posterior border of the upper extremity of the ilium (see Fig. 14–2). The **ischial spine,** which is a projection from the dorsal surface of the ischial body, is located at the lower boundary of the greater sciatic notch. The **ischial tuberosity** is the inferior roughened expansion of the ischial body that supports the weight of the body in a sitting position.

▲ Pelvic Ligaments

The appendicular pelvic bone is bound to the axial skeleton by tough fibrocartilaginous ligaments

The articulation between the auricular surface on the sacropelvic aspect of the ilium and the lateral alar mass of the sacrum is a synovial joint. The articular capsule of the joint is buried within three strong ligaments (Fig. 14–3). These are

- ♦ the **ventral sacroiliac ligament;**
- ♦ the massive dorsal **interosseous sacroiliac ligament,** which fills the spaces between the sacrum and iliac bones; and
- ♦ the **dorsal sacroiliac ligament,** which covers the interosseous sacroiliac ligament.

The space between these latter two dorsal ligaments is large enough to allow the dorsal rami of sacral nerves and blood vessels to pass through it.

A series of tough **vertebropelvic ligaments** also binds the pelvis to the axial skeleton (Fig. 14–3). There are three complexes:

- ♦ **iliolumbar ligaments,**
- ♦ **sacrotuberous ligaments,** and
- ♦ **sacrospinous ligaments.**

The **iliolumbar ligaments** are oriented horizontally and bind the transverse processes of vertebra L5 to the iliac crests. The **sacrotuberous ligaments** course from the posterior surface of the iliac tuberosities to the ischial tuberosities and are also firmly attached to the posterior superior and inferior iliac spines. The **sacrospinous ligaments** are attached to the ischial

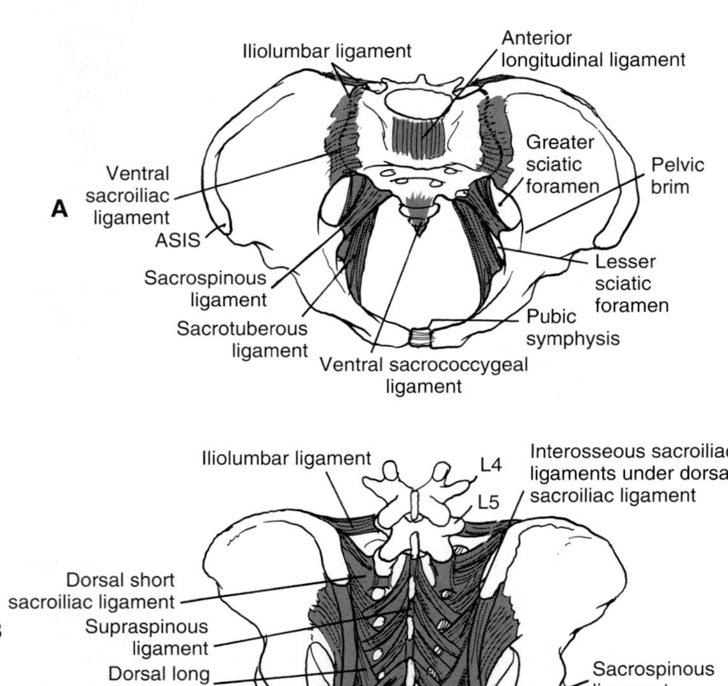

FIGURE 14–3

Ligaments of the pelvis. **A.** Anterior view shows iliolumbar, ventral sacroiliac, sacrospinous, and sacrotuberous ligaments. **B.** Posterior view shows iliolumbar, dorsal sacroiliac, sacrospinous, sacrotuberous, and supraspinous ligaments.

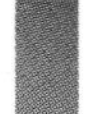

TABLE 14–1
Structures that Pass Into, Through, or Out of the Pelvis

Site of Entry or Egress	Structure
Pelvic inlet	Rectum, ureters, pregnant uterus, gonadal vessels, common iliac vessels, lumbosacral trunk, obturator nerve
Pelvic outlet	Rectum, anus; urethra; uterus, vagina, vestibule; vas deferens; internal pudendal vessels, pudendal nerve
Obturator canal	Obturator vessels, obturator nerve
Greater sciatic foramen	Superior and inferior gluteal vessels, superior and inferior gluteal nerves, piriformis muscle, sciatic nerve, internal pudendal vessels, pudendal nerve
Lesser sciatic foramen	Obturator internus muscle, internal pudendal vessels, pudendal nerve
Over anterior pelvic brim to exit false pelvis	External iliac to femoral vessels, iliopsoas tendon, femoral nerve, femoral and genital branches of genitofemoral nerve, ilioinguinal nerve, lateral femoral cutaneous nerve, round ligament of uterus, spermatic cord

spine (laterally) and the ventral surface of the sacrum and coccyx (medially). Each ligament passes at an oblique angle across the ventral surface of the sacrotuberous ligament and divides the aperture created by the sacrotuberous ligament into a superior **greater sciatic foramen** and an inferior **lesser sciatic foramen.**

▲ Pelvic Apertures and Foramina

The pelvis is perforated by apertures and foramina through which important visceral structures pass from the abdominal and pelvic cavities to the perineum or lower extremity

The pelvis transports muscles, nerves, and blood vessels from superior parts of the trunk to the external genitalia, anal canal, and lower extremities. Strategic openings within the pelvic bone are required for the transmission of these structures from the pelvic cavity to the **perineum, gluteal region, or anterior, posterior, or medial compartments** of the **thigh** (Table 14–1 and see below).

Chapter 12 describes how the pelvic brim demarcates the boundary between the false pelvis superiorly and the true pelvis inferiorly. The aperture between these cavities (at the level of the pelvic brim) is the **superior aperture of the pelvis (pelvic inlet).** This opening may be heart-shaped or oval. The heart-shaped opening is known as the **android opening,** meaning "to resemble a man." The inlet may have three different oval-shaped configurations: (1) the **anthropoid opening,** also meaning "to resemble a man," which is an oval shape with a larger dorsoventral diameter; the **gynecoid opening,** meaning "to resemble a woman," which is a slightly oval shape with a larger transverse diameter; or a **platypelloid opening,** meaning "to resemble a bowl," which is a more extreme, transversely disposed oval shape (Fig. 14–4). Obviously, the anthropoid and android shapes are most common in males and the platypelloid and gynecoid shapes are most common in females.

It should be apparent that the shapes of both the superior and inferior apertures of the female pelvis are advantageous for childbirth

In contrast to the superior aperture of the pelvis, the **inferior aperture (pelvic outlet)** is more irregular in shape with a larger dorsoventral diameter in males and a larger transverse diameter in females. It is bounded anteriorly by the puboischial rami, laterally by the ischial tuberosities and sacrotuberous ligaments, and posteriorly by the coccyx (Fig. 14–4).

Several structures of the gastrointestinal and genitourinary tracts traverse both of these apertures as they course between the abdomen and the perineum. For example, the rectum and associated vessels and nerves pass through both apertures to terminate in the posterior part of the perineum (within the anal triangle). In addition, the male and female urinary tracts pass through both apertures to terminate in the anterior region of the perineum (within the urogenital triangle). Finally, the male and female genital structures within the true pelvis traverse the inferior aperture only to terminate within the urogenital triangle of the perineum. However, the superior part of the uterus extends into the abdominal cavity during pregnancy so that most of the fetus traverses both the superior and inferior apertures of the pelvis during childbirth (see below and Chapter 15).

The anterior **obturator foramen,** which was described above (Fig. 14–5 and see Fig. 14–1), is mostly covered by the **obturator membrane,** except for a small superior opening called the **obturator canal.** The obturator canal provides a conduit for the transmission of the **obturator artery, obturator vein,** and **obturator nerve,** which serve the **medial,** or **adductor, compartment** of the **thigh** (see Chapter 18).

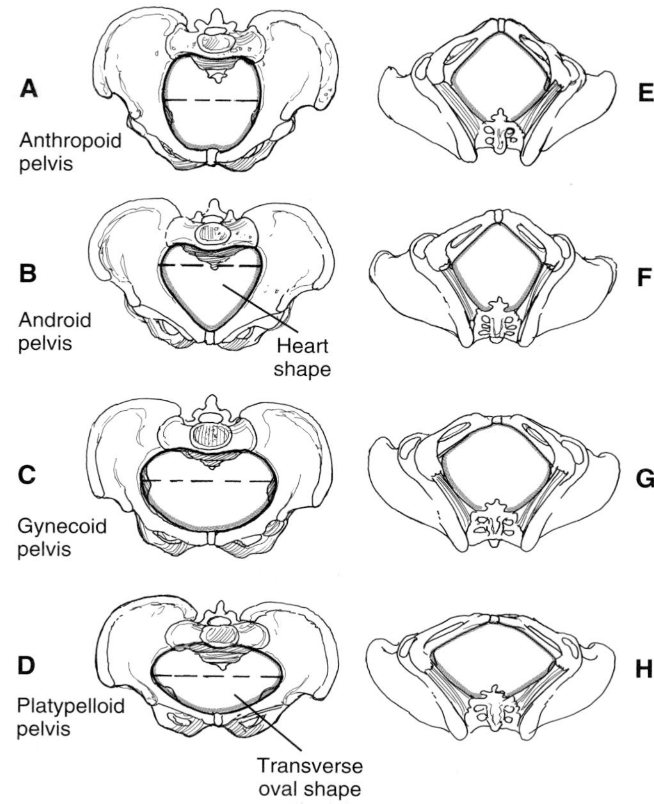

FIGURE 14–4
Shapes of the pelvis. The dorsoventral diameter is relatively elongated in the anthropoid and android pelves. The transverse diameter is relatively elongated in the gynecoid and platypelloid pelves.

The **greater** and **lesser (ischiadic) sciatic foramina,** also described above (see Figs. 14–3 and 14–5*B*), transmit nerves and vessels from the pelvis to the gluteal region and perineum. Several branches of the posterior divisions of the internal iliac vessels and nerves of the lumbosacral plexus issue from the pelvis through the greater sciatic foramen to provide vasculature and innervation of the **gluteal region (superior** and **inferior gluteal vessels** and **nerves)** and **lower extremities (sciatic nerves).** The **pudendal vessels** and **nerves** exit the pelvis from the greater sciatic foramen but immediately pass back through the lesser sciatic foramen. The rectal branches enter the anal triangle to serve the inferior region of the rectum. Other branches, continuations of the **pudendal vessels** and **nerves,** enter the **pudendal canal,** which is a fascial tunnel located on the medial surface of the ischial ramus. Upon exiting the pudendal canal, they enter the urogenital triangle to provide the vasculature and innervation of the external genitalia (see Chapter 15).

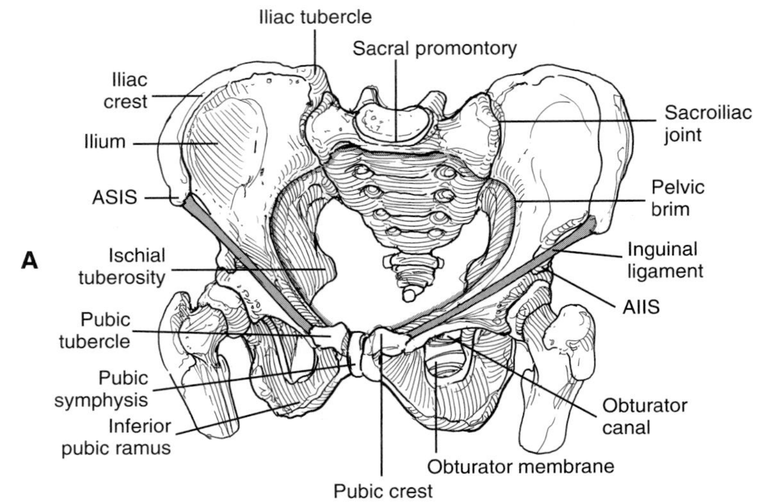

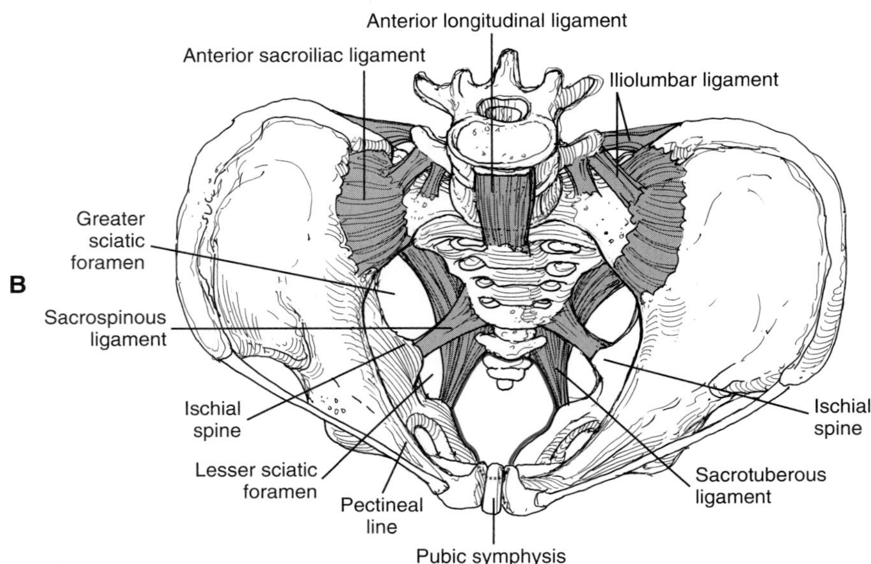

FIGURE 14–5

Landmarks of the pelvis. **A.** The pubic symphysis and pubic crests can be palpated just above the root of the penis in males and root of the clitoris in females. The palpable anterior superior iliac spines and pubic tubercles anchor the inguinal ligaments. The anterior inferior iliac spines are the origins of the rectus femoris muscles. The upper edge of the ilium is the palpable iliac crest, which serves as an attachment site for the abdominal and quadratus lumborum muscles. The widened posterior part of the iliac crest, or iliac tubercles (tuberosities), anchors the erector spinae muscles. The inferior ischial tuberosities support the trunk when a person is sitting. The pelvic brim defines the pelvic inlet and the boundary between the abdominal cavity above and pelvic cavity below. **B.** The pelvic outlet is defined by the coccyx (posteriorly), ischial tuberosities and sacrotuberous ligaments (laterally), and puboischial rami (anteriorly). The greater and lesser sciatic foramina are separated by the sacrospinous ligament.

Not all of the structures that exit the peritoneal cavity gain access to the lower extremities or perineum through the apertures just described. Some structures that serve the urogenital triangle and anterior and lateral compartments of the thigh **exit the false pelvis** by coursing over the anterosuperior edge of the pelvic brim. The **iliopsoas muscle** exits the false pelvis over the superior edge of the anterior pelvic brim to insert upon the lesser tubercle of the femur (see Chapter 17). The **ilioinguinal nerve** exits the body wall via the inguinal canal and passes over the pubic crest through the superficial ring to innervate the anterosuperior integument of the external genitalia and medial thigh (see Chapters 11 and 13). The **round ligament of the uterus** in females and the **spermatic cord** in males follow a similar course from their retroperitoneal positions within the abdominal cavity through the inguinal canal and then into the labia majora or scrotum. The **genital branch of the genitofemoral nerve** courses within the inguinal canal and out through the superficial ring as it innervates the cremaster muscle (cremasteric fascia) in males. The **lateral femoral cutaneous nerve** of the lumbar plexus passes over the anterior lip of the pelvic brim by coursing under the inguinal ligament just anterior to the anterior superior iliac spine (ASIS) to innervate the integument of the lateral thigh (see Chapter 13). The **femoral nerve, femoral branch of the genitofemoral nerve,** and **external iliac vessels** also pass under the inguinal ligament, but over the superior edge of the pecten pubis, to gain access to the anterior compartment of the thigh (Fig. 14–5).

▲ Palpable Bony Landmarks of the Pelvis

Many of the specialized structures and extremities of the pubic, iliac, and ischial bones described above can be palpated to help the physician make a clinical diagnosis or identify a site for making an incision

The **pubic symphysis** and **pubic crests** form a hard ridge just superior to the root of the penis in males and clitoris in females (see Figs. 14–1, 14–2, and 14–5). The more lateral anterior superior iliac spines (ASIS) and posterior iliac tubercles (tuberosities) are prominent extensions of the iliac crest, most of which can be palpated. One often becomes aware of the presence and location of the ischial tuberosities after one sits on a hard surface for a length of time. The sacrum and coccyx of the axial skeleton are palpable in the posterior midline. Because the coccyx extends so prominently, it is often fractured in falls on the buttocks.

VISCERA OF THE PELVIC CAVITY

Embryonic Development of the Pelvic Viscera

Anatomic relationships of definitive pelvic gastrointestinal and urogenital organs are explained by their coordinated development

The embryonic hindgut of males and females is a large expanded region called the **cloaca** (from the Latin, meaning *sewer*). By the end of the embryonic period, the cloaca is divided by the urorectal septum into an anterior **primitive urogenital sinus** and a posterior **rectum** (Fig. 14–6*A* and *B* and see Chapter 12). In females, the primitive urogenital sinus gives rise to the **bladder,**

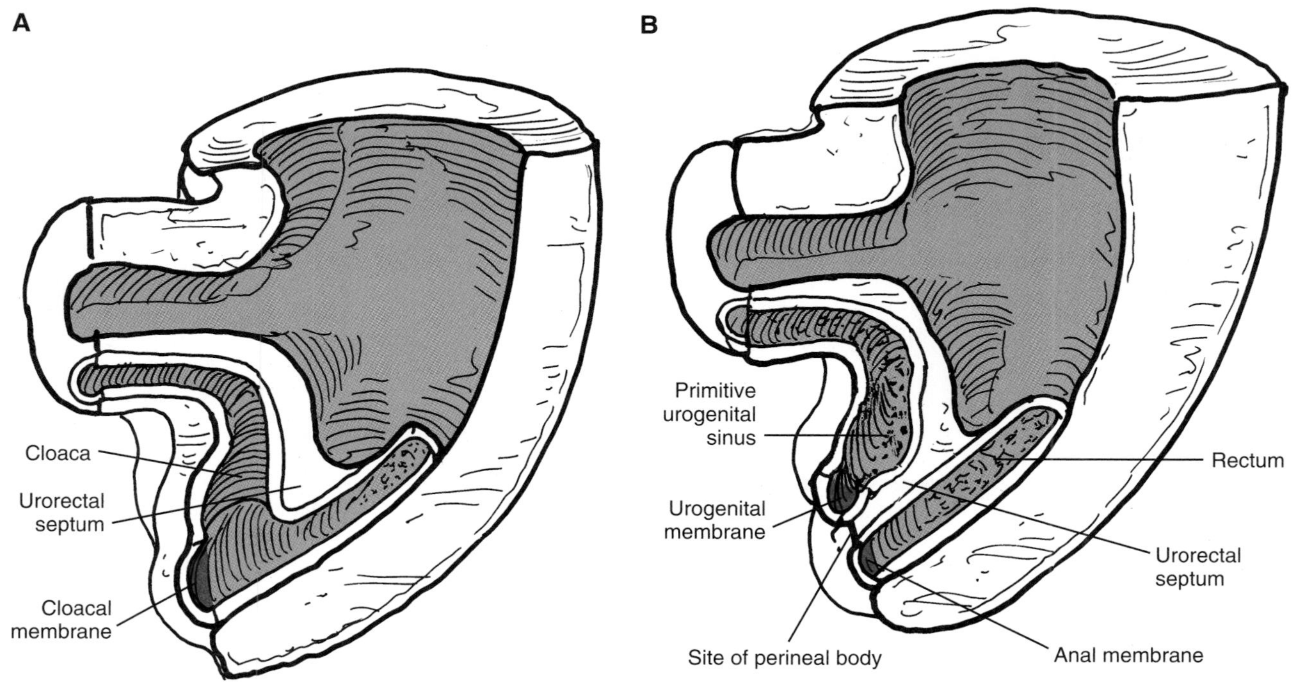

FIGURE 14–6

Pouches, fossae, and recesses of the pelvic cavity. **A.** The urorectal septum begins to divide the cloaca in the fourth week. **B.** By the end of the seventh week, the cloaca has been split into an anterior primitive urogenital sinus and a posterior rectum. The primitive urogenital sinus will form the urachus, bladder, pelvic urethra, and definitive urogenital sinus. The pelvic urethra forms the membranous urethra in females and the prostatic and membranous urethras in males. The definitive urogenital sinus forms the vestibule of the vagina in females and the penile urethra in males.

Continued

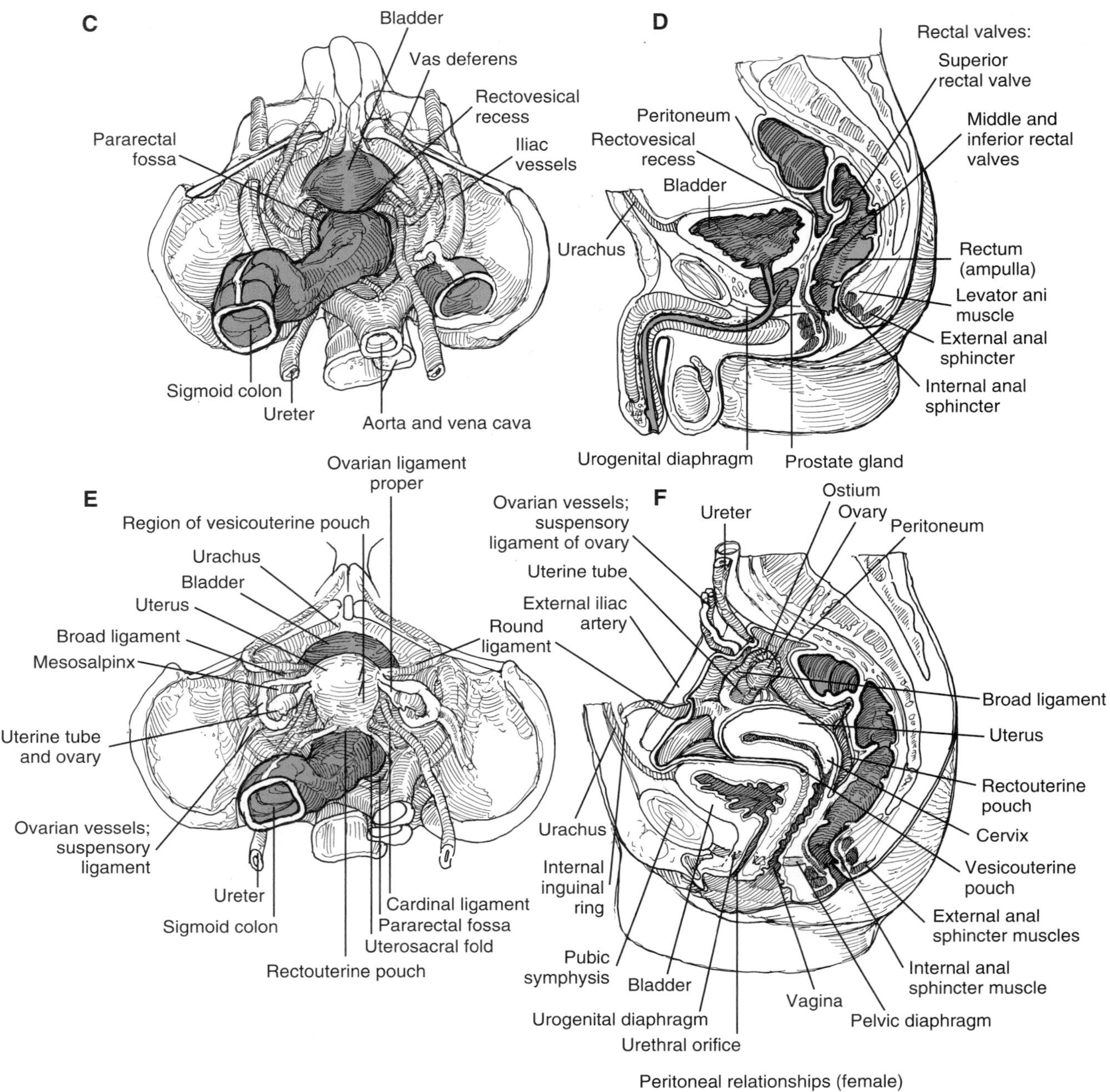

FIGURE 14–6, cont'd

C. Superior view of the male pelvic cavity. The vesicorectal recess is located between the bladder and the rectum. It is contiguous with the lateral pararectal fossae. **D.** A sagittal section shows that the vesicorectal recess is the lowest excursion of the peritoneal cavity in males and is located about the length of an index finger from the anal orifice. **E.** A superior view of the female pelvic cavity shows the region of the vesicouterine pouch and the rectouterine pouch (pouch of Douglas). **F.** A sagittal section shows that the rectouterine pouch is the lowest excursion of the peritoneum in females.

membranous urethra, and **vestibule of the vagina.** In males, the primitive urogenital sinus forms the **bladder, membranous** and **prostatic urethras,** and **penile urethra** (see Chapter 15). Thus, the bladder is a retroperitoneal organ of the ventral wall of the pelvic cavity, and the rectum is a retroperitoneal organ of the dorsal wall of the pelvic cavity. Because the embryonic urinary system, bladder, and urethra develop in close association with the genital system, the formation of these organs will be briefly described together.

Development of the Genital and Urinary Duct Systems

Early development of male and female genital and urinary duct systems is the same

The intermediate mesoderm of the thoracolumbar region in male and female embryos gives rise to the

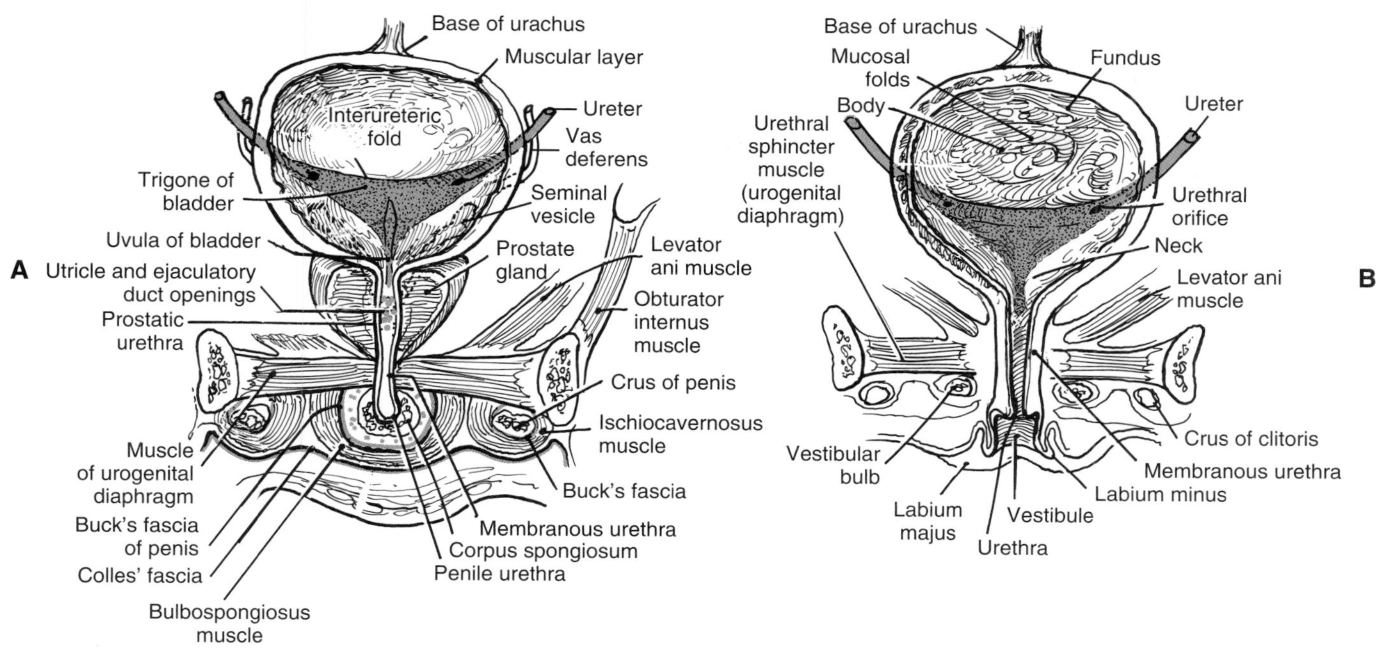

FIGURE 14–7
The bladder has a fundus, body, and neck. The trigone is a triangular area on the posterior wall defined by the orifices of both ureters and the boundary between the neck of the ureter and the urethra. **A.** Male structures. **B.** Female structures.

paired embryonic kidneys, or **mesonephroi,** in the fifth week. These kidneys are functional in both sexes for the next 5 weeks. They drain urine through a pair of **mesonephric ducts.** The ducts first become connected to the lateral walls of the cloaca and then become emplaced on the posterior bladder wall once it becomes separated from the rectum. The definitive kidneys, or **metanephroi,** begin to form during the latter part of the fifth week as **ureteric buds** sprout from the mesonephric ducts into the intermediate mesoderm in the sacral region. The ureteric buds give rise to the collecting system of the definitive kidneys and become emplaced on the posterior bladder wall as the lower ends of the mesonephric ducts exstrophy and are incorporated into the bladder to form the **trigone.** As the metanephroi ascend into the superior lumbar region, the ureteric buds elongate to form the **ureters.** In adults, the ureters course between the kidneys and bladder within the subserous fascia of the posterior body wall (Fig. 14–6*C* and *E* and see Chapter 13).

During the second month of development, a second set of ducts develops within the connective tissue investments of the mesonephric ducts. These are the **paramesonephric ducts.** Their inferior ends become connected to the posterior midline of the bladder (between the two mesonephric ducts) inferiorly. Their superior ends become associated with the gonads. It is at this point in development, at about the seventh week, that the development of the male and female urogenital systems diverges from this common **ambisexual (indifferent) stage** of genital development.

Differentiation of Male and Female Pelvic Viscera

The genital viscera begin to differentiate as male or female after the seventh week

In **males,** the constricted pelvic urethra at the base of the bladder becomes elongated and enveloped by the **prostate gland,** which is a pelvic organ (Fig. 14–6*D*). The **vasa deferentia,** which arise from the mesonephric ducts, terminate within the substance of the prostate at an expansion of the prostatic urethra called the **prostatic utricle.** Paired **seminal vesicles** sprout from inferior segments of the **vasa deferentia, or spermatic ducts,** just outside the posterolateral walls of the prostate gland, and so the short segment of each vas deferens between the root of the seminal vesicle and prostatic utricle is called the **ejaculatory duct** (see Fig. 14–11 and Chapter 15). The thin muscular sphincteric **urogenital diaphragm** forms just inferior to the prostate and regulates the release of urine from the more superior bladder and the release of seminal fluid during ejaculation (Fig. 14–7*A* and see Fig. 14–6*C* and *D*).

The constricted pelvic urethra of the **female** is short and enveloped only by the muscular sphincteric urogenital diaphragm (Fig. 14–7*B*). In addition, the mesonephric ducts regress while the paramesonephric ducts differentiate into the paired **uterine tubes (fallopian tubes,** or **oviducts), uterus,** and **superior end of the vagina** (see Fig. 14–6*E* and *F*).

Peritoneal Recesses in Males

Male pelvic viscera are related to pelvic peritoneal recesses

As has been described above, the coronal urorectal septum divides the cloaca into the bladder, which is an anterior structure, and the rectum, which is a posterior structure (see Fig. 14–6). There are no structures situated between the bladder and rectum in males, and so the depression that forms between these two organs is the **rectovesical recess,** or **space.** This recess is the most inferior region of the male pelvic cavity. The rectovesical recess is continuous with the **pararectal fossae,** which are depressions within the pelvic floor just lateral to the rectum. The lowest region of the rectovesical recess extends to within about 7.5 cm of the anus (approximately the length of the index finger).

Therefore, structures at the bases of the rectum and bladder in males, including the seminal vesicles and prostate gland, can be readily palpated via the anorectal canal.

Because the rectovesical space is the lowest excursion of the peritoneum in males, infectious agents or cancer cells may accumulate within it, eroding the peritoneum, bladder, and rectal walls to form connections, or fistulas, between the bladder and rectum (see below).

Peritoneal Recesses in Females

Female pelvic viscera are also related to pelvic peritoneal recesses

In females, the paramesonephric ducts initially attach to the posterior midline of the presumptive bladder. The superior end of the vagina and uterus then form as the ducts fuse together from their inferior ends. As the inferior end of the vagina becomes attached to the **vestibule of the vagina,** the vagina and uterus become interposed between the bladder and rectum (see Fig. 14–6). The inferior excursion of the peritoneum just posterior to the bladder is, thus, called a **vesicouterine pouch (recess,** or **space).** The inferior space between the uterus and rectum becomes the **rectouterine pouch,** or **pouch (cul-de-sac) of Douglas.** The rectouterine pouch is continuous with the **pararectal fossae** on both sides of the rectum.

The rectouterine pouch is the most inferior recess of the female pelvic cavity, extending to within 5.5 cm of the anus. As in the male, infectious agents and cancer cells may accumulate at this site. Erosion of the peritoneum, bladder, and uterine or vaginal walls by these agents may cause fistulas to develop between the bladder and vagina or uterus.

■ COMMON AND UNIQUE STRUCTURES OF THE MALE AND FEMALE PELVIC CAVITIES

Many of the pelvic viscera are common to males and females

The pelvic cavities of both sexes contain many of the same vital organs, including the **rectum** of the gastrointestinal tract and several **urogenital organs.** At the point where the **abdominal sigmoid colon** bends inferiorly, it becomes the **rectum.** The rectum enters the pelvic cavity in the region of the sacral promontory, courses just anterior to the sacrum, and exits the pelvic cavity via an opening in the levator ani muscle just ventral to the coccyx. The opening in the levator ani muscle marks the boundary between the rectum and anal canal, and so the anal canal lies outside of the pelvis within the **anal compartment of the perineum** (see Fig. 14–9 and Chapters 12 and 15).

In both sexes, the **bladder** lies upon the inner surface of the anterior wall of the pelvic cavity. It is located somewhat superior and posterior to the symphysis pubis and is also posterior to the pubic bones (see Fig. 14–6*D* and *F*). The ureters, which are attached to the posterior wall of the bladder, course superiorly from the true pelvis as they rise up and over the pelvic brim in the region of the sacroiliac joints. They continue to course within the subserous fascia of the posterior body wall on either side of the vertebral column in a superior direction to the kidneys. Other pelvic organs present in both males and females include a variety of structures of the lateral and posterior pelvic walls, such as branches of the **internal** and **external iliac arteries** and **veins, branches** of the **lumbosacral plexus,** and **parasympathetic nerves (pelvic splanchnic nerves)** and **sympathetic nerves (inferior hypogastric plexus)** of the autonomic nervous system (see below).

Many pelvic structures are uniquely male or female

Genital organs of the male and female pelvis are distinct. These include the genital duct systems (vasa deferentia in males; oviducts, uterus, and vagina in females) and numerous accessory glands.

The anatomy of these structures, in turn, leads to differences in the anatomy of structures otherwise common to both sexes. For example, the pelvic urethra of males also includes a prostatic region not present in females. The pelvic diaphragm in females is uniquely modified to accommodate the support and function of the vagina. In addition, the anatomy of the peritoneal recesses is different in males and females (see above).

▲ Rectum and Anal Canal

The rectum is the pelvic terminus of the hindgut

As the gastrointestinal tract bends inferiorly to enter the true pelvis, the structure and peritoneal relationships characteristic of the **sigmoid colon** abruptly change into those characteristic of the most terminal region of the rectum. For example, the rectum is never suspended by mesentery and, therefore, is a retroperitoneal organ. It is embedded within the posterior body wall adjacent to vertebrae S3 to S5 and the coccygeal vertebrae. The rectum is attached to the anterior wall of the sacrum by loose connective tissue, which also encloses vessels and nerves (see Fig. 14–6 and below). The rectum is about 5 inches (15 to 20 cm) long, and its diameter is approximately the same as that of the sigmoid colon, except at a slightly expanded inferior region called the **rectal ampulla** (see Fig. 12–21). In addition, the haustra (sacculi) that are characteristic of the sigmoid colon are absent from the rectum. However, alternating infolds of the rectal wall (most superior on the left, then on the right, and then on the left) form the so-called **superior, middle,** and **inferior rectal valves** (see Fig. 14–6). The anterior and lateral surfaces of the upper two thirds of the rectum have a serosal layer. However, only the anterior surface of the lower one third of the rectum is invested by peritoneum. The subserosal layer of rectal connective tissue is not unlike that in other regions of the gastrointestinal tract, but the longitudinal layer of deep muscle is organized in a unique manner. Just above the junction of the sigmoid colon and rectum, the taeniae coli widen to form an anterior and posterior longitudinal band within the rectal wall that courses throughout the full length of the rectum. Some of the deepest longitudinal muscle fibers diverge to join the circular muscle layer. The circular muscle is uniformly distributed throughout most of the rectal wall but is significantly thickened at the terminus of the rectum (i.e., the boundary of the rectum and **anal canal)** (see also Chapters 12 and 15). This thickened region of circular muscle is the **internal anal sphincter (sphincter ani internus).** It surrounds the upper three fourths of the anal canal (see Figs. 14–6 and 14–16 and Chapter 12).

The **anal canal** arises from an ectodermal invagination called the **anal pit.** Its vascularization and innervation are distinct from that of the upper two thirds of the anorectal canal (rectum). (See also the discussion of the portal system, below, and in Chapter 15.) The diameter of the anal canal is regulated by the thickened smooth muscle of the internal anal sphincter and a complex of striated muscles, including the **external anal sphincter** and **puborectalis muscle** of the **pelvic diaphragm** (see below and Chapters 12 and 15). The external anal sphincter surrounds the entire length of the anal canal but is typically divided into three parts. The most superior (deepest) part is the **deep external anal sphincter;** the middle part, the **superficial external anal sphincter;** and the most inferior part, the **subcutaneous external anal sphincter** (see Figs. 14–6*D* and *F* and 14–16*C*). This lowest region of the external anal sphincter is partitioned by fascicles of smooth muscle emanating from the longitudinal layer of the anorectal wall, or **corrugator cutis ani muscle.**

The anatomy and functions of the pelvic diaphragm, including the puborectalis muscles, are described below.

▲ Bladder and Ureters

The bladder and ureters are retroperitoneal structures

In both males and females, the **bladder** lies just behind the pubic bones within the anterior pelvic wall (see Fig. 14–6). The bladder of a newborn infant holds 20 to 50 ml of urine, and the bladder of an adult holds 150 to 600 ml of urine. When the bladder is full, its superior apex extends slightly above the pubic crest and symphysis in both sexes.

The lumen of the bladder can be surgically entered through the lower abdominal wall with a **high,** or **suprapubic, lithotomy.** (The term *lithotomy* literally means to "cut for stone," or to make an incision for the purpose of removing a calculus.) This incision is sometimes made to remove small tumors or concretions that have precipitated within the urinary tract. Because of its location and accessibility, the bladder is prone to rupture from traumatic injury to the abdomen or anterior pelvis (see below).

The **urinary bladder** has three parts: a lower **neck,** an expanded **body,** and a superior **fundus** (see Figs. 14–6 and 14–7). The neck encloses the **orifice of the urethra.** The superior extension of the bladder is the **urachus,** which is located within the **median umbilical fold** (see also Chapter 11).

This vestige of the embryonic allantois rarely remains patent. If it is patent, urine may be expressed in the region of the umbilicus.

Only the superior surface of the bladder is covered by peritoneum. The other surfaces are embedded within the pelvic subserous fascia. Most of the bladder wall has three layers of smooth muscle: an inner and an outer layer of longitudinal fibers and an intermediate circular layer. The inner surface of the bladder is covered with a loose layer of mucosa, which develops folds when the bladder is empty. However, a smooth, tightly fused mucous membrane is present in a distinct triangular region on the posterior bladder wall just superior to the neck of the bladder. This is the **trigone of the bladder,** which is formed during embryonic life when the roots of the mesonephric ducts expand to become incorporated into the posterior wall of the presumptive bladder, resulting in emplacement of the roots of the **ureters** at the superolateral apices of the trigone (see Fig. 14–7). The definitive ureters course from these points of attachment into the subserous fascia and out of the pelvic cavity over the posterior pelvic brim within the posterior abdominal wall to the kidneys (see Chapter 13 for a discussion of nerves and blood vessels of the ureters in the abdomen).

Inflammation of the Bladder

Inflammation of the urinary bladder is more common in females but occurs in both sexes

In females, the relatively short urethra allows infectious agents to easily reach the bladder. In males, bladder infection is most often the result of urinary retention associated with prostatic disease (see below). Symptoms of urinary inflammation include frequent and painful urination, urgency, pain above the pubic region, and blood in the urine.

Cancer of the Bladder

Cancer of the bladder is not diagnosed as frequently as some other cancers, but it affects approximately 20,000 individuals and results in approximately 10,000 deaths in the United States each year. About 66% of patients are male, and 34% of patients are female. Like many other cancers, early diagnosis is the key to successful treatment. About 85% of patients survive for 5 years following diagnosis and surgical removal of tumors that have not spread to other organs. When tumors have spread, the outcome of treatment (i.e., surgical removal and chemotherapy) is less successful, and less than 50% of patients survive for 5 years. Symptoms include blood in the urine and urinary tract infection. Treatment ranges from surgical removal of the tumor and surrounding tissue to complete removal of the bladder, prostate gland, and seminal vesicles in males and removal of the bladder, uterus, uterine tubes, ovaries, anterior vagina, and urethra in females, followed by chemotherapy.

Injury to the Bladder

Injury to the urinary bladder usually occurs following pelvic fracture

In adults, blunt abdominal trauma that does not result in pelvic fracture causes the bladder to rupture only if the bladder is full. In children, bladder rupture is more common because the bladder extends more prominently into the abdomen, particularly when it is full and distended. Rupture of the urinary bladder is more common when there is a true fracture of the pelvis, particularly if the fracture involves the pubic bones. Extravasation of urine into the peritoneal space is most likely when the rupture occurs across the superior aspect of the bladder (e.g., as the consequence of a penetrating wound or trauma that does not cause a pelvic fracture). Extravasation of urine into the extraperitoneal space tends to occur following rupture in the anterior or inferior region of the bladder as a result of pelvic fracture. In all cases, the bladder must be surgically repaired.

▲ Urethra and Ligaments of the Bladder

The urethra is also a retroperitoneal structure

The urethra, at the base of the bladder, drains urine to the outside of the body (see Figs. 14–6 and 14–7). In males, the urethra has three parts: the **prostatic urethra, membranous urethra,** and **penile urethra.** In females, the urethra has only one segment, the **membranous urethra,** which is about as long as the prostatic and membranous urethras combined in males.

For this reason, calculi or small tumors may be more easily removed from the female bladder via the urethra.

Various specialized forms of subserous fascia provide support for the base of the bladder (Fig. 14–8). These include thickened bands on both sides of the bladder, which are the **puboprostatic ligaments** in males and **pubovesical ligaments** in females. The so-called **false ligaments** of the bladder include the **median umbilical fold** and **medial umbilical folds,** which contain the obliterated umbilical arteries (see Chapter 11 and below). In contrast to the puboprostatic or pubovesical ligaments, these false ligaments are not considered to provide functional support for the bladder.

▲ Pelvic Diaphragm

The muscular pelvic diaphragm lines the floor of the pelvic cavity

The inferior boundary of the pelvic cavity (just inferior to the inner layer of deep pelvic fascia) is a muscular sheet called the **pelvic diaphragm** (Fig. 14–9). This sheet of striated muscle is suspended from the coccyx posteriorly, from a specialized tendinous arch of the obturator internus muscle laterally, and from the inner surface of the bodies and superior rami of the pubic bones anteriorly. The pelvic diaphragm can be divided into two parts: the **coccygeus muscles,** which constitute the posterior part and course from the lateral edges of the lower sacrum and coccyx laterally to the ischial spines, and the **levator ani muscle,** which is the anterolateral part. The levator ani muscle can be divided into the lateral **iliococcygeus muscle** and anteromedial **pubococcygeus muscle.** The iliococcygeus muscles arise from the lateral inner surface of the coccyx and from a midline aponeurosis called the **levator plate (median raphe of the levator ani muscle).** The pubococcygeus muscles arise from the medial inner surface of the coccyx and sacrum, the anterior sacrococcygeal ligament, and the levator plate. Both of these muscles insert into an anterolateral **specialized tendinous arch of the levator ani muscle,** which is suspended from the inner surface of the superior pubic ramus anteriorly and from the ischial spine posterolaterally. The tendinous arch of the levator ani muscle courses deep to the **obturator internus muscle** and inferior to the lateral region of the iliopectineal line of the pelvic brim and the **obturator canal.**

The pubococcygeus muscle also includes a distinct medial subregion called the **puborectalis muscle (puborectal sling)** (Fig. 14–9). The fibers of the puborectal sling arise from the posterior surface of the bodies of the pubic bones and course in a posterior direction. They swing around the **anorectal hiatus,** which is the opening in the levator ani muscle for the gastrointestinal tract at about the level of the boundary between the rectum and anal canal (see Fig. 14–7). The levator ani muscle functions in the conscious control of defecation

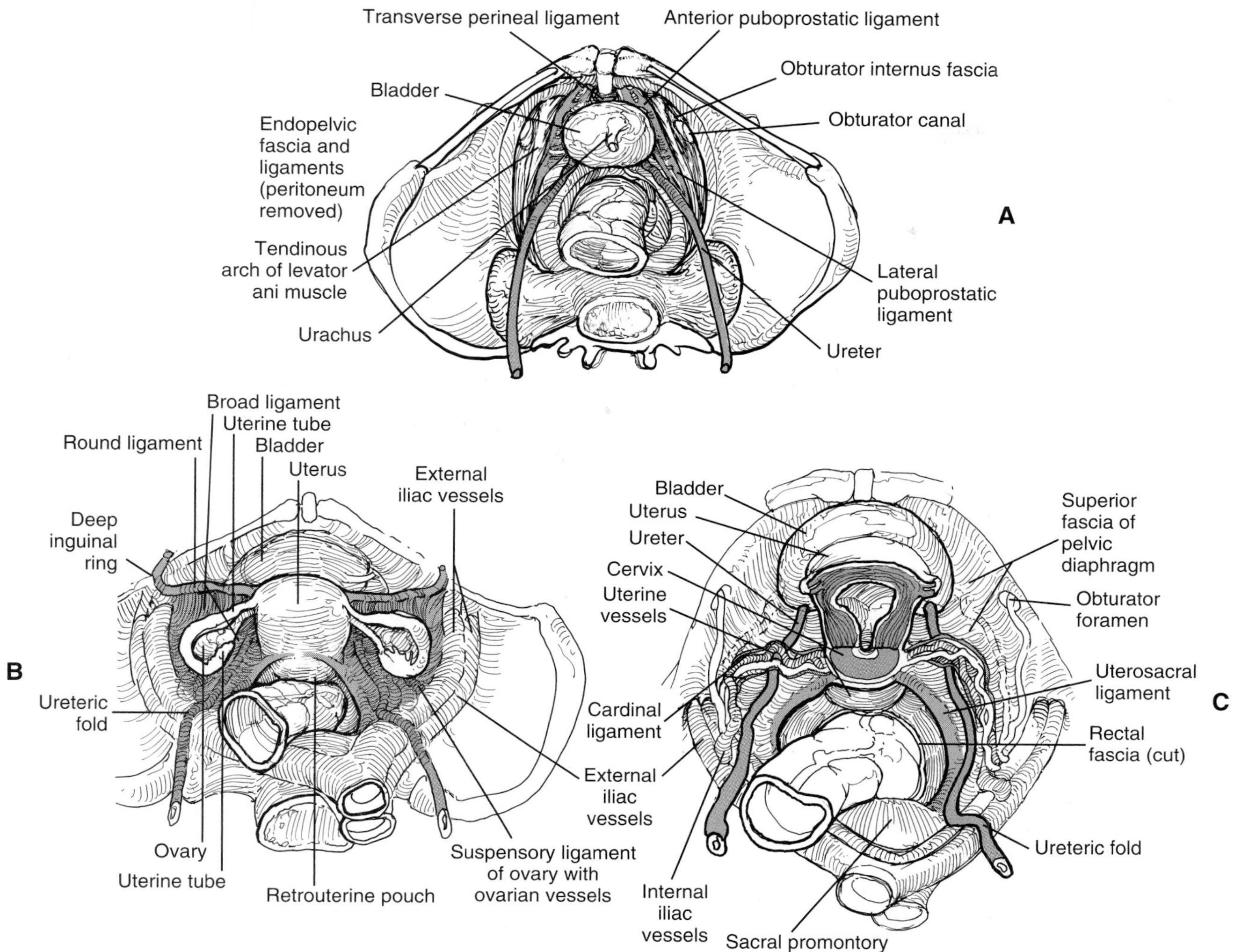

FIGURE 14–8
Specializations of subserous fascia in the pelvic floor. **A.** The puboprostatic ligaments support the bladder and the prostate gland in males. **B** and **C.** The pubovesical ligaments support the bladder in females. The vesicouterine ligaments, uterosacral ligaments, and transverse cervical ligaments (cardinal ligaments) support the uterus.

through contraction and relaxation of its striated fibers (see Chapter 15).

It should be noted that there is little difference in the anatomic structure of the male and female pelvic diaphragms (compare Fig. 14–9*A* and *B* with Fig. 14–9*C* and *D*). In both sexes, the pelvic diaphragm has a relatively large anterior hiatus. In males, the hiatus is traversed by the deep dorsal veins of the penis and the urethra. In females, however, it is traversed by the deep dorsal veins of the clitoris, the urethra, and the vagina.

Other muscles that are present within the floor of the pelvis in both sexes are the **obturator internus** and **piriformis muscles** (Fig. 14–9). These are muscles of the lower limb, which function in **locomotion** (see Chapter 17). Both muscles arise from the inner surfaces of the pelvic bones and exit the pelvis to insert on the femur. The obturator internus muscles arise from the inner edges of the obturator foramina (from the inner surfaces of the pubic bodies and superior and inferior pubic rami) (see Figs. 14–2*B* and 14–9*A* and *C*). These muscles exit the pelvis through the lesser sciatic foramina to insert upon the greater trochanter of each femur (see Chapters 16 and 17). Similarly, each **piriformis muscle** arises from the inner surface of the lower part of the sacral ala and exits the pelvis via the greater sciatic foramen. The piriformis muscle inserts just above the insertion of the obturator internus muscle on the greater trochanter of the femur.

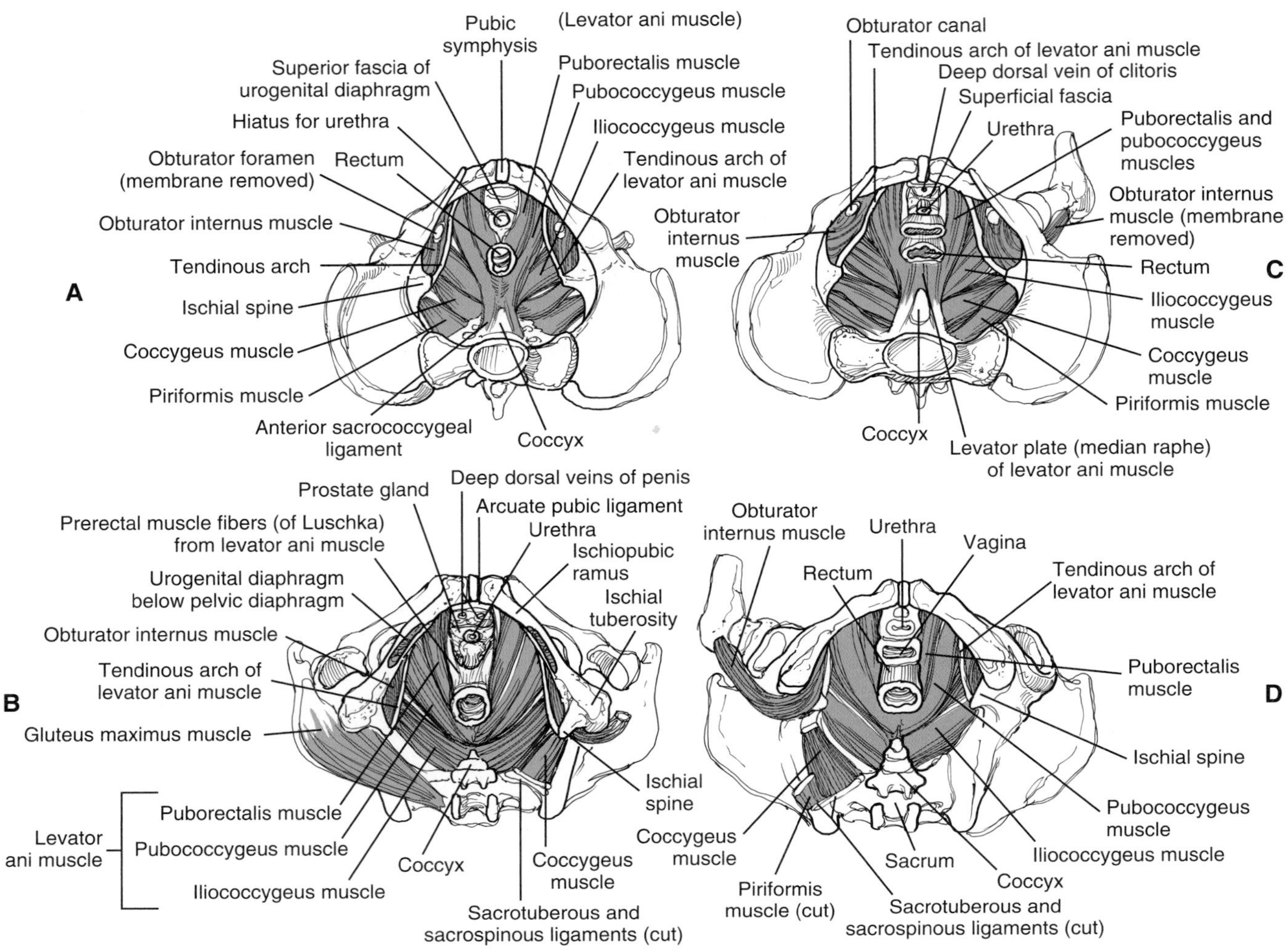

FIGURE 14–9
A. Superior view of the pelvic diaphragm in males. **B.** Inferior view of the pelvic diaphragm in males. **C.** Superior view of the pelvic diaphragm in females. **D.** Inferior view of the pelvic diaphragm in females.

▲ Sacral Plexus

The sacral plexus lies upon the floor of the pelvic cavity and provides innervation primarily to the lower extremity

Large nerves issue from the **ventral sacral foramina** to serve the ventral rami of spinal nerves S1 to S4. They join with the large lumbosacral trunk (spinal nerves L4 and L5) and ventral rami of spinal nerves S5 and Co1 to form the **sacral** and **coccygeal plexuses** (Fig. 14–10). The nerves formed within the sacral plexus course over the piriformis muscle (and behind the branches of the internal iliac vessels). They exit the pelvic cavity via the greater sciatic foramen. Although a few small branches contributed by fibers from spinal nerves S4, S5, and Co1 innervate muscles of the pelvic diaphragm (see below), most of the nerve fibers within the sacral plexus (along with the nerves of the lumbar plexus) innervate structures within the perineum and lower extremities. Their distribution and function is described in detail in Chapters 15 and 18.

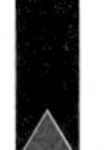

ANATOMY OF SPECIALIZED MALE PELVIC ORGANS

Prostate Gland

The prostate gland is a male genital gland

The **prostate gland** is located at the base of the bladder and surrounds the urethra. It has large **left** and **right lateral lobes;** a **middle (median) lobe,** which is interposed between the urethra and the ejaculatory ducts; and a **posterior lobe,** which is interposed between the posterior surface of the gland and the ejaculatory ducts (Fig. 14–11). The **isthmus of the prostate** is a band of fibromuscular tissue just deep to the anterior surface of the prostate that connects the right and left lateral lobes. The **ejaculatory ducts** are distal segments

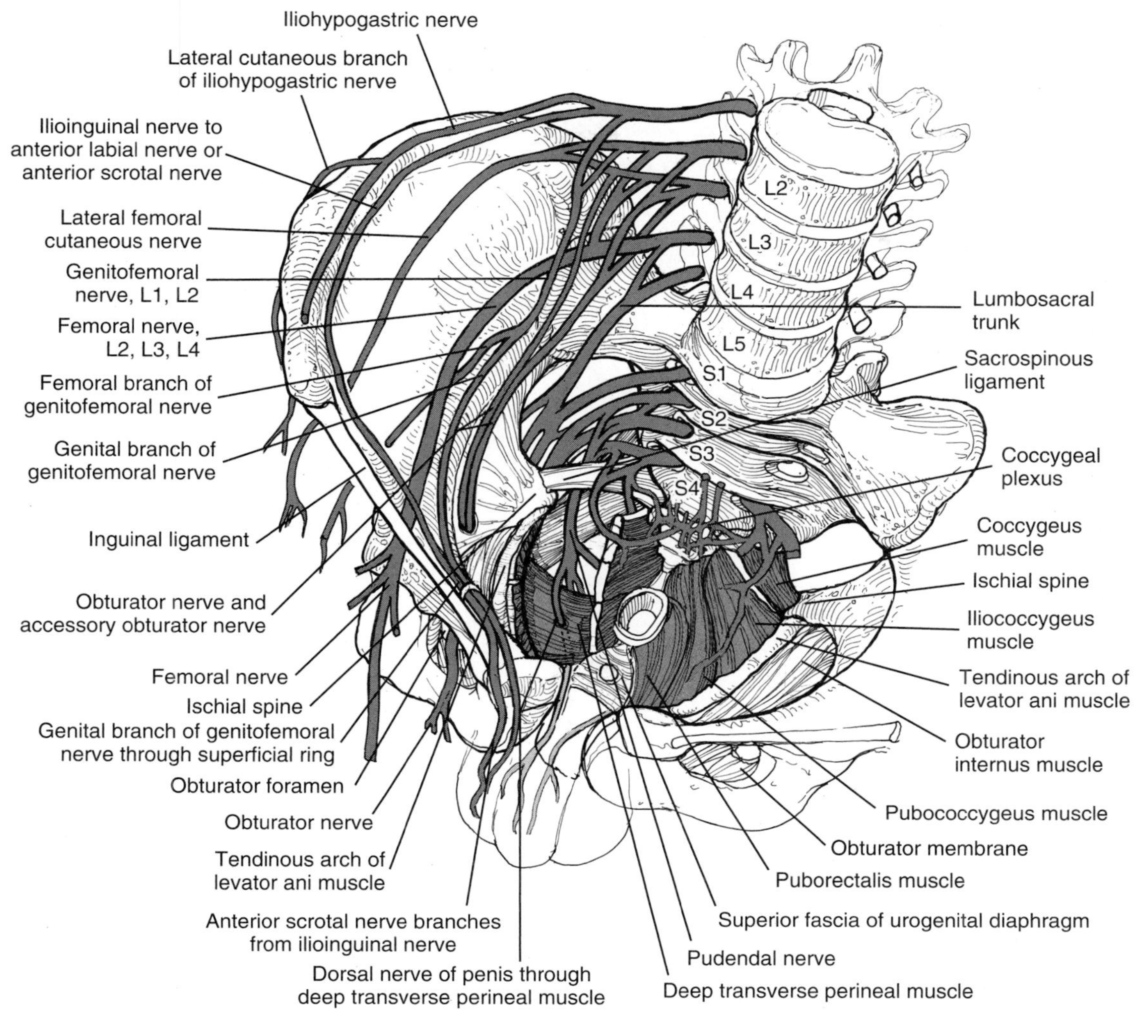

FIGURE 14–10

Sacral plexus and coccygeal plexus on the floor of the pelvic cavity. The sacral plexus consists of the ventral rami of spinal nerves S1 to S5 and contributions from the lumbosacral trunk (spinal nerves L4 and L5). The coccygeal plexus consists of the ventral ramus of spinal nerve Co1 and contributions from spinal nerve S5.

of the vasa deferentia, which are situated between the seminal vesicles and prostatic urethra. They course within the substance of the prostate after entering its superoposterior surface. They open into an expansion of the prostatic urethra called the **urethral sinus,** which surrounds an appendage called the **prostatic utricle.** The prostatic utricle protrudes from the floor (posterior side) of the prostatic urethra.

The prostate gland is invested by a thin capsule, which is derived from the pelvic subserous fascia. The **prostatic stroma** consists of connective tissue and smooth muscle, which invests the **glandular tissue** of the prostate. An outer circular layer of smooth muscle also surrounds the prostate gland, and another inner circular layer surrounds the prostatic urethra. This inner smooth muscle layer is continuous with the innermost smooth muscle layer of the bladder. The contraction of these fibers may prevent the escape of urine and the reflux of seminal fluid into the lumen of the bladder during ejaculation (see Chapter 15). Secretions of the prostate and seminal vesicles form most of the seminal fluid of the ejaculate.

Prostatitis. Disorders of the prostate gland are among the most common disorders of the male pelvic organs. Prostatitis is inflammation of the prostate gland. The cause is unknown or unclear in approximately 95% of cases. This condition affects about 50% of adult males at some time following puberty. The prostate gland becomes swollen and tender, causing pain in the superior pubic region and symptoms of

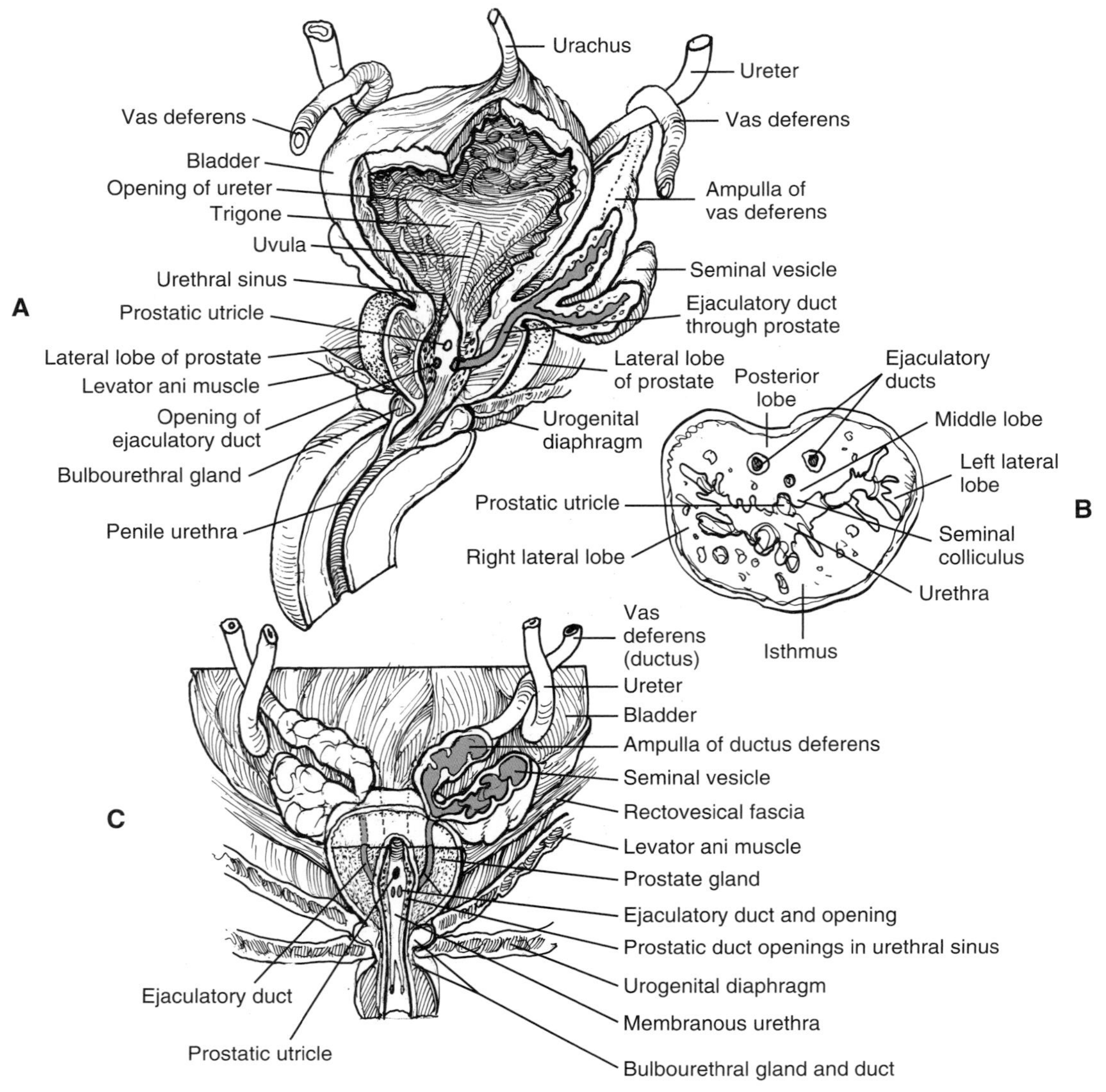

FIGURE 14–11
Accessory sexual glands of the male. **A.** The prostate gland and seminal vesicles are in close apposition to the base of the bladder. The seminal vesicles are buds of the vas deferens. They empty their secretions into the ejaculatory duct. **B.** The ejaculatory ducts penetrate the substance of the prostate gland to empty into the prostatic urethra. **C.** The prostate gland empties its secretions through small openings into the urethral sinus of the prostatic urethra.

urethral obstruction. These include difficulty in initiating urinary flow, decreased force and caliber of flow, urinary retention (i.e., the urinary bladder does not empty completely), and excessive dribbling after the flow has ceased. Retention of urine in the bladder leads to irritation, including frequent urination, particularly at night, an increased sense of urgency to urinate, and pain during urination. Bacterial infection may cause fever and urinary tract inflammation. This type of infection is often successfully treated with antibiotic therapy.

Benign Prostatic Hypertrophy. The symptoms of benign prostatic hypertrophy mimic those of prostatitis. Benign prostatic hypertrophy tends to occur in older males (over age 60 years). Patients do not have pain in the pubic region or fever, and the urinary flow rate is slower than in prostatitis. Patients suffering from benign prostatic hypertrophy are most commonly treated by surgical removal of a portion of the prostate.

Carcinoma of the Prostate Gland. Like benign prostatic hypertrophy, carcinoma of the prostate most frequently affects older males (55 years of age or older). It is the second most common cancer diagnosed in males in the United States and the third most common cause of death from cancer. The venous plexus that covers the prostate (see above) is the usual pathway for the spread of metastatic cells. Carcinoma of the prostate is often asymptomatic until it has spread to the urethra, when it produces symptoms similar to those of benign prostatic hypertrophy; to the skeleton, when it produces pain or fractures; or to the ureters, when it produces uremia (i.e., excessive nitrogenous waste in the blood). Treatment is based on the spread of the disease. If the tumor is confined to the prostate gland, the most common treatment is surgical removal of the gland. This treatment is very successful (there is no difference in the mean survival rates of these patients and age-matched control patients). There are complications, however, which include urinary incontinence (in 5% of patients) and impotence (in 30%). If the disease has spread significantly and surgical treatment is not a viable option, radiation therapy or antitestosterone drugs designed to inhibit the growth of the tumor are used. The success of these treatments is limited.

▲ Spermatic Cords

A segment of each vas deferens is located within the pelvis

During embryonic life, the **mesonephric ducts** drain urine from the thoracolumbar mesonephroi (embryonic kidneys) into the cloaca (presumptive bladder) through inferior connections in the lateral cloacal walls. Later, the mesonephric ducts of males differentiate into the **vasa deferentia,** and their connections to the presumptive bladder migrate inferiorly to the region of the prostatic urethra (see above), where they expand to form the **ampullae** of the vasa deferentia before emptying into the prostatic utricle (Fig. 14–11). The student will recall that the testes descend during fetal life. This results from the shortening of connective tissue ligaments called **gubernacula.** As the gubernaculum on each side shortens, it pulls the testis through the inguinal canal and into the scrotum. In this definitive configuration, the vasa deferentia course from the prostatic urethra at the base of the bladder upward upon the anterior pelvic wall and over the external iliac vessels. They then loop laterally around the inferior epigastric vessels to enter the deep ring of the inguinal canal (see Fig. 11–19*A* and Chapters 11 and 15). The testicular vessels of the spermatic cord do not enter the pelvis. Instead, they course within the posterior abdominal wall and along the lateral side of the iliac vessels within the iliac fossa to enter the deep ring with the vas deferens just lateral to the inferior epigastric vessels.

▲ Seminal Vesicles

Seminal vesicles are outgrowths of the mesonephric ducts

The **seminal vesicles** sprout from the male mesonephric ducts in the tenth week of development. In the definitive condition, each seminal vesicle is a single-coiled tube that folds back upon itself. Each gland is appressed to the posterior wall of the bladder just lateral to the ampulla of the vas deferens and extends superiorly to the distal end of the ureter (see Fig. 14–11*A* and *C*). The seminal vesicles are embedded within the pelvic fascia between the bladder and the rectum inferior to the rectovesical recess. They can be palpated via the anorectal canal.

The wall of the seminal vesicle consists of an outer layer of connective tissue, a middle layer of longitudinal and circular muscle fibers, and an internal layer of mucosal tissue.

Function of the Seminal Vesicles. The seminal vesicles are glands that produce a fructose-laden fluid, which provides an energy source for spermatozoa and constitutes most of the volume of the ejaculate (see Chapter 15).

■ ANATOMY OF SPECIALIZED FEMALE PELVIC ORGANS

The uterus, superior region of the vagina, and broad ligaments of the uterus are interposed between the bladder and the rectum within the pelvis in females

The superior end of the **vagina, uterus,** and **ovarian ducts (fallopian tubes, oviducts)** are derived from the **paramesonephric (müllerian) ducts,** which originally course from the midline of the posterior bladder wall in a superior direction to the developing ovaries within the posterior body wall. These ducts form in both male and female embryos but degenerate in male embryos under the influence of antimüllerian hormone.

In females, the paramesonephric ducts continue to grow and develop because antimüllerian hormone is absent. The ducts fuse during the second trimester. Fusion begins at their inferior ends and continues in a superior direction (like a zipper) to form the superior end of the vagina and the uterus. At the same time, the inferior attachment site of the fused müllerian duct is translocated to the roof of the presumptive **vestibule of the vagina (definitive urogenital sinus).**

In female embryos, the gubernaculum on each side courses from the labioscrotal folds (presumptive labia majora) inferiorly to the ovary superiorly. Within the posterior peritoneal wall, however, the gubernaculum becomes attached to each paramesonephric duct. Since the paramesonephric ducts are translocated medially as they fuse to form the vagina and uterus, they pull the gubernacula medially. As a consequence, the ovaries are pulled from their superior position within the posterior thoracic wall into the **broad ligaments of the uterus** (Fig. 14–12*A* and see Fig. 14–6*E*). Each definitive broad ligament then contains an **ovarian ligament,** a segment of the gubernaculum that courses from the ovary to the uterus, and a **round ligament of the uterus,** an inferior segment that courses from the uterus, through the inguinal canal, and into the labium majus. The combined length of the ovarian ligament and the round ligament of the uterus is approximately 15 inches. These ligaments are approximately $^1/_4$ inch in diameter (Fig. 14–12 and see Chapter 15).

The two broad ligaments and the uterus separate the true pelvis in females into an anterior compartment containing the bladder and a posterior compartment containing the rectum (see Figs. 14–6*E* and 14–12*A*). The roots of the broad ligaments originate from the lat-

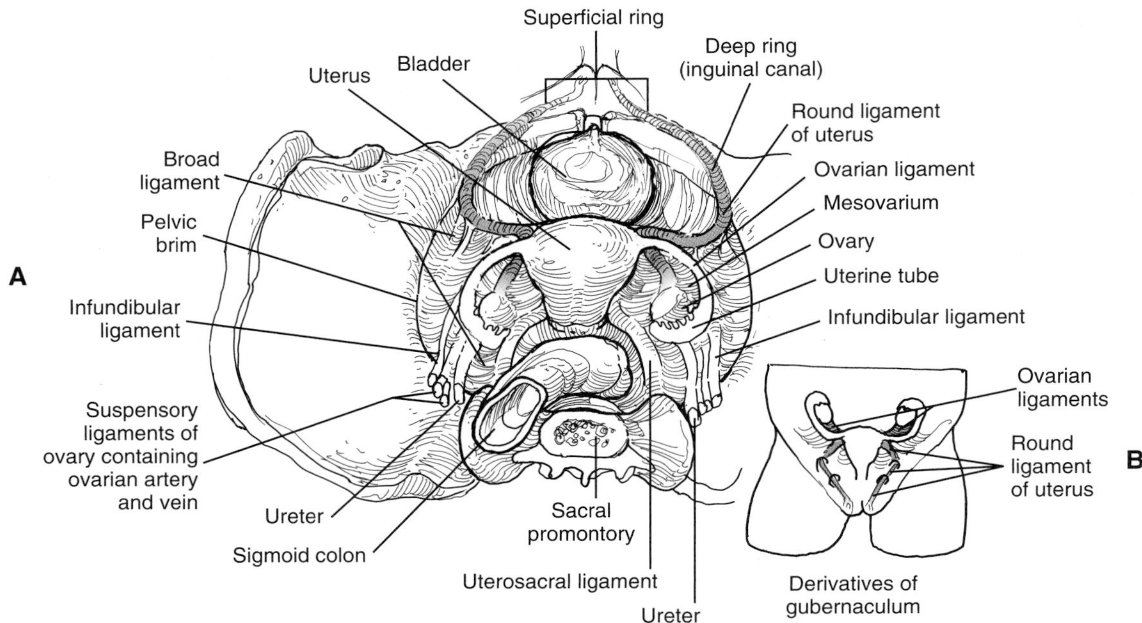

FIGURE 14–12
Female genital organs in the pelvic cavity. **A.** The uterus is between the bladder and the rectum, supported by specializations of the pelvic subserous fascia and by the broad ligaments of the uterus. The ovaries are suspended by a mesovarium from the posterior side of the broad ligaments, by suspensory ligaments of the ovary (which contain the ovarian vessels), and by the ovarian ligament. The ovarian ligament is attached to the lateral surface of the uterus and is continuous with the round ligament of the uterus, which traverses the inguinal canal, exits through the superficial ring, and inserts into the labium majus. **B.** The round ligaments of the uterus and ovarian ligaments are vestiges of the gubernaculum.

eral body walls of the pelvis and from the pelvic floor just superior to the pelvic diaphragm. As a consequence, the fascia enclosed between the anterior and posterior mesothelium of the broad ligaments contains the arteries, veins, and nerves of the uterus, vagina, and ovarian ducts; the ovaries; the ovarian ligaments; and the superior ends of the round ligaments of the uterus (Figs. 14–12*A* and 14–13*A* and *B* and see Fig. 14–17*B*).

The subserous fascia within the pelvic floor is thickened to form ligaments that provide additional support for the vagina and uterus. The **supportive ligaments of the uterus** include the anterior vesicouterine ligaments, posterior uterosacral ligaments, and lateral transverse cervical ligaments (ligaments of Mackenrodt, cardinal ligaments) (see Fig. 14–8*B*). The **vesicouterine ligaments** are thickened bands of subserous fascia that course from the lateral walls of the base of the uterus to the base of the bladder. The **uterosacral ligaments** are thickened bands of subserous fascia and muscle fibers that course from the base of the uterus to the sacrum. These ligaments are enclosed within the lateral **uterosacral folds,** which form the lateral borders of the **pararectal fossae** within the pelvic floor (see Figs. 14–6, 14–8*B*, and 14–12*A*). The **transverse cervical ligaments** are thickened bands of subserous fascia that course within the inferior roots of the broad ligaments. They connect the lateral walls of the base of the uterus to the pelvis in the regions of the sacroiliac joints at the medial surfaces of the psoas muscles. In this lateral region, the internal iliac vessels give off the **uterine artery** and **vein,** which vascularize the uterus (Fig. 14–13*B* and see below). In addition to the subserous ligaments just described, the uterus is supported to some degree by fibers of the levator ani muscle, the urogenital diaphragm, and the transverse perineal muscles and perineal body (see Chapter 15).

▲ Ovaries and Oviducts

Female genital ducts course from the ovaries to the vestibule of the vagina

As has been discussed above, the paired paramesonephric ducts fuse together to form the **superior end of the vagina** (including the **cervix)** and the **uterus.** The more superior unfused regions form the **oviducts (fallopian tubes, uterine tubes).** The lower end of the genital duct system, including the **inferior end of the vagina** and **vestibule of the vagina,** arises from the anterior region of the cloaca, which is the primitive urogenital sinus. The inferior segment of the vagina forms from an elongating diverticulum of the pelvic urethra (sinusal tubercle) near the base of the presumptive bladder. The vestibule of the vagina arises directly from the definitive urogenital sinus.

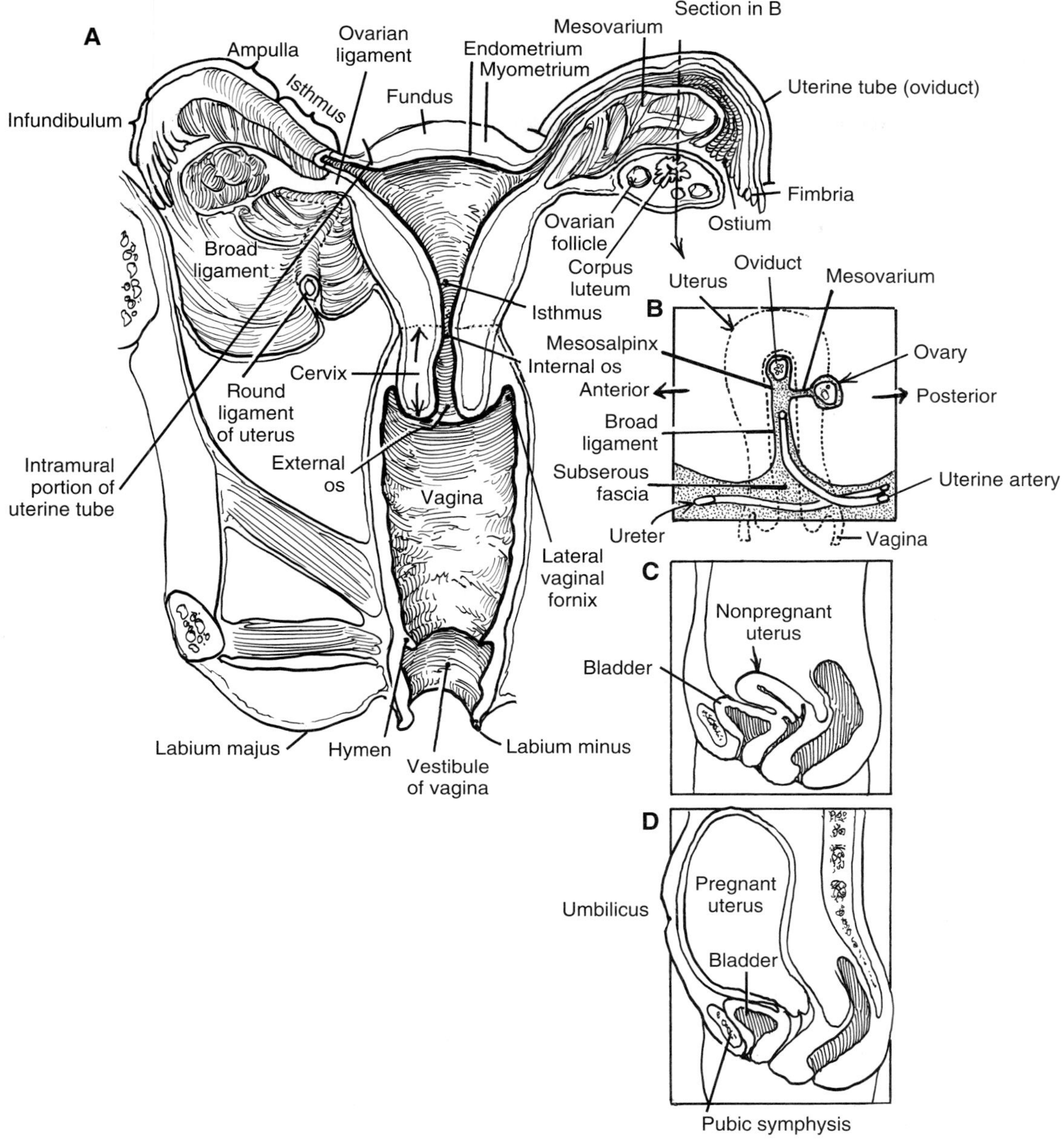

FIGURE 14–13
Relationships of the vagina, uterus, oviducts, ovaries, and supporting ligaments and mesenteries. **A.** Frontal section of left ovary, oviduct, uterus, and vagina. **B.** Parasagittal section of the broad ligament, showing its relationship to the mesovarium, ovary, mesosalpinx, and oviduct. **C.** Disposition of normal nonpregnant uterus. **D.** Disposition of normal pregnant uterus.

Each of the paired **ovaries** first develops in the lower thoracic and upper lumbar region of the posterior body wall and is then pulled into the true pelvis by the gubernaculum as the paramesonephric ducts fuse together (see above). The inferior **uterine extremity** of the ovary is suspended from the uterus by the round ligament of the ovary. The superior **tubal extremity** of the ovary is suspended from the surface of the psoas muscle by a fold of peritoneum called the **suspensory ligament** of the ovary. Ovarian vessels and nerves pass into the ovary through the suspensory ligament. The suspensory ligament also helps hold the ovary near the open end of the oviduct. The anterior surface, or **mesovarian border,** of the ovary is directly attached to the posterior surface of the **broad ligament of the uterus** by a fold of mesentery called the **mesovarium** (Figs. 14–12 and 14–13).

Each **oviduct** is enclosed within a mesentery **mesosalpinx,** which extends from the anterosuperior border of the broad ligament. The mouth, the **ostium,** of the oviduct is surrounded by scalloped projections called **fimbria.** The expanded region just distal to the fimbria is called the **infundibulum.** Just distal to the infundibulum is the **ampulla** (about halfway along the length of the oviduct). The ampulla narrows into an **isthmus** before coursing through the uterine wall as the **intramural segment of the oviduct.**

▲ Uterus and Vagina

In adult females who are nulliparous (i.e., have never borne children), the **uterus** is about 3 inches long and 2 inches wide and is completely contained within the true pelvis. It is shaped like an inverted pear. The large superior **body** of the uterus includes a **fundus,** a dome-shaped region above the openings of the oviducts (Fig. 14–13). The uterus narrows near its base into a short segment called the **isthmus** and a more inferior segment called the **cervix.** The cervix is slightly over 1 inch long. It has an internal constriction called the **internal os** and an external opening called the **external os.** The internal os marks the boundary between the isthmus and the cervix.

The inferior part of the cervix projects into the vagina, forming the **vaginal region** of the cervix. The superior region of the cervix is the **supravaginal region** of the cervix. The projection of the vaginal region of the cervix into the vagina creates the **vaginal fornix,** which is a continuous circumferential recess at the superior end of the vagina. It may be subdivided into **anterior, posterior,** and **lateral fornices** (Fig. 14–13*A*).

The **uterine cavity** is almost nonexistent in nulliparous adult females because it is compressed by the thick uterine walls. The uterine walls have an outer serous layer; a muscular layer, which consists of an outer longitudinal layer and an inner circular layer of myometrial smooth muscle; and an inner uterine mucosal layer, which consists of a connective tissue stroma containing many uterine glands and blood vessels and ciliated columnar **endometrium** lining the uterine cavity.

During pregnancy, the uterus enlarges so that the superior part of the body extends into the abdominal cavity and may even reach the epigastric region (Fig. 14–13*D* and see below). As the uterus enlarges, the uterine cavity expands and the uterine wall becomes very thin. The uterus also enlarges somewhat and is more highly vascularized during menstruation.

In normal adult females, disposition of the nonpregnant uterus varies somewhat depending on the fullness of the bladder. When the bladder is empty, the anterior (vesical) surface of the uterus lies on the superoposterior bladder wall. The uterus is, thus, disposed in a normal **retroverted** position (Figs. 14–13 and 14–14*A*). As the bladder fills, the uterus is displaced posteriorly. If the displacement is extreme, the uterus is cradled by the concave curvature of the sacrum and rectum. Even in this position, the anterior surface of the normal uterus retains its concave shape.

In some cases, however, the uterus is severely bent anteriorly (anteflexion) or posteriorly (retroflexion). Infrequently, the base of the uterus may be displaced posteriorly by the base of the bladder (retrocession). Abnormal anteflexion or retroflexion of the uterus may result in painful menstruation (dysmenorrhea).

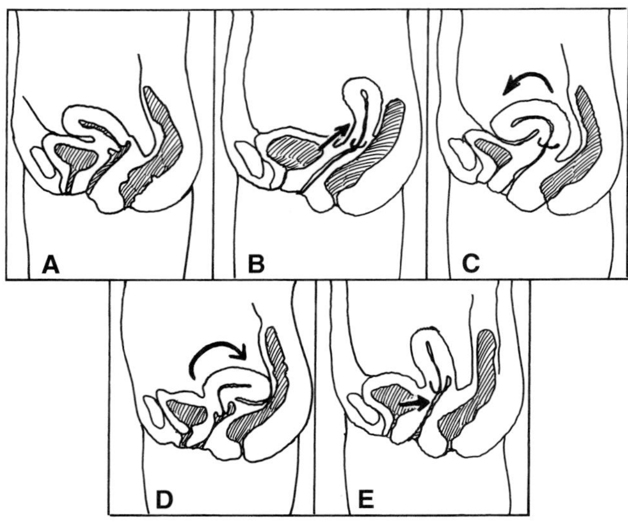

FIGURE 14–14
Normal and abnormal dispositions of the uterus. **A.** Normal retroverted uterus. **B.** Extreme retroversion of the uterus with a full bladder. **C.** Anteflexion of the uterus. **D.** Retroflexion of the uterus. **E.** Retrocession of the uterus.

The **vagina** connects the uterus with the **vestibule of the vagina** (Fig. 14–13*A*). The vagina is suspended from above by the supporting ligaments of the uterus (uterosacral and cardinal [transverse cervical] ligaments), levator ani muscles, urogenital diaphragm, and transverse perineal muscles. The vagina is 3 to 4 inches long. It is slightly wider above than below and slightly constricted at its inferior boundary with the vestibule by remnants of the **hymen.**

The **vestibule of the vagina** is a small cavity about 1 inch long, which technically lies within the **perineum.** It lies inferior to the pelvic cavity and between the labia minora of the external genitalia (see Fig. 14–13*A* and Chapter 15).

Female Sexual Response

Reflexes of the female sexual response ensure that the male ejaculate will be trapped by the vagina and uterus

Psychogenic factors and mechanical stimulation of the sensory endings of the pudendal nerve, which innervates the external female genitalia, initiate the **excitation phase** of the female sexual response. Reflex feedback via the **parasympathetic** nerves (i.e., the pelvic splanchnic nerves at S2 to S4; see below) results in expansion and elongation of the vagina, vasodilatation of the external genitalia, and stimulation of secretory activity by the greater and lesser vestibular glands (see

Chapter 15). The secretions lubricate the vaginal canal to facilitate intercourse. The **plateau phase** of the female sexual response is characterized by further vascular congestion and enlargement of the external genitalia and retraction of the clitoris toward the pubic symphysis. As **orgasm** is initiated, the outer one third of the vagina contracts in response to the **sympathetic** reflex activity of the lumbar splanchnic nerves (see below). At the same time, coordinated somatic motor reflexes cause the pelvic diaphragm to contract, particularly the puborectal sling, which receives reflex stimulation through fibers from the sacral plexus at S4. This elevates the uterus and cervix, producing a reservoir for deposition of the ejaculate in the region of the posterior fornix of the vagina. In addition, the genital canal of the cervix opens slightly to facilitate the entry of sperm into the uterus. The **resolution phase** is characterized by the gradual draining away of blood from the genital organs. The cervix remains open for approximately 30 minutes following orgasm, and a slight negative pressure within the uterine lumen is maintained to further facilitate the entry of sperm into the uterine canal.

Pregnancy and Childbirth

The uterus contracts synchronously and autonomously during labor and childbirth

When an oocyte is released from an ovary, the follicle is converted to a **corpus luteum,** which begins to secrete the steroid hormone progesterone. Elevated levels of progesterone circulate to the uterus, causing the endometrium to thicken in preparation for implantation of the embryo about 6 days later. If the oocyte is not fertilized and fails to become implanted, the corpus luteum degenerates (usually by about 11 days after ovulation), progesterone levels fall, and the endometrial lining is sloughed, along with the unfertilized oocyte, during the menstrual phase of the menstrual cycle.

If the oocyte is fertilized and becomes implanted, feedback from the uterus maintains the corpus luteum for approximately 6 weeks. At this point, the developing trophoblastic membranes of the placenta begin to secrete large quantities of progesterone, which maintain the nutritive, quiescent uterine state of pregnancy until about 38 weeks, when labor begins.

The signals that initiate labor in humans are not fully understood, but **hormonal factors** are thought to be more prominent than **neurogenic factors.** One theory is that endocrine signals from the fetal brain may cause the placenta to produce estrogen, which increases uterine contractility and initiates labor. In many species, such as sheep, rats, and rabbits, a distinct primary signal for the initiation of parturition is a decrease in levels of uterine progesterone. Evidence of progesterone withdrawal has not been obtained in humans or other primates. It is known, however, that high levels of progesterone are required to maintain pregnancy in humans. In addition, the artificial reduction of or interference with the action of progesterone in humans (e.g., by administration of the progesterone antagonist RU486) results in premature initiation of labor.

It is clear that significant secondary hormonal signals at parturition are provided by the pituitary peptide oxytocin and uterine prostaglandins. It is also well documented that the exogenous administration of oxytocin stimulates contractions of the uterus near the end of pregnancy and that the exogenous administration of prostaglandins PGE_2 or PGF_2 stimulates contractions and expulsion of the fetus at virtually any stage of pregnancy. Initiation of the normal, effective synchronous contractions of labor and childbirth in humans seems to require the well-regulated, coordinated secretion of many specific prostaglandins, cytokines such as interleukin-1, oxytocin, peptide hormones, and nitric oxide.

Cervical ripening (softening) must also precede effective labor to facilitate the dilatation and effacement of the cervical opening. This process is thought to depend on many of the same signals that prepare the uterus for contractile activity. However, contractile activity of the cervical smooth muscle does not play a role in cervical ripening. Ripening, instead, appears to primarily require the **degradation of collagen** within the cervical extracellular matrix along with an **increase in cervical hyaluronic acid.**

The process of labor occurs in three stages. The **first stage** is dilation of the cervix to about 10 cm. In normal labor, the head of the fetus passes into the vagina during this stage. The **second stage** is the delivery of the infant. The **third stage** is the delivery of the placenta.

As labor progresses, the uterus develops two segments: an **active upper segment,** consisting of the fundus, and a **passive lower segment,** consisting of the isthmus and cervix. During the three stages of labor, the walls of the active upper segment thicken because the muscle fibers do not relax to their original length following each contraction. At the same time, the uterine cavity becomes progressively smaller. As the upper active segment pushes down on the fetus, like the end of a shortening sock, it pushes more of the fetus into the passive lower segment. This causes the myometrial muscle fibers of the lower segment to stretch and the walls to become progressively thinner. The continued shortening of the upper active segment finally pushes the entire fetus into the vagina and out through the vestibule.

Pain and fear during labor may initiate sympathetic stimulation of the vagina, causing vaginal contractions to develop. This creates more resistance to the passage of the fetus and increases the mother's pain and frustration. The combination of these factors may create a positive feedback cycle that continues to stimulate vaginal contractions. As a consequence, the birth process may be prolonged until the muscles of the birth canal are fatigued enough to allow delivery to proceed.

Muscles of the abdominal wall play an important role in the second phase of labor because they increase the intraabdominal pressure. The muscles used are the diaphragm, external and internal oblique muscles, and transversus abdominis muscles. These are the same muscles used to increase intraabdominal pressure in defecation, urination, and vomiting. In all of these processes, the intraabdominal pressure is regulated by the interplay of contraction and relaxation of muscles of the abdominal wall and diaphragm. However, the forces generated by the abdominal musculature during childbirth are much greater than in the other processes. The essential role played by the abdominal muscles in childbirth is illustrated by the difficulties experienced by paraplegic women during labor.

In 8% to 10% of births in the United States, the signals initiating labor occur prematurely. About 250,000 preterm infants are born each year. Preterm labor may have devastating consequences. It is estimated that over 80% of the perinatal deaths that do not result from congenital disease result from preterm labor. Infection probably plays a significant role in the premature induction of many of the secondary signals, but current knowledge is inadequate for the design of truly effective preventive strategies.

Infection of the Female Reproductive Tract

The female reproductive tract is especially prone to infection

Infection of the female reproductive organs is common. **Vaginitis** may result from protozoan, bacterial, viral, or fungal infections. *Candida albicans* is a common fungal agent. Vaginitis is more irritating than it is life threatening. It is associated with the use of oral contraceptives or antibiotics. **Cervicitis** is among the most common lesions treated by gynecologists. It is characterized by a discharge in the absence of pain. If it is left untreated, cervicitis may lead to **pelvic inflammatory disease,** which is a more serious condition in which infection spreads to the lining of the uterus, oviducts, and pelvic peritoneum. The symptoms of pelvic inflammatory disease mimic those of acute appendicitis, with fever and abdominal pain that becomes intense when the abdomen is palpated. Diagnosis of pelvic inflammatory disease is based on the results of a cervical smear.

Disorders of the Female Reproductive Ligaments

Childbirth may stretch the supportive ligaments of the female reproductive tract

The fascial condensations and perineal muscles that support the vagina, urinary bladder, and uterus (see above) may become stretched over time, particularly after a woman has given birth a number of times. **Cystocele** (bladder herniation) occurs when the floor of the urinary bladder herniates into the anterior vaginal wall. **Urethrocele** (urethral herniation into the anterior vaginal wall) often occurs at the same time. These disorders result in recurring urinary bladder infections and incontinence. Surgical repair of the hernia must be performed to correct the condition. **Uterine prolapse** occurs when the supporting ligaments become weak and allow the uterus to herniate into the vagina. There are varying degrees of prolapse, the most severe of which is complete evagination of the uterus into the vagina. The symptoms of uterine prolapse include lower back pain, vaginal bleeding, feelings of pelvic pressure, and protrusion of the uterus from the vaginal opening. The only successful treatment is surgery, which may include repair of the pelvic diaphragm and hysterectomy (removal of the uterus).

Cancer of the Female Reproductive Organs

Cancer of the female reproductive organs is common

Endometrial cancer is the most common cancer of the female reproductive tract. It occurs primarily in postmenopausal women 50 to 70 years of age. Uterine bleeding is the classic symptom. Treatment usually involves surgical removal of the uterus and is very successful if it is done early in the course of the disease. If the cancer has spread to adjacent organs, radiation therapy is administered following surgery.

Cervical cancer is the second most common cancer of the female reproductive tract. It accounts for 15% of all cancers in women. Unlike endometrial cancer, cervical cancer tends to affect women in their 30s and 40s. It is asymptomatic at the stage when it would be most treatable. Therefore, the key to cure of this disease is early detection, typically by a Papanicolaou (Pap) smear. In its early stages, cervical carcinoma can be treated conservatively by electrocautery or surgical excision of the lesion. Treatment of cervical cancer that has spread to adjacent tissues is highly individualized. It may involve surgical removal of the upper portion of the vagina, cervix, uterus, and the pelvic lymph nodes or radiation therapy.

Although **ovarian cancer** (cancer of the ovarian mesothelium) is far less common (5% of all cases of malignant disease in women), its prognosis is the bleakest. Even if it is detected at an early stage, one third of patients do not survive beyond 5 years. Women who have not borne children, who have undergone pelvic irradiation, who have a history of benign ovarian tumors, or who have a family history of cancer are more at risk for developing ovarian cancer than others. The mean age of onset is 51 years, with 58% of these patients being postmenopausal. Abdominal pain and swelling are the most common symptoms. Less common symptoms are irregular bleeding, weight loss of 10 pounds or more, accumulation of ascites (serous fluid within the peritoneal cavity), or pleural effusion (see Chapter 8). The treatment is total hysterectomy, including removal of the uterine tubes and ovaries, and partial removal of the greater omentum. Lymph node sampling and washing of the abdominal cavity are done to assess the spread of the disease.

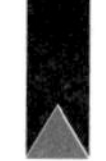

SYSTEMS THAT INTEGRATE PELVIC STRUCTURES

Pelvic Arteries

Pelvic walls and viscera are supplied by internal iliac arteries

The **common iliac arteries** bifurcate from the dorsal aorta on the left side of the vertebral column at the

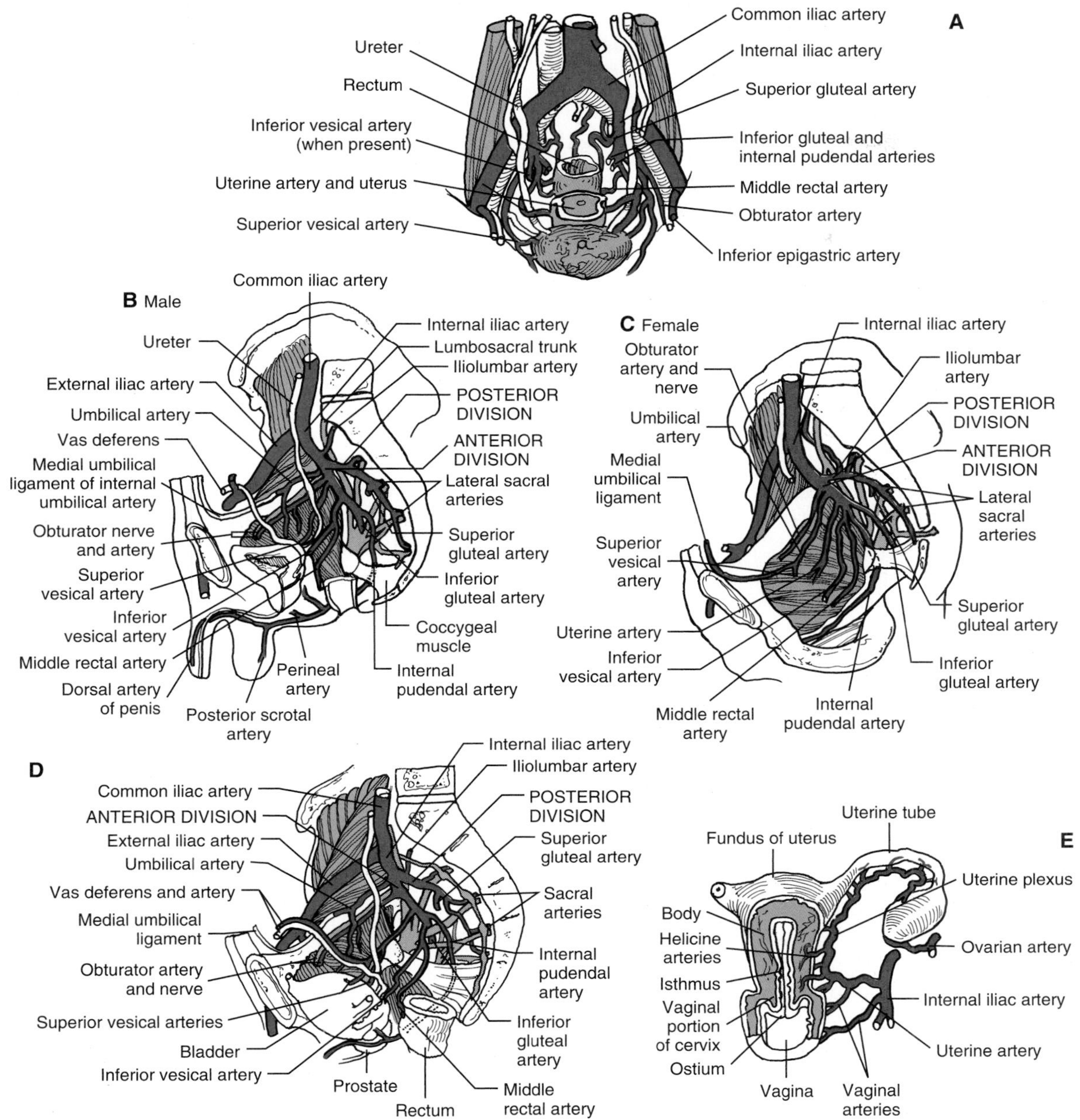

FIGURE 14–15
Arteries of the pelvis. **A.** Overview of pelvic arteries in the female. **B.** Overview of pelvic arteries in the male. **C.** Obturator artery shown as first anterior division branch. **D.** Prostatic and vesicular arteries in the male. **E.** Specialized ovarian, uterine, vaginal, and vesicular arteries in the female.

level of the disc between vertebrae L4 and L5 (Fig. 14–15*A* and *B*). The right branch is slightly longer than the left branch. Each of these large vessels divides into an **external** and **internal iliac artery.** The **external iliac arteries** do not enter the true pelvis. They skirt the pelvic brim, exit the iliac fossa, and enter the anterior thigh by coursing under the inguinal ligament and over the anterior pelvic brim in the region of the pecten pubis (see above and Chapter 18).

Almost immediately after the **common iliac arteries** bifurcate into the **internal iliac** and **external iliac arteries,** the internal iliac arteries branch into an **anterior**

division (trunk) and a **posterior division (trunk).** The posterior division supplies blood to the posterior and lateral walls of the pelvis, iliac crest, and gluteal region. The anterior division supplies blood to the pelvic viscera, perineum (see Chapter 15), and gluteal region. The branches of the posterior division are located primarily within the lateral regions of the pelvic cavity and the pelvic wall, while the branches of the anterior division typically course more medially to supply the pelvic and perineal viscera (Fig. 14–15*B* and *C*).

Posterior Division of the Internal Iliac Artery

The posterior division of the internal iliac artery usually has only three major branches

Two branches of each **posterior division of the internal iliac artery** supply the pelvic wall. These are the **iliolumbar** and **lateral sacral arteries.** A third branch, the **superior gluteal artery,** exits the greater sciatic foramen to supply the gluteal muscles of the gluteal region (Fig. 14–15*B* and *C*).

The iliolumbar artery supplies blood to the pelvic wall

The **iliolumbar artery** branches just anterior to the sacroiliac joint, ascends to the medial border of the psoas muscle (Fig. 14–15*B* and *C*), and splits into **lumbar** and **iliac branches.** The **lumbar branch of the iliolumbar artery** supplies the lower regions of the psoas and quadratus lumborum muscles and anastomoses with the fourth lumbar artery (see Chapters 13 and 18). It also emits a small branch that supplies the cauda equina by entering the vertebral canal through the intervertebral foramen between vertebra L4 and the sacrum. The **iliac branch of the iliolumbar artery** provides blood to the iliacus muscle. It courses along the **iliac crest** to supply the ilium, inferior fibers of the abdominal muscles, and superior fibers of the gluteal muscles along their apposed boundaries in the region of the crest. The iliac branch also provides important collateral circulation to the gluteal region because it anastomoses with the **superior gluteal artery,** to the anterior abdominal wall because it anastomoses with the **superficial** and **deep circumflex iliac arteries,** and to the hip joint at its terminal anastomoses with the **lateral femoral circumflex artery.**

Lateral sacral arteries supply the sacrum and structures within the vertebral canal

The lateral sacral arteries usually branch from the posterior division of the internal iliac artery within the shallow fossa between the lumbosacral trunk and the root of the first sacral nerve (Fig. 14–15*B* and *C*). Each artery descends along a line that connects the **ventral sacral foramina,** giving off branches that enter each sacral foramen to vascularize the bone and contents of the sacral canal. Continuations of each branch escape the sacral canal by coursing posteriorly through each **dorsal sacral foramen** to provide blood to the muscles and skin of the dorsal sacrum. The terminal branches may anastomose with the **superior gluteal artery** (see Chapter 18).

The superior gluteal artery is the largest branch of the internal iliac artery

The third major branch of the posterior division of the internal iliac artery is the **superior gluteal artery.** It continues beyond the lateral sacral branch of the posterior division. It exits the pelvis almost immediately through the greater sciatic foramen just above the superior edge of the **piriformis muscle** (Fig. 14–15*B* and *C* and see Chapter 18). Within the pelvis, small branches may supply the obturator internus and piriformis muscles. Once the artery passes into the gluteal region, it splits into **superficial** and **deep branches.** The **superficial branch of the superior gluteal artery** penetrates the deep surface of the **gluteus maximus muscle.** Several of its branches supply the muscle and others emerge from its superficial surface to supply the skin over the sacrum. Some of these branches may anastomose with superficial branches of the lateral sacral arteries (see above). The superficial branch of the superior gluteal artery may also anastomose with the **inferior gluteal artery.** The **deep branch of the superior gluteal artery** divides to supply the **gluteus medius** and **gluteus minimus muscles.** Branches may also anastomose with the **deep circumflex iliac, lateral** and **medial femoral circumflex,** and **inferior gluteal arteries** (see Chapter 18).

Branches of the posterior division of the internal iliac artery, their fields of vascularization, and their collateral connections are listed in Table 14–2.

Anterior Division of the Internal Iliac Artery

The anterior division of the internal iliac artery provides most of the blood supply to the pelvic viscera and perineum

In both sexes, the **obturator artery** is usually the first branch of the anterior division of the internal iliac artery (Fig. 14–15*C*). This artery courses along the lateral pelvic wall just inferior to the pelvic brim and exits the pelvic cavity via the **obturator canal.** It may be joined by or completely replaced by an **accessory obturator arterial branch** from the external iliac artery. The obturator and accessory obturator arteries supply the muscles of the medial compartment of the thigh.

The next branch of the anterior division of the internal iliac artery in both sexes is the **umbilical artery** (Fig. 14–15*C*). This artery courses anteriorly and medially just lateral to the base of the uterus in females and onto the inferior lateral wall of the bladder in both sexes. In the fetus, the artery carries deoxygenated blood back to the placenta. However, the termini of the umbilical arteries are obliterated at birth, and remnants of the arteries form the **medial umbilical ligaments,** which are enclosed within the **medial umbilical folds.** Nonetheless, the proximal regions of the umbilical arteries remain patent in adults and provide blood to their **superior vesical branches,** which supply the body and fundus of the bladder (Fig. 14–15*D*).

In **males,** a small branch of the superior vesical artery may supply the ductus deferens (see Fig. 13–5). The **artery to the ductus deferens** follows the ductus deferens through the inguinal canal and anastomoses with the **testicular artery** within the scrotum (see Chapter 15).

In **females,** the **uterine artery** branches from the anterior division of the internal iliac artery as the first of an array of terminal branches (Fig. 14–15*A* and *E*). It crosses over the top of the ureter to intercept the uterus at the lateral fornix of the vagina. At this point, the artery bifurcates. One branch ascends along the lateral wall of the uterus within the broad ligament, and the other descends along the lateral wall of the vagina within the thickened subserous fascia.

The **ascending branch of the uterine artery** remains closely apposed to the uterus until it reaches the oviduct. It then courses out along the oviduct to the hilus of the ovary where it anastomoses with the **ovarian artery** (Fig. 14–15*E*). The ovarian artery branches directly from the descending aorta and reaches the ovary via the suspensory ligament of the ovary (see Chapter 13). Its branches also supply the round ligament of the uterus. Because branches of the uterine artery that supply the uterine muscle are highly convoluted, they are called the **helicine** (from the Greek, meaning *coiled*) **arteries of the uterus.**

The **descending branch of the uterine artery** supplies the cervix of the uterus. It then descends upon the wall of the vagina (Fig. 14–15*E*). At this point, the uterine artery anastomoses with branches of the **vaginal artery,** which may originally branch from the same stem as the uterine artery or from a more distal stem of the anterior division of the internal iliac artery. Anastomoses of the uterine and vaginal arterial branches are collectively known as the **azygos arteries of the vagina.**

As was noted above, the **vaginal artery** may branch from the same stem of the anterior division of the internal iliac artery as the uterine artery or from another stem. If two or three vaginal arteries exist on each side of the vagina, both patterns may be apparent in the same individual. The inferior vesical artery of the female may also arise from one of the branches of the vaginal artery. The vaginal arteries supply the vagina and may have branches that supply the vestibular bulbs (see Chapter 15).

In males, the **inferior vesical artery** branches from the anterior division of the internal iliac artery just distal to the umbilical artery (Fig. 14–15*D*). It is sometimes a separate branch, and it sometimes branches from the same stem as the **middle rectal artery** (see below). Similar branches may be found in females (Fig. 14–15*C*). The inferior vesical arteries of males, in addition to supplying the fundus of the bladder, supply the distal end of the ureter, seminal vesicles, and prostate gland. The inferior vesical artery of females supplies only the fundus of the bladder.

The **middle rectal artery** in both sexes usually arises from the same stem as the inferior vesical artery or may branch separately from the anterior division of the internal iliac artery (Fig. 14–15*B* to *D*). It may supply several organs of the pelvis, including the bladder, prostate gland, and seminal vesicles. The chief function of the terminal branch of the middle rectal artery, however, is to supply the distal end of the rectum.

Unlike the previously described branches of the anterior division of the internal iliac artery, the **internal pudendal artery** in both sexes escapes the pelvis via the **greater sciatic foramen** (Fig. 14–15*B* and *C* and see Chapter 15). It immediately passes back through the **lesser sciatic foramen** and enters a fascial canal on the medial surface of the ischium called the **pudendal canal (Alcock's canal).** However, shortly after it enters the pudendal canal, the internal pudendal artery gives off its first branch. This is the **inferior rectal artery,** which supplies the inferior one third of the anorectal canal. The internal pudendal artery courses anteriorly through the pudendal canal, emerging at its anterior end just posterior to the point where the transverse perineal muscles are attached to the ischium. The branches of the internal pudendal artery supply the perineum.

Like the internal pudendal artery, the **inferior gluteal artery** escapes the pelvis to vascularize extrapelvic structures (Fig. 14–15*B* to *D* and see Chapter 18). To accomplish this, this large branch usually passes between the third and fourth sacral ventral rami, just inferior to the lower edge of the piriformis muscle, over the upper edge of the coccygeus muscle, and into the gluteal region via the greater sciatic foramen. The inferior gluteal artery courses inferiorly just deep to the gluteus maximus muscle, which it supplies. Other branches of the inferior gluteal artery supply the obturator internus muscle, superior and inferior gemelli muscles, superior regions of the rectus femoris muscle, and hamstring muscles. A sciatic branch supplies the sciatic nerve. Once the inferior gluteal artery emerges from under the lower edge of the gluteus maximus muscle, it gives off cutaneous branches, which supply the skin of the posterior thigh. The terminal branches of the inferior gluteal artery may anastomose with the superficial branch of the superior gluteal artery and the ascending branch of the lateral femoral circumflex artery (see Chapter 18).

The branches of the anterior division of the internal iliac artery and their major fields of vascularization are listed in Table 14–2.

▲ Pelvic Veins

Venous drainage of the pelvic viscera, pelvic wall, and gluteal region follows a pattern similar to that of the arterial supply

The pattern of venous drainage of the internal iliac branches has more variations than the corresponding arterial supply, including some specialized regions that must be mentioned (Fig. 14–16*A* and *B*). In addition, veins draining the bladder and prostate, uterus, and in-

TABLE 14–2
Branches of the Posterior and Anterior Divisions of the Internal Iliac Arteries

Artery	Organ or Tissue Supplied
POSTERIOR DIVISION	
Iliolumbar artery	Psoas, iliacus, and quadratus lumborum muscles; superior gluteal muscle over iliac crest; cauda equina
Lateral sacral artery	Bone and contents of sacral canal, skin and muscle of dorsal sacrum
Superior gluteal artery	Obturator internus, piriformis, gluteus maximus, gluteus medius, and gluteus minimus muscles
ANTERIOR DIVISION	
Obturator artery	Medial thigh
Umbilical artery	Superior bladder, vas deferens
Uterine artery	Uterus, vagina
Vaginal artery	Vagina, inferior bladder
Inferior vesical artery	Inferior bladder
Middle rectal artery	Distal end of rectum, prostate, seminal vesicles
Internal pudendal artery	Anal canal, structures of perineum (see Chapter 15)
Inferior gluteal artery	Gluteus maximus muscle, skin of posterior thigh, obturator internus and gemelli muscles, superior end of rectus femoris muscle, hamstring muscles

ferior end of the anorectal canal form complex plexuses. In females, veins may anastomose with branches of the **vaginal plexus,** which is located on the lateral walls of the vagina. The vaginal plexus also communicates with the **uterine plexus,** which communicates with the **ovarian plexus.** The vaginal and uterine plexuses are drained by the vaginal and uterine veins. The **prostatic plexus** is located just anterior and lateral to the prostate gland. It receives blood from the prostate and **dorsal vein of the penis** (Fig. 14–16*B* and see Chapter 15). The **vesical plexus** is located at the base of the bladder. In males, it anastomoses with branches of the prostatic plexus. The prostatic and vesical plexuses are drained chiefly by the inferior vesical vein. All of these veins empty into the internal iliac veins.

The **rectal plexus** invests the rectum (Fig. 14–16*C*). It is comprised of branches of the **superior, middle,** and **inferior rectal veins.** The **external rectal plexus** is comprised of branches of all three major veins, but the **internal rectal plexus,** which lies within the anorectal mucosa, is comprised only of branches of the superior and inferior rectal veins. The external and internal rectal plexuses communicate with each other, draining blood back into the systemic venous system via the middle and inferior rectal veins or into the portal system via the superior rectal veins. The terminal branches of the rectal plexus are invested by very loose connective tissue, which provides little support for the plexus.

Because portal veins have no valves, portal blood may flow into the systemic veins of the rectal plexus in cases of portal obstruction. These features predispose the veins of the rectal plexus to dilation and the formation of varicoceles called **hemorrhoids** (see Chapters 12 and 15).

▲ Pelvic Lymphatics

As in other regions of the trunk, the **lymphatic vessels** and **lymph nodes** of the pelvis follow the course of the arterial system. Therefore, lymph is drained from the pelvic viscera, gluteal region, and perineum via branches of the internal iliac lymph vessels. It drains back to the common iliac vessels and lumbar vessels and nodes, particularly those of the **lateral** and **preaortic regions** (Fig. 14–17). These vessels drain into the cisterna chyli and thoracic duct, which empties into the venous circulation near the junction of the left jugular and subclavian veins (see Chapters 10 and 13). Lymph draining from the gluteal region and perineum may also drain into the external lymphatic vessels and nodes that accompany branches of the **external pudendal, superficial epigastric,** and **superficial circumflex iliac arteries** (see Chapters 15 and 18).

▲ Pelvic Nerves

Somatic motor and sensory fibers of the sacral plexus innervate the pelvic diaphragm

The levator ani muscles are innervated by nerve fibers from the ventral rami of spinal nerve S4 (see Fig. 14–10). The fibers branch from the ventral ramus just anterior to the ventral sacral foramen and course anteriorly, parallel, and inferiorly to the pelvic splanchnic nerves. A small branch of the sacral plexus comprised of fibers derived from spinal nerves S4, S5, and Co1 inner-

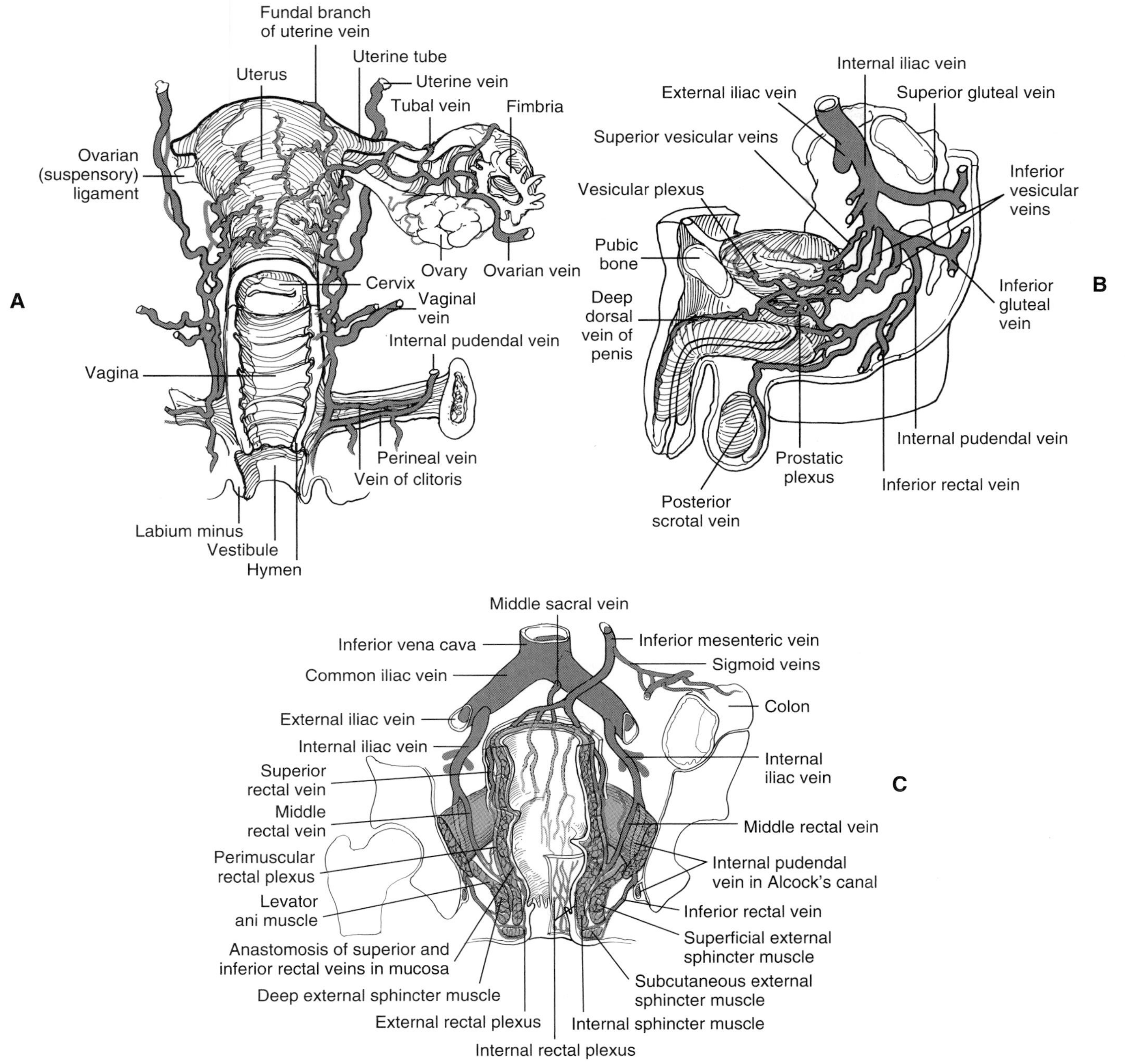

FIGURE 14–16
Veins of the pelvis. **A.** Specialized ovarian, uterine, vaginal, and vesicular veins in the female. **B.** Prostatic and vesicular veins of the male. **C.** Rectal plexus.

vates the coccygeus muscle. The actions of the levator ani muscles are described in Chapter 15.

Superior and Inferior Hypogastric Plexuses

Sympathetic and parasympathetic fibers of the superior and inferior hypogastric plexuses innervate the pelvic viscera

The pelvic viscera receive preganglionic sympathetic fibers from **thoracic, lumbar,** and **sacral splanchnic nerves** and from the **aortic (intermesenteric) plexus** via the **superior** and **inferior hypogastric plexuses** (Fig. 14–18). The sympathetic fibers may be from spinal levels T10 and T11 (i.e., the lesser splanchnic nerves to the ovaries or testes) or T10 to L2 (i.e., the lesser splanchnic, least splanchnic, and lumbar splanchnic nerves to the oviducts). The **hypogastric nerves** are the preganglionic sympathetic fibers and visceral afferent fibers from thoracic, lumbar, and sacral splanchnic nerves (and some ascending preganglionic parasympathetic fibers from the pelvic splanchnic nerves; see below) that connect the superior and inferior hypogastric plexuses.

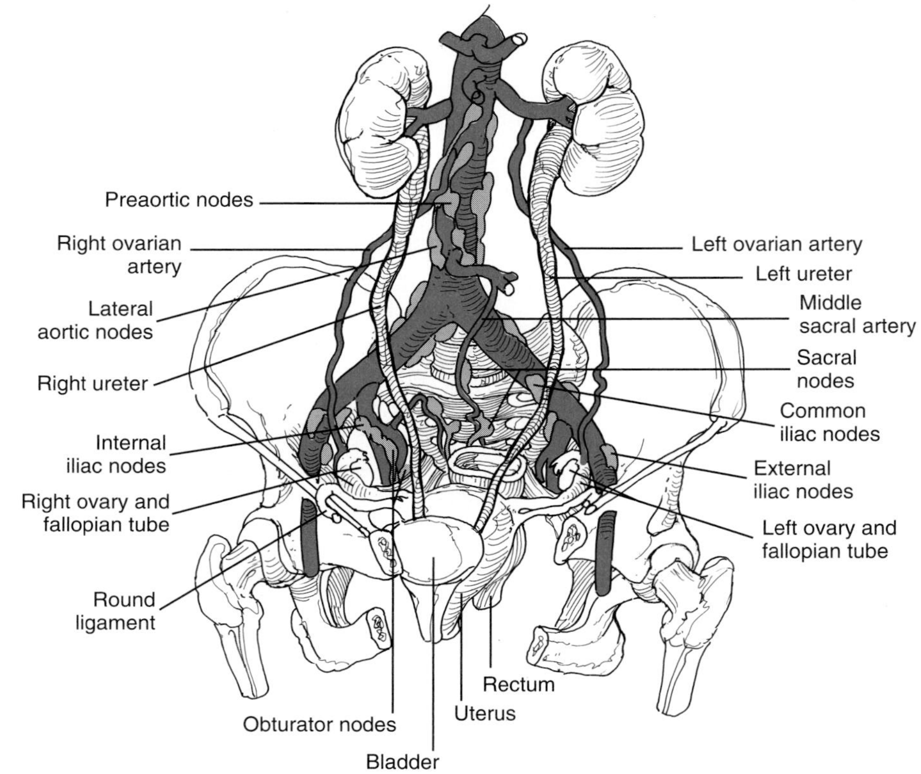

FIGURE 14–17

Lymphatic drainage of the pelvic viscera in the female. Lymphatic vessels follow the course of the pelvic arteries. Lymph is ultimately drained into lateral and preaortic nodes and then into the cisterna chyli and thoracic duct.

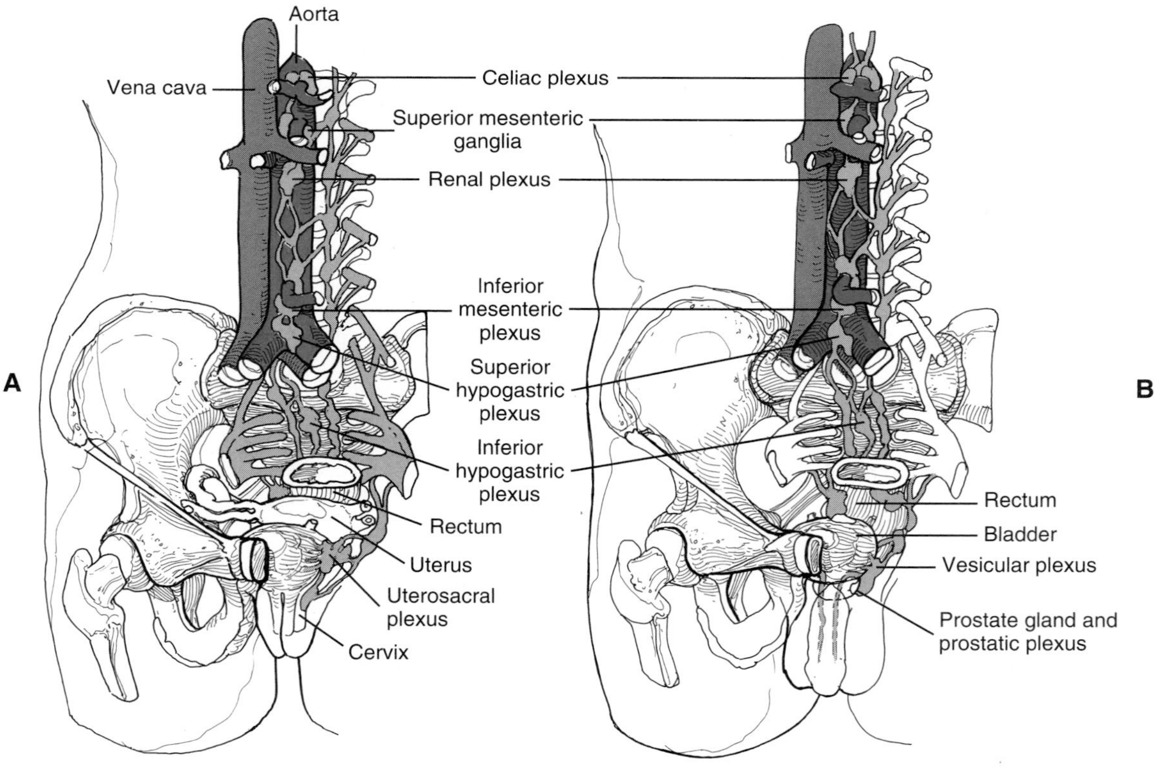

FIGURE 14–18

Pelvic nerves. The superior hypogastric plexus contains sympathetic preganglionic fibers arising at spinal cord levels T10 to L2. The inferior hypogastric plexus contains neurons or small collections of neurons, which are innervated by these preganglionic fibers and which emit postganglionic fibers that innervate pelvic and perineal urogenital organs (see Chapter 15). The inferior hypogastric plexuses also contain parasympathetic preganglionic fibers of the pelvic splanchnic nerves that arise from spinal cord levels S2 to S4. These fibers innervate the hindgut and the urogenital pelvic and perineal viscera.

TABLE 14–3
Origin of Pelvic Sympathetic Nerves that Arise from the Spinal Cord

Organ Supplied	Nerve	Level of Origin
Testis or ovary	Lesser splanchnic	T10, T11
Spermatic duct	Lesser splanchnic Least splanchnic	 T12
Oviduct	Lesser splanchnic Least splanchnic Lumbar splanchnic	T10, T11 T12 L1
Prostate	Lesser splanchnic Least splanchnic Lumbar splanchnic	T11 T12 L1
Ureter	Lesser splanchnic Least splanchnic Lumbar splanchnic	T11 T12 L1
Bladder	Lesser splanchnic Least splanchnic Lumbar splanchnic	T11 T12 L1, L2
Seminal vesicle	Least splanchnic	T12
Uterus	Least splanchnic Lumbar splanchnic	T12 L1
Vagina	Lumbar splanchnic	L1, L2
Unknown	Sacral splanchnic	L1, L2

The **superior hypogastric plexuses** contain preganglionic sympathetic fibers, which originate within the spinal cord at the level of T10 to L2, and visceral afferent fibers, which synapse with association neurons within the spinal cord at these same levels (Fig. 14–18). Interestingly, the peripheral ganglia of these sympathetic nerves are distributed more like the peripheral ganglia of the parasympathetic nerves (i.e., they are located in the vicinity of the target organ within the **inferior hypogastric [pelvic] plexuses** of nerves that ramify upon the walls of the pelvic visceral organs). The sympathetic innervation of the pelvic viscera is summarized in Table 14–3.

The **preganglionic parasympathetic fibers** of the pelvic viscera are provided by **pelvic splanchnic nerves,** which originate within the intermediolateral columns of the spinal cord at the level of S2 to S4 (Fig. 14–18). These fibers exit the cord via the ventral roots of these nerves and combine to form the **nervi erigentes,** or **pelvic splanchnic nerves.** The pelvic splanchnic nerves join the preganglionic and postganglionic sympathetic fibers of the inferior hypogastric plexuses and are then distributed to the pelvic viscera. Like the preganglionic parasympathetic fibers of the vagus nerve, the preganglionic parasympathetic fibers of the pelvic splanchnic nerves synapse with ganglia embedded within the walls of their target organs.

The function and coordination of the autonomic innervation of many of the pelvic viscera (including the rectum and bladder) and perineal viscera and the coordination of the autonomic and somatic systems are described in detail in Chapter 15.

15 The Perineum

The **perineum** and its contents cover and partially fill the inferior aperture of the bony pelvis. Thus, the bony circumferential boundaries of the perineum are the inner edges of the **pelvic outlet,** consisting of the pubic arch anteriorly; the pubic and ischial rami, ischial tuberosities, and sacrotuberous ligaments laterally; and the coccyx posteriorly (Fig. 15–1). If an imaginary plane were drawn intersecting the circumference of the pelvic outlet, it would be diamond shaped and could be subdivided into a posterior anal triangle and an anterior urogenital triangle by a transverse line connecting the ischial tuberosities (Fig. 15–1). The **anal triangle** defines the **anal compartment** of the perineum, which contains structures that assist in defecation, including the fatty tissues of the ischiorectal fossae, the inferior one third of the anorectal canal (anal canal) and its sphincteral muscles, and associated vessels and nerves (Table 15–1). The **urogenital triangle** defines the **urogenital compartment** of the perineum, which contains structures assisting in micturition and sexual function. This compartment is subdivided into a **superficial space,** which contains structures related primarily to the external genitalia, and a **deep space,** which contains only the urogenital diaphragm and a few accessory structures. Many of the structures within these compartments are small and delicate and may not be readily or easily appreciated in the dissecting laboratory. An exception is the major vessels and nerves supplying these structures, which are consistently present and easily identifiable: the paired internal pudendal vessels and their branches and the paired pudendal nerves (from spinal nerves S2 to S4) and their branches (see Chapter 14 and below). Unfortunately, it is a common human tendency to be somewhat repulsed or embarrassed by this region of the body. It must be emphasized, however, that the normal functioning of structures within the perineum is very important for the maintenance of an acceptable **quality of life.** Clearly, therapeutic interventions by the physician that repairs disruptions of the mechanisms of urination, defecation, and sexual function are essential to normal human activity.

EMBRYOLOGIC DEVELOPMENT OF THE PERINEUM

Structures within the anal and urogenital compartments form between weeks 4 and 7 of development as the **urorectal septum** divides the cloaca into an anterior **primitive urogenital sinus** and a posterior **rectum** (Fig. 15–2 and see Chapter 14). As this process is completed, the urorectal septum fuses with the cloacal membrane in the region of the presumptive superficial transverse perineal muscle and perineal body (Fig. 15–2*B* and *D*). The **cloacal membrane,** which is the inferior boundary of the cloaca, is thus divided into an anterior **urogenital membrane** and a posterior **anal membrane.** The anal membrane defines the inferior boundary of the rectum, while the urogenital membrane defines the inferior boundary of the primitive urogenital sinus (Fig. 15–2*B* and *D*).

BONY AND FASCIAL BOUNDARIES OF THE PERINEUM

As has been noted above, the bony boundary of the perineum is established by the diamond-shaped configuration of the pelvic outlet. More specifically, the pelvic outlet is defined by the **pubic arcuate ligament,** the bony rim of the inferior pelvic aperture (pubic and ischial rami and ischial tuberosities), the **sacrotuberous ligament,** and the **coccyx** (see Fig. 15–1*A* to *C*). In both males and females, a thin **superficial transverse perineal muscle** courses medially from each of the ischial tuberosities to insert into a midline knot of fibromuscular tissue called the **perineal body** (see Fig. 15–1*B* and *C*). These superficial transverse perineal muscles divide the diamond-shaped area into the posterior anal triangle and anterior urogenital triangle (much like the imaginary plane intersecting the pelvic brim, which defines the boundary between the false pelvis and the true pelvis).

The perineum also has fascial boundaries. It is lined with fascia and is bounded anteriorly by the **arcuate ligament** of the pubic arch (see Fig. 15–1*A*), laterally by the fascia of the medial surface of the obturator internus muscles; posteriorly by the deep inferomedial fascia of the gluteus maximus muscles; superiorly by the fascia of the pelvic diaphragm (levator ani and coc-

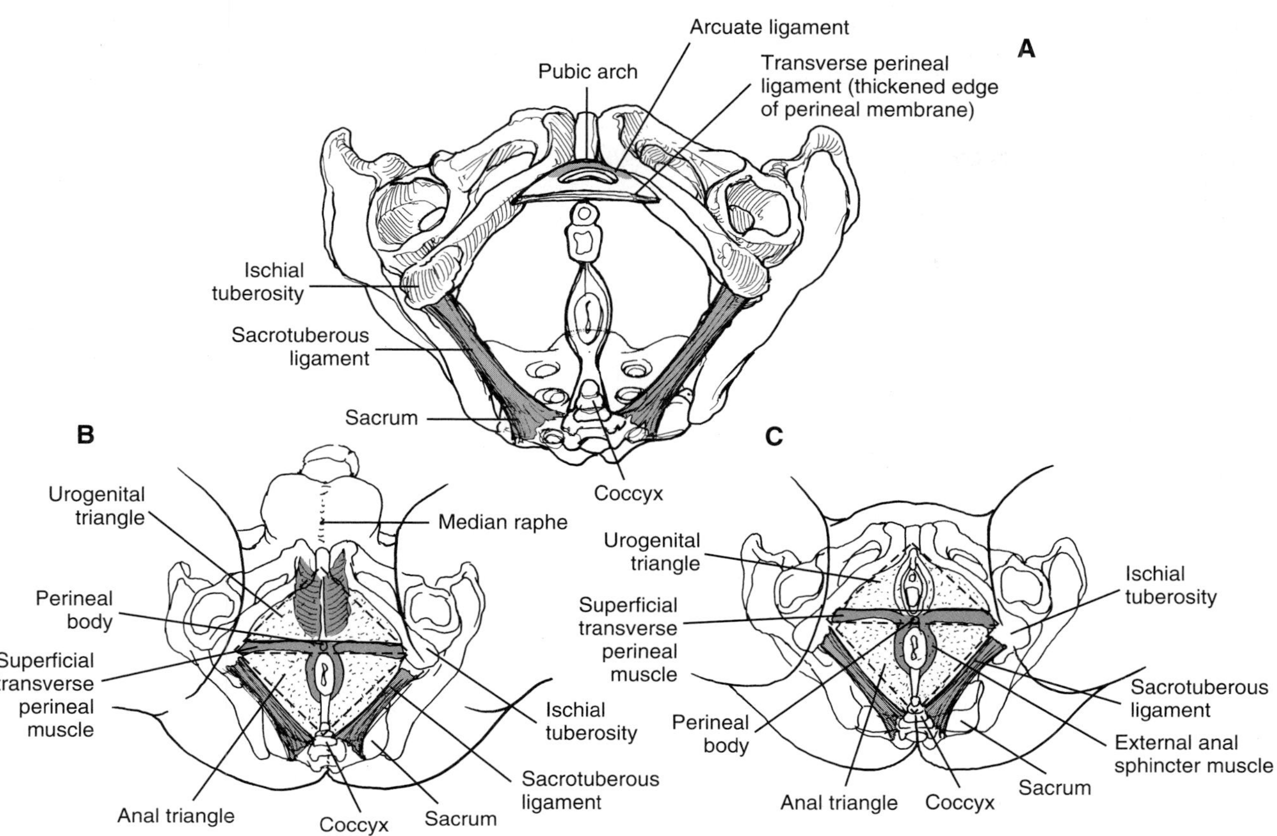

FIGURE 15–1
Boundaries of the perineum and the anal and urogenital triangles. **A.** Circumferential bony and connective tissue boundaries of the perineum include the pubic arch, arcuate ligament, and transverse perineal ligament anteriorly; the ischiopubic rami and sacrotuberous ligaments laterally; and the coccyx posteriorly. **B.** The anal and urogenital triangles in males are separated by the transverse perineal muscles and perineal body. **C.** The anal and urogenital triangles in females are separated by the transverse perineal muscles and perineal body.

TABLE 15–1
Structures of the Anal Compartment

Female	Male
Fat within ischiorectal fossae	Fat within ischiorectal fossae
Anorectal canal inferior to pelvic diaphragm	Anorectal canal inferior to pelvic diaphragm
Pudendal nerve and branches to levator ani muscles and external anal sphincters (inferior rectal branches)	Pudendal nerve and branches to levator ani muscles and external anal sphincters (inferior rectal branches)
Internal pudendal vessels and inferior rectal branches	Internal pudendal vessels and inferior rectal branches
Internal pudendal branches to anterior region of external sphincter	Internal pudendal branches to anterior region of external sphincter

cygeus muscles); and inferiorly by the perineal skin and its associated superficial fascia (Figs. 15–3 and 15–4).

▲ Skin of the Perineum

The perineum in both sexes is covered by skin within the circumferential boundaries defined by the pubic arch anteriorly, the median boundary of the thighs laterally, and the posteromedial boundary of the buttocks and the coccyx posteriorly. Within this margin, the integument is reflected onto the penis and scrotum in males or onto the clitoris, labia majora, and labia minora in females (see Fig. 15–3). In the anal region, the perineal skin is perforated by the anus in both sexes. In the urogenital region, the skin is perforated by the vestibule of

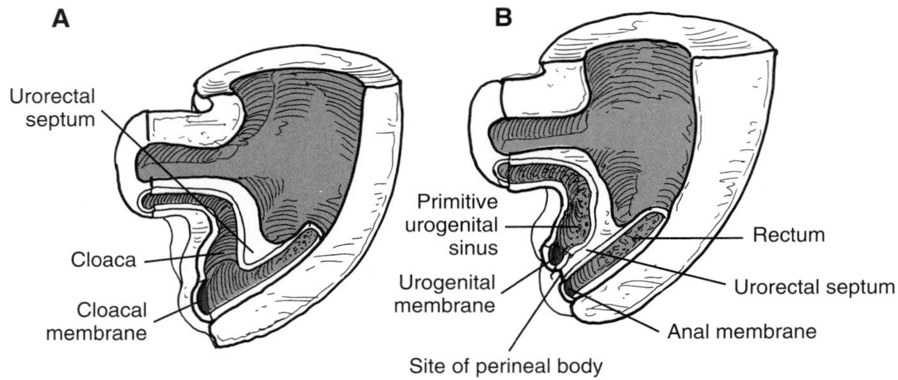

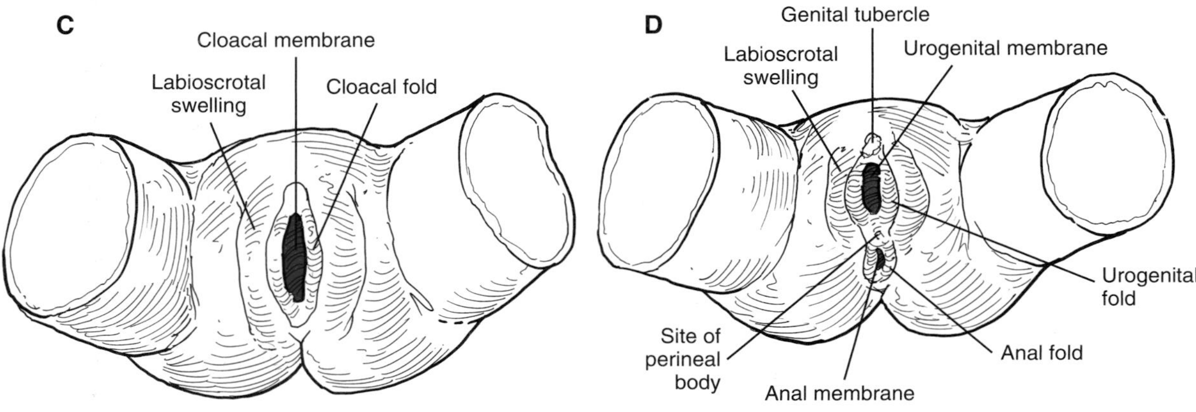

FIGURE 15–2

Embryonic origin of the perineum. The mesodermal urorectal septum **(A)** migrates inferiorly to separate the cloaca into an anterior primitive urogenital sinus and a posterior rectum **(B)**. **C.** Before development of the septum is complete, the inferior boundary of the cloaca is the cloacal membrane. **D.** Once development of the septum is complete, the cloacal membrane is divided into an anterior urogenital membrane (now the inferior boundary of the primitive urogenital sinus) and an anal membrane (now the inferior boundary of the gastrointestinal tract).

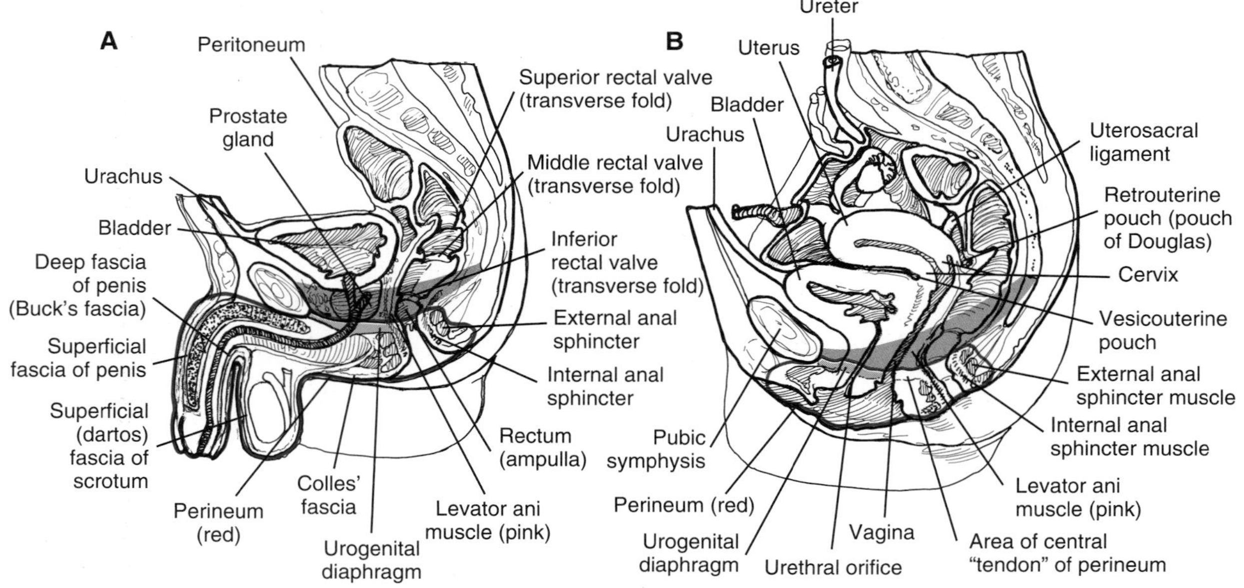

FIGURE 15–3

The inferior boundary of the perineum is the skin and superficial fascia surrounding the anus and covering the external genitalia. The superior boundary of the perineum is the pelvic diaphragm (posteriorly and laterally) and the superior layer of deep fascia covering the urogenital diaphragm anteriorly and medially. **A.** Male. **B.** Female.

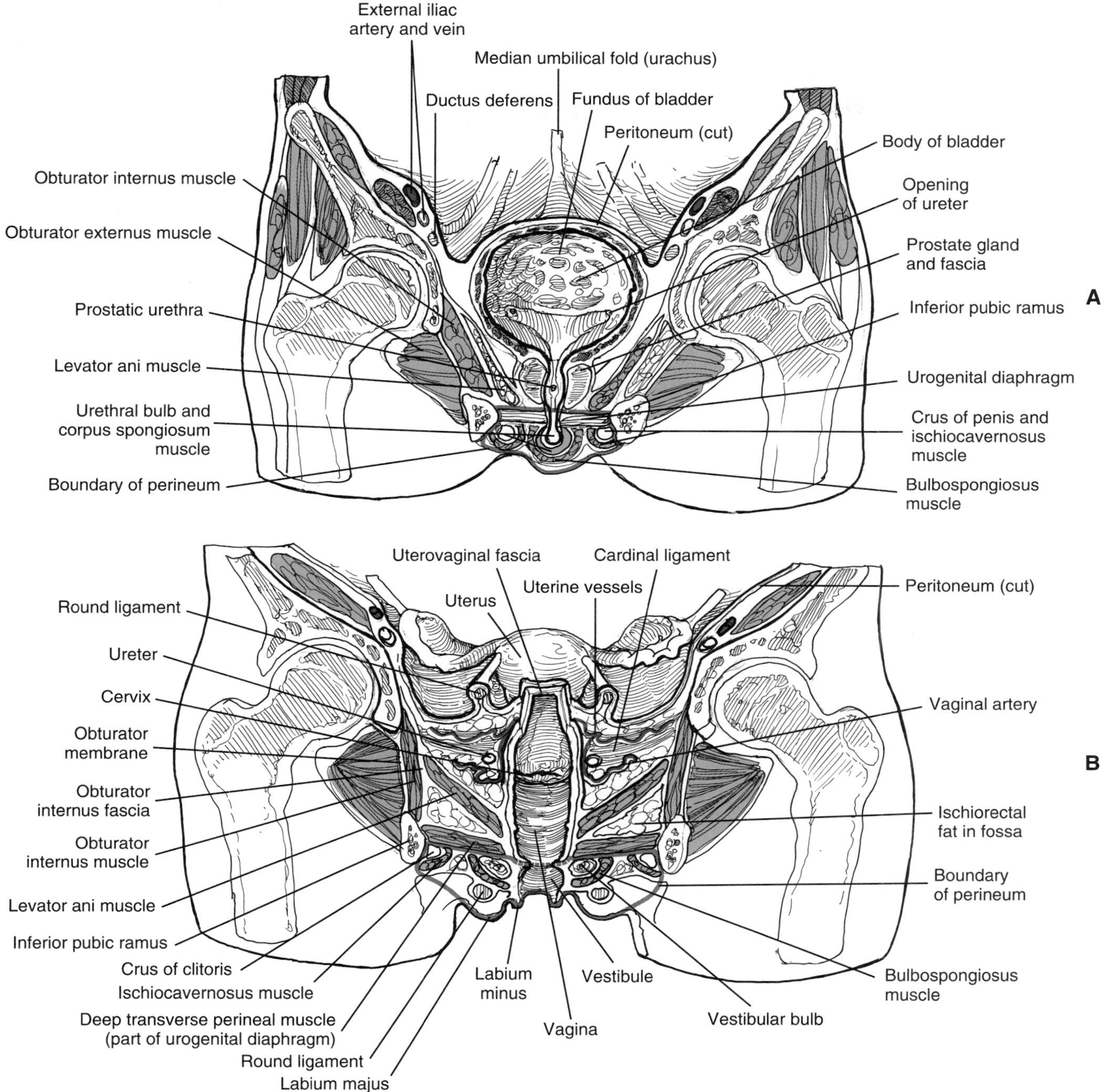

FIGURE 15–4
Coronal sections of the perineum in the male **(A)** and the female **(B)**, showing superior, inferior, and lateral boundaries of the perineal compartments. Note that part of the ischiorectal fossae (containing ischiorectal fat) is superior to the urogenital diaphragm in the posterolateral region of the urogenital triangle (see also Fig. 14–6*A*).

the vagina in females or by the diminutive penile urethra at the tip of the penis in males (see Fig. 15–3).

▲ Superficial Fascia of the Perineum

The superficial fascia of the perineum is located just deep to the skin, as in other regions of the body, and is continuous throughout the perineum. In various regions of the perineum, this fascia is modified and given distinctive names (see Fig. 15–3*A* and *B*).

The fatty layer of superficial fascia underlying the skin in the anal region has become significantly thickened to form extended fatty wedges **(ischiorectal fat)**, which fill regions of the ischiorectal fossae on both sides of the anorectal canal (see Fig. 15–4 and 15–6).

The superficial fascia of the urogenital region (excluding that of the scrotum in males) consists of both fatty and membranous layers. The **membranous fascia of the urogenital triangle (superficial perineal fascia;** or **Colles' fascia)** is continuous with the superficial fascia of the anterior abdominal wall and is fused tightly to the deep fascia of the thighs and the transverse perineal muscles (see below). It also invests the penis in males (superficial penile fascia) and the clitoris in females. The superficial fascia of the scrotum is modified as the **dartos tunic,** which contains smooth muscle fibers (see Fig. 15–3*A*). The tunica dartos also forms a septum, which divides the scrotal cavity into two compartments. Its location is indicated by a median raphe on the surface of the scrotum (see Fig. 15–1*B*). In females, the superficial fascia of the labia majora contains adipose tissue intermixed with smooth muscle fibers similar to those of the tunica dartos in males.

▲ Compartments of the Perineum

The fascia investing the posterior surface of the superficial and deep transverse perineal muscles subdivides the perineum into the anterior **urogenital compartment** and posterior **anal compartment.** The urogenital compartment is further subdivided by the **perineal membrane** into **superficial** and **deep spaces (compartments)** (see below).

ANAL COMPARTMENT OF THE PERINEUM

Structures that function in the process of defecation fill the anal compartment

The anal compartment consists of lateral communicating fascia-lined cavities that are completely filled with fat surrounding the inferior one third of the anorectal canal. As has been noted above, the superior boundary of the anal compartment is the fascia investing the inferior surface of the pelvic diaphragm, and the lateral boundaries are delimited by fascia covering the medial walls of the obturator internus muscles. It is more appropriate to think of the skin of the anal region as the inferior boundary of the anal compartment because the fatty layer of superficial fascia in this region has become thickened into large wedges of **ischiorectal fat,** which are defined, by convention, to fill the left and right compartments of the **ischiorectal fossae** (see below).

▲ Embryologic Development of the Rectum and Anorectal Canal

The separate embryologic origins of the inferior one third and superior two thirds of the anorectal canal are clinically relevant

As has been described above, following fusion of the urorectal septum with the cloacal membrane, the endodermal rectum ends blindly at the anal membrane. However, proliferation of ectoderm around the anal membrane at the end of the second month of development produces an indentation called the **anal pit,** or **proctodeum** (Fig. 15–5*A*). The anal pit forms the distal one third of the anorectal canal, which remains separated from the superior two-thirds (the rectum) by the anal membrane until week 7, when the membrane breaks down. Several vertical mucosal folds **(anal columns)** form within the most inferior segment of the rectum (Fig. 15–5*B* and *C*). These vertical folds are connected at their inferior ends by crescent-shaped folds, the **anal valves,** which form at the site where the anal membrane breaks down (pectinate line) (Fig. 15–5*B*). The developmental origins of the rectum and the lower one third of the anorectal canal result in differences in vascularization and innervation.

▲ Fat Within the Ischiorectal Fossae

The fat of the ischiorectal fossae is specialized to assist in the process of defecation

The fatty tissue filling the ischiorectal fossae defines the boundaries of the anal compartment, including its two anterior recesses superior to the lateral regions of the urogenital diaphragm (Fig. 15–6 and see Fig. 15–4). The composition and structure of the **ischiorectal fat** allows the inferior one third of the anorectal canal to change shape, facilitating passage of stool during defecation. However, this property and the large amount and extent of the ischiorectal fossae also contribute to the ease with which infectious agents may spread within the boundaries of the fossae (see below).

▲ Muscles of the Anal Compartment

Fibers of the **levator ani muscles** suspend the rectum at the level of the anorectal junction (see Figs. 15–3 to 15–5) and, along with the internal anal sphincter, prevent movement of feces from the dilated area of the lower rectum (ampulla of the rectum) into the anorectal canal. The **internal anal sphincter** is formed by a thickening of circular smooth muscle fibers within the wall of the anorectal canal at the level of the pectinate line (see Fig. 15–5*B* and *C*). These smooth muscles are innervated by **autonomic pelvic splanchnic nerves** (S2 to S4) via the inferior hypogastric plexus (see below). In addition, the lower region of the anorectal canal is surrounded by striated muscles **(external anal sphincter).** These muscles consist of **subcutaneous, superficial,** and **deep parts,** although these areas are not easily discriminated (see Fig. 15–5*C*). Anteriorly, the external anal sphincter is attached to the perineal body by a tough fibromuscular septum. Posteriorly, it is anchored to the coccyx by the fibromuscular anococcygeal ligament (see Figs. 15–5*C* and 15–6*A*). Striated muscle fibers of the external anal sphincter are innervated by the **somatic inferior rectal nerve** (S2 to S4) and, anteriorly, by a branch of the **somatic perineal nerve** (S4) (see below).

▲ Structures that Integrate the Anal Compartment of the Perineum

Vascularization of the Anal Compartment

The **middle rectal (hemorrhoidal) branches** of the internal iliac arteries and veins vascularize the

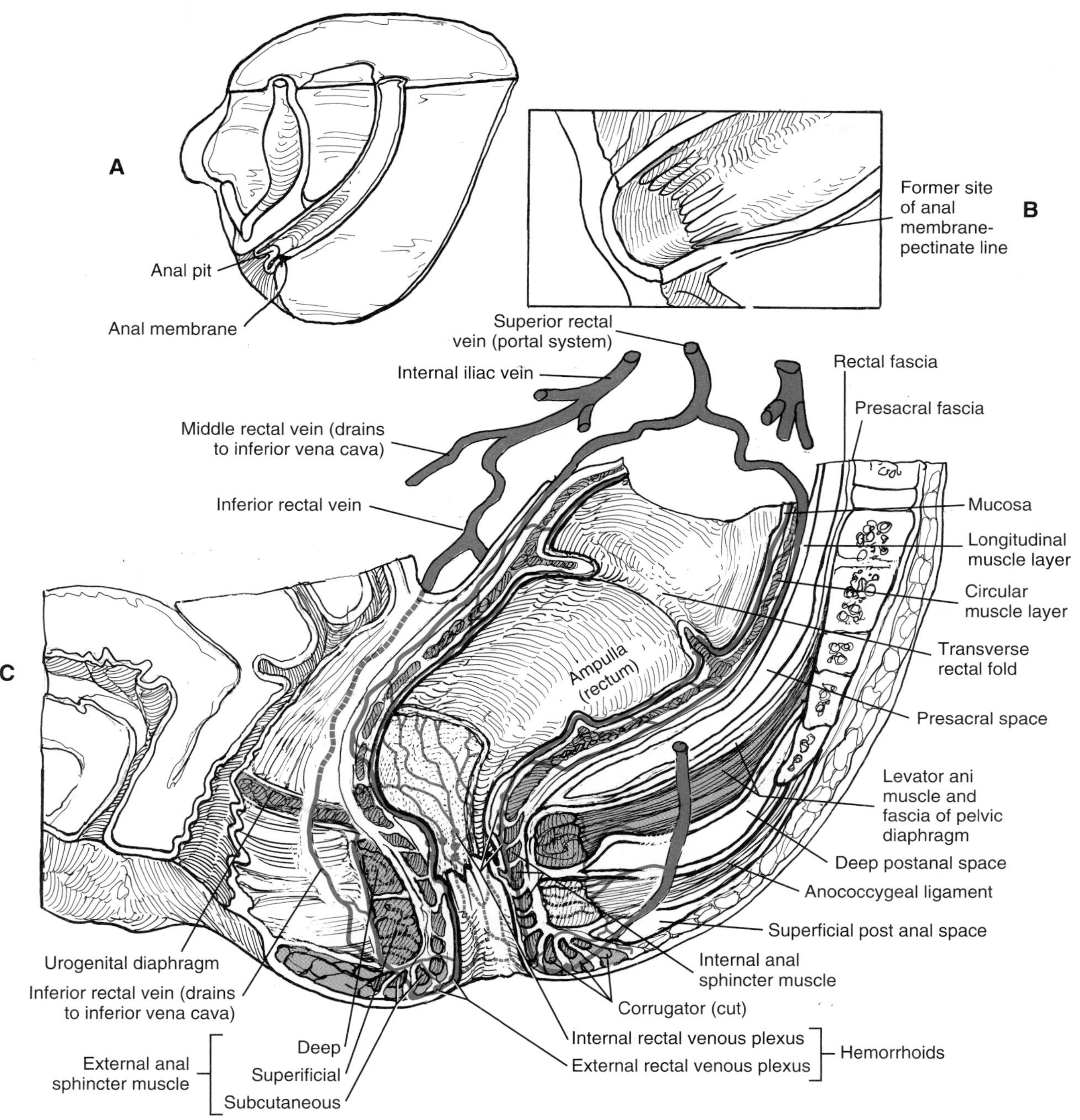

FIGURE 15–5
Anorectal canal. **A.** The lower third of the anorectal canal arises by proliferation of ectoderm around the orifice of the rectum, which results in the formation of the anal pit. **B.** The anal membrane separates the anal pit (the presumptive lower one third of the anorectal canal) from the rectum (the upper two thirds of the anorectal canal) at the level of the pectinate line. **C.** Muscles of the anorectal canal include the internal anal sphincter (a specialization of the circular smooth muscle of the rectum) and the external anal sphincter (striated muscle). Three different regions of the external anal sphincter can be distinguished: namely, the deep, superficial, and subcutaneous parts.

musculature of the superior end of the inferior one third of the anorectal canal by penetrating the wall of the rectum within the pelvic cavity (Fig. 15–7A). These vessels do not vascularize the mucosa of the anorectal canal to any appreciable degree and form only limited anastomoses with superior and inferior rectal vessels.

Structures of the anal compartment are primarily vascularized by branches of the internal pudendal vessels

The most significant vessels of the anal compartment branch from the internal pudendal artery and vein. The internal pudendal vessels exit the pelvic cavity through the greater sciatic foramen and then course inferiorly through the lesser sciatic foramen between the

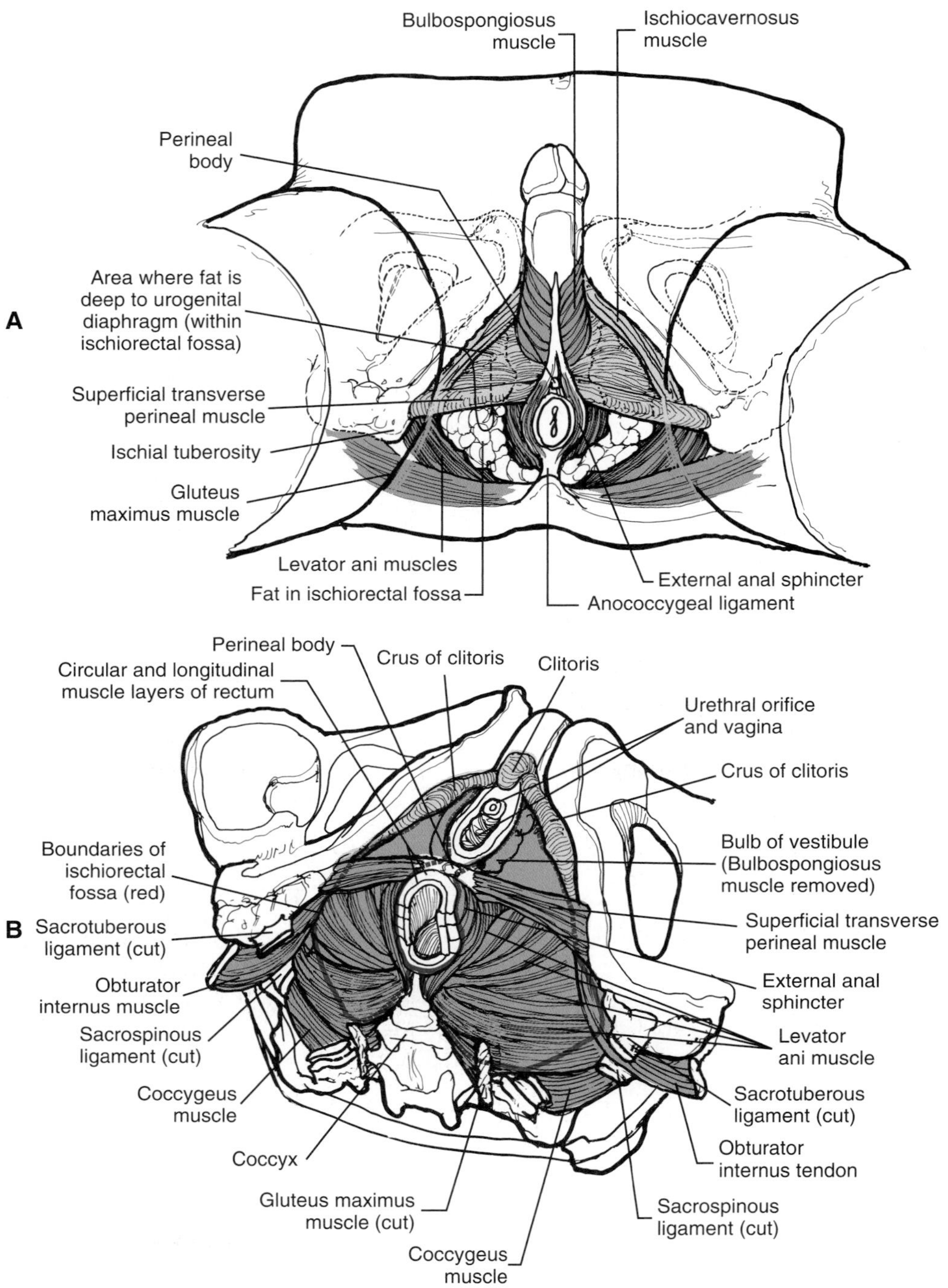

FIGURE 15–6

Ischiorectal fossae. **A.** Male. The ischiorectal fossa on either side of the rectum is bounded superiorly by the pelvic diaphragm. These fossae are communicating compartments that contain fat. The fat extends anteriorly (into anterior recesses of the ischiorectal fossa) into the region of the urogenital triangle between the urogenital diaphragm and pelvic diaphragm. **B.** Female. The fat is removed from the ischiorectal fossa in this illustration. Outlines of the fossa are shown in red, including their extensions into anterior recesses superior to the urogenital diaphragm.

sacrotuberous and sacrospinous ligaments to enter the anal compartment (Fig. 15–7*A* and *B*). Just inferior to the ischial spine, however, the internal pudendal vessels enter the **pudendal canal (Alcock's canal),** a fibrous connective tissue tunnel within the connective tissue of the inferomedial surface of the obturator internus muscle, which is located on the medial side of the ischial ramus (Figs. 15–7*B* and 15–8). Just after entering the pudendal canal, they give off **inferior rectal (hemorrhoidal) branches,** which course through the fat of

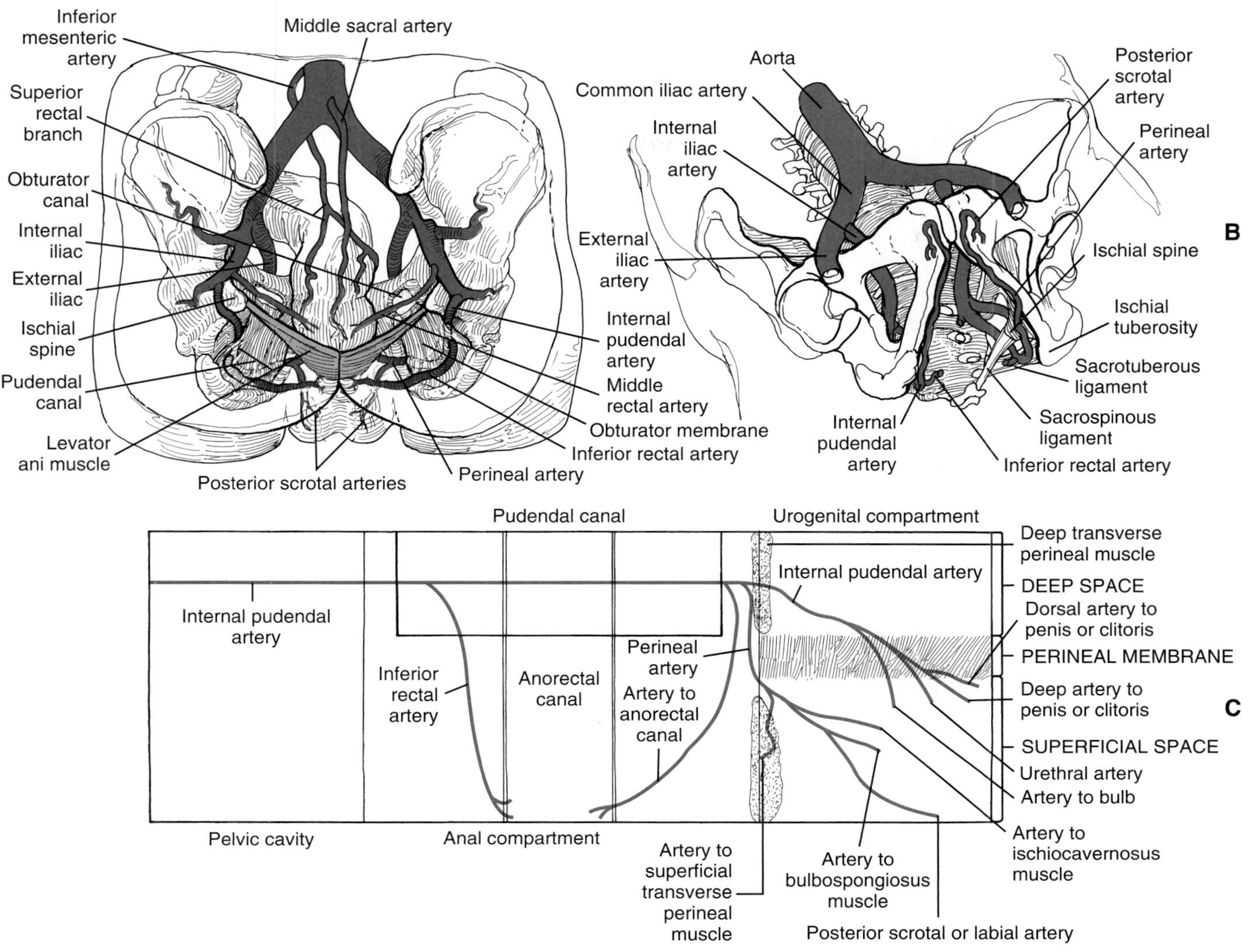

FIGURE 15–7
Arterial supply to the anal and urogenital compartments. **A.** Posterior view showing relationships of internal pudendal, inferior rectal, and perineal arteries in the anal compartment. **B.** Anterior view showing relationships of internal pudendal and perineal arteries in the urogenital compartment. **C.** Diagram showing relationships of internal pudendal arteries and their branches to structures of the pelvis, pudendal canal, anal compartment, and deep and superficial spaces of the urogenital compartment.

the ischiorectal fossae to vascularize the external anal sphincter and the skin just posterior and lateral to the anus (Figs. 15–7*B* and 15–8).

The main trunks of the internal pudendal arteries and veins then course anteriorly within the pudendal canal (see Chapter 14). These vessels exit the pudendal canal and enter the anterior region of the ischiorectal fossae where they give off branches that course through the ischiorectal fat to vascularize the anterior aspect of the anorectal canal and perineal skin. The internal pudendal arteries and veins then give off **perineal branches** before entering the deep space of the urogenital compartment (Fig. 15–7*C*). The perineal artery and vein are described in the discussion of the urogenital compartment below.

Lymphatic Drainage of the Anal Compartment

Lymphatic vessels and nodes of the anal compartment are associated with arteries that vascularize this region

Lymphatic drainage of the inferior one third of the anorectal canal is via vessels and nodes accompanying the arteries that supply this segment of the gastrointestinal tract (i.e., the inferior rectal, internal pudendal, internal iliac, and common iliac arteries and the descending aorta) (see Fig. 15–7). Lymph nodes involved in the drainage of the inferior segment of the anorectal canal include **internal pudendal nodes, common iliac nodes,** and **paraaortic nodes** (i.e., **preaortic** and **lateral aortic nodes**). Some lymph from the most inferior end of the anorectal canal drains into **superficial inguinal nodes** just inferior to the inguinal ligament via lym-

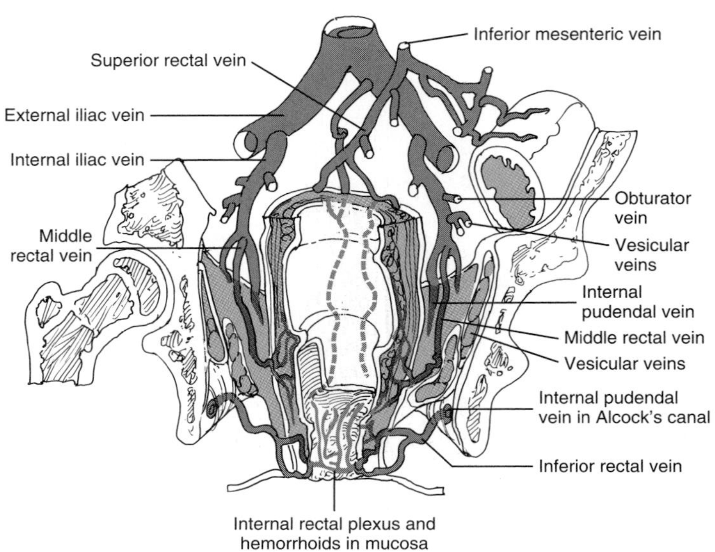

FIGURE 15–8
Venous drainage of the anal compartment occurs mainly via inferior rectal veins and veins that drain the anterior region of the anorectal canal and adjacent skin and superficial fascia.

phatic vessels accompanying branches of the external pudendal arteries (see Fig. 15–17 and the discussion of the vasculature of the urogenital compartment below).

Innervation of the Anal Compartment

The major innervation of the anal compartment is provided by the inferior rectal branches of the pudendal nerve (S2 to S4)

Primary innervation of the structures within the anal compartment is provided by the **pudendal nerve** (S2 to S4), which follows the course of the internal pudendal vessels (Fig. 15–9). After exiting the pelvis via the greater sciatic foramen and passing through the lesser sciatic foramen, the pudendal nerve gives off an **inferior rectal branch,** which courses through the ischiorectal fat to innervate the wall of the anorectal canal and the skin around the anus. After giving off this inferior rectal branch, the pudendal nerve enters the pudendal canal and splits into its two terminal branches: the **perineal nerve** and the **dorsal nerve of the penis** or **clitoris.** These two branches course onward through the pudendal canal, exiting from its anterior boundary into the ischiorectal fossa before entering the urogenital compartment (Fig. 15–9). Upon exiting the pudendal canal, the perineal nerve branches within the anterior region of the ischiorectal fossae to provide innervation to anterior muscles of the **external anal sphincter** (Fig. 15–9) and the skin overlying the anterior region of the anal compartment (S4).

Minor cutaneous branches of the coccygeal nerve (at spinal cord level Co1) innervate the skin between the coccyx and anus. A perineal branch of the posterior femoral cutaneous nerve (from spinal cord levels S1 to S3) provides cutaneous innervation to the lateral edge of the anal triangle.

Parasympathetic and sympathetic innervation of smooth muscles in the wall of the inferior one third of the anorectal canal is supplied by nerves emanating from the **inferior hypogastric (pelvic) plexus** (Fig. 15–10). Preganglionic parasympathetic fibers within these nerves originate from the pelvic splanchnic nerves (S2 to S4). Postganglionic sympathetic fibers within these nerves are innervated by preganglionic fibers originating from levels T10 to L2 of the spinal cord (Fig. 15–10). These autonomic fibers may course to the anorectal canal independently or may be carried by the middle rectal artery.

Function of Defecation

Defecation is a multistep process requiring coordination between voluntary and involuntary mechanisms

Reflex arcs that control the activity of structures within the anal compartment are involved in a complex interplay between afferent and efferent elements of both the somatic and autonomic nervous systems. For example, filling of the inferior end of the rectum, a dilated area called the **rectal ampulla,** with feces from the sigmoid colon stimulates stretch receptors within the walls of the rectum. Sensory impulses traveling to the central nervous system via afferent fibers that follow the pelvic splanchnic nerves to spinal cord level S2 to S4 are then relayed to higher cortical centers, resulting in a conscious sensation of rectal filling. When convenient, defecation can be consciously initiated by relaxation of the **puborectal sling** (nerve to the levator ani muscle [S3 and S4]), allowing feces to escape the rectal ampulla to enter the lower one third of the anorectal canal. This action is enhanced by conscious contraction of the **abdominal musculature** (spinal nerves T7 to L1) and the **diaphragm** (phrenic nerve [C3 to C5]), resulting in increased intraabdominal pressure and stimulation of stretch receptors within the wall of the anorectal canal. Activation of these stretch receptors stimulates afferent fibers that accompany the **autonomic pelvic splanchnic nerves** back to levels S2 to S4 of the spinal cord. These sensations result in reflex motor activity of the parasympathetic fibers of the pelvic splanchnic nerves (S2 to S4) via the inferior hypogastric plexus, and this causes relaxation of the **internal anal sphincter** and stimulation of contraction of circular muscle fibers in the wall of the anorectal canal, forcing feces toward the anus.

Conscious relaxation of the **external anal sphincter** (inferior rectal nerve [S2 to S4]), subsequent contraction of the **longitudinal muscle of the anorectal canal** (pelvic splanchnic nerves [S2 to S4]), and elevation of the rectum by the levator ani muscle (nerve to levator ani muscle [S3 and S4]) result in ejection of stool.

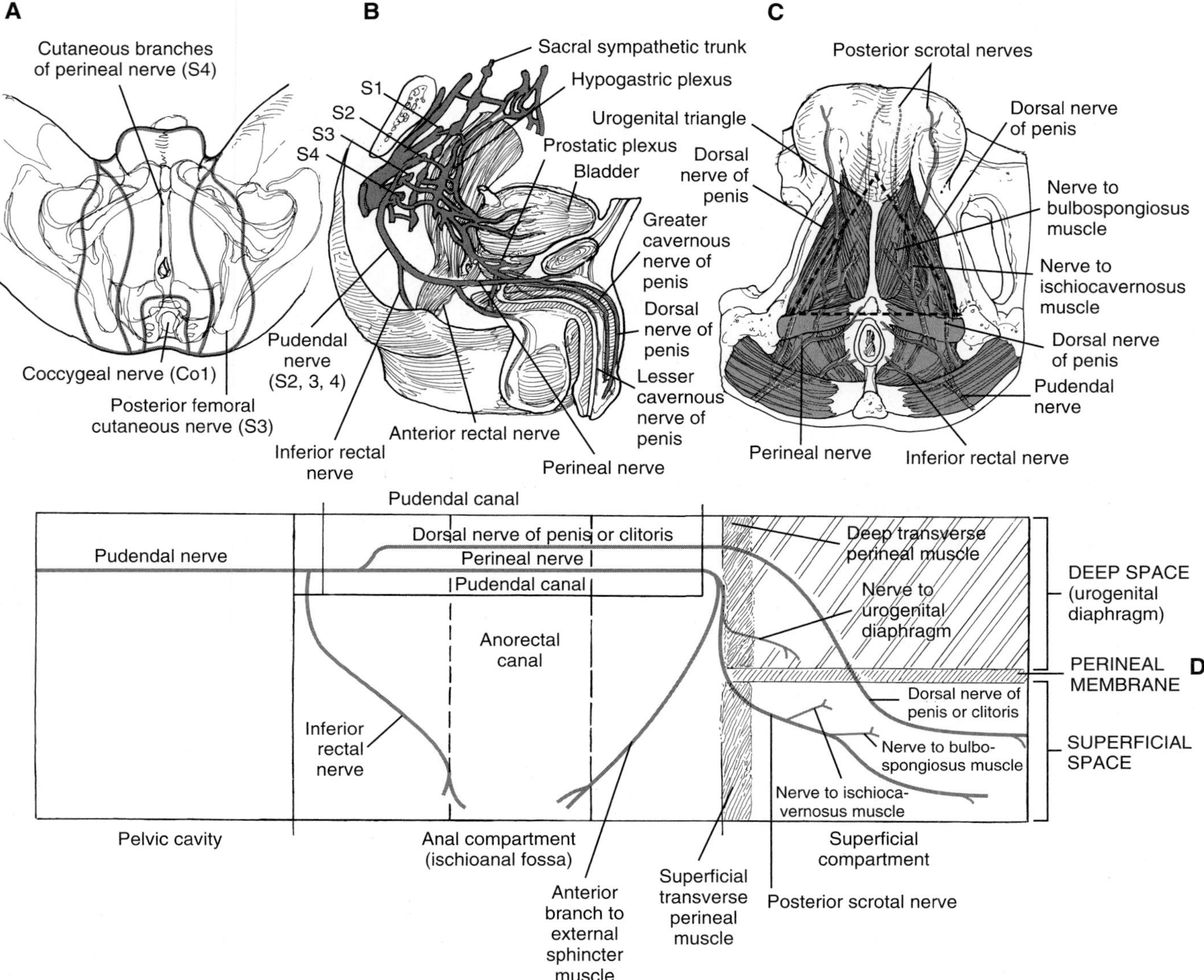

FIGURE 15–9
Innervation of the perineum. **A,** Inferior view showing territories of cutaneous innervation. **B,** Sagittal view showing the courses of the pudendal nerve and its branches and their relationships to the inferior hypogastric plexus. **C,** Inferior view showing the courses and targets of two main terminal branches of the pudendal nerve, the perineal nerves, and the deep dorsal nerve of the penis or clitoris. **D,** Diagram showing relationships of the pudendal nerve, perineal nerve, and deep dorsal nerve of the penis or clitoris and their branches to the pelvis, pudendal canal, and structures of the anal compartment and the deep and superficial spaces of the urogenital compartment.

Following ejection of stool, sympathetic activity via the inferior hypogastric plexus (T10 to L2) results in relaxation of smooth muscle in the walls of the anorectal canal and constriction of the internal anal sphincter. Conscious activity of the inferior rectal nerve (S2 to S4) again constricts the external anal sphincter.

Fecal Incontinence
Functional disruption of reflex arcs that control defecation may result in fecal incontinence

At birth, the young child's external anal sphincter is weak and cannot be consciously controlled. Thus, defecation in infants is solely a reflexive act. Many parents have observed that the need for a diaper change often occurs shortly after feeding, and this is a practical illustration of the **gastrocolic reflex!** During the toddler years (age 1 to 3 years), the external sphincter becomes stronger as the child learns how to regulate the contraction and relaxation of this muscle.

Some **weakening of the external anal sphincter** commonly occurs as part of the aging process, but normally the muscle retains sufficient strength to maintain continence. This

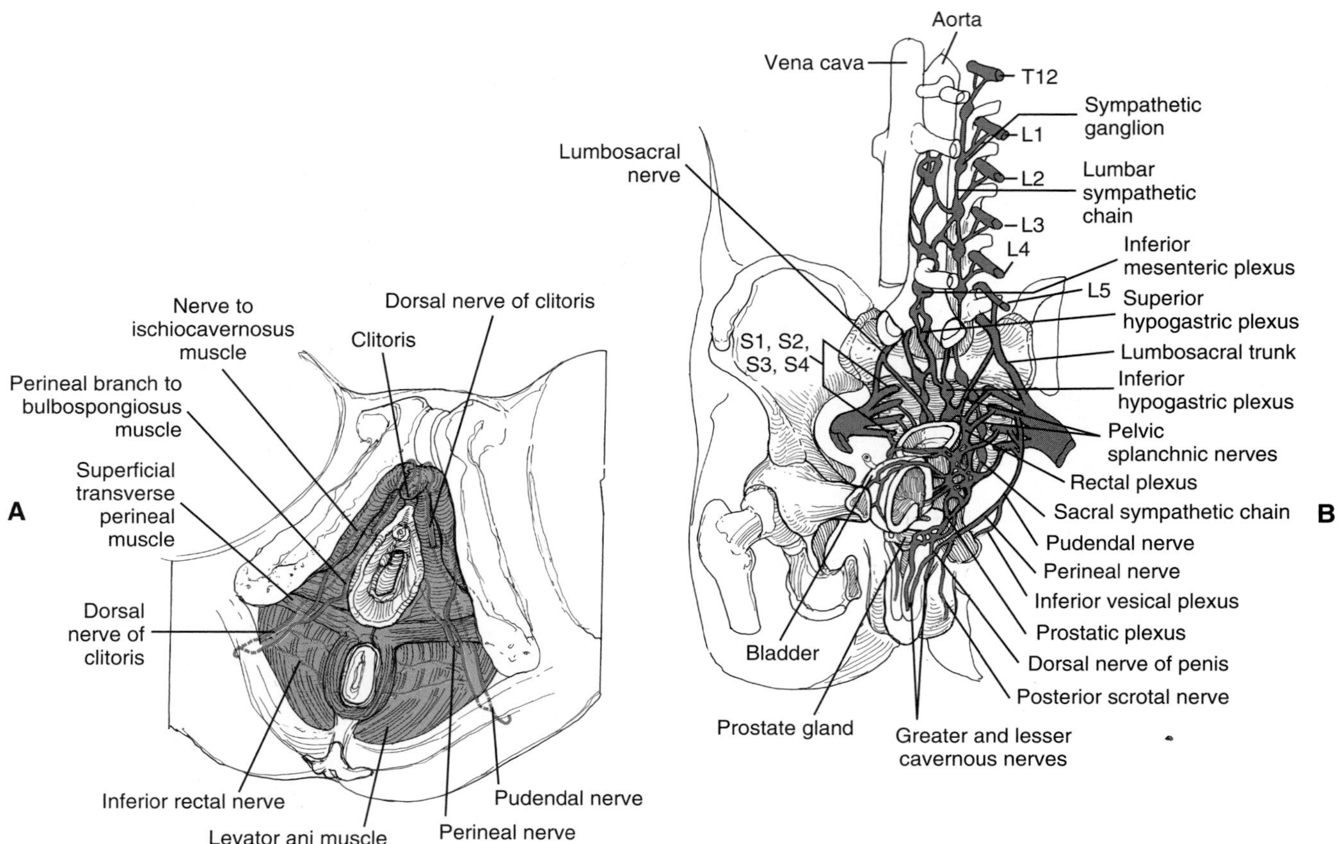

FIGURE 15–10
Nerves of the perineum. The innervation of structures of the perineum is both somatic (pudendal nerve from spinal cord level S2 to S4) and autonomic (sympathetic innervation via the hypogastric plexus by splanchnic nerves from spinal cord level T10 to L2 [parasympathetic innervation by pelvic splanchnic nerves from spinal cord level S2 to S4]).

normal age-related decrease in sphincter tone may occasionally give rise to fecal incontinence occurring secondary to a gastrointestinal tract disturbance (e.g., diarrhea may result in incontinence in elderly individuals, but when it resolves, continence returns).

The most typical underlying cause of the advanced weakening of the internal and external sphincters associated with incontinence is neurologic, involving the pudendal nerve (from spinal cord level S2 to S4). The nerve may be stretched as a consequence of excessive straining during defecation or may become entrapped as it traverses the pudendal canal (e.g., following true hip fracture). This condition is often accompanied by prolapse of the rectum.

In severe cases of chronic loss of tone of the external anal sphincter, the rectum may relax so much that it has an **everted** or **prolapsed configuration.** This condition occurs most frequently in older females who have not borne children (nulliparous women). A likely cause is dysfunction of the inferior rectal or pudendal nerve, but the increased incidence in nulliparous women does not support the hypothesis that the neuropathy results from childbirth.

Direct trauma or **injury** to the sphincters themselves, such as the anterior tearing of the external anal sphincter that may occur during childbirth, may also result in incontinence. More commonly, however, fecal retention is due to interference with the reflexes associated with defecation. In geriatric patients, stretch receptors in the wall of the rectum and afferent neurons may lose their function. A greater degree of rectal distention is required to stimulate a desire to defecate and bring about relaxation of the internal sphincter. Individuals may ignore the urge to defecate, causing stretch receptors to become less responsive. Increasing dependence on self-administered laxatives along with complete loss of stretch receptor function or afferent neuronal function (or both) may result in **constipation** or **fecal impaction.**

Infection of the Ischiorectal Fossae

Infections may spread throughout the ischiorectal fossae following a perineal abscess or the development of anal fistulas

Infections of the ischiorectal fossae most often result from perianal abscess or anal fistula. Infections arising from a

perianal abscess may originate within the wall of the anorectal canal between the internal and external anal sphincters (see Fig. 15–5). If left untreated, the abscess can spread into the ischiorectal fossae vertically, gaining access to the fossae from the region of the superior border of the external anal sphincter. Alternatively, the abscess may spread horizontally, penetrating the external anal sphincter to enter the ischiorectal fossae (see Fig. 15–6).

Anal fistulas often form as epithelium-lined communications between the anorectal canal and the perianal skin. Usually, these fistulas follow the fascial plane between the internal and external anal sphincters. In approximately 30% of cases, the fistula enters the ischiorectal fossae, allowing fecal material to enter this space, giving rise to an ischiorectal abscess.

Regardless of the mechanism, once an infection has formed within the ischiorectal fossae, it may spread rapidly throughout the fossa and to the fossa on the other side of the rectum. Patients experience fever and pain associated with defecation. Once diagnosed, the abscess must be drained and any infected tissue removed. If the infection spreads to the fascia of the anal or urogenital compartments, the condition can become life threatening and requires substantial surgical intervention.

Hemorrhoids

The different embryonic origins of the rectum and anorectal canal are the basis for the development of hemorrhoids

Superior rectal veins of the portal system within the mucosa of the superior two thirds of the anorectal canal form anastomotic connections with inferior rectal branches of the systemic system (see Fig. 15–8). Because portal veins lack valves, obstructions of the portal system may force blood to flow backward through the superior rectal veins of the portal system, into the inferior rectal veins, and into the internal pudendal and internal iliac veins of the systemic vasculature. If the portal obstruction is of sufficient duration, the rectal (hemorrhoidal) veins in the region of the anastomosis enlarge to produce **hemorrhoidal varicoceles (hemorrhoids).** Those occurring in the inferior aspect of the anorectal canal often cause the **anal mucosa** to **prolapse** through the anal orifice **(external hemorrhoids).** Those occurring in the region of the anal columns may cause the mucosa to prolapse downward into the **anorectal canal (internal hemorrhoids).** More extensive prolapse of internal hemorrhoids through the anal orifice may occur in conjunction with weakness of the external anal sphincter.

Portal obstructions leading to hemorrhoids may result from obesity, pregnancy, or diseases of the liver, including cirrhosis or cancer (see Chapter 12).

Childbirth Injury Affecting the Anal Compartment

Injury to muscles and fascial structures during childbirth may have a significant impact on the quality of daily life

During the birth of a first child, the perineum is often torn as the infant's head passes through the vagina. Infection of the superficial or deep compartment of the urogenital region may occur. The infection will spread along the fascial planes of these compartments or into the fascia themselves **(fasciitis).** This latter condition may be life threatening. It often requires **surgical debridement** (excision of dead tissue and foreign matter) of the area, which may result in disfigurement or urinary and fecal incontinence. Perineal infections may also result in formation of an **anovaginal fistula,** leading to incontinence of flatus or fecal material via the vaginal orifice.

Some physicians elect to make an **incision in the perineum (episiotomy)** when tearing is anticipated. The incision is usually made in the midline, from the vaginal opening posteriorly to the perineal body. In extreme cases, the physician may bisect the perineal body as well. There is little bleeding from this incision. Episiotomy has fallen out of favor with many practitioners, however.

UROGENITAL COMPARTMENT OF THE PERINEUM

Structures that are specialized for micturition and reproduction fill the superficial and deep spaces of the urogenital compartment

Superficial Space of the Urogenital Compartment

The inferior boundary of the superficial space is the superficial fascia and skin, and the superior boundary is the perineal membrane

The reflection of skin and superficial fascia onto the penis or clitoris and the scrotum or labial folds produces an irregular three-dimensional inferior boundary of the **superficial space of the urogenital compartment** (see Figs. 15–2 and 15–3). Although this **superficial perineal fascia (Colles' fascia)** is firmly fused with the fascia of the posterior surface of the superficial transverse perineal muscles and perineal body and with the fascia lata of the thighs (see Fig. 11–6), it is only loosely adherent to most of the structures lying just beneath it. In addition, anterior excursions of the superficial fascia investing the urogenital compartment are continuous with the superficial fascia of the anterior abdominal wall. Regions of fusion of Colles' fascia are clinically important because they limit the movement of extravasated blood or urine or of infectious agents just deep to the membranous fascia by preventing leakage into the thighs or anal compartment (see Fig. 11–6 and below).

The superior (internal) boundary of the superficial space is formed by the **perineal membrane,** a layer of thickened deep fascia investing the inferior surface of a muscular sheet called the **urogenital diaphragm** (see below). This tough connective tissue substratum provides a firm foundation for the attachment of the **bulb of the penis** in males and the **vestibular bulbs** in females (see below).

▲ Male and Female Genitalia

The external genitalia are the main structures in the superficial space of the urogenital compartment

The spongy and muscular tissues of the penis, the superficial transverse perineal muscles, the testes, and the distal end of the spermatic cord are the chief structures of the superficial space in males (see Fig. 15–12 and Table 15–2). The spongy and muscular tissues of the clitoris, the superficial transverse perineal muscles, the vestibular bulb, and the vestibular glands are the chief structures of the superficial space in females (see Fig. 15–14 and Table 15–2).

Embryonic Development of Male and Female Genitalia

The definitive male and female genitalia are strikingly different but arise from the same embryonic precursors

The **external genitalia** of males and females arise from common embryologic precursors that are similar in appearance to the mature female genitalia. These precursors include the **genital tubercle** and the **urogenital** and **labioscrotal folds** (Fig. 15–11*A*). The presence of a Y chromosome in males, with its **sex-determining region (SRY),** initiates a male developmental cascade at about the seventh week of embryogenesis, resulting in growth of the **penile tubercle** and fusion of the **urogenital (urethral) folds** to form the **penis** and its enclosed **penile urethra.** The **labioscrotal folds** fuse together to form the **scrotum** (this area of fusion is indicated by the **median raphe** evident in the midline of the scrotum) (Fig. 15–11*B*). These changes occur largely in response to the androgenic hormone dihydrotestosterone. In the absence of a Y chromosome (in females), the fundamental program encoded within the presumptive genitalia is followed, resulting in development of the **clitoris** from the **penile tubercle,** the **labia minora** from the **urogenital folds,** and the **labia majora** from the **labioscrotal folds** (Fig. 15–11*C*).

The Penis

The penis of males consists of a single median body (corpus spongiosum) and two lateral bodies of spongy tissue (corpora cavernosa) (Fig. 15–12). The proximal end of the **corpus spongiosum** forms the **bulb of the penis,** which lies just superficial to the perineal membrane, while the distal end forms the **glans penis.** The corpus spongiosum encloses the entire length of the penile (spongy) urethra (Fig. 15–12*A*, *C*, and *E*). The **penile urethra** of males arises from the **definitive urogenital sinus** and is homologous to the **vestibule of the vagina** in females.

The proximal end of each **corpus cavernosum** of the penis is made up of a crus, which is attached to the medial surface of the ischial and pubic rami (Fig. 15–12*D*). These left and right crura join the corpus spongiosum in the region of the pubic arch, and their distal ends extend to the base of the glans penis to form superolateral compartments of the **shaft of the penis.**

The spongy tissues of each corpus cavernosum and the corpus spongiosum are individually enclosed within a thick connective tissue layer (tunica albuginea) (Fig. 15–12*D*). In addition, in the region of the shaft of the penis, a layer of deep connective tissue (deep perineal fascia [Buck's fascia]) overlies the tunica albuginea to enclose all three spongy elements and the deep dorsal vein, dorsal arteries, and dorsal nerve within a common compartment (Fig. 15–12*D*). A layer of superficial perineal fascia (superficial penile fascia [Colles' fascia]) and skin invests the Buck's fascia of the shaft and glans of the penis and also encloses the superficial dorsal vein and lateral superficial veins of the penis (Fig. 15–12*D*). The penile skin is unusually thin. A fold of skin at the distal end of the penile shaft (prepuce) extends over the corona of the glans penis (Fig. 15–12*C*). This skin is often removed shortly after birth **(circumcision).**

The **bulb of the penis** is invested by a thin sheet of **bulbospongiosus muscle** (Fig. 15–12*A* and *C*). The two halves of this muscle arise from the perineal body and a median raphe. The most posterior fibers of the bulbospongiosus muscle insert on the perineal membrane, and its more anterior fibers blend with the deep fascia at the proximal end of the penile shaft (Fig. 15–12*A*). The **ischiocavernosus muscles** invest the **crura** of the corpora cavernosa. These thin sheets of skeletal muscle arise from the ischium and ischial rami at the base of the crura and insert into fascia on the lateral sides of the proximal end of the penile shaft (Fig. 15–12*A* and *C*).

The penis is suspended by a **fundiform ligament,** which consists of specially modified superficial fascia arising from the linea alba and attaching to the lateral sides of the base of the penis (Fig. 15–13). The penis is also suspended by a **suspensory ligament,** which is also specially modified fascial tissue, connecting the dorsum of the penis to the skin and connective tissue overlying the pubic symphysis (Fig. 15–13).

The Clitoris

The clitoris of females lies within the superficial space and is homologous to the penis of males (Fig. 15–14 and see Table 15–2). The root of the clitoris is formed from the two lateral **crura of the corpora cavernosa** and the paired piriform **vestibular bulbs of the corpus spongiosum** (Fig. 15–14*B* and *C*). The crura are attached to the medial surfaces of the ischial and pubic rami like the crura of the penis and are invested by fibers of the **ischiocavernosus muscle** (Fig. 15–14*A*). The vestibular bulbs lie deep to the **labia majora** and are separated by the **vestibule of the vagina** (Fig. 15–14*B* and *C*). They are invested by thin skeletal muscle fibers of the **bulbospongiosus muscles,** which arise from the perineal body and insert on fascia covering the root of the clitoris (Fig. 15–14*B*). The vestibular bulbs are united anteriorly by a small commissure, which is continuous with erectile tissue

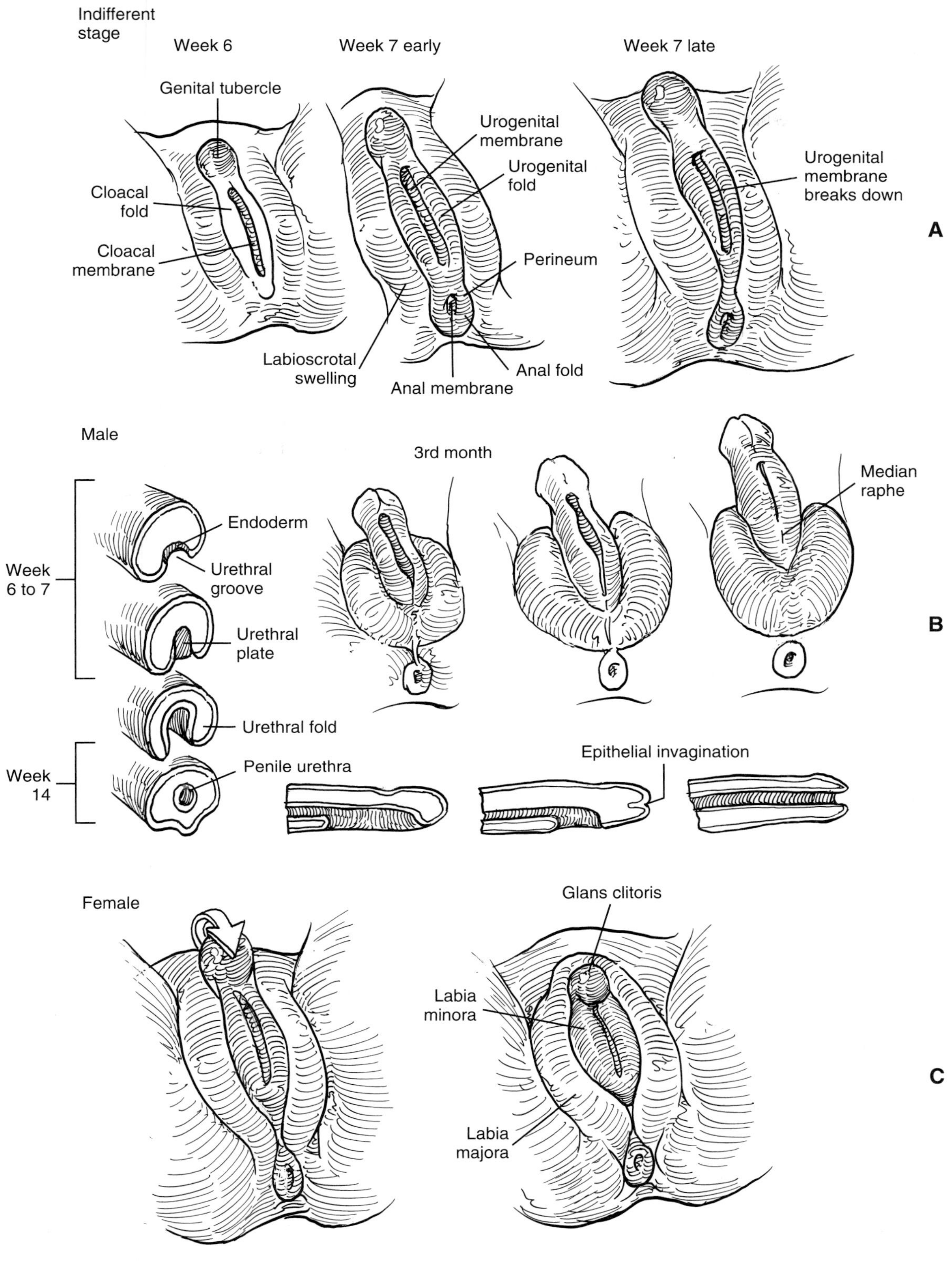

FIGURE 15–11

A. Initial development of the external genitalia in both sexes. Cloacal folds surround the cloacal membrane, and a genital tubercle develops at the anterior end of the cloacal membrane (week 6). The urorectal septum fuses with the cloacal membrane (week 7). The external genitalia now consist of a pair of urogenital folds, a pair of labioscrotal swellings, and a genital tubercle. The urogenital membrane breaks down (week 7). **B.** Development of the male genitalia. The genital tubercle elongates to form the shaft and glans of the penis. Fusion of the urogenital folds contributes to formation of the penile shaft and penile urethra, and the labioscrotal swellings fuse to form the scrotum. **C.** Development of the female external genitalia. The genital tubercle bends to form the clitoris. The urogenital folds become the labia minora, and the labioscrotal swellings become the labia majora.

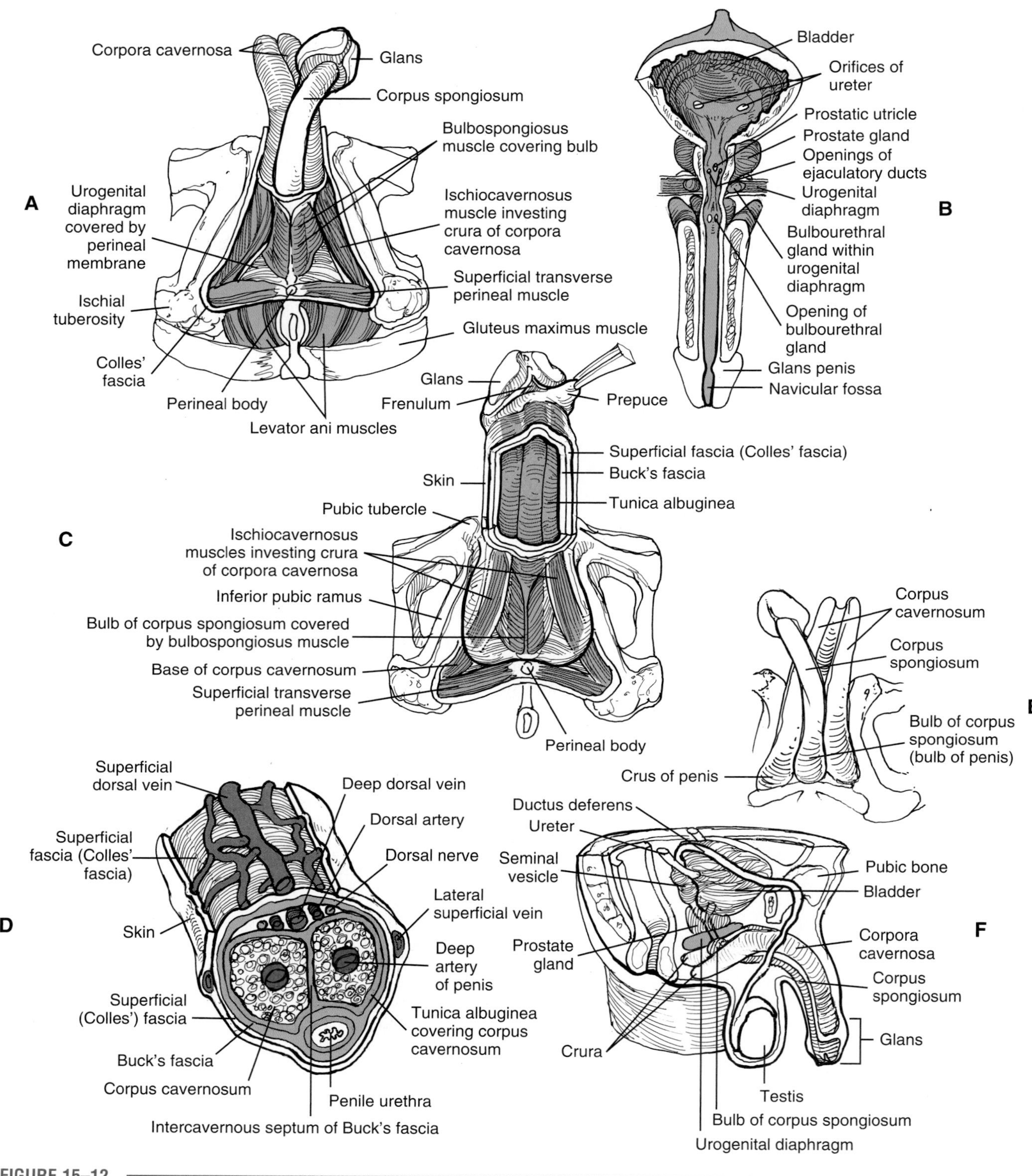

FIGURE 15–12
Structures of the superficial space of the urogenital compartment of the male.

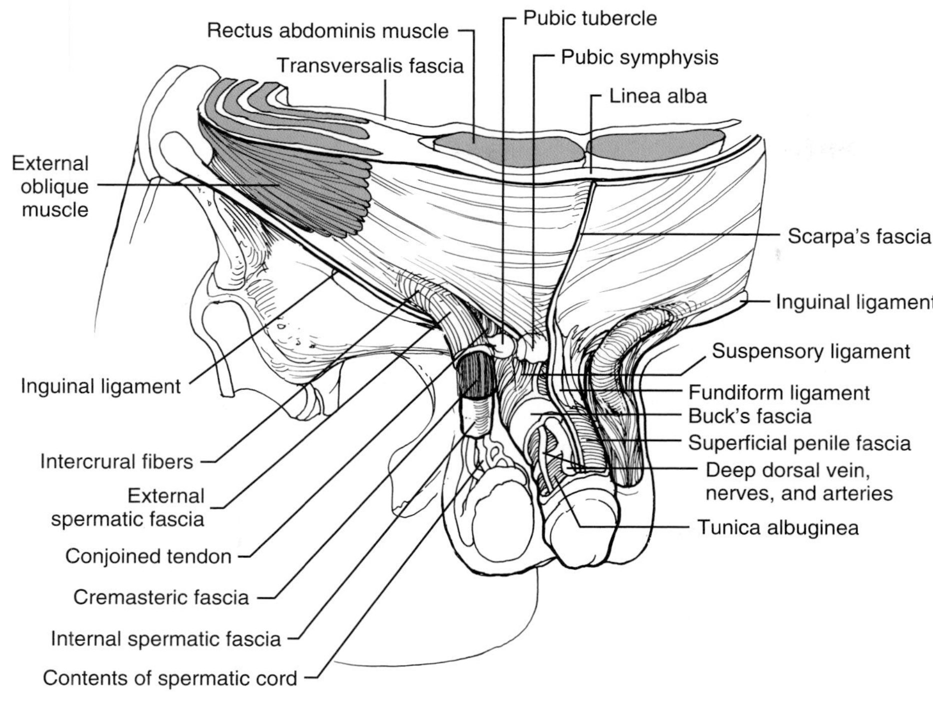

FIGURE 15–13
Fundiform and suspensory ligaments of the penis.

that joins with the distal ends of the corpora cavernosa to form the **shaft of the clitoris** (Fig. 15–14*C* and *inset*). The distal end of the corpus spongiosum forms the **glans clitoris,** which is also covered by an anterior fold of skin from the clitoral shaft called the **prepuce.** The base of the clitoris is stabilized by **fundiform** and **suspensory ligaments** like those which stabilize the base of the penis (Fig. 15–14*B* and *C*).

A significant difference between the penis and the clitoris is that the corpus spongiosum within the clitoris does not enclose a segment of the urethra. Instead, the urogenital folds of the female remain separated to form the **labia minora** located at the margins of the **vestibule of the vagina,** which is the homolog of the male penile urethra. These folds also enclose the distal end of the clitoris with its glans. The **urethra** in females thus empties directly into the vestibule of the vagina. Its relatively short length has clinical consequences (see below).

Other Male and Female Structures of the Superficial Space

The **superficial transverse perineal muscles** in males and females are also located in the superficial space. These muscles originate from the medial surface of the ischial tuberosities and insert into the fibromuscular **perineal body,** defining the boundary between the anal and urogenital triangles (see Figs. 15–12A and C and 15–14*A* and *B*).

In males, the superficial space also contains the testes and distal ends of the spermatic cords (see Fig. 15–12*E*), while in females, it also contains a pair of **greater vestibular glands (Bartholin's glands)** (Table 15–2 and see Fig. 15–14*B*). These glands are located just posterior to the vestibular bulbs within the **labia majora.** They are homologous to the bulbourethral glands of males. Their secretions empty into and lubricate the vestibule of the vagina. The numerous **lesser vestibular glands (Skene's glands)** are located within the walls of the vestibule (medial walls of the labia minora) between the terminus of the urethra and orifice of the vagina. These glands produce a moisturizing mucoid secretion.

▲ Deep Space of the Urogenital Compartment

The deep space of the urogenital compartment is bounded by the fascia investing the urogenital diaphragm

As has been noted above, the boundary between the superficial and deep spaces is made up of specially modified **deep fascia on the inferior side of the urogenital diaphragm (perineal membrane)** (see Figs. 15–12*A* and 15–14*B*). This thickened membrane is firmly attached to the medial surfaces of the pubic rami and the anterior surfaces of the ischial rami. An especially thick area in the most anterior region of the perineal membrane is the **transverse perineal ligament.** The superior boundary of the deep space is the superior layer of deep connective tissue investing the urogenital

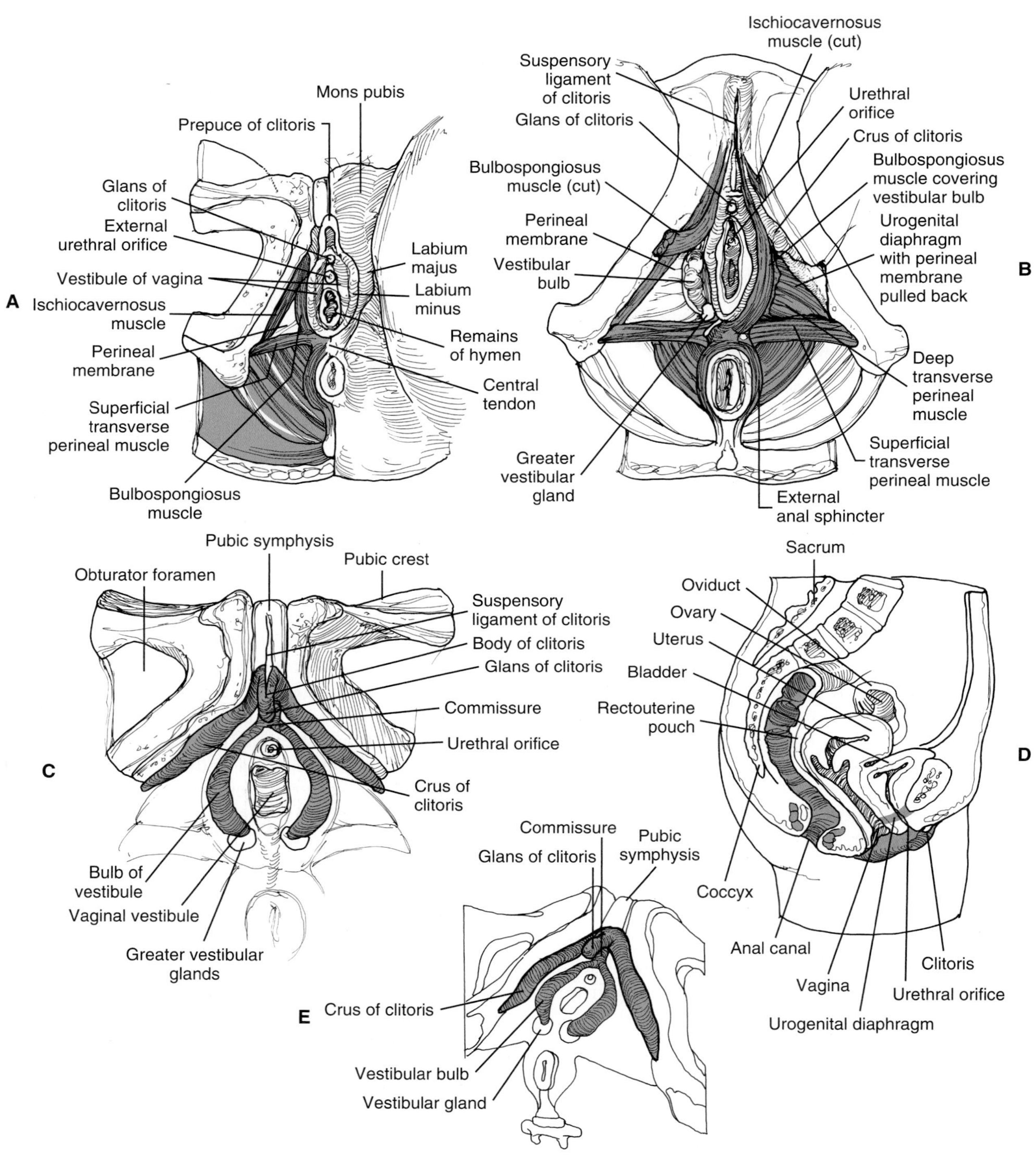

FIGURE 15–14
Structures of the superficial space of the urogenital compartment of the female.

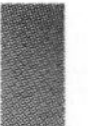

TABLE 15–2
Structures of the Superficial Space of the Urogenital Compartment

Female	Male
Vestibular bulbs, including corpus spongiosum and bulbospongiosus muscles	Bulb of penis, including corpus spongiosum and bulbospongiosus muscles
Body and crura of clitoris, including corpora cavernosa and ischiocavernosus muscles	Body and crura of penis, including corpora cavernosa and ischiocavernosus muscles
Superficial transverse perineal muscles Greater vestibular gland	Superficial transverse perineal muscles
Branches of internal pudendal artery, including artery to vestibular bulb, dorsal artery of clitoris, and deep artery of clitoris	Branches of internal pudendal artery, including artery to bulb, dorsal artery to penis, and deep artery of penis
Deep dorsal vein of clitoris (drains into vesicle plexus and internal pudendal vein)	Deep dorsal vein of penis(drains into prostatic plexus and internal pudendal vein)
Superficial dorsal vein of clitoris (branch of external pudendal vein)	Superficial dorsal vein of penis (branch of external pudendal vein)
Perineal artery and vein and branches to muscles (superficial transverse perineal, ischiocavernosus, and bulbospongiosus muscles) and to skin of perineum, including posterior labial vessels	Perineal artery and vein and branches to muscles (superficial transverse perineal, ischiocavernosus, and bulbospongiosus muscles) and to skin of perineum, including posterior scrotal vessels
Perineal nerve and branches to muscles (superficial transverse perineal, bulbospongiosus, and ischiocavernosus muscles) and to skin of perineum, including posterior labial nerves	Perineal nerve and branches to muscles (superficial transverse perineal, bulbospongiosus, and ischiocavernosus muscles) and to skin of perineum, including posterior scrotal nerves
Dorsal nerve of clitoris	Dorsal nerve of penis Testes and distal end of spermatic cord

diaphragm, which is the major structure located in the deep space (Fig. 15–15).

Urogenital Diaphragm

The main structure within the deep space in males and females is the urogenital diaphragm, which is a thin, triangular sheet of muscle

In both sexes, the urogenital diaphragm and its investing fascia are perforated by the membranous urethra (Table 15–3 and see Figs. 15–11*B* and 15–15). Contraction of fibers of the urogenital diaphragm surrounding the membranous urethra controls urination. These fibers are collectively called the **sphincter urethrae.** Bands of muscle fibers within the thickened posterior edge of the urogenital diaphragm are the **deep transverse perineal muscles** (Fig. 15–15). These muscles, like the superficial transverse perineal muscles, arise from the medial surfaces of the ischial rami and insert into the perineal body. The deep and superficial transverse perineal muscles function together to stabilize the perineal body. In females, the vagina also perforates the urogenital diaphragm, thus muscular fibers within the urogenital diaphragm in this region are called the **sphincter vaginae** (Fig. 15–15*B*). This muscle, along with the pubovaginalis (anterior fibers of the levator ani muscle) and bulbospongiosus muscles, may function to compress the vagina.

Other Structures of the Deep Space

The deep space of the urogenital compartment in both males and females also contains short segments of internal pudendal vessels, the deep dorsal nerve of the penis or clitoris, and the perineal nerve and its branches to the urogenital diaphragm.

Structures unique to the deep space in males are the **bulbourethral glands,** which bud from the membranous urethra (see Fig. 15–15*A* and Table 15–3). These glands produce secretions that empty into the prostatic urethra to mix with secretions of the seminal vesicles and prostate glands, producing the seminal fluid that protects and nourishes the ejaculated sperm.

▲ Structures that Integrate the Urogenital Compartment of the Perineum

Vascularization of the Urogenital Compartment

Branches of the internal pudendal artery provide the primary vascular supply to structures of the urogenital compartment

As has been noted above in the discussion of the anal compartment, after the internal pudendal artery emerges from the pudendal canal, it gives off branches that supply structures associated with the anterior side of the anorectal canal. It then gives off a **perineal artery** (see Fig. 15–7 and Fig. 15–16*A* to *C*). In the vicinity of the posterior boundary of the urogenital compartment, the main trunk of the perineal artery first gives rise to a

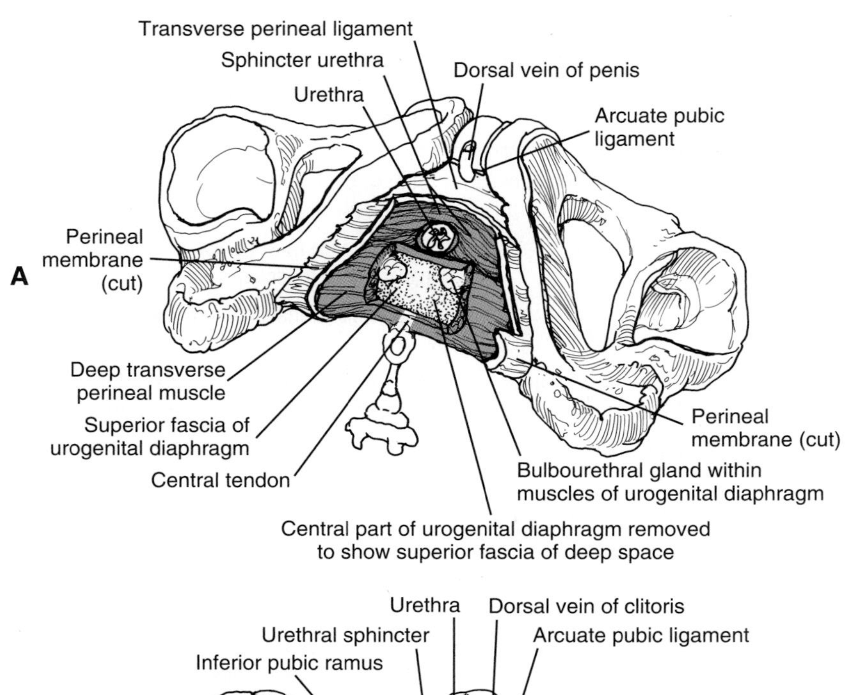

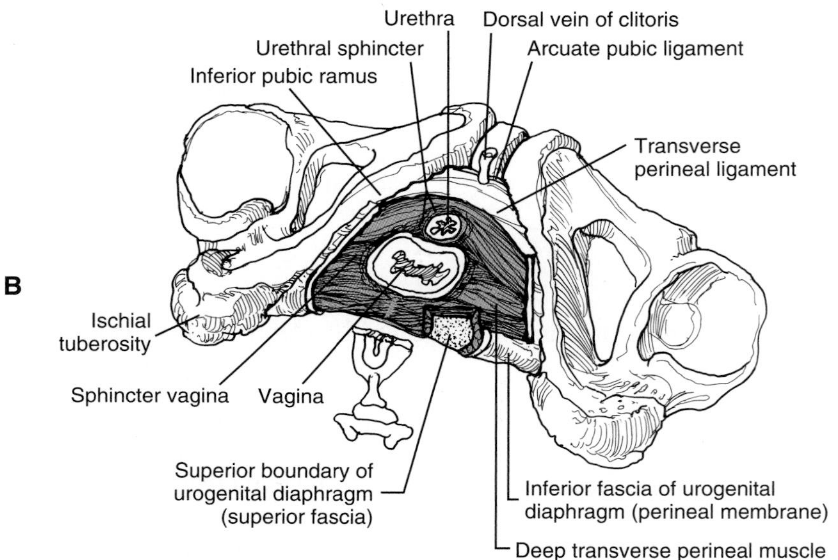

FIGURE 15–15

Deep space of the urogenital compartment. The urogenital diaphragm is a thin triangular muscle sandwiched between its inferior perineal membrane fascia and its superior fascial border. **A.** In males, the deep space of the urogenital compartment contains the sphincter urethra (urogenital diaphragm) and bulbourethral glands. The urogenital diaphragm is penetrated by the urethra. **B.** In females, the deep space of the urogenital compartment contains the sphincter urethra and sphincter vagina (urogenital diaphragm), which is penetrated by the urethra and vagina. Muscle fibers in the posterior portion of the urogenital diaphragm are called the deep transverse perineal muscles.

transverse perineal branch, which supplies the superficial transverse perineal muscle (Figs. 15–16 and 15–17). The perineal artery then gains access to the superficial space by coursing between the superficial and deep transverse perineal muscles (Fig. 15–16). While coursing just superficial to the perineal membrane, it splits into branches that supply the muscles of the superficial compartment (i.e., the superficial transverse perineal, bulbospongiosus, and ischiocavernosus muscles). Cutaneous branches are also given off by the perineal artery to supply the superficial fascia and skin of the posterior scrotum **(posterior scrotal arteries)** in males and the posterior region of the labia **(posterior labial arteries)** in females (Fig. 15–16*A* and *C*).

After giving off the perineal artery, the internal pudendal artery penetrates the posterior fascia that forms the boundary of the deep space (i.e., the fascia of the deep transverse perineal muscle). The internal puden-

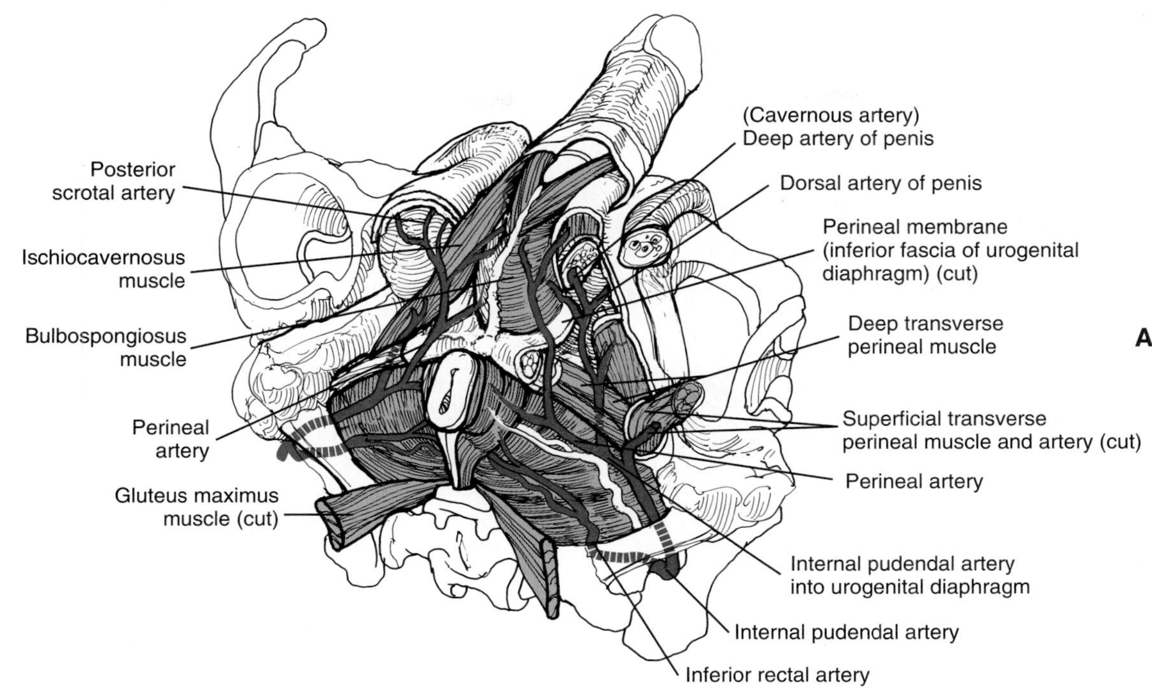

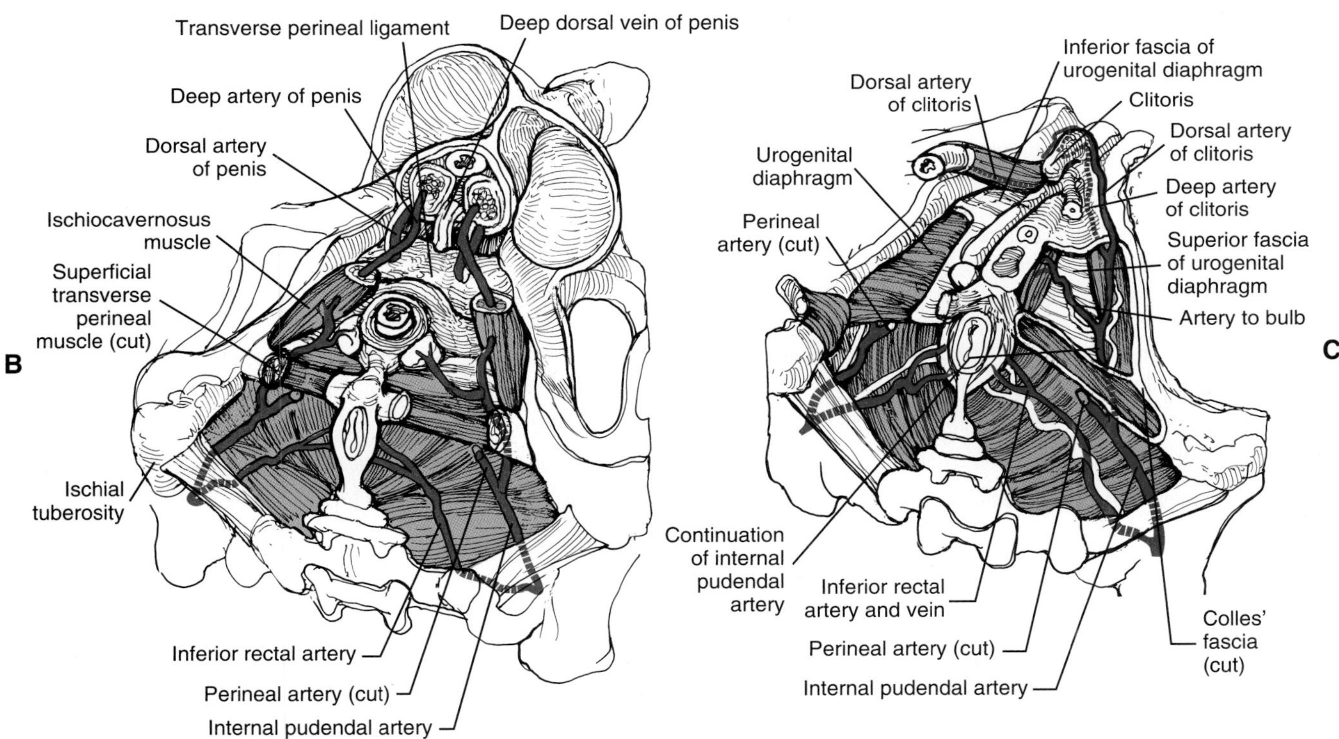

FIGURE 15–16
Arterial supply to the urogenital triangle from the internal pudendal artery. **A** and **B.** Male. **C.** Female.

dal artery then courses anteriorly just deep to the perineal membrane (Fig. 15–16*A* and see Fig. 15–7). In males, it gives off a branch to the bulbourethral gland and almost immediately pierces the perineal membrane to enter the superficial space. Once it is in the superficial space, it gives off the **artery to the bulb,** which supplies the spongy tissue of the bulb of the penis in males and the vestibular bulb in females. In females, the internal pudendal artery then gives off a branch that supplies the greater vestibular glands. In both

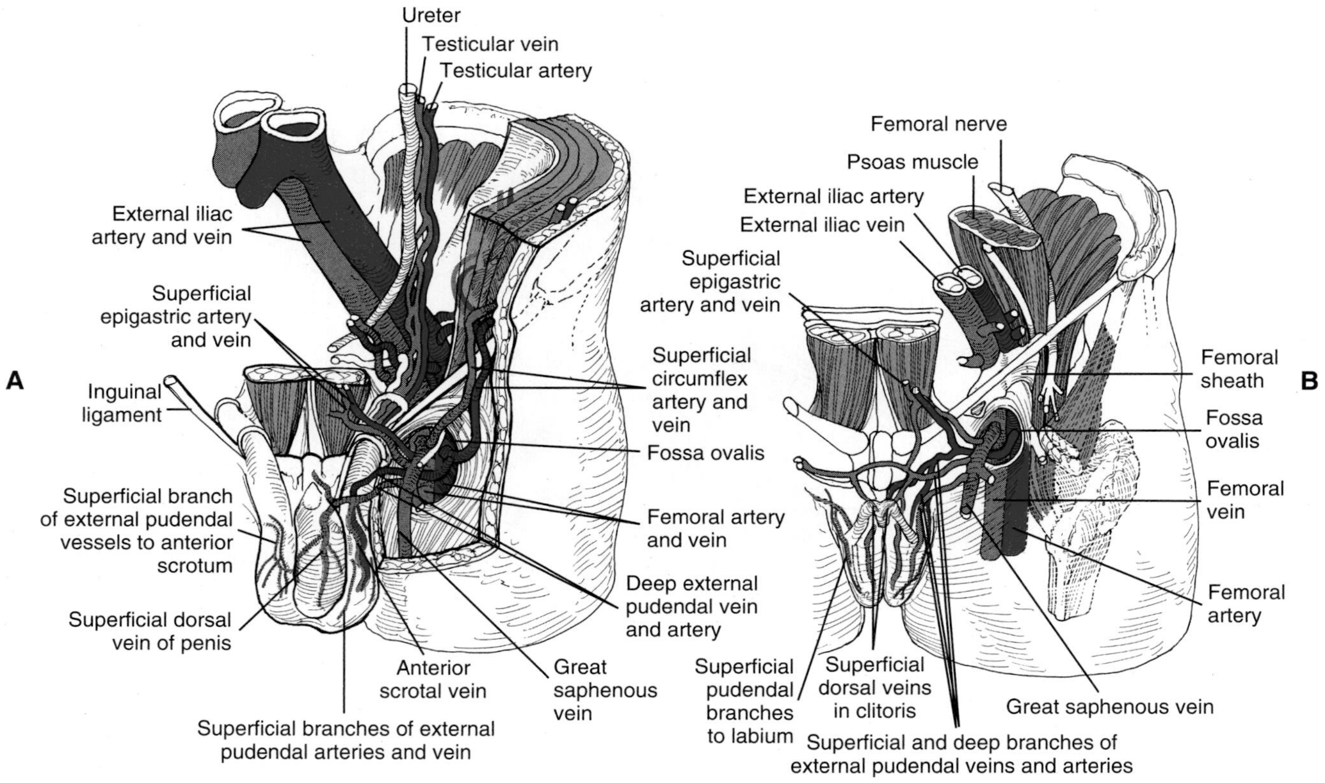

FIGURE 15–17
Arterial supply to structures of the superficial space of the urogenital triangle. **A.** Male. **B.** Female.

TABLE 15–3
Structures of the Deep Space of the Urogenital Compartment

Female	Male
Urogenital diaphragm, including sphincter urethrae, deep transverse perineal muscle, and sphincter vaginae muscle	Urogenital diaphragm, including sphincter urethrae and deep transverse perineal muscles
	Bulbourethral glands
Internal pudendal artery and vein	Internal pudendal artery and vein
Branches of perineal nerve to urogenital diaphragm	Branches of perineal nerve to urogenital diaphragm

sexes, it also gives off a **urethral artery,** which courses through the corpus spongiosum to supply the glans penis in males and the glans clitoris in females (Fig. 15–16*C* and *D*).

After continuing anteriorly within the superficial space, the internal pudendal artery branches into the **deep** and **dorsal arteries of the penis** or **clitoris** (Fig. 15–16 and see Fig. 15–7). The dorsal artery supplies superficial tissues (including the skin) of the penis or clitoris. It also provides deeper branches that assist the artery to the bulb and the deep artery of the penis or clitoris to supply the spongy erectile tissue of the external genitalia. When the penis or clitoris is flaccid, the deep arteries, **helicine arteries,** are coiled.

The skin of the penis or clitoris is also supplied by superficial external pudendal arteries, which branch from the external pudendal arteries. The external pudendal arteries branch from the femoral arteries (Fig. 15–17). The superficial external pudendal branches anastomose with branches of the dorsal artery of the penis in males (Fig. 15–17*A*) or clitoris in females (Fig. 15–17*B*). The external pudendal arteries also give off **deep external pudendal branches,** which supply the skin of the anterior scrotal wall or the anterior regions

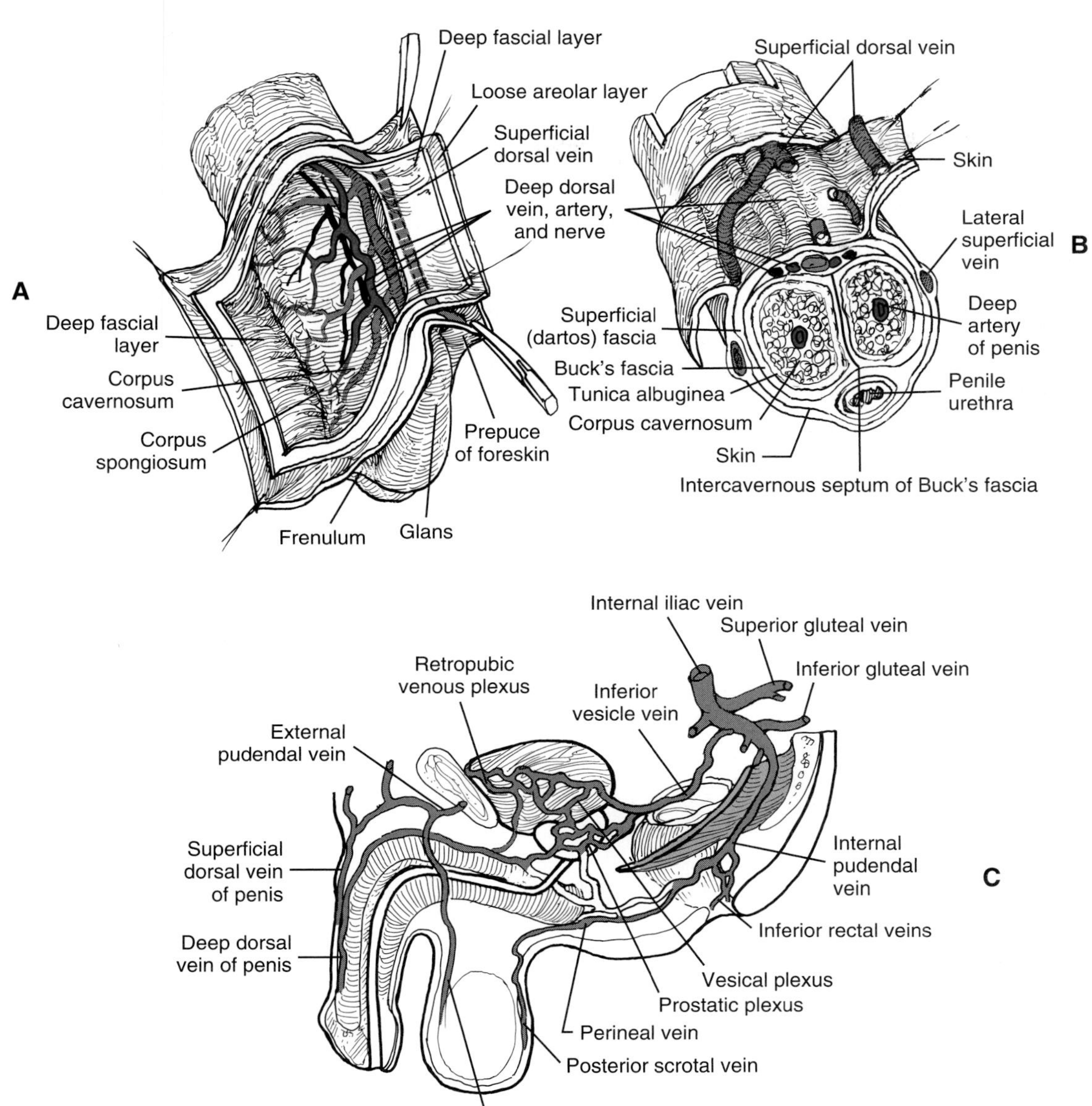

FIGURE 15–18
Venous drainage of the external genitalia in the superficial space of the male. **A.** Superficial vein pattern. **B.** Cross-section through body of penis. **C.** Sagittal section.

of the labia through **anterior scrotal** or **labial branches,** respectively (Fig. 15–17). The anterior scrotal or labial arteries anastomose with posterior scrotal or labial branches of the internal pudendal arteries.

Venous blood of the urogenital compartment drains into internal pudendal veins, under the pubic symphysis into a plexus of veins within the pelvis, and into external pudendal veins

Venous blood of the urogenital compartment drains back to the inferior vena cava via three different routes. It drains into the internal pudendal veins, under the pubic symphysis into a plexus of veins within the pelvis, and into the external pudendal veins. The internal pudendal vein terminates as the **deep dorsal vein of the penis** or **clitoris** (Fig. 15–18). This vein accompanies the dorsal artery and dorsal nerve of the penis or clitoris just deep to the deep fascia (Buck's fascia) (see Fig. 15–16*B* and *C*). These veins drain blood from the cavities within the spongy tissues of the penis or clitoris, including blood within the corpus spongiosum and corpora cavernosa (Fig. 15–18). Although blood may drain into the internal pudendal veins, their primary drainage is directly under the pubic arch (between the pubic arcuate ligament and transverse perineal ligament) into a **prostatic plexus** at the base of the prostate gland in males and into a **vesicular plexus** at the base of the bladder in females (Fig. 15–18*C*). These plexuses, in turn, drain into the internal iliac veins within the pelvic cavity.

The skin and superficial fascia of the penis are drained by a prominent **superficial dorsal vein of the penis** (just superficial to the deep fascia of the penis), which is formed by fusion of paired branches of the external pudendal veins (Fig. 15–17*A*). These, therefore, drain primarily into the femoral vein (Fig. 15–17*A*). A comparable vein called the **superficial dorsal vein of the clitoris** is present in females (see Fig. 15–17*B*).

Lymphatic Drainage of the Urogenital Compartment

Lymph vessels within the urogenital compartment accompany the perineal and internal pudendal blood vessels

Lymph vessels draining structures within the urogenital compartment tend to follow the blood vessels that vascularize these tissues (see Figs. 15–16 and 15–17). Lymphatic vessels accompanying the perineal and internal pudendal vessels drain the corpora cavernosa, corpus spongiosum, urogenital diaphragm, and muscles of the superficial space in both sexes and the penile urethra of the male. Lymph continues to drain back through lymphatic vessels accompanying internal and common iliac vessels and the descending aorta via **internal** and **common iliac** and **paraaortic nodes** (see Fig. 14–17). The skin of the penis and scrotum or clitoris and labia majora is drained via lymphatic vessels that accompany the external pudendal vessels to the **superficial inguinal nodes** (see Fig. 18–16). Lymphatic drainage from the glans penis or glans clitoris is via the **deep inguinal** and **external iliac nodes** (see Chapter 18).

Lymphatics draining the testes accompany the testicular vessels. Lymph then drains into paraaortic (upper lumbar) nodes. Drainage of the vasa deferentia (spermatic ducts) is into external iliac nodes. Lymph from the seminal vesicles drains into vessels that accompany both internal and external iliac arteries and veins (see Chapter 11).

Innervation of the Urogenital Compartment

Terminal branches of the pudendal nerve in the urogenital compartment include the perineal nerve and dorsal nerve of the penis or clitoris

Just after giving off an inferior rectal branch within the ischiorectal fossae, the pudendal nerve enters the pudendal canal and splits into its two terminal branches: the perineal nerve and dorsal nerve of the penis or clitoris (Fig. 15–19). After emerging from the pudendal canal, the perineal nerve gives off branches to anterior fibers of the external anal sphincter (S4) and cutaneous branches to the skin covering the anterior region of the

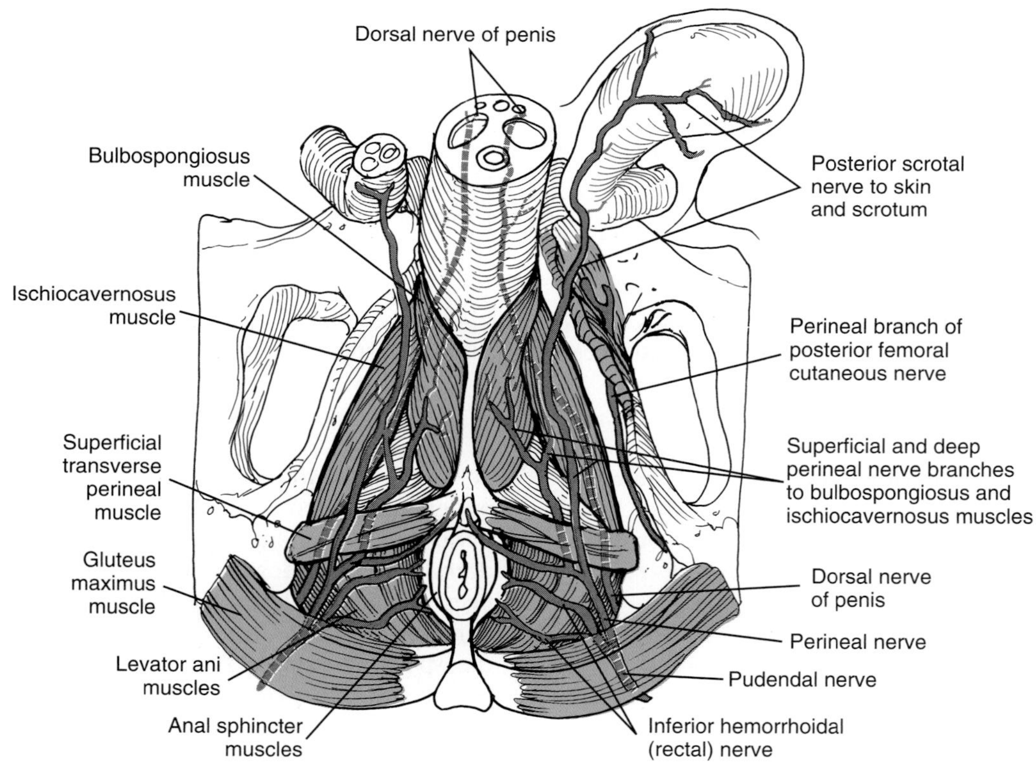

FIGURE 15–19
Territories and targets of the pudendal nerve and its terminal branches.

anal compartment. The **perineal nerve** then gives off several motor branches to muscles within the urogenital compartment (S2 to S4). These are the muscles of the urogenital diaphragm within the deep space, and the muscles of the superficial space, including the superficial transverse perineal, bulbospongiosus, and ischiocavernosus muscles. The perineal nerve also branches into cutaneous posterior scrotal nerves (S4) in males, and posterior labial nerves (S4) in females (Fig. 15–19).

The other terminal branch of the pudendal nerve, the **dorsal nerve of the penis** or **clitoris,** emerges from the anterior end of the pudendal canal and initially accompanies the internal pudendal artery into the deep space (Fig. 15–19 and see Figs. 15–7 and 15–9). It pierces the perineal membrane with the internal pudendal artery, entering the superficial space to innervate the dorsum of the penis or clitoris and providing sensory innervation to the skin of these organs.

Additional contributors to the rich sensory innervation of the urogenital region include perineal branches of the posterior femoral cutaneous nerve (S3) and the ilioinguinal nerve (L1). **Perineal branches of the posterior femoral cutaneous nerves** innervate the lateral skin of the urogenital region and the root of the penis or clitoris (Fig. 15–19). The **ilioinguinal nerve** provides innervation to the skin just superior and lateral to the penis and clitoris and to the skin of the anterior scrotum and anterior labia (see Chapter 11).

The autonomic innervation of genital structures is via the cavernous nerves of the inferior hypogastric plexus

Cavernous nerves from the inferior hypogastric plexus provide autonomic innervation to structures within the urogenital compartment. Postganglionic sympathetic fibers within the cavernous nerves are innervated by preganglionic fibers from T10 to L2, and preganglionic parasympathetic fibers of the cavernous nerves are supplied by the pelvic splanchnic nerves from S2 to S4 (see Figs. 15–10 and 15–21). In males, these nerves emanate from the vicinity of the prostate to innervate the vas deferens, seminal vesicles, and prostate gland. Other fibers pass under the pubic arch (between the arcuate and transverse perineal ligaments) to innervate the bulbourethral glands and smooth muscle of vessels within the erectile tissues of the penis (see Figs. 15–9 and 15–21). In females, the cavernous nerves originate from a region of the inferior hypogastric plexus near the base of the bladder. They pass under the pubic arch to innervate the greater vestibular glands and smooth muscle of the erectile tissues of the clitoris (see Figs. 15–10 and 15–22).

Autonomic innervation of the bladder and its sphincter is also via the nerves that emanate from the inferior hypogastric plexus

Autonomic fibers arising from the anterior region of the inferior hypogastric plexus innervate the smooth muscle within the walls of the bladder (excluding the trigone) and a thickened sphincteric region, which consists of specially modified fibers of smooth muscle, at the base of the bladder (see Fig. 14–7). Preganglionic parasympathetic fibers originate from pelvic splanchnic nerves from spinal cord level S2 to S4, and postganglionic sympathetic fibers within these nerves come from preganglionic sympathetic fibers originating from spinal cord level T11 to L2. The smooth muscle of the bladder wall (excluding the trigone) is called the **detrusor muscle** (see below).

Stretch receptors are located within the bladder wall. Their afferent fibers accompany the pelvic splanchnic nerves to return sensation to spinal cord level S2 to S4.

▲ Function of Structures Within the Urogenital Compartment

Micturition

Micturition is controlled largely by synergism between the sympathetic and parasympathetic nervous systems

Normally, urine is prevented from escaping from the bladder by elastic fibers that constrict the urethra at the base of the bladder and by continuous contraction of the sphincter urethrae muscle of the **urogenital diaphragm** (perineal nerve [S2 to S4]) (Fig. 15–20). Although the bladder may hold as much as 500 ml of urine, a sensation of fullness usually occurs when it is about half full. The **"full bladder reflex"** is initiated when stretch receptors in the bladder wall stimulate afferent fibers associated with the pelvic splanchnic nerves (S2 to S4). Reflex activity induced in these nerves stimulates the smooth muscle of the bladder wall, or **detrusor muscle,** widening and shortening the urethra at the bladder base. This opening of the urethra is also aided by relaxation of the **pubovesicle fibers** of the levator ani muscle (pelvic diaphragm) (see Fig. 14–7).

If urination is not convenient, constant contraction of the **sphincter urethrae** via branches of the perineal nerve (S2 to S4) prevents micturition. When micturition is desired, the sphincter urethrae relaxes. The **detrusor muscle, abdominal muscles** (spinal nerves [T7 to L1]), and **diaphragm** (phrenic nerve [C3 to C5]), which increase intraabdominal pressure, can then expel the urine. The final drops of urine may be expelled from the spongy urethra in males by contraction of the **bulbospongiosus muscle** (perineal nerve, a branch of the pudendal nerve [S2 to S4]).

At the conclusion of micturition, sympathetic activity via the hypogastric plexus (or by sacral splanchnic nerves) relaxes the detrusor muscle (T10 to L2). The urethra becomes constricted once again by contraction of the pubovesicle fibers (nerve to the levator ani muscle [S3 and S4]) of the pelvic diaphragm and the sphincter urethrae (perineal nerve [S2 to S4]), with the aid of elastic fibers at the base of the bladder.

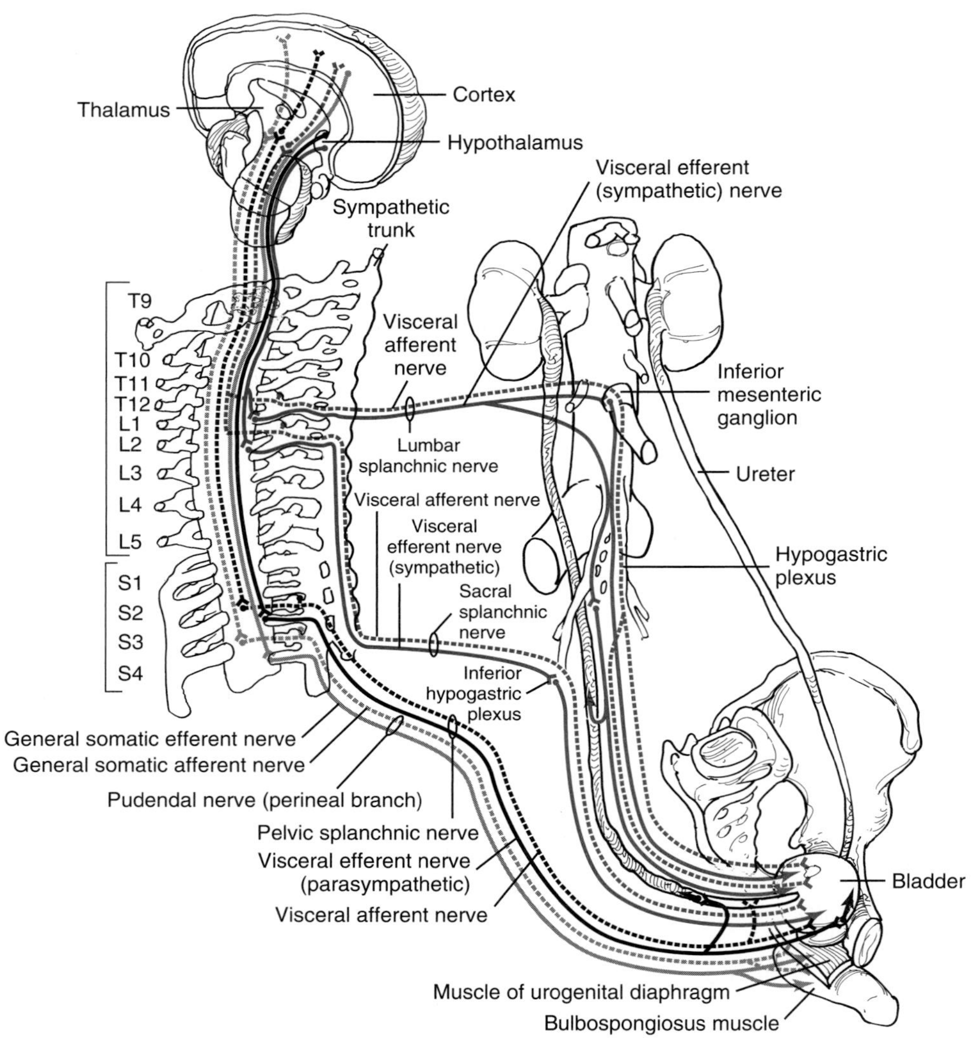

FIGURE 15-20

Pathways in micturition. Normally, continuous contraction of the sphincter urethrae muscle of the urogenital diaphragm prevents urine from escaping (perineal nerve [S2 to S4]). When bladder is about half full, stretch receptors in the bladder wall initiate a complex reflex involving both sympathetic and parasympathetic innervation and spinal nerves. Pelvic splanchnic nerves S2 to S4 can stimulate smooth muscle of the bladder to relax, or the perineal nerve can prevent micturition if urination is not convenient. When desired, the phrenic nerve acts on the diaphragm and spinal nerves T7 to L1 act on detrusor and abdominal muscles to expel urine. *Dotted lines,* Afferent nerves; *solid lines,* efferent nerves.

Urinary Incontinence

Clinically significant urinary incontinence is most common in geriatric patients

Urinary incontinence can be defined as failure to store urine. It is a symptom of a variety of conditions. It is a common problem in geriatric patients and has significant social consequences. Urinary incontinence is most often related to problems associated with the urinary bladder or its outlet, or both. It may also result from **urinary bladder fistula** formation or **congenital ectopic ureter** (see Chapter 15).

In **bladder-related incontinence,** the smooth muscle of the bladder wall becomes hyperactive. In this condition, contraction of the smooth muscle in the bladder wall is initiated (pelvic splanchnic nerves [S2 to S4]) with little or no afferent stimulation (pudendal nerve [S2 to S4]).

Interruption of the nerves innervating the internal urinary sphincter of the bladder wall (pelvic splanchnic nerves) or urogenital diaphragm (pudendal nerve) resulting from trauma or surgery (e.g., radical prostatectomy) results in **outlet-related urinary incontinence.** This is particularly common in elderly patients following loss of internal sphincter elasticity, thus necessitating retention of urine by conscious control of the urogenital diaphragm. When coupled with bladder wall hyperactivity, this condition frequently results in incontinence.

Sexual Function

Sexual arousal and erection of the penis or clitoris incorporates four distinct elements: sensory, psychological, learned, and environmental components. Tactile stimulation of the genital organs results in reflexive erection involving the somatic and parasympathetic systems. Frequently, however, erection is not the result of sensory stimulation but rather of mental imagery. This is illustrated by the observation that patients suffering lower motor neuron loss are frequently unable to attain erection as the result of physical stimulation but are capable of achieving erection as the result of mental arousal. The opposite is true in patients suffering from upper motor neuron deficits. Learning and the environment also contribute to the process of erection, but although the significance of these factors is well documented, their mechanism of action is poorly understood.

Typically, **erotic thoughts** or **tactile stimulation** of the penis or clitoris (primarily via sensory receptors of afferent fibers within the **dorsal nerve of the penis** or **clitoris** [S2 to S4]) results in reflex activity of parasympathetic fibers of the **cavernous nerves** (pelvic splanchnic nerves [S2 to S4]). The ganglia within the penis or clitoris innervated by the pelvic splanchnic nerves relax the smooth muscle fibers within the fibrous trabeculae surrounding the **cavernous erectile tissue.** Relaxation of this smooth muscle results in straightening of the **helicine arteries** and increased flow of blood into the **cavernous spaces.** (The new anti-impotence drug sildenafil citrate [Viagra] contains a smooth muscle relaxant.) Simultaneously, contraction of the **bulbospongiosus** and **ischiocavernosus muscles** (via the perineal nerve [S2 to S4]) obstructs venous drainage of the cavernous spaces, although this process is of lesser importance than the increased vascular inflow. The combination of increased arterial inflow and impeded drainage results in engorgement of the cavernous spaces (20 to 50 ml of blood in the male) and the consequent erection of the penis or clitoris (see Figs. 15–16 to 15–18).

Male Sexual Function

In males, erection may be accompanied by emission and ejaculation of semen

The **emission of semen** is a coordinated process involving the movement of spermatozoa through the vas deferens and the addition of secretions from the **seminal vesicles, prostate gland,** and **bulbourethral glands.** Peristaltic activity of the vas deferens and contraction of smooth muscle fibers of the seminal vesicles mix spermatozoa and secretions of the seminal vesicles within the ejaculatory ducts. This mixture is further modified within the prostatic urethra by additions of secretions from the prostate and bulbourethral glands. Peristalsis of the vas deferens and contraction of smooth muscle fibers within the walls of the seminal vesicles, prostate, and bulbourethral glands are stimulated through sympathetic innervation via the cavernous nerves (T10 and L2). This reflex is usually initiated by tactile stimulation of sensory receptors of the glans penis (via the dorsal nerve of the penis) (Fig. 15–21).

Ejaculation of semen is also initiated by stimulation of sensory receptors of the glans penis (via the dorsal nerve of the penis [S2 to S4]), resulting in reflex activation of parasympathetic nerves to the urethra (pelvic splanchnic nerves [S2 to S4]) and contraction of urethral smooth muscle. Coordinated contraction of the bulbospongiosus muscle through stimulation of the perineal nerve (S2 to S4) results in the pulsatile ejection of semen from the external urethral meatus. Reflux of semen into the bladder is prevented by constriction of sphincteric smooth muscle at the base of the bladder, which is innervated by postganglionic sympathetic fibers from the inferior hypogastric (pelvic) plexus (T10 to L2).

Impotence

Impotence may arise from a wide variety of causes

Although erection of the penis may occur before puberty, erection plays a fundamental role in sexual function in mature males. Inability to achieve erection and, therefore, to function sexually may arise from many different causes, and its specific anatomic or psychological cause must be correctly diagnosed in order for treatment to be successful. Impotence can be defined as the inability to achieve and maintain an erection. Major factors that contribute to impotence include neurologic disorders, vascular disruption, endocrine disorders, surgical and traumatic causes, therapeutic medications, and psychological factors.

Neurologic disorders such as **multiple sclerosis** and **stroke** may disrupt the reflex pathways controlling erection. Other diseases of the nervous system have also been associated with impotence, including **Parkinson's disease** and **Huntington's chorea.** The relative degree to which these latter conditions interfere with specific reflexes regulating erection or with desire arising in cortical centers, however, is unknown.

Disruption of vasculature to the perineum may interfere with the process of erection. Thus, **atherosclerosis** resulting in narrowing or partial occlusion of the abdominal aorta, common or internal iliac artery, or internal pudendal arteries will contribute to impotence. Likewise, **Leriche's syndrome,** a sudden thrombotic occlusion of the common iliac arteries at the point of their bifurcation from the aorta, may result in impotence.

Diabetes mellitus may result in neuropathy of peripheral nerves involved in the reflex controlling erection and is the most typical endocrine disorder associated with impotence. Additionally, **disorders affecting the production of testosterone**

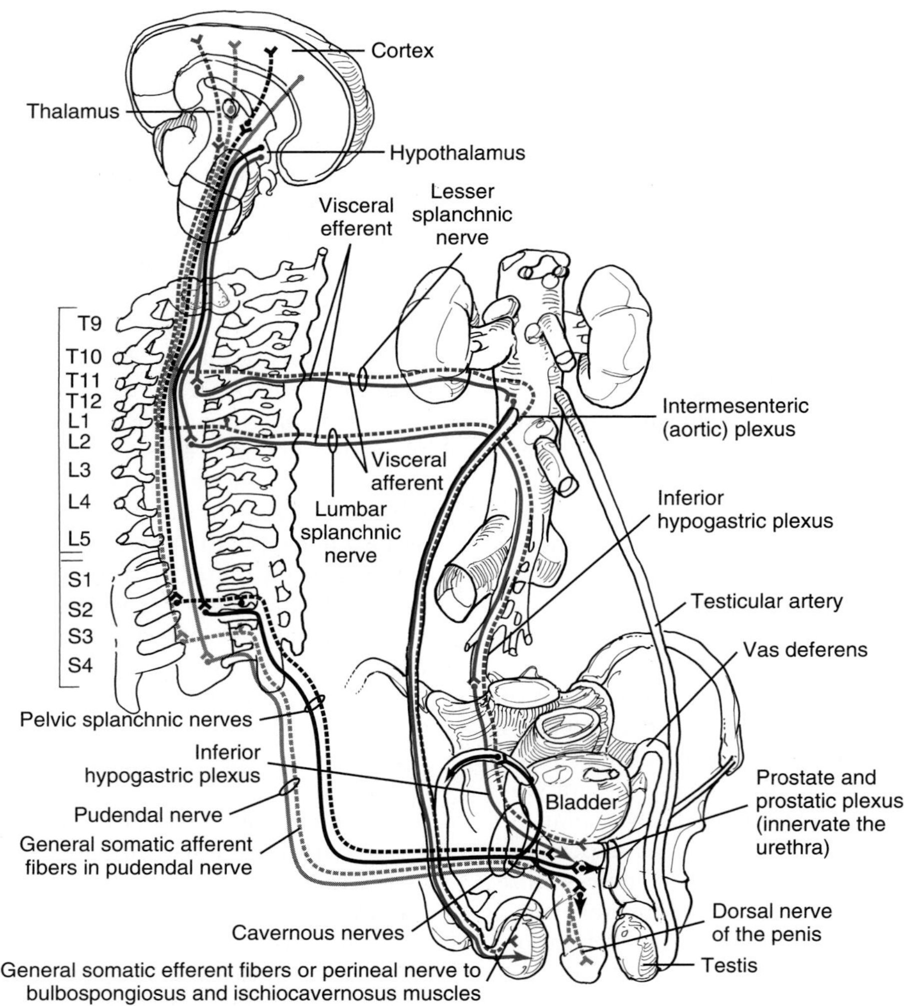

FIGURE 15-21
Pathways in male sexual function. Autonomic innervation of the vas deferens, seminal vesicles, prostate gland, bulbourethral glands, and erectile tissues of the penis is via the cavernous nerves of the inferior hypogastric plexus emanating from the vicinity of the prostate gland. Postganglionic sympathetic fibers originating from T10 to L2 join preganglionic parasympathetic fibers from S2 to S4 **(pelvic splanchnic nerves).** Tactile stimulation of the dorsal nerve of the penis (S2 to S4) or mental imagery results in reflex activity of parasympathetic fibers of cavernous nerves, resulting in relaxation of smooth muscle and increased flow of blood to erectile tissues. A combination of sympathetic and parasympathetic innervation coordinates emission and ejaculation of semen. *Dotted lines,* Afferent nerves; *solid lines,* efferent nerves.

can result in impotence (i.e., disorders affecting the production or release of luteinizing hormone by the anterior pituitary gland or the release of gonadotropin-releasing hormone by the hypothalamus). **Hyperthyroidism** (overproduction of thyroxine) and **hyperprolactinemia** (overproduction of prolactin) have also been implicated in the development of impotence.

Traumatic injury to relevant neuronal elements, particularly the pudendal nerves (at spinal cord level S2 to S4) and pelvic splanchnic nerves (at spinal cord level S2 to S4) may lead to impotence. Injury to these nerves may result from **pelvic fracture** or **gunshot or stab wounds** or may occur during **surgery.** Likewise, **spinal cord trauma** resulting in injury of reflex pathways that control erection may result in impotence. In the past, **radical prostatectomy** (complete removal of the prostate) often led to impotence resulting from interruption of the pelvic splanchnic nerves surrounding this organ. **Vascular surgery** of the inferior aorta and common iliac arteries may also result in destruction of neuronal pathways within the hypogastric plexus and may thus result in impotence. Recent improvements in surgical techniques, however, have resulted in a reduced incidence of postsurgical impotence. **Frontal lobotomy** and **electroshock therapy** may result in impotence, but the degree to which these procedures directly or indirectly influence the erectile reflexes is not known.

Administration of **therapeutic medications** may be the single most significant factor resulting in impotence in men. **Antihypertensive drugs** and **antidepressant drugs** are implicated more frequently than others. Examples include alpha- and beta-adrenergic blocking agents, tricyclic antidepressants, and monoamine oxidase inhibitors.

Psychological factors may also cause impotence, frequently contributing to disturbances of peripheral reflex control of erection. Males suffering from **primary psychogenic impotence** (impotence where there is no discernible organic causative factor) frequently come from family or cultural backgrounds where discussions of sexual activity were nonexistent or primarily negative. These individuals may suffer from excitement inhibition or desire inhibition. In **excitement inhibition,** erection is frequently achieved but cannot be maintained to climax, whereas individuals suffering from **desire inhibition** fail to achieve erection at any time. In both cases, extensive psychological therapy is indicated. The prognosis is more positive for those suffering from excitement inhibition than for those suffering from desire inhibition.

Female Sexual Function

In females, erection of the clitoris may be accompanied by secretions of the greater vestibular gland

In females, tactile stimulation of the glans clitoris (via the dorsal nerve of the clitoris [S2 to S4]) may initiate a reflex that activates parasympathetic stimulation (pelvic splanchnic nerves [S2 to S4]) of cavernous nerves to the **greater vestibular glands** (Fig. 15–22 and see Fig. 15–14*B*). These glands (and the lesser vestibular glands) produce secretions that lubricate the vestibule and vagina.

Resolution, or **detumescence,** is the return of the penis or clitoris to the flaccid state. This occurs as the flow of blood into the cavernous spaces is once again restricted by contraction of smooth muscle in the spongy tissue, which creates bends or spirals in the **helicine arteries.** Contraction of these muscles is stimulated by sympathetic fibers carried within the cavernous nerves (T10 to L2). In addition, relaxation of the bulbospongiosus and ischiocavernosus muscles (innervated by the perineal nerve [S2 to S4]) allows relaxation of veins within the spongy tissues and release of blood from the cavernous spaces via the deep dorsal vein of the clitoris (Fig. 15–22). Other aspects of the female sexual response, including reflexes of the vagina, cervix, and puborectal sling, are described in Chapter 14.

Gender-Related Disorders of the Urogenital Compartment

Disorders of the urogenital compartment may be gender related

Fundamental gender-related differences in the perineal anatomy influence the relative incidence of specific clinical problems in males and females. Urinary bladder infections are far more common in females as a consequence of the comparatively short urethra. The larger, less protected external genitalia of males have increased susceptibility to traumatic injuries, such as torsion (twisting) of the testicular artery or rupture of blood vessels, erectile tissue, or the urethra.

Extravasation of Urine or Blood and Spread of Infection

Extravasation of urine or blood and spread of infection within the urogenital compartment may be limited by fascial boundaries

Extravasation of urine into the superficial or deep space is most often the result of **trauma to the urethra** following fracture of the pelvis (see Fig. 11–6). Gunshot or stab wounds and straddle injuries may result in urethral rupture. Rupture of the membranous urethra allows urine to enter the deep space, where it may be confined. However, if this condition is left untreated, increased pressure may rupture the fascial boundaries of the deep space, as may the original rupture, allowing urine to enter the superficial space as well. Because Colles' fascia is fused with the deep fascia of the transverse perineal muscles and the fascia lata, urine seeping into the superficial space may not enter the anal triangle or medial thighs. However, because Colles' fascia is continuous with Scarpa's fascia of the anterior abdominal wall, blood, urine, or infectious agents within the superficial space may escape the region of the urogenital triangle by seeping anterosuperiorly just deep to the membranous fascia of the anterior abdominal wall (see Fig. 11–6). The blood supply to the urogenital compartment in both sexes is extensive, and bleeding from traumatic injuries to this region may be severe.

Sexually Transmitted Disease of the Urogenital Compartment

Sexually transmitted infection may cause pathogenic lesions of perineal structures

The perineal anatomy is frequently distorted as the result of **sexually transmitted disease.** The more commonly observed diseases in the United States include **chlamydial** and **gonorrheal** (bacterial) **infections, syphilis** (spirochetal infection), and **genital warts** and **herpesvirus infection** (viral infections).

Chlamydial infection can result indirectly in the formation of genital ulcers in both sexes. The prostate, seminal vesicles, and testes can be affected in the male and the vestibular glands, cervix, and uterus in the female.

Gonorrhea does not produce obvious lesions of genital structures but may infect the greater vestibular glands as described below, resulting in their swelling and distention. When patients present with this condition, they are often screened for gonococcal infections and other sexually transmitted diseases.

Syphilis results in formation of chancres as well as flat, wartlike, red mucocutaneous lesions in the perineum.

Genital warts appear as raised skin-colored, cauliflower-like growths on the cervix, vagina, vulva, penis, or perianal areas, while **herpesvirus infection** is characterized by painful clusters of vesicular lesions filled with clear fluid.

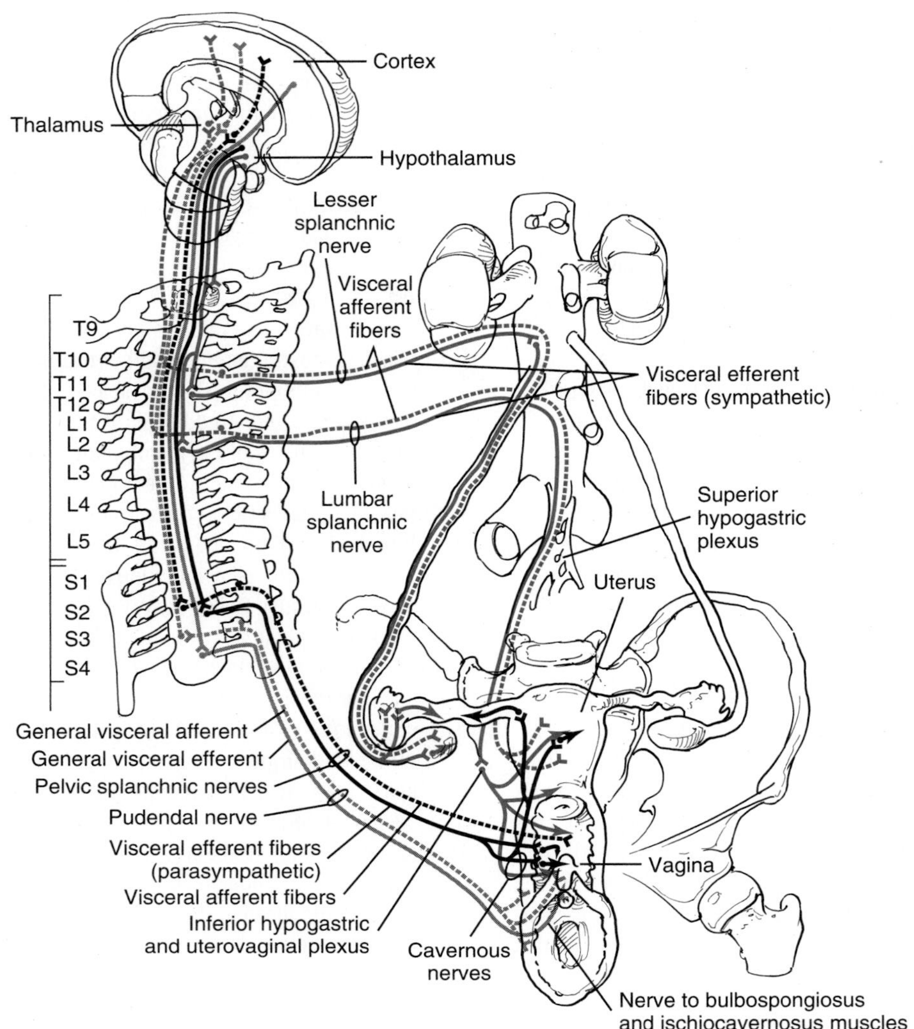

FIGURE 15-22

Pathways in female sexual function. Cavernous nerves from the region of the inferior hypogastric plexus near the base of the bladder innervate the greater vestibular glands and smooth muscle that controls the flow of blood to the erectile tissues of the clitoris. Stimulation of the glans clitoris via the dorsal nerve of the clitoris (S2 to S4) may initiate parasympathetic stimulation of greater vestibular glands, producing secretions that lubricate the vestibule and vagina as well as increased flow of blood to the erectile tissue. *Dotted lines,* Afferent nerves; *solid lines,* efferent nerves.

Chlamydial infection, gonorrhea, syphilis, and genital warts can be treated, but there is no known treatment for genital herpesvirus infection.

Disorders of Aging in Females

Many clinical disorders of the urogenital compartment occur in conjunction with aging

Pubertal development in females is initiated at age 7 or 8 years, when growth is accelerated. Other physical changes occur over the next 4 to 5 years, including breast development, growth of pubic hair, and menarche (onset of the menstrual cycle). The development of pulsatile secretions by the hypothalamus and pituitary gland stimulates ovarian estrogen secretion, which is responsible for developmental changes of the perineum associated with puberty. The vaginal orifice enlarges, and the vaginal mucosa thickens. The greater and lesser vestibular glands also become functional, and the labial folds enlarge relative to the clitoris. There is little further change until menopause (the final menstrual cycle), when many of these alterations are reversed. The vaginal opening shrinks, and the mucosa thins. Secretions of the vestibular glands diminish significantly or cease altogether. These transformations are problematic for postmenopausal females who remain sexually active. Estrogen replacement therapy, however, is frequently prescribed.

Disorders of the Female Urogenital Compartment Caused by Pregnancy or Childbirth

Pregnancy and childbirth may stretch and weaken the fascia and supporting structures associated with the perineum. As a result, the vagina and, in more extreme cases, the uterus may **prolapse.** Pregnant women are customarily taught to exercise the perineal musculature to prevent weakening of the fascia separating the anal and urogenital compartments. Weakening of this fascia may result in fecal retention. Childbirth may also result in injury to structures within the anal compartment, including the external anal sphincter (see above).

Inflammation of the Vestibular Glands

Inflammation of the vestibular glands is a common gynecologic problem

The vestibular glands of sexually active females produce copious amounts of mucous secretions. Occasionally, the duct draining the greater vestibular gland may become occluded or constricted, resulting in swelling and inflammation of the gland. This condition is painful and may recur. In such cases, surgical intervention is often required.

Misdiagnosis of Cryptorchidism in Males

Although the **onset of puberty in males** is more difficult to define than in females, it is usually initiated about 2 years later than in females. The penis, testes, and scrotum enlarge under the influence of testosterone. The skin of the glans penis and scrotum becomes darker, and the skin of the scrotum also becomes wrinkled as a consequence of development and stimulation of the tunica dartos. As in the female, hair grows on the genitalia as well as the surrounding pubic skin. The cremaster muscle is quite active in children, holding the testes close to the body. It is not uncommon for the novice practitioner to misdiagnose **cryptorchidism** (undescended testis) in children. The cremaster muscle becomes progressively weaker during adulthood, resulting in stretching of the scrotum and spermatic cord.

SECTION 2 THE EXTREMITIES

16 Bones and Joints of the Lower Extremities

The anatomy and function of the lower limbs are described in this chapter and the following two chapters. This chapter describes the development of the lower limbs and discusses principles that underlie lower limb structure and function. It also describes the skeleton and joints of the lower extremities in a way that allows these features to be used as a framework for understanding the attachments of muscles and muscle functions.

Chapter 17 describes the anatomy of lower extremity musculature; muscle attachments to the skeleton; functional relationships of muscles to lower extremity joints; and mechanisms of standing, walking, and running.

Chapter 18 describes the vasculature and innervation of lower limb tissues and provides both vascular and neural frameworks for integrating the details of lower limb anatomy and function. Pathologic disorders of the lower limbs are described where relevant in all three chapters.

DEVELOPMENT OF THE LOWER EXTREMITIES

The lower limbs arise as paddle-shaped buds of the lateral flank

The **upper** and **lower limbs** begin to develop during the fourth week of embryonic life as small buds of mesoderm covered by a cap of ectoderm. The upper **limb buds** arise from the lateral flank in the region of vertebrae C4 to T1 and the lower limb buds from the lateral flank in the region of vertebrae L4 to S5 (Fig. 16–1*A*). Proliferation of limb bud mesoderm is stimulated by a thickened distal ridge of ectoderm, the **apical ectodermal ridge.** As the limb bud grows outward, it differentiates along three major axes: the craniocaudal, dorsoventral, and proximodistal axes (Fig. 16–1*B*). The sequential expression and actions of growth factors, transcription factors, and other regulatory genes direct the development of the limb along each axis of the limb bud. The first to fifth digits develop along the craniocaudal axis, the extensor and flexor muscles of the limbs develop in the dorsoventral axis, and the limb segments develop along the proximodistal axis. The expression of HOX genes in sequential combination regulates the differentiation of elements or segments along all three axes. For example, with respect to the proximodistal axis, the differentiation of the pelvis is regulated by the expression of HOX9 genes; the thigh by genes HOX9 and HOX10; the leg by genes HOX9 to HOX11; the proximal tarsals by genes HOX9 to HOX12; and the distal tarsals, metatarsals, and phalanges by genes HOX9 to HOX13 (see Fig. 1–3).

It is now apparent that disruptions of HOX genes in the limbs may result in human congenital limb malformations characterized by partial transformations of one limb segment into another (see discussion of homeotic transformations of limbs below).

Tissues and structures of the limb are derived from diverse precursors

Skin arises from the ectoderm, and pigment cells of the skin are derived from neural crest cells. The lateral plate mesoderm of the limb buds differentiates into bones, tendons, and connective tissues. The mesenchymal precursor of the long bones is, at first, a single unsegmented structure. As differentiation proceeds, however, **interzones** appear and differentiate into joints, separating the unsegmented mesenchyme into the segments that will form the individual bones. The joints thus anatomically and functionally distinguish the **gluteal region** from the **thigh,** the thigh from the **leg,** and the leg from the **foot** (see Fig. 16–3). The foot is further divided by many joints. In addition, each segment of the lower extremity is divided into **compartments** by fascial sheets or septa (see Chapter 17). The fascial septa isolate functional muscle groups. The muscles develop from invading somitic myoblasts. As the muscles differentiate, they secrete tropic substances that attract the growth cones of specific nerves of the lumbar and sacral plexuses so that the muscles of individual compartments become appropriately innervated (see Chapter 18). The vessels to each lower extremity muscle compartment branch from a simple axis artery, which

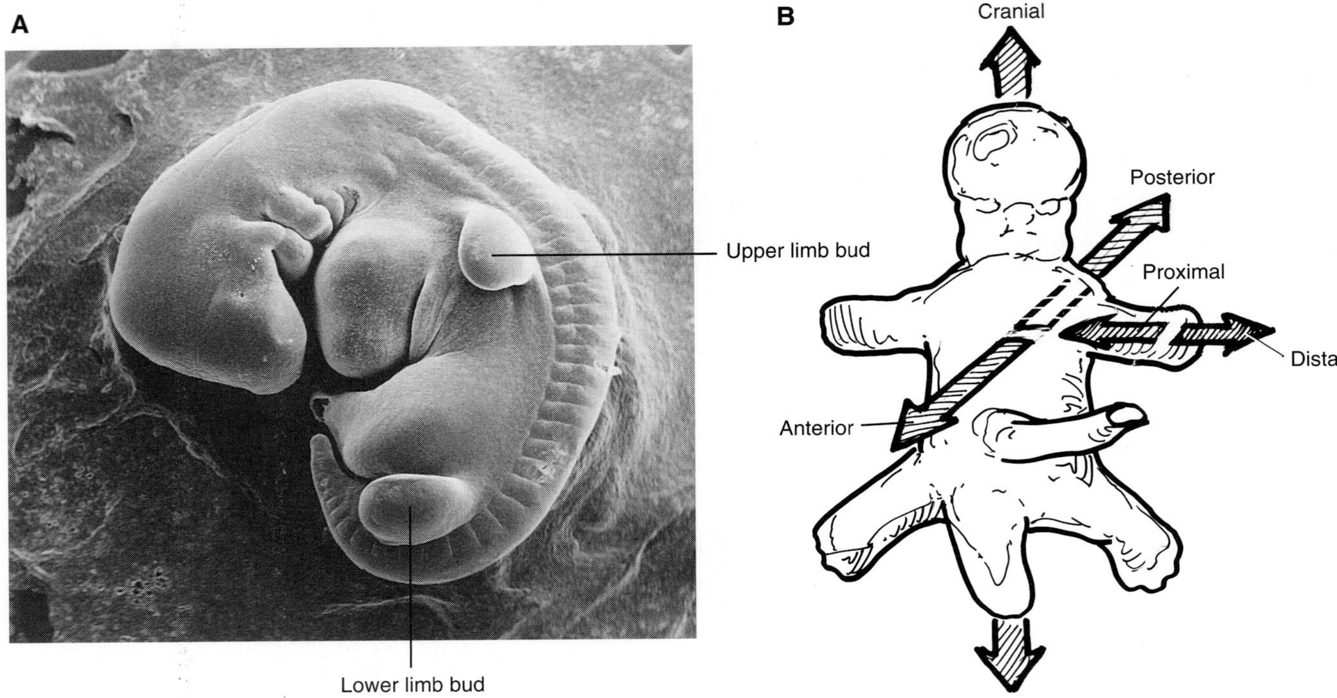

FIGURE 16–1
A. Scanning electron micrograph of 5-week-old human embryo. Upper and lower limb buds are adjacent to the segmental somites. **B.** The limb buds develop along three axes: the craniocaudal axis (digits), dorsoventral axis (flexors and extensors), and proximodistal axis (segments of the limb).

originates from embryonic intersegmental artery L5 (see Chapter 18).

Development of upper limb buds precedes that of lower limb buds by several days, but by the eighth week, the definitive forms of both upper and lower extremities are apparent. The characteristic vasculature and innervation of the limbs have also developed by this time. Ossification of most of the bony elements begins by the twelfth week. For some skeletal elements, such as carpals (of the wrist) and tarsals (of the ankle), ossification does not begin until early childhood.

The lower limb buds twist medially during development; this explains the distribution of the lower extremity nerves and the orientation of the lower limb muscle compartments in the thigh, leg, and foot

The paddle-shaped lower limb buds twist 180 degrees in a medial direction between the fourth and eighth weeks of development. During the fourth week, the presumptive big toe occupies the most superior region of the limb bud, but by the end of the eighth week, the differentiated big toe is located at the medial aspect of the foot (Fig. 16–2). The most superior nerve fibers (at spinal nerve L4), which innervate the presumptive big toe are twisted in a medial direction down the lower extremity to innervate the big toe and medial side of the foot (Fig. 16–2). Nerves such as S1 and S2, which initially innervate inferior aspects of the presumptive distal lower limb bud (e.g., the presumptive small toe), are also twisted medially to innervate the lateral side of the foot and small toe.

The twisting of the lower limb bud results in other peculiarities of anatomic organization, as well. For example, in anatomic position, the **knee** (unlike the elbow) faces ventrally, while its corresponding concavity, the **popliteal fossa,** faces dorsally (Fig. 16–2). The dorsal surface of the presumptive foot is turned so that it faces anteriorly (and superiorly). For this reason, the top of the foot is called the **dorsum of the foot** and the reduction of the angle of the ankle joint (in which the toes are raised toward the anterior surface of the leg) is given the unique name of **dorsiflexion.** The ventral surface of the presumptive foot becomes the inferior **plantar surface** of the definitive foot. The movement that opens the angle of the ankle joint (referred to as extension in other joints) is, therefore, called **plantarflexion.**

▲ Congenital Malformations

Many defects of the upper and lower limbs occur in humans. They may be caused by genetic defects, the actions of teratogens, or physical disruptions during development. Genetic defects may involve autosomal or sex-linked mutations or may be associated with specific chromosomal anomalies, such as trisomy 18. Several environmental and therapeutic

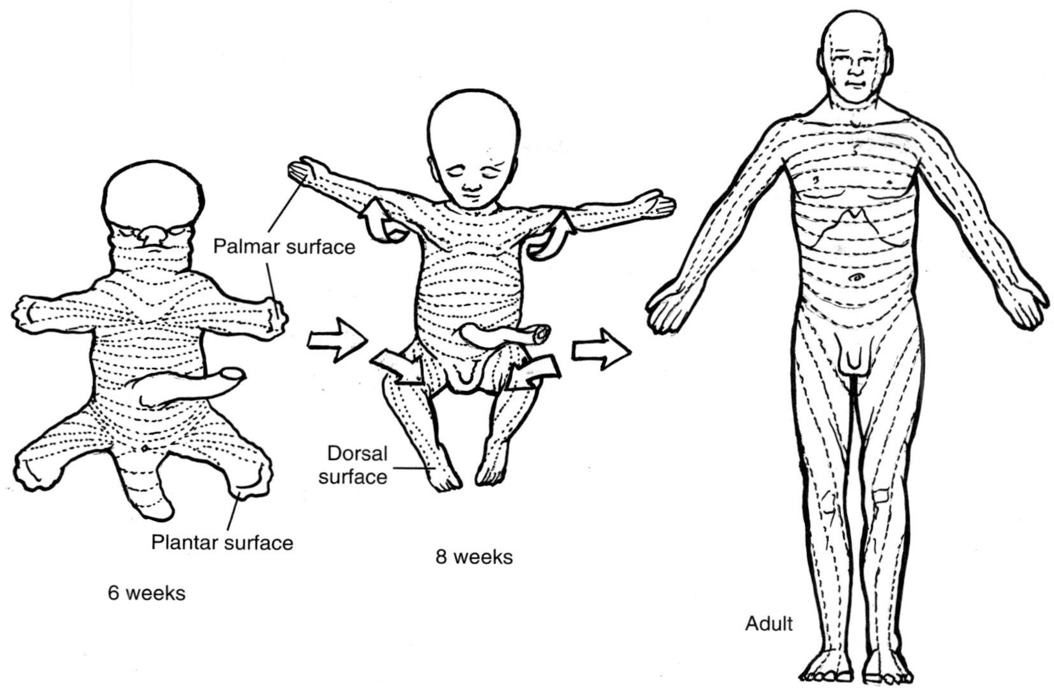

FIGURE 16–2
The lower extremity limb buds rotate about 180 degrees medially during development. The dorsal surface of the lower extremity limb bud rotates to face ventrally in the definitive limb. The dermatomes, which are horizontal in the limb bud, spiral medially down the definitive lower limb. Only a slight amount of lateral rotation occurs in the upper extremity limb buds during development.

teratogens are notorious disrupters of limb development, including thalidomide, cadmium, acetazolamide, and retinoic acid. Physical disruptions may also result from reduced amounts of amniotic fluid, interruption of the local vasculature, or constriction of a limb by loosened bands of amniotic membrane.

The severity of congenital limb defects may range from the complete absence of a limb (amelia) to partial absence of a limb (meromelia) to conditions such as **syndactyly** (fusion of digits) or **polydactyly** (an excessive number of digits).

Disruption of the HOX gene code has been found to underlie the disruption of limb development. Disruption of the HOXD13 or HOXA13 genes results in partial **homeotic transformations** of the metatarsophalangeal segment of the hand and foot. Metacarpals, metatarsals, and phalanges are shortened so that they resemble the distal carpal or tarsal bones (see Fig. 1–3). In addition, these shortened carpal-like or tarsal-like phalanges tend to be fused (syndactyly).

A woman who takes retinoic acid for acne while she is pregnant may have a child with limb malformations. The cause is thought to be disruption of the craniocaudal expression and distribution of the morphogens responsible for specification of the digits. The result is a **reduction in the number of digits, fusion of the digits,** and other anomalies of the limbs. Thalidomide is a spasmolytic that was given to pregnant women to reduce nausea and is now used in the treatment of autoimmune and other diseases. It may disrupt the vasculature of the growing limb bud in the fetus, causing a wide variety of malformations including reduced growth, or **hypoplasia,** of digits and **syndactyly.** Both the upper and the lower limbs are vulnerable to the effects of teratogens during the fourth to eighth weeks of embryonic life.

STRUCTURE OF THE DEFINITIVE LOWER LIMB

Surface Anatomy

The integument of the lower extremity consists of epidermis and dermis. It is underlaid by a fatty hypodermis (superficial fascia). The integument and fascia play significant roles in the function and stability of the lower extremity.

Deep to the hypodermis, the deep fascia of the thigh, the **fascia lata,** is especially thick. This tough fascia serves as an anchor for several muscles of the gluteal region and thigh (see Chapter 17). In addition, the deep fascia and integument provide a tight investment for underlying muscles and help stabilize the joints (see below). The integument bulges where it passes over bones, ligaments, or muscles (Fig. 16–3). Other obvious features of the surface anatomy are the major superficial veins. These veins play a special role in returning blood from the lower extremities (see function of lower extremity vasculature in Chapter 18). The superficial veins do not have a corresponding system of arteries.

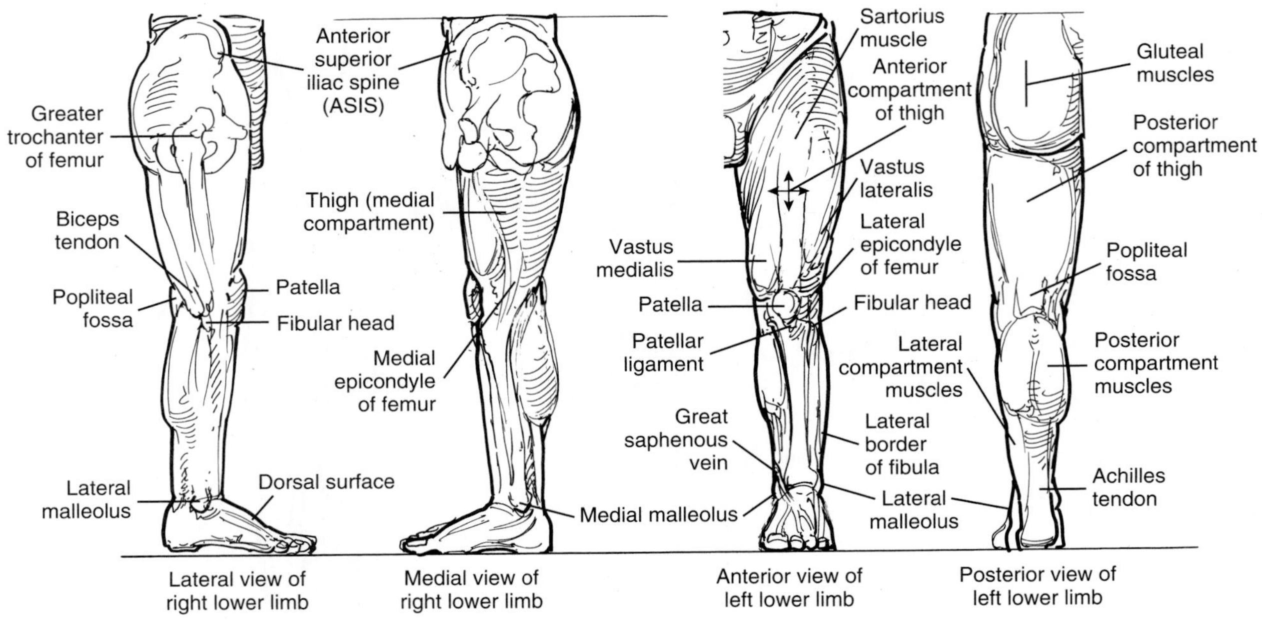

FIGURE 16–3
Surface features of the definitive lower extremity. Obvious bony landmarks of the definitive lower extremity include the anterior superior iliac spine (ASIS), greater trochanter, lateral and medial epicondyles of the femur, patella, anterior border and tuberosity of the tibia, head and lateral border of the fibula, and lateral and medial malleoli. Palpable tendons include the biceps, quadriceps, and Achilles tendons. Obvious muscles include the gluteus, sartorius, vastus, and gastrocnemius muscles.

▲ Structural and Functional Relationships of the Definitive Limbs

The lower extremity has become a stable structure at the expense of its mobility

The upper and lower extremities can be characterized as a **series of sequential platforms** that act together to emplace their most distal elements (the hands and fingers or the feet and toes) in the desired location. In the upper extremity, synergistic movements of the shoulder, first, and then the arm, forearm, and wrist move the hand and fingers precisely to grasp an object. The sequential actions of these contiguous platforms can be visualized as one reaches into a grocery bag to grasp an object and places it on a kitchen shelf. In the lower extremity, the movements of the pelvis, thigh, leg, ankle, foot, and toes place the foot upon the substratum when a person is walking or running (Fig. 16–3 and see the discussion of walking and running in Chapter 17). One can visualize the changing positions of lower extremity segments as a person runs diagonally down and back up a hill with an uneven surface. In these examples, the final position of the most distal element of the upper or lower extremity is determined by the sum of the movements of all moveable segments of the extremity.

Lower extremity joints have been designed for weight bearing while the body is standing, walking, or running

Joints of the upper extremity are designed primarily for a prehensile (grasping) function. They are not strongly reinforced and are relatively mobile. In contrast, the major function of the lower extremity is to support the upper body while a person is standing or during bipedal locomotion. For this reason, lower extremity joints are strongly reinforced and have a restricted range of motion. For example, the **tibiofibular joints** and **interosseous membrane** bind the tibia and fibula so firmly that, unlike the ulna and radius, these leg bones act as a single unit rather than as relatively separate or interactive units. The **articulating surfaces** of lower extremity joints are deeply sculpted so that they fit snugly together. For example, the deep acetabulum and closely fitting lunate cartilage of the hip joint firmly entrap the head of the femur. In contrast, the shoulder joint is designed for mobility and the more diminutive humeral head lies loosely against the glenoid (shallow) fossa. Indeed, in several instances, the security of lower extremity joints is further enhanced by the presence of cartilaginous elements such as the lunate cartilage of the hip joint just mentioned or the medial and lateral menisci of the tibia. In addition, the size, extent, and strength of lower extremity **ligaments** and associated **fibrous capsules** are consistent with the load-bearing requirements of lower extremity joints.

Differences in the relative stability and mobility of the hip and shoulder joints explain differences in clinical problems associated with these joints. For example, because the femoral head is retained within the acetabulum by femoral-pelvic ligaments and the fibrous capsule of the hip, the femur tends to **fracture** at the femoral neck, particularly in elderly persons (see Fig. 16–7B). In the shoulder, the very lax capsule and ligaments enclose the humeral head loosely, and, thus, when disruptive (particularly downward) forces are exerted upon the joint, the **humerus is often dislocated** from the glenoid fossa of the scapula (see Chapter 19).

In another example, ligaments so tightly enclose the ankle joint that they significantly curtail eversion and inversion. Disruptive forces at this joint often result in **injury to a ligament** or **avulsion of the bone** at the point of ligamentous attachment rather than dislocation (see Fig. 16–26).

Locomotory functions of the lower extremity depend on the architecture of the joint and on the actions of related muscles

The movements of the lower limbs are dictated by (1) the mechanical degree of freedom allowed by the bony architecture of the joints; (2) the restrictions of motion imposed by the ligaments, fibrous capsules, and integument; and (3) the relationship of the longitudinal axis of specific muscle fibers to the fibers' points of attachment to skeletal elements of the lower extremity (see Chapter 17). The specific skeletal and arthrologic (joint) frameworks that underlie coordinated movements of the lower limbs are described below.

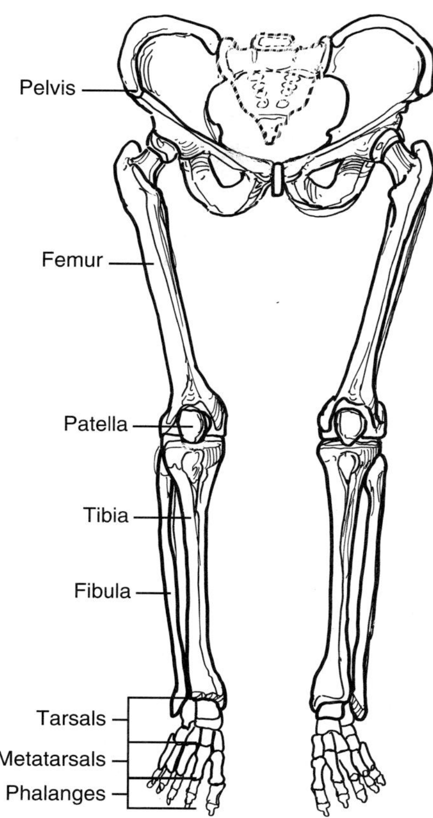

FIGURE 16–4
The skeleton of the lower extremity includes the pelvis, femur, tibia, fibula, tarsals, metatarsals, phalanges, and sesamoid bones. The sesamoid bones are the patella and about 20 bones in the foot.

SKELETAL FRAMEWORK AND JOINTS OF THE LOWER EXTREMITY

Bones and joints of the lower extremity are strong and well stabilized

Understanding the anatomy of bones and joints of the lower extremities provides a framework for learning about the structures and relationships of lower extremity muscles, vessels, and nerves, as well as their functions. The appendicular skeleton of the lower extremities will be described in a superior-to-inferior sequence, and the major joints will then be described.

The bones of the lower extremity include the **pelvis, femur, tibia, fibula, tarsals, metatarsals,** and **phalanges** (Fig. 16–4). The joints include the **hip, knee, tibiofibular, ankle, foot,** and **toe joints.**

Skeleton of the Pelvic Girdle: The Pelvic Bone and Acetabulum

The anatomy of the pelvic bone is described in detail in Chapter 14. Each half of the pelvic bone is formed by the fusion of three bones: the **pubis, ischium,** and **ilium.** The posterior edge of each half of the pelvic bone is joined to the sacrum by a synovial sacroiliac joint, which has very limited movement. The anterior edges of the two halves of the pelvic bone are joined to each other by a syndesmosis called the *pubic symphysis,* which is almost totally immovable (see Chapter 14). The pubic bone provides many sites for the attachments of ligaments and muscles of the trunk and lower extremities. These are listed and described in Table 16–1 and illustrated in Chapter 17. The pelvis provides a stable platform for the support of the rest of the lower extremity skeleton. The stability comes from the secure "ball-and-socket" mechanism at the hip joint and numerous muscle attachments and connective tissue investments. The socket of the hip joint is the **acetabulum** (vinegar cup) of the pelvis. It is formed by the three bones (pubis, ilium, and ischium) that make up each half of the pelvis (Fig. 16–5 and see Fig. 16–15). The acetabulum is, thus, a deep socket, which provides an articulation for the "ball" of the joint, which is the **head** of the **femur.** The **acetabular margin (limbus)** is prominent from the six o'clock to the five o'clock positions but is interrupted by an **acetabular notch** in the five o'clock to six o'clock region of its circumference.

The head of the femur articulates with the moon-shaped **lunate surface** of the acetabulum. The depth of the acetabulum and its investment of the head of the femur provide stability for the hip joint but limit the range of motion of the femur (see below).

Skeleton of the Thigh

Femur

The proximal end of the femur consists of a large, smooth, round **head** that fits into the acetabulum of

TABLE 16–1
Specialized Skeletal Processes of the Lower Extremity and Major Attachments and Articulations

Bone	Skeletal Process	Attachments or Articulations
Pelvis	Posterior gluteal line	Gluteus maximus muscle
	Iliac crest	Gluteus maximus, tensor fascia latae muscles
	Ischial spine	Superior gemellus muscle; sacrospinous ligament
	Ischial tuberosity	Inferior gemellus muscle, long head of biceps femoris muscle, semimembranous and semitendinosus muscles
	Pecten pubis	Psoas minor muscle
	Pectineal line	Pectineus muscle
	Iliac fossa	Iliacus muscle
	Acetabular notch	Round ligament of femur
	Anterior superior iliac spine (ASIS)	Sartorius, rectus femoris muscles
Femur	Fovea	Round ligament of femur
	Greater trochanter	Iliofemoral ligament; gluteus medius, gluteus minimus, piriformis, obturator internus, superior gemellus, inferior gemellus muscles
	Trochanteric fossa	Pubofemoral, iliofemoral, ischiofemoral ligaments; obturator externus muscle
	Lesser trochanter	Psoas major muscle
	Gluteal tuberosity	Gluteus maximus, adductor magnus muscles
	Intertrochanteric crest	Ischiofemoral ligament; quadratus femoris muscle
	Intertrochanteric line	Iliofemoral ligament; vastus lateralis muscle
	Quadrate tubercle	Quadratus lumborum muscle
	Lateral supracondylar line	Plantaris muscle
	Medial supracondylar line	Vastus medialis muscle
	Linea aspera	Adductor longus and adductor magnus muscles, short head of biceps femoris muscle
	Lateral condyle	Articulates with lateral condyle of tibia; anterior cruciate ligament; capsule of knee joint
	Medial condyle	Articulates with medial condyle of tibia; posterior cruciate and posterior meniscofemoral ligaments; capsule of knee joint; and popliteus muscle
	Adductor tubercle	Tibial (medial) collateral muscle; distal tendon of adductor magnus muscle
	Lateral epicondyle	Fibular collateral ligament
	Medial epicondyle	Tibial collateral ligament
Tibia	Oblique line of tibia	Iliotibial tract
	Gerdy's tubercle	Iliotibial tract
	Tuberosity of tibia	Quadriceps-patellar tendon
	Medial condyle	Articulates with medial condyle of femur; tibial collateral ligament; capsule of knee joint
	Lateral condyle	Articulates with lateral condyle of femur; anterior cruciate ligament, anterior and posterior ligaments of head of fibula; capsule of knee joint
	Intercondylar surface	Posterior cruciate ligament
	Soleal line	Soleus muscle
	Medial malleolus	Articulates with trochlea of talus; deltoid, tibionavicular, tibiocalcaneal ligaments
Fibula	Lateral malleolus	Articulates with tibia and trochlea of talus; anterior talofibular, posterior talofibular, and calcaneofibular ligaments
Talus	Trochlea	Articulates with tibia and fibula
	Sinus tarsi	Cervical and talocalcaneal ligaments
	Posterior process	Posterior talofibular ligament
	Medial process (tubercle)	Posterior tibiotalar ligament
	Lateral process (tubercle)	Posterior talofibular ligament

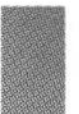

TABLE 16–1, cont'd
Specialized Skeletal Processes of the Lower Extremity and Major Attachments and Articulations

Bone	Skeletal Process	Attachments or Articulations
Calcaneus	Tuberosity of calcaneus	Calcaneal (Achilles) tendon; abductor hallucis, abductor digiti minimi, flexor digitorum brevis muscles
	Lateral process	Calcaneofibular ligament
	Sustentaculum tali	Articulates with talus; tibiocalcaneal, medial talocalcaneal, plantar calcaneonavicular (spring) ligaments
Navicular bone	Navicular tuberosity	Tibionavicular ligament; tendon of tibialis posterior muscle

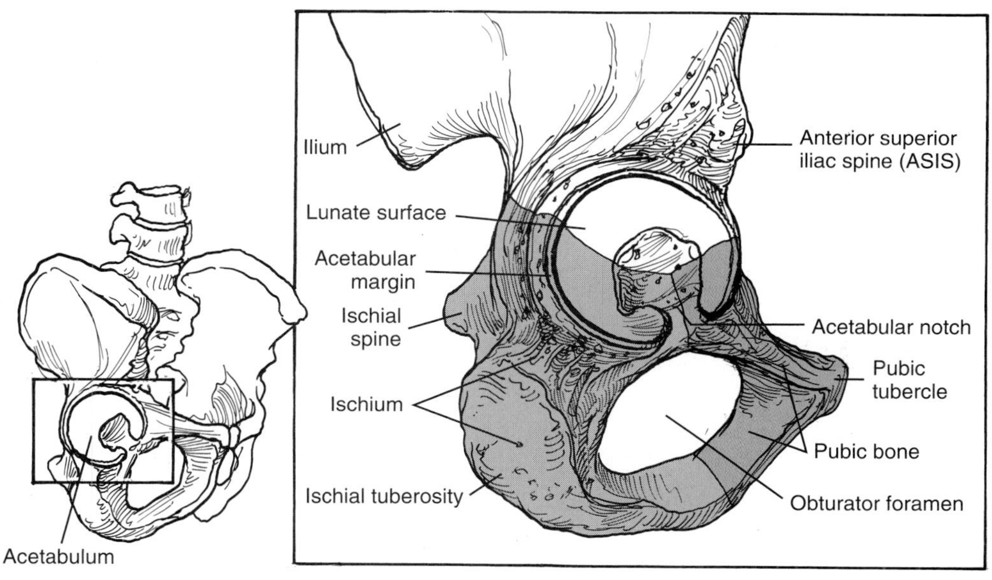

FIGURE 16–5
The pelvis is formed by the paired ilium, ischium, and pubic bones. Each hip joint socket is formed by the convergence of one ilium, one ischium, and one pubic bone.

the pelvis. A roughened depression at approximately the **center of the femur (fovea)** serves as an attachment site for the apex of the **round ligament of the femur (ligamentum capitis femoris).** The base of the round ligament is attached to the rim of the **acetabular notch** (see Fig. 16–5) and the **transverse acetabular ligament** (see Fig. 16–15). A thick fibrous capsule encloses the joint cavity and the head and neck of the femur within and is attached to the rim of the acetabulum, floor of the acetabular notch, and transverse acetabular ligament.

The head of the femur is attached to the **shaft** of the femur by an angled **neck** about 2 inches long (Fig. 16–6). An angle of about 120 degrees between the shaft and the neck allows the shaft to clear the pelvis during walking.

The junction of the neck and the shaft of the femur is marked by a large superolateral projection called the **greater trochanter of the femur** and a smaller inferomedial projection, the **lesser trochanter of the femur** (Fig. 16–6). An **intertrochanteric line** on the anterior surface of the femur (Fig. 16–6*A*) and **intertrochanteric crest** on the posterior surface (Fig. 16–6*B*) demarcate the anterior and posterior junctions of the neck and shaft of the femur. The intertrochanteric crest provides an attachment site for the ischiofemoral ligament and part of the distal tendon of the quadratus femoris muscle, whereas the anterior intertrochanteric line serves as an attachment site for the iliofemoral ligament and part of the proximal tendon of the vastus lateralis muscle (Table 16–1). The lesser trochanter provides an attachment site for the psoas major muscle. The greater trochanter provides an attachment site for part of the capsule of the hip joint and several deep lateral rotator muscles of the gluteal region. A small projection at the superior end of the intertrochanteric crest called the **quadrate tubercle** provides a site for attachment of the quadratus femoris muscle (Fig. 16–6*B* and Table 16–1).

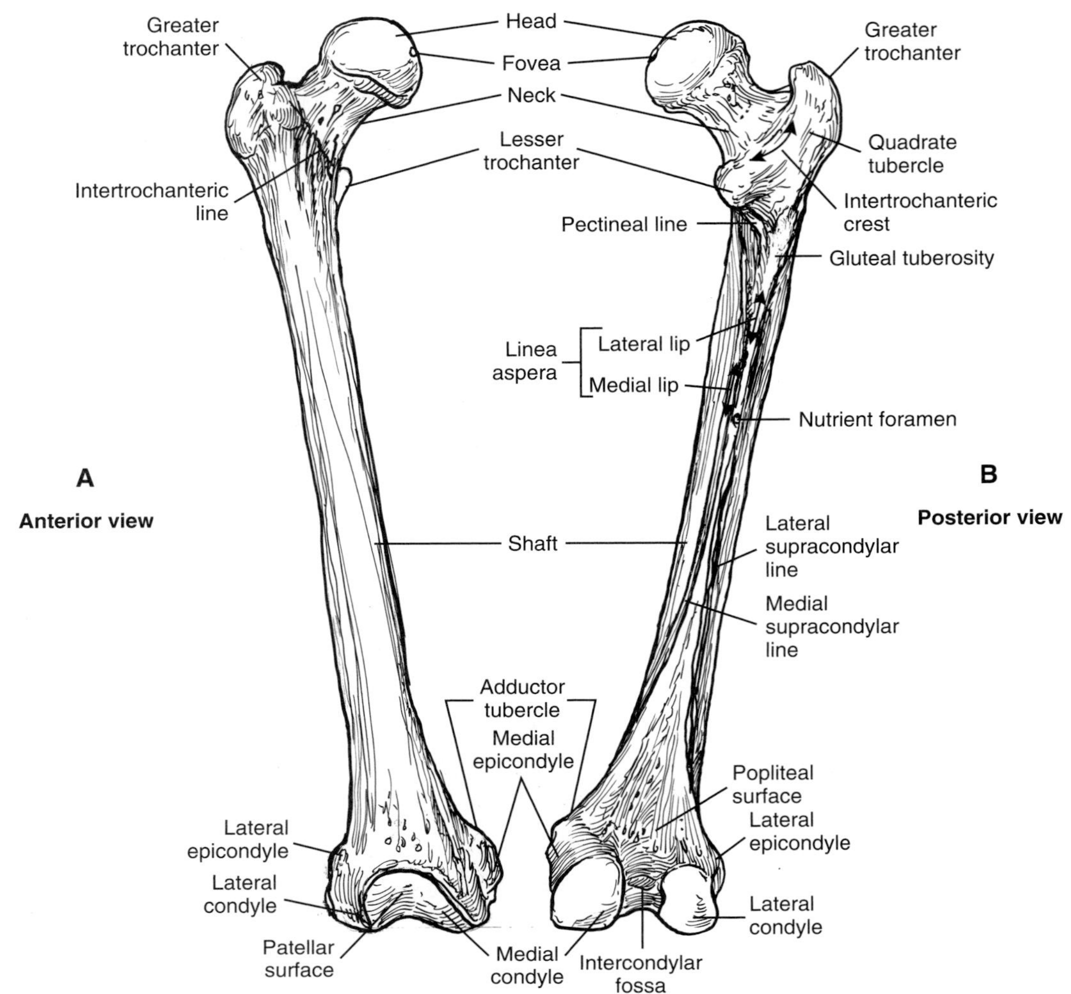

FIGURE 16–6
The femur. The proximal head of the femur is connected to the shaft by the neck. The femoral head articulates with the acetabulum of the pelvis, while the lateral and medial condyles at the distal end of the shaft articulate with the tibia. Many prominent processes serve as attachment points for muscle tendons, ligaments, and capsular connective tissue elements. These processes include the greater and lesser trochanters, trochanteric fossa, intertrochanteric line, intertrochanteric crest, pectineal line, linea aspera, and lateral and medial epicondyles.

From the neck of the femur, the **shaft** is angled in a medial direction toward the knee, transposing the body's center of gravity toward the midline (see Fig. 16–4 and Chapter 17). The shaft is narrowest in the middle and widens slightly toward both ends. Its anterior and lateral surfaces are rounded and relatively smooth (Fig. 16–6). The middle part of its posterior surface has a raised ridge, the **linea aspera.** Its medial and lateral lips provide attachment sites for muscles of the posterior and medial compartments of the thigh (Fig. 16–6*B* and Table 16–1). The lateral lip widens into a **gluteal tuberosity,** which is an attachment site for the gluteus maximus and adductor magnus muscles (see Table 16–1). Inferiorly, the linea aspera flares into diverging medial and lateral supracondylar lines, which enclose the triangular **popliteal surface** of the femur (Fig. 16–6*B*).

The large **lateral** and **medial condyles** at the inferior end of the femur provide large **articular surfaces,** which interact with the **tibia** inferiorly **(tibial surface)** and the **patella** anteriorly **(patellar surface)** (Fig. 16–6). These condyles are also attachment sites for muscles and ligaments of the knee joint (Table 16–1). Posteriorly, the condyles are separated by a deep groove **(intercondylar fossa [notch])** (Fig. 16–6*B*). The lateral condyle is larger than the medial condyle. Because of the position and mass of the lateral condyle, it probably plays a larger role in supporting the body weight than the medial condyle. The lateral surface of the lateral condyle has a palpable projection **(lateral epicondyle),** which provides an attachment site for the fibular (lateral) collateral ligament. A medial projection of the medial condyle, the **medial epicondyle,** serves as an attachment site for the tibial (medial) collateral ligament

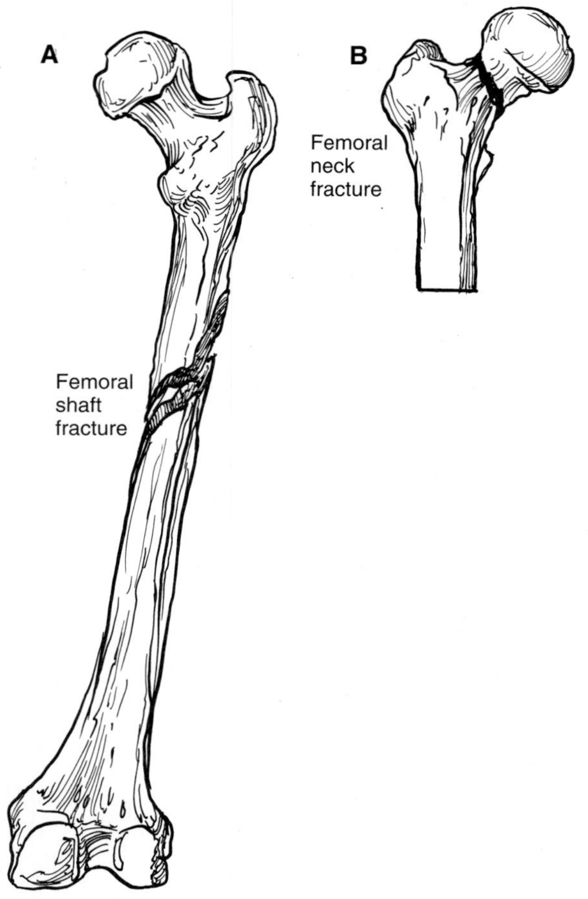

FIGURE 16–7
Fractures of the femur. **A.** Femoral shaft fracture. **B.** Femoral neck fracture.

of the knee joint (Fig. 16–6 and Table 16–1 and see below). The superior edge of the medial epicondyle also has a small projection, the **adductor tubercle,** which serves as an attachment site for the distal tendon of the adductor magnus muscle and tibial collateral ligament (Fig. 16–6 and Table 16–2).

> Bones of the lower limb may fracture in spite of their innate strength and stability. **Fracture of the femoral shaft** caused by trauma is especially common in children, adolescents, and young adults (Fig. 16–7*A*). Elderly individuals, particularly women suffering from **osteoporosis,** more commonly suffer fractures of the **femoral neck** (fracture of the hip) (Fig. 16–7*B*). These fractures occur most typically when an individual steps off a curb or into a hole. Fractures of the femoral neck are commonly treated by replacing the head and neck of the femur with a prosthesis (Fig. 16–8).

Patella

The patella is a **sesamoid bone** (i.e., shaped like a sesame seed) as are several much smaller bones of the foot (see below) and hand (see Chapter 19). The patella is actually shaped somewhat like a heart, with its **apex** extending inferiorly. It has a rough **anterior surface;** a **posterior surface** (which articulates with the anterior patellar surface of the femur); and **superior, medial,** and **lateral borders** (Fig. 16–9*A* and *B*). When a person is standing, the tip of the apex of the patella lies just superior to the knee joint. The patella is held in place by a tendon, which extends inferiorly from the superior complex of **quadriceps femoris muscles** (see below), passes over the patella, and attaches to the **tuberosity of the tibia.** The patella is attached to the quadriceps tendon at its superior, lateral, and medial borders; anterior surface; and apex. The inferior extension of the tendon of the quadriceps femoris muscle, which courses between the patellar apex and the tuberosity of the tibia, is often called the **patellar ligament** (Fig. 16–9*A* and see Chapter 17).

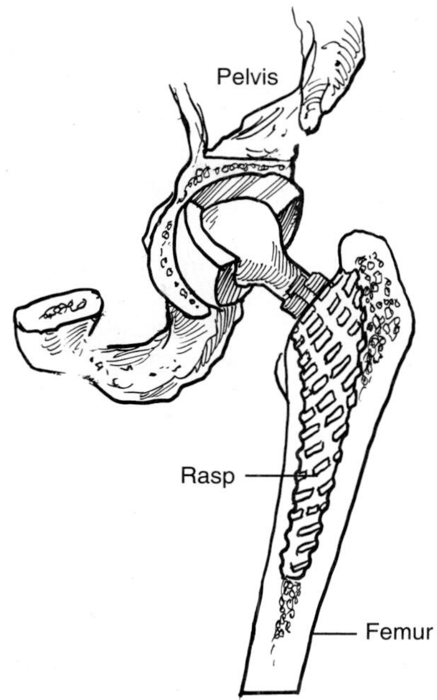

FIGURE 16–8
Total hip replacement.

> The patella may be fractured by trauma to the region of the knee. Patellar fractures may even result from violent contraction of the quadriceps femoris muscle.

▲ Skeleton of the Leg

Tibia

The **tibia** is the strongest bone of the leg and provides the main structural support within it. The tibia articulates exclusively with the femur superiorly. The inferior end of the tibia forms the major portion of the articulation of the ankle joint as it interacts with the superior surface of the talus, a large tarsal bone.

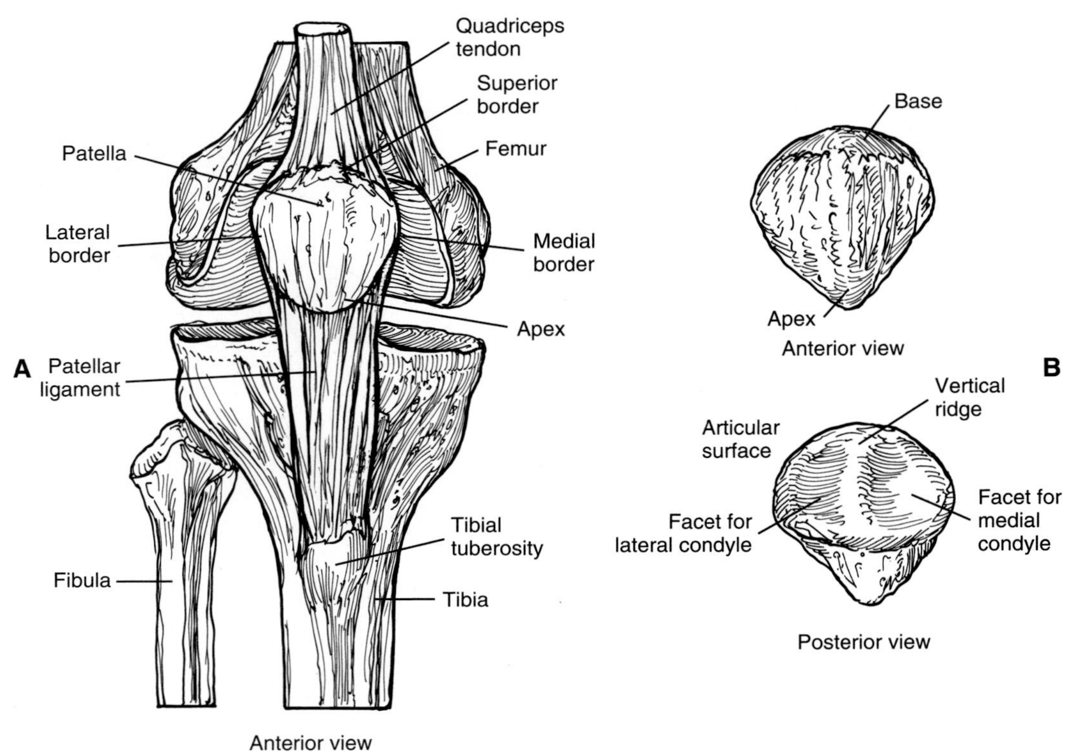

FIGURE 16–9
Patella. The patella is a heart-shaped sesamoid bone connected to the quadriceps muscles above and to the tibia below.

The **superior end of the tibia** flares into a broad plateau, widening in a medial direction as the **medial condyle** and in a lateral direction as the **lateral condyle** (Fig. 16–10*A* to *D*). The somewhat concave **articular surfaces** of the medial and lateral condyles articulate with the medial and lateral condyles of the femur and provide attachment sites for ligaments of the knee joint (see Table 16–1). These articular surfaces are separated by an **intercondylar area** consisting of two protrusions, the **medial** and **lateral intercondylar tubercles,** which are separated by a depression (Fig. 16–10*C* and *D*). This intercondylar area also provides an attachment site for cruciate ligaments of the knee joint. The slightly concave articular surfaces are deepened somewhat by the cartilaginous **medial** and **lateral menisci** (see Fig. 16–17 and discussion of knee joint below).

The **anterior surface** of the superior end of the tibia just beneath the lateral condyle is marked by a tubercle, which provides an attachment site for the iliotibial tract called **Gerdy's tubercle** (Fig. 16–10*A* and *C*). At the lateral boundary of Gerdy's tubercle, an oblique line leads downward in a medial direction to the prominent **tibial tuberosity** (Fig. 16–10*A* and *C* and see Table 16–1 and above). Just inferior to the medial condyle, the anterior surface of the tibia is smooth, but the lower medial boundary of the medial condyle provides attachment sites for the **gracilis, sartorius,** and **semitendinosus muscles.** The tibial tuberosity demarcates the inferior apex of this triangular area. The lower rough part of the tibial tuberosity can be palpated because it is separated from the skin only by an **infrapatellar bursa** (see discussion of knee joint below). The upper smooth part of the tibial tuberosity is the specific site of attachment of the patellar tendon.

The **posterior surface** of the superior end of the tibia just beneath the lateral condyle is somewhat depressed, but in its most lateral region, it elaborates an articular facet for the **fibula (fibular facet)** (Fig. 16–10). The posterior surface of the superior end of the tibia just beneath the lateral condyle also provides a roughened attachment site for the semimembranosus muscle.

The **shaft of the tibia** is triangular in section and has **posterior, lateral,** and **medial surfaces.** The three apices of a triangular transverse section of the tibia constitute its **anterior, lateral,** and **medial borders** (Fig. 16–10*A* and *B*). The **anterior border** is a sharp crest of bone that courses inferiorly from just below the tibial tuberosity and veers medially toward a distinct specialization at the inferior end of the shaft called the **medial malleolus** (Fig. 16–10*A* and see below). This crest is readily palpated in living humans. The **lateral border** of the tibial shaft is called the **interosseous border** because it is attached to a tough connective tissue **in-**

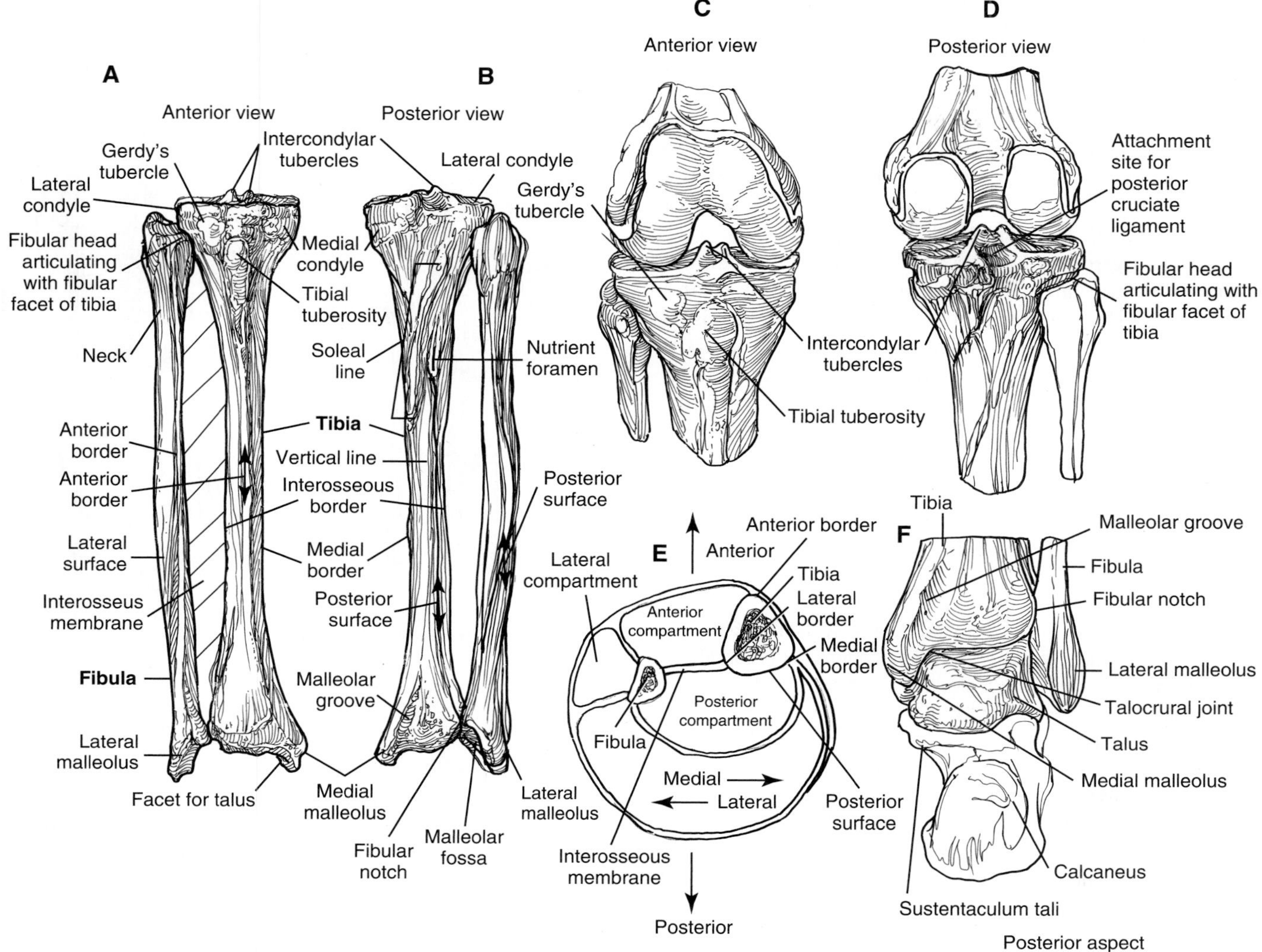

FIGURE 16–10

The tibia and fibula are so tightly bound together that they act as a single unit. However, the tibia is the main structural support of the leg. Both bones have prominent borders and surfaces. **A.** Anterior view. **B.** Posterior view. **C.** Anterior view of articulating surfaces of femur and tibia. **D.** Posterior view of articulating surfaces of femur and tibia. **E.** Section of leg showing relationships of surfaces and borders of tibia and fibula with the interosseous membrane and intermuscular septa. **F.** Posterior view showing relationship of tibia, fibula, and talus.

terosseous membrane, which ties the tibia to the more laterally located **fibula** (Fig. 16–10*E*). The **medial border,** which courses from the medial condyle superiorly to the medial malleolus inferiorly, lies just under the skin for most of its length and can also be palpated in living individuals (Fig. 16–10*A* to *E*). The **medial malleolus** articulates with the medial articulating surface of the **talus bone** of the ankle and serves as an attachment site for several ligaments of the ankle joint (Fig. 16–10*F* and see Table 16–1 and discussion of the ankle joint, below). The lateral surface of the inferior end of the tibia has a groove that accommodates the **fibula (fibular notch)** (Fig. 16–10*B* and *F*). Grooves on the posterior surface of the lower end of the tibia accommodate tendons of muscles that course from the leg to the plantar surface of the foot (Fig. 16–10*F* and see Fig. 16–22).

The large, flat **inferior articular surface of the tibia** sits squarely on the top of the talus bone of the ankle (Fig. 16–10*F* and discussion of talocrural joint, below).

Fibula

The **fibula** is a long, slender bone on the lateral side of the leg. The fibula does not play much of a role in directly supporting the body, but its surfaces provide sites for attachments of many muscles. The effects of its breakage, however, are significant (see below).

The **superior end of the fibula** consists of a rounded **head** connected to a shaft by a tapered **neck** (Fig. 16–10*A* and *B*). The top of the head is slightly pointed to form an **apex.** The medial side of the head articulates with the **fibular facet** of the lateral condyle of the tibia.

The **shaft of the fibula,** like that of the tibia, is triangular in shape, with lateral, medial, and anterior surfaces. The anterior and medial borders, however, are closely apposed. The medial border is also called the **interosseous border** because it is the site of attachment of the **interosseous membrane,** which binds the fibula to the tibia (Fig. 16–10*E*). The **posterior border of the fibula** is most clearly demarcated in the lower half of the fibular shaft (Fig. 16–10*B*).

The **inferior end of the fibula** flares into an expansion called the **lateral malleolus** (Fig. 16–10*A, B,* and *F*). The posterior surface of the lateral malleolus is marked by a depression, or **fossa of the lateral malleolus,** which carries tendons of muscles that course from the lateral compartment of the leg to the plantar compartment of the foot (see Chapter 17). The medial **articular surface of the lateral malleolus** articulates with the lateral articulating surface of the **talus bone** of the ankle (see Fig. 16–21). In addition, the lateral malleolus serves as an attachment site for several ligaments of the ankle joint (see Table 16–1 and Fig. 16–22*A*).

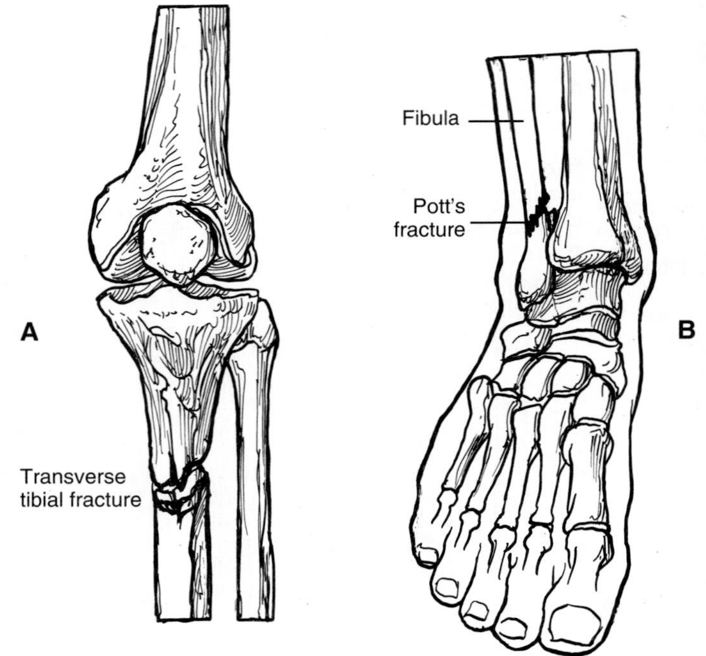

FIGURE 16–11
A. Tibial fracture. **B.** Fibular fracture.

Tibial fractures, including superior transverse fractures, are often complicated by the proximity of the tibia to the surface of the leg and, thus, may protrude through the skin (compound fracture) (Fig. 16–11*A*).

Fractures of the fibula may occur during forced eversion or inversion of the ankle. These fractures are proximal to the lateral malleolus (Pott's fractures) (Fig. 16–11*B*). In spite of the minor involvement of the fibula in weight bearing, these fractures result in significant instability of the ankle joint and typically require reduction (realignment of the fibular fragments).

▲ Skeleton of the Foot

The skeleton of the foot includes the proximal **tarsal bones, metatarsal bones,** and distal **phalanges** (Fig. 16–12). There are 7 tarsal bones, 5 metatarsal bones, and 14 phalanges. About 20 small ovoid **sesamoid bones** are also found throughout the foot, typically in association with articulations.

Tarsal Bones

The seven tarsal bones constitute the proximal skeleton of the foot (Fig. 16–12). The most proximal tarsal bone is the **talus bone,** which articulates directly with the tibia and fibula at the **talocrural (ankle) joint** (see below). Just below and somewhat lateral to the talus is the **calcaneus bone.** The talus and calcaneus together make up a **proximal row** of tarsal bones. The **distal row** of tarsal bones is comprised of four bones: the **medial, intermediate,** and **lateral cuneiform bones** and a **cuboid bone.** Laterally, the calcaneus articulates directly with the cuboid bone, but medially, a seventh intermediate tarsal bone, the **navicular bone,** is interposed between the talus and the three cuneiform bones.

The **talus bone** provides an articular connection between the distal leg and more proximal elements of the foot (Figs 16–12*A* and 16–13*A*). Although it is bound to other bones by many ligaments (see discussion of ankle joint, below), it does not have any attachments for muscles (see Chapter 17). The **head of the talus** is its distal end, which is specialized to articulate with the more distal **navicular bone** and inferior **calcaneus bone** (Figs. 16–12*C* and 16–13*B* and *C*). The **neck of the talus** is a constricted roughened section connecting the head and body. It functions mainly as an attachment site for ligaments. Its medial surface has a deep groove called the **tarsal sinus (sinus tarsi),** which, in living persons, accommodates the talocalcaneal and cervical ligaments (Fig. 16–12*C* and see below). The **body of the talus** is a cuboidal expansion of bone posterior to the neck. The surfaces of the tarsal body are specially formed to articulate with neighboring skeletal elements. Its superior **trochlear surface** articulates with the tibia and fibula above it (Figs. 16–12*A* and 16–13*A* and see Table 16–1); its lateral surface with the lateral malleolus of the fibula (see Fig. 16–13*C*); its medial surface with the medial malleolus of the tibia (Figs. 16–12*C* and 16–13*C*); and its inferior surface with the calcaneus bone (Figs. 16–12*B* and 16–13*B*). Roughened regions of the body of the talus include a **posterior process,** which consists of lateral and medial tubercles separated by a smooth groove normally occupied by the tendon of the flexor hallucis longus muscle (Fig. 16–12*B* and *C*). A rough-

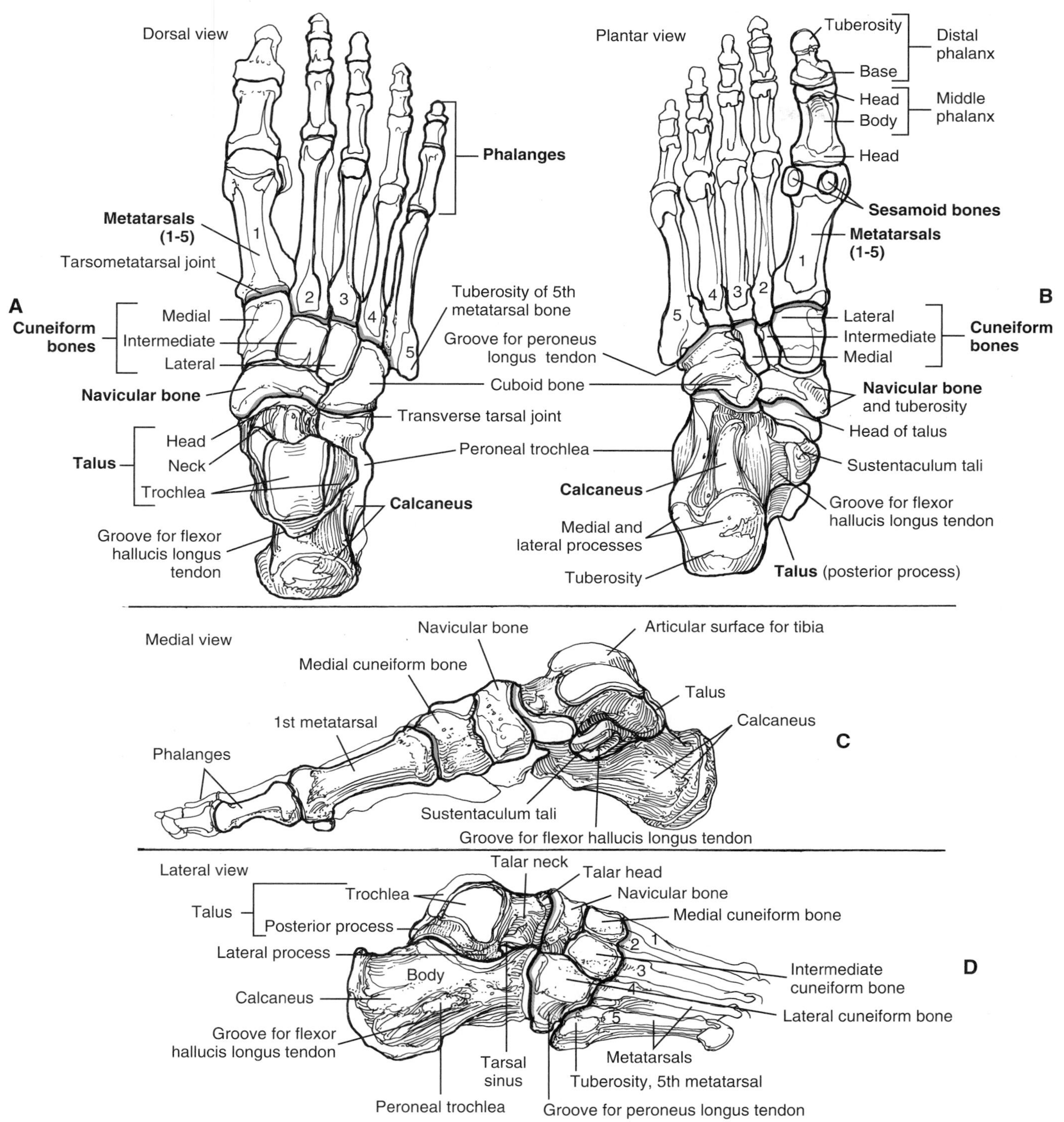

FIGURE 16–12

Bones of the foot. Tarsal bones include the talus, calcaneus, navicular, cuboid, and medial, intermediate, and lateral cuneiform bones. Five metatarsal bones serve as bases for the phalanges of the five toes. Toes 2 to 5 have three phalanges each, and toe 1 (hallux) has two phalanges. **A.** Dorsal view of the right foot. **B.** Plantar view of the right foot. **C.** Medial view of the right foot. **D.** Lateral view of the right foot.

ened **medial process** provides an attachment site for part of the deltoid ligament (see Fig. 16–22). A roughened **lateral process** is located just inferior to the articulation for the lateral malleolus. This lateral process provides an attachment site for the posterior talofibular ligament (Fig. 16–12*C* and see Table 16–1).

The **calcaneus bone** is the largest tarsal bone. It is best described by noting specializations of its superior, plantar, lateral, medial, posterior, and anterior surfaces. Its **superior surface** is specialized primarily to articulate with the talus through anterior, middle, and posterior articulating facets (Figs. 16–12*D* and 16–13*E*). The anterior and middle facets may be combined and tend to be flattened or concave, while the posterior facet is convex. The superior surface of the posterior extension, however, is roughened (Figs. 16–12*A, C,* and *D* and 16–13*E* and *F*). Indeed, all of the **plantar, lateral,** and **medial surfaces** of the calcaneus are roughened (Figs. 16–12 and 16–13*E* to *H*). Each of these latter surfaces has one or two specialized structures on it: an **anterior tubercle** on the plantar surface, a **peroneal trochlea** and **lateral process** on the lateral surface, and the **sustentaculum tali** and **medial process** on the medial surface (Figs. 16–12*C* and *D* and 16–13*G* and *H*). The plantar surface of the sustentaculum tali has a groove for the flexor hallucis longus muscle (Figs. 16–12*B* and *C* and 16–13*F*). The dorsal surface of the sustentaculum tali articulates with (and suspends) the talus bone (hence its name). Its roughened areas provide attachment sites for several ligaments (Figs. 16–13*F* and 16-22 and Table 16–1). The **anterior surface** of the calcaneus is completely covered by an articular facet for the **cuboid bone** (Fig. 16–13*G*). The **posterior surface** of the **calcaneal tuberosity** has three parts: (1) a smooth superior region covered by a bursa, which separates it from the **tendo calcaneus** (tendon of calf muscles) (see below); (2) a roughened middle region for attachment of the tendo calcaneus; and (3) a striated lower weight-bearing region (Fig. 16–13*E* and *F*). The calcaneal tuberosity provides attachment sites for the abductor hallucis muscle (medially), the abductor digiti minimi muscle (laterally), and the flexor digitorum brevis muscle and tendo calcaneus (Achilles tendon) (see Table 16–1 and Chapter 17).

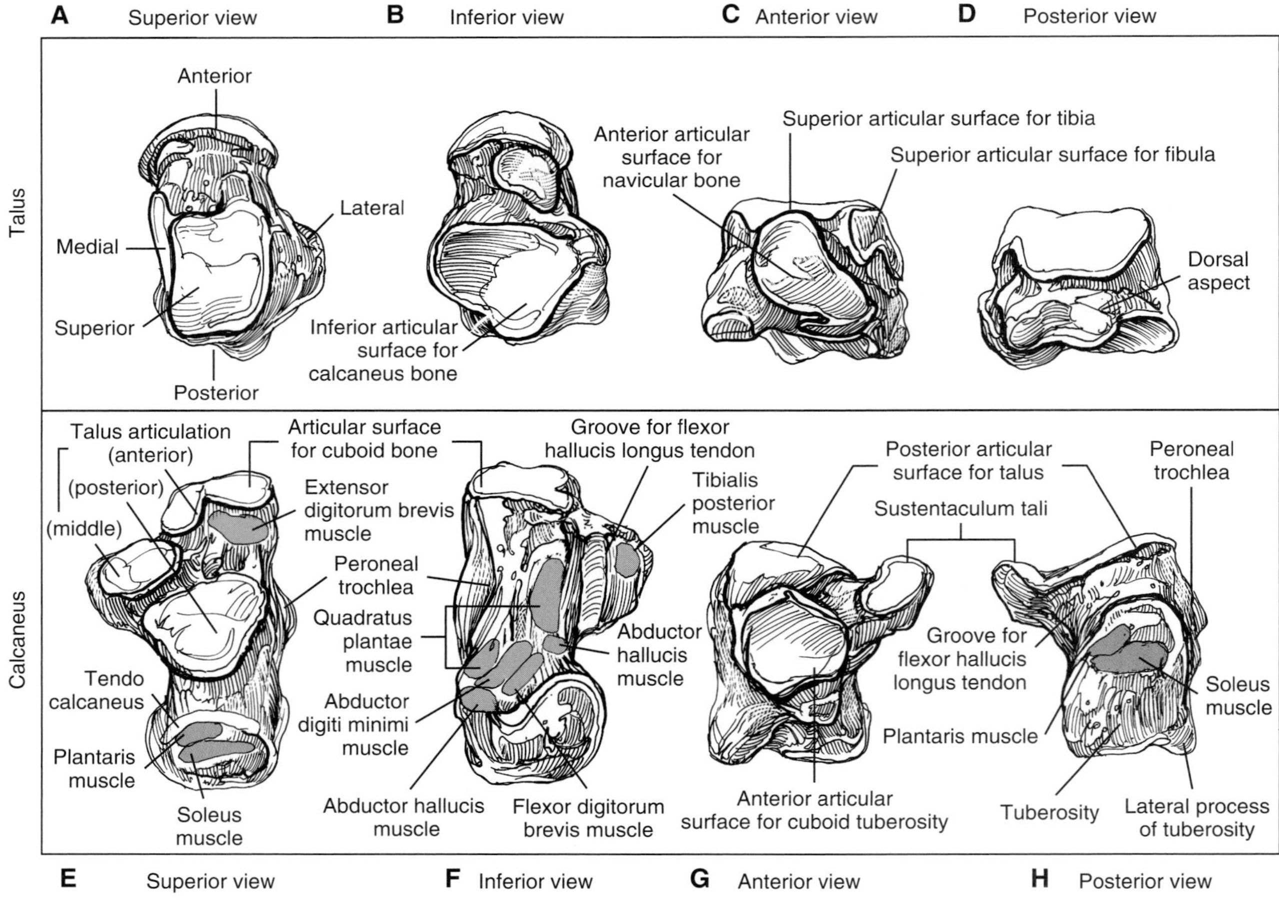

FIGURE 16–13
Talus and calcaneus bones. Superior view, **(A)**; inferior view, **(B)**; anterior view, **(C)**; and posterior view, **(D)** of talus. Superior view, **(E)**; inferior view, **(F)**; anterior view, **(G)**; and posterior view, **(H)** of calcaneus.

The **navicular bone** articulates with all three **cuneiform bones** at its distal aspect and with the **talus bone** at its proximal aspect (Fig. 16–12). A **tuberosity** on its medial surface provides an attachment site for the tibionavicular ligament and the tendon of the tibialis posterior muscle (see Fig. 16–12 and Table 16–1).

The wedge-shaped **medial, intermediate,** and **lateral cuneiform bones** are interposed between the talus and the **first, second,** and **third metatarsal bones.** In contrast, the **cuboid bone** articulates with the calcaneus proximally and with the **fourth** and **fifth metatarsal bones** distally.

Fractures of the talus or **calcaneus** most commonly occur when a person lands on the feet after falling or jumping from a great height (Fig. 16–14). Fractures of the talus may also occur during forced dorsiflexion. The most common **tarsal fractures** are stress fractures caused by running or walking for long distances. These **"march fractures"** are most common in runners, backpackers, and soldiers.

Metatarsal Bones

Each of the five **metatarsal bones** has a **base,** which articulates with a tarsal bone; a **shaft;** and a **head,** which articulates with one of the **phalanges.** The metatarsals are numbered one through five, beginning on the medial side of the foot. The first metatarsal articulates with the medial cuneiform bone; the second metatarsal with the intermediate cuneiform bone; the third metatarsal with the lateral cuneiform bone; and the fourth and fifth metatarsals with the cuboid bone (see Fig. 16–12).

Phalanges

The **phalanges** of the foot are much shorter than those of the hand. There are 14 phalanges among the 5 digits. The big toe (digit 1) has 2 phalanges, and each of the remaining toes (digits 2 to 5) has 3 (see Fig. 16–12).

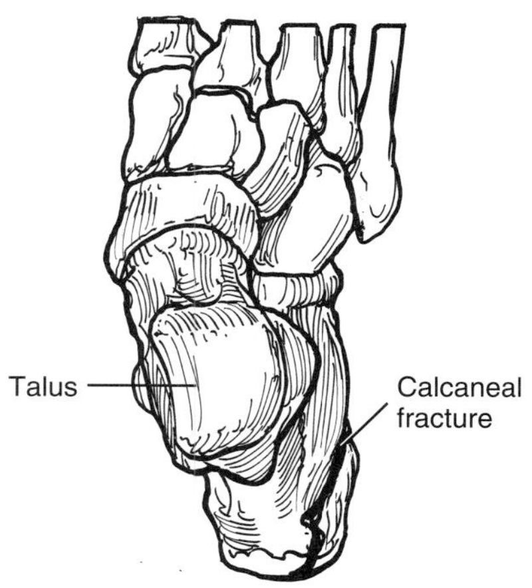

FIGURE 16–14
"March fracture" of calcaneus.

The big toe is also called the **hallux,** and the little toe is called the **digitus minimus pedis.**

Sesamoid Bones

The foot has about 20 **sesamoid bones.** Each one may be directly associated with an articulation (e.g., two sesamoid bones are almost always associated with the metatarsophalangeal joint and tendon of the flexor hallucis longus muscle of the big toe (see Fig. 16–12*B* and *C*). Some of the sesamoid bones are embedded in tendons if the tendons are deflected around a bony process (e.g., as where the tendon of the tibialis posterior muscle courses around the medial surface of the talus bone).

▲ Joints of the Lower Extremity

General Features of Lower Extremity Joints

The appendicular skeleton of the lower extremity has only one joint that is a **symphysis** (a nonsynovial cartilaginous joint): the **symphysis pubis.** The symphysis pubis joins the pubic bones along the anterior midline of the pelvis (see Chapter 14). This **cartilaginous synarthrosis** has the following arrangement of bone and connective tissue:

Bone ⟷ Hyaline growth cartilage ⟷
Fibrocartilaginous disc ⟷ Hyaline growth cartilage ⟷ Bone

Most of the joints of the lower extremity are **diarthroses (synovial joints)** in which bone is connected to bone via cavitated connective tissue. Synovial joints join the sacrum to the pelvis and connect most of the bones of the lower extremity to each other. These joints are organized in the following manner:

Bone ⟷ Articular hyaline cartilage ⟷ Cavity lined
by synovial membrane containing synovial fluid ⟷
Articular hyaline cartilage ⟷ Bone

The lower extremity has a large number of synovial joints because such joints create little friction between bones during bipedal locomotion. The coefficient of friction resulting from the interspersion of synovial fluid between articular cartilages is similar to that of ice moving over ice. The viscosity of the synovial fluid is greater when the bones move slowly past each other than it is when they move rapidly. The fluid is secreted by synovial membranes as a dialysate of blood, but it contains a high concentration of hyaluronic acid.

Synovial joints of the lower extremity may be classified as **simple,** with only one set of articulating surfaces, or **compound,** with two or more sets of articulating surfaces. They may also be classified as **complex** if an intracapsular cartilaginous meniscus (disc) is present. Such discs may deepen and more firmly secure the articulation. In the hip and knee joints, discs absorb forces induced by gravity during walking or running.

Extracapsular **synovial bursas** may also be associated with synovial joints of the lower extremity. A bursa is a fluid-filled sac lined by a synovial membrane. The bursa is positioned to reduce the friction of muscle or tendon sliding over bone. In some cases, the cavity of the extracapsular bursa is continuous with the synovial cavity of the joint, providing a conduit for the spread of infection.

Other bones of the lower extremity are connected by the following arrangement of bone and connective tissue:

Bone ⟷ Collagenous interosseous element ⟷ Bone

This arrangement occurs in the dorsal region of the sacroiliac joint (see Chapter 14) and inferior region of the tibiofibular joint (see below). It also characterizes the joining of the tibia to the fibula via the **crural interosseous membrane** (see below). Such a joint is a **fibrous type of synarthrosis** called a **syndesmosis.**

Arthritis

Because most joints of the upper and lower extremities are cartilaginous joints, they may be affected by arthritis. Arthritis is a condition that results in degeneration of the cartilaginous lining of the joint or bone, or both.

Osteoarthritis (degenerative arthritis) is the most common form of arthritis. It typically occurs after age 45 years. It tends to affect weight-bearing joints and joints of the fingers in both men and women. It is treated with antiinflammatory drugs and exercise. In severe cases, surgery and joint replacement may be required.

Rheumatoid arthritis is an autoimmune disease that affects 1 in 7 persons in the United States. It is more common in women than men and may have a familial pattern. This disease most commonly affects weight-bearing joints on both sides of the body. It requires life-long treatment. Antiinflammatory drugs, including glucocorticoids, may be injected directly into the affected joint. **Disease-modifying antirheumatic drugs** are used to reduce the rate of joint destruction. One such drug, **methotrexate,** an anticancer drug, has been used since the 1980s. Immunosuppressive drugs such as **cyclosporine** have also been used to treat very severe cases of rheumatoid arthritis, but a risk of kidney damage has limited their use for this disorder. A new generation of drugs specifically interferes with the cells of the immune system.

Hip Joint

The head of the femur fits snugly into the acetabulum of the pelvis, forming a **simple synovial joint.** In the hip joint, an **articular cartilage** covers the head of the femur and a **lunate cartilage** partially covers the inner surface of the acetabulum (Fig. 16–15*A*). A synovial membrane lines the joint cavity, except where surfaces are covered by cartilage (see Fig. 16–6*B*). Friction is reduced between these elements by **synovial fluid,** which is secreted by the **synovial membrane.**

The hip joint is stabilized by several strong ligaments. The head of the femur is directly attached to the floor of the acetabular notch and to the **transverse acetabular ligament** by a tough **round ligament (ligamentum capitis femoris).** This ligament is attached to the femoral head at the **fovea** (Fig. 16–15*A* and *B*). The entire joint is also invested by three tough, fibrous ligaments: the **pubofemoral, iliofemoral,** and **ischiofemoral ligaments** (Fig. 16–16). Pelvic attachments of these three ligaments are to the pubic, iliac, or ischial bones at the margin of the acetabulum. In this region, their fibers blend with the cartilaginous articular disc that covers the lunate surface of the acetabulum to form the tough **fibrocartilaginous labrum** of the acetabulum (Fig. 16–6*A*). The femoral attachment of the pubofemoral ligament is in the region of the **trochanteric fossa.** The femoral attachment of the iliofemoral ligament is on the superior aspect of the greater trochanter and along a line joining the anterior edges of the **greater** and **lesser trochanters,** which includes the **intertrochanteric line** (Fig. 16–16*A*). The femoral attachment of the ischiofemoral ligament is along an **intertrochanteric crest** joining the posterior aspects of the greater and lesser trochanters (Fig. 16–16*B*).

The pubofemoral, iliofemoral, and ischiofemoral ligaments are intimately invested by a tough fibrous **capsule** comprised of longitudinal and circular fibers. The longitudinal fibers are disposed mostly over the anterior surface of the iliofemoral ligament. The circular fibers form a loose collar, the **zona orbicularis,** around the neck of the femur (Fig. 16–16*B*).

The **synovial cavity** of the hip joint extends beyond the edge of the capsule posteriorly, protruding slightly beyond the zona orbicularis (Fig. 16–16*B*). Anteriorly, an external extension of the synovial cavity forms a subtendinous **iliopectineal bursa,** which covers the gap between the pubofemoral and iliofemoral ligaments and separates the tendon of the psoas muscle from the pubic bone and capsule of the hip joint (Fig. 16–16*A*). The cavity of the iliopectineal bursa may or may not communicate with the synovial cavity within the hip joint. Other **trochanteric bursae** are also associated with the hip joint (see Chapter 17).

The hip joint receives additional stability from muscle tendons (see Chapter 17), fascia, and integument.

Movements of the Hip Joint

The range of motion of the hip joint is limited but varied. The femur can be **flexed, extended, abducted, adducted, circumducted,** and **medially** and **laterally rotated** (Fig. 16–17). All of these movements are limited by the intimate encapsulation of the head of the femur by the acetabulum, external ligaments of the hip joint, and joint capsule. The flexibility of the hip joint can be greatly increased by exercise and stretching, as has been shown by dancers and gymnasts.

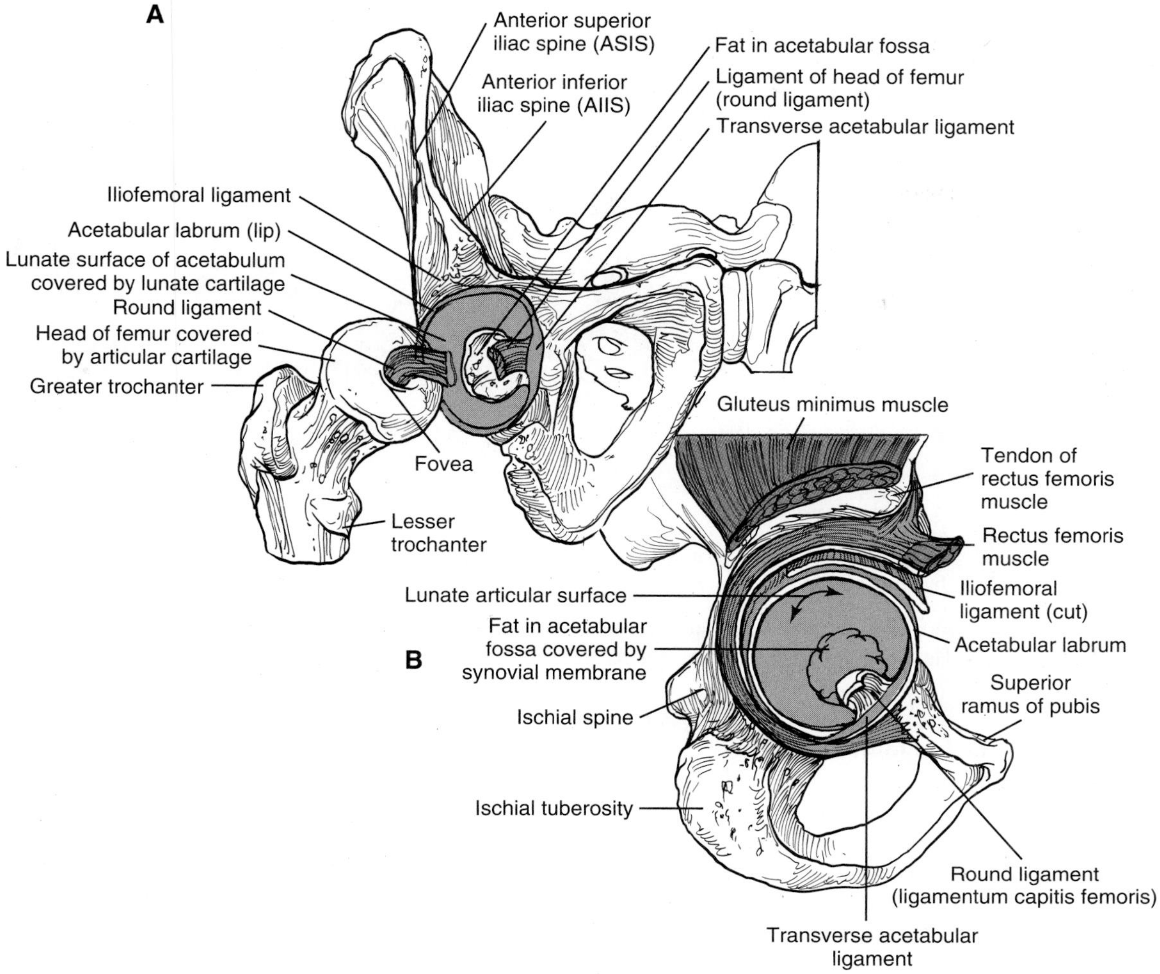

A
Anterior superior
iliac spine (ASIS)
Anterior inferior
iliac spine (AIIS)
Fat in acetabular fossa
Ligament of head of femur
(round ligament)
Transverse acetabular ligament
Iliofemoral ligament
Acetabular labrum (lip)
Lunate surface of acetabulum
covered by lunate cartilage
Round ligament
Head of femur covered
by articular cartilage
Greater trochanter
Fovea
Lesser
trochanter
Gluteus minimus muscle
Tendon of
rectus femoris
muscle
Rectus femoris
muscle
Lunate articular surface
Iliofemoral
ligament (cut)
Fat in acetabular
fossa covered by
synovial membrane
B
Acetabular labrum
Superior
ramus of pubis
Ischial spine
Ischial tuberosity
Round ligament
(ligamentum capitis femoris)
Transverse acetabular
ligament

FIGURE 16–15
Hip joint. Note that specializations of the hip joint are designed to enhance stability of the joint.

Anterior superior
iliac spine (ASIS)
Anterior inferior
iliac spine (AIIS)
A
Iliofemoral ligament
(Y ligament of Bigelow)
Greater trochanter
Iliopectineal
bursa
Intertrochanteric line
Femur
Lesser
trochanter
Obturator
crest
Pubofemoral
ligament
Superior pubic
ramus
Iliofemoral
ligament
B
Intertrochanteric
crest
Region of zona
orbicularis
Ischiofemoral
ligament

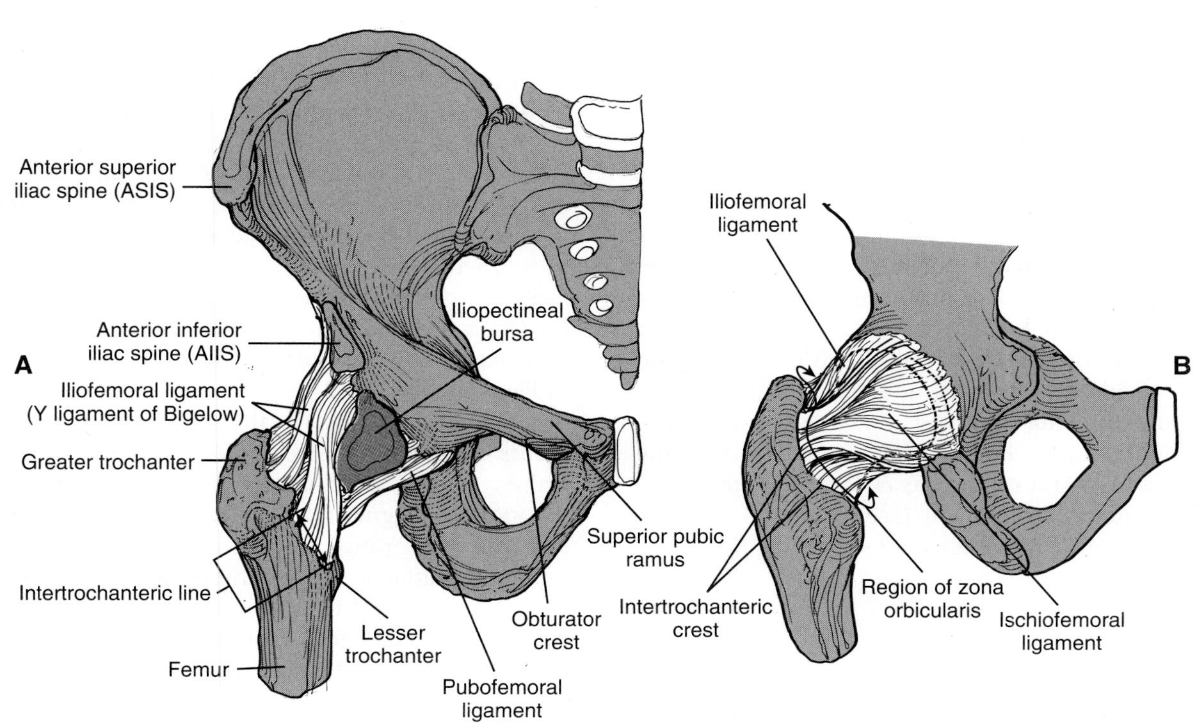

FIGURE 16–16
The pubofemoral, iliofemoral, and ischiofemoral ligaments constitute the capsule of the hip joint. **A,** Anterior. **B,** Posterior.

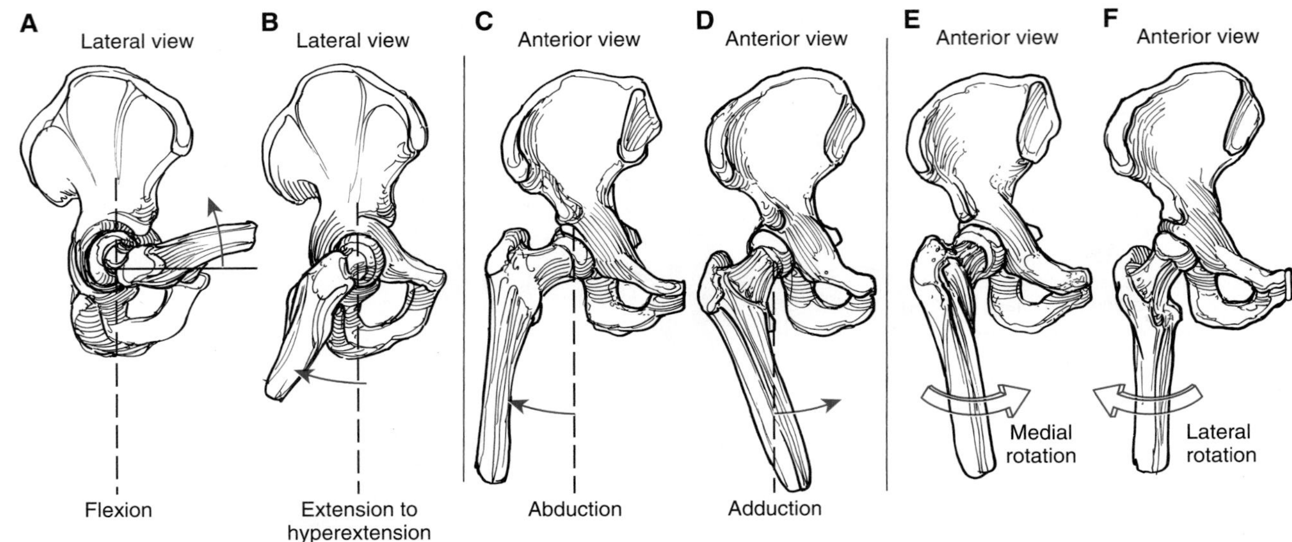

FIGURE 16–17
Movements of the hip joint. **A.** Flexion. **B.** Extension to hyperextension. **C.** Abduction. **D.** Adduction. **E.** Medial rotation. **F.** Lateral rotation.

Muscles that flex the hip joint include several muscles of the anterior compartment of the thigh (Table 16–2 and see Table 17–1). Flexion of the thigh is checked by gravity and extensor actions during walking or running (see below). Muscles that extend the hip joint include the gluteal muscles and muscles of the posterior compartment of the thigh. Extension is checked by passive forces arising from the innate architecture of the joint, which is in closely packed configuration during hyperextension. Extreme extension is also countered by flexors of the hip joint. Adduction of the thigh is performed by muscles of the medial compartment of the thigh. Abduction is performed by deep gluteal muscles, the tensor fasciae latae muscle, and the sartorius muscle. Thus, adduction is checked by the abductors, the lateral region of the iliofemoral ligament, and the round ligament of the femur. Abduction is checked by the adductors, the pubofemoral ligament, and the medial region of the iliofemoral ligament. Medial rotation is executed by the most anterior regions of the gluteus medius, gluteus minimus, and tensor fasciae latae muscles, while lateral rotation is produced by the obturator externus and internus, gemellus superior and inferior, quadratus femoris, gluteus maximus, piriformis, and sartorius muscles. Medial rotation is primarily checked by the lateral rotators and ischiofemoral ligament, and lateral rotation is checked by the adductors and iliofemoral ligament (see Chapter 17 for detailed discussions of muscle actions).

Injury of the Hip Joint

The extreme stability of the hip joint tends to preclude its dislocation unless force is brought against the distal end of the femur when the thigh is flexed, adducted, and medially rotated (Fig. 16–18). Under these circumstances, the head of the femur may be driven from the acetabular fossa onto the posterior surface of the ilium (posterior dislocation) or onto the anterior surface of the ilium (anterior dislocation). Posterior dislocation may result in injury to the sciatic nerve, while the obturator nerve may be injured in anterior dislocation.

Knee Joint

Like the hip joint, the knee joint is a synovial diarthrosis. Articular cartilages of the **lateral** and **medial condyles of the femur** articulate with articular cartilages of the **lateral** and **medial condyles of the tibia** within a synovial cavity (Fig. 16–19*A* to *H*). The flattened, somewhat concave surfaces of the tibial condyles are deepened by semilunar cartilages called the **lateral** and **medial menisci** (Fig. 16–19*A* and *G*). These menisci are deficient in the center. The lateral meniscus is thickened at its lateral edge and the medial meniscus at its medial edge. Friction between the articular surfaces is reduced by synovial fluid, which is secreted by the synovial membrane that lines the synovial cavity. Attachments of the lateral and medial menisci are shown in Fig. 16–19*H*.

The knee joint is stabilized by specialized ligaments, a capsule, muscle tendons, and integument. Together, these structures provide an extraordinary amount of integrity for the joint, but also they allow a relatively wide range of motion. The **anterior cruciate ligament** is attached to the anteromedial edge of the lateral condyle of the tibia and to the posteromedial surface of the lateral condyle of the femur (Fig. 16–19*A*, *B*, and *F* to *H*). This ligament "checks" the anterior movement of the tibia with respect to the femur or the pos-

TABLE 16–2
Movements of Lower Extremity Joints

Joint	Movement	Primary Muscles	Accessory Muscles
Hip joint	Flexion	Psoas major, iliacus, pectineus, rectus femoris, sartorius	Adductor longus, adductor brevis, adductor magnus
	Extension	Gluteus maximus, biceps femoris, semitendinosus, semimembranosus	
	Adduction	Adductor longus, adductor brevis, adductor magnus	Pectineus, gracilis
	Abduction	Gluteus medius, gluteus minimus	Tensor fasciae latae, sartorius
	Medial rotation	Tensor fasciae latae, gluteus medius (anterior), gluteus minimus (anterior)	
	Lateral rotation	Obturator externus, obturator internus, gemellus superior, gemellus inferior, quadratus femoris	Piriformis, gluteus maximus, sartorius
Knee joint	Flexion	Biceps femoris, semitendinosus, semimembranosus	Gracilis, sartorius, popliteus, gastrocnemius, plantaris
	Extension	Biceps femoris, semitendinosus, semimembranosus	Tensor fasciae latae
	Medial rotation (of leg when flexed)	Popliteus, semimembranosus, semitendinosus	Sartorius, gracilis
	Lateral rotation (of leg when flexed)	Biceps femoris	
Tibiofibular joint	Minimal		
Talocrural (ankle) joint	Dorsiflexion	Tibialis anterior	Extensor digitorum longus, extensor hallucis longus, peroneus tertius
	Plantarflexion	Gastrocnemius, soleus	Plantaris, tibialis posterior, flexor digitorum longus, flexorhallucis longus
Talocalcaneal (subtalar) joint	Inversion	Tibialis anterior, tibialis posterior	
Talocalcaneonavicular joint	Eversion	Peroneus longus, peroneus brevis	
Cuboideonavicular, intercuneiform, cuneocuboid joints	Minimal gliding assisting in pronation and supination		
Tarsometatarsal joint	Minimal gliding assisting in pronation and supination		
Intermetatarsal joint	Minimal gliding		
Metatarsophalangeal joint	Flexion	Flexor digitorum brevis, lumbricals, interossei, flexor digiti minimi, flexor hallucis longus, flexor hallucis brevis	Flexor digitorum longus, flexor accessorius
	Extension	Extensor digitorum longus, extensor hallucis longus, extensor digitorum brevis	
	Adduction	Adductor hallucis; first, second, third plantar interosseous	
	Abduction	Abductor hallucis; first, second, third, fourth dorsal interosseous; abductor digiti minimi	
Interphalangeal joint	Flexion	Flexor digitorum longus, flexor hallucis longus, flexor digitorum brevis, flexor accessorius	
	Extension	Extensor digitorum longus, extensor hallucis longus, extensor digitorum brevis	

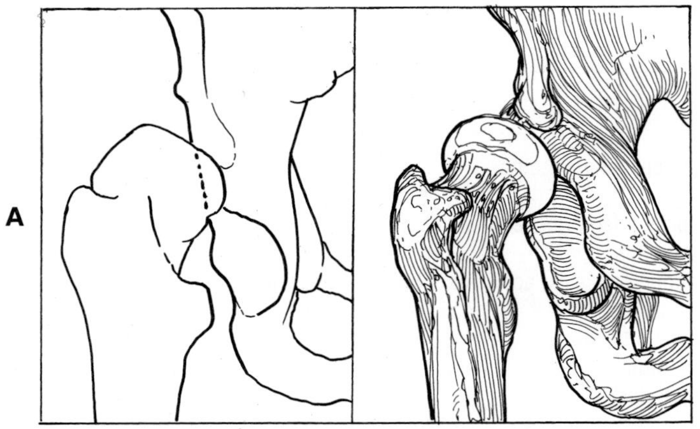

FIGURE 16–18
Posterior dislocation of the hip joint. **A.** Schematic drawing of x-ray. **B.** The head of the femur has been driven onto the posterior surface of the ilium.

terior movement of the femur with respect to the tibia (Fig. 16–19*I*). The **posterior cruciate ligament** is attached to the posterior intercondylar surface of the tibia and to the lateral surface of the medial condyle of the femur (Fig. 16–19*A, B,* and *F* to *H*). This ligament "checks" the posterior movement of the tibia with respect to the femur or the anterior movement of the femur with respect to the tibia at the knee joint (Fig. 16–19*J* and discussions of function and pathologic conditions of the knee joint below). The synovial membrane of the knee joint is reflected just anterior to the cruciate ligaments so that this central posterior region of the joint is excluded from the joint cavity. The cruciate ligaments are, therefore, not enclosed within the synovial cavity but are located within the joint capsule.

The knee joint is further strengthened by several other ligaments and a fibrous capsule. The **fibular (lateral) collateral ligament** courses from the lateral epicondyle of the femur to the head of the fibula (Fig. 16–19*A* to *C* and *E* to *G*). The **tibial (medial) collateral ligament** is attached superiorly to the medial epicondyle of the femur, and it courses inferiorly to attach to the medial condyle of the tibia. It is partially attached to the medial edge of the medial meniscus (Fig. 16–19*A* to *C, F,* and *G*). These ligaments play a major role in checking adduction and abduction of the knee joint (see discussions of function and pathologic conditions of the knee joint below). The **transverse ligament** joins the anteromedial edge of the medial meniscus to the entire anterior edge of the lateral meniscus (Fig. 16–19*D*). The **posterior meniscofemoral ligament** is composed of fibers that emerge from the posterior edge of the lateral meniscus and course along the posterior surface of the posterior cruciate ligament to attach to the medial condyle of the femur (Fig. 16–19*B*).

The **fibrous capsule** of the knee joint is complicated by connections to accessory structures and the presence of several significant deficiencies. In the posterior region, the capsule is a simple sheath, which connects the medial and lateral condyles of the femur with the medial and lateral condyles of the tibia. The sheath covers the attachment of the superior end of the **popliteus muscle** to the lateral condyle of the femur, but a small hiatus allows the distal end of the popliteus muscle to escape and attach to the medioposterior surface of the tibia (Fig. 16–19*E*). Medially, fibers of the capsule blend with the posterior edge of the medial (tibial) collateral ligament, and laterally, the capsule courses just deep to the lateral (fibular) collateral ligament. Although the capsule is connected to all of the exposed edges of the medial and lateral menisci, it is deficient in the anterior region beneath the patella (Fig. 16–19*G*). However, capsular fibers fan out from the medial and lateral boundaries of the patella to form the **medial** and **lateral patellar retinacula** (Fig. 16–19*C* and *F*). The capsule is also deficient just superior to the patella, where a hiatus allows communication between the synovial cavity and the **suprapatellar bursa** (Fig. 16–19*D*). The suprapatellar bursa helps cushion the movements of the patella on the femur. In addition, an **infrapatellar fat pad** cushions the movements of the inferior patella and patellar tendon upon the tibia. Three bursas associated with the knee joint usually communicate directly with the main synovial cavity: the **popliteal bursa** (between the popliteal muscle and the lateral femoral condyle); **semimembranous bursa** (between the semimembranosus tendon and the medial tibial condyle); and **gastrocnemius bursa** (between the medial head of the gastrocnemius muscle and the joint capsule). Three other bursas are not usually connected to the synovial cavity: the **prepatellar bursa** (between the skin and the inferior patella); **superficial infrapatellar bursa** (between the skin and the patellar ligament); and **deep infrapatellar bursa** (between the patellar ligament and the infrapatellar fat pad).

The stabilizing function of the ligaments and fibrous capsule is reinforced by many **muscle tendons** and the **integument** covering the knee joint (see discussion of function of the knee joint, below).

Movements of the Knee Joint

The movements of the knee joint are more limited than those of the hip joint. The most typical movements are **flexion** and **extension,** which, of course, occur most often in walking or running (Fig. 16–20). However, the knee is not a simple "hinge" joint. Its motion is more complex because the axis upon which flexion and extension occur is not fixed. Because of the contours of the articulating surfaces, the axis moves backward during flexion and forward during extension. In addition, the final 30 degrees of extension (with the foot firmly planted) also involves a prominent medial rotation of the femur upon the tibia (Fig. 16–20*B*). As the full weight of the body is planted upon the fully extended

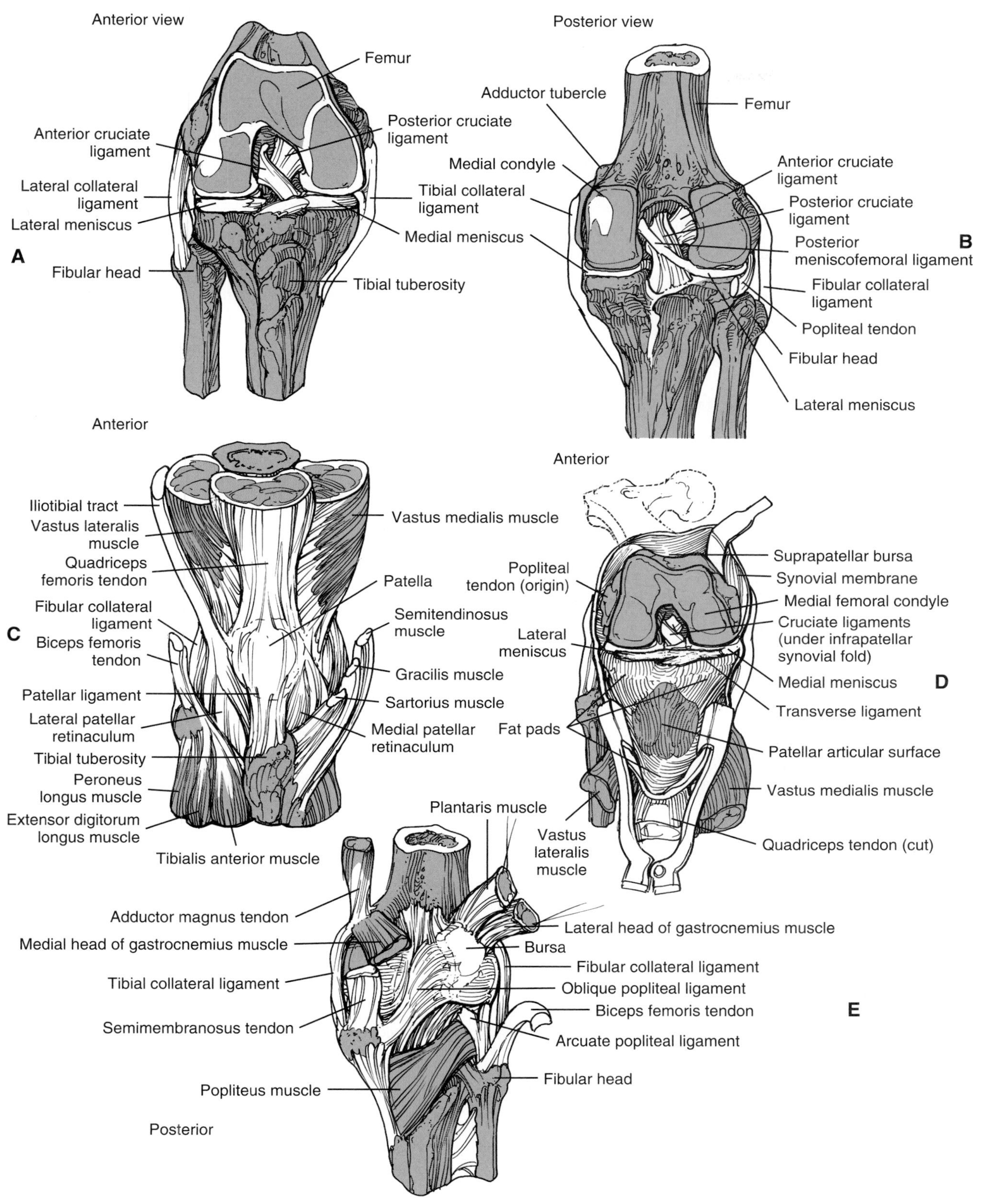

FIGURE 16–19

Knee joint. **A.** Anterior view with capsule completely removed. **B.** Posterior view with capsule completely removed. **C.** Anterior view with capsule intact. **D.** Anterior view with patella reflected. **E.** Posterior view with plantaris and gastrocnemius muscles reflected. *Continued*

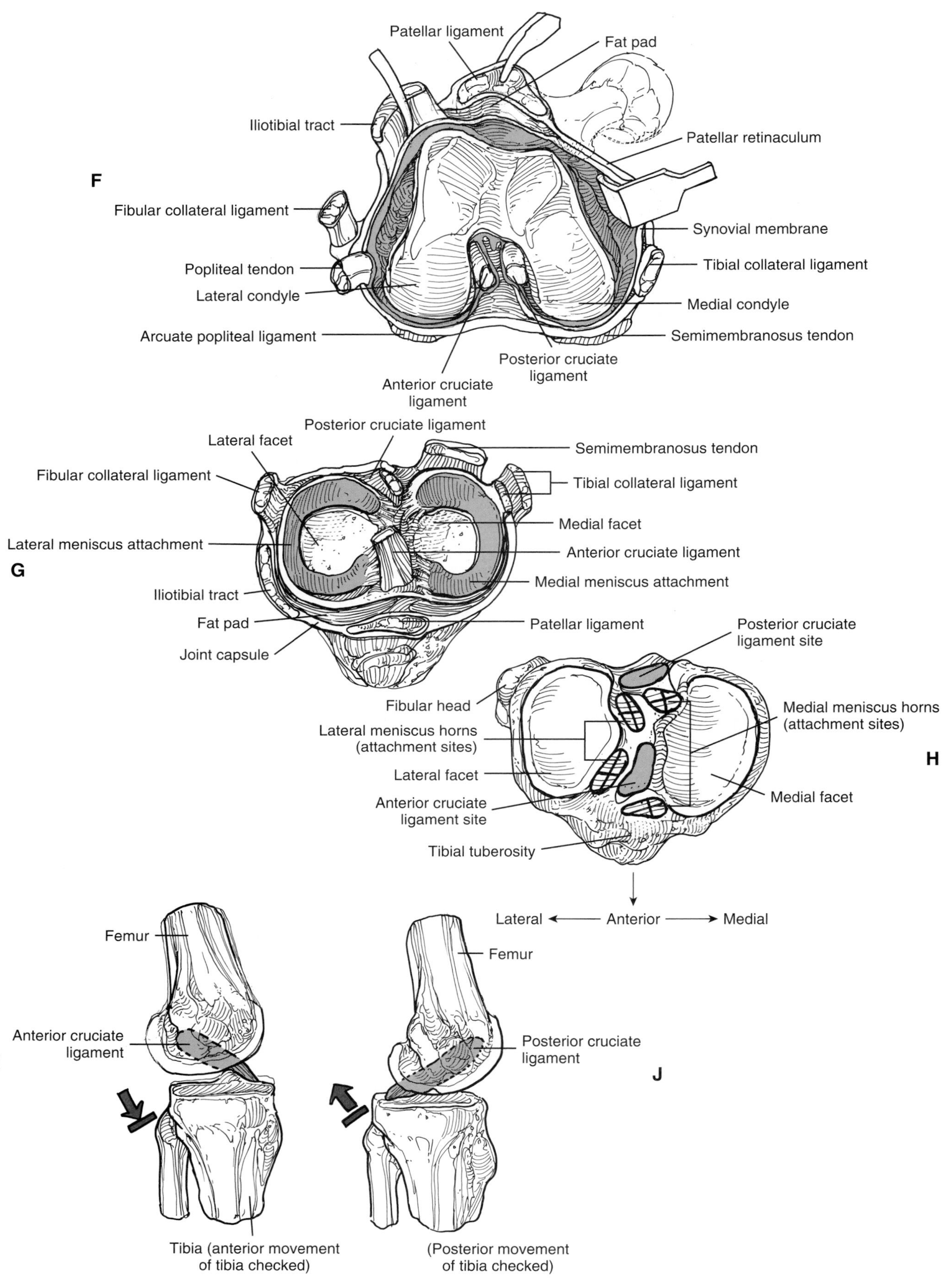

FIGURE 16–19, cont'd

F. Inferior view of lateral and medial condyles of femur. **G.** Superior view of articular facets and menisci of tibia. **H.** Superior view of articular facets of tibia, showing attachment sites of menisci. **I.** The anterior cruciate ligament checks the forward movement of the tibia with respect to the femur. **J.** The posterior cruciate ligament checks the posterior movement of the tibia with respect to the femur.

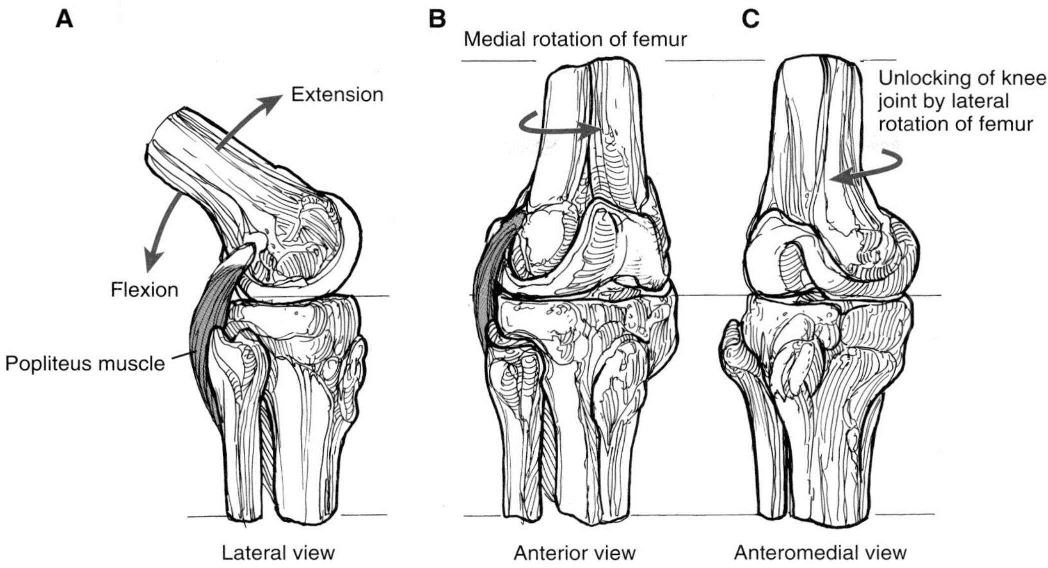

FIGURE 16–20
Movements of the knee joint. **A.** Flexion and extension. **B.** Medial rotation. **C.** Lateral rotation.

knee joint, the articular surfaces assume their most congruent, closely packed configuration. Further extension is limited by the cruciate and collateral ligaments and the capsule and skin of the knee, which are now taut. This balance between the forces that extend the knee (extensor muscles and gravity) and the forces that resist extension (ligaments, capsule, and skin) lock the knee joint. This provides an efficient mechanism, which stabilizes the joint as it supports the full weight of the body while the other leg swings forward in the next step (see Chapter 17).

The extended knee joint must be unlocked to initiate the flexion required for the next stride. This begins while the foot is still planted, as the **popliteus muscle** contracts to laterally rotate the femur upon the tibia (Fig. 16–20*C*). This action should be apparent if one pictures the foot planted and then thinks about the attachments and course of the popliteus muscle from the lateral epicondyle of the femur to the medial two thirds of the posterior surface of the femur just superior to the **soleal line** (see Fig. 16–10*B*). (It should also be obvious that the popliteus muscle medially will rotate the tibia, with respect to the femur, when the femur is fixed and the tibia is free.) Once the popliteus muscle unlocks the joint, flexion is initiated by the gastrocnemius muscle (assisted by the plantaris muscle). Once flexion is initiated and the foot is lifted, further flexion is effected by the hamstring and gracilis muscles (see Table 16–2, Chapter 17, and Table 17–1). Maximal flexion is checked by contact of the calf with the posterior thigh.

Because the ligaments, capsule, and skin are taut and, thus, most restrictive of movement of the leg when it is in the fully extended position, it should not be surprising that the range of motion of the semiflexed leg is somewhat greater. For example, there is no adduction or abduction of the knee when the leg is extended. Slight adduction and abduction of the knee is possible, however, when the leg is partially flexed and the tension of the collateral ligaments is decreased. In semiflexion, the tibia can also glide forward and backward on the femur, and slight rotational movements are possible.

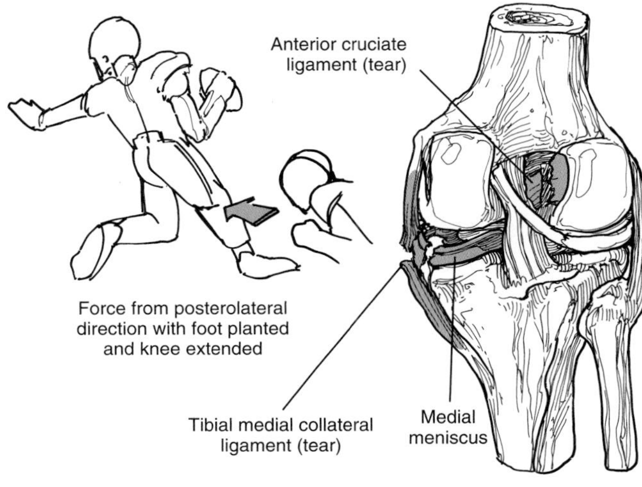

FIGURE 16–21
Injury of the "unholy triad" (the tibial [medial] collateral ligament, medial meniscus, and anterior cruciate ligament).

Flexors, extensors, and medial and lateral rotators of the knee are listed in Tables 16–2 and 17–1.

Injury of the Knee Joint

The relative instability of the knee joint may predispose it to injury and dislocation. Injury generally results from trauma directed from a posterolateral direction when the knee is extended and the foot planted (especially when one is wearing athletic shoes with cleats) (Fig. 16–21). This forces the medial condyle of the femur to separate from the medial tibial condyle (plateau), rupturing the anterior cruciate and tibial (medial) collateral ligaments and simultaneously tearing the medial meniscus from the medial tibial condyle (Fig. 16–21). Together, the anterior cruciate ligament, medial collateral ligament, and medial meniscus are called the "unholy triad." Injuries to any of these elements are common in contact sports such as football, soccer, and basketball.

Tibiofibular Joints

The tibia and fibula articulate directly with each other at their superior and inferior ends. Their shafts are bound to each other by a tough **interosseous ligament.**

The superior **tibiofibular joint** is a synovial joint. Therefore, articulating surfaces of the tibia and fibula are covered with cartilages, the joint is enclosed within a fibrous capsule, and the tibia and fibula are bound by tough ligaments. The head of the fibula is bound to the lateral condyle of the tibia by **anterior** and **posterior ligaments of the head of the fibula** (Fig. 16–22*A* and *B*). The anterior region of the **fibrous capsule** is thick. The capsule is attached to the margins of the articulating surfaces of both bones

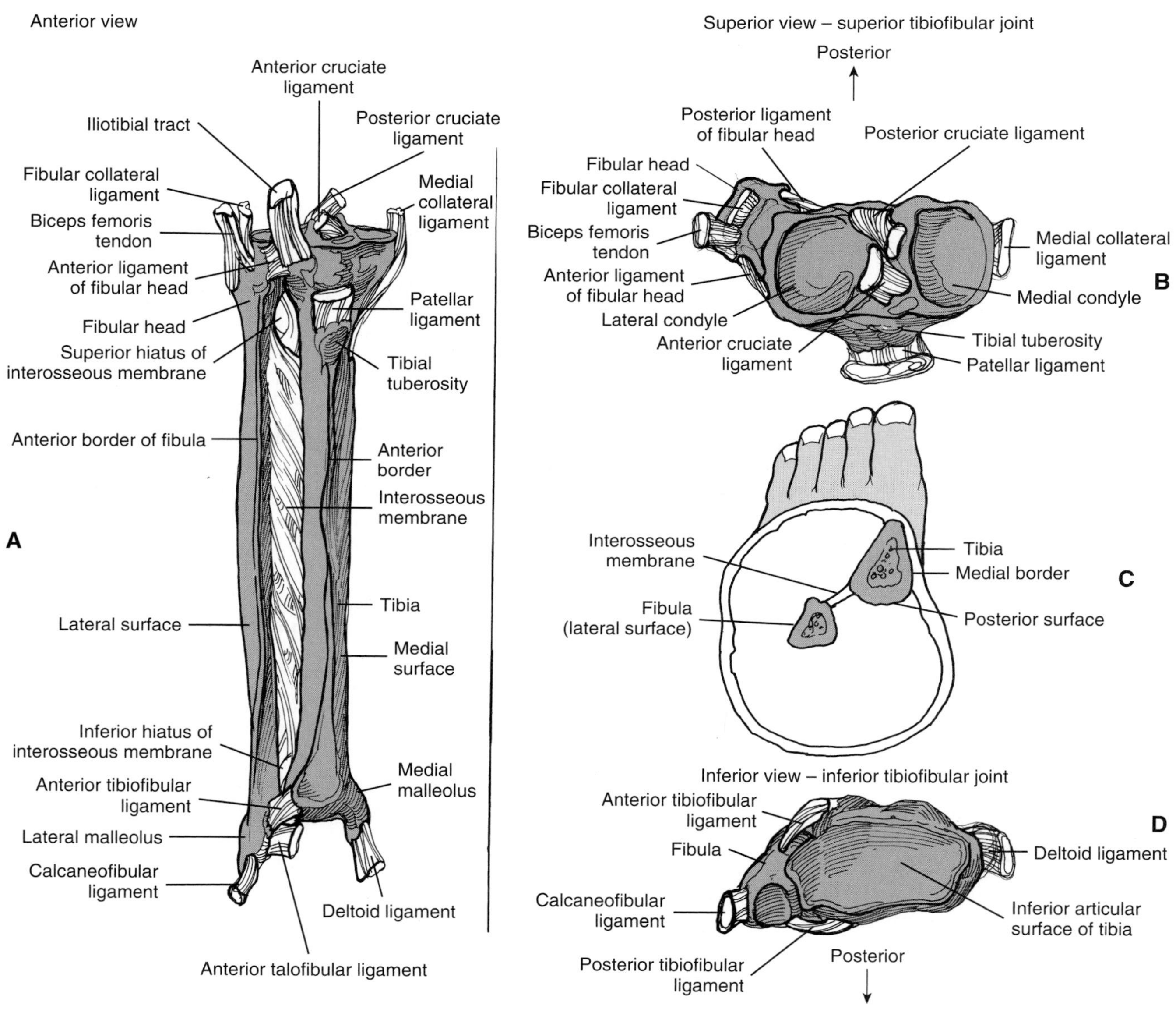

FIGURE 16–22
Tibiofibular joint. The tibia and fibula are bound tightly together by strong ligaments and capsular elements at both ends of their shafts and by the interosseous membrane. Anterior and posterior tibiofibular ligaments make up the lateral ligament of the ankle joint. **A.** Anterior view of the tibia and fibula of the right leg. **B.** Superior view of the superior tibiofibular joint. **C.** Superior view of section of the leg showing the interosseous membrane connecting the tibia and the fibula. **D.** Inferior view of the inferior tibiofibular joint.

around the entire circumference of the joint. In a small percentage of individuals, the synovial cavity of the superior tibiofibular joint is continuous with that of the knee joint.

The interosseous borders of the tibial and fibular shafts (see Fig. 16–10*E*) are connected to each other by a tough **interosseous membrane** (Fig. 16–22*A*). This membrane separates the muscles in the anterior and posterior compartments of the leg, except at two points where openings allow communication between the two compartments. A superior hiatus allows the anterior interosseous artery to pass into the anterior compartment from the popliteal fossa (behind the knee) as it branches from the popliteal artery (Fig. 16–22*A* and see Chapter 18). The inferior hiatus transports the perforating branch of the peroneal (fibular) artery to the ventral side of the ankle.

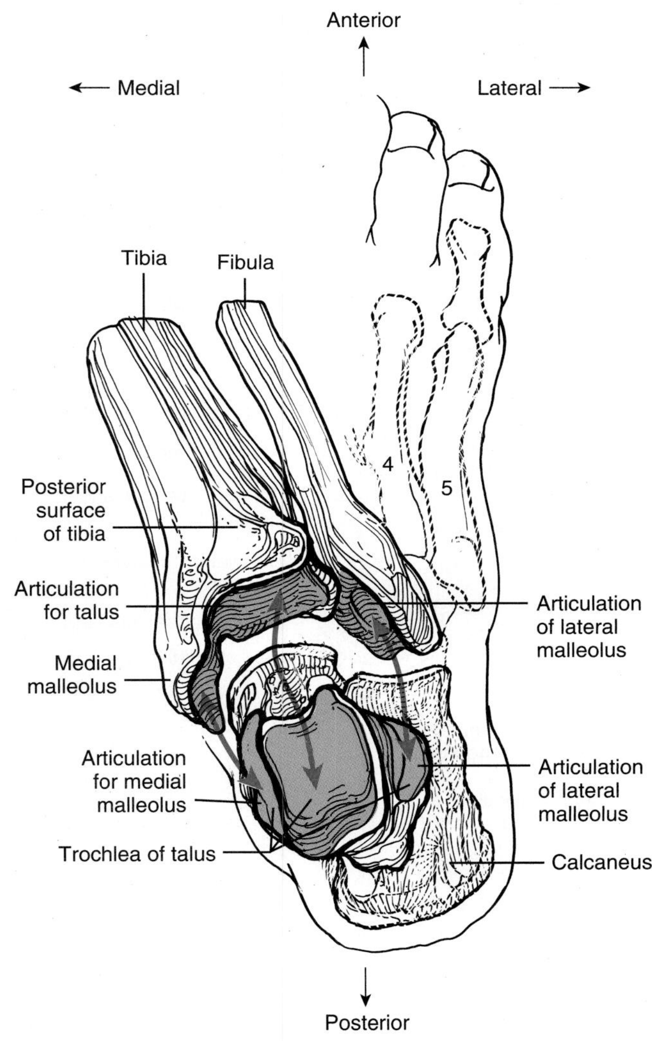

FIGURE 16–23
Talocrural joint. View of opened joint reveals the articulating surfaces of the tibia, fibula, and talus.

The **inferior tibiofibular joint** is a syndesmosis, except for a small inferior area (which is more accurately described as an extension of the joint between the tibia, fibula, and talus bone), which is a synovial joint. Therefore, most of the rough articulating surfaces of the tibia and lateral malleolus articulate via a thin fibrocartilaginous matrix. This joint is further strengthened by **anterior** and **posterior tibiofibular ligaments** (Fig. 16–22*A* and *D*).

Movements of the Tibiofibular Joints

The range of motion of the tibiofibular joints is restricted. Only very slight rotational movements of the fibula are possible with respect to the tibia.

Talocrural Joint

The talocrural (ankle) joint is the joint between the talus bone of the foot (see below), tibia, and fibula. It is a synovial joint. The large inferior articular surface of the tibia and lateral articular surface of the medial malleolus of the tibia articulate with the large superior and medial surfaces of the talus (Fig. 16–23). The medial articulating surface of the lateral malleolus (of the fibula) articulates with the lateral articulating surface of the talus (Fig. 16–23). These lateral, superior, and medial articulating surfaces of the talus are collectively called the **trochlea of the talus** (Fig. 16–23 and see Fig. 16–13*C*). Articulating surfaces of the joint are covered by cartilage and separated by a synovial cavity containing synovial fluid. Bones of the ankle joint are further bound by ligaments and a tough fibrous capsule.

Ligaments of the ankle joint include the composite medial **deltoid ligament** and composite **lateral ligament of the ankle joint** (Fig. 16–24).

At the **lateral aspect of the ankle joint,** the lateral malleolus is joined to the talus and calcaneus bones by the **lateral ligament of the ankle joint.** The lateral ligament is a composite structure consisting of an **anterior talofibular ligament,** which courses from the anterior boundary of the lateral (fibular) malleolus to the neck of the talus just anterior to the lateral articular facet of the trochlea (Fig. 16–24*A*); a **posterior talofibular ligament,** which courses from the posterior boundary of the lateral (fibular) malleolus to the **posterior process** of the talus; and, between these two, a **calcaneofibular ligament,** which courses inferoposteriorly from the apex of the lateral malleolus to a tubercle on the lateral surface of the calcaneus (Fig. 16–24*A* and see Fig. 16–22*A* and *D*).

At the **medial aspect of the ankle joint,** the medial malleolus of the tibia is joined to the talus, navicular, and calcaneus bones of the foot by the **deltoid (medial collateral) ligament** of the ankle joint (Fig. 16–24*B*). The deltoid ligament is a triangular structure consisting of **superficial** and **deep fibers,** which arise from the medial (tibial) malleolus. The superfi-

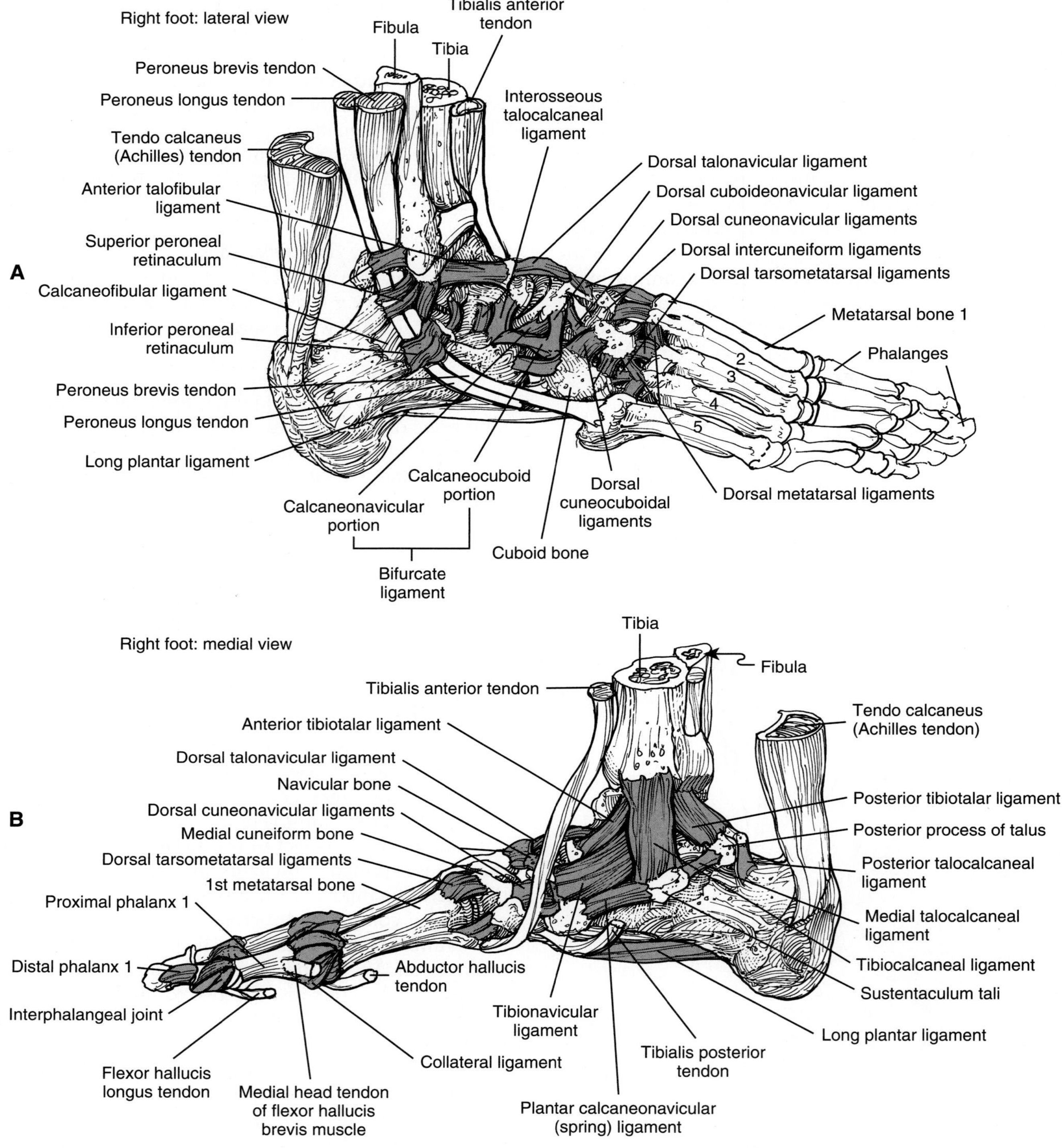

FIGURE 16–24

Ankle joint. **A.** Lateral view. **B.** Medial view. The anterior tibiotalar, tibionavicular, middle tibiocalcaneal, and posterior tibiotalar ligaments constitute the deltoid ligament. The calcaneonavicular and calcaneocuboid ligaments make up the bifurcate ligament.

cial fibers include anterior fibers, which attach the anterior border of the medial malleolus to the talus bone **(anterior tibiotalar ligament)** or to the **tuberosity of the navicular bone (tibionavicular ligament);** middle fibers, which course inferiorly to attach the medial malleolus to the **sustentaculum tali of the calcaneus (tibiocalcaneal ligament);** and posterior fibers **(posterior tibiotalar ligament),** which sweep posteriorly to attach the posterior border of the medial malleolus to the medial tubercle of the talus (Fig. 16–24*B*). **Deep fibers of the deltoid ligament** are attached superiorly to the tip of the medial malle-

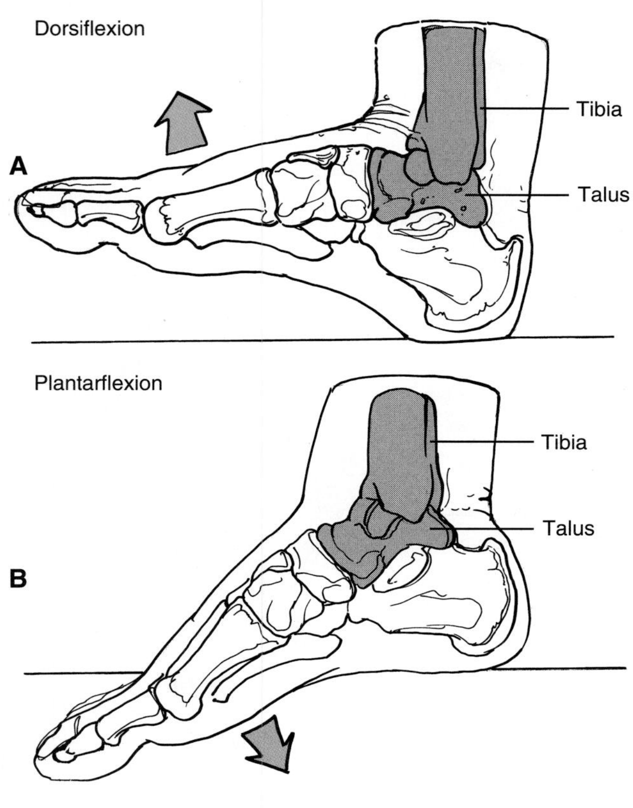

FIGURE 16–25
Movements of the ankle joint. **A.** Dorsiflexion. **B.** Plantarflexion.

olus and inferiorly to the lateral (nonarticulating) process of the talus bone.

The **capsule of the ankle joint** is relatively thin in the anterior and posterior regions. Its medial and lateral regions, however, are strengthened by the many ligaments described above. The capsule is lined by a synovial membrane, which may extend into a recess between the lower ends of the tibia and fibula.

Movements of the Ankle Joint

The movements of the talocrural joint are primarily **plantarflexion** and **dorsiflexion** (Fig. 16–25). However, when the foot is plantarflexed, slight **side-to-side gliding, abduction, adduction,** and **rotation** may also occur. In contrast, the talocrural joint is most stable in dorsiflexion because additional movements are impeded by maximum ligamentous tension and close packing of bony elements. It is from the most dorsiflexed position that forward propulsion begins during locomotory movements (see Chapter 18). Dorsiflexion is facilitated by the tibialis anterior muscle and assisted by the extensor digitorum longus, extensor hallucis longus, and peroneus tertius muscles (see Tables 16–2 and 17–1). Dorsiflexion is countered by the ligaments, capsule, and bony architecture of the ankle joint, as well as the plantarflexors of the joint, which include the soleus, gastrocnemius, plantaris, tibialis posterior, flexor digitorum longus, and flexor hallucis longus muscles (see Table 16–2 and 17–1). Plantarflexion is checked primarily by the actions of the dorsiflexors just listed.

> ***Injury of the Ankle Joint.*** Ankle joint injuries typically involve **stretching** or **tearing of ankle joint ligaments.** The laxity and weakness of lateral ankle ligaments predispose them more commonly to injury. Conversely, the relative strength of the medial ligaments, including the deltoid ligament, tends to prevent them from being injured. Indeed, the medial malleolus typically becomes avulsed before its associated ligaments will tear (Fig. 16–26). Twisting of the joint when the foot is planted or when it is everted or inverted while bearing weight may also lead to injury. Minor forces may result in **ankle sprain,** while more significant forces may result in **fracture** of the fibula or medial (tibial) malleolus.

Joints of the Arch of the Foot. The **intertarsal joints** include the subtalar (talocalcaneal), talocalcaneonavicular, calcaneocuboid, cuneonavicular, cuboideonavicular, intercuneiform, and cuneocuboid joints.

The **subtalar (talocalcaneal) joint** is a synovial articulation between the concave facet on the plantar surface of the talus and the superior (dorsal) convex facet of the calcaneus (Fig. 16–27). The joint is strengthened by **lateral, medial, interosseous,** and **cervical ligaments** and a **capsule** consisting of a few short fibrous slips and a thin fibrous sheath (see Fig. 16–24A). The enclosed synovial cavity does not communicate with other synovial cavities of the tarsus. The capsule and ligaments mainly check the rotational and gliding movements that allow **inversion** and **eversion** of the main part of the foot with respect to the talus. These movements are especially useful when one firmly **plants the foot** on the substratum when one is walking or running.

The **talocalcaneonavicular joint** is a multiaxial synovial joint in which (1) the anterior and middle facets of the superior surface of the calcaneus articulate with the plantar facets of the talus and (2) the pronounced convex facet of the rounded head of the talus articulates with the concave posterior facet of the navicular bone (Fig. 16–27). Movements of this joint are checked by the **interosseous, talonavicular,** and **bifurcate ligaments,** as well as by an incomplete fibrous capsule (see Fig. 16–24). The capsule is better developed in the posterior region than the anterior region. Movements at the talocalcaneonavicular joint include slight pronation (downward rotation of the medial border of the foot) and supination (downward rotation of the lateral border of the foot) of the distal tarsus with respect to the calcaneus and talus. These movements are elements of inversion and eversion, which are performed together by this joint and the subtalar joint (see above).

The **calcaneocuboid joint** is a synovial articulation between the convex anteromedial facet of the calcaneus

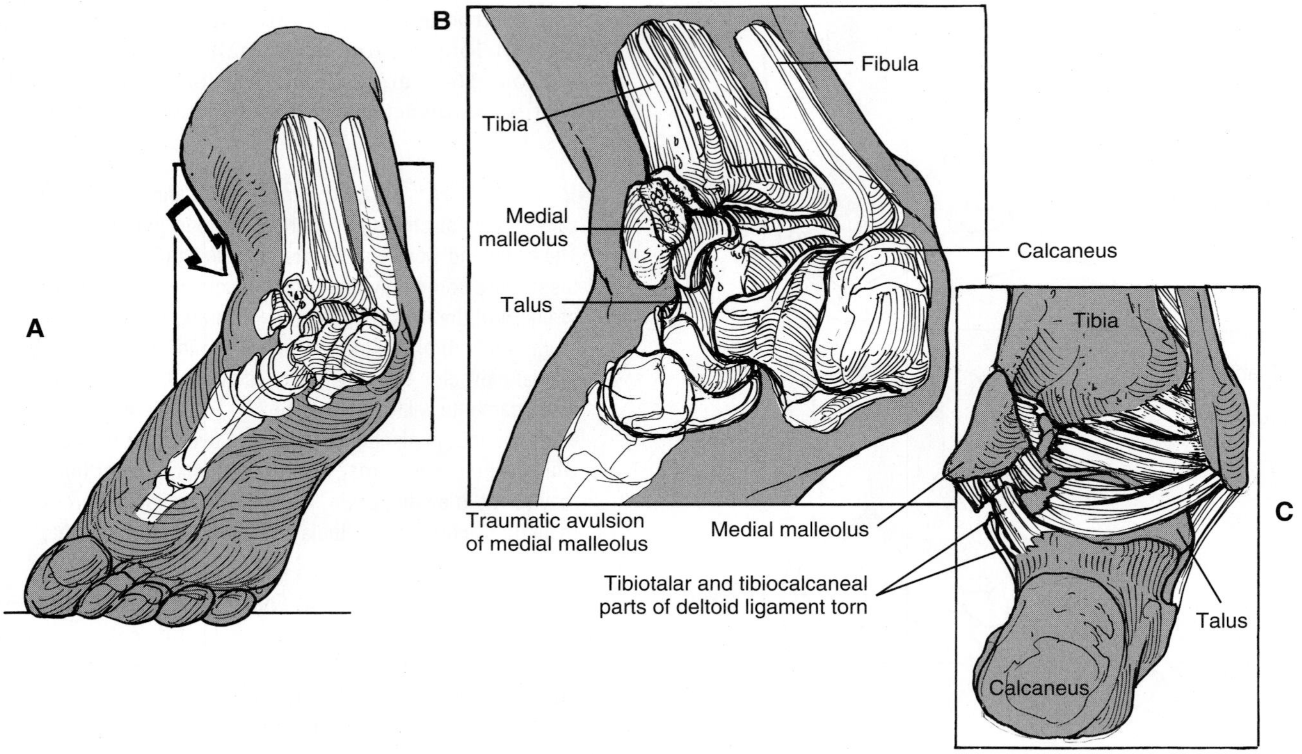

FIGURE 16–26
Injuries of the ankle joint. **A.** Fracture of the medial malleolus. **B.** Avulsion of the medial malleolus. **C.** Tearing of the tibiotalar and tibiocalcaneal parts of the deltoid ligament.

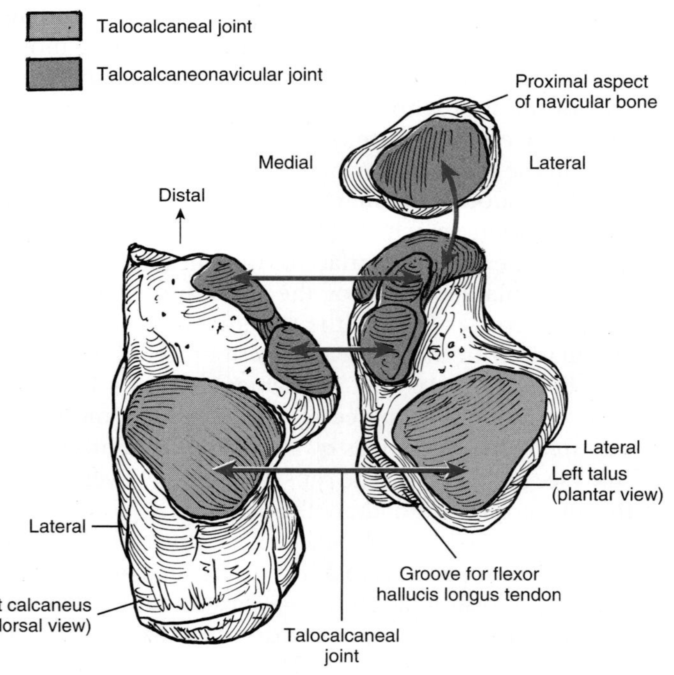

FIGURE 16–27
Talocalcaneal and talocalcaneonavicular (intertarsal) joints. View of opened joints reveals articulating surfaces.

and the posterolateral articulation of the cuboid bone (Fig. 16–28). Rotational and gliding movements of this joint also contribute to inversion, eversion, pronation, and supination of the foot (see above). However, these movements are significantly checked by three strong ligaments, the **bifurcate, long plantar,** and **plantar calcaneocuboid (short plantar) ligaments,** and a fibrous capsule (Figs. 16–29 and 16–30 and see Fig. 16–24*A*). The long and short plantar ligaments span the lateral side of the arch created by the articulation of the tarsal bones. These two ligaments, along with the deeper, more medial **plantar calcaneonavicular (spring) ligament** and **tendon of the peroneus longus muscle,** help prevent collapse of the arch of the foot (see below).

The **cuneonavicular joint** is a synovial joint, which provides an articulation between the anterior surface of the navicular bone and the posterior surfaces of the three **cuneiform bones** (Fig. 16–28). The joint is strengthened by **dorsal** and **plantar ligaments** and a fibrous capsule, which encloses a synovial cavity that is continuous with the synovial cavities of the intercuneiform and cuneocuboid joints (Fig. 16–30 and see Fig. 16–24 and below).

In most persons, the **cuboideonavicular joint** is a fibrous joint (syndesmosis) connected by **dorsal, interosseous,** and **plantar ligaments** (Figs. 16–28 to

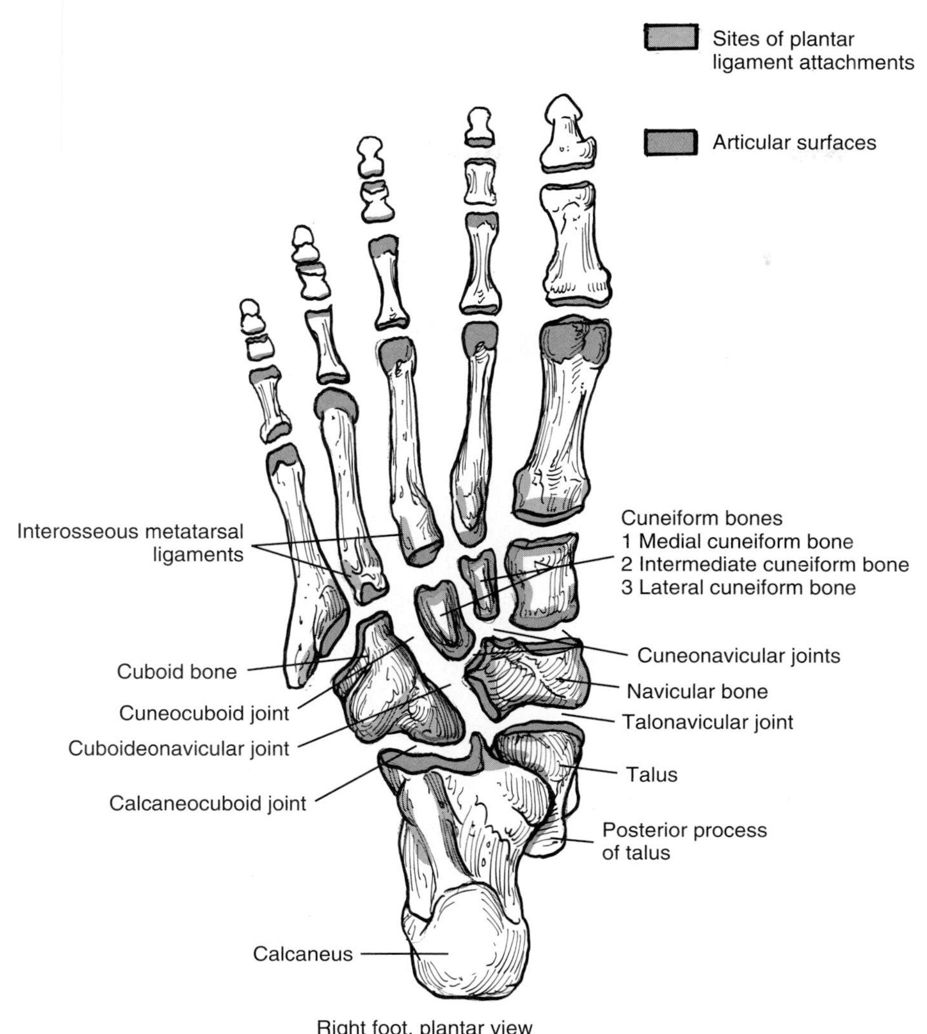

FIGURE 16–28
Other intertarsal joints and tarsometatarsal, metatarsophalangeal, and interphalangeal joints of the foot.

16–30). In some persons, it is a planar synovial articulation and its synovial cavity is continuous with the synovial cavities of the cuneonavicular, intercuneiform, and cuneocuboid joints.

The **intercuneiform** and **cuneocuboid joints** are synovial joints, which are strengthened by **dorsal, interosseous,** and **plantar ligaments** (Figs. 16–28 to 16–30). The bones form a planar unit, or slight side-to-side arch. Their relative movements are minimal but aid in supination and pronation when the foot is planted.

Motions of the Intertarsal Joints. The motions of the intertarsal joints are largely of a **gliding** or **rotational** type so that when a person is walking or running, the elevated foot may be inverted and slightly plantarflexed (as it swings forward) and then everted as it is dorsiflexed (as it is planted and begins to push off). These movements occur largely at the talocalcaneal and talocalcaneonavicular joints. **Inversion** at the more proximal talocalcaneal and talocalcaneonavicular joints is largely a function of the tibialis anterior and tibialis posterior muscles (see Tables 16–2 and Table 17–1). Inversion at these joints is checked by the lateral peroneal muscles and interosseous talocalcaneal ligament. **Eversion** at the talocalcaneal and talocalcaneonavicular joints is a function of the peroneus longus and peroneus brevis muscles (see Table 16–2 and see Table 17–1). This motion is checked by the medial tibialis anterior and tibialis posterior muscles and deltoid ligament. When the load on the everted foot is extreme, the medial malleolus may be avulsed (plucked out) because the tough deltoid ligament fails to tear (see below).

The more distal intertarsal joints as well as the **tarsometatarsal joints** allow slight gliding and rotational movements so that the foot may be **supinated** or **pronated** to maintain the sole of the foot in maximum contact with the substratum during locomotory move-

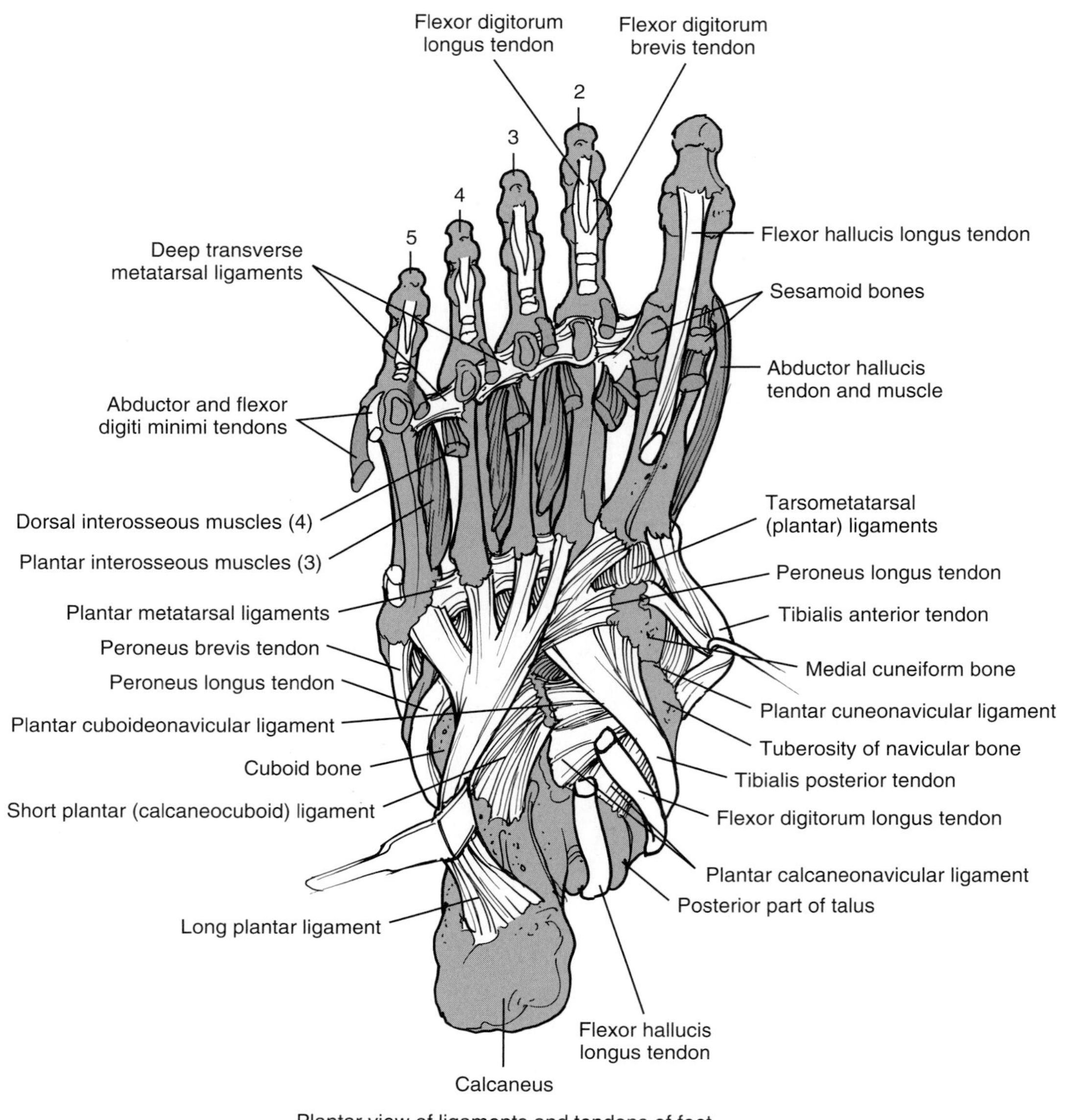

FIGURE 16–29
Inferior view of superficial plantar ligaments of the foot.

ments on uneven surfaces. (Pronation and supination are twisting of the distal part of the foot with respect to the proximal part of the foot.)

The **tarsometatarsal joints** include synovial articulations between (1) the first metatarsal and medial cuneiform bones, (2) the second metatarsal and medial, intermediate, and lateral cuneiform bones, (3) the third metatarsal and lateral cuneiform bones, (4) the fourth metatarsal and lateral cuneiform and cuboid bones, and (5) the fifth metatarsal and cuboid bones. The tarsometatarsal joints are strengthened by **dorsal, interosseous,** and **plantar ligaments** (Fig. 16–28).

The tarsometatarsal joints assist in planting of the foot by contributing to the foot's ability to pronate and supinate.

The **intermetatarsal joints** are found at the bases of the second and third, third and fourth, and fourth and fifth metatarsal bones. These bones form synovial articulations, which are strengthened by **dorsal, interosseous,** and **plantar ligaments** (Figs. 16–28 to 16–30). The head (distal end) of each metatarsal is connected to the adjacent metatarsals by **deep transverse metatarsal ligaments.**

The intermetatarsal joints make only slight gliding movements when the foot is under heavy load.

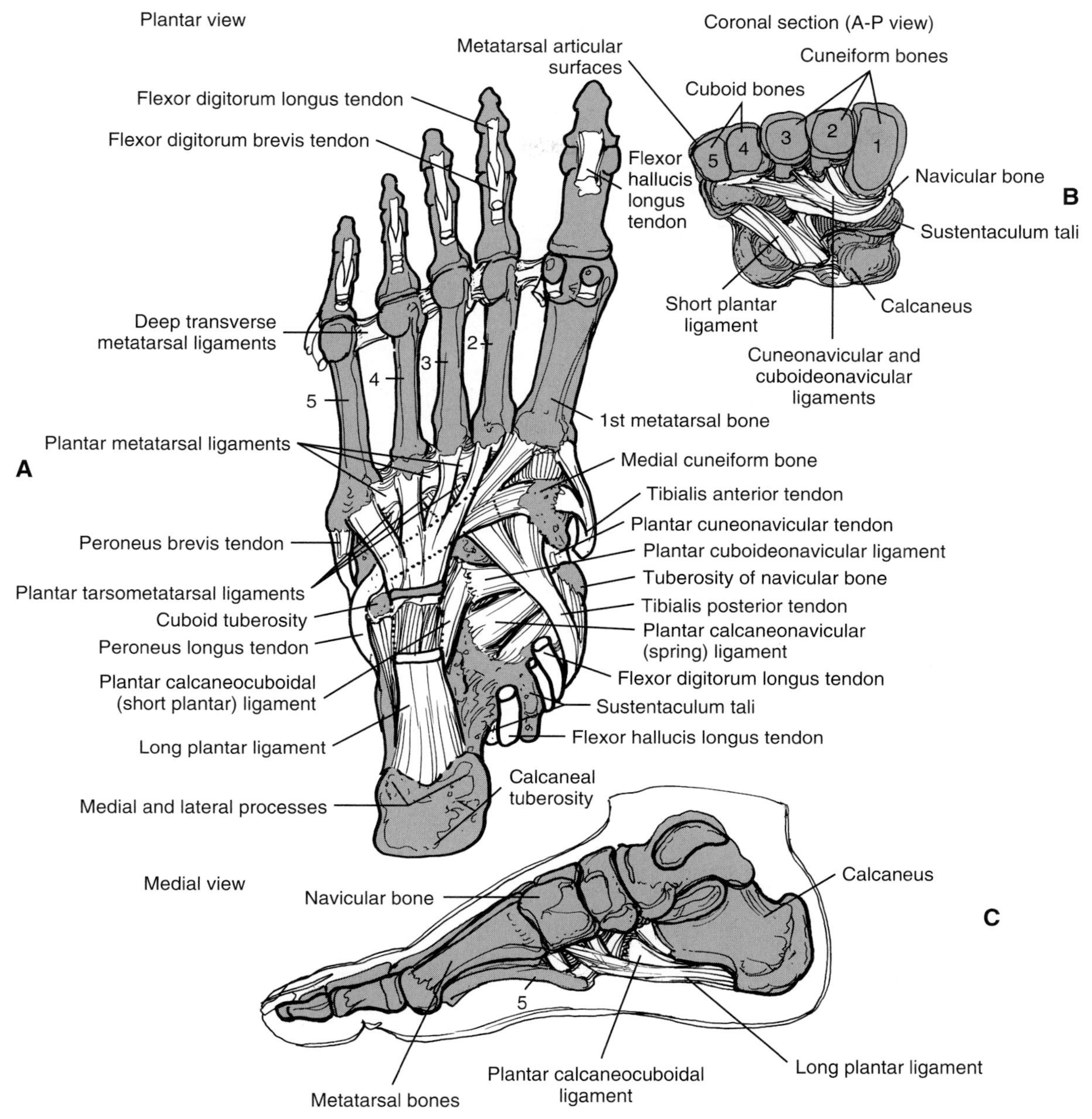

FIGURE 16–30
Deeper plantar ligaments of the foot. **A.** Plantar view. **B.** Anteroposterior view of coronal section. **C.** Medial view.

Injury to the Arch of the Foot

The foot is a technically sophisticated functional tripod as well as a flexible lever (see discussion of standing and walking in Chapter 17). Unfortunately, these anatomic characteristics may predispose the foot to a variety of pathologic conditions that affect the gait. The normal foot makes contact with the substratum at three points: (1) the head of the first metatarsal, (2) the head of the fifth metatarsal, and (3) the calcaneus (Fig. 16–31). The rest of the plantar surface does not normally make contact because it is arched both horizontally (medially) and longitudinally between these three points (see above).

When the arches collapse **(flatfoot; pes planus),** the entire plantar surface of the foot may come into contact with the substratum as the forefoot (anterior to the talus) deviates laterally and becomes everted (Fig. 16–32). The foot is unable to respond to changes in the terrain and to act as a flexible lever. Flattening or collapse of the arches occurs most frequently in obese middle-aged or elderly individuals, those who stand for long periods in a stationary position, or those who carry heavy loads. The arches collapse as their supporting ligaments, particularly the calcaneonavicular ligaments, stretch and lengthen. As this occurs, the shapes of the tarsal bones

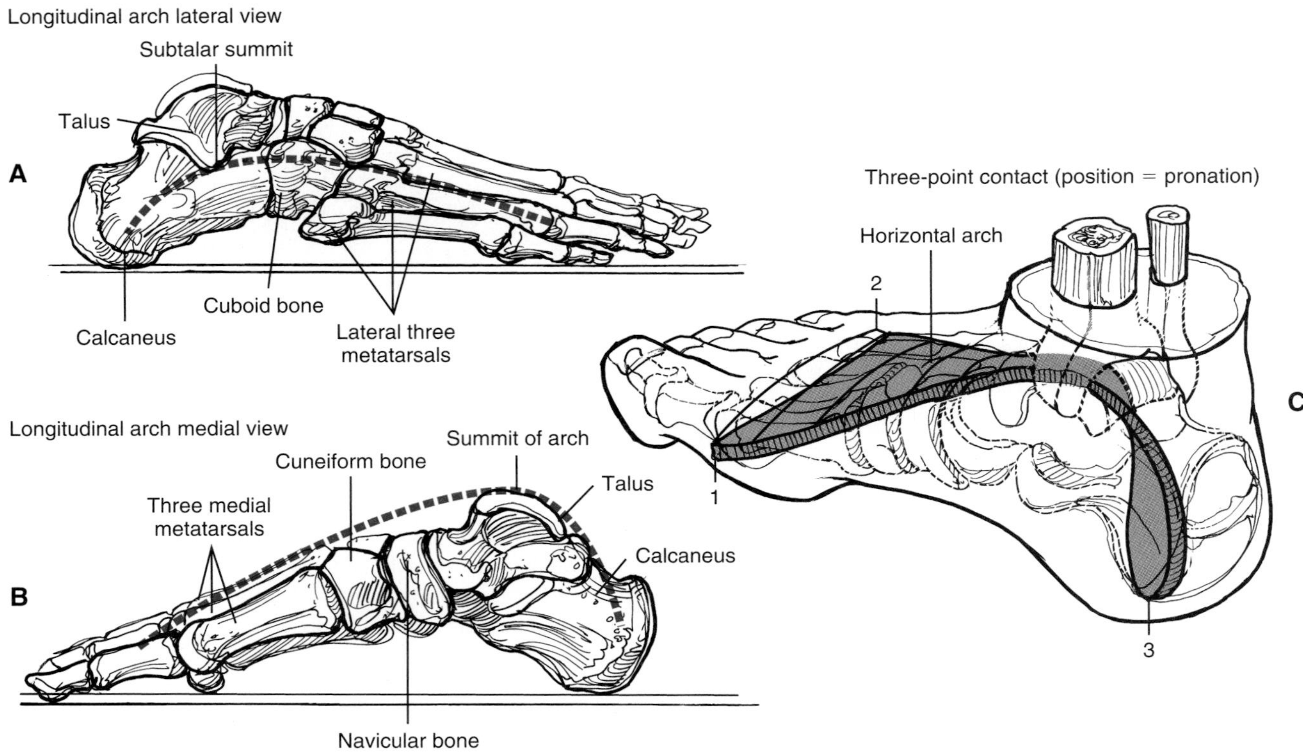

FIGURE 16–31
Arches of the foot. **A.** Longitudinal arch (lateral view). **B.** Longitudinal arch (medial view). **C.** Three-dimensional view of arch, showing three points of contact of foot.

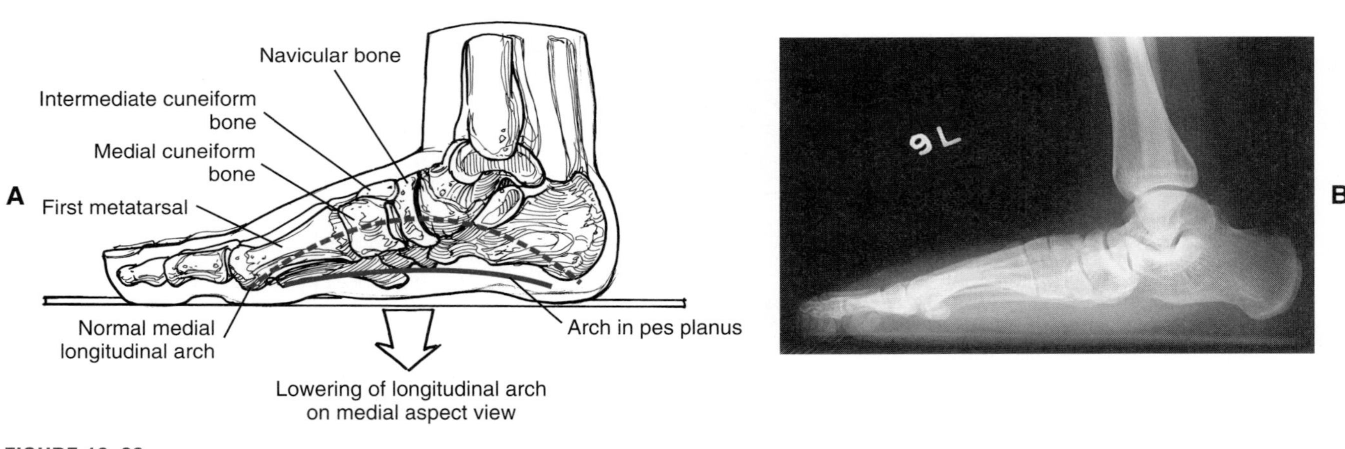

FIGURE 16–32
Flatfoot. **A.** Diagram showing collapse of arch. **B.** X-ray showing pes planus.

may change and the talus may slip in a medial direction, resulting in enlargement of the medial malleolus. This puts pressure on structures in the vicinity of the sustentaculum tali. This enlargement of the medial malleolus and flattening of the arches puts increased tension on muscles and tendons of the deep posterior compartment of the leg. This may result in cramping while a person is walking or standing (see Chapter 17).

Joints of the Toes

The **metatarsophalangeal joints** consist of convex plantar and distal facets of the metatarsal heads, which form synovial articulations with the concave facets of the most proximal phalanges (see Fig. 16–28). Each of these articulations incorporates two sesamoid bones, which fit into longitudinal grooves in the lateral and medial aspects of the plantar sur-

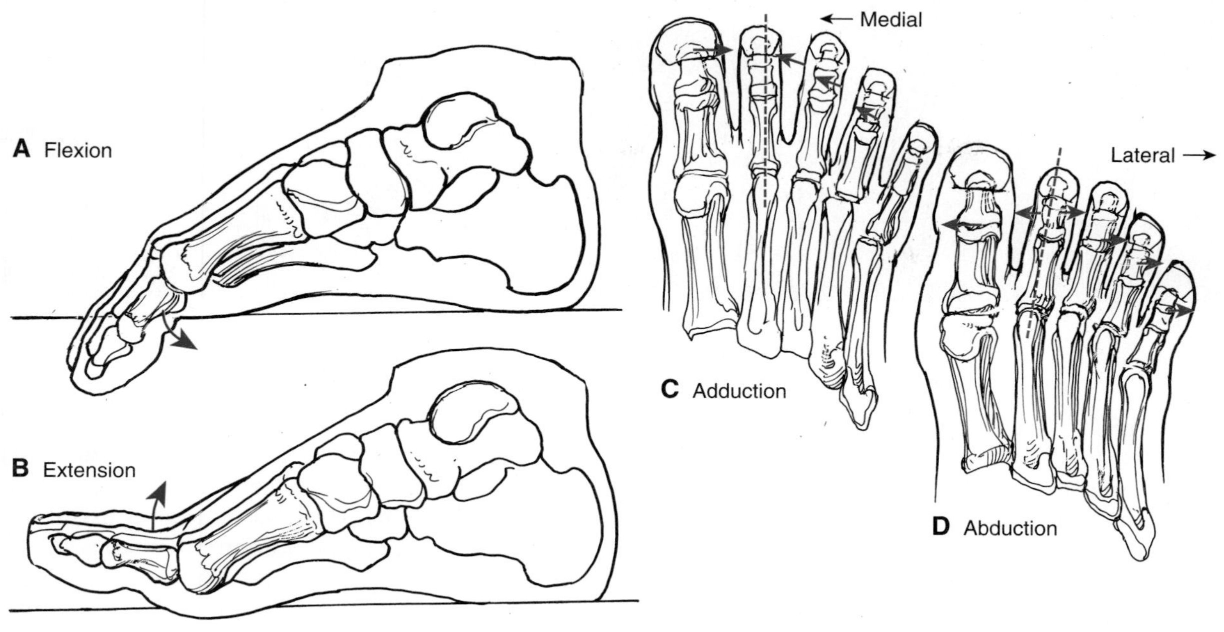

FIGURE 16–33
Movements of the metatarsophalangeal joints. **A.** Flexion. **B.** Extension. **C.** Adduction. **D.** Abduction.

face of the facet of the metatarsal head. Movements at these joints are limited by **deep transverse metatarsal** and **collateral ligaments** and a **fibrous capsule,** which is strengthened at its plantar surface (see Figs. 16–29 and 16–30).

Movements of the Metatarsophalangeal Joints. The movements of the metatarsophalangeal joints of the foot include significant extension (as much as 90 degrees) and limited flexion (Fig. 16–33*A* and *B*). This is in direct contrast to these movements in the hand. Some accessory gliding and rotational movements of the phalanges of the foot are also possible at these joints. **Flexion** is facilitated by the flexor digitorum brevis, lumbrical, interossei, flexor digitorum longus, quadratus plantae (flexor accessorius), flexor hallucis longus, flexor hallucis brevis, and flexor digiti minimi muscles. **Extension** is performed by the extensor digitorum longus, extensor hallucis longus, and extensor digitorum brevis muscles. **Adduction** is performed by the adductor hallucis and first, second, and third plantar interosseous muscles (see above). **Abduction** is performed by the abductor hallucis; third, fourth, and fifth interosseous; and abductor digiti minimi muscles (see Tables 16–2 and 17–4). The axis of reference for abduction and adduction is the second digit (Fig. 16–33*C* and *D*).

The **interphalangeal joints** are synovial hinge joints between the middle and distal phalanges. They are similar in structure to the metatarsophalangeal joints (see Fig. 16–28). The joints are strengthened by **collateral ligaments** and a **fibrous capsule,** which is thickened in the plantar region.

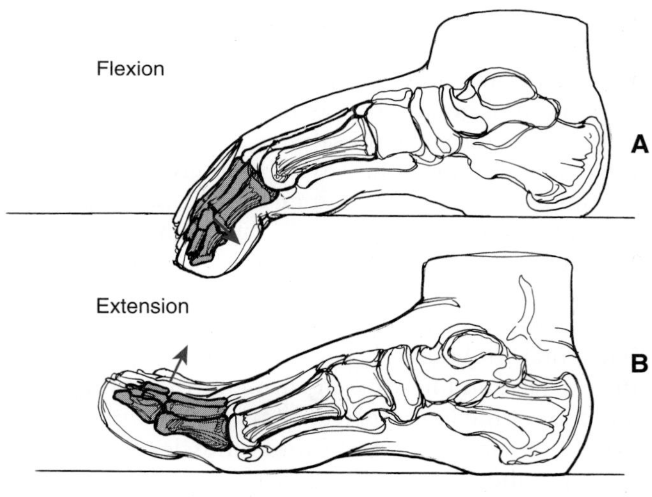

FIGURE 16–34
Movements of the interphalangeal joints. **A.** Flexion. **B.** Extension.

The movements of the metatarsophalangeal joints of the foot are similar to that of the hand. More flexion than extension is possible, with some adduction occurring with flexion and some abduction occurring with extension (Fig. 16–34). **Flexion** at these joints is a function of the long and short flexors (see Tables 16–2 and 17–1). **Extension** is a function of the long extensors of the anterior compartment of the leg and a short flexor on the dorsum of the foot (see Figs. 16–2 and 17–4 and Tables 17–3 and 17–4).

17 Muscles of the Lower Extremities

MUSCLES OF THE LOWER LIMB

Embryonic Origin of Lower Limb Musculature

As has been discussed in Chapters 2 and 16, the muscles of the limbs arise from myoblasts, which migrate from somites into the limb bud. In the lower extremity, the muscles develop from myoblasts that originate within somites at levels L2 to S2. These myoblasts migrate into the lower limb buds to form two masses of muscle precursors: the **dorsal muscle mass** and the **ventral muscle mass** (Fig. 17–1). In general, the most proximal muscles of the upper and lower limbs are formed by myoblasts within the dorsal muscle masses. Thus, muscles of the scapular region of the upper extremity and superficial muscles of the gluteal region of the lower extremity have similar origins and are considered to be **homologous** (Box 17–1). In more distal regions of the extremities, the dorsal muscle masses of both the upper and lower extremity limb buds give rise to extensor muscles, whereas the ventral muscle masses give rise to flexor muscles. However, as has been discussed in Chapter 16, the lower limb bud rotates 180 degrees medially between the fourth and eighth weeks of embryologic development, whereas the upper extremity limb buds rotate only slightly laterally. Thus, the positions of the extensor and flexor compartments in the thigh, leg, and foot of the lower extremity are reversed in comparison with the positions of these muscles in the arm, forearm, and hand of the upper extremity (Box 17–1 and see Fig. 16–2). The dramatic rotation of the lower extremity limb bud also affects the distribution of nerves to the skin and muscles of the lower limb (see Chapter 18).

Organization of Definitive Lower Extremity Muscles

Muscles of the lower extremity can be classified as **gluteal muscles, femoral (thigh) muscles, crural (leg) muscles,** or **intrinsic muscles of the foot** (see also Chapter 16). Each class of muscles correlates with a segment of the limb. Groups of muscles in each segment may be separated into compartments by thickened sheets of deep fascia called **fascial septa.** Thus, in each segment of the lower extremity, muscles may be classified according to the **specific compartment** in which they are located (e.g., anterior, posterior, or medial compartment of the thigh) or as **superficial** or **deep** (e.g., superficial gluteal muscles, deep lateral rotator muscles of the gluteal region). This classification is useful not only for learning names and locations of muscles, but also for learning muscle functions because muscles in a particular group may have the same function. For example, anterior thigh muscles tend to be extensors of the knee, whereas posterior thigh muscles tend to be flexors. In addition, the intermuscular septa, through their connections to skeletal elements and the fascia lata, provide integrity and stability of the lower extremity (see discussion of standing below). The septa also provide attachments for muscles and carry and protect deep vessels and nerves (see below and Chapter 18).

The **gluteal region** has only one compartment but contains both superficial and deep groups of muscles. The **thigh** (between the hip and knee joints) has **medial, anterior,** and **posterior compartments.** The **leg** (between the knee and ankle joints) has **lateral, anterior,** and **posterior compartments.** The posterior compartment contains superficial and deep groups of muscles. The **foot** (inferior to the ankle joint) has **dorsal** and **plantar compartments.**

As in the case of muscles described elsewhere (e.g., those of the trunk), muscles of the lower extremity may be active in dynamic movements such as walking or running or in the static maintenance of posture. Indeed, the controlled movements of a segment are possible only because of the coordinated activity of opposing muscle groups (see discussion of walking and running below and in Chapter 18). For example, muscles of the **gluteal compartment abduct, extend,** or **laterally rotate** the thigh, and muscles of the **medial compartment of the thigh adduct, flex,** or **medially rotate** the thigh (Fig. 17–2). This allows the thigh to return to any position from which it has moved, and, as in other regions of the body (see Chapters 5, 6, and 11), the dynamic actions of one muscle group work against the resistance provided by an opposing muscle group or by gravity, or both. In another example, **anterior compartment thigh muscles** such as the **psoas** and **sartorius muscles** cross the hip joint to **flex** the thigh, countering the actions of

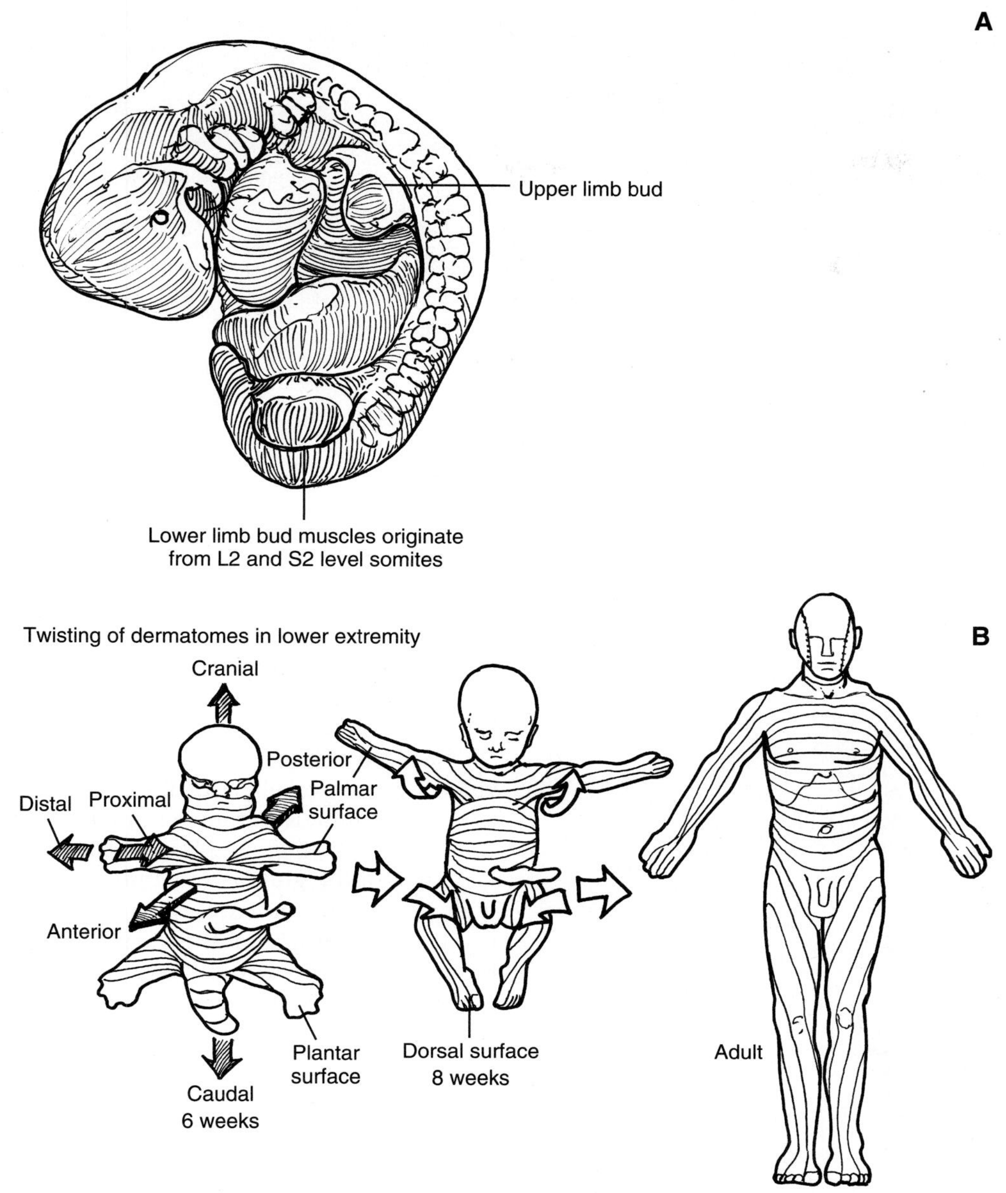

FIGURE 17–1
Embryonic origin of lower limb musculature.

extensors (hamstrings) located in the **posterior compartment of the thigh** (see Fig. 17–4).

Many muscles of the lower extremity **cross two joints** and have more than one function. The rectus femoris muscle flexes the hip joint and crosses the knee to extend the knee joint. The hamstrings extend the hip joint and flex the knee joint. The sartorius muscle of the anterior thigh compartment has three major functions: (1) it flexes the hip joint, (2) it extends the knee joint, and (3) it rotates the thigh in a lateral direction. Similar examples could be cited for muscles of the leg and foot.

The following description of lower extremity muscles is organized from superior to inferior (i.e., from the gluteal region to the foot) and by location within specific **muscle compartments** or layers.

▲ Specific Muscles of the Lower Extremities

Muscles of the Gluteal Region (Buttock)

Muscles of the gluteal region are located in only one compartment, the gluteal compartment. However, they may be characterized either as a superficial group of extensors and abductors of the hip (gluteus maximus, gluteus medius, and gluteus minimus muscles) or as a deeper group of lateral rotators (piriformis, obturator internus and externus, gemellus superior and inferior, and quadratus femoris muscles) (Fig. 17–3). Although

BOX 17–1
MUSCLES OF THE DORSAL AND VENTRAL MUSCLE MASSES

Dorsal Muscle Mass		Ventral Muscle Mass	
Upper Limb	**Lower Limb**	**Upper Limb**	**Lower Limb**
Levator scapulae, rhomboids, supraspinatus, infraspinatus, teres major and minor, latissimus dorsi, subscapularis, deltoid, serratus anterior, posterior compartment muscles of arm and forearm, lateral compartment muscles of forearm and hand	Gluteus maximus, gluteus medius, gluteus minimus, piriformis, psoas, iliacus, anterior compartment muscles of thigh and leg, short head of biceps femoris, tensor fasciae latae, lateral compartment muscles of leg, muscles of dorsum of foot	Anterior compartment muscles of arm and forearm, all muscles of palmar side of hand	Obturator internus, gemellus superior and inferior, medial compartment muscles of thigh, posterior compartment muscles of thigh and leg, all muscles of plantar side of foot

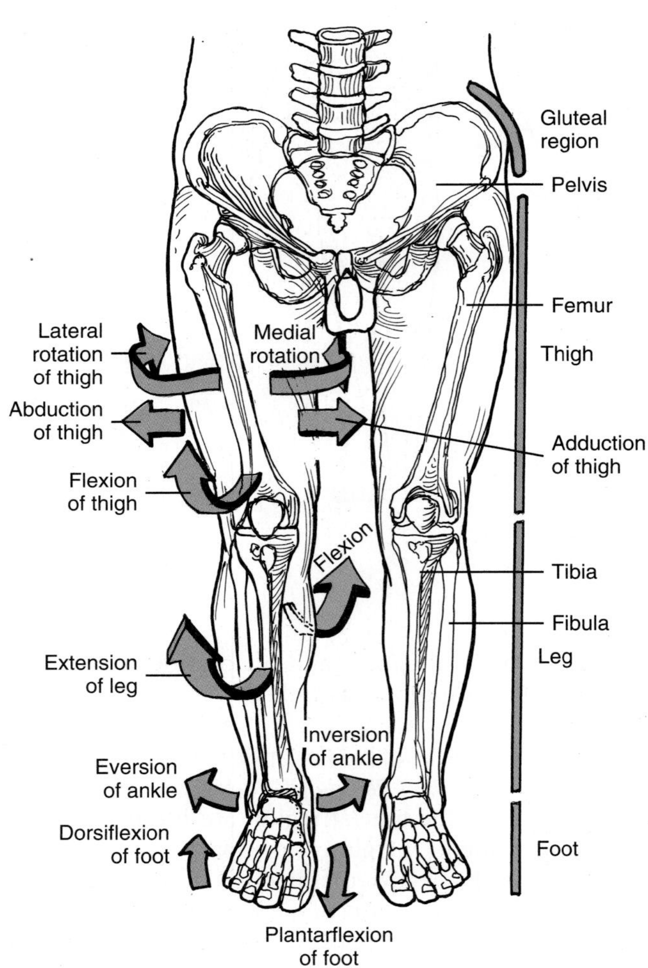

FIGURE 17–2
Opposing muscle groups allow controlled lower limb movement.

the obturator externus muscle arises from the anterior surface of the pelvis, its tendon passes posterior to the hip joint. Therefore, it is classified here as a gluteal muscle (see also below). Some medial rotation is also provided by anterior fibers of the gluteus medius muscle and by the gluteus minimus muscle (see below).

Superficial Gluteal Muscle. The prominence and large size of the **gluteus maximus muscle** is consistent with its primary function of raising the weight of the trunk to an upright position (Fig. 17–3*A* to *C*). This broad muscle arises from

- the posterior gluteal line and iliac crest in the medial region of the dorsal surface of the ilium (see Table 16–1),
- the lateral region of the dorsal surface of the sacrum,
- the aponeurosis of the erector spinae muscles (see Chapter 5),
- the superomedial region of the sacrotuberous ligament, and
- the fascia covering the gluteus medius muscle, which lies just deep to the gluteus maximus muscle (Figs. 17–3 and 17–4*A*).

The fibers of the gluteus maximus muscle course inferiorly and laterally over the greater trochanter of the femur as the inferomedial end of the muscle forms a short, wide tendon. The more superficial fibers of the tendon are attached to the superoposterior edge of the **iliotibial tract** (a thickened lateral band of deep fascia; see below), while deeper fibers of the tendon are attached to the posterior surface of the femur between the attachment sites of the adductor magnus and vastus lateralis muscles (Figs. 17–3 and 17–4*A*).

Movements of the gluteus maximus muscle over underlying structures are cushioned by the **trochanteric bursa,** which lies between the gluteus maximus muscle

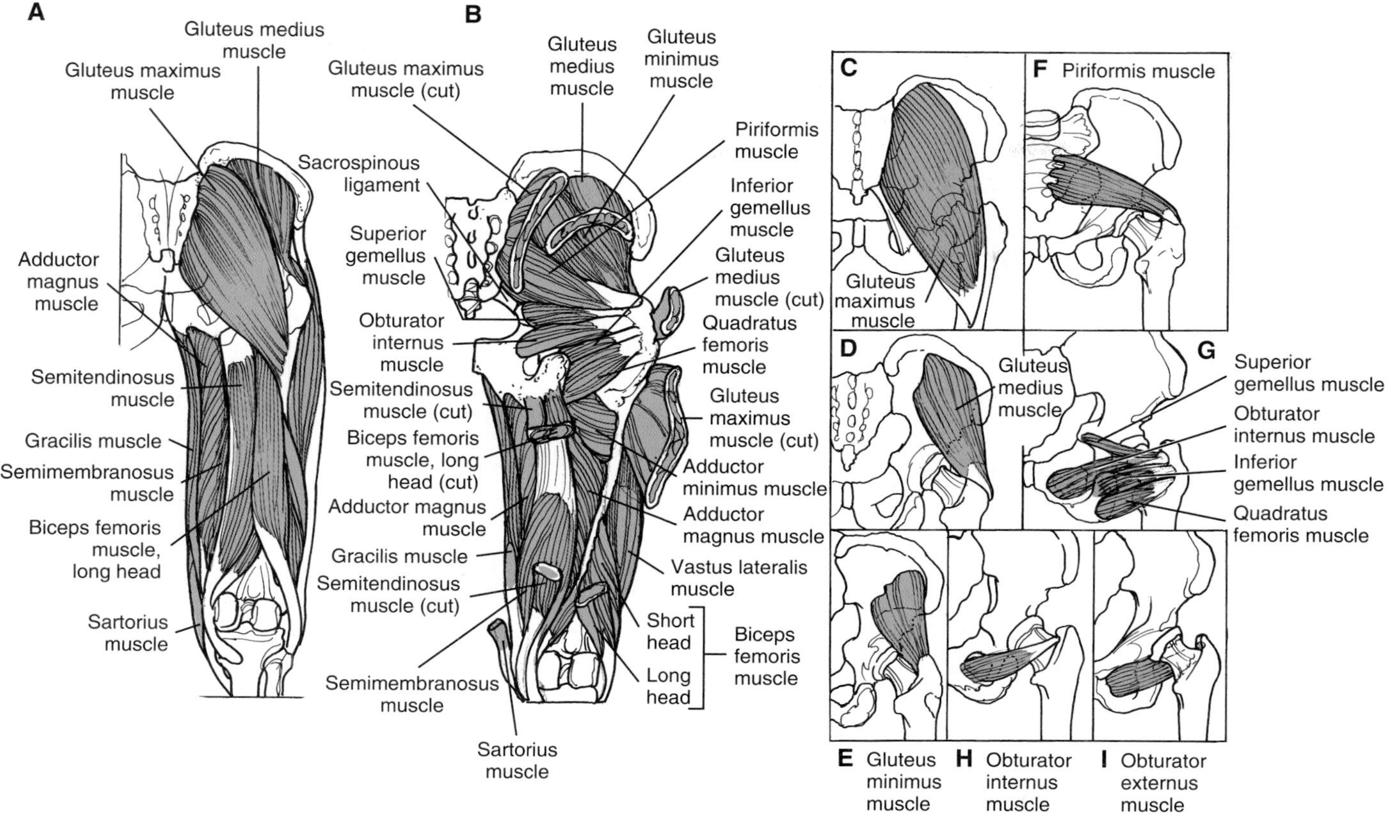

FIGURE 17–3
Posterior views of the muscles of the gluteal region. **A.** Superficial gluteal muscles. **B.** Deep gluteal muscles. **C** to **E.** Individual superficial muscles. **F** to **I.** Individual deep muscles.

and greater trochanter; the **gluteofemoral bursa,** which lies between lateral fibers of the gluteus maximus muscle (attached to the iliotibial tract) and the vastus lateralis muscle; and the **ischial bursa,** which lies between the gluteus maximus muscle and the ischium.

The most significant action of the gluteus maximus muscle is to extend the trunk when the thigh is flexed, as when one rises from a sitting or stooping position (Fig. 17–5*A* and Table 17–1). Its action also prevents the flexion of the trunk that would occur if the forward momentum of the trunk generated by walking were to remain unchecked. The gluteus maximus muscle is a strong lateral rotator of the thigh (Fig. 17–5*B* and see Fig. 17–2), and its superior fibers are strong abductors of the thigh (Fig. 17–5*C* and Table 17–1 and see Fig. 17–2). It indirectly stabilizes the knee joint when one is standing by augmenting the tension of the iliotibial tract.

The pelvic attachment of the **gluteus medius muscle** is extensive. The gluteus medius muscle arises from the superior part of the dorsal surface of the ilium just lateral to the attachment of the gluteus maximus muscle (Figs. 17–3*A*, *B*, and *D* and 17–4*A*). As a consequence, its medial one third is covered by the gluteus maximus muscle and its lateral two thirds is uncovered (Fig. 17–3*A*). Its fibers course inferiorly and laterally. Its convergent inferior fibers form a tendon, which is attached to the lateral surface of the greater trochanter. The movements of the gluteus medius muscle over the greater trochanter are cushioned by the **trochanteric bursa of the gluteus medius muscle.**

The main action of the gluteus medius muscle is to abduct the thigh (Fig. 17–5*C* and see Fig. 17–2), but its anterior fibers also rotate the thigh in a medial direction (Fig. 17–5*D* and Table 17–1 and see Fig. 17–2).

The **gluteus minimus muscle** is completely covered by the gluteus medius muscle, and, therefore, its origin from the dorsal surface of the ilium is located directly inferior to that of the gluteus medius muscle (Fig. 17–3*B* and *E*). Its fibers course inferolaterally, converging to form a tendon, which is attached to the anterior surface of the greater trochanter of the femur (Figs. 17–3*B* and 17–4*B*). The muscle's movements over the trochanter are cushioned by the **trochanteric bursa of the gluteus minimus muscle.**

The gluteus minimus muscle acts in conjunction with the gluteus medius muscle to abduct and rotate the

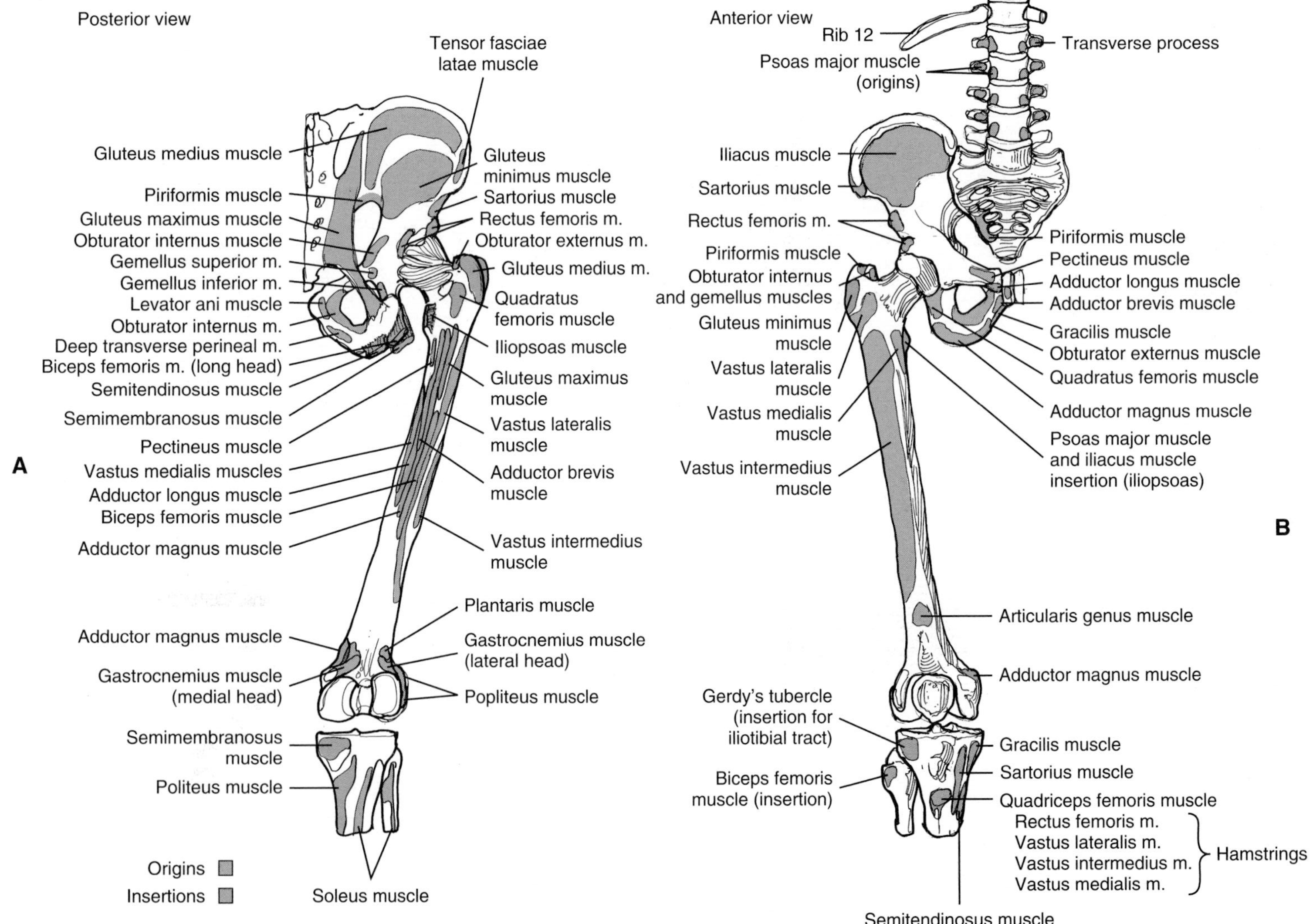

FIGURE 17–4
Origins and insertions of gluteal muscles. **A,** Posterior view. **B,** Anterior view.

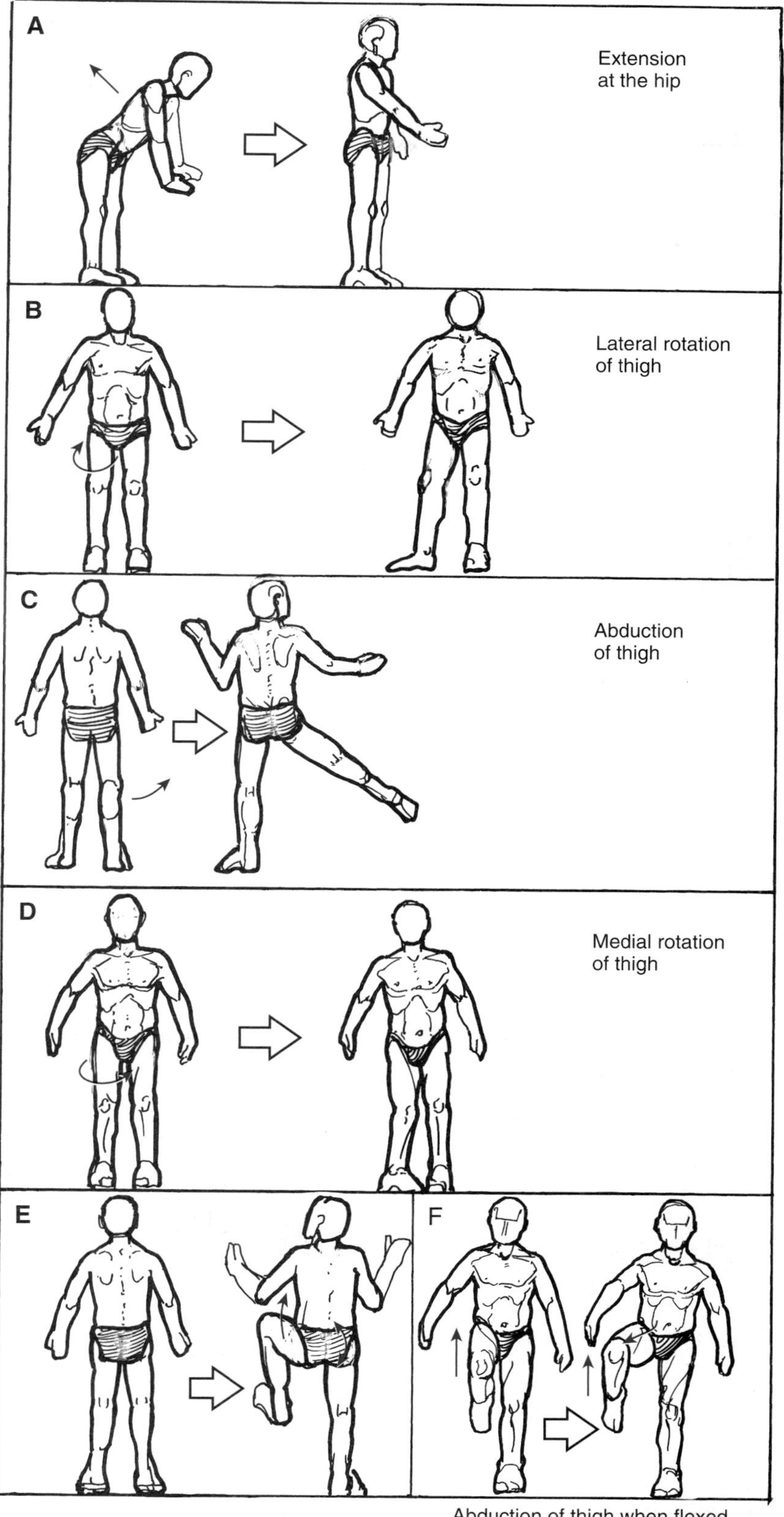

FIGURE 17–5

Actions of gluteal muscles. **A.** Extension of the hip. **B.** Lateral rotation of the thigh. **C.** Abduction of the thigh. **D.** Medial rotation of the thigh. **E** and **F.** Abduction of the thigh when flexed.

TABLE 17–1
Attachments and Actions of Gluteal Muscles

Muscle Group	Individual Muscle	Proximal Attachment	Distal Attachment	Action
Superficial gluteal muscles	Gluteus maximus	Posterior gluteal line and iliac crest of medial ilium; lateral region of dorsal surface of sacrum; aponeurosis of erector spinae muscle; sacrotuberous ligament; fascia of gluteus medius muscle	Iliotibial tract; posterior surface of proximal shaft of femur	Extension of trunk when thigh is flexed; lateral rotation of thigh; abduction of thigh; stabilization of knee joint
	Gluteus medius	Superior part of dorsal surface of ilium	Lateral surface of greater trochanter of femur	Abduction of thigh; medial rotation of thigh
	Gluteus minimus	Dorsal surface of ilium	Anterior surface of greater trochanter of femur	Abduction of thigh; medial rotation of thigh
Deep lateral rotators of gluteal region	Piriformis	Inner surface of sacrum	Superior boundary of greater trochanter of femur	Lateral rotation of thigh when extended; abduction of thigh when flexed
	Obturator internus	Inner border of obturator foramen and obturator membrane	Medial surface of greater trochanter of femur	Lateral rotation of thigh when extended; abduction of thigh when flexed
	Superior gemellus	Dorsal surface of ischial spine	Medial surface of greater trochanter of femur	Lateral rotation of thigh when extended; abduction of thigh when flexed
	Inferior gemellus	Ischial tuberosity	Medial surface of greater trochanter of femur	Lateral rotation of thigh when extended; abduction of thigh when flexed
	Quadratus femoris	Posterior surface of ischial body	Intertrochanteric crest and quadrate tubercle on posterior surface of femur	Lateral rotation of thigh
	Obturator externus	Outer border of obturator foramen; medial region of obturator membrane	Trochanteric fossa on medial side of greater trochanter	Lateral rotation of thigh

thigh in a medial direction (Fig. 17–5*C* and *D* and Table 17–1 and see Fig. 17–2). The most significant action of these two muscles, however, is to support the hip when the foot on the same side is raised from the substratum during walking or running (Fig. 17–5*E* and Table 17–1 and see discussion of locomotion at the end of this chapter).

Deep Lateral Rotators of the Gluteal Region. The **piriformis muscle** arises within the pelvis from the inner surface of the sacrum between the sacral foramina (Fig. 17–3*D*). Its body passes laterally and anteriorly through the greater sciatic (ischiatic) foramen. Its tendon attaches to the superior boundary of the greater trochanter of the femur (Figs. 17–3*B* and *F* and 17–4*B*). Its distal tendon may be partially consolidated with tendons of the gemellus superior, gemellus inferior, and obturator internus muscles (Fig. 17–3*B*).

Actions of the piriformis muscle include rotation of the thigh in a lateral direction when it is extended (Fig. 17–5*B* and see Fig. 17–2) and abduction of the thigh when it is flexed (Fig. 17–5*F* and Table 17–1).

The **obturator internus muscle** also originates from the inner surface of the pelvis, from the bone that forms the boundary of the obturator foramen, and from the inner surface of the obturator membrane (Figs. 17–3*B*, *G*, and *H* and 17–4*A*). This fan-shaped muscle narrows as its fibers join to form its distal tendon, which exits the pelvis via the lesser sciatic foramen (Fig. 17–3*B*). As the obturator internus tendon exits the lesser sciatic foramen, it loops around a groove between the ischial spine and ischial tuberosity. The tendon courses over the hip joint capsule and inserts within an anterior groove of the medial surface of the greater trochanter of the femur (Figs. 17–3*B*, *G*, and *H* and 17–4*B*).

The obturator internus muscle acts with the gemellus superior, gemellus inferior, and piriformis muscles to laterally rotate the extended thigh (Fig. 17–5*B* and see Fig. 17–2) and to abduct the thigh when it is flexed (Fig. 17–5*C* and Table 17–1 and see Fig. 17–2).

The **superior** and **inferior gemellus muscles** are located along the superior and inferior boundaries of the obturator internus tendon (Fig. 17–3*B* and *G*). The

superior gemellus muscle arises from the dorsal surface of the ischial spine. Its tendon joins with the obturator internus tendon to insert into the medial surface of the greater trochanter of the femur (Figs. 17–3*B* and 17–4*B*). The **inferior gemellus muscle** arises from the ischial tuberosity adjacent to the lower border of the obturator internus muscle. Its tendon also joins with the obturator internus tendon to insert into the medial surface of the greater trochanter (Figs. 17–3*B* and *G* and 17–4*B*).

The actions of both of these muscles include assisting the obturator internus muscle in both rotating the extended thigh in a lateral direction (Fig. 17–5*B* and see Fig. 17–2) and in abducting the thigh when it is flexed (Fig. 17–5*B* and Table 17–1 and see Fig. 17–2).

The **quadratus femoris muscle** is a flattened quadrilateral muscle arising from the posterior surface of the ischial body just beneath the acetabulum (Fig. 17–3*B* and *G*). It courses in a lateral direction to insert upon the intertrochanteric crest on the posterior surface of the femur (Fig. 17–4*A*).

The quadratus femoris muscle thus acts as a lateral rotator of the thigh (Fig. 17–5*B* and Table 17–1 and see Fig. 17–2).

As has been noted above, the **obturator externus muscle** arises from bone that forms the anterior boundary of the obturator foramen and from the medial region of the obturator membrane. It essentially mirrors the obturator internus muscle (Fig. 17–3*B* and *I* and above). It is classified as a gluteal muscle, however, because its fibers course laterally and around the posterior side of the neck of the femur to insert into the trochanteric fossa on the medial side of the greater trochanter (Fig. 17–3*I*).

The obturator externus muscle acts to assist the quadratus femoris muscle in the lateral rotation of the thigh (Fig. 17–5*B* and see Fig. 17–2).

Muscles of the Thigh (Femoral Muscles)

Muscles of the thigh are located in anterior, medial, and posterior compartments, which are separated from each other by thick intermuscular septa. A thick **lateral intermuscular septum** separates muscles of the anterior and posterior compartments, and a thinner **medial intermuscular septum** separates muscles of the anterior and medial compartments (Fig. 17–6). The muscles of the medial and posterior compartments are separated by an unnamed fascial septum.

Muscles of the Anterior Compartment of the Thigh. These muscles act upon the hip and knee joints. The main functions of these muscles are to flex the hip joint and extend the knee joint (see Table 17–2 and Fig. 17–8*A*). Other functions are also served by these muscles (see Fig. 17–8). Muscles of this compartment include the tensor fasciae latae, sartorius, and quadriceps femoris muscles (including the rectus femoris and three vastus muscles). The main parts of the bodies of the psoas major and iliacus muscles are located within the peritoneal cavity and are, therefore, usually described with muscles of the posterior abdomen (see Chapters 13 and 14). However, the tendons of the psoas major and iliacus muscles exit the false pelvis to cross the hip joint, acting as flexors of the thigh and trunk. Therefore, they are described with muscles of the anterior compartment of the thigh.

As has been noted in Chapters 13 and 14, the **psoas major muscle** arises from all five lumbar vertebral transverse processes and from five muscle slips, each of which is attached to the lateral surfaces of two vertebral bodies and their intervening disc (Fig. 17–7*A* and *B*). The body of the psoas major muscle courses inferiorly within the true pelvis, just adjacent to the pelvic brim, and exits the pelvis under the inguinal ligament to enter the anterior compartment of the thigh. The inferior tendon of the psoas major muscle joins with the tendon of the iliacus muscle. The consolidated tendons pass anterior to the hip joint capsule and attach to the lesser trochanter of the femur (Fig. 17–7 and see Fig. 17–4*B*). The psoas-iliacus tendon is separated from the hip joint capsule by the **iliopectineal bursa.**

Because the psoas major muscle crosses between the lumbar vertebrae and sacrum as well as near the hip joint, its primary action is flexion of the trunk or thigh, or both, when one is lying in a supine position as when one is doing sit-ups (Fig. 17–8*B* and Table 17–2). The muscle may also function in walking but, apparently, only when it is consciously activated (Fig. 17–8*A*). The psoas major muscle also laterally rotates the thigh as it pulls the lesser trochanter on the medial femur forward (Figs. 17–8*C* and 17–9).

The **psoas minor muscle,** when present, originates from a slip attached to vertebral bodies T12 and L1 and their intervening disc.

The distal tendon of the psoas minor muscle is attached to the pecten pubis (Fig. 17–7*A*), and so the muscle acts only weakly to flex the trunk but not the thigh (Fig. 17–8*B* and Table 17–2).

The **iliacus muscle** arises from the iliac fossa and upper region of the sacroiliac joint and sacrum (Fig. 17–7*B*). Its most anterior and lateral fibers originate from the outer surface of the pelvis in the region of the anterior superior iliac spine (ASIS) and anterior inferior iliac spine (AIIS). The fan-shaped iliacus muscle narrows as it passes under the inguinal ligament. Its tendon courses inferiorly, lateral to the tendon of the psoas major muscle, which it joins (Fig. 17–7*B* and see above).

The iliacus muscle acts in concert with the psoas major muscle (see above). However, because the iliacus muscle originates within the pelvis and does not cross any of the intervertebral joints, it acts only in flexing and laterally rotating the thigh (Fig. 17–8*B* and *C* and Table 17–2).

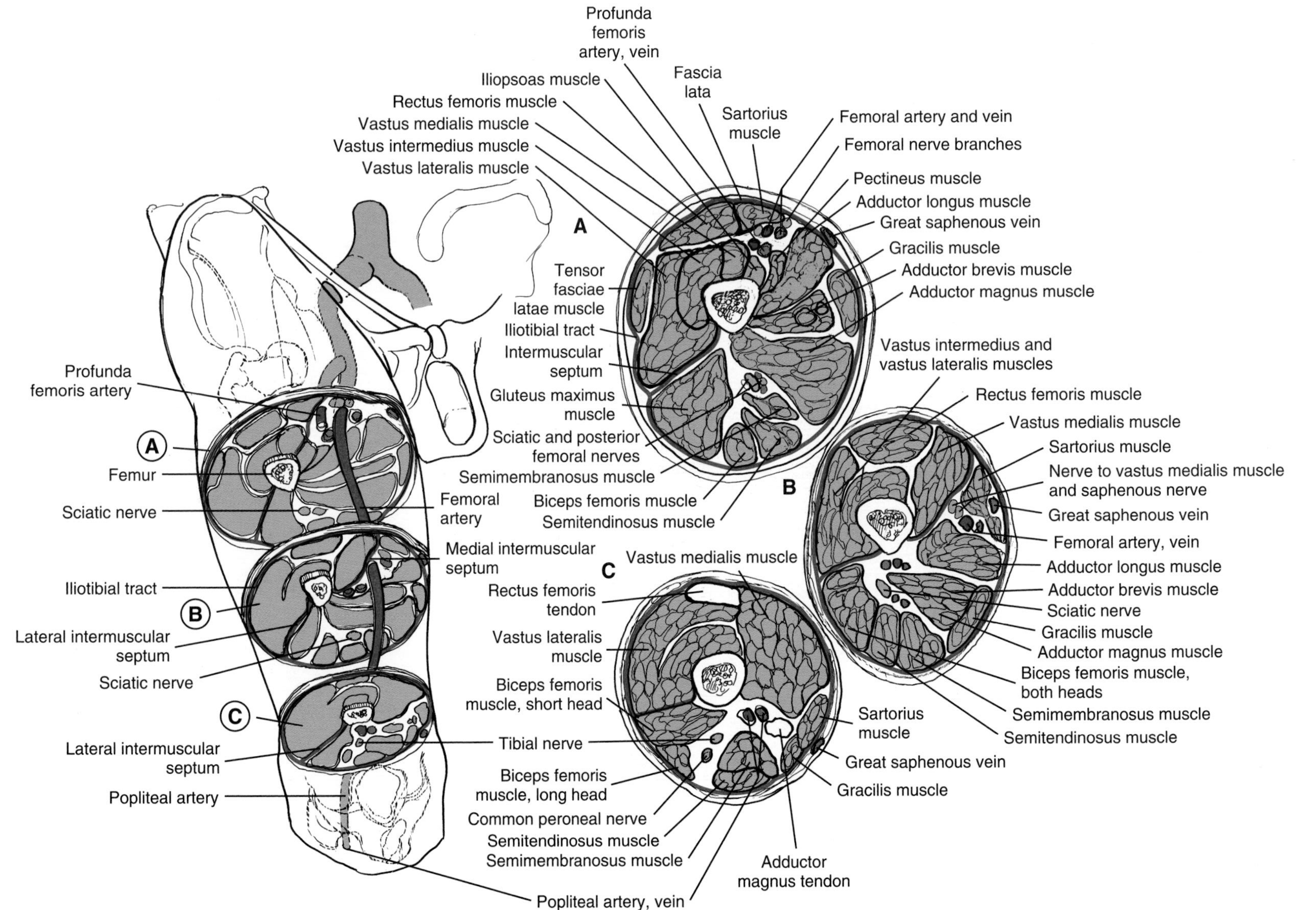

FIGURE 17–6

The drawing at the left shows the muscles of the thigh organized into compartments, as an orientation view for parts A, B, and C. **A.** Cross section showing muscles of the upper thigh. **B.** Cross section showing muscles of the mid thigh. **C.** Cross section showing muscles above the knee.

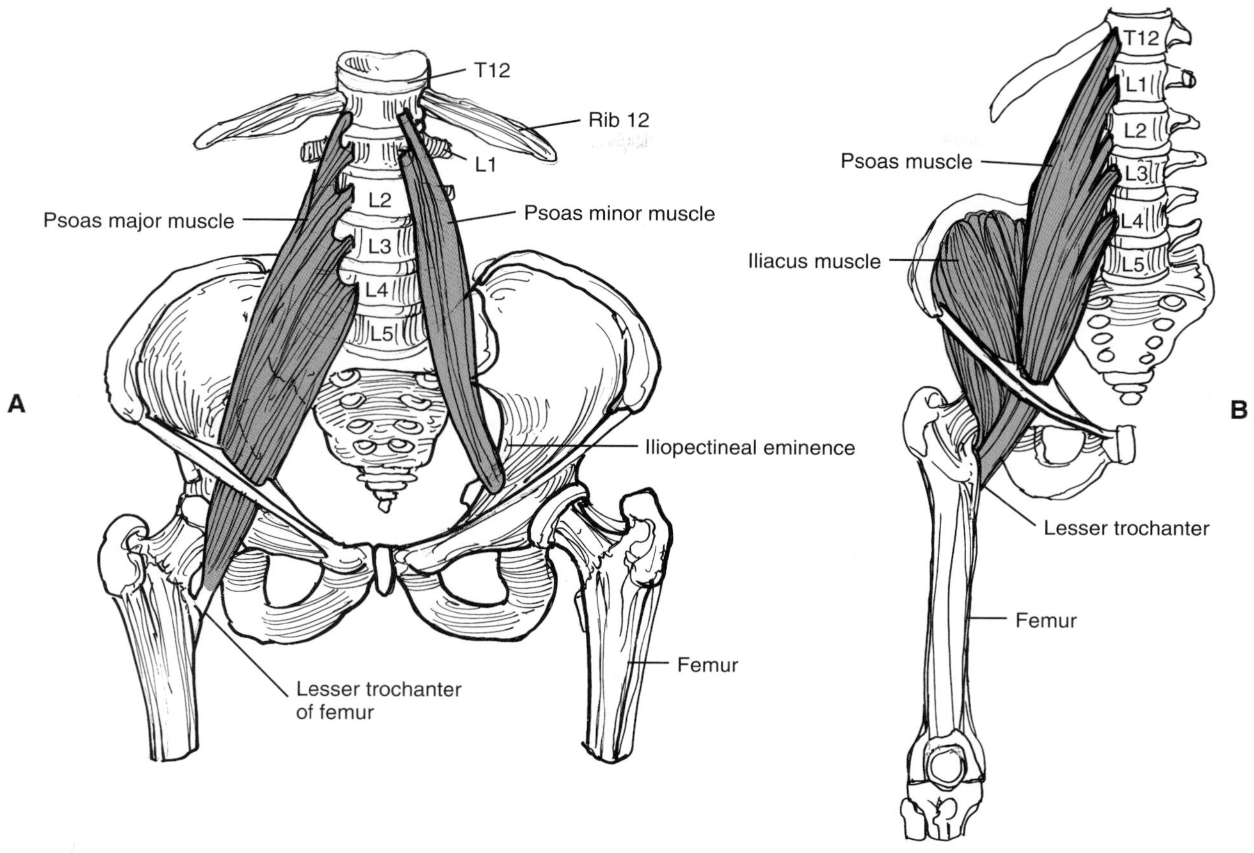

FIGURE 17–7
A, Psoas major and minor muscles. **B,** Iliacus muscles.

The remaining muscles of the anterior thigh compartment cross both the hip and knee joints or the knee joint only. These muscles include the tensor fasciae latae, sartorius, rectus femoris, and vastus muscles (Figs. 17–10 and 17–11).

The superior end of the **tensor fasciae latae muscle** arises from a small posterolateral region of the iliac crest, just superior to the ASIS, and from the deep surface of the fascia lata (Fig. 17–10). Its inferior end attaches to the iliotibial tract near the boundary between the upper and middle thirds of the thigh. The iliotibial tract courses inferiorly to attach to Gerdy's tubercle just inferior to the lateral condyle on the anterior surface of the tibia (Fig. 17–10 and see Fig. 17–4*B* and below).

The tensor fasciae latae muscle and its distal tendon thus cross two joints, the hip and knee joints, and so their chief actions are to flex (Fig. 17–8*A*) and medially rotate the thigh (Fig. 17–8*D*) and to extend (Fig. 17–8*A*) and laterally rotate the leg (Fig. 17–8*E* and Table 17–2).

The **sartorius muscle** also crosses both the hip and knee joints. Because it courses from the anterior tip of the anterior surface of the ASIS to the anteromedial surface of the tibia, its actions are relatively complex (Figs. 17–10*B* and 17–11).

The sartorius muscle acts to flex the hip and knee joints while it abducts and laterally rotates the thigh (see Fig. 17–8*H* and Table 17–2). This occurs when a person sits down and places the lateral surface of one ankle on the contralateral knee (as would a tailor while mending a garment).

The sartorius muscle also forms one of the boundaries of the **femoral triangle.** This landmark of the thigh is formed by the medial edge of the sartorius muscle (inferolateral boundary), lateral edge of the adductor longus muscle (inferomedial boundary) (see below), and inguinal ligament (superior boundary) (Figs. 17–10*B* and 17–11). Several significant anatomic structures are located within the femoral triangle, namely, the femoral sheath and its contents, including the femoral artery, vein, lymphatics, and nerve.

The **quadriceps femoris muscle** is a compound muscle made up of (1) the **rectus femoris,** (2) **vastus lateralis,** (3) **vastus intermedius,** and (4) **vastus medialis muscles** (Figs. 17–10*B* and 17–11). The superior ends of the four heads of the quadriceps femoris muscle

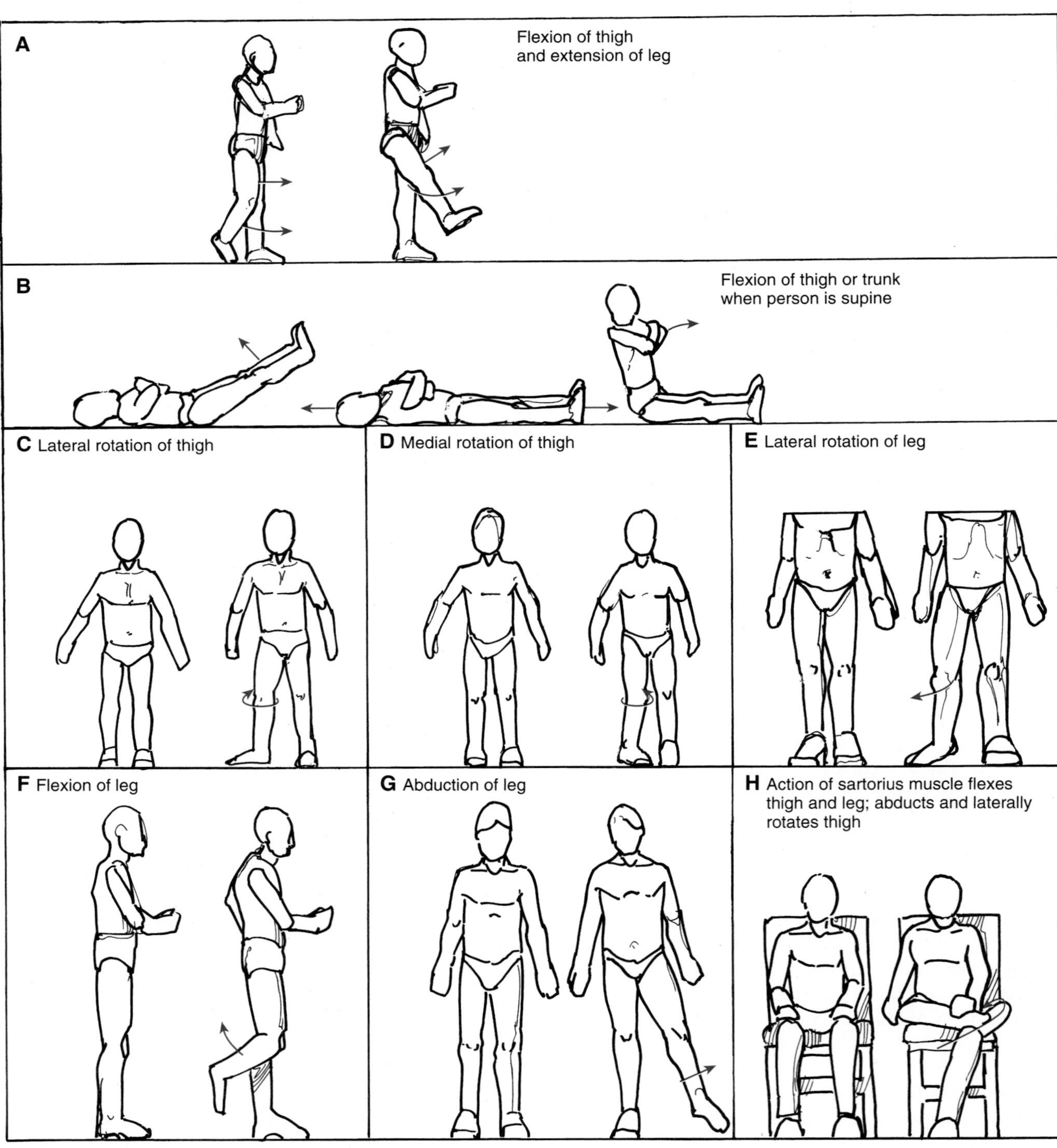

FIGURE 17–8

Lower limb movements governed by the muscles of the thigh.

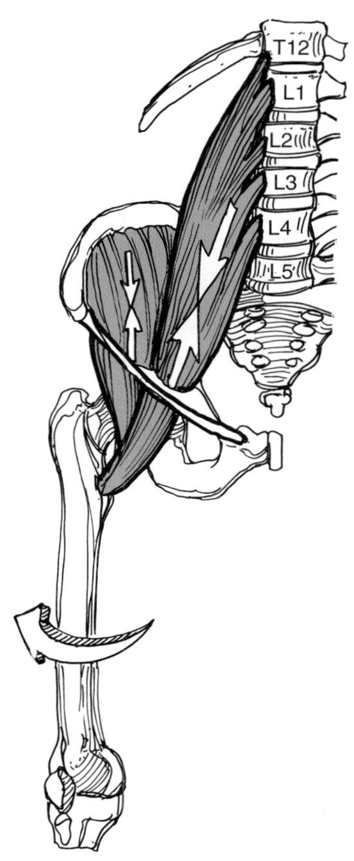

FIGURE 17–9
Lateral rotation of the thigh by the psoas major muscle.

arise from different points, but their inferior tendons merge to form the **quadriceps ligament,** which courses over the patella and continues as the **patellar ligament** (Figs. 17–10 and 17–11). The patellar tendon is attached to the **tibial tuberosity** on the anterior surface of the tibia (Fig. 17–11). The **rectus femoris muscle** arises from the AIIS and an adjacent site on the acetabular labrum (lip) and thus crosses both the hip and knee joints (Fig. 17–11*B* and see Fig. 17–4*B*). The **rest of the muscles of the quadriceps complex** arise from the shaft of the femur. The vastus lateralis muscle arises from the intertrochanteric line, the vastus intermedius muscle from a large region of the anterolateral shaft of the femur, and the vastus medialis muscle from a small region just anterior to the lesser trochanter of the femur (see Fig. 17–4*B*).

The rectus femoris muscle acts to flex the thigh and, with the vastus muscles, to extend the leg at the knee (Fig. 17–8*A*). The quadriceps muscle also prevents lateral displacement of the patella from its groove on the patellar surface of the femur. This could easily happen if the muscle did not shorten during the final phase of extension at the knee.

The diminutive **articularis genus muscle** is technically a fifth member of the quadriceps femoris group. It lies deep to the vastus intermedius muscle and arises from the anterior surface of the distal end of the femur (Fig. 17–11*E* and see Fig. 17–4*B*).

The articularis genus muscle inserts onto a superior extension of the synovial membrane of the subpatellar bursa and acts to pull the bursa superiorly during extension of the knee joint.

Muscles of the Medial Compartment of the Thigh. These muscles include the gracilis, pectineus, adductor longus, adductor brevis, and adductor magnus muscles (Fig. 17–12). The gracilis muscle crosses both the hip and knee joints, but the other muscles cross the hip joint only.

The **gracilis muscle** originates from the anterior surface and inferior edge of the inferior pubic ramus (Fig. 17–12). This long flat muscle courses inferiorly, curves around the medial aspect of the knee joint, and inserts upon the anterior surface of the tibia just inferior to the medial tibial condyle (Figs. 17–11*B* and 17–12 and see Fig. 17–4*B*).

The actions of the gracilis muscle include flexion of the leg (Fig. 17–13*A*) and medial rotation of the leg (Fig. 17–13*B* and Table 17–2).

The **pectineus muscle** lies just medial to the psoas major muscle in the superior thigh. It arises from the pectineal line and anterior surface of the superior pubic ramus (Fig. 17–11 and 17–12 and see Fig. 17–4*B*). This fan-shaped muscle narrows as it courses inferiorly, laterally, and posteriorly to insert upon the medial lip of the linea aspera, just inferior to the lesser tubercle of the femur (Fig. 17–12*B* and see Fig. 17–4*A*). The pectineus muscle is sometimes split into superficial and deep layers, which are innervated by branches of the femoral and obturator nerves (see below).

The pectineus muscle acts to adduct the thigh (Fig. 17–13*C*).

The **adductor longus muscle** is the most anterior of the three adductor muscles. It lies just medial to the pectineus muscle (Figs. 17–11*A* to *C* and 17–12). This fan-shaped muscle arises from the midregion of the anterior surface of the pubic body (Fig. 17–12*B* and see Fig. 17–4*B*). It narrows as it courses inferiorly and laterally and sweeps posteriorly around the shaft of the femur to insert upon the lower part of the linea aspera (Fig. 17–12 and see Fig. 17–4*A*).

The adductor longus muscle acts in a synergistic way to control gait and maintain posture by adducting and flexing the thigh (Fig. 17–13*C* and *D* and Table 17–2).

The **adductor brevis muscle** lies posterior to the pectineus and adductor longus muscles (Fig. 17–12). This short triangular muscle arises from the anterior surfaces of the pubic body and its inferior ramus (see Fig. 17–4*B*). The adductor brevis muscle narrows as it

TABLE 17–2
Attachments and Actions of Femoral (Thigh) Muscles

Muscle Group	Individual Muscle	Proximal Attachment	Distal Attachment	Action
Muscles of anterior compartment of thigh	Psoas major	All five lumbar transverse processes; lateral surfaces of all five lumbar vertebrae and intervening discs	Lesser trochanter of femur	Flexes trunk when one is lying supine (strong)
	Psoas minor	Bodies of vertebrae T12 and L1	Pecten pubis	Flexes trunk (weak)
	Iliacus	Iliac fossa; upper region of sacroiliac joint; upper region of inner surface of sacrum	Joins tendon of psoas major muscle to insert on lesser trochanter of femur	Flexes thigh and acts in concert with psoas major muscle
	Tensor fasciae latae	Posterolateral iliac crest	Iliotibial tract, which, in turn, attaches to Gerdy's tubercle just inferior to lateral condyle anterior surface of tibia	Flexes and medially rotates thigh; extends and laterally rotates leg
	Sartorius	ASIS	Anteromedial surface of proximal tibia	Flexes, abducts, and laterally rotates thigh; flexes leg
	Rectus femoris	ASIS	Tibial tuberosity on anterior tibia as part of patellar tendon	Flexes thigh; extends leg
	Vastus lateralis	Intertrochanteric line of femur	Tibial tuberosity on anterior tibia as part of patellar tendon	Extends leg
	Vastus intermedius	Anterolateral shaft of femur	Tibial tuberosity on anterior tibia as part of patellar tendon	Extends leg
	Vastus medialis	Region just anterior to lesser trochanter of femur	Tibial tuberosity on anterior tibia as part of patellar tendon	Extends leg
	Articularis genus	Anterior surface of distal end of femur	Superior end of subpatellar bursa	Pulls subpatellar bursa superiorly when leg is extended
Muscles of medial compartment of thigh	Gracilis	Anterior surface and inferior edge of pubic ramus	Anterior surface of tibia just inferior to its medial epicondyle	Flexes and medially rotates leg
	Pectineus	Pectineal line; anterior surface of superior pubic ramus	Medial lip of linea aspera just inferior to lesser trochanter of femur	Adducts thigh
	Adductor longus	Midregion of anterior surface of pubic body	Lower part of linea aspera	Adducts and flexes thigh
	Adductor brevis	Anterior surface of pubic body and inferior pubic ramus	Posterior surface of femur between greater trochanter and linea aspera	Adducts and flexes thigh
Muscles of posterior compartment of thigh	Biceps femoris	Long head arises from midregion of ischial tuberosity and inferior part of sacrotuberous ligament; short head arises from lateral lip of linea aspera and superior part of supracondylar ridge of femur	Lateral surface of head of fibula	Long head extends thigh and flexes leg; short head flexes leg
	Semitendinosus	Midregion of ischial tuberosity	Medial side of anterior surface of tibia	Extends thigh; flexes leg; pulls body upright when bent forward; medially rotates leg

ASIS, Anterior superior iliac spine.

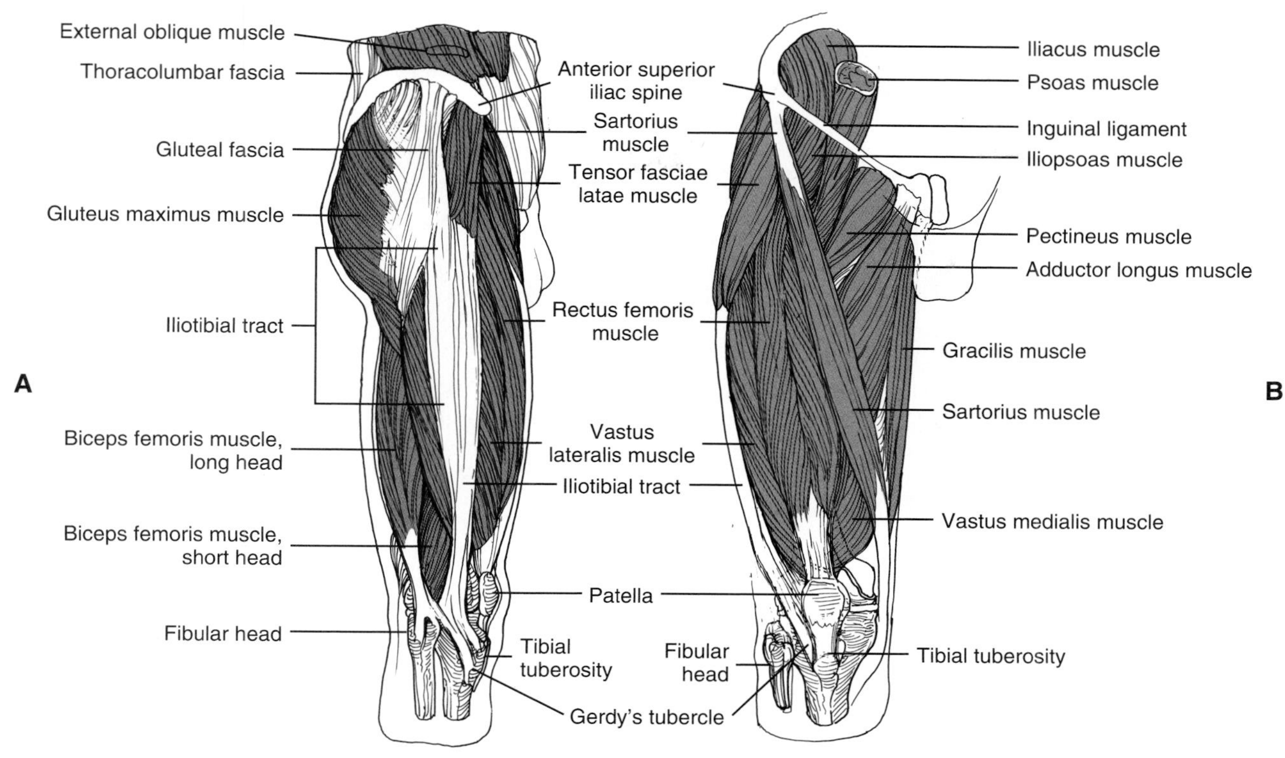

FIGURE 17–10
Lateral **(A)** and anterior **(B)** views of the femoral muscles.

courses posterolaterally to insert upon the posterior surface of the femur between the lesser trochanter and the superior end of the linea aspera.

The adductor brevis muscle acts to adduct (Fig. 17–13*C*) and flex (Fig. 17–13*D*) the thigh in concert with other adductors when one is standing, walking, or running (Table 17–2).

The **adductor magnus muscle** is the largest and most medially positioned of the three adductor muscles (Figs. 17–11*C* and 17–12). This fan-shaped muscle arises from the inferior part of the puboischial ramus (see Fig. 17–4*B*). It narrows as it descends posterolaterally to its extensive insertion on the linea aspera (just lateral to attachments of the adductor brevis and adductor longus muscles) and on the superior part of the medial supracondylar line of the femur (see Fig. 17–4*B*). The muscle's more medial fibers insert upon the adductor tubercle, just above the medial epicondyle of the femur. An opening in the lower border of the adductor magnus muscle, the **adductor hiatus,** allows the femoral artery and vein to cross from the anterior thigh compartment to the popliteal fossa (posterior to the knee) (see Chapter 18). In addition, the adductor magnus muscle has three or four other openings in more superior regions for the transport of **perforating branches** of the **arteria profunda femoris (deep femoral artery).** These vessels of the anterior compartment thus gain access to the posterior femoral compartment (see below).

The adductor magnus muscle contributes to the actions of adduction (Fig. 17–13*C*) and flexion (Fig. 17–13*D*) of the thigh when one is standing, walking, or running (Table 17–2).

Muscles of the Posterior Compartment of the Thigh. These include the biceps femoris, semitendinosus, and semimembranosus muscles. These muscles (except for the short head of the biceps femoris muscle) cross the hip and knee joints. They may act on just one of these joints if the other joint is fixed by counteracting muscle action or gravitational forces (Table 17–2). Like the muscles of the gluteal region, the posterior compartment muscles are most active during movement and only minimally active during standing. However, when the upper body bends forward, they become activated to counteract the force of gravity. This group of muscles is commonly called the **hamstrings.**

The **biceps femoris muscle** has **long** and **short heads** (Fig. 17–14). The long head arises from the middle of the ischial tuberosity and inferior part of the sacrotuberous ligament (Fig. 17–14*B*). This fusiform muscle courses inferiorly, joining with the short head, which arises from the lateral lip of the linea aspera and superior part of the lateral supracondylar line just lat-

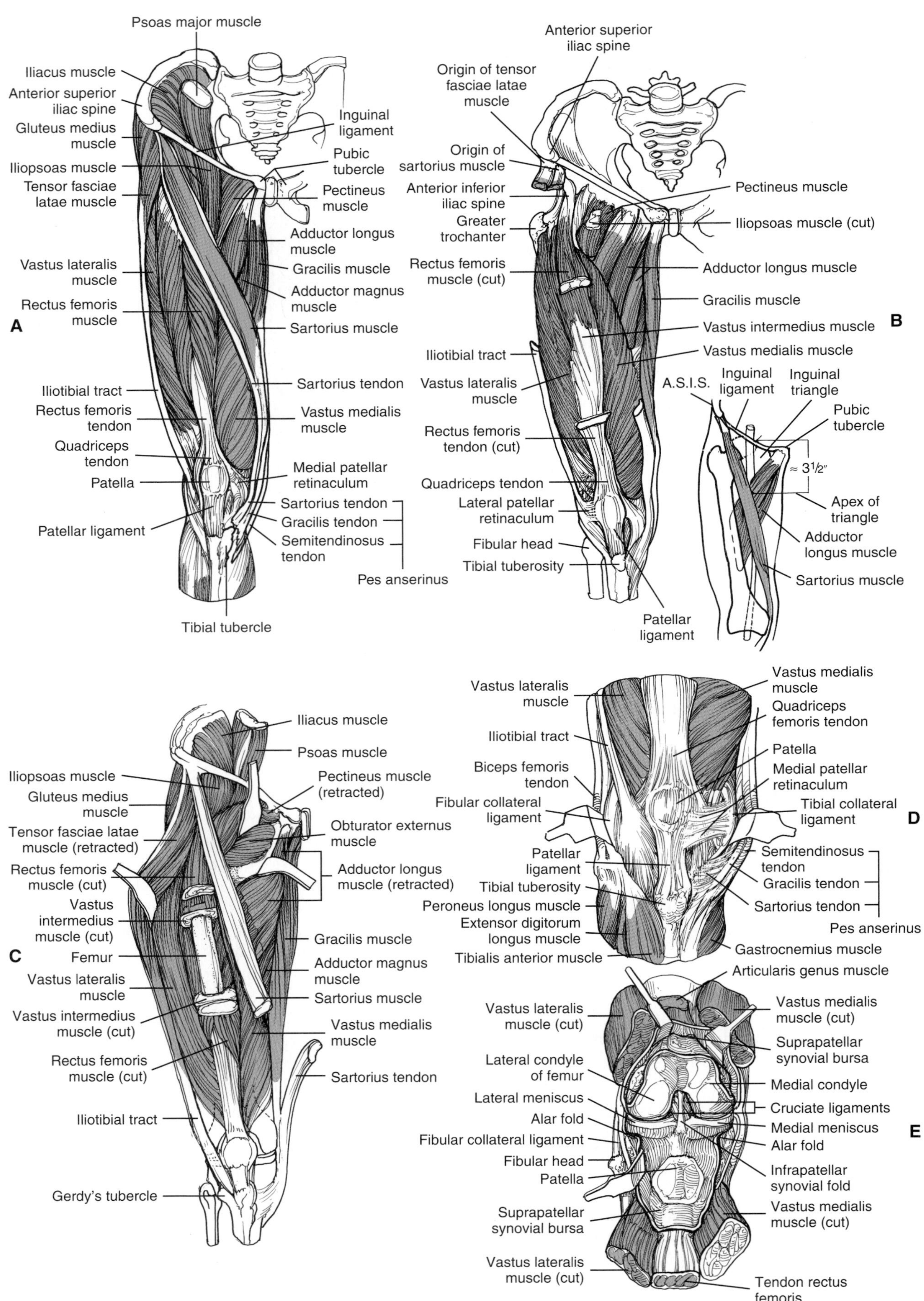

FIGURE 17–11
Muscles of the anterior compartment of the thigh.

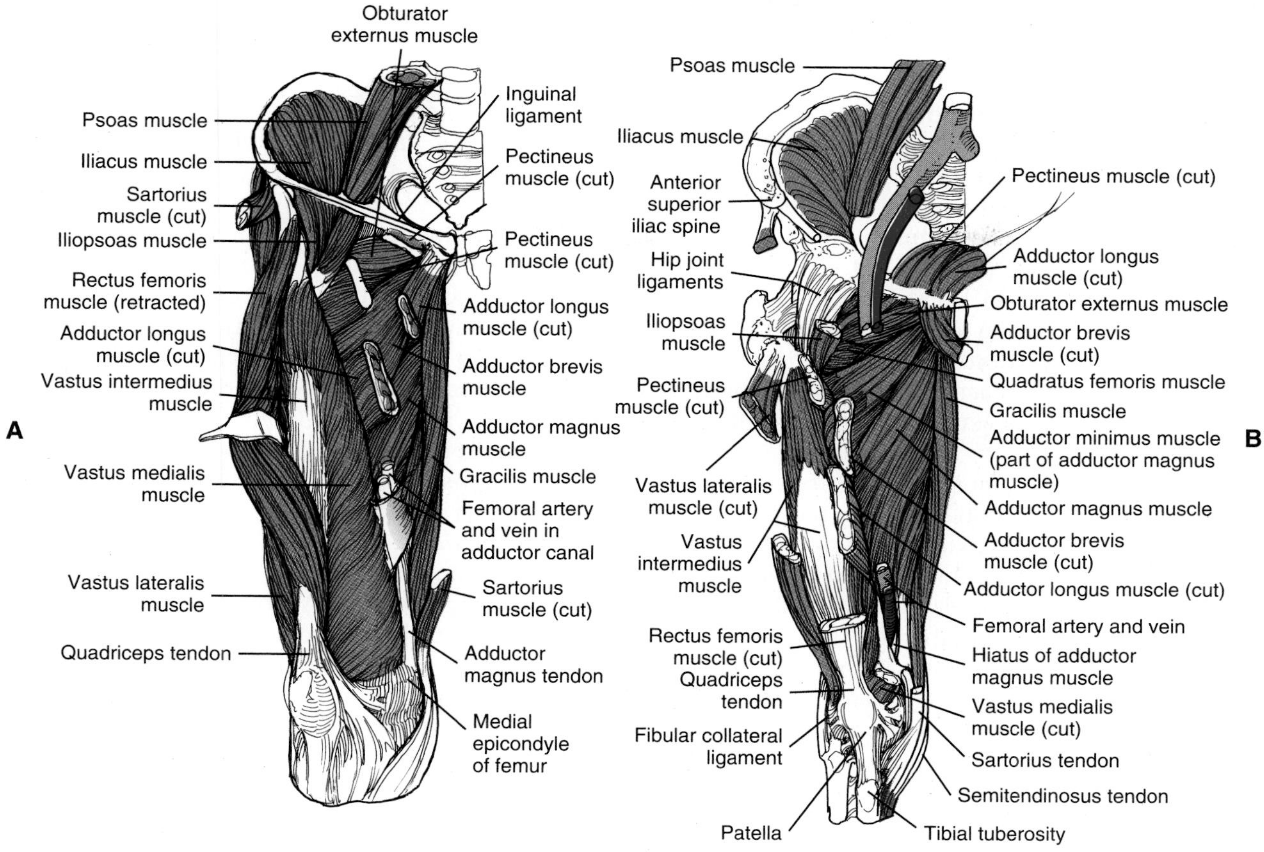

FIGURE 17–12
Muscles of the medial compartment of the thigh.

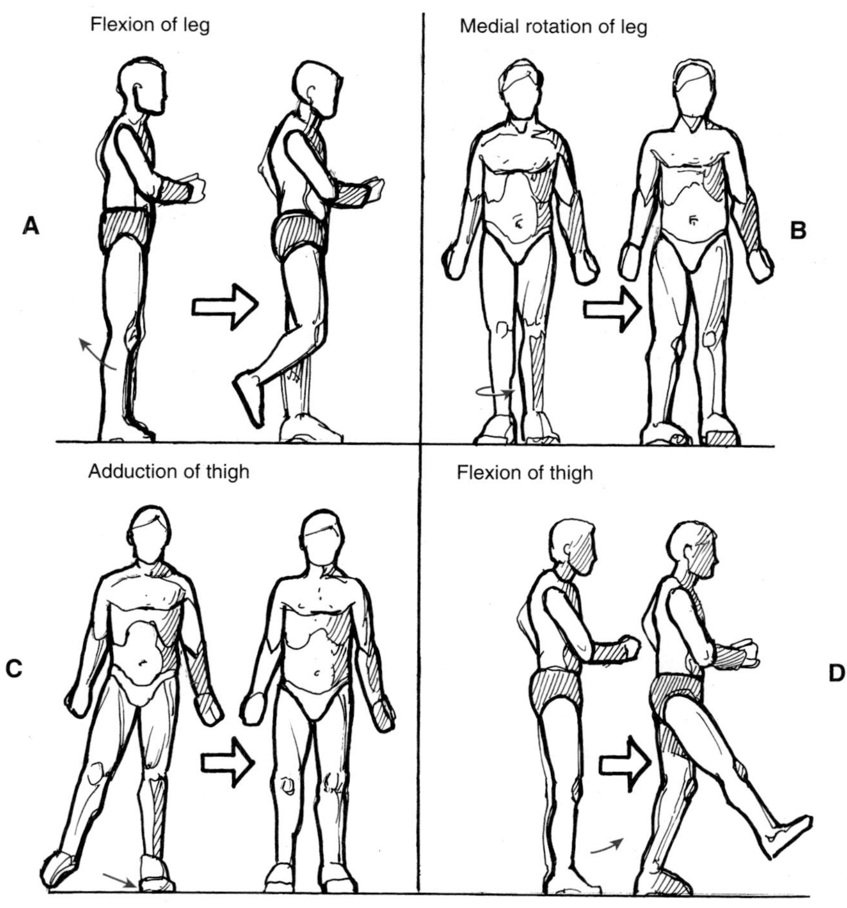

FIGURE 17–13
Actions of muscles of the medial compartment of the thigh.

eral to the origin of the adductor magnus muscle (Fig. 17–14*B* and see Fig. 17–4*A*). The fused inferior part of the muscle narrows into a tendon (or lateral hamstring) that passes inferiorly over the lateral part of the posterior surface of the knee joint to insert upon the lateral surface of the fibular head (Fig. 17–14).

The long head of the biceps femoris muscle acts to extend the hip and flex the knee joint (Fig. 17–15*A*). The short head flexes only the knee joint (Fig. 17–15*B*). Both heads are active in lateral rotation of the leg when the knee is extended (Fig. 17–15*C* and Table 17–2).

The **semitendinosus muscle** arises from a tendon that it shares with the long head of the biceps muscle and semimembranosus muscle (Fig. 17–14*B* and see Fig. 17–4*A*). It therefore originates from the posterior surface of the midregion of the ischial tuberosity and inferior aspect of the sacrotuberous ligament (Fig. 17–14*B*). This long fusiform muscle courses inferiorly along the posterior surface of the semimembranosus muscle (see below). Its inferior tendon begins near the boundary between the middle and lower thirds of the thigh (Fig. 17–14*A*). The tendon sweeps inferolaterally around the medial tibial condyle and attaches to the medial side of the anterior tibial surface just beneath the attachment for the gracilis muscle and medial to the attachment for the sartorius muscle.

The semitendinosus muscle acts with other hamstring muscles to extend the thigh, flex the leg (Fig. 17–15*A*), and pull the upper body upright against the forces of gravity when the body is bent forward (Fig. 17–15*D*). In contrast to the biceps femoris muscle, the semitendinosus muscle rotates the leg in a medial direction (Fig. 17–15*E* and Table 17–2).

The superior tendon of the **semimembranosus muscle** arises from the lateral surface of the ischial tuberosity (Fig. 17–14*B*). This long, flattened muscle courses inferiorly just anterior to the semitendinosus muscle for most of its length (Fig. 17–14). The inferior tendon of the semimembranosus muscle begins just superior to the medial condyle of the femur and crosses the knee joint to insert upon the posteromedial surface of the tibia, just beneath the medial tibial condyle (Fig. 17–14*B* and see Fig. 17–4*B*). Other tendinous slips attach to surrounding fascia and ligaments on the medial side of the knee.

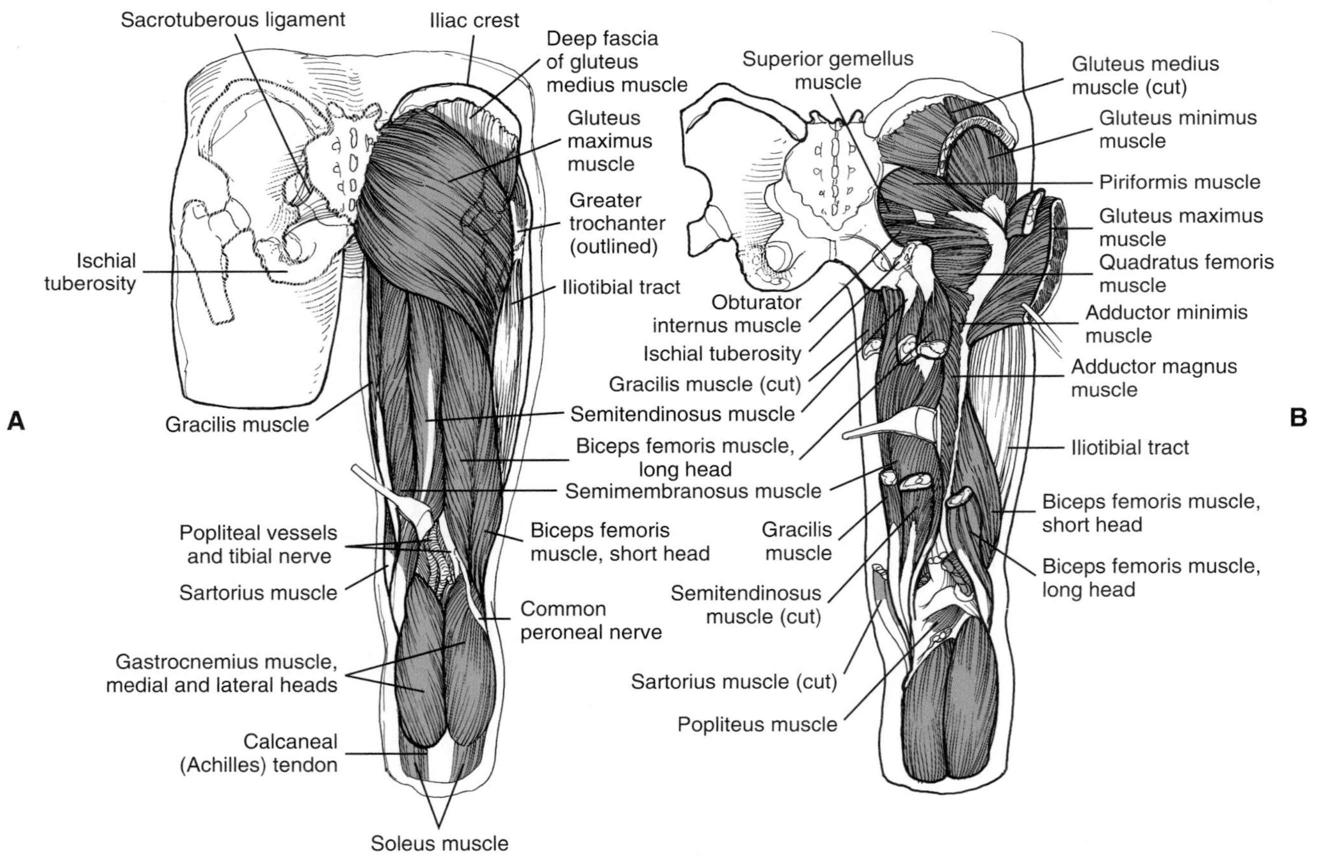

FIGURE 17–14
Muscles of the posterior compartment of the thigh.

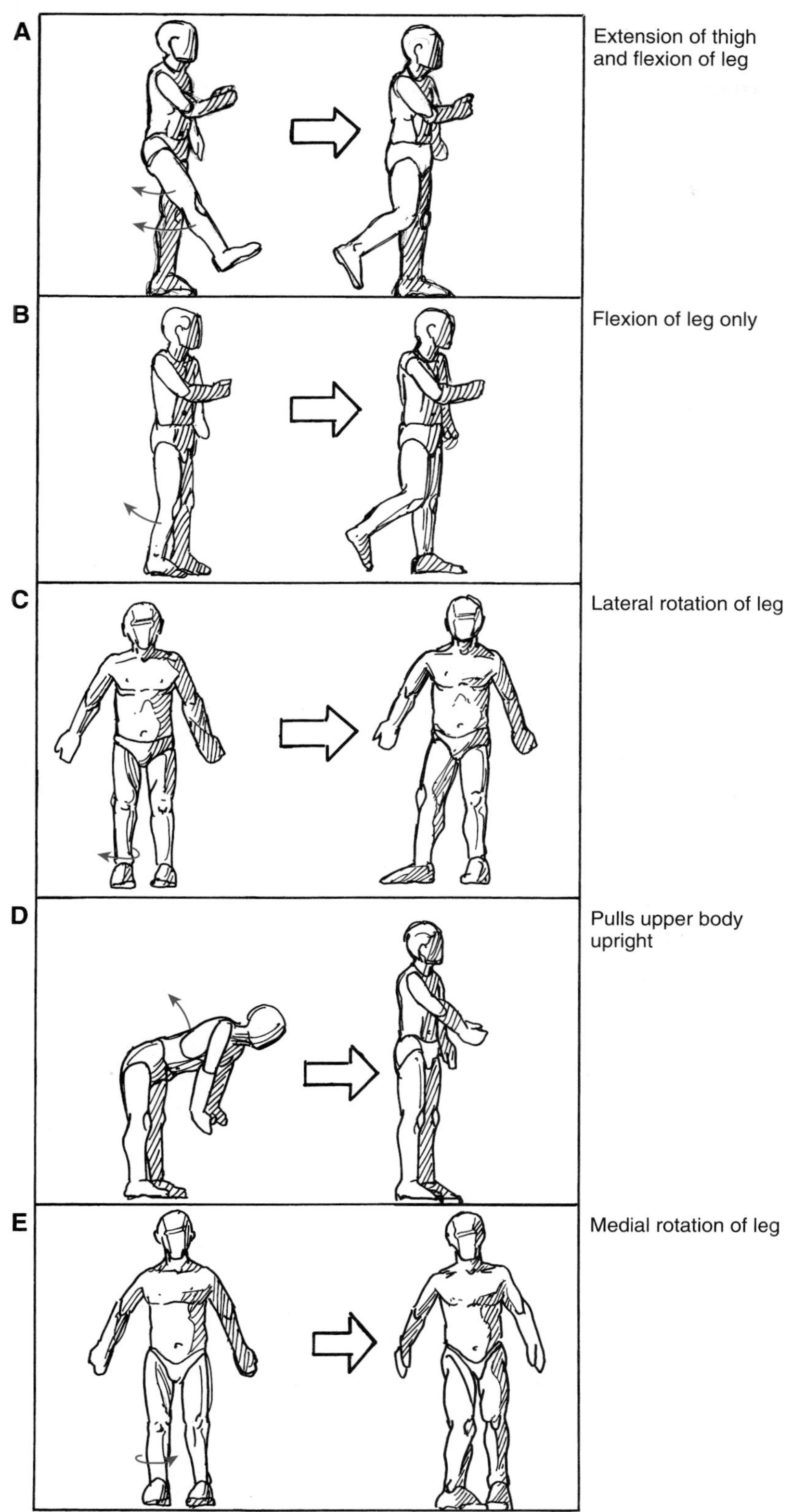

FIGURE 17–15
Actions of muscles of the posterior compartment of the thigh.

The semimembranosus muscle acts to extend the hip, to flex the knee (Fig. 17–15*A*), and, with the semitendinosus muscle, to rotate the leg in a medial direction (Fig. 17–15*E* and Table 17–2).

Muscles of the Leg (Crural Muscles)

Crural muscles (muscles of the leg) are organized in three major groups: extensors of the anterior compartment, flexors of the posterior compartment, and muscles of the lateral compartment (Fig. 17–16 and Table 17–3). Anterior, posterior, and lateral (peroneal) compartments of the leg are separated by thick fascial septa. For example, the anterior and posterior compartments are separated by the **interosseous membrane** that joins the tibia and fibula (Fig. 17–16 and see discussion of the tibiofibular joint in Chapter 16). The lateral compartment is separated from the anterior compartment by an **anterior intermuscular septum** and from the posterior compartment by a **posterior intermuscular septum.**

Because the upper and lower limbs rotate in opposite directions during embryogenesis, the positions and, thus, the actions of the anterior and posterior compartment muscles of the leg are reversed. Anterior muscles of the leg are extensors (Table 17–3 and see above), whereas anterior muscles of the forearm are flexors (see Chapter 20). Posterior muscles of the leg are flexors (see Fig. 17–24), whereas posterior muscles of the forearm are extensors (see Chapter 20).

Muscles of the Posterior Compartment of the Leg. The **posterior crural compartment** is divided into a **superficial posterior compartment,** which contains the gastrocnemius, soleus, and plantaris muscles and a **deep posterior compartment,** which contains the popliteus, flexor hallucis longus, flexor digitorum

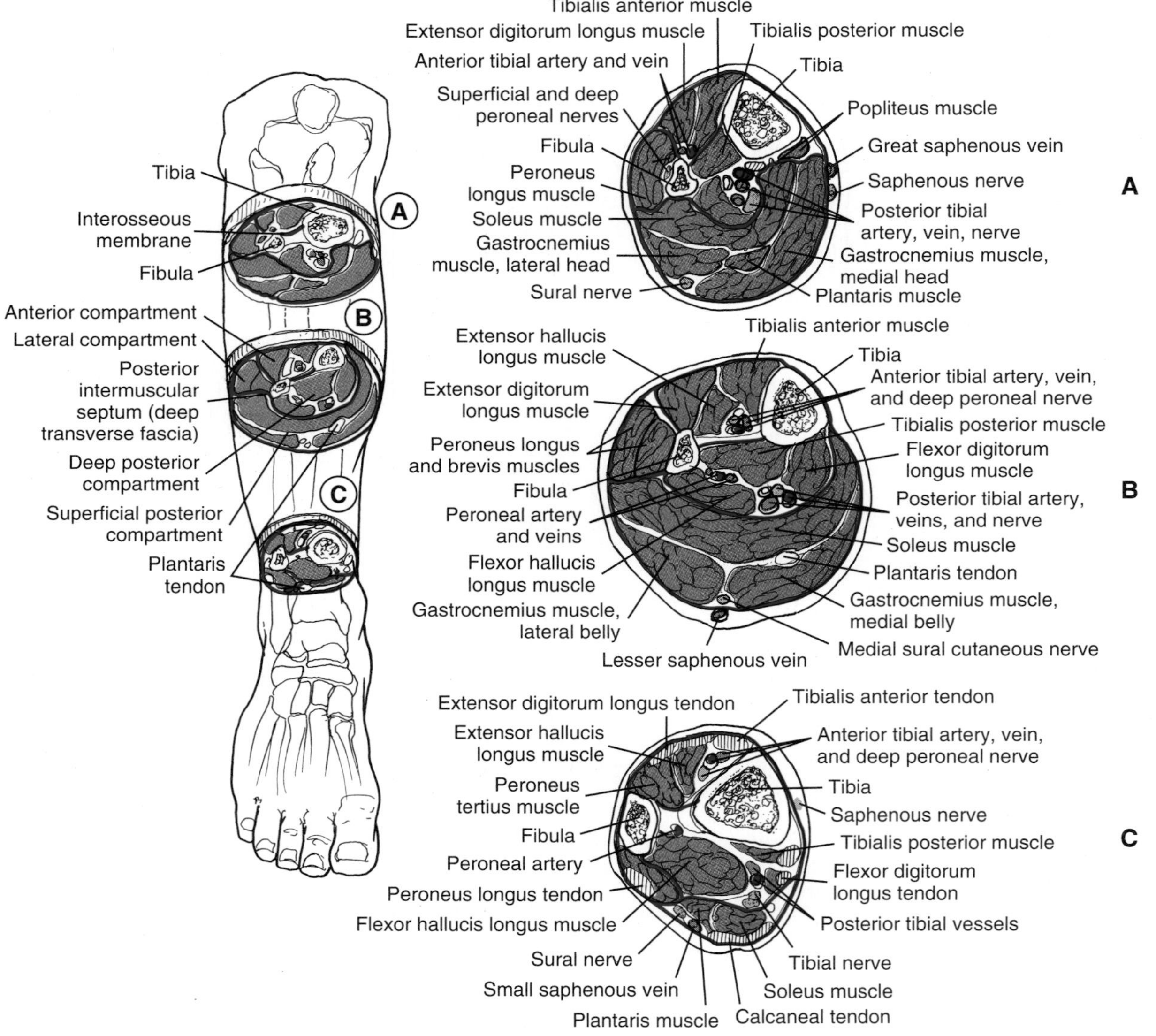

FIGURE 17–16
Organization of muscles of the lower leg. Anterior view *(left)* showing orientation of cross sectional views at right.

longus, and tibialis posterior muscles (Fig. 17–16). The superficial and deep muscles are separated by a thick fibrous septum called the **deep transverse fascia of the leg.** Posterior crural muscles contribute to movements of the leg, foot, and toes (see Table 17–4).

Superficial Muscles of the Posterior Compartment of the Leg. These include two muscles that act upon the knee and ankle joints (gastrocnemius and plantaris muscles) and one that acts upon the ankle joint only (soleus muscle).

The **gastrocnemius muscle** is the most superficial and obvious of the three superficial calf muscles. The muscle forms the prominent bulge of the calf and is readily palpated. It has medial and lateral heads (Figs. 17–17 and 17–18 and see Fig. 17–19), both of which are attached to the posterior surface of the femur just above its medial and lateral condyles (Figs. 17–17 and 17–18 and see Fig. 17–21). The large fleshy bodies of the muscle course inferiorly, joining into a common tendon, the **tendo calcaneus,** about halfway down the leg (Figs. 17–17 and 17–18). This is the largest, strongest tendon of the body. It is attached to the middle roughened part of the posterior surface of the calcaneus (see Figs. 16–13*E* and 17–21). This roughened area also serves as an attachment site for tendons of the plantaris and soleus muscles (see Fig. 16–13*E*). The tendo

TABLE 17–3
Attachments and Actions of Crural (Leg) Muscles

Muscle Group	Individual Muscle	Proximal Attachment	Distal Attachment	Action
Superficial muscles of posterior crural compartment	Gastrocnemius	Posterior surface of femur just medial and lateral to condyles	Tendo calcaneus attached to posterior calcaneus	Flexes leg; plantarflexes foot
	Plantaris	Lateral supracondylar line of femur	Tendo calcaneus attached to posterior calcaneus	Assists gastrocnemius muscle in flexion of leg and plantarflexion of foot
	Soleus	Posterior surface of head and upper third of fibula; soleal line on upper third of tibia	Tendo calcaneus attached to posterior calcaneus	Assists gastrocnemius muscle in plantarflexion of foot
Deep muscles of posterior crural compartment	Popliteus	Lateral surface of lateral condyle of femur	Posterior surface of tibia just superior to soleal line	Unlocks knee joint
Muscles of lateral (peroneal) compartment of leg	Flexor hallucis longus	Posterior surface of middle third of fibula	Courses under sustentaculum tali to attach to plantar surface of distal end of most proximal phalanx of big toe	Plantarflexes foot; flexes big toe
	Flexor digitorum longus	Posterior surface of middle third of tibia	Plantar surfaces of distal phalanges of toes 2 to 5	Flexes toes 2 to 5; assists in plantarflexion of foot
	Tibialis posterior	Posterolateral surface of upper third of tibia; posteromedial surface of upper third of fibula	Lateral side of plantar surface of navicular bone; plantar surfaces of medial, intermediate, and lateral cuneiform bones; plantar surfaces of bases of second, third, and fourth metatarsals	Plantarflexes foot; inverts foot
Muscles of anterior compartment of leg	Peroneus longus	Anterior and lateral surfaces of upper half of fibula	Lateral sides of plantar surfaces of medial cuneiform bone and first metatarsal	Everts foot
	Peroneus brevis	Anterior and lateral surfaces of lower half of fibula	Medial surface of base of fifth metatarsal	Assists peroneus longus muscle in eversion of foot
	Extensor digitorum longus	Anterior surface of superior two thirds of fibula and superolateral surface of interosseous membrane	Four distal tendons elaborated into dorsal digital expansions that cover metatarsophalangeal joints of digits 2 to 5	Extends phalanges 2 to 5; dorsiflexes foot
	Peroneus tertius	Anterior surface of lower fibula	Dorsal surface of base of fifth metatarsal	Assists in dorsiflexion of foot; assists in eversion of foot

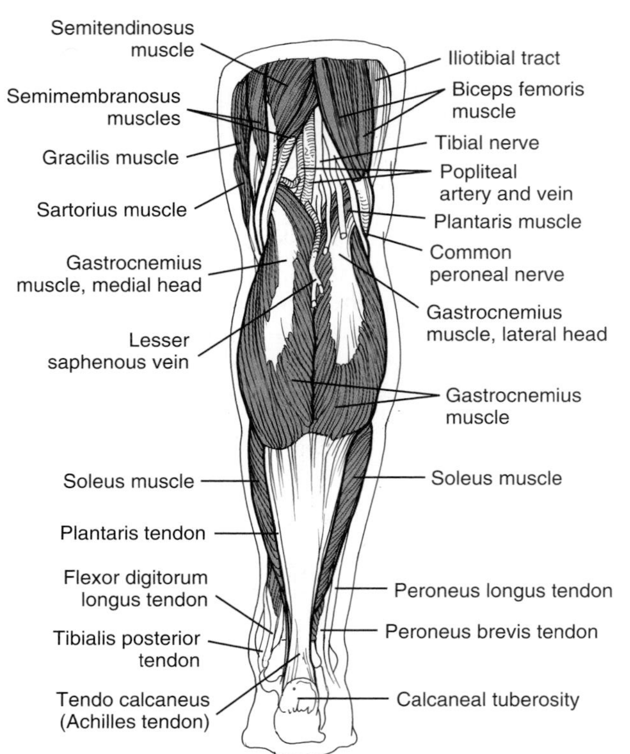

FIGURE 17–17
Superficial muscles of the posterior compartment.

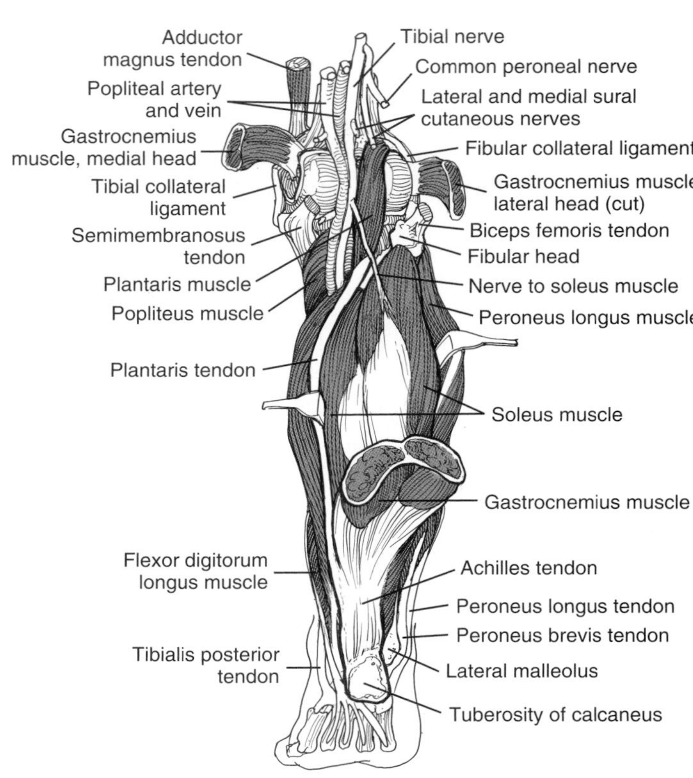

FIGURE 17–19
Deep dissection of the muscles of the posterior compartment.

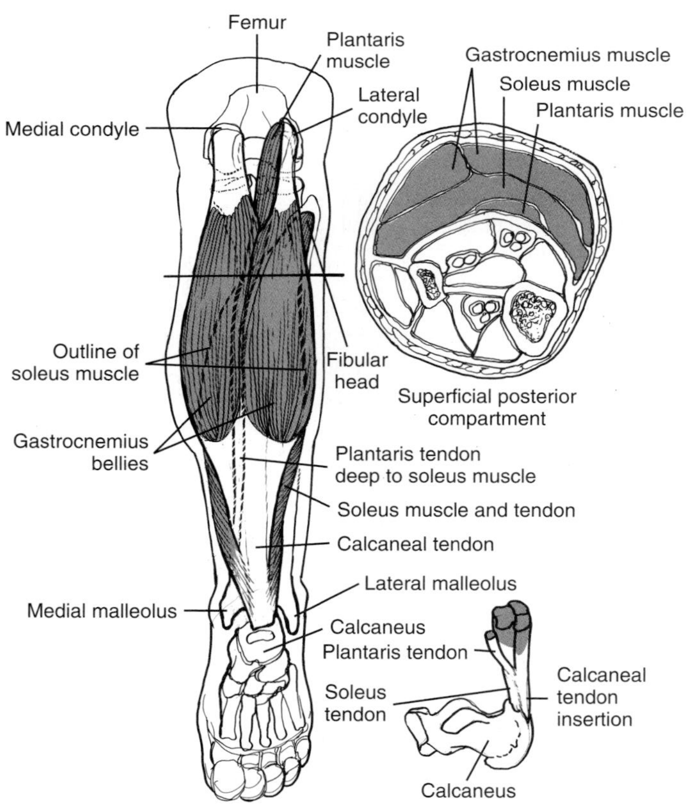

FIGURE 17–18
Dissection of superficial muscles of the posterior compartment.

calcaneus is separated from the smooth superior region of the posterior surface of the calcaneus by a synovial bursa.

The gastrocnemius muscle acts to powerfully flex the knee (see Fig. 17–20*A*) or to plantarflex (extend) the foot (Table 17–3 and see Fig. 17–20*B*).

The diminutive **plantaris muscle** arises from the lateral supracondylar line just superior to the origin of the lateral head of the gastrocnemius muscle (Figs. 17–18 and 17–18 and see Fig. 17–21). Its small body quickly gives way to an inferior (distal) tendon as it courses inferiorly and medially over the posterior surface of the knee joint (Fig. 17–19). The long, slender, inferior tendon courses between the medial head of the gastrocnemius muscle and the soleus muscle and merges with the medial edge of the tendo calcaneus just above the ankle (Fig. 17–18).

The action of the plantaris muscle is to assist the gastrocnemius muscle (Fig. 17–20*A* and *B* and Table 17–3). However, the role it plays is relatively insignificant because it seems to be a vestigial remnant of a much larger muscle. Indeed, its distal tendon may snap when the foot is excessively dorsiflexed, but this results in little or no reduction in the strength of plantarflexion.

The **soleus muscle** arises from the posterior surface of the head and upper one third of the fibula and from the soleal line on the posterior surface of the upper tibia (Figs. 17–19 and 17–21). Between these two bony at-

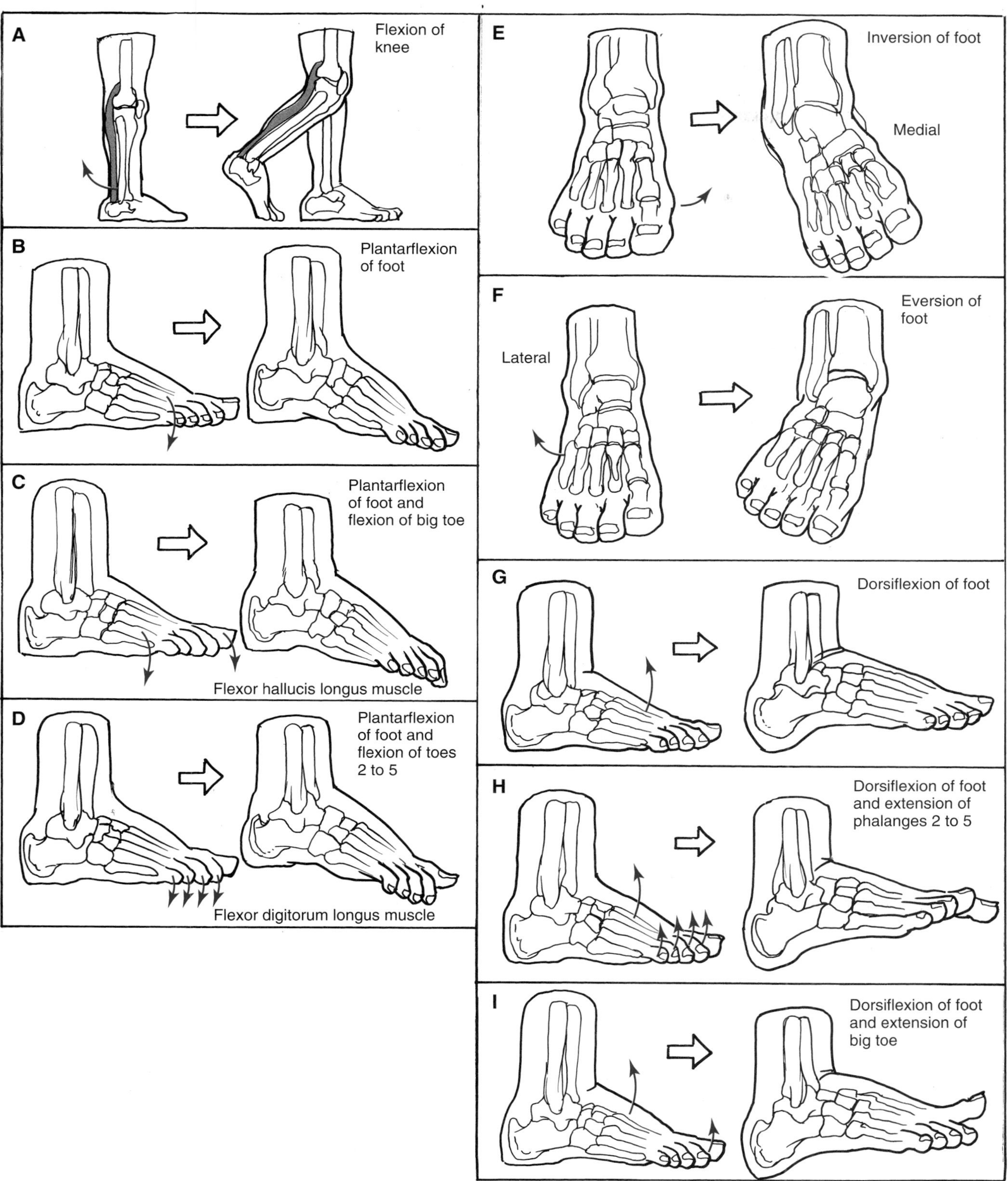

FIGURE 17–20
Actions of the muscles of the leg.

tachments, the muscle originates from a fascial layer overlying the popliteal vessels and tibial branch of the sciatic nerve. The muscle forms a **tendinous arch** through which the popliteal and tibial vessels pass into the deep posterior compartment of the leg (Fig. 17–19). Much of the central region of the superior part of the soleus muscle has a tendinous structure, but its lateral and medial regions are fleshy. The entire inferior end of the muscle narrows to become a tendon about halfway down the calf. This tendon fuses with the anterior surface of the distal gastrocnemius tendon to form the tendo calcaneus.

The soleus muscle thus acts to assist the gastrocnemius muscle in plantarflexion of the foot (Fig. 17–20*B* and Table 17–3).

Deep Muscles of the Posterior Compartment of the Leg. These include the popliteus, flexor hallucis longus, flexor digitorum longus, and tibialis posterior muscles

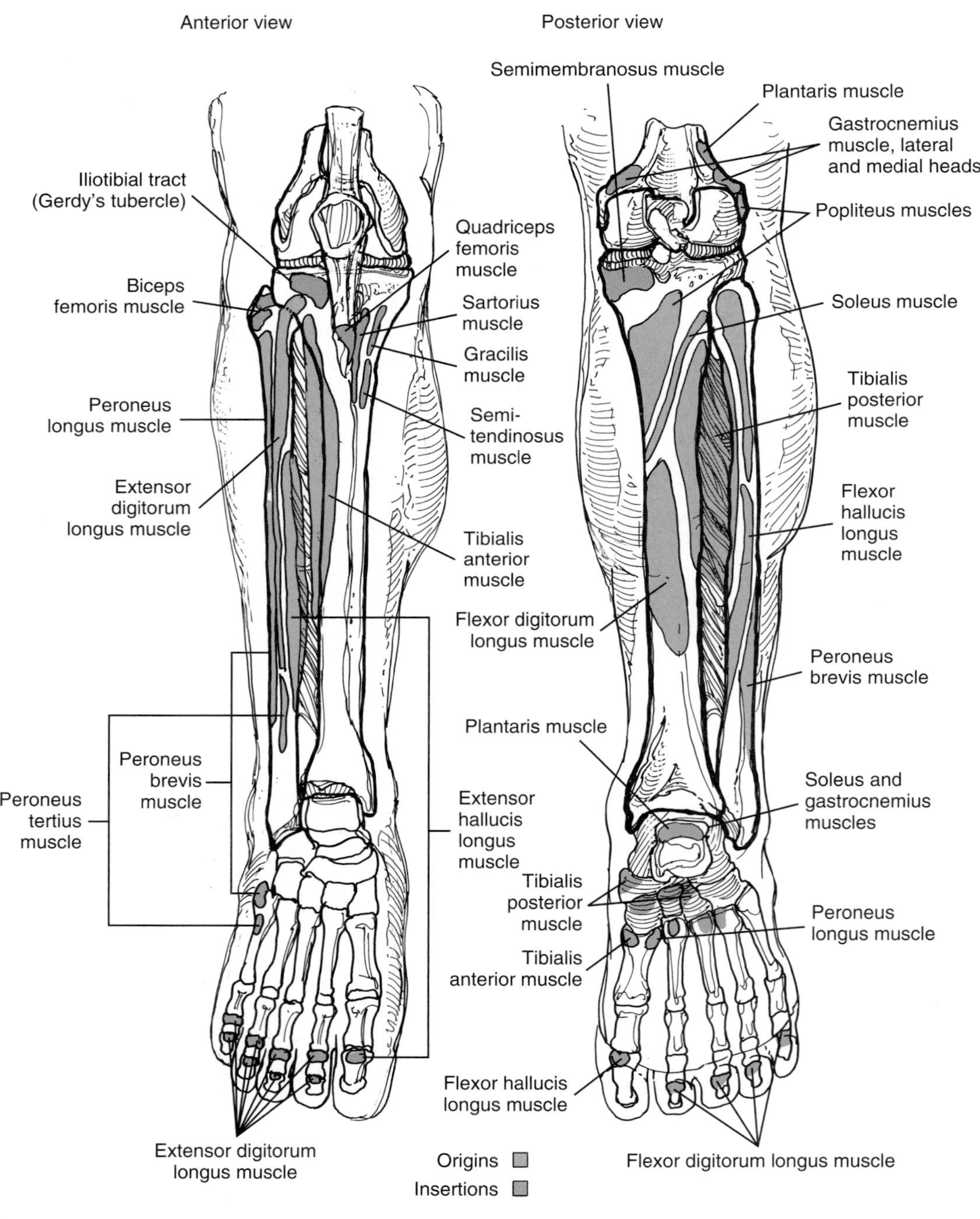

FIGURE 17–21
Origins and insertions of the muscles of the leg.

(Fig. 17–16). The popliteus muscle is a diminutive muscle that crosses the posterior surface of the knee joint. The remaining muscles of the deep posterior crural compartment are long muscles that have their origins in the leg. Their distal tendons cross the ankle joint on its medial side to insert within the plantar compartment of the foot. The long flexor muscles act synergistically with short flexors and other muscles of the sole (Table 17–3 and see below).

The superior end of the **popliteus muscle** is attached to the lateral surface of the lateral condyle of the femur (Fig. 17–21). Its body courses inferomedially so that its distal tendon may attach to the posterior surface of the tibia just superior to the soleal line. The popliteal muscle forms much of the floor of the popliteal fossa.

The flat, triangular popliteus muscle is only a few inches long, but its action "unlocks" the knee joint. This action is required before the knee can be flexed as in walking or running (Table 17–3 and see below).

The **flexor hallucis longus muscle** originates from the posterior surface of the middle third of the fibula. Its body descends toward the ankle just deep to the soleus muscle and tendo calcaneus where its tendon runs through a groove at the lower end of the tibia (see Fig. 16–10*B*). As the tendon sweeps medially around the ankle joint, it enters a synovial capsule (Fig. 17–22), which passes over the posterior surface of the talus and under a thickened band of connective tissue called the **flexor retinaculum** (see discussion of the flexor retinaculum below). The flexor retinaculum acts as a pulley, confining and directing the actions of the flexor hallucis longus, flexor digitorum longus, and tibialis posterior muscles so that the muscles function properly at the ankle joint and in the foot. If the tendons of these muscles were not bound down at the ankle joint, they would slip out of position when they contracted and would be unable to perform useful work.

Once the distal tendon of the flexor hallucis longus muscle emerges from the flexor retinaculum, the tendon courses within a groove on the inferior surface of the sustentaculum tali, which also acts as a pulley (Fig. 17–22 and see Fig. 16–12*B*). This tendon then courses anteriorly to attach to the inferior surface of the distal end of the most distal of the two phalanges of the big toe (see Fig. 17–32).

The flexor hallucis longus muscle acts as a powerful plantarflexor of the ankle (Fig. 17–20*B*) and flexor of the big toe (Fig. 17–20*C* and Table 17–3).

The **flexor digitorum longus muscle** arises from the posterior surface of the middle third of the tibia. Its body courses inferomedially. Its distal tendon crosses over the tendon of the tibialis posterior muscle (Figs. 17–21 and 17–22). These two tendons (of which the flexor digitorum longus tendon is now the most posterior) pass just behind the medial malleolus, over the medial surface of the sustentaculum tali, and under the **flexor retinaculum** (Fig. 17–22). Although the distal flexor digitorum longus tendon is closely associated with the distal tibialis posterior tendon in the medial foot, the structures are embedded within different synovial capsules. After emerging from its synovial capsule, the distal flexor digitorum longus tendon courses into the **second muscle layer** (of four layers) of the sole (plantar compartment of the foot). It splays into four separate tendons, which attach to the plantar surfaces of the distal phalanges of toes 2 to 5 (Figs. 17–21 and 17–22). Because the flexor digitorum longus tendon gains access to the toes from the medial side of the foot, its logical action would be to pull the toes medially as it flexed them. However, a diminutive muscle of the second layer of the plantar compartment, the flexor accessorius (quadratus plantae) muscle, is attached to the flexor tendons within the sole and acts with the flexor digitorum longus tendon to alter the vectors of the flexor tendons so that the tendons pull in a more posterior direction (Fig. 17–20*D* and see Fig. 17–32). The flexor digitorum longus muscle also acts to assist in plantarflexion of the foot (Fig. 17–22*B*).

The proximal tendon of the **tibialis posterior muscle** is attached to the posterolateral surface of the superior half of the tibia, the superior half of the interosseous membrane, and the posteromedial surface of the upper half of the fibula (Figs. 17–21 and 17–22). The body of the tibialis posterior muscle courses inferomedially to form a distal tendon, which crosses under the flexor digitorum longus tendon (Fig. 17–22). This distal tendon passes just posterior to the medial malleolus of the tibia, within its own synovial capsule, under the flexor retinaculum, and over the surface of the sustentaculum tali. It divides into seven slips, which insert on the lateral side of the plantar surface of the navicular bone; on the plantar surfaces of the medial, intermediate, and lateral cuneiform bones; and on the plantar surfaces of the bases of the second, third, and fourth metatarsal bones.

The tibialis posterior muscle is, therefore, well positioned to act in plantarflexion of the foot (Fig. 17–20*B*) and inversion of the foot (Fig. 17–20*E*).

The **flexor retinaculum** lies upon the medial aspect of the foot. This specialization of deep fascia is attached superiorly to the end of the medial malleolus and inferiorly to the medial surface of the calcaneus and the plantar aponeurosis. From superior to inferior, it binds down tendons of the tibialis posterior, flexor digitorum, and flexor hallucis longus muscles (Fig. 17–23). In addition, the posterior tibial vessels and tibial nerve are bound down between the tendons of the flexor digitorum and flexor hallucis longus muscles.

Deep fascia of the ankle also form the superior and inferior extensor retinacula and superior and inferior peroneal retinacula (Figs. 17–23 and 17–24 and see Figs. 17–26*A* and 17–28*A* and below).

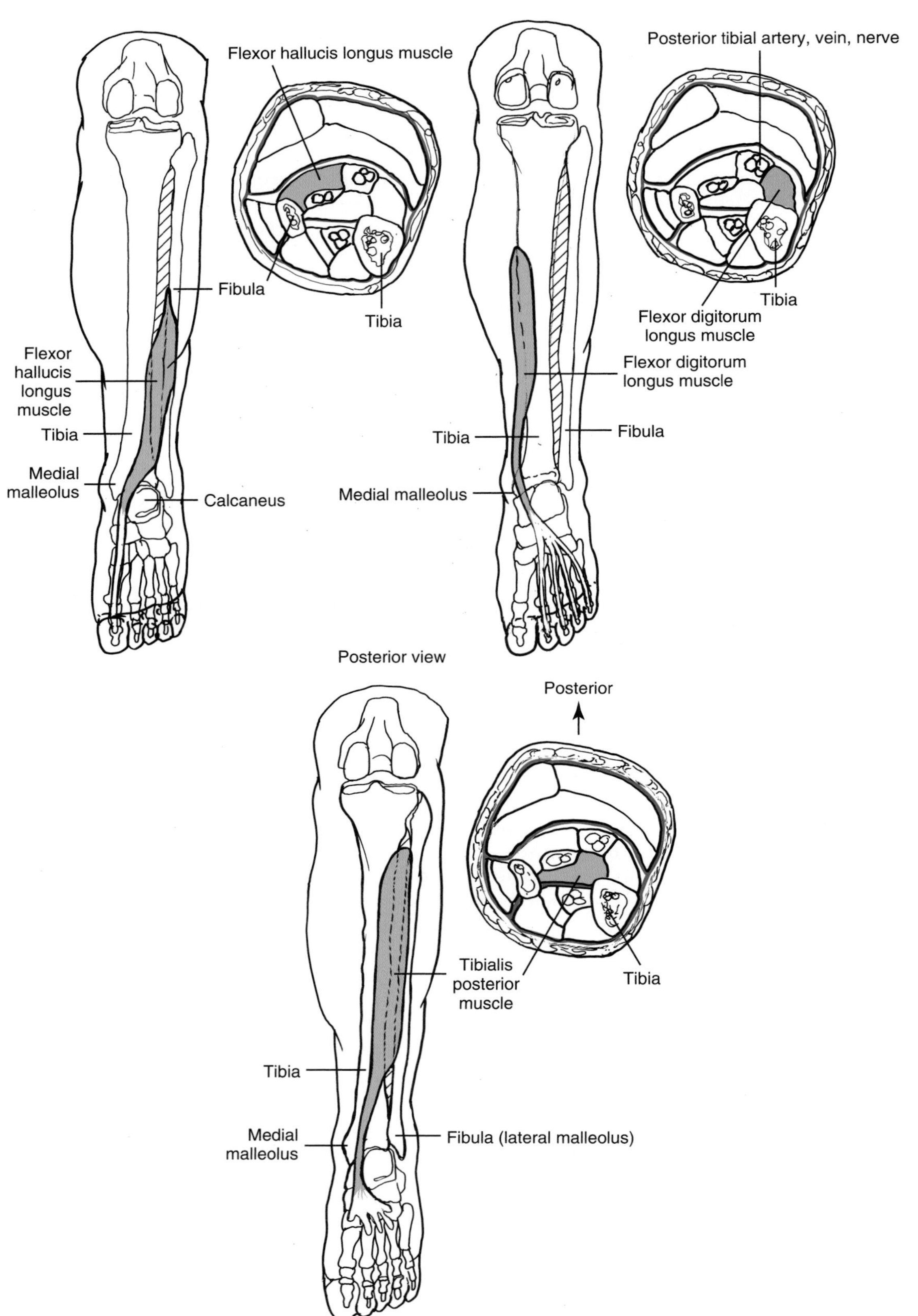

FIGURE 17–22
Deep muscles of the posterior crural compartment.

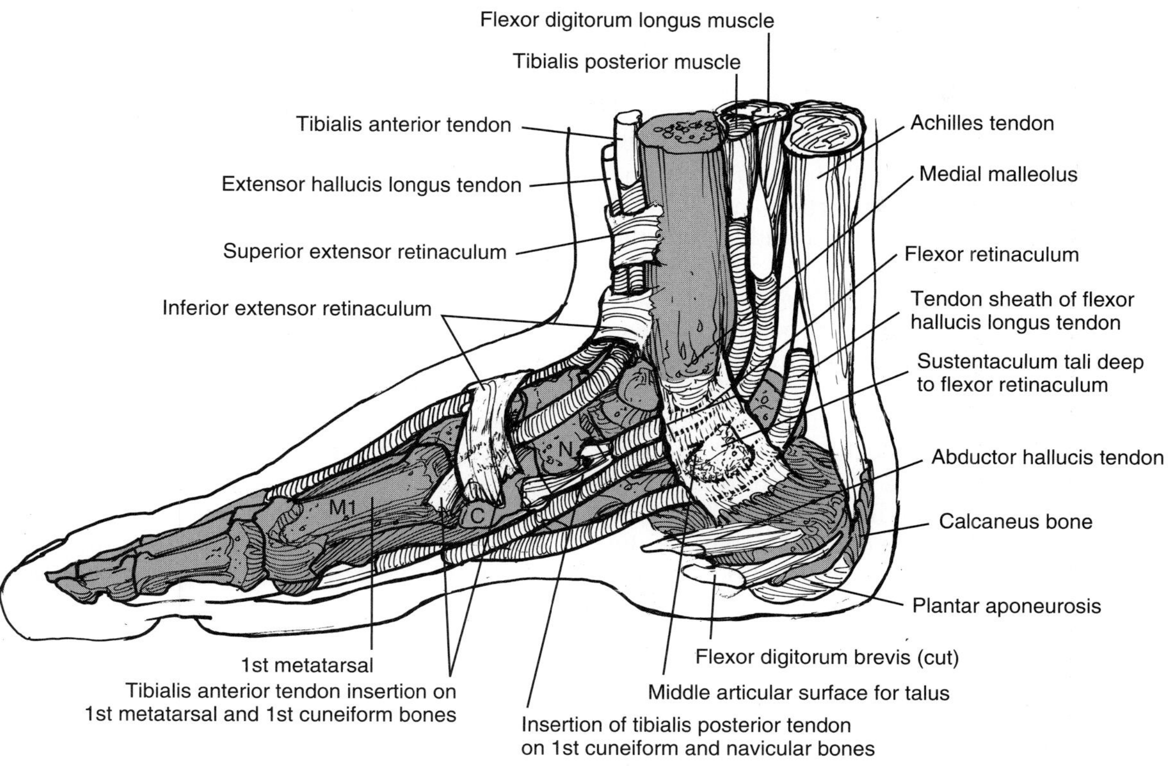

FIGURE 17–23
Medial view of the ankle showing tendons of the deep muscles of the leg.

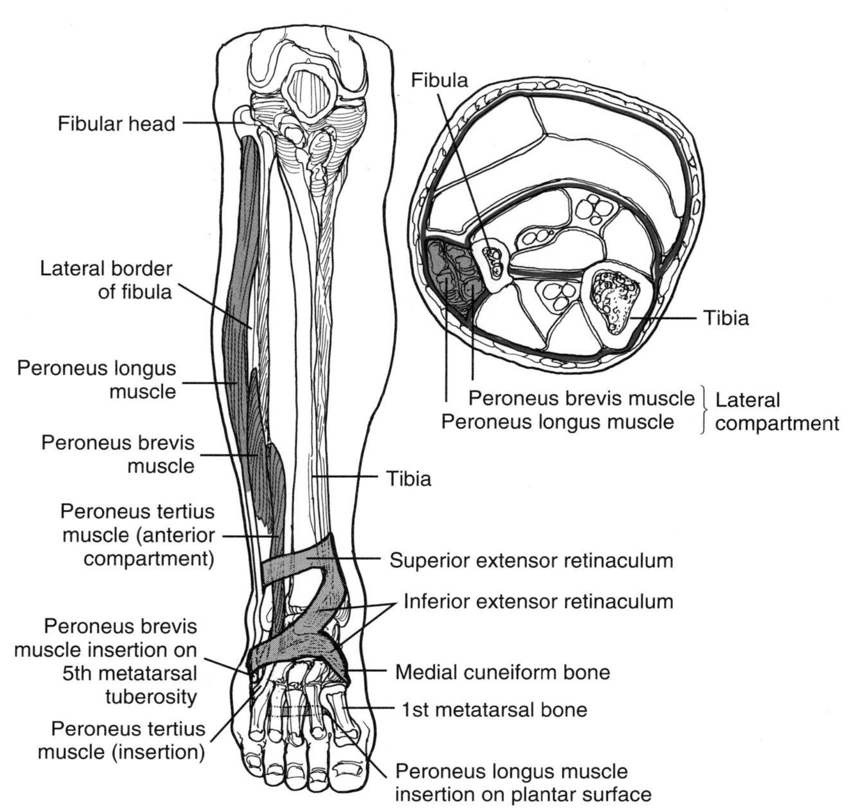

FIGURE 17–24
Lateral compartment muscles of the leg.

Synovial tendon sheaths play an important role in the mechanisms of the retinacula. The tendons of the long extensor, long and short peroneal, and long flexor muscles are invested by synovial sheaths lined by a fluid-secreting synovial membrane (Fig. 17–22). Thus, synovial fluid lubricates the articulating surfaces of the tendon and its sheath, decreasing friction and allowing the tendon to slip easily through the sheath so that the retinaculum may act as a pulley.

Muscles of the Lateral Compartment of the Leg. These are the peroneus longus and peroneus brevis muscles. These muscles function in everting the foot or in resisting inversion.

The belly of the **peroneus longus muscle** can be palpated in the upper third of the lateral part of the leg. The superior end of the muscle is attached to the anterior and lateral surfaces of the upper half of the fibula (Figs. 17–21 and 17–24). Fibers of the long belly of the muscle converge to form its distal tendon about halfway down the leg. This tendon descends to sweep around (from back to front) and under the lateral malleolus of the fibula, passing under two connective tissue bands called the **superior** and **inferior peroneal retinacula** and over the lateral sides of the calcaneus and cuboid bones (Figs. 17–24 and 17–25 and see discussion of the superior and inferior peroneal retinacula below). The tendon passes inferior to the plantar surface of the cuboid bone and lateral and intermediate cuneiform bones and inserts upon the lateral sides of the plantar surfaces of the medial cuneiform and first metatarsal bones (Figs. 17–21 and 17–25). As the tendon passes under the superior and inferior peroneal retinacula, it is enveloped within a synovial sheath, which it shares with the peroneus brevis muscle (Fig. 17–25). An additional synovial sheath envelops the tendon within the sole of the foot (see Fig. 17–33). The peroneus longus muscle acts as a strong everter of the foot (Fig. 17–20*F* and Table 17–3).

The **peroneus brevis muscle** is attached to the anterior and lateral surfaces of the lower half of the fibula (Fig. 17–24). Its short belly descends deep and slightly anterior to the tendon of the peroneus longus muscle. The distal peroneus brevis tendon sweeps around (from back to front) and under the lateral malleolus of the fibula and passes under the superior and inferior retinacula within a synovial sheath, which it shares with the peroneus longus tendon (Figs. 17–24 and 17–25). The distal peroneus brevis tendon inserts upon the medial surface of the base of the fifth metatarsal (Fig. 17–21 and see 17–32).

The peroneus brevis muscle acts with the peroneus longus muscle to evert the foot (Fig. 17–20*F*). However,

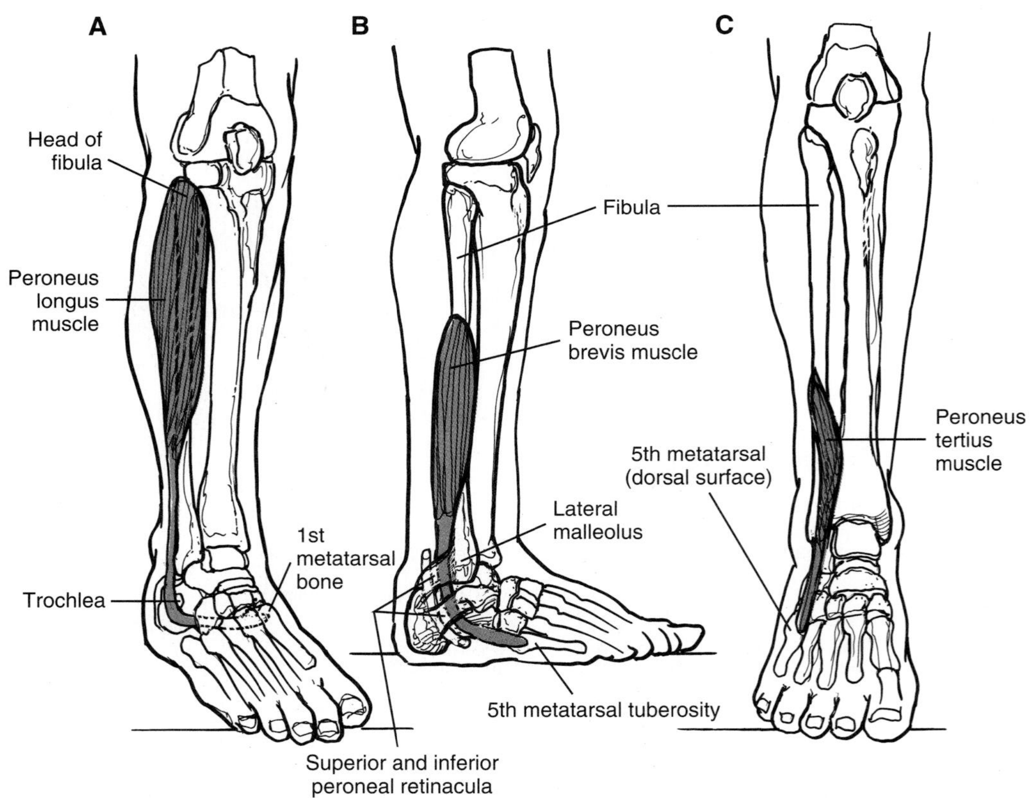

FIGURE 17–25
Muscles of the lateral (peroneal) compartment of the leg.

it is thought that its chief function is to counteract forces tending to invert the foot (Table 17–3).

The **superior peroneal retinaculum** is attached laterally to the posterior surface of the lateral malleolus and medially to the lateral surface of the calcaneus (Fig. 17–25). From lateral to medial, it binds down the tendons of the peroneus longus and peroneus brevis muscles. The **inferior peroneal retinaculum** is bound laterally to the lateral calcaneal surface, while medially, its fibers are continuous with those of the inferior extensor retinaculum. From lateral to medial, the inferior peroneal retinaculum binds down the distal regions of the peroneus longus and peroneus brevis tendons.

Muscles of the Anterior Compartment. These include the tibialis anterior, extensor digitorum longus, peroneus tertius, and extensor hallucis longus muscles. Their main functions are dorsiflexion and eversion of the foot and extension of the toes. Long extensor muscles function synergistically with short extensors and other muscles of the dorsum of the foot (see below).

The **tibialis anterior muscle** is the most superficial muscle of the anterior compartment of the leg. Its belly can be palpated in the upper third of the leg just lateral to the tibial tuberosity and anterior border of the tibia. The superior end of the tibialis anterior muscle arises from the lateral surface of the upper third of the tibia and from an adjacent region of the interosseous membrane (see Fig. 17–21). The muscle descends inferiorly and medially to form a tendon that courses along the anterior border of the lowest third of the tibial shaft (Fig. 17–26). It passes deep to the **superior** and **inferior extensor retinacula,** sweeping forward within its synovial sheath to attach to the medial half of the plantar surface of the medial cuneiform bone and adjacent surface of the first metatarsal (Fig. 17–21 and see Fig. 17–32 and discussion of superior and inferior extensor below).

The tibialis anterior muscle acts to dorsiflex the foot (Fig. 17–20*G*). It also antagonizes the action of the tibialis posterior muscle by inverting the foot (Fig. 17–20*E*). It is especially active when one is walking (Table 17–3).

The belly of the **extensor digitorum longus muscle** lies just lateral to the belly of the tibialis anterior muscle (Fig. 17–26). This pennate (feather-shaped) muscle arises from the anterior surface of the superior two thirds of the fibula and the superolateral surface of the interosseous membrane (Fig. 17–21). The muscle's belly descends inferiorly to form a tendon that courses under the medial part of the superior and inferior retinacula within a synovial sheath. This synovial sheath also encloses the distal tendon of the peroneus tertius muscle (Fig. 17–26). The distal tendon of the extensor digitorum longus muscle splits into four slips on the dorsum of the foot. Each slip forms a **dorsal digital expansion (extensor expansion),** which is elaborated in its distal region as an expanded sheath over the dorsal surface of the metatarsophalangeal joint of digits 2 to 5 (Fig. 17–26 and see Figs. 17–27 and 17–28*B*). These expansions provide attachment sites for the diminutive lumbrical and interosseous muscles (see below). As each of these expansions courses proximally onto the dorsal surface of a toe, it splits into three slips. The center slip attaches to the dorsal surface of the base of the middle phalanx, whereas the outer two slips reunite to insert upon the dorsal surface of the base of the most proximal phalanx. These dorsal digital expansions closely resemble those formed in the hands (see Chapter 20).

The extensor digitorum longus muscle acts to extend the second to fifth phalanges and dorsiflexes the foot (Fig. 17–20 and Table 17–3).

The **peroneus tertius muscle** can be considered a lateral component of the extensor digitorum longus muscle (Figs. 17–26 and 17–27*B*). Its muscle belly narrows to form a fifth tendon lying lateral to the extensor digitorum longus tendon to the fifth toe (Fig. 17–24). It arises from the anterior surface of the lower fibula and courses inferiorly, deep to the superior and inferior extensor retinacula (Figs. 17–21 and 17–24).

The distal tendon of the peroneus tertius muscle is attached to the dorsal surface of the base of the fifth metatarsal (Fig. 17–21). It contributes to the actions of

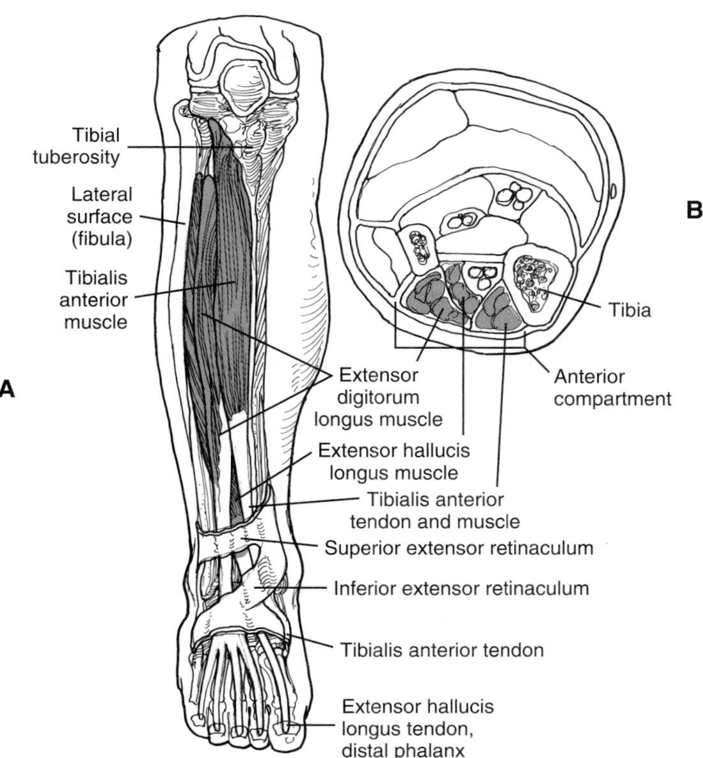

FIGURE 17–26
Muscles of the anterior compartment of the leg.

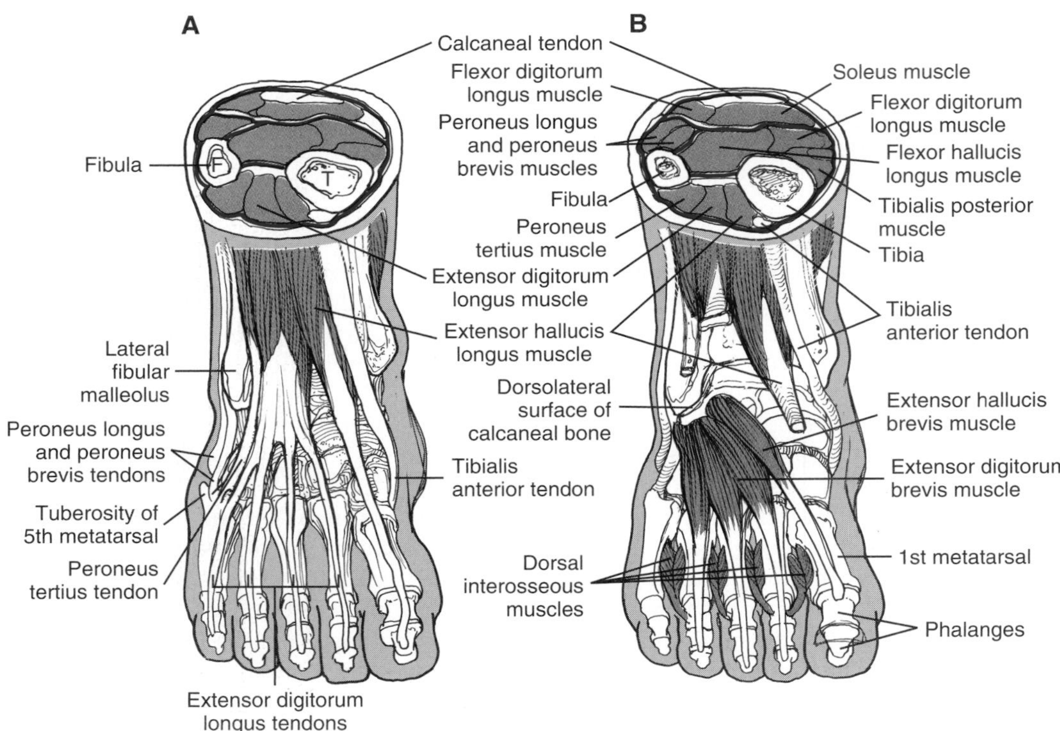

FIGURE 17–27
Overview of the muscles of the foot.

dorsiflexion (Fig. 17–20*G*) and eversion of the foot (Fig. 17–20*F* and Table 17–3).

The belly of the **extensor hallucis longus muscle** lies between the bellies of the tibialis anterior and extensor digitorum longus muscles (Fig. 17–26). Its superior half also lies deep to these adjacent muscles. The extensor hallucis longus muscle arises from the medial surface of the middle third of the fibula and adjacent interosseous membrane. The muscle courses inferiorly to become a distal tendon that passes deep to the superior and inferior extensor retinacula within its own synovial sheath (Fig. 17–26*A*). It sweeps medially onto the dorsal surface of the big toe, where it widens into a dorsal digital expansion that covers the metatarsophalangeal joint. One tendinous slip extends distally from this expansion to insert upon the dorsal surface of the base of the distal phalanx of the big toe (Figs. 17–26 to 17–28).

The extensor hallucis longus muscle acts to extend the big toe (Fig. 17–20*I*) and to dorsiflex the foot (Fig. 17–20G and Table 17–3).

The **superior extensor retinaculum** is a band of thickened deep fascia bound to the anterior surface of the fibula (laterally) and the anterior surface of the tibia (Figs. 17–26 and 17–28*A*). From the lateral to the medial side of the ankle, this retinaculum holds down the tendons of the peroneus tertius, extensor digitorum longus, extensor hallucis longus, and tibialis anterior muscles. It also invests the deep peroneal nerve and anterior tibial artery and vein. The **inferior extensor retinaculum** is attached laterally to the lateral surface of the calcaneus and medially to the tibial (medial) malleolus and tough connective tissue on the plantar aspect of the foot (plantar aponeurosis) (Fig. 17–28*A*). From lateral to medial, the inferior extensor retinaculum binds down the tendons of the peroneus tertius, extensor digitorum longus, extensor hallucis longus, and tibialis anterior muscles and also the dorsal nerves and vessels.

Muscles of the Foot

Muscles of the foot reside within dorsal or plantar compartments. The single short dorsal muscle assists long muscles of the anterior compartment of the leg in extending the toes, whereas short muscles of the plantar compartment assist long muscles of the posterior compartment of the leg in flexing the toes. Some muscles of the plantar compartment also adduct or abduct the digits.

Muscles of the Dorsal Compartment of the Foot. The **dorsum of the foot** contains a single muscle, the **extensor digitorum brevis muscle,** which arises from the dorsolateral surface of the calcaneus (see Figs. 17–27*B* and 17–28). As the thin belly of the muscle courses distally just deep to the tendons of the extensor digitorum longus muscle, it sweeps medially to form four tendons. Three of the tendons attach to the lateral sides of the long flexor tendons of the second to fourth digits in the region of the metatarsophalangeal joint. The fourth ten-

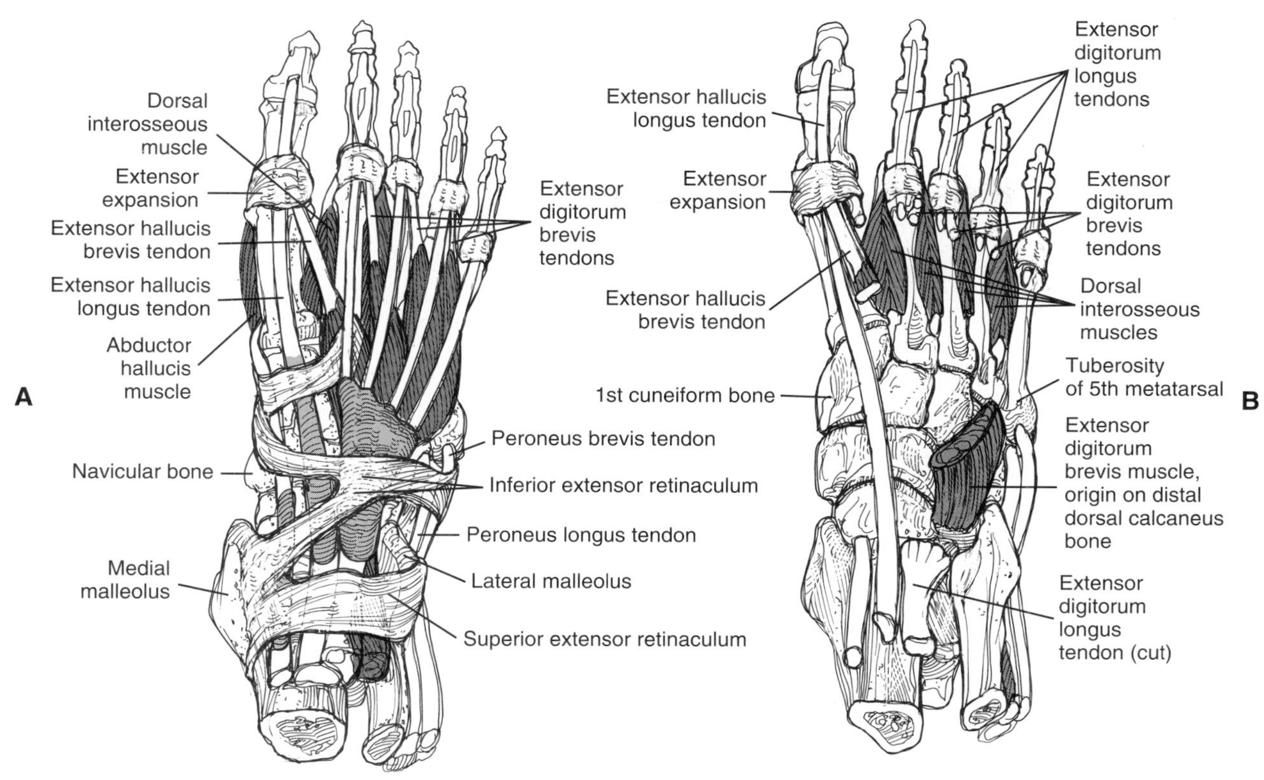

FIGURE 17–28
Superficial dissection, **(A)**, and deep dissection, **(B)**, of the dorsal compartment of the foot.

don attaches to the base of the proximal phalanx of the first toe (see Fig. 17–27*B*).

The small extensor digitorum brevis muscle acts to extend digits 1 to 4 (Fig. 17–29*A*). The medial region of the muscle and the tendon attached to the big toe are also called the **extensor hallucis brevis muscle.**

Muscles of the Plantar Compartment of the Foot. **Muscles and other structures within the plantar compartment of the foot** are organized in four layers. Other, more functional groupings are described below. The first, most superficial layer contains three muscles whose primary function is to maintain the longitudinal arch of the foot. The second layer contains a muscle that assists the flexor digitorum longus muscle in flexing digits 2 to 4 and four small wormlike lumbrical muscles that flex the distal phalanx while they extend the proximal phalanges of digits 2 to 4. The third layer contains short flexors of the big and little toes and a short adductor of the big toe. The fourth and deepest layer contains small proximal interosseous muscles, which are further characterized as dorsal abductors or plantar adductors.

The **first and most superficial layer of the plantar compartment** is covered by a thick connective tissue investment called the **plantar aponeurosis** (Fig. 17–30 and see discussion below). The plantar aponeurosis must be cut away to reveal the three muscles within the first layer (Fig. 17–31). The wider, more prominent flexor digitorum brevis muscle lies between the medial abductor hallucis muscle and the lateral abductor digiti minimi muscle. The three muscles arise from the tuberosity of the calcaneus (Fig. 17–31). It should be pointed out for further discussion that abduction and adduction of the toes are considered to occur with reference to the axis of the second digit (i.e., a toe is abducted when it moves away from the second toe and adducted when it moves toward the second toe). In contrast, the axis of abduction and adduction of the fingers is the third finger (see Chapter 20).

The **abductor hallucis muscle** arises from the medial side of the tuberosity of the calcaneus, courses along the medial side of the foot, and forms a distal tendon, which inserts upon the medial side of the base of the proximal phalanx of the big toe (Fig. 17–31).

Actions of the abductor hallucis muscle include abduction of the big toe (Fig. 17–29*B*) and assistance in flexion of the big toe (Fig. 17–29*C* and Table 17–4).

The **abductor digiti minimi muscle** arises from the lateral surface of the calcaneal tuberosity and courses along the lateral side of the foot to form a distal tendon that attaches to the lateral side of the base of the proximal phalanx of the small toe (Figs. 17–31 and 17–32).

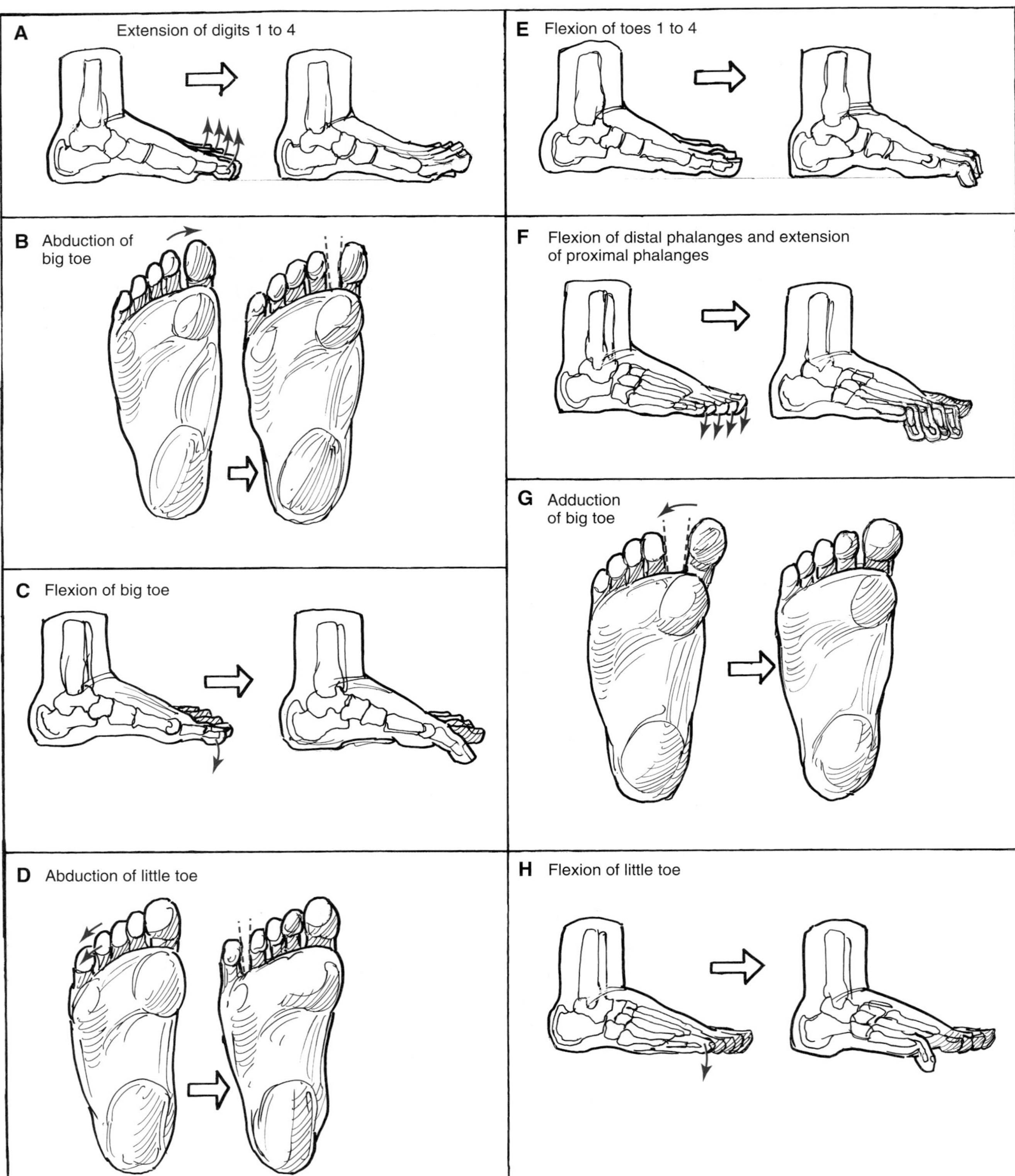

FIGURE 17–29
Actions of the muscles of the foot.

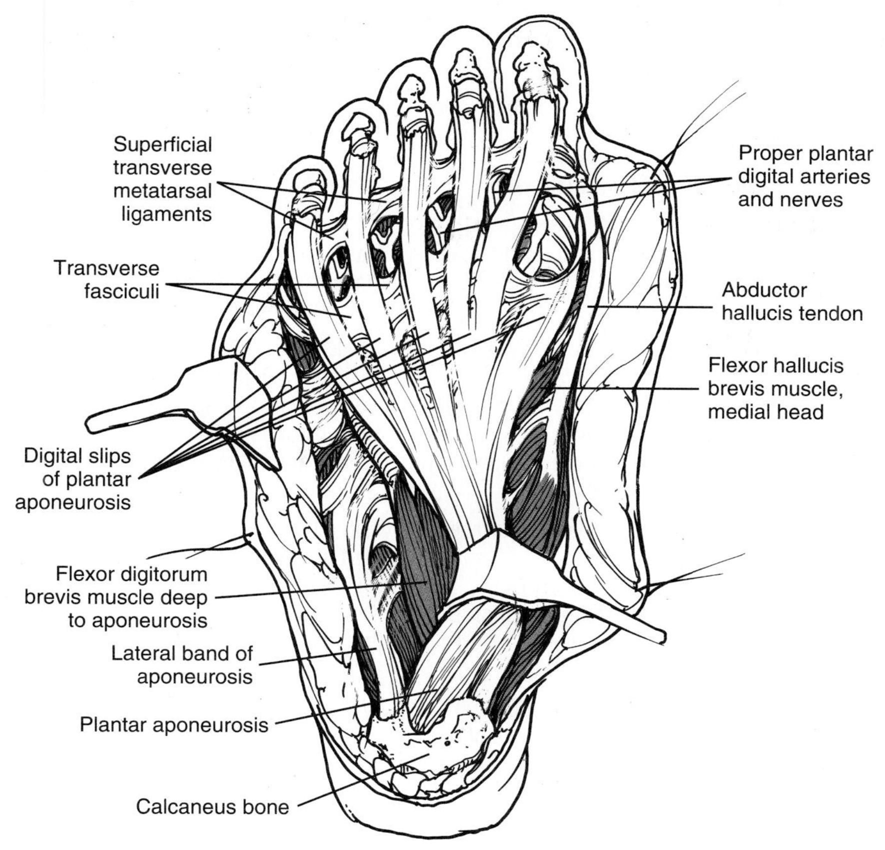

FIGURE 17–30
Muscles of the plantar compartment of the foot.

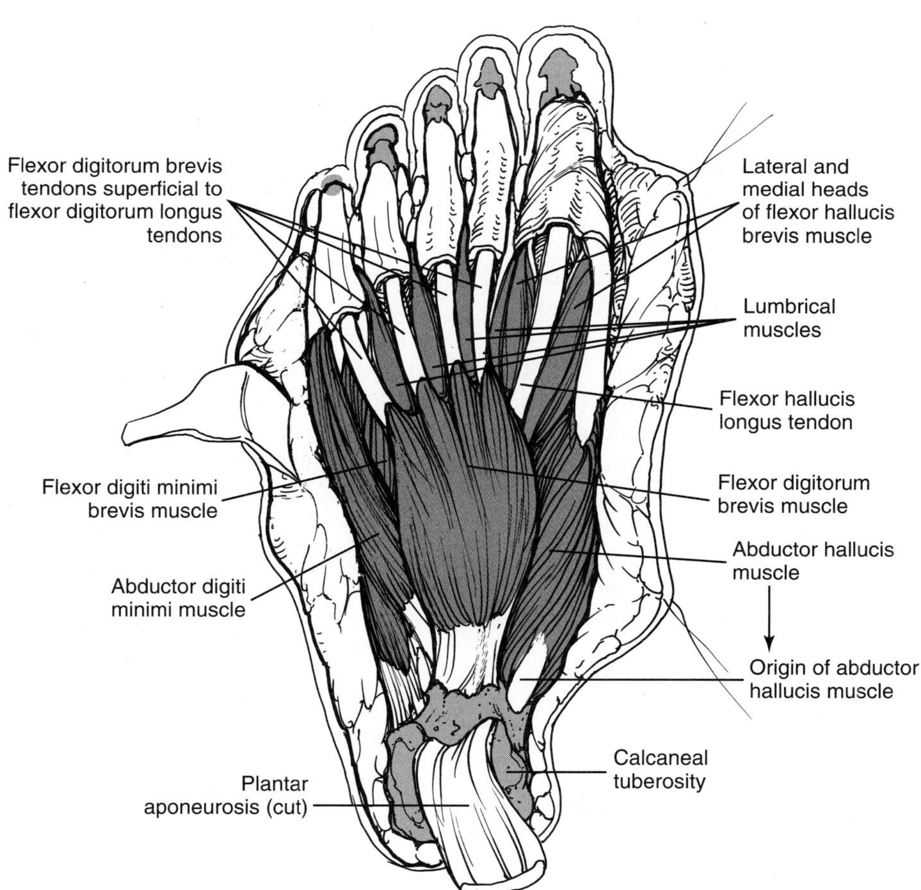

FIGURE 17–31
Superficial dissection of the plantar compartment or first layer of the plantar muscles of the foot.

TABLE 17–4
Attachments and Actions of Muscles of the Foot

Muscle Group	Individual Muscle	Proximal Attachment	Distal Attachment	Action
Muscles of dorsal compartment of foot	Extensor digitorum brevis	Dorsolateral surface of calcaneus	Lateral sides of long flexor tendons of digits 2 to 4; base of proximal phalanx of digit 1	Assists in extension of digits 1 to 4
First layer of plantar muscles	Abductor hallucis	Medial side of tuberosity of calcaneus	Medial side of base of proximal phalanx of digit 1	Abducts digit 1; assists in flexion of digit 1
	Abductor digiti minimi	Lateral surface of tuberosity of calcaneus	Lateral side of base of proximal phalanx of digit 5	Abducts digit 5; assists in flexion of digit 5
	Flexor digitorum brevis	Plantar surface of tuberosity of calcaneus	Medial and lateral sides of middle phalanges of digits 1 to 4	Flexes all phalanges of digits 1 to 4
Second layer of plantar muscles	Quadratus plantae	Medial and lateral surfaces of calcaneus	Lateral boundary of common part of tendon of flexor digitorum longus muscle	"Corrects" oblique vector of flexor digitorum longus muscle
	Four lumbricals	Medial sides of each of four distal tendons of flexor digitorum longus muscle	Dorsal digital expansions of digits 2 to 4	Flexes distal phalanx of digits 2 to 4; extends proximal phalanges of digits 2 to 4
Third layer of plantar muscles	Flexor hallucis brevis	Plantar surface of cuboid bone; plantar surface of lateral cuneiform bone; tibialis posterior tendon	Medial and lateral sides of proximal phalanx of digit 1	Assists in flexion of digit 1
	Adductor hallucis	Ligaments of metatarsophalangeal joints of digits 3 to 5; plantar surfaces of bases of metatarsals 2 to 4	Base of proximal phalanx of digit 1	Adducts digit 1
	Flexor digiti minimi	Medial plantar surface of base of metatarsal 5	Lateral surface of base of proximal phalanx of digit 5	Flexes digit 5; assists in abduction of digit 5
Fourth layer of plantar muscles	Four dorsal interosseous	Bases and shafts of metatarsals of digits 2 to 4	Bases of proximal phalanges of digits 2 to 4	Abduct digits 2 to 4
	Three plantar interosseous	Bases and shafts of metatarsals of digits 3 to 5	Bases of proximal phalanges of digits 3 to 5	Adduct digits 3 to 5

The abductor digiti minimi muscle acts to abduct the small toe (Fig. 17–29*D*), and it also assists in flexion of the small toe (Fig. 17–29*H*).

The **flexor digitorum brevis muscle** arises from the plantar surface of the calcaneal tuberosity and expands into a fleshy belly as it courses distally to split into four tendons (Fig. 17–31). As each of these tendons reaches the base of its most proximal phalanx, it splits into two slips that reunite to form a tunnel through which the distal tendons of the long flexors may pass (Figs. 17–32 and 17–33). The tendon splits again to attach to the medial and lateral sides of each intermediate phalangeal shaft.

The flexor digitorum brevis muscle acts to flex the metatarsophalangeal and interphalangeal joints of digits 1 to 4 (Fig. 17–29*E* and *F* and Table 17–4).

The skin and superficial fascia of the sole of the foot are bound firmly by connections to a thickened band of deep fascia called the **plantar aponeurosis.** This tough band of connective tissue is attached posteriorly to the plantar surface of the calcaneal tuberosity. As the plantar aponeurosis courses distally, it splits into five bands (one for each toe). The distal end of each band is attached to the base of the phalanx and associated ligaments and tendons. The proximal and distal ends of each band are also connected by transverse bands of deep fascia (Fig. 17–30). The plantar aponeurosis is especially effective in protecting the integument from shearing and impact forces generated by walking and running. It also binds down plantar muscles and tendons and protects plantar vessels and nerves from compression.

Plantar fasciitis is a painful condition resulting from inflammation of the plantar aponeurosis. Pain is localized along the medial aspect of the plantar surface of the foot just distal to the calcaneus. This condition usually occurs in long-distance runners or walkers. The treatment is rest and use of an orthotic shoe insert that elevates the medial aspect of the heel. In extreme cases, the medial aspect of the plantar aponeurosis may be surgically incised.

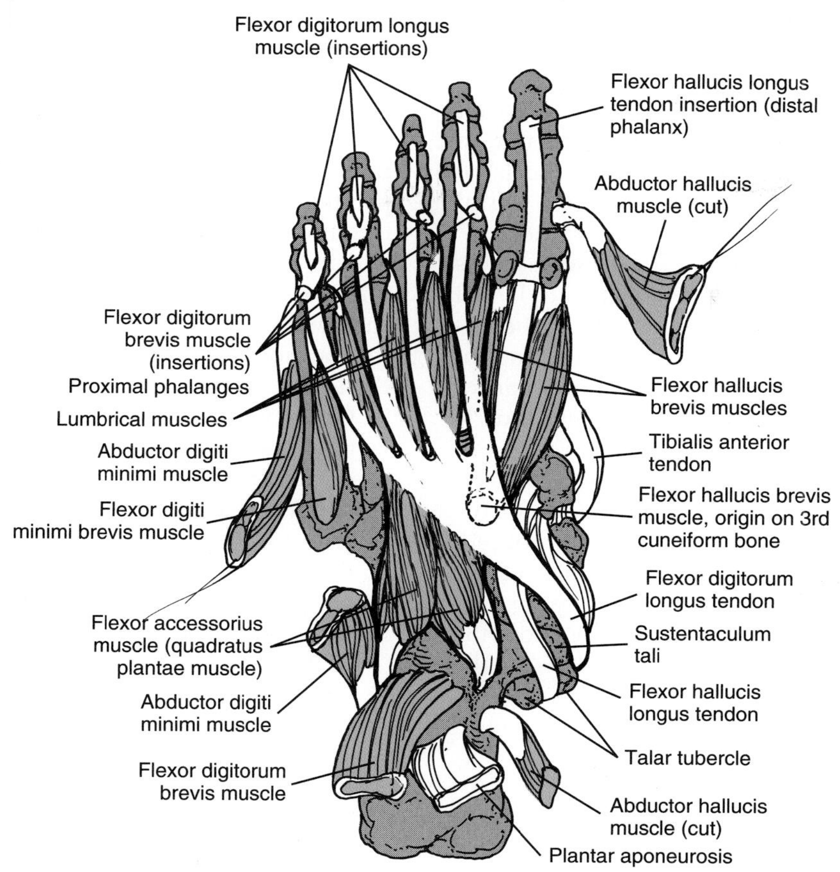

FIGURE 17–32
Second layer of the plantar muscles.

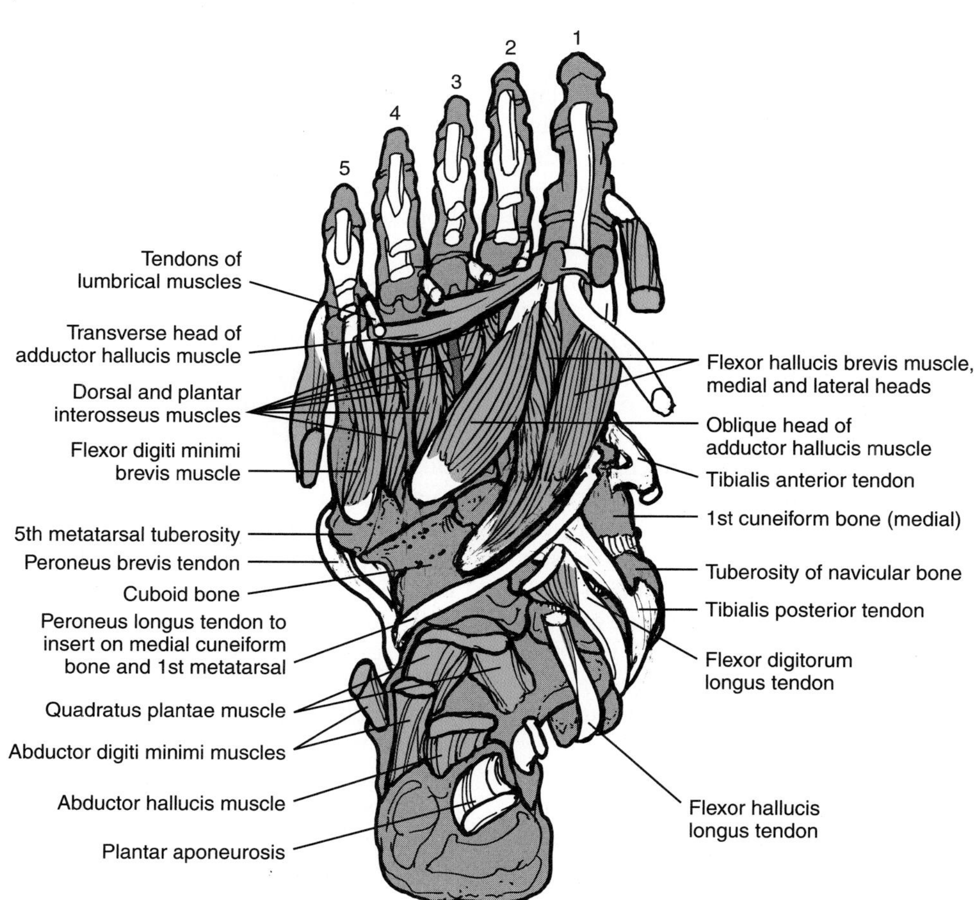

FIGURE 17–33
Third layer of the plantar muscles with ligaments removed.

The **second layer of plantar muscles of the foot** consists of a short flexor, which assists in digital flexion through its attachment to the distal tendon of the flexor digitorum longus muscle, and four diminutive wormlike muscles, which originate from this same tendon.

The short flexor muscle is the **flexor accessorius (quadratus plantae) muscle.** Its medial and lateral heads arise from medial and lateral surfaces of the calcaneus (see Fig. 17–32). The heads usually fuse and insert upon the lateral boundary of the common part of the distal tendon of the flexor digitorum longus muscle (Fig. 17–32).

The position and consequent action of this accessory flexor muscle "correct" the oblique vector of the flexor digitorum longus muscle so that it does not pull the toes in a medial direction when it contracts (Table 17–4).

Each of the four **lumbrical muscles** arises from the medial side of one of the four distal tendons of the flexor digitorum longus muscle (Fig. 17–32). One lumbrical muscle courses along the medial side of digits 2 to 5 to insert upon the dorsal digital expansion (Fig. 17–32).

The action of the lumbrical muscles results in flexion of the distal phalanx and extension of the proximal phalanges (Fig. 17–29F and Table 17–4).

The **third layer of plantar muscles of the foot** contains the short intrinsic flexors of the big and little toes and an adductor of the big toe.

The two-headed **flexor hallucis brevis muscle** arises from the plantar surface of the cuboid bone, lateral cuneiform bone, and tibialis posterior tendon (Fig. 17–33). Its two distal tendons attach to opposite sides of the base of the most proximal phalanx of the big toe (Fig. 17–32).

The flexor hallucis brevis muscle acts to assist in flexion of the hallux (Fig. 17–29*C* and Table 17–4).

The **adductor hallucis muscle** also has two heads, a **transverse** and an **oblique head** (Fig. 17–33). The transverse head arises from ligaments associated with the metatarsophalangeal joints of the third to fifth digits. The oblique head arises from the plantar surfaces of the bases of the second to fourth metatarsals. The fibers of both heads converge to form a single distal tendon, which inserts upon the base of the proximal phalanx of the big toe.

As its name suggests, the adductor hallucis muscle acts to adduct the big toe (Fig. 17–29*G* and Table 17–4).

The **flexor digiti minimi brevis muscle** arises from the medial plantar surface of the base of the fifth metatarsal. Its distal tendon inserts upon the lateral surface of the base of the proximal phalanx of the little toe (Fig. 17–33).

The main action of the flexor digiti minimi brevis muscle is to flex the fifth digit (Fig. 17–29*H*), but it may also assist in abduction of the digit (Fig. 17–29*D* and Table 17–4).

The **deepest muscles of the foot** are the seven **interosseous muscles** (Figs. 17–34 and 17–35). Four of these are dorsal abductors of the toes (Fig. 17–34*A*), and three are plantar adductors (Fig. 17–34*B*). The muscles arise from the bases and shafts of metatarsal bones and insert upon the bases of the proximal phalanges. The insertion is on the same side as that from which each muscle originates (Fig. 17–34). One way to deduce the locations and actions of these muscles is to consider the following facts:

1. Of the five toes, digits one, three, four, and five have an adductor and an abductor. Digit two has two abductors and no adductors (because movements of abduction and adduction are relative to its own axis) (Fig. 17–34). Therefore, the five digits share four adductors and six abductors.
2. An abductor of the big toe and an abductor of the little toe are located in the first layer, and an adductor of the big toe is located in the third layer. This leaves seven interosseous muscles to provide the remaining four abductors and three adductors.
3. The big toe, therefore, has its own adductor and abductor; the second toe has two dorsal interosseous abductors; the third and fourth toes each have a dorsal interosseous abductor and a plantar interosseus adductor; and the fifth toe has a plantar interosseous adductor and an abductor in the first layer (Fig. 17–35).

▲ Mechanisms of Standing (Weight Bearing) and Bipedal Locomotion

Standing is largely a passive function of the intrinsic architecture of bones, joints, ligaments, and fascia

When a person is in the **standing position,** the body's center of gravity is located about 1 cm dorsal to the sacral promontory. The vector of the center of gravity is along a line directed vertically downward just posterior to the fulcrum of the hip joint and just anterior to the fulcrum of the knee joint and then to a point just anterior to the ankle joints. Therefore, the weight of the body forces hyperextension of the hip and knee joints. This brings the articulating surfaces into their most closely packed configuration and forces the knee joint to assume a **"locked" position.** Further hyperextension of the knee and hip joints is checked by the architecture, ligaments, and surrounding fasciae and integument of the joints (see above). In contrast, passive dorsiflexion at the ankle joints is checked by contraction of the powerful soleus muscle via its attachment to the calcaneus (Fig. 17–36*A*). The passive role of the iliotibial tract and associated connective tissue septa is also important because the femoral-tibial axis is not strictly vertical (i.e., the inferior ends of the femurs and superior ends of the tibias slant medially) (Fig. 17–36*B*). The condylar planes of the femur and tibia are also angled with respect to the long axes of these bones to bring them into

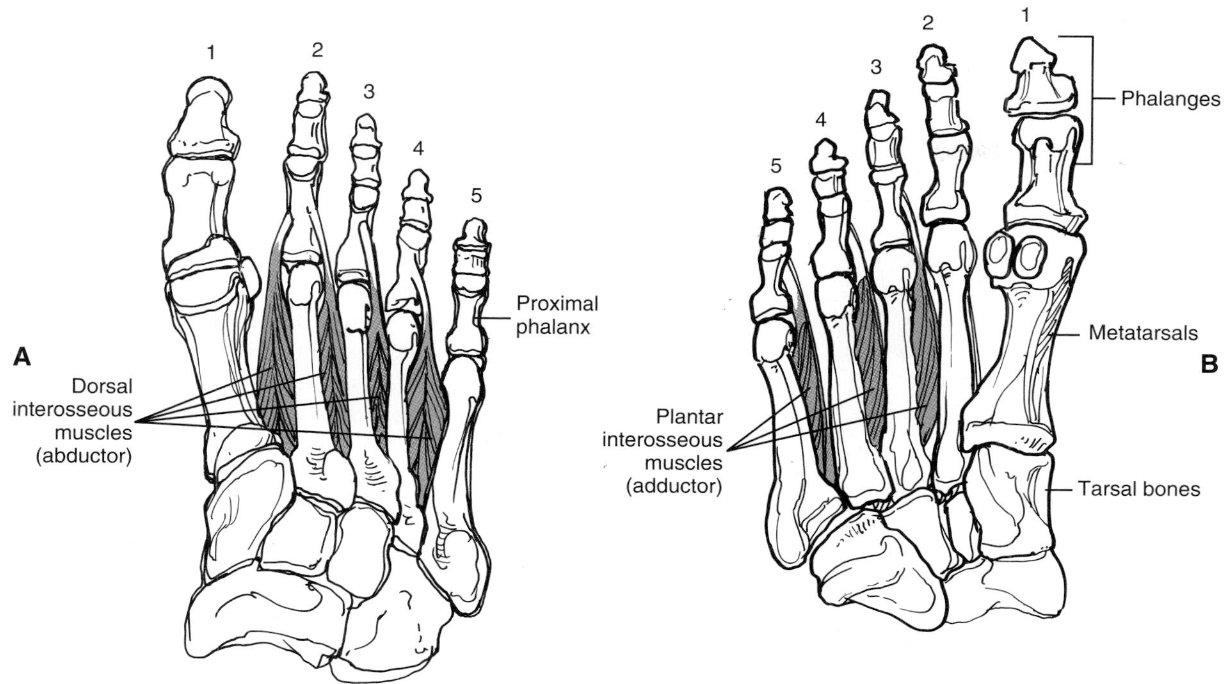

FIGURE 17–34
Fourth layer of the plantar muscles (interosseous muscles).

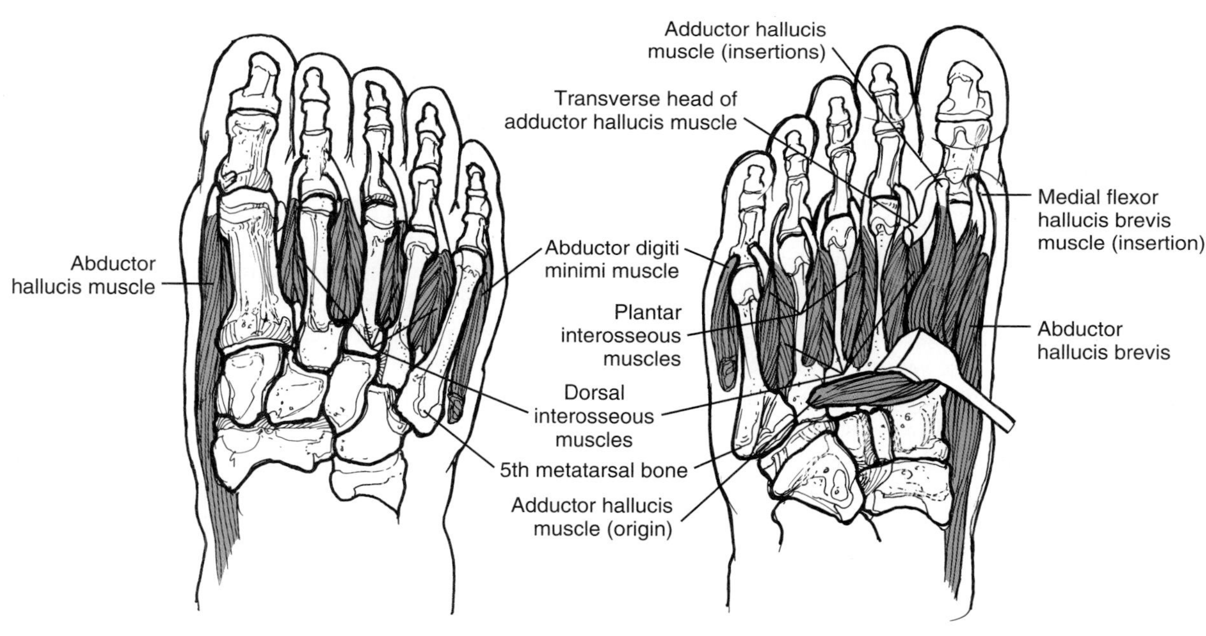

FIGURE 17–35
Adductors and abductors of the toes from all layers shown together.

a horizontal plane (Fig. 17–36*B*). The resulting closely fitting articulations of the extended knee joint, especially the strong ligaments, capsule, and iliotibial tract, tend to prevent gravity-induced abduction of the tibia. Slight swaying of the body is checked by rapid muscle contractions, which last only moments within the lower extremity and trunk (erector spinae and transversospinal muscles). If a person has been standing for a long time, he or she may shift the body's weight from foot to foot. One leg will be slightly flexed to act as a prop that allows most of the weight to be supported by the other leg.

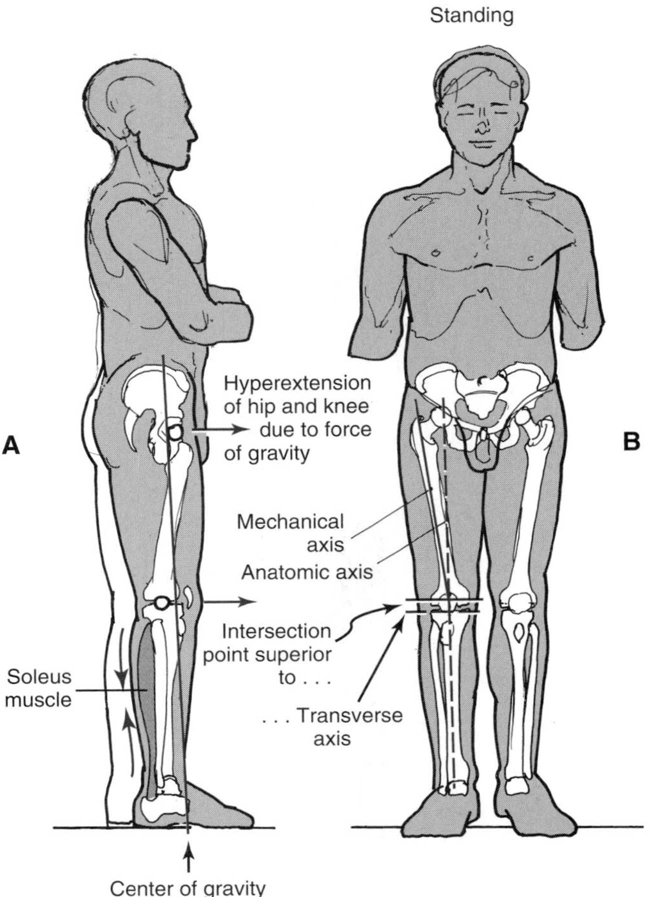

FIGURE 17-36
Mechanisms of weight bearing in a standing position. **A.** Center of gravity is behind fulcrum of hip joint, anterior to knee and ankle joints. Position maintained by soleus muscle and iliotibial tract. **B.** Anterior view showing medial slant of femoral tibial axis.

The **fascia lata** (see discussions of gluteal and anterior thigh muscles above) also provides significant stability to the hip and knee joints when a person is standing with the thigh and leg fully extended. The fascia lata is attached superiorly to the sacrum, iliac crest, ischial tuberosity, and superior and inferior pubic rami. As the fascia lata courses from these points, it splits into two layers, which invest the deep and superficial surfaces of the gluteus maximus muscle. The deep layer is firmly connected to the capsule of the hip joint. The superficial and deep layers fuse at the lower border of the gluteus maximus muscle to form the **iliotibial tract.** This tough band of deep fascia receives an insertion at its superoposterior edge from the gluteus maximus muscle (see above). In the superolateral region of the thigh, the iliotibial tract also encloses the tensor fasciae latae muscle (see above). The tract descends to attach to all of the bony projections of the femoral, tibial, and fibular condyles. It is continuous with the thick lateral intermuscular septum of the thigh, which is attached to the linea aspera. It is also attached to the medial intermuscular septum of the thigh. This tough, extensive, integrated system of fascia steadies the pelvis upon the head of the femur and the femoral condyles upon the tibial condyles. Thus, when a person is standing, extension of the leg causes the fascia lata and skin to become taut, preventing abduction or adduction of the knee joint.

Tendons, ligaments, and **muscles** within the **plantar compartment** of the foot play an integral role in maintaining the **arch of the foot** during standing, walking, running, and jumping. The arch is created by the architecture of the tarsus and metatarsus, their joints, and their supporting ligaments, tendons, and muscles. The arch of the foot has transverse and longitudinal curvatures. The **transverse curvature** is a half dome, which rises to its pinnacle on the medial side of the foot. For the purpose of functional discussions, it is useful to divide the **longitudinal curvature** into medial and lateral longitudinal arches. The **medial longitudinal arch** is created by the calcaneus, talus, and navicular bones; the middle, intermediate, and lateral cuneiform bones; and the three most medial metatarsal bones (see below and Chapter 16). This part of the longitudinal arch is always elevated from the substratum in healthy individuals and plays a critical role in standing and weight bearing. The **lateral longitudinal arch** is created by the calcaneus bone, cuboid bone, and fourth and fifth (lateral) metatarsals. It is not elevated as much as the medial arch and plays a more crucial role in locomotion (see below and Chapter 16). Thus, when a person is standing with the muscles of the foot relaxed, the medial arch is maintained by (1) the shapes of the calcaneal, talar, cuneiform, and metatarsal bones and their articulating surfaces; (2) the intrinsic and extrinsic ligaments of these bones; and (3) the plantar aponeurosis (see Fig. 17–30). Maintenance of this region of the longitudinal arch (and also, to some degree, of the lateral longitudinal and transverse arches) when a person is standing sustains the foot's three-point contact with the substratum. This configuration also allows for various degrees of supination or pronation of the foot so that the foot can make the most secure contact possible with the substratum no matter how steep the gradient may be or whether the individual is standing with the feet together or apart.

Mechanisms of Walking and Running

In contrast to standing, walking and running require the expenditure of a significant amount of muscle energy

To understand the mechanisms employed in **walking** and **running,** it is important to define several key terms. A single **walking cycle** is the period between the impact of one heel with the substratum and the impact of the other heel with the substratum (Fig. 17–37*A*). As the heel is planted, the extremity enters the **stance phase.** It remains in the stance phase until the toes leave

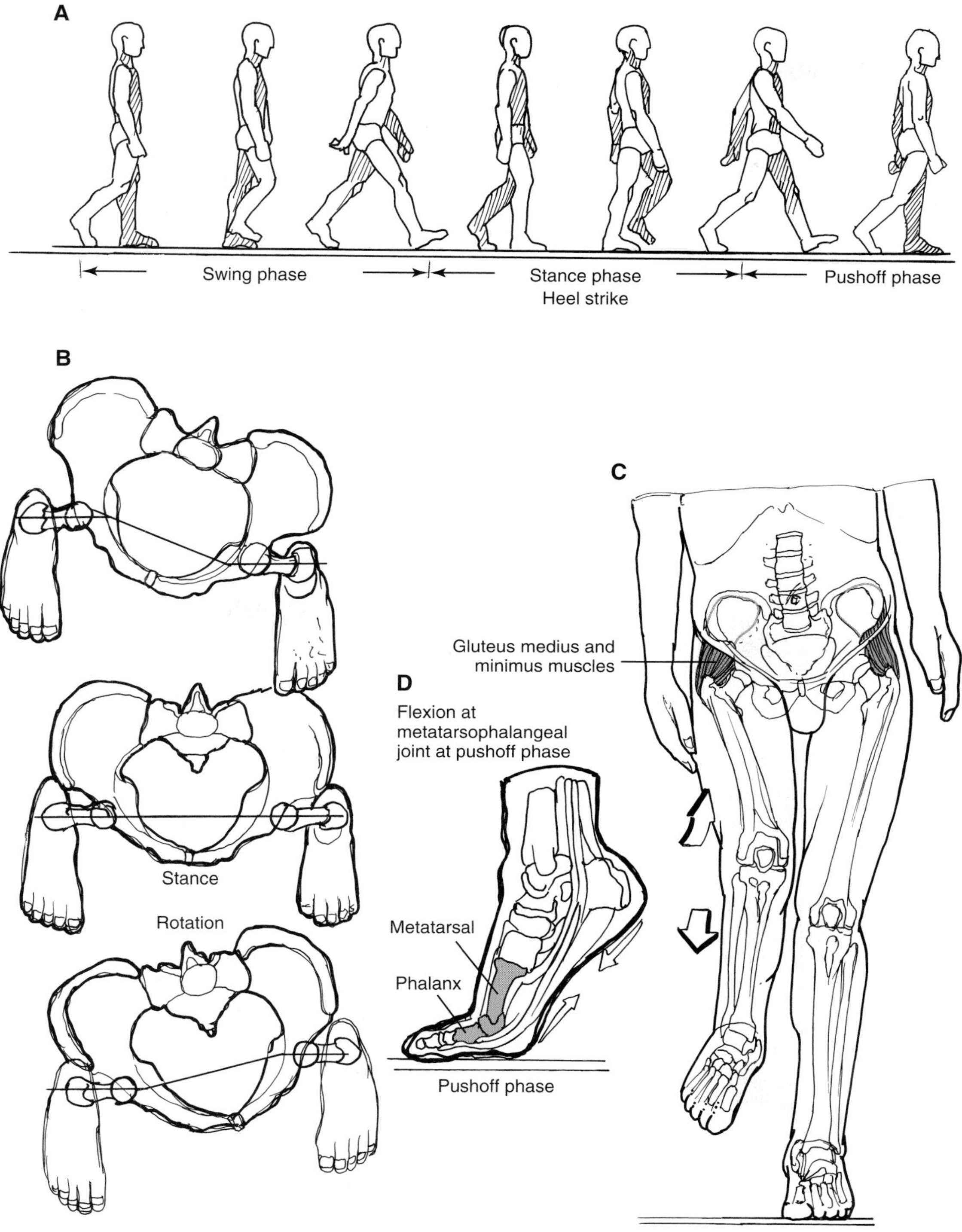

FIGURE 17-37

Elements of the walking cycle. **A.** Two walking cycles: stance phase with heel planted and swing phase as toes leave the ground. **B.** Rotation of pelvis in relation to forward movement of the body. **C.** Medial rotation of pelvis counters lateral motion of femur and tibia. Gluteus medius and gluteus minimus muscles support pelvis on the unsupported side. **D.** During flexion of the metatarsophalangeal joints at push off, phalanges remain in extension, maintaining stability and maximum contact with the substratum.

the ground during the initiation of the next walking cycle. As the toes of the foot break contact with the substratum, the extremity enters the **swing phase.** The extremity remains in the swing phase until the heel again makes contact with the substratum. Each walking cycle begins as one foot enters the stance phase and the other foot simultaneously enters the swing phase.

Walking. When the heel is planted during the stance phase, the weight of the entire body is shifted to this planted extremity as the body sways laterally to that side. After the heel is planted and as the body is propelled forward, the lateral edge of the foot makes a rolling, progressive contact with the substratum, and the body weight is continuously shifted from the heel to the toes. This transfer of body weight tends to flatten the arches of the foot, but flattening of the sole is countered not only by the passive resistance of the bony architecture and intrinsic and extrinsic plantar ligaments, but also by tendons of the activated intrinsic flexor muscles of the foot and long flexor muscles of the posterior compartment of the leg. In addition, the forward movement of the body over the planted foot increases the dorsiflexion of the ankle joint so that the arches become even more accentuated. As the planted foot continues to dorsiflex, the tibia rotates medially with respect to the talus, and the femur rotates medially with respect to the pelvis (Fig. 17–37*B*). As the extremity in the stance phase completes the final 30 degrees of extension, the femur (because of the weight of gravity) medially rotates upon the tibia to "lock" the knee joint. These medial rotations are countered by lateral rotation of the pelvis as the contralateral side of the body is thrust forward. The interplay between the long and short flexors of the toes maintains the phalanges in extension while allowing flexion of the proximal interphalangeal joints and metatarsophalangeal joints (Fig. 17–37*D*). As weight is shifted to the distal end of the planted foot, the foot is supinated. The integration of all of these actions results in (1) maximum stability of the knee and hip joints, (2) generation of tautness in the foot and accentuation of the arches, (3) maintenance of the toes in maximum contact with the substratum, and (4) stabilization of the weight-bearing function of the balls of the feet (metatarsal heads). This is important because it is from the metatarsal heads that forward thrust is initiated to propel the body forward during the next walking cycle.

The forward thrust during "takeoff" from the ball of the foot at the end of the stance phase is largely generated by the long flexors of the posterior crural (leg) compartment. The gastrocnemius and tibialis posterior muscles play a particularly important role in generating forward thrust. The consequence of their actions is the initiation of plantarflexion along with pronation to transfer the final pushoff thrust to the big toe as the heel is lifted. As the toes finally leave the substratum (at the same time that the heel of the other foot is planted), the hip is flexed and the limb enters the swing phase (Fig. 17–37*A*). As the tibia is freed from bearing weight, it rotates laterally with respect to the talus and the femur rotates laterally with respect to the pelvis (Fig. 17–37*B*). The tibia is also medially rotated with respect to the femur (unlocking the knee joint) through the action of the popliteus muscle. Overall, the lateral rotation of the tibia (with respect to the talus) and femur (with respect to the tibia) is accompanied by flexion of the knee and further flexion of the hip to raise the foot. The lateral rotations of the femur and tibia are countered by the medial rotation of the pelvis on that side of the body. In addition, sagging of this unsupported side of the pelvis is countered by contraction of the contralateral gluteus medius and gluteus minimus muscles (Fig. 17–37*C*). Finally, as the body is propelled forward, extensors of the anterior compartments of the thigh and leg contract, at first inverting and slightly dorsiflexing the foot and then bringing the heel into contact with the substratum and initiating the next stance phase (Fig. 17–38*A*).

Muscular elements also play an important role in maintaining the arches during locomotion. As the foot is planted during walking, the heel first makes contact with the substratum. As the foot is plantarflexed and supinated during the stance phase (see above), the arches (especially the lateral longitudinal arch) tend to flatten to maximize contact with the substratum. As the weight of the body bears directly upon the planted foot, further flattening of the arches is countered by the bones, ligaments, and connective tissues. As the foot plantarflexes and the heel is lifted to initiate the next step, curvatures of the longitudinal arches are restored or enhanced by contractions of the tibialis posterior, flexor digitorum longus, flexor hallucis longus, and intrinsic plantar muscles. During the push-off, or thrust, phase of the stride, these plantar muscles and tendons behave as dynamic struts, which pull the calcaneus and distal metatarsals together (Fig. 17–39). In addition, the peroneus longus and peroneus brevis muscles act to slightly evert the foot during push off (Fig. 17–38*B*). Some anatomists believe that the tibialis anterior muscle may be a "suspender" of the arch. However, this muscle is quiescent during standing. Moreover, if the muscle were activated during the pushoff phase, when it would be most needed, its action would paradoxically antagonize the plantarflexion that generates forward thrust.

Running. Running is similar to walking, except that the heel does not touch the ground. Only the metatarsus and phalanges make contact with the substratum. However, once the forefoot is planted, the controlled, balanced action of plantarflexors and dorsiflexors gently lowers the heel toward the substratum. This minimizes shock and establishes a more dorsiflexed, closely packed configuration of the foot to maximize the thrust generated by plantarflexors at the next pushoff. Moreover, the knee is not extended, medially rotated, and

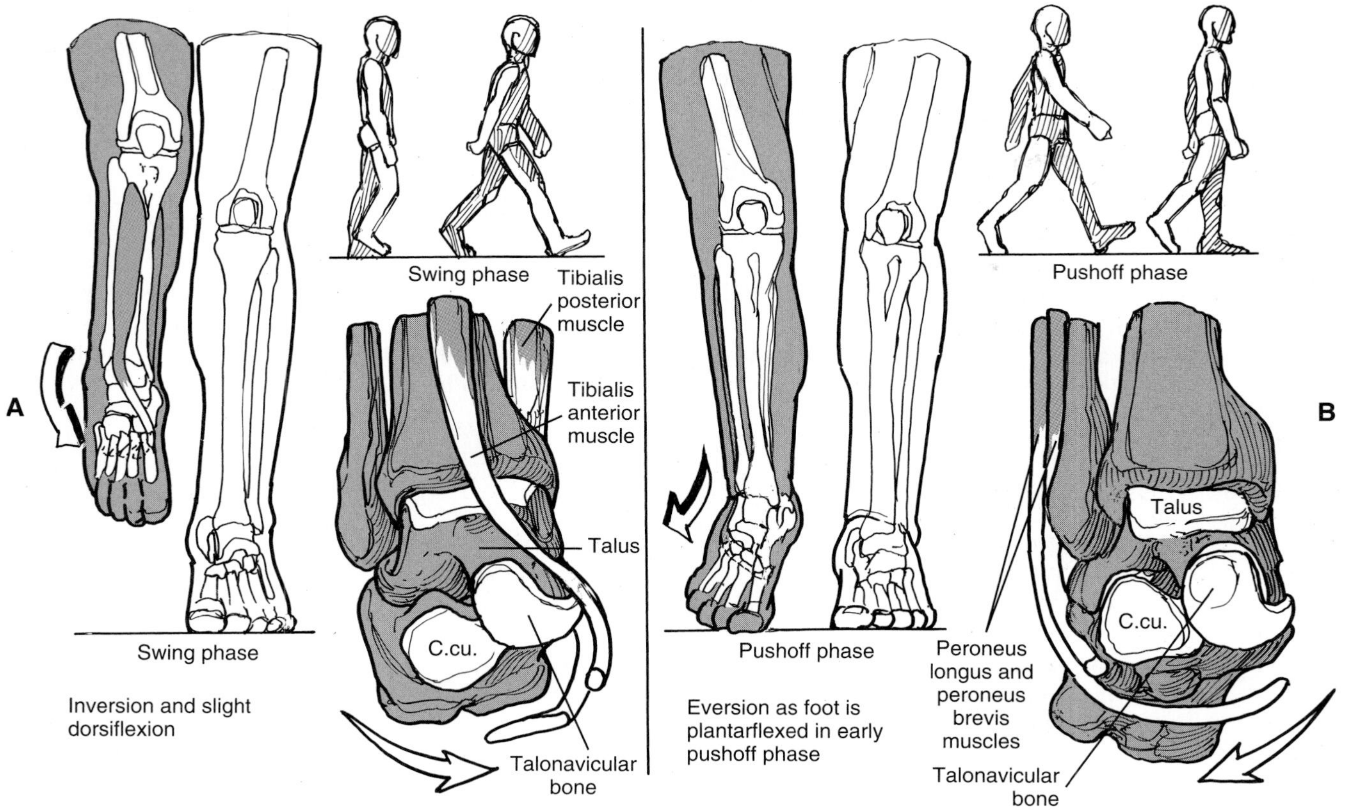

FIGURE 17-38
Muscles acting on the feet during locomotion. **A.** Inversion of the foot by anterior extensor and tibialis anterior muscles. **B.** Eversion of the foot by lateral compartment muscles, peroneus longus and peroneus brevis.

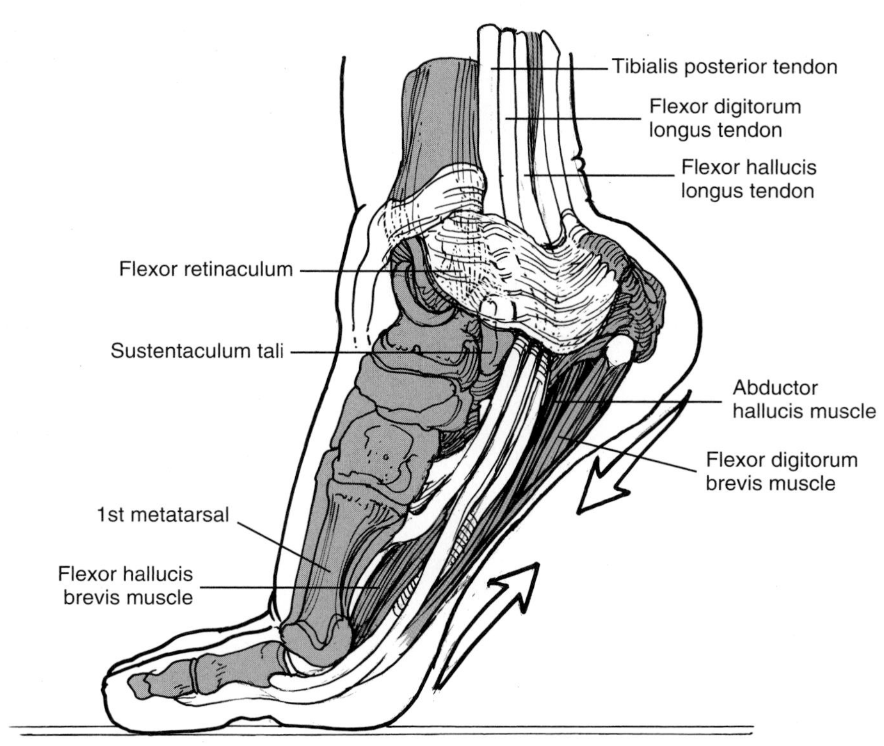

FIGURE 17–39
Muscles maintaining foot arches during locomotion.

locked in the weight-bearing extremity until the moment that thrust is generated by plantarflexion at pushoff. In addition, forward movement of the body occurs unsupported in the interval between pushoff from one foot and planting of the other.

Other Parts of the Body Used in Locomotion. As the body weight shifts from one extremity to the other during forward movement, balance is maintained by the swinging of the arm contralateral to the extremity in swing phase and by the swaying of the trunk laterally over the extremity in stance phase.

These activities are not so pronounced in humans as they are in other primates that walk on their hind legs. Part of the reason for this difference is the configuration of the human femur and tibia, which emplaces both knees medially and closer to a point immediately beneath the body's center of gravity (see Fig. 17–36*B*). As weight is shifted from one foot to the other, balance can be maintained by small lateral shifts of the upper body (which are required to position the center of gravity directly above the extremity in stance phase). The femoral-tibial axis of apes is almost vertical, requiring pronounced upper body swaying and arm swinging to maintain the center of gravity above the supporting extremity when the ape is walking on two legs.

18 Vessels and Nerves of the Lower Extremities

This chapter describes the vasculature and innervation of the lower extremity and provides an opportunity for the review and integration of other lower limb structures such as bones, joints, and muscles. To support these objectives, each major vessel and nerve is described from its origin to its terminus. Several figures in this chapter illustrate the entire course of each vessel or nerve so that the progression of the vessel or nerve from one compartment to another and the comprehensive distribution of the vessel or nerve may be seen on a single page.

Because the lower extremity is so definitively divided into compartments by deep fascial barriers, strategically placed foramina are required to transport vessels and nerves between compartments. These specialized apertures include those in the femoral sheath and cribriform fascia and the following conduits: the obturator canal; the adductor (subsartorial) canal; smaller adductor perforations; a superior hiatus, or tendinous arch, at the upper boundary of the soleus muscle; a superior hiatus within the interosseous membrane; and an inferior hiatus within the interosseous membrane.

These apertures are described in detail where appropriate (see specific vessel and nerve distributions below).

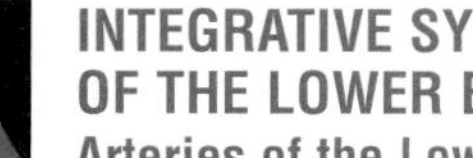

INTEGRATIVE SYSTEMS OF THE LOWER EXTREMITY

Arteries of the Lower Extremity

The femoral artery provides the major blood supply to the lower limb but is aided by other vessels

Most of the lower extremity is vascularized by the **femoral artery** and its branches. Smaller vessels such as the **superior** and **inferior gluteal vessels** serve the gluteal compartment, and the **obturator artery** contributes to the vasculature of the medial compartment of the thigh. Branches of all of these vessels communicate with one another, providing an extensive collateral circulatory system within the lower extremity (Fig. 18–1). Each major vessel and its branches are described in turn.

Femoral Artery and Its Branches and Associated Structures

The large femoral artery first descends from the level of the inguinal ligament into the anterior compartment of the thigh (Fig. 18–1*A*). It courses inferiorly at the border of the anterior and medial compartments, giving off branches to anterior and posterior compartment muscles. It escapes posteriorly into the popliteal fossa (behind the knee); branches into vessels that serve the anterior, posterior, and lateral compartments of the leg; and finally branches into vessels that serve the dorsum and plantar compartment of the foot (Fig. 18–1).

Femoral Sheath. *The femoral sheath transports vessels from the posterior abdominal wall to the anterior compartment of the thigh.* Both the **femoral artery** and **femoral vein** gain access to the anterior thigh as they course under the medial portion of the inguinal ligament and over the pelvic brim. Because these vessels are not located within the peritoneal cavity and are, therefore, retroperitoneal vessels, there is no need for them to pierce the peritoneum. However, the vessels are invested by posterior and anterior layers of deep fascia as they course under the inguinal ligament (Fig. 18–2*B* and *C*). In the false pelvis, femoral vessels course within the subserous fascia and, thus, lie upon the iliac fascia. The **iliac fascia** remains located posterior to the femoral vessels as they exit the false pelvis and enter the anterior thigh. In addition, the **fascia transversalis (transverse fascia)** extends downward from the anterior body wall about $1\frac{1}{2}$ to 2 inches (3 to 4 cm) to form an anterior covering for the femoral vessels in the superior thigh. Together, the posterior and anterior fascial investments of the femoral vessels form a funnel-shaped structure called the **femoral sheath** (Fig. 18–2*B* and *C*). It is wide at the level of the inguinal ligament and narrow below this level, where the transverse fascia is fused tightly to the fascia of the vessels as they pierce the sheath to descend further into the thigh. The femoral sheath is, therefore, located in the superior region of the femoral triangle (Fig. 18–2*B* and *C*).

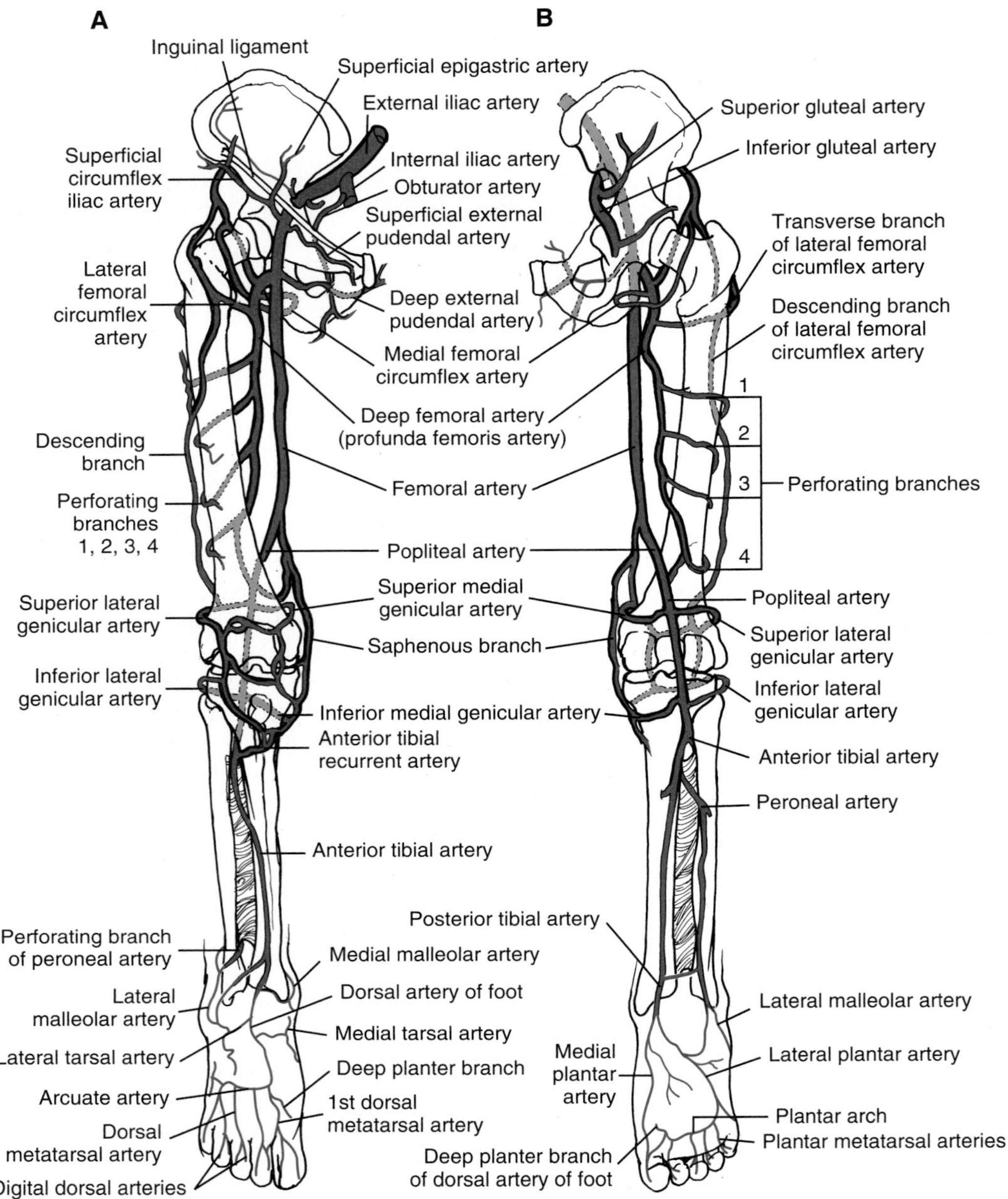

FIGURE 18–1
Arteries of the lower extremity. **A.** Anterior view. **B.** Posterior view

The femoral sheath is divided into three vertical compartments (Fig. 18–2*B*). From lateral to medial, the compartments contain the femoral branch of the genitofemoral nerve, femoral artery, femoral vein, and lymphatic vessels. The medial compartment, containing the lymphatic vessels, is the smallest of the three and is called the **femoral canal** (Fig. 18–2*B*). Its superior entrance is the **femoral ring** (Fig. 18–2*C*). Unlike the femoral vessels that course anterior to the iliac fascia, which constitutes the posterior wall of the sheath, the more laterally placed **femoral nerve** courses under the inguinal ligament posterior to the iliopsoas fascia between the fascia and the iliopsoas muscle. Therefore, it is excluded from the femoral sheath (Fig. 18–2). As the femoral nerve enters the thigh after passing under the inguinal ligament, it branches into many muscular and cutaneous branches, which serve structures of the anterior compartment of the thigh (see below).

Just before passing beneath the inguinal ligament, the femoral sheath is perforated laterally by the **femoral branch of the genitofemoral nerve.** In the superior region of the femoral triangle, the sheath is penetrated medially by **lymphatic vessels** and the **superficial great saphenous vein** as it joins with the

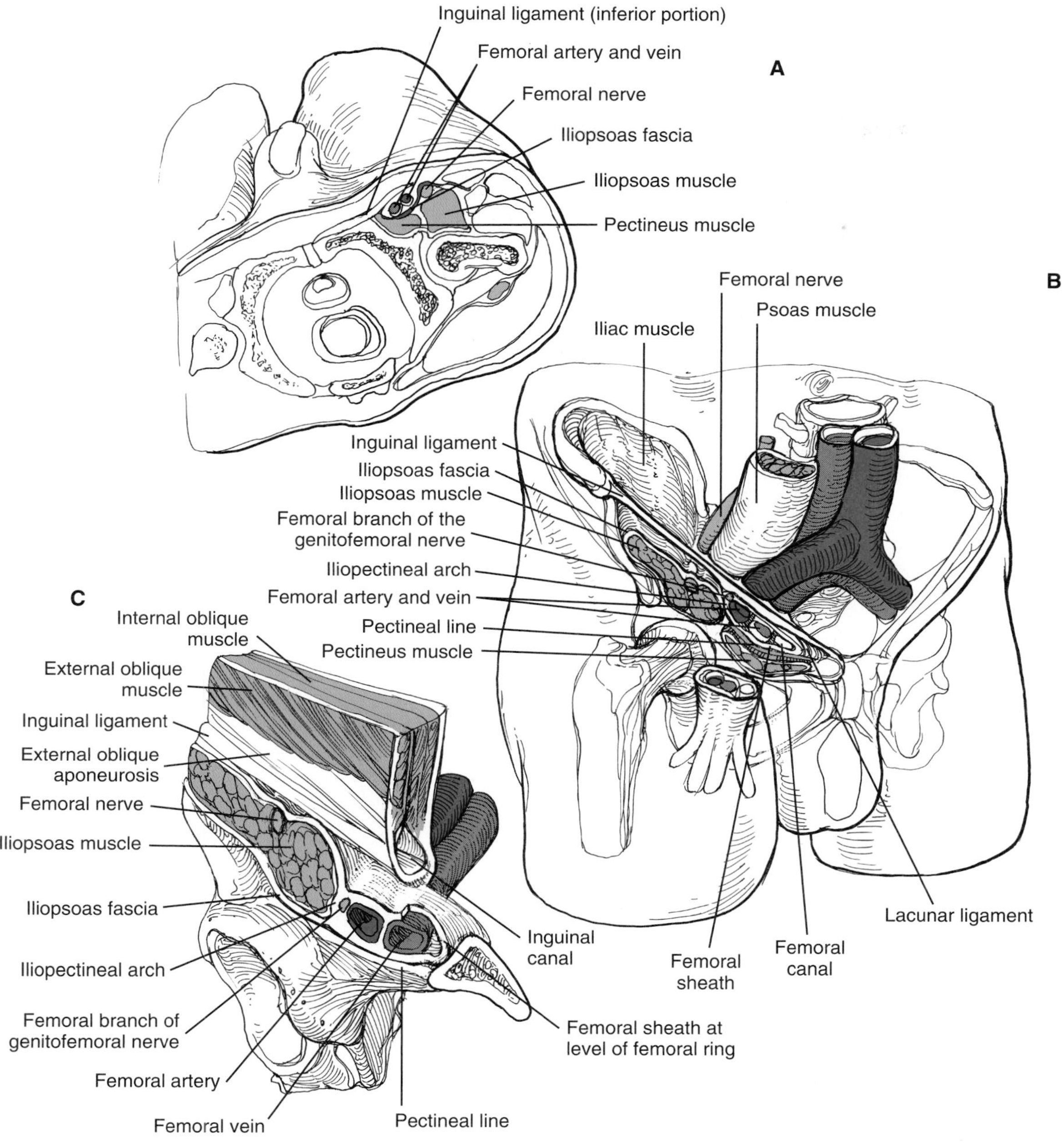

FIGURE 18–2
Compartments and vessels of the femoral sheath. **A.** Superior cross-sectional view. **B.** Anterior lateral view showing femoral artery and vein under the inguinal ligament as they enter the anterior thigh. **C.** Close-up view of the femoral sheath showing iliopsoas and transversalis fascia, the posterior and anterior fascia covering femoral vessels that, together, form the femoral sheath.

femoral vein (Fig. 18–3). Because the great saphenous vein courses within the superficial fascia of the thigh as it ascends to the level of the femoral sheath, it must also penetrate the fascia lata (the thickened deep fascia of the thigh) to gain access to the sheath. It does this through a hiatus in the fascia lata called the **saphenous opening,** or **hiatus** (Fig. 18–3*A* and *C*). The thin layer of superficial fascia covering the saphenous hiatus is called the **cribriform fascia** because, just like a sieve, it is penetrated by many small lymphatic vessels (Fig. 18–3*A*).

Once the skin and fascia have been removed from the thigh, the femoral vessels and nerve can be seen passing into the thigh in a region bounded by the in-

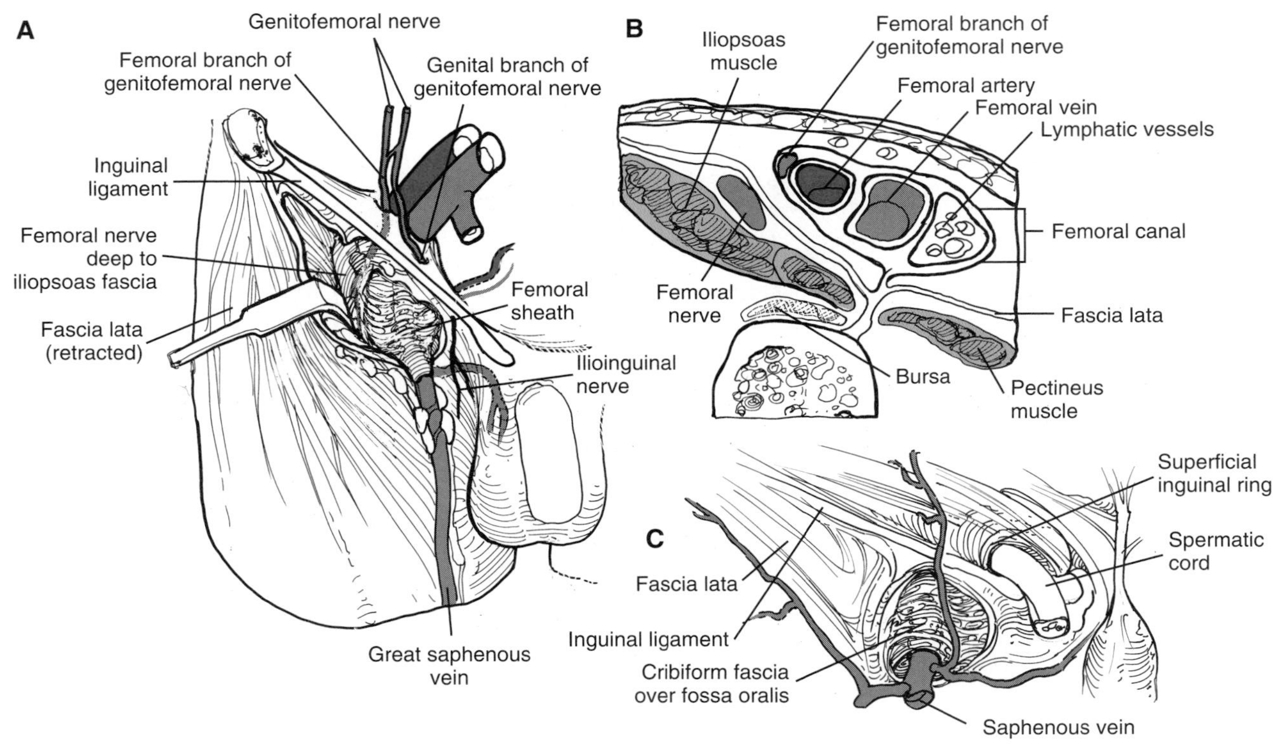

FIGURE 18–3
Perforations of the femoral sheath. **A.** Superior to inguinal ligament, femoral branch of genitofemoral nerve perforates femoral sheath laterally. Inferior to inguinal ligament, ascending lymphatic vessels and great saphenous vein penetrate fascia lata as the vein joins the femoral vein in the medial portion of femoral sheath. **B.** Cross section of femoral sheath showing relationships of fascia, nerves, and vessels. **C.** Detail of cribriform fascia over saphenous opening.

guinal ligament superiorly, the medial edge of the sartorius muscle laterally, and the lateral border of the adductor longus muscle medially. The region defined by these boundaries is the **femoral triangle** (see Fig. 17–11*A*).

Because this collection of major vessels is unprotected, injury to the femoral triangle can be life-threatening.

As soon as the femoral artery passes under the inguinal ligament, it gives rise to three small branches: the **superficial circumflex iliac artery, superficial epigastric artery,** and **superficial external pudendal artery** (Fig. 18–4 and see Fig. 18–1*A*). The arteries course within the superficial fascia to supply the skin and hypodermis of the anterolateral body wall (see Chapter 11). Just below the superficial external pudendal artery, the femoral artery gives rise to the large **deep femoral artery (arteria profunda femoris)** and the diminutive **deep external pudendal artery** (see Figs. 18–1*A* and 18–4). The external pudendal arteries supply the skin of the perineum and the anterior scrotum or labium majus (see Chapter 15). Typically, veins of the same names accompany these arteries (see below).

The **deep femoral artery** usually branches from the lateral side of the femoral artery just below the lower end of the femoral sheath (see Figs. 18–1*A* and 18–4). It descends between the pectineus and the adductor longus muscles, the adductor longus and the adductor brevis muscles, and the adductor longus and the adductor magnus muscles (Fig. 18–5).

Lateral Femoral Circumflex Branch. *The deep femoral artery first gives off a lateral femoral circumflex branch.* The deep femoral artery usually first gives off a small **lateral femoral circumflex artery,** which courses laterally and immediately splits into three branches: the ascending, transverse, and descending branches (see Figs. 18–1*A* and 18–4).

The **ascending branch** courses superiorly and laterally to supply the greater trochanter of the femur and the tensor fasciae latae and iliopsoas muscles. It continues around the hip joint to anastomose with the **superior gluteal artery** and transverse branch of the **medial femoral circumflex artery** (see Fig. 18–4). These anastomoses provide a significant system of collateral circulation in the region of the hip joint (see Figs. 18–1*A* and 18–4). The **transverse branch,** which is the smallest branch, supplies the superior end of the vastus intermedius muscle. The **descending branch,** which is the largest branch, courses inferiorly just behind the rectus femoris muscle and just anterior to the vastus lateralis muscle, supplying both muscles

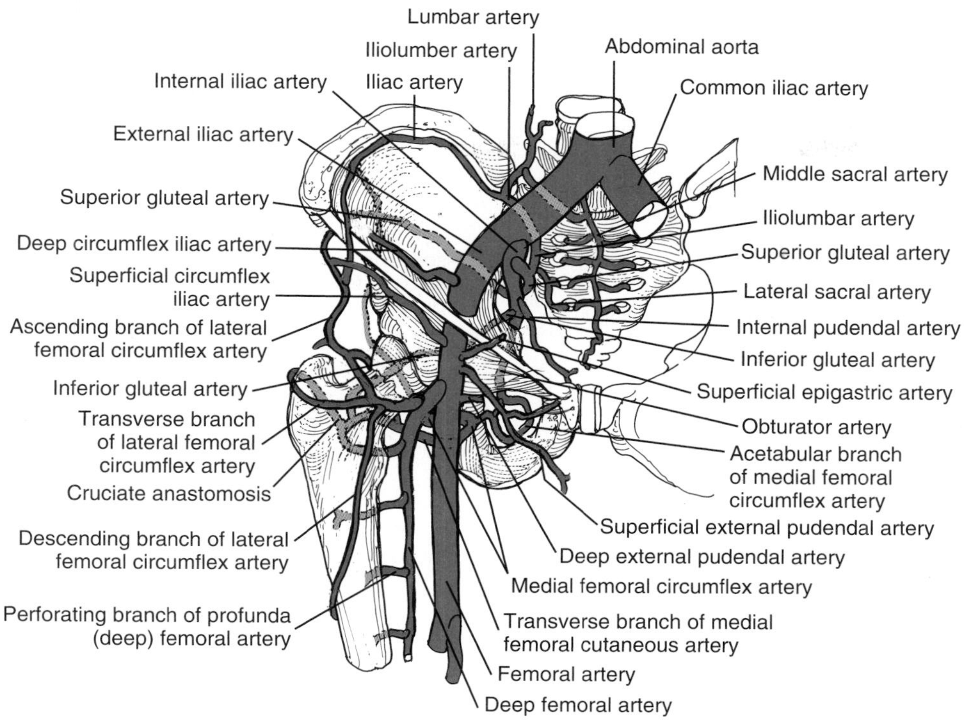

FIGURE 18–4
Branches of the femoral artery.

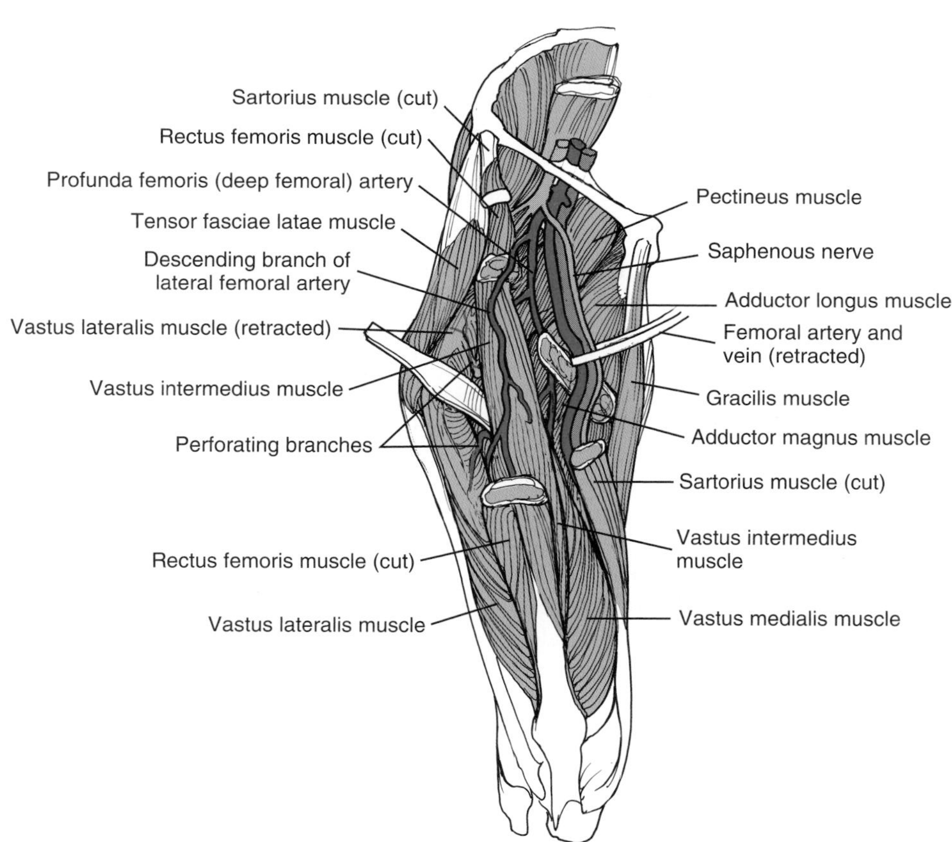

FIGURE 18–5
Path of the deep femoral artery.

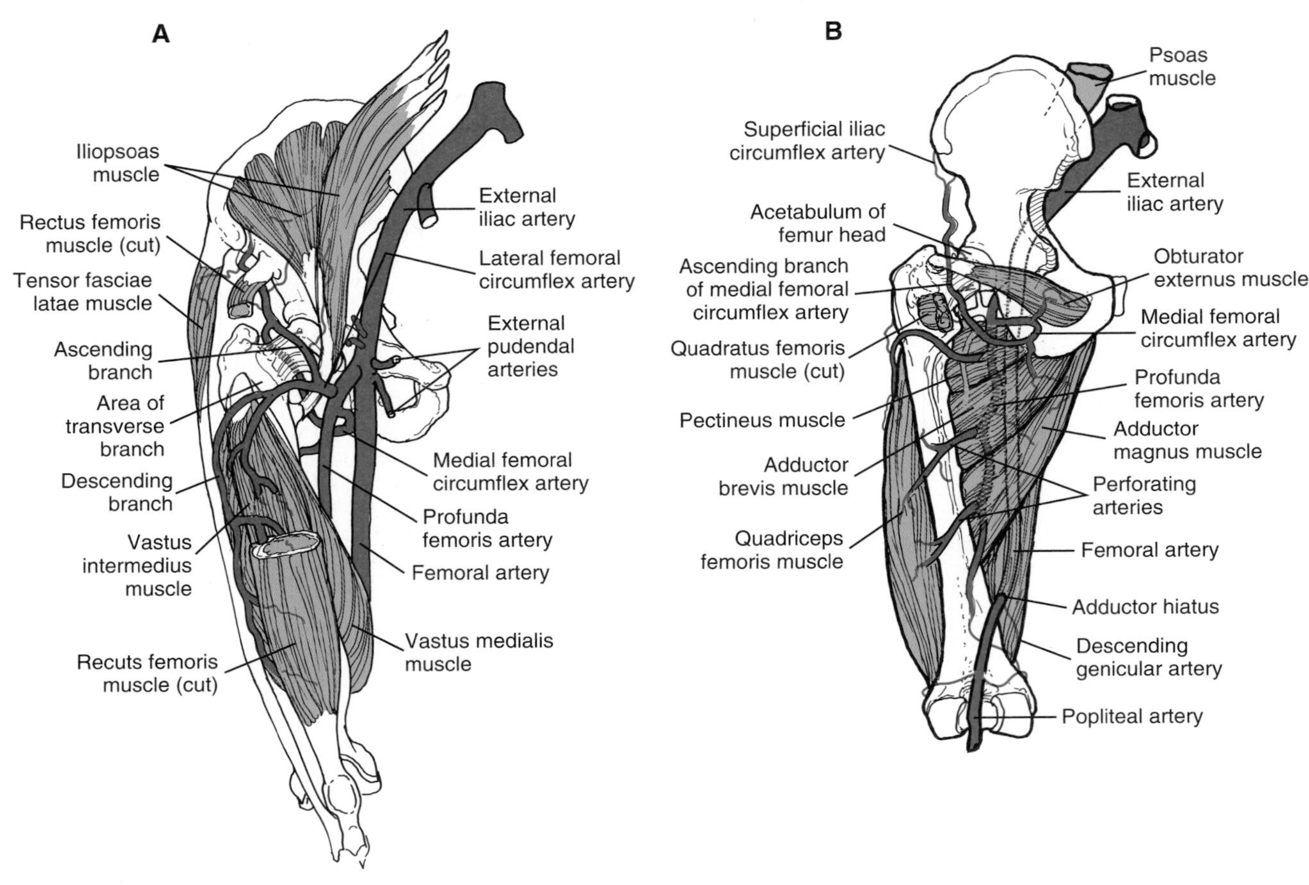

FIGURE 18–6
A. Branches of the lateral femoral circumflex artery, anterior view. **B.** Branches of the medial femoral circumflex artery, posterior view.

(Fig. 18–6*A* and Table 18–1). The descending branch finally anastomoses with the **superior genicular branch of the popliteal artery** just above the knee (see Fig. 18–9). Veins of the same names usually accompany these arteries.

Medial Femoral Circumflex Branch. *Typically, a medial femoral circumflex branch also arises from the deep femoral artery.* A small artery branching from the medial side of the deep femoral artery is typically present at about the same level as the lateral femoral circumflex artery, although it may sometimes branch from the femoral artery. The **medial femoral circumflex artery** courses medially between the psoas and the pectineus muscles, the obturator externus and the adductor brevis muscles, and the quadratus femoris and the adductor magnus muscles. Here, it splits into transverse and ascending branches (see Figs. 18–1*A*, 18–4, and 18–6*B*). The **transverse branch** continues around the posterior thigh to anastomose with the inferior gluteal artery, the ascending branch of the lateral femoral circumflex artery, and the first perforating branch of the deep femoral artery (see Figs. 18–1*A* and 18–4). This complex anastomosis is the **cruciate anastomosis** (see Fig. 18–4). The **ascending branch** of the medial femoral circumflex artery also continues posteriorly to anastomose with branches of the inferior gluteal and lateral femoral circumflex arteries (see Figs. 18–1*A* and 18–4). Veins of the same names typically accompany these arteries (see below).

Perforating Branches of Deep Femoral Artery. *Perforating branches of the deep femoral artery must penetrate the insertion of the adductor magnus muscle in order to enter the posterior compartment of the thigh.* As the deep femoral artery continues to descend within the thigh, it gives off **three perforating branches,** which course posteriorly to approach the insertion of the adductor magnus muscle along the linea aspera (see Figs. 18–1*A* and 18–4). The first of these arteries penetrates the adductor magnus muscle insertion to enter the posterior compartment by coursing around the superolateral border of the adductor brevis muscle. The second artery must penetrate the adductor brevis muscle. The third artery courses under

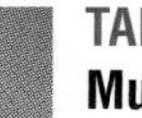

TABLE 18–1
Muscles and Other Structures Supplied by the Femoral Artery and Its Branches

Artery	Muscles Supplied	Other Regions or Structures Supplied
FEMORAL ARTERY		
Superficial epigastric artery	Abdominal muscles	Abdominal skin and superficial fascia to umbilicus
Superficial circumflex iliac	Abdominal muscles	Skin and superficial fascia of flank artery
External pudendal artery		Lower abdominal, penile or clitoral, scrotal or labial skin
Muscular branches	Sartorius, vastus medialis, femoral adductor muscles	
Cutaneous branches		Skin over anterior thigh
DEEP FEMORAL ARTERY		
Lateral femoral circumflex artery	Vastus lateralis, vastus intermedius, rectus femoris, tensor fasciae latae muscles	Skin over hip and lateral thigh
Medial femoral circumflex artery	Femoral adductor muscles	Acetabulum and head of femur
PERFORATING BRANCHES OF FEMORAL ARTERY		
First perforating branch	Adductor brevis, adductor magnus, biceps femoris, gluteus maximus muscles	
Second perforating branch	Posterior femoral muscles	Nutrient artery to femur
Third perforating branch	Posterior femoral muscles	Diaphyseal nutrient artery
Terminal perforating branches	Posterior femoral muscles	
Muscular branches	Adductor and flexor muscles of thigh	
POPLITEAL ARTERY		
Superior muscular artery	Adductor magnus muscle and posterior flexors of thigh	
Sural (muscular) artery	Gastrocnemius and soleus muscles	
Cutaneous branches		Posterior surface of leg
Superior genicular artery	Vastus medialis and vastus lateralis muscles	
Middle genicular artery		Cruciate ligaments and synovial membrane of knee joint
Inferior genicular artery	Popliteus muscle	Bone and articular structures of ankle
POSTERIOR TIBIAL ARTERY		
Circumflex fibular artery		Bone and articular structures of ankle
Muscular branches	Soleus muscle and deep flexors of leg	
Nutrient artery		Tibia
Medial malleolar artery		Tibial malleolus
Calcaneal artery	Muscles on lateral side of sole	Fat and skin around tendo calcaneus
Lateral plantar artery	Plantar muscles of sole and toes	Skin and connective tissue of lateral sole and toes
Medial plantar artery	Plantar muscles of sole and toes	Skin and connective tissue of medial sole and toes
PERONEAL ARTERY		
Muscular branches	Soleus, tibialis posterior, flexor hallucis longus, peroneus longus, peroneus brevis, peroneus tertius muscles	
Nutrient artery		Fibula

Continued

TABLE 18–1, cont'd
Muscles and Other Structures Supplied by the Femoral Artery and Its Branches

Artery	Muscles Supplied	Other Regions or Structures Supplied
ANTERIOR TIBIAL ARTERY		
Anterior tibial recurrent artery		Knee joint
Muscular branches	Anterior extensor muscles	
Anterior medial and lateral malleolar arteries		Ankle joint
Arteria dorsalis pedis	Extensor digitorum brevis muscles; dorsal muscles of toes	Skin of dorsum of foot; tarsal and metatarsal phalanges

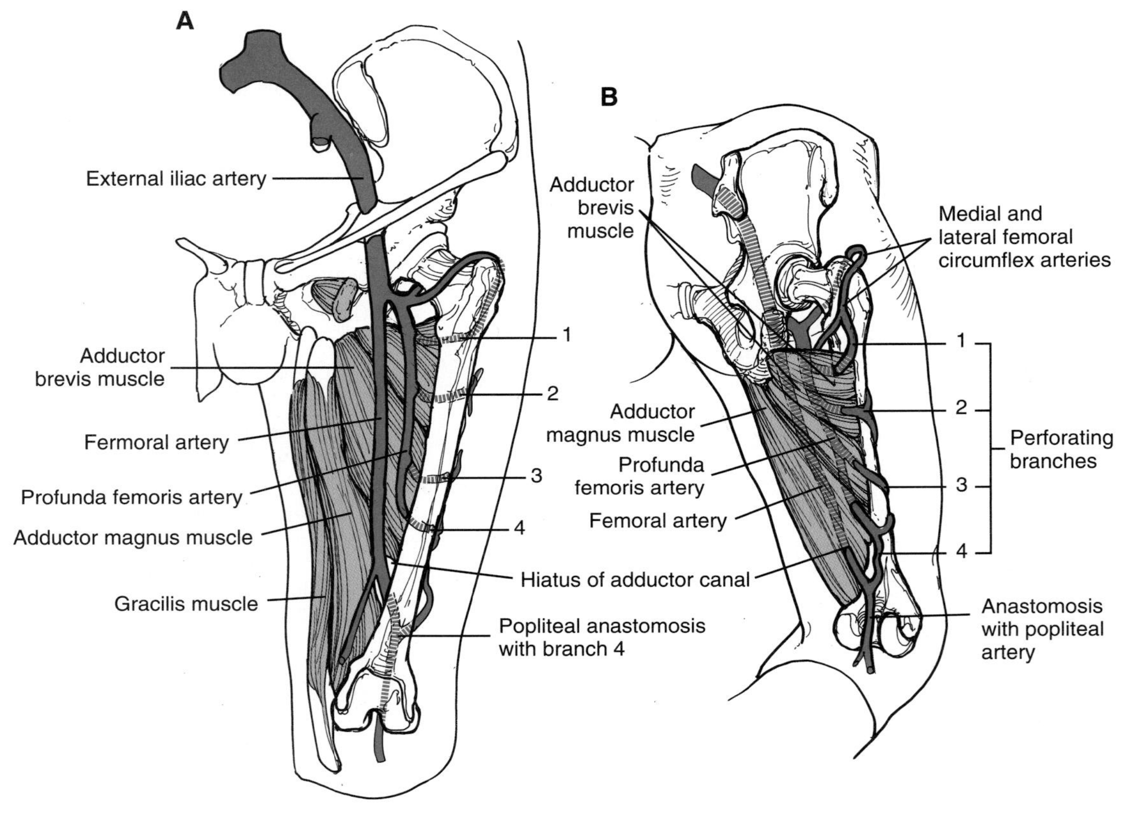

FIGURE 18–7
Perforating branches of the deep femoral artery. **A.** Anterior view. **B.** Posterior view.

the inferomedial border of the adductor brevis muscle (Fig. 18–7). The terminal branch of the deep femoral artery (sometimes called a **fourth perforating branch**) anastomoses with superior muscular branches of the **popliteal artery,** a continuation of the femoral artery (see Fig. 18–1). The deep femoral artery and its circumflex and perforating branches provide the main blood supply to extensors, flexors, and adductors of the thigh (see Table 18–1). Generally, these arteries are accompanied by veins of the same names.

Subsartorial (Adductor) Canal. *The femoral artery exits the femoral sheath to enter an aponeurotic tunnel called the subsartorial (adductor) canal.* Once the femoral artery exits the femoral sheath, it descends within the thigh just deep to the sartorius muscle within a tunnel called the **subsartorial (adductor) canal** (Fig. 18–8). The adductor canal is triangular in cross section, with the sartorius muscle forming the anterior wall, the adductor longus and adductor magnus muscles forming the posterior wall, and the vastus medialis muscle forming the anterolateral

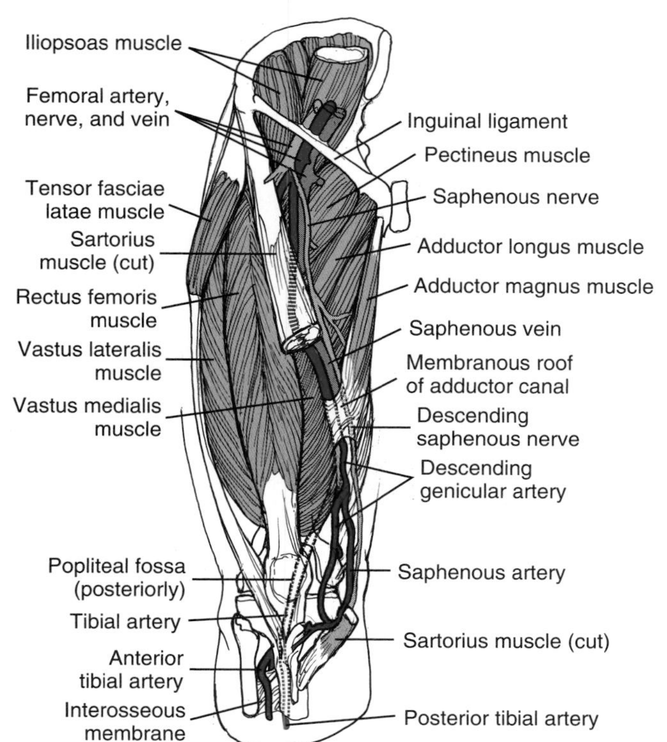

FIGURE 18–8
Subsartorial (adductor) canal and popliteal fossa.

wall. As the femoral artery descends, it gives off small branches to these surrounding muscles (see Table 18–1). The **femoral vein** and a branch of the femoral nerve, the **saphenous nerve,** accompany the femoral artery within the adductor canal (see below).

Popliteal Fossa and Adductor Hiatus. *The femoral artery leaves the adductor compartment of the thigh through a perforation in the tendon of the adductor magnus muscle to gain access to the popliteal fossa (behind the knee).* At the point where the lower end of the adductor magnus muscle narrows to form its inferior tendon, the femoral artery and vein penetrate the tendon through an opening called the **adductor hiatus** to enter a compartment posterior to the knee called the **popliteal fossa** (see Figs. 18–6*B* and 18–7). Once the femoral artery gains access to the popliteal fossa, it is called the **popliteal artery** (see Figs. 18–6*B* and 18–7). The femoral and popliteal veins follow the same course as the arteries (see below).

In the region of the adductor hiatus, the adductor canal is covered by a membranous "roof," which bridges the gap between the adductor magnus and the vastus medialis muscles (Fig. 18–8). The saphenous nerve and a branch of the femoral artery, the **descending genicular branch,** penetrate this membrane rather than the adductor hiatus as they course inferiorly to enter the popliteal fossa with the femoral artery and vein (see Fig. 18–8). The descending genicular artery quickly gives rise to a **saphenous branch,** which continues inferiorly and superficially with the saphenous nerve. A second **articular branch** penetrates the vastus medialis muscle to emerge just lateral to the patella, where it anastomoses with lateral and medial genicular arteries to form a patellar plexus (Fig. 18–9). It should be noted that the greater and lesser (small) saphenous veins are **superficial veins,** which course within the superficial fascia. The greater saphenous vein courses along the medial side of the lower extremity and is joined below the knee by the saphenous nerve and saphenous branch of the superior genicular artery (see discussion of venous system below). The lesser saphenous vein courses within the superficial fascia of the posterior leg. Its course is not related to that of the saphenous nerve and artery and greater saphenous vein. The word *saphenous* comes from the Greek root "saphena," which means "manifest" or "clearly visible."

Popliteal Artery. *The popliteal artery crosses the popliteal fossa and enters the leg by piercing the tendon of the soleus muscle.* The popliteal artery crosses the popliteal fossa between the femoral condyles and superficial to the popliteus muscle (Fig. 18–10). The popliteal artery lies deep within the popliteal fossa, with the popliteal vein superficial to it.

Between its entrance to the adductor hiatus and its division into **anterior** and **posterior tibial arteries** after it has left the popliteal fossa, the popliteal artery gives off a series of genicular branches that supply the knee joint, as well as some muscular branches (see Figs. 18–1 and 18–9). The **medial** and **lateral genicular arteries** arise at the lower end of the femur. The single **middle genicular artery** runs anteriorly to supply the knee joint and structures within the joint. The **inferior medial** and **lateral genicular arteries** encircle the upper end of the tibia. The largest muscular branches are the paired **sural arteries,** which arise just before the popliteal artery divides. They are the chief arterial supply to the gastrocnemius and soleus muscles. These genicular and muscular branches participate in a complex, extensive, and somewhat variable anastomosis surrounding the knee joint (see below).

After spanning the knee joint, the popliteal artery passes through a superior **tendinous arch** of the soleus muscle to gain access to a plane between the superficial and deep muscles of the posterior crural (leg) compartment. At this point, the artery divides into the **posterior** and **anterior tibial arteries.** The anterior tibial artery pierces a hiatus at the upper border of the interosseous membrane to gain access to the anterior compartment of the leg (see Figs. 18–1, 18–9, and 18–10). After giving off a small **anterior tibial recurrent artery,** which courses superior to the

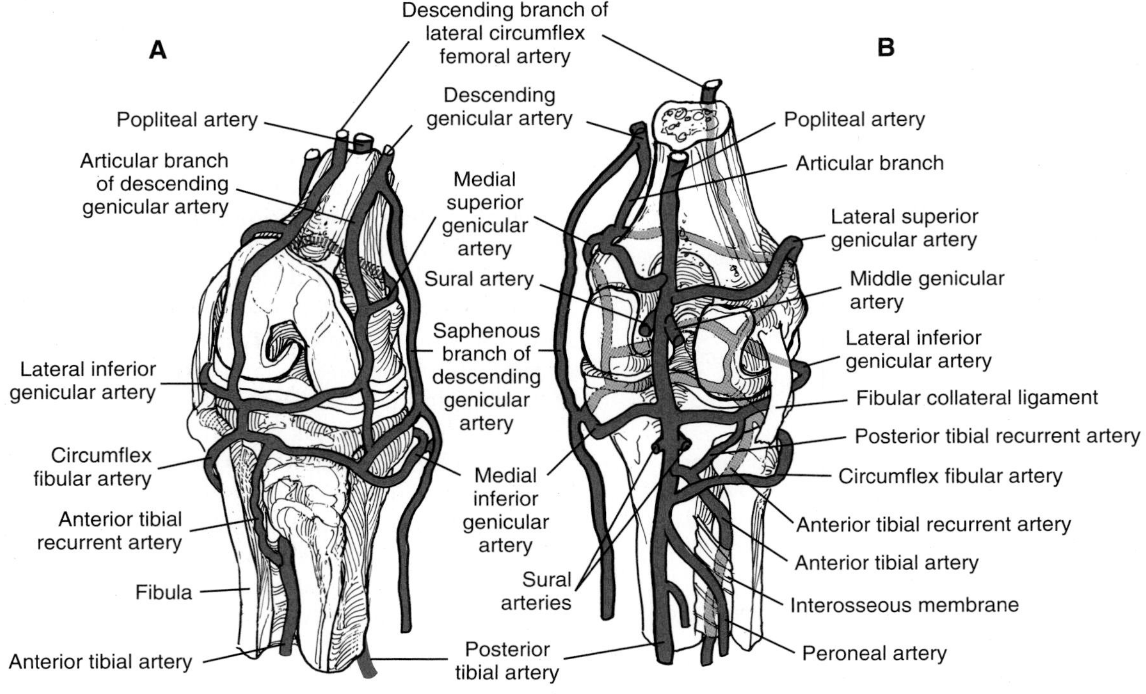

FIGURE 18–9
Vessels surrounding the knee joint. **A.** Anterior view. **B.** Posterior view.

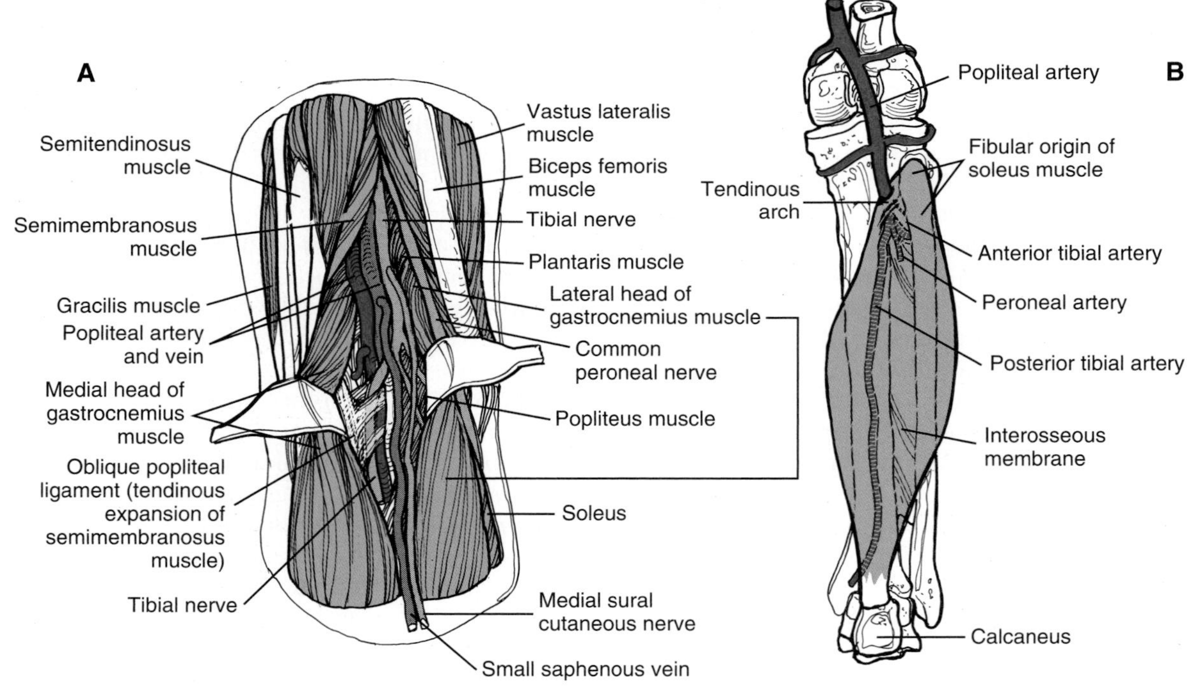

FIGURE 18–10
Popliteal artery and its branches. **A.** Popliteal artery at point it pierces tendon of soleus muscle to enter leg. **B.** Course of popliteal artery between femoral condyles through tendinous arch of soleus muscle showing arterial branches within the leg.

knee, the main trunk of the anterior tibial artery descends between the extensor digitorum longus and tibialis anterior muscles, giving off small branches to these muscles as well as to the somewhat deeper, more inferior extensor hallucis longus muscle (see Figs. 18–9 and 18–10 and Table 18–1). Typically, veins of the same names accompany these arteries (see below).

Anterior Tibial Artery. *Terminal branches of the anterior tibial artery supply the dorsal compartment of the foot.* Finally, the anterior tibial artery gives off small branches in the region of the ankle and continues on to the dorsum of the foot as the **arteria dorsalis pedis (dorsal artery of the foot)** (Fig. 18–11*A* and see Table 18–1). The dorsal artery gives off lateral and medial tarsal branches, while its main trunk forms an **arcuate artery.** The arcuate artery gives rise to 6 dorsal metatarsal arteries, which give rise to 10 dorsal digital arteries (Fig. 18–12 and see Table 18–1). Generally, veins with corresponding names parallel the arteries just described (see below).

Posterior Tibial Artery. *The posterior tibial artery gives rise to branches that serve the posterior and lateral crural compartments.* Once the posterior tibial artery gains access to the plane between the superficial and deep layers of the posterior crural compartment, the **peroneal artery** splits off to supply the lateral (peroneal) compartment of the leg (see Fig. 18–11*B* and Table 18–1). However, the main trunk of the peroneal artery courses between the flexor hallucis longus muscle and the deeper tibialis posterior muscle just medial to the fibula within the deep posterior compartment of the leg (see Fig. 18–11*B*). Branches arise from the peroneal artery to course posteriorly around the fibula, gaining access to the lateral compartment to supply the peroneal muscles (see Fig. 18–11*B* and Table 18–1). Veins of the same names accompany the posterior tibial artery and its branches (see below).

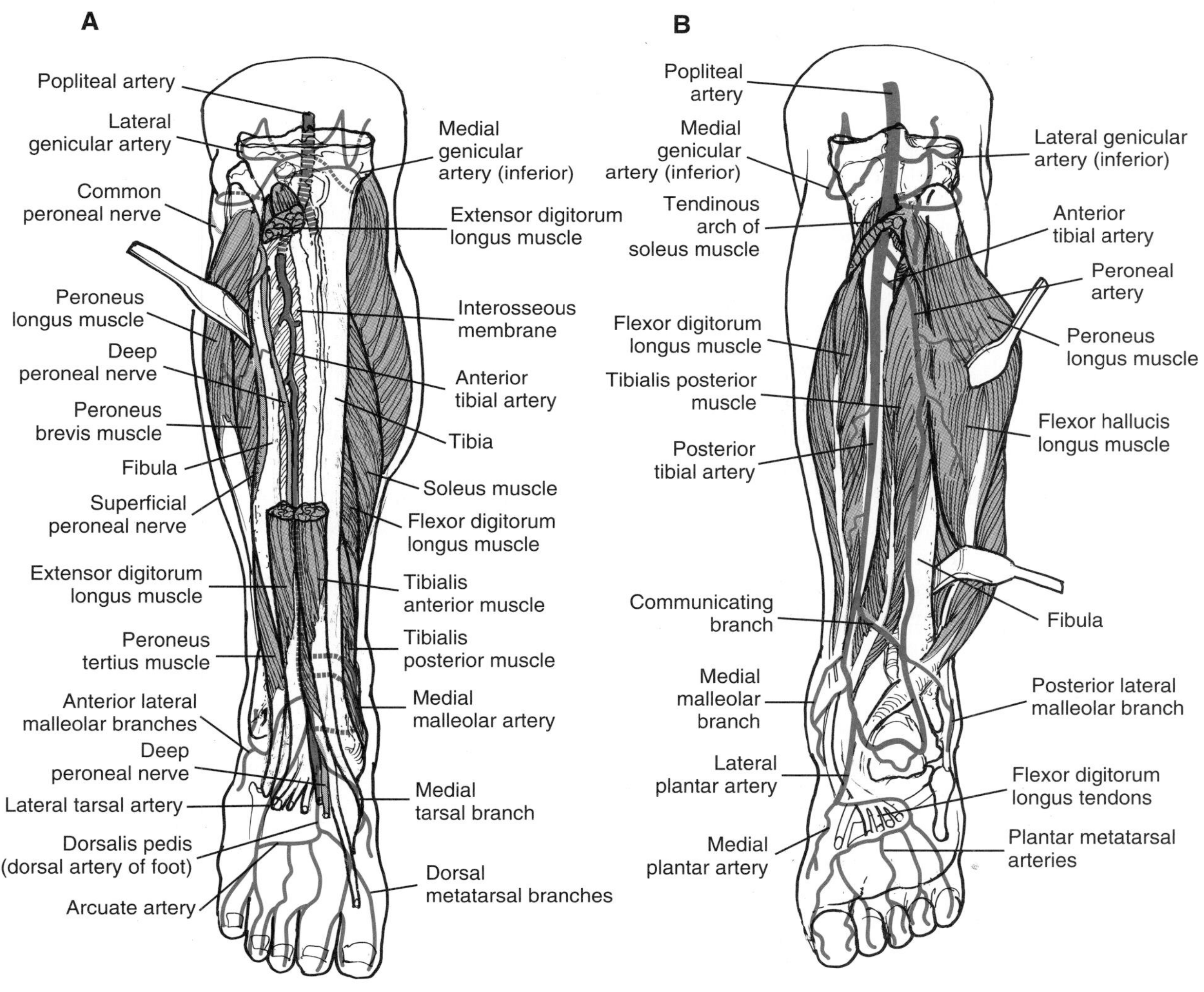

FIGURE 18–11
Vessels of the leg in relation to muscles. **A.** Branches of the anterior tibial artery. **B.** Branches of the posterior tibial artery.

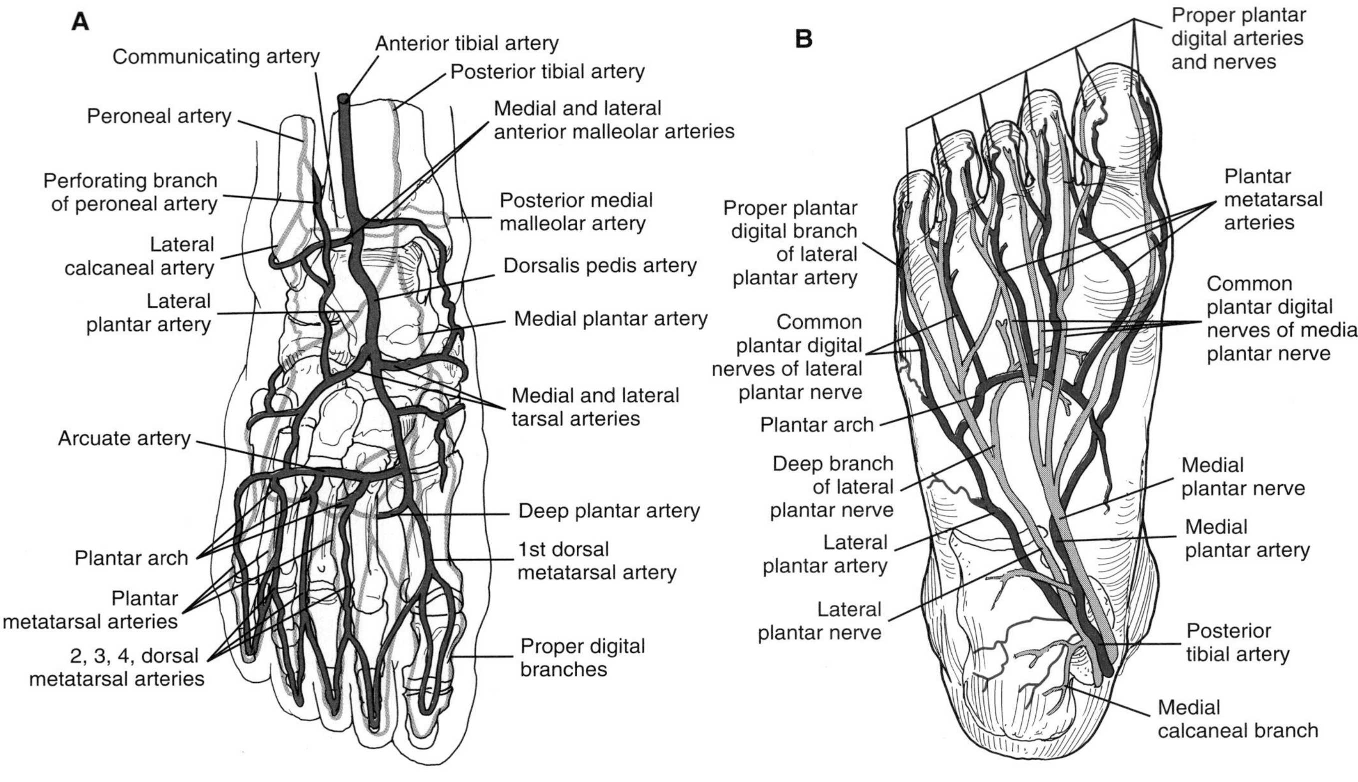

FIGURE 18–12
Arterial anastomosis at the ankle and arteries of the plantar compartment of the foot. **A.** Ankle and foot arteries. **B.** Plantar region of foot showing arteries and nerves.

Arterial Anastomosis at the Ankle. *The main trunks of the posterior tibial, peroneal, and anterior tibial arteries reunite at the ankle.* As the posterior tibial artery reaches the ankle, it gives off a **communicating branch** that anastomoses with the main trunk of the peroneal artery just posterior to the lateral malleolus (see Fig. 18–12). Just proximal to this anastomosis, the peroneal artery gives off a **perforating branch** that traverses an opening at the lower edge of the interosseous membrane. It anastomoses with the anterior lateral malleolar artery that branches from the anterior tibial artery (see Figs. 18–11*A* and 18–12).

Arteries of the Plantar Compartment of the Foot. *Terminal branches of the posterior tibial artery (mainly) and peroneal artery (to a minor degree) supply the plantar compartment of the foot.* The main arterial supply to the plantar compartment of the foot is the posterior tibial artery (see Table 18–1). This artery gains access to the compartment by sweeping posteriorly and inferiorly to the medial malleolus and coursing deep to the flexor retinaculum (see Fig. 18–12). Before emerging from the flexor retinaculum, the posterior tibial artery gives off a small medial calcaneal branch, which anastomoses with lateral calcaneal branches of the peroneal artery (see Fig. 18–12).

As the posterior tibial artery emerges from the flexor retinaculum, it splits into lateral and medial plantar arteries. The **lateral plantar artery** passes between the abductor hallucis and the quadratus plantae (flexor accessorius) muscles and gives rise to the **deep plantar arterial arch** (see Fig. 18–12). The deep plantar arterial arch gives rise to four plantar metatarsal arteries, which terminate as **plantar digital arteries** (see Fig. 18–12). After giving rise to the deep plantar arterial arch, the lateral plantar artery continues to the base of the lateral side of the small toe where it terminates as a **proper plantar digital branch of the lateral plantar artery** (see Fig. 18–12). The **medial plantar artery** passes between the abductor hallucis muscle and lateral head of the flexor hallucis brevis muscle and continues to the medial side of the big toe where it anastomoses with the deep plantar arterial arch and terminates as a **proper plantar digital branch of the medial plantar artery** (see Fig. 18–12 and Table 18–1). In general, veins of the same names accompany the arteries just described (see below).

Superior Gluteal Artery and Its Branches and Associated Structures

Branches of the superior gluteal artery supply muscles and skin of the gluteal region and anastomose with a branch of the femoral artery

The **superior gluteal artery** is the largest branch of the posterior division of the internal iliac artery. It exits the pelvic cavity between the lumbosacral trunk and the ventral ramus of spinal nerve S1 or between the ventral rami of spinal nerves S1 and S2 as a continuation of the posterior trunk of the internal iliac artery (Fig. 18–13 and see Fig. 18–4 and Chapter 14). The superior gluteal artery courses into the gluteal region via the greater sciatic foramen just superior to the piriformis muscle where it splits into superficial and deep branches (Fig. 18–13). The **superficial branch** penetrates the deep surface of the gluteus maximus muscle as it splits into several muscular branches (Fig. 18–13 and see Table 18–2). Some of these branches completely penetrate the gluteus maximus muscle to supply superficial fascia and integument overlying the sacrum (see Table 18–2). The **deep branch** first courses between the gluteus medius muscle and the pelvic bone and then splits into superior and inferior rami. The superior ramus supplies the gluteus minimus muscle and anastomoses with the lateral femoral circumflex artery (Fig. 18–13 and see Table 18–2). The inferior ramus supplies the gluteus minimus and gluteus medius muscles and anastomoses with the medial and lateral femoral circumflex arteries (see Table 18–2). Veins of the same names typically accompany the arteries just described (see below).

Inferior Gluteal Artery and Its Branches and Associated Structures

Branches of the inferior gluteal artery supply muscles and skin of the gluteal region and anastomose with branches of the femoral artery

The inferior gluteal artery is a large terminal branch of the anterior division of the internal iliac artery. It usually passes from the pelvis between the ventral rami of spinal nerves S2 and S3 (see Chapter 14) and through the lower part of the greater sciatic foramen just inferior to the piriformis muscle (Fig. 18–13). The initial branches supply the gluteus maximus and obturator internus muscles (Fig. 18–13 and see Table 18–2). Once the inferior gluteal artery has entered the gluteal region, its main trunk courses laterally toward the greater trochanter of the femur as it gives off branches that supply the piriformis, gemellus superior and inferior, quadratus femoris, and superior hamstring muscles (Fig. 18–13 and see Table 18–2). Its terminal branches anastomose with the superior gluteal artery, medial femoral circumflex artery, and first perforating artery of the deep femoral artery (see Fig. 18–4). Veins of the same names accompany the branches just described (see below).

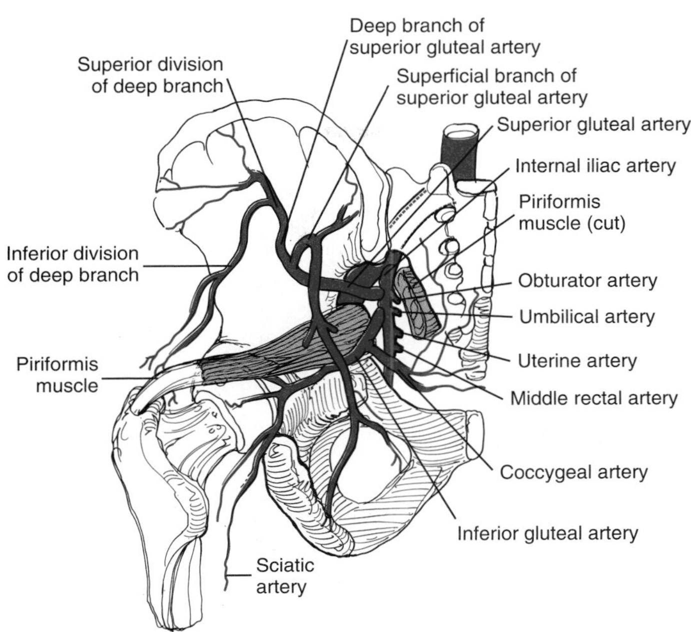

FIGURE 18–13
Superior gluteal artery and its branches.

Obturator Artery and Its Branches and Associated Structures

The obturator artery escapes the pelvis via the obturator canal to supply the medial (adductor) compartment of the thigh

As the **obturator artery** exits the pelvis via the obturator canal, it splits into anterior and posterior branches (Fig. 18–14). The **anterior branch** supplies the obturator externus muscle, pectineus muscle, medial adductor muscles of the thigh, and gracilis muscle (Fig. 18–14*A* and Table 18–2). It anastomoses with the medial femoral circumflex artery (Fig. 18–14*B*). The **posterior branch** supplies muscles associated with the ischial tuberosity and anastomoses with the inferior gluteal artery (Fig. 18–14*B*). Its branches also supply the acetabulum and round ligament of the femur (Fig. 18–14*B* and Table 18–2).

Collateral Arteries of Lower Extremity Joints

Extensive collateral arteries within the lower extremity joints provide supplemental blood supplies to safeguard these active, functionally important "machines."

Collateral Arteries of the Hip Joint. *Branches of the inferior and superior gluteal, obturator, and deep femoral arteries unite around the hip joint.* The hip joint and surrounding structures are well vascularized by branches of several major arteries. A unique anastomosis **(cruciate [cross-shaped] anastomosis)** between some of these vessels is located just posterior to the hip joint (see Fig. 18–4*A*). In this region, the confluence of the **medial and lateral circumflex iliac arteries** is joined by a **branch of the inferior gluteal artery** (from above) and a **branch of the**

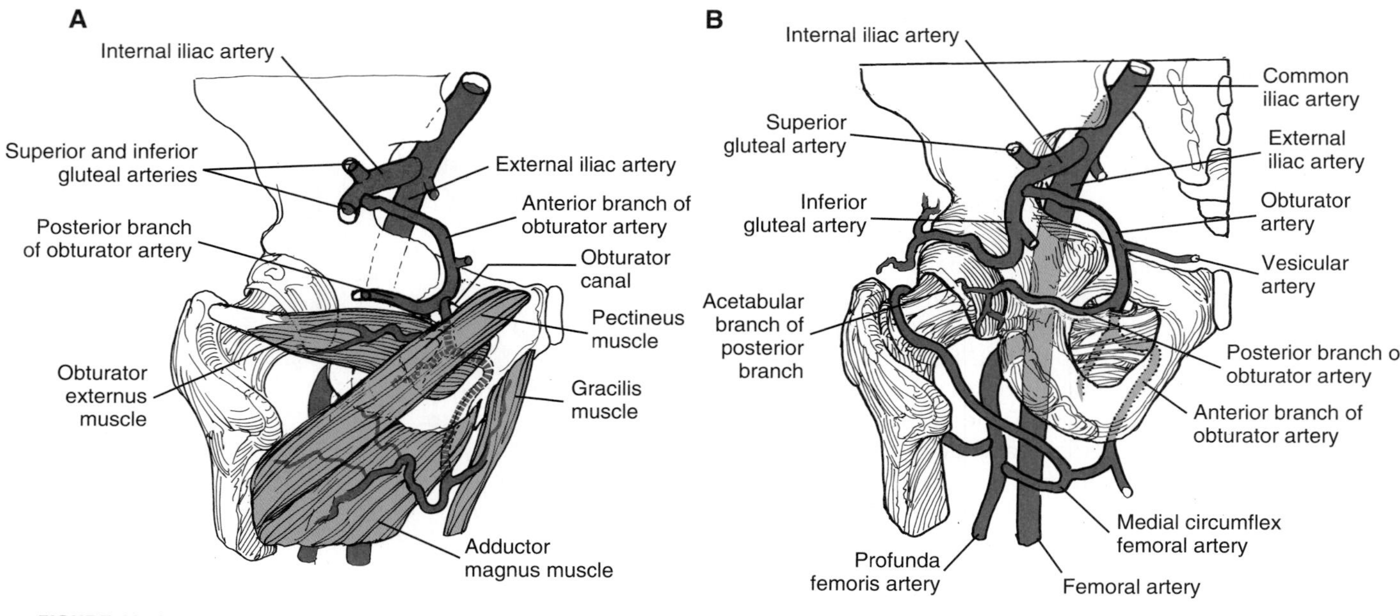

FIGURE 18–14
Obturator artery and its branches and associated structures. **A.** Anterior branch. **B.** Posterior branch.

TABLE 18–2
Muscles and Other Structures Supplied by the Superior and Inferior Gluteal and Obturator Arteries

Artery	Muscles Supplied	Other Regions or Structures Supplied
SUPERIOR GLUTEAL ARTERY		
Superficial branch	Gluteus maximus muscle	Skin over sacrum
Deep branch	Gluteus medius and gluteus minimus muscles	Hip joint
INFERIOR GLUTEAL ARTERY	Gluteus maximus, obturator internus, piriformis, gemellus superior and inferior, quadratus femoris, and superior hamstring muscles	
OBTURATOR ARTERY		
Anterior branch	Obturator externus, pectineus, femoral adductor, and gracilis muscles	
Posterior branch	Muscles associated with ischial tuberosity	Acetabulum and round ligament of femur

first perforating artery of the deep femoral artery (from below) to form a cross-shaped anastomosis (see Fig. 18–4*A*). Other vessels also contribute to the anastomotic network surrounding the hip joint. These include branches of the superior gluteal artery, iliac artery (from the iliac crest), deep circumflex iliac artery, obturator artery, and ascending branch of the lateral femoral circumflex artery. Together, these vessels supply the skin, fascia, ligaments, and capsule surrounding the hip joint. **Retinacular branches** penetrate the hip joint capsule to supply the head of the femur. Typically, a **foveolar branch** of the obturator artery supplies the acetabulum and round ligament of the femur (see Fig. 18–14*B*).

Collateral Arteries of the Knee Joint. *Branches of the femoral, deep femoral, popliteal, and anterior and posterior tibial arteries unite around the knee joint.* The knee joint is invested by a complex anastomotic network of arterial branches derived from several major arteries. Superiorly, a descending genicular branch of the femoral artery branches into articular and saphenous branches, which contribute to the network (see Fig. 18–9). An additional superior contribution is made by the descending branch of the lateral femoral circumflex artery (see Fig. 18–9). Medial and lateral superior genicular, middle genicular, and medial and lateral inferior genicular branches are contributed by the popliteal artery. Inferiorly, the ante-

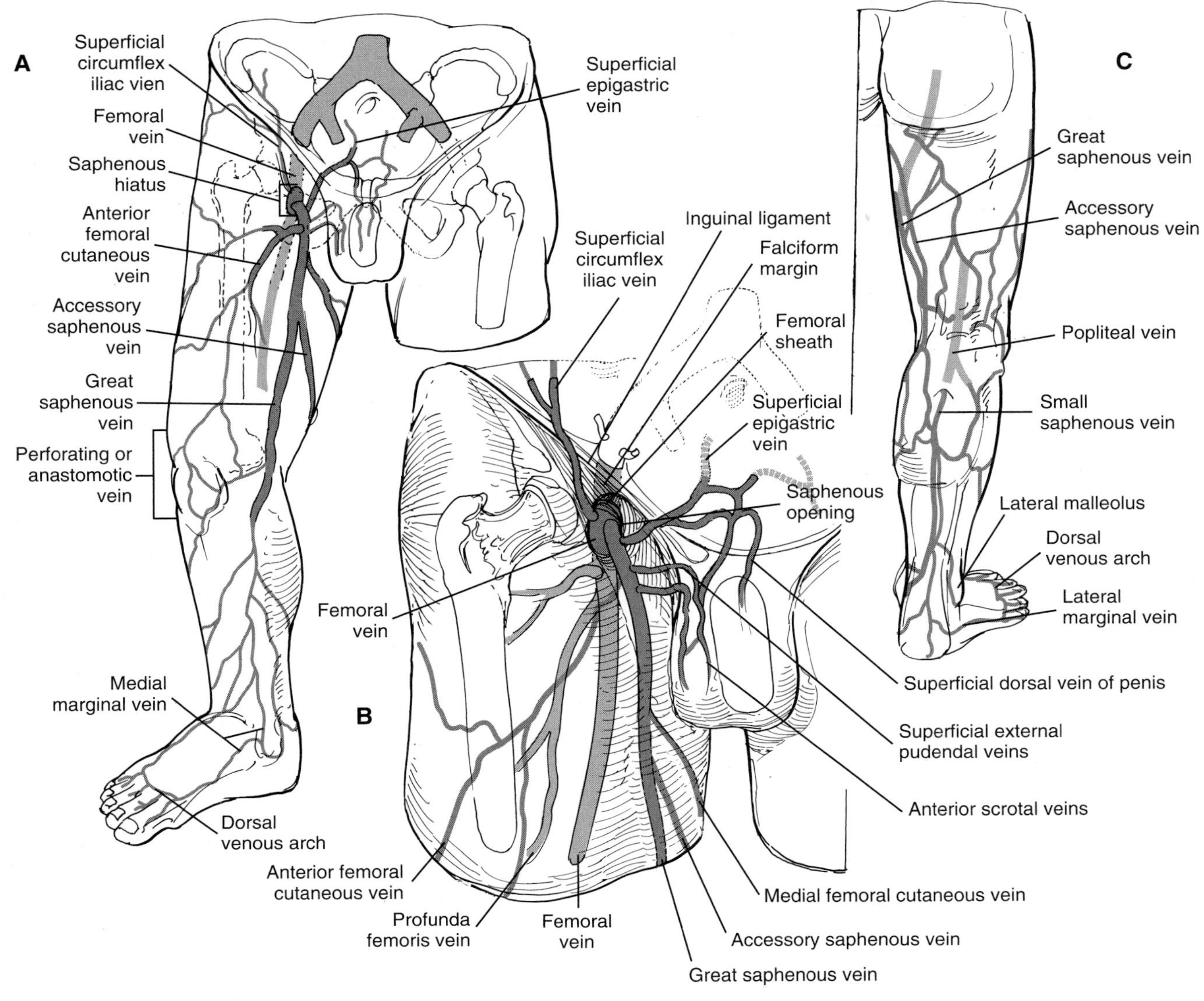

FIGURE 18–15
Veins of the lower extremity. **A.** Anterior view. **B.** Femoral sheath region. **C.** Posterior view.

rior tibial artery may contribute posterior recurrent tibial, circumflex fibular, and anterior recurrent tibial branches to the genicular (knee) anastomosis (see Fig. 18–9). A **superficial network** derived from these vessels supplies the skin, connective tissue of the knee joint, and patella and its associated tendons **(patellar plexus).** A **deep network** supplies the marrow, articular capsule, cruciate ligaments, and articular capsule.

Collateral Arteries of the Ankle Joint. *Branches of the anterior and posterior tibial and peroneal arteries unite around the ankle joint.* Superior contributions to the arterial anastomosis of the ankle include a posterior medial malleolar branch of the posterior tibial artery, an anterior lateral malleolar branch of the anterior tibial artery, and a perforating branch of the peroneal artery (see Fig. 18–12). The extensive plexus arising from this anastomotic network supplies the skin, fascia, ligaments, and articulations of the ankle, tarsal, and tarsometatarsal joints.

▲ Veins of the Lower Extremity

The venous system of the lower extremity is composed of deep and superficial veins

In the discussion of the arterial system, above, it was noted that deep arteries of the lower extremities are typically accompanied by **deep veins** of the same names. A system of **superficial veins** within the superficial fascia is also present. The superficial veins drain into the deep veins because of the orientation of valves in the two systems (see below). There are two main named superficial veins of the lower extremity: the great (long) saphenous vein and the small (short) saphenous vein (Fig. 18–15*A* and *C*).

Great Saphenous Vein

The great saphenous vein courses from the medial side of the foot as a continuation of the **medial marginal vein** just anterior to the medial malleolus and along the medial aspect of the tibia. It passes alongside the medial border of the knee and thigh and pierces the femoral sheath superiorly via the **saphenous opening** to empty into the femoral vein (Fig. 18–15*A* and *B*). Many unnamed tributaries drain into the great saphenous vein from the dorsum of the foot and the anterior, lateral, and posterior aspects of the leg and thigh. In addition to its connection with the femoral vein within the femoral sheath, the great saphenous vein has many connections to deep veins throughout the lower extremity, particularly in the leg. The great saphenous vein is often duplicated and typically has about 20 valves.

Small Saphenous Vein

The small saphenous vein courses from the lateral aspect of the foot as a continuation of the **lateral marginal vein** and continues posteriorly around the lateral malleolus (Fig. 18–15*C*). It ascends along the posterior aspect of the leg, between the heads of the gastrocnemius muscle, and pierces the underlying deep fascia to connect with the popliteal vein and other deep veins of the leg. Many unnamed tributarial veins of the foot and leg empty into the small saphenous vein. The small and great saphenous veins may also be connected to one another. Blood flows from superficial to deep regions and is regulated by 10 to 20 valves.

Circulatory Function of Lower Extremity Vasculature

Superficial veins unaccompanied by arteries are required for efficient drainage of the extremities

As noted above, the upper and lower limbs have both deep veins accompanied by arteries and superficial veins not accompanied by arteries. Venous return in the upper and lower extremities requires the combined functions of deep and superficial veins and their perforating vein connections. As the calf muscles contract, the deep veins are compressed and blood is squeezed upward into deep veins of the thigh and regions superior to the thigh. At the same time, valves within the perforating veins prevent the blood from flowing from deep veins to superficial veins. As the muscles relax, the deep vessels of the calf re-expand. The expansion of these vessels and the actions of their valves cause blood to be aspirated from the superficial veins via the perforating veins into the deep veins. A continuous cycle of contraction and relaxation of the calf muscles pumps blood from superficial veins to deep veins and upward.

Clinical Disorders of Lower Extremity Vessels

Interruptions of the blood supply may affect gait

As has been described in Chapter 17, functionally related muscles of the lower limb are enclosed within compartments defined by thick layers of fascia. As a consequence of the unyielding quality of this fascia, vessels running within the muscle compartments may be subject to compression following pathologic swelling of muscles. This condition occurs most commonly in the anterior and deep posterior compartments of the leg. Swelling of muscles within the anterior compartment **(anterior compartment syndrome)** tends to result from activities requiring repeated dorsiflexion such as cross-country skiing or snowshoeing. The condition is treated by surgical release of the crural fascia.

The **competence of valves within the perforating veins** is very important for proper drainage of the lower extremity. When these valves become dysfunctional, blood may pool within the superficial veins, producing **varicosities** that may require surgical removal.

▲ Lymphatics of the Lower Extremity

Three main groups of lymph nodes filter lymph from the lower extremity, anterior abdominal wall, and perineal region

Lymphatic vessels of the lower extremity converge upon three groups of lymph nodes in the proximal thigh: **proximal** and **distal groups of superficial nodes** and a **group of deep nodes.** The proximal group of about five superficial nodes is located just inferior to the inguinal ligament. The distal group of about five superficial nodes is located in the vicinity of the saphenous opening (Fig. 18–16). The deep inguinal nodes (usually three) are located within the femoral canal. Lymphatic vessels draining into the proximal group of superficial nodes follow the external pudendal arteries, draining the external genitalia, the inferior anal canal and perianal region, the adjoining anterior abdominal wall, and the round ligament of the uterus. The distal group of superficial nodes drains the superficial fascia of the entire lower extremity, except for the posterolateral quadrant of the calf and lateral foot. The posterolateral quadrant of the calf and lateral foot drain into **popliteal nodes,** which also drain lymphatic fluid from the knee joint. The popliteal nodes drain into lymph vessels accompanying the popliteal and femoral arteries and then into deep inguinal lymph nodes (Fig. 18–16*C*). The gluteal region and superior part of the posterior compartment of the thigh are also drained by lymphatic vessels and nodes that accompany the superior and inferior gluteal arteries (see Table 18–3).

Lymph filtered by the superficial and deep inguinal lymph nodes drains into vessels associated with the external iliac artery, common iliac artery, and aorta and finally into the thoracic duct (see Chapter 10).

▲ Innervation of the Lower Extremity

The lower extremity is innervated by nerves of the lumbar and sacral plexuses

The lumbar and sacral plexuses are described in Chapters 13 and 14. Many of the named nerves emerg-

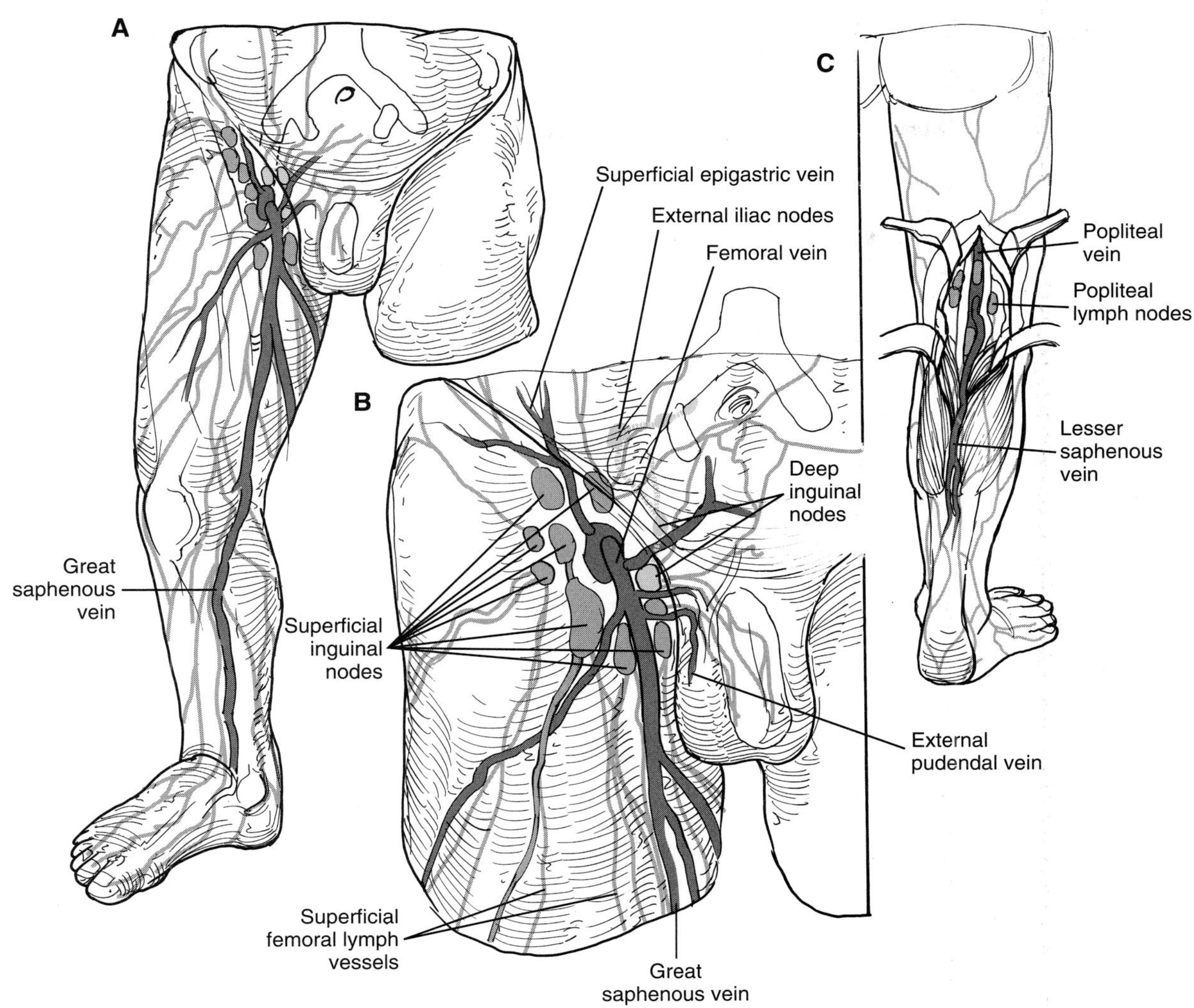

FIGURE 18–16

Lymphatics of the lower extremity. **A.** Proximal and distal superficial lymph nodes in the proximal area of thigh. **B.** Detail showing deep nodes within femoral canal. **C.** Popliteal lymph nodes drain lymphatic fluid from knee, posterolateral quadrant of calf, and lateral foot.

TABLE 18–3
Lymphatics of the Lower Extremity

Group of Lymph Nodes	Structures Drained*
SUPERFICIAL INGUINAL NODES	
Proximal group	External genitalia, inferior anal canal, perianal region, anterior abdominal wall, region of umbilicus, round ligament of uterus, superficial lateral thigh, inferior gluteal region
Distal group	Superficial lower extremity, except for posterolateral region of leg and lateral foot
Deep inguinal nodes	All deep tissues of lower extremity; posterolateral leg, lateral foot, and knee joint via popliteal nodes; ankle and foot joints
Superior gluteal nodes	Gluteus maximus, gluteus medius, and gluteus minimus muscles; skin over sacrum and hip joint
Inferior gluteal nodes	Gluteus maximus, lateral rotator, and superior hamstring muscles

*If the structures become infected, the lymph nodes may swell.

ing from these plexuses of spinal nerve ventral rami innervate the muscles and skin of the lower extremity.

Development of Nerves of the Lower Limb

The general distribution of spinal nerves in the lower extremity can be understood by considering the development of the lower limb buds

In early development, the dermatomes of the limb buds are organized horizontally because they are in adjacent regions of the trunk. During development, the lower extremity limb buds twist 180 degrees in a medial direction. When development is complete, the dermatomes have become twisted along the length of the lower extremity in a corkscrew fashion (Fig. 18–17). The distribution of sensory nerves reflects the twisting of the spinal nerves. The twisting causes the sensory nerves to innervate specific spiral-shaped territories. For example, the ilioinguinal nerve, which contains fibers from spinal nerve L1, innervates the superomedial thigh; the genitofemoral nerve, which is composed of fibers from spinal nerves L1 and L2, innervates the slightly more inferior skin of the medial thigh; and the cutaneous branches of the obturator nerve, which are derived from spinal nerves L2 to L4, innervate even more inferior regions of the medial thigh. Twisting of the lower extremity causes cutaneous branches of the femoral nerve (which is derived from spinal nerves L2 and L3) to be distributed to the anterior skin of the thigh and causes branches of the sural nerve (derived from fibers of spinal nerves L5, S1, and S2) to be distributed to the posterior surface of the lower leg (Fig. 18–17). This scheme is complicated somewhat by the encroachment of adjacent nerves during development. Therefore, distribution of a cutaneous nerve may not cover an entire dermatome but only a specific region or regions within the dermatome (Fig. 18–17*B* and *C*).

The innervation of the musculature within the lower extremity is generally consistent with the definitive distribution of dermatomes and spinal nerve territories of sensory innervation. For example, the anterior muscles of the thigh are innervated by the femoral nerve, which contains fibers from spinal nerves L2 to L4. The lateral and anterior muscles of the leg are innervated by branches of the common peroneal nerve, which contains fibers from spinal nerves L4, L5, S1, and S2 (Fig. 18–17*B* and *C*).

Specific Nerves of the Lower Extremity

Lumbar Plexus. Several lower extremity nerves are formed by the lumbar plexus (Fig. 18–18 and see Table 18–4). These include the **ilioinguinal nerve,** which is a branch of the ventral ramus of spinal nerve L1 (see Chapters 11 and 13). The ventral ramus of spinal nerve L1 bifurcates to form the ilioinguinal nerve and the iliohypogastric nerve at varying points within the posterior or lateral body wall (see Chapter 13). Once the ilioinguinal nerve reaches the anterior abdominal wall, it courses medially and inferiorly within a plane between the transversus abdominis and the internal oblique muscles, providing innervation to muscles of the most inferior region of the anterior abdominal wall. As the ilioinguinal nerve enters the region of the inguinal canal, it courses between the transverse fascia and internal oblique muscle because the transversus abdominis muscle is deficient in this area (see Chapter 11). The ilioinguinal nerve emerges from the superficial ring of the inguinal canal and enters the superficial fascia to supply the skin of the anterior scrotum or labium majorum and the medial thigh.

The **femoral branch of the genitofemoral nerve** is composed of ventral rami from spinal nerves L1 and L2. These fibers provide cutaneous innervation to the superior region of the anterior thigh after they emerge from the false pelvis and course over the pelvic brim and under the inguinal ligament (Fig. 18–18*A* and Table 18–4).

The **lateral femoral cutaneous nerve** is composed of ventral rami from segmental nerves L2 and L3. These fibers provide cutaneous innervation to the lateral thigh (Fig. 18–18*A* and Table 18–4). The course of this nerve is distinctive. It emerges from the false pelvis by coursing behind or through the inguinal ligament on the medial side of the anterior superior iliac spine and into the superficial fascia of the lateral thigh (Fig. 18–18*A*).

> **Paresthesia** (a tingling sensation) or **hypothesia** (reduced sensation) of the lateral thigh may be experienced by obese individuals as a consequence of crushing of the lateral femoral cutaneous nerve by the overlying inguinal ligament or by a low-slung belt.

The **femoral nerve** combines fibers from ventral rami of spinal nerves L2, L3, and L4. It provides motor innervation to muscles within the posterior body wall (i.e., psoas and iliacus muscles) and muscles of the anterior thigh (Fig. 18–18*A* and Table 18–4). Within the false pelvis, the femoral nerve courses between the iliacus and psoas muscles. The femoral nerve remains within the plane of the deep fascia of the iliopsoas muscle as it passes under the inguinal ligament and into the thigh. The femoral nerve gives off small branches to the iliacus muscle within the false pelvis and a **branch to the pectineus muscle** in the region of the inguinal ligament. It then splits into anterior and posterior divisions. The anterior division gives off a motor **branch to the sartorius muscle.** Beginning about 3 inches (8 cm) inferior to the inguinal ligament, the **first anterior cutaneous branches** of the femoral nerve pierce the deep fascia of the thigh (fascia lata) to supply the **skin of the anterior thigh.** Other branches of the anterior division cross the apex of the femoral sheath to supply the skin of the medial thigh. A deep branch descends within the

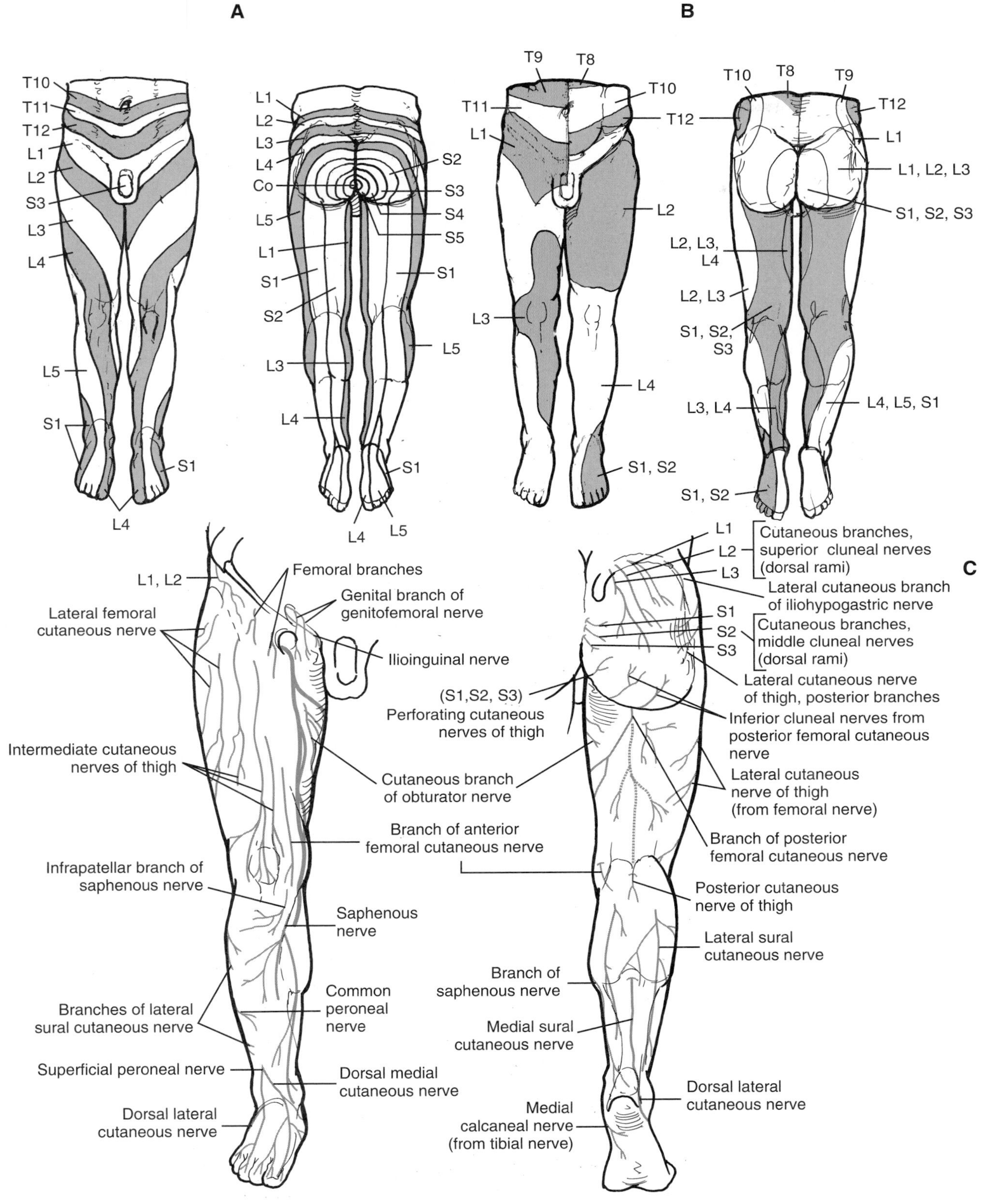

FIGURE 18–17

Development of nerves of the lower limbs. **A.** Dermatomes. **B.** Named nerve territories. **C.** Nerves.

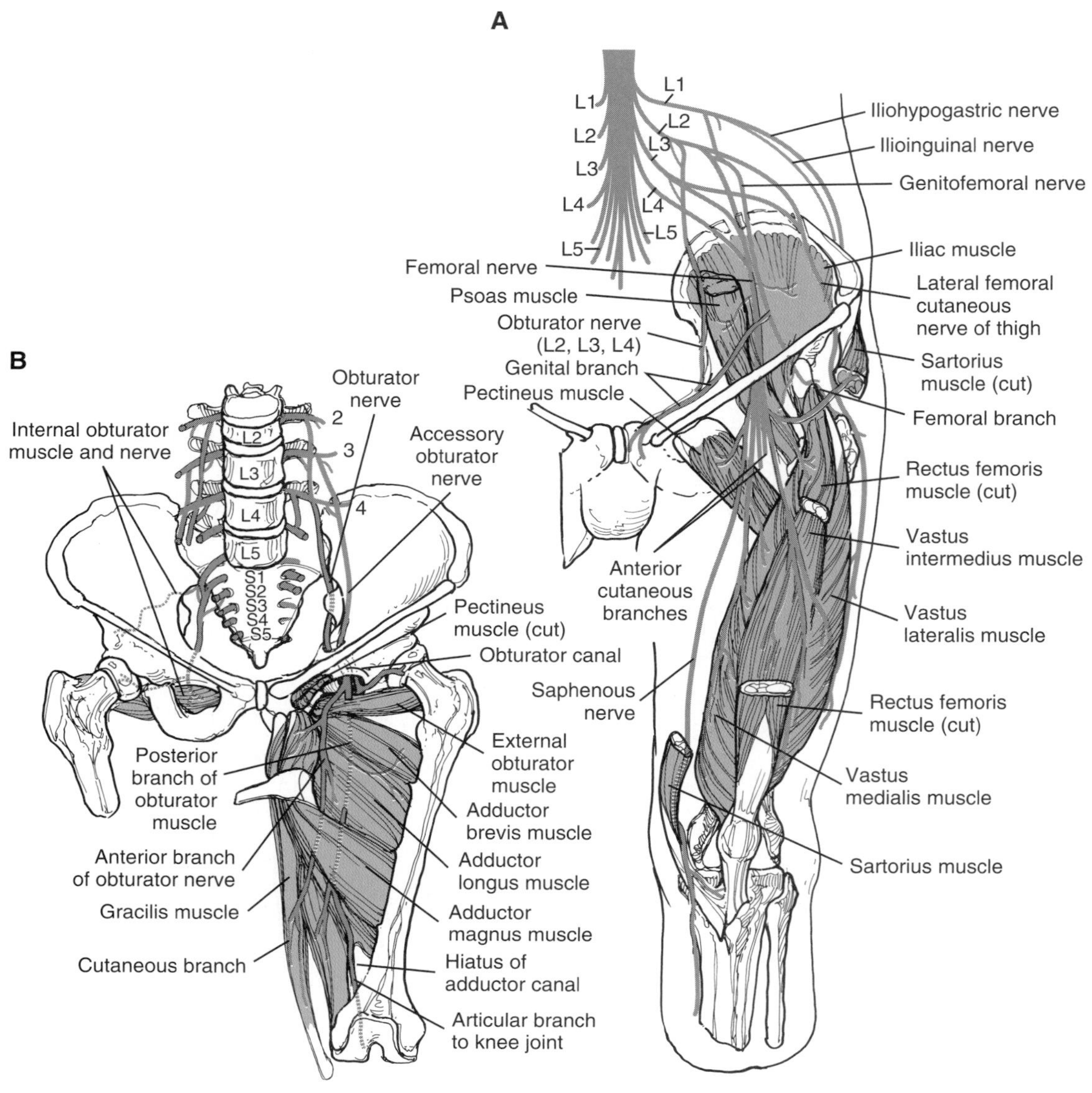

FIGURE 18–18
Nerves of the lumbar plexus and the muscles they innervate. **A.** Femoral nerve. **B.** Obturator nerve.

thigh along the posterior border of the sartorius muscle to supply the skin of the medial side of the knee and leg. The posterior division of the femoral nerve gives rise to the **saphenous nerve,** which descends within the thigh just lateral to the femoral artery within the adductor (subsartorial) canal. It pierces the fascia lata between the sartorius and gracilis tendons to supply the anteromedial knee, leg, and foot (Fig. 18–18*A* and Table 18-4). **Muscular branches** of the posterior division descend within the thigh to supply all of the quadriceps femoris muscles, the articularis genu muscle, and the knee joint.

Femoral nerve damage often occurs with penetrating wounds of the femoral triangle, resulting in inability to extend the knee. A person may compensate for this condition by forcefully hyperextending the knee (usually with the hand) and vaulting over the hyperextended knee.

The **obturator nerve** is also formed by fibers from spinal nerves L2, L3, and L4, but it provides motor innervation to the medial (adductor) compartment of the thigh and cutaneous innervation to a small patch of skin covering the medial thigh (Fig. 18–18*B* and Table 18–4). The obturator nerve exits the true pelvis via the obturator canal and splits into anterior and posterior branches. The anterior branch descends within the medial thigh between the adductor brevis and the pectineus muscles. A small branch innervates the hip joint, and other branches supply the adductor longus, gracilis, adductor brevis, and

TABLE 18–4
Nerves of the Lumbar Plexus

Nerve	Origin	Structures Innervated
Nerves to quadratus lumborum muscle	T12, L1, L2, L3	Quadratus lumborum muscle
Iliohypogastric nerve	L1	
Muscular branches		External oblique, internal oblique, transversus abdominis muscles in iliac and hypogastric regions of anterior abdominal wall
Cutaneous branches		Skin of iliac and hypogastric regions of anterior abdominal wall; lateral cutaneous branch innervates skin of superior gluteal region
Ilioinguinal nerve	L1	
Muscular branches		External oblique, internal oblique, transversus abdominis muscles in inferior iliac and hypogastric regions of anterior abdominal wall
Cutaneous branches		Inferior iliac and hypogastric regions of anterior abdominal wall and skin of anterior root of phallus, anterior labium majus or scrotum, medial thigh
Genitofemoral nerve	L1, L2	
Genital branch		
Muscular branches		Cremaster muscle
Cutaneous branches		Skin of scrotum or labium majus and medial thigh
Femoral branch		
Cutaneous branches		Skin of anterior thigh in superior part of femoral triangle
Lateral femoral cutaneous nerve	L2, L3	Lateral skin of thigh to knee
Nerves to psoas and iliacus muscles	L2, L3, L4	Psoas and iliacus muscles
Femoral nerve	L2, L3, L4	
Muscular branches		Iliacus, pectineus, sartorius, rectus femoris, vastus lateralis, vastus intermedius, articularis genu muscles; nerves to psoas and iliacus muscles may accompany femoral nerve
Cutaneous branches		
Intermediate femoral cutaneous nerve		Skin of anterior thigh to knee
Medial femoral cutaneous nerve		Skin of medial thigh, medial knee, and lateral patella; arises in common with nerve to sartorius muscle
Saphenous nerve		Medial side of knee and leg, ankle, and foot to metatarsophalangeal joints
Articular branches		Knee joint
Obturator nerve	L2, L3, L4	
Muscular branches		Adductor longus, gracilis, adductor brevis muscles; often pectineus, obturator externus, and adductor magnus muscles
Cutaneous branches		Skin of medial thigh
Articular branches		Hip and knee joints
Accessory obturator nerve	L3, L4	Inconstant
Muscular branches		Pectineus and adductor longus muscles
Articular branches		Hip joint
Lumbosacral trunk	L4, L5	Sacral plexus (see Table 16–5)

pectineus muscles. Sensory fibers supply the skin of the medial thigh (Fig. 18–18*B*). The posterior branch pierces and supplies the obturator externus muscle. It passes inferiorly between the adductor magnus and adductor brevis muscles, supplying both of them (Fig. 18–18*B* and Table 18–4). An inferior branch supplies the knee joint. As has been noted in Chapter 13, the **accessory obturator nerve,** when present, follows the course of the obturator nerve but includes branches of spinal nerves L3 and L4 only. It may supply the hip joint and pectineus muscle (Fig. 18–18*B* and Table 18–4).

Injuries of the obturator nerve are uncommon but may occur secondary to other overriding conditions such as dislocation of the hip. Disruption of the obturator nerve results in loss of the ability to adduct the thigh and pelvic stability during walking.

Sacral Plexus. The sacral plexus provides innervation to the pelvic diaphragm, perineum, posterior thigh, all compartments of the leg, and the dorsal and plantar compartments of the foot (Fig. 18–19 and Table 18–5). The sacral plexus and its innervation of the pelvic diaphragm were described in Chapter 14. Its innervation

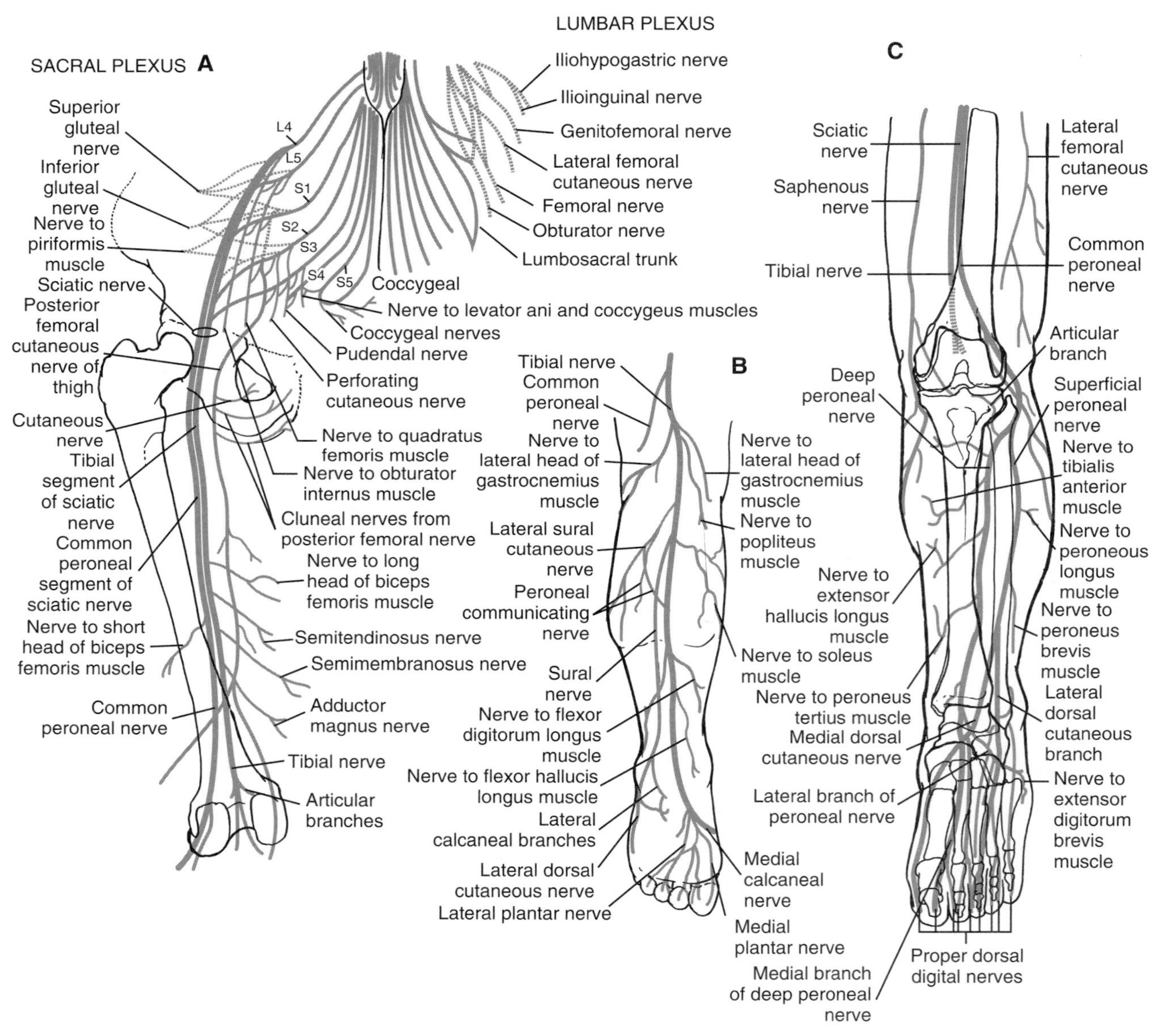

FIGURE 18–19

Nerves of the sacral plexus composed of ventral rami of spinal nerves L4, L5, and S1 to S4. **A.** Overview of major proximal nerve branches of sacral plexus. **B.** Common peroneal nerve and its branches innervating skin and major branches of tibial nerve. **C.** Course of superficial and deep peroneal nerve branches.

TABLE 18–5
Nerves of the Sacral Plexus

Nerve	Origin	Structures Innervated
Nerve to quadratus femoris and inferior gemellus muscles	L4, L5, S1	Quadratus femoris and inferior gemellus muscles
Articular branches		Hip joint
Superior gluteal nerve	L4, L5, S1	Gluteus medius, gluteus minimus, tensor fasciae latae muscles
Sciatic nerve	L4, L5, S1, S2, S3	
Common peroneal (fibular) nerve	L4, L5, S1, S2	
Muscular branches		Short head of biceps muscle
Lateral sural nerve		Lateral, anterior, medial skin of superior leg
Communicating sural nerve		Skin over head of fibula
Articular branches		Knee joint
Deep peroneal (anterior tibial) nerve		
Muscular branches		Tibialis anterior, extensor digitorum longus, extensor hallucis longus, peroneus tertius, extensor digitorum brevis, first and second dorsal interosseous muscles
Cutaneous branches		Skin of adjacent sides of big toe and second toe
Articular branches		Ankle joint, tarsal and metatarsophalangeal joints of toes 1 to 4
Superficial peroneal nerve		
Muscular branches		Peroneus longus, peroneus brevis muscles
Cutaneous branches		Skin of lower leg; medial side of big toe and adjacent surfaces of toes 2 and 3; adjacent surfaces of toes 3 and 4, 4 and 5 and lateral ankle; dorsum of foot; dorsal skin of all toes
Tibial nerve	L4, L5, S1, S2, S3	
Muscular branches		Semitendinosus muscle; long head of biceps muscle; adductor magnus, semimembranosus, soleus, gastrocnemius, popliteus, plantaris, tibialis posterior, flexor digitorum longus, flexor hallucis longus muscles
Cutaneous branches		
Sural nerve		Skin of posterior and lateral lower third of leg; skin between big toe and second toe
Median calcaneal nerve		Skin of heel and medial sole
Articular branches		Knee, tibiofibular, ankle joints
Medial plantar nerve		
Muscular branches		Adductor hallucis, flexor digitorum brevis, flexor hallucis brevis, first lumbrical muscles
Cutaneous branches		Skin of medial sole; medial side of big toe; between toes 1 and 2, 2 and 3, 3 and 4; balls of toes 1 to 4
Articular branches		Tarsal and metatarsal joints
Lateral plantar nerve		
Muscular branches		All muscles of plantar compartment of foot that are not innervated by medial plantar nerve
Cutaneous branches		Skin of lateral sole, lateral side of toe 5, between toes 4 and 5, ball of toe 5
Inferior gluteal nerve	L5, S1, S2	Gluteus maximus muscle
Nerve to obturator internus and superior gemellus muscles	L5, S1, S2	Obturator internus and superior gemellus muscles
Nerve to piriformis muscle	S1, S2	Piriformis muscle

Continued

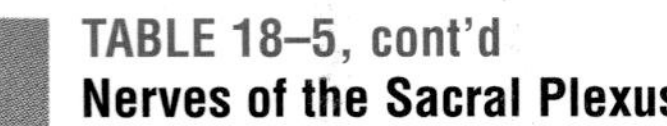

TABLE 18–5, cont'd
Nerves of the Sacral Plexus

Nerve	Origin	Structures Innervated
Posterior femoral cutaneous nerve	S1, S2, S3	Cutaneous branches to gluteal region, perineum, posterior thigh and leg
Perforating cutaneous nerve	S2, S3	Skin over inferomedial part of gluteus maximus muscle
Pudendal nerve	S2, S3, S4	See Chapter 15
Sacral nerve		
Visceral branches	S2, S3, S4	Pelvic viscera
Muscular branches	S4	Levator ani, coccygeus muscles; anal sphincter
Cutaneous branches	S4	Skin between anus and coccyx

of the perineum via the pudendal nerve was described in Chapter 15. Its innervation of the lower extremity will be discussed here.

The sacral plexus is comprised of ventral rami of spinal nerves L4, L5, and S1 to S4. The sacral plexus lies upon the piriformis muscle on the posterior pelvic wall. The ventral rami that make up the plexus issue from ventral foramina of the sacrum and course laterally to converge in the vicinity of the greater sciatic foramen (see Fig. 18–19*A*). The nerves arising from the plexus, their relationships, and their targets are described in a superior to inferior order. Some of this information is summarized in Table 18–5.

The **nerve to the quadratus femoris and gemellus inferior muscles** is composed of fibers from spinal nerves L4, L5, and S1. The nerve exits the pelvis via the greater sciatic foramen just inferior to the lower border of the piriformis muscle. It descends in close contact with the ischium to innervate the quadratus femoris and gemellus inferior muscles and hip joint (Table 18–5).

The **superior gluteal nerve** is composed of fibers from spinal nerves L4, L5, and S1. It exits the pelvis via the greater sciatic foramen superior to the piriformis muscle with the superior gluteal vessels (see above). It splits into a **superior branch,** which innervates the gluteus medius and gluteus minimus muscles and an **inferior branch,** which innervates the gluteus medius, gluteus minimus, and tensor fasciae latae muscles (Fig. 18–19*A* and Table 18–5).

Injury of the superior gluteal nerve as it exits the pelvis results in a characteristic pelvic tilt. As has been discussed in Chapter 17, when the foot is raised in the swing phase, the gluteus medius and gluteus minimus muscles on the contralateral side of the body contract to prevent the unsupported side of the pelvis (directly over the raised lower limb) from sagging. Injury to the superior gluteal nerve results in paralysis of the gluteus medius and gluteus minimus muscles and consequent sagging of the pelvis and a "lurching" gait during walking or running. This is called the **Trendelenburg sign.** The Trendelenburg sign may also be observed in individuals with congenital dislocation of the hip joint or in those who have had a fracture of the neck of the femur that has healed improperly.

The **sciatic nerve** is a large nerve of fibers from spinal nerves L4, L5, and S1 to S3. It exits the pelvis via the greater sciatic foramen just inferior to the piriformis muscle and descends under the gluteus maximus muscle into the posterior thigh (Fig. 18–19*A* and *C*). It crosses the gemellus superior and inferior muscles, obturator internus tendon, and quadratus femoris muscle posteriorly and descends within the posterior compartment just posterior to the adductor magnus muscle and deep to the long head of the biceps femoris muscle. It typically splits within the popliteal fossa into two distinctive nerves: the **common peroneal nerve** (with fibers from spinal nerves L4, L5, S1, and S2) and **tibial nerve** (with fibers from spinal nerves L4, L5, and S1 to S3) (Fig. 18–19). The separation of the common peroneal and tibial nerves may occur at a more superior level, sometimes even within the gluteal region. The tibial nerve is the larger of the two.

The **sciatic nerve may be injured** by penetrating wounds of the posterior thigh or gluteal region. Herniations of the lumbar intervertebral discs may also disrupt specific components of the sciatic nerve, leading to denervation of muscles within the posterior compartment of the thigh and all compartments of the leg. Complete interruption of the sciatic nerve results in severe disability. Braces or other devices are usually needed to compensate for the loss of function.

The **common peroneal nerve** typically splits from the sciatic nerve within the superolateral region of the popliteal fossa. It immediately innervates the short head of the biceps muscle and gives rise to the **lateral sural nerve,** which innervates the skin of the lateral leg, and **peroneal communicating nerves,** which innervate the skin over the superior head of the fibula (Fig. 18–19*B*). Before leaving the popliteal fossa, the common peroneal nerve produces an articular branch that innervates the knee joint. The common peroneal nerve then courses laterally around the head of the fibula. At this point, it is vulnerable to injury (see below). As the common peroneal nerve rounds the fibula, it bifurcates into a **deep peroneal nerve,** which serves the anterior compartment of the leg, and a **superficial peroneal nerve,** which serves the lateral compartment of the leg (Fig. 18–19*C*).

Damage to the common peroneal nerve is more frequent because of its vulnerability as it loops around the head of the fibula. For example, fractures of the fibular head may result in severing of the common peroneal nerve, which causes denervation of the anterior leg muscles. This results in **footdrop** (inability to dorsiflex the foot). The individual compensates by lifting the affected foot much higher than normal and slapping it to the ground at the end of the swing phase **(steppage gait).** The patient is typically fitted with a spring-loaded device that repositions the foot at the beginning of each swing phase.

The **superficial peroneal nerve** arises from the common peroneal nerve just after it rounds the lateral aspect of the fibula and courses just deep to the tendon of the peroneus longus muscle (Fig. 18–19*C*). The superficial peroneal nerve courses inferiorly between the heads of the peroneus longus and the extensor digitorum longus muscles, innervating the peroneus longus and peroneus brevis muscles and skin of the lateral leg (Fig. 18–19*C* and Table 18–5). The superficial peroneal nerve courses over the anterior surface of the extensor retinacula and divides into medial and lateral branches. The medial branch descends to innervate the medial side of the big toe and adjacent skin of the second and third toes (Fig. 18–19*C*). The lateral branch courses over the dorsal side of the foot to supply the skin between the third, fourth, and fifth toes and the skin of the lateral ankle (Fig. 18–19*C* and Table 18–5).

The **deep peroneal nerve** is also called the **anterior tibial nerve.** This name is certain to confuse the student of anatomy because the nerve is clearly not a branch of the tibial nerve (see below). The common peroneal nerve, however, courses inferiorly within the anterior compartment of the leg along with the anterior tibial artery (Fig. 18–19*C*). It joins this artery just below the knee after it passes deep to the tendons of the peroneus longus and extensor digitorum muscles. The common peroneal nerve supplies the tibialis anterior, extensor digitorum longus, extensor hallucis longus, and peroneus tertius muscles. It also sends a branch to the ankle joint (Fig. 18–19*C* and Table 18–5). The main trunk of the deep peroneal nerve descends to the anterior surface of the ankle under the superior and inferior extensor retinacula (see below) where it splits into lateral and medial branches (Fig. 18–19*C*). The **lateral branch** supplies the extensor digitorum brevis muscle, the tarsal and metatarsophalangeal joints of the middle three toes, and the second dorsal interosseous muscle. The **medial branch** courses anteriorly upon the dorsum of the foot to supply the skin between the big toe and the second toe, the first tarsal and the metatarsophalangeal joints, and the first dorsal interosseous muscle.

The **tibial nerve** is also called the **medial popliteal nerve.** It is composed of fibers from ventral rami of spinal nerves L4, L5, and S1 to S3. It innervates the semimembranosus muscle, semitendinosus muscle, and long head of the biceps muscle within the posterior compartment of the thigh and the adductor magnus muscle within the medial compartment of the thigh (Fig. 18–19*A*). After branching from the sciatic nerve in the superior region of the popliteal fossa, the tibial nerve descends between the lateral and medial condyles of the femur and tibia to the inferior border of the popliteus muscle. Here, it innervates the popliteus and plantaris muscles, knee joint, and superior tibiofibular joint. Descending branches innervate the soleus and gastrocnemius muscles (Fig. 18–19*B* and Table 18–5). The **sural nerve** also branches from the tibial nerve within the popliteal fossa to innervate the lateral and posterior skin of the lower third of the leg and the skin between the big toe and the second toe (Fig. 18–19*B*). The main trunk of the tibial nerve pierces the tendinous arch of the soleus muscle along with the popliteal artery. It descends within the posterior compartment of the leg just superficial to the boundary between the flexor digitorum longus and the tibialis posterior muscles to innervate the flexor digitorum longus, flexor hallucis longus, and tibialis posterior muscles (Fig. 18–19*B* and Table 18–5). It courses inferiorly, just posterior to the medial malleolus muscle and inferior to the flexor digitorum longus tendon. As it passes medial to the tuberosity of the calcaneus, the tibial nerve lies deep to the flexor retinaculum, giving rise to a **medial calcaneal branch,** which innervates the skin of the heel and medial sole. It then splits into lateral and medial plantar nerves. The **medial plantar nerve** passes between and innervates the abductor hallucis and the flexor digitorum brevis muscles and courses distally to innervate the flexor hallucis brevis and first lumbrical muscles (Fig. 18–19*B* and Table 18–5). Cutaneous branches innervate the skin of the medial sole; medial side of the big toe; skin between toes 1 to 4; and the balls of toes 1 to 4. Articular branches innervate joints of the tarsus

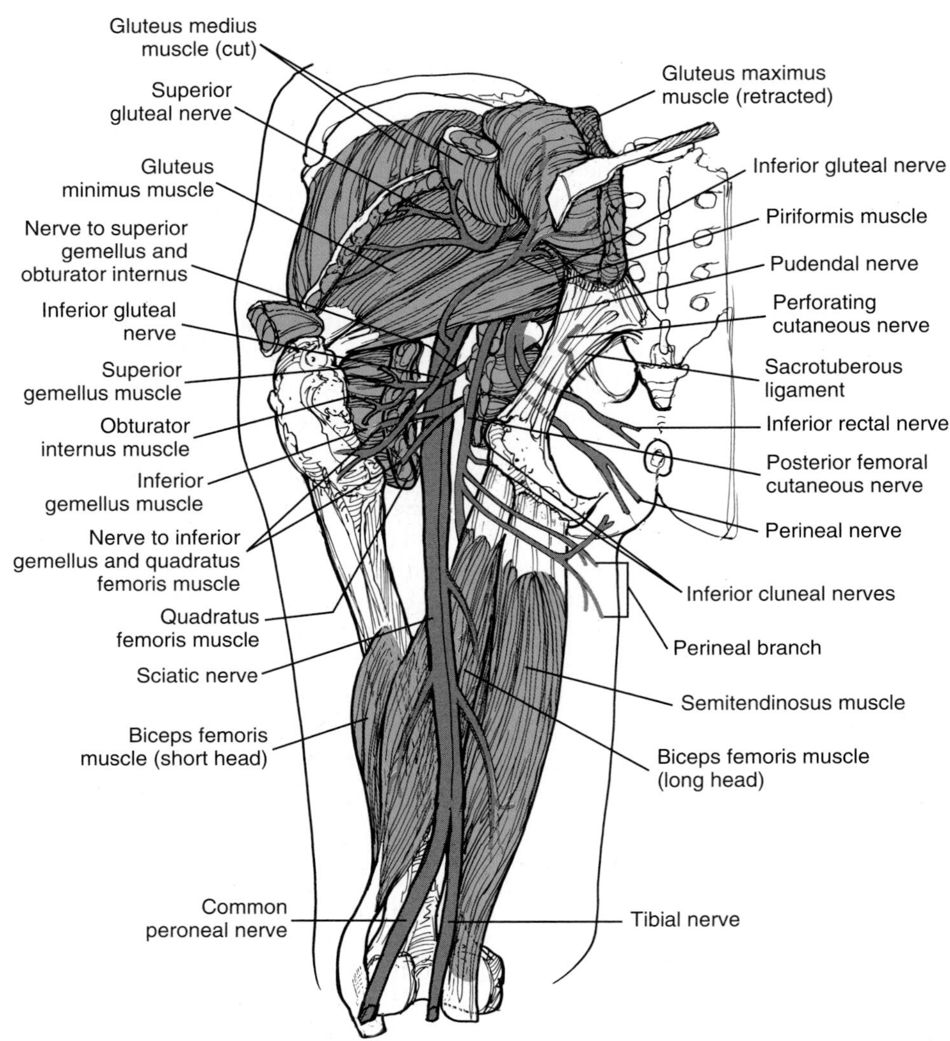

FIGURE 18–20
Nerves of the sacral plexus and the muscles they supply.

and metatarsus. The **lateral plantar nerve** passes laterally and distally between the flexor digitorum brevis and the flexor accessorius (quadratus plantae) muscles to the lateral side of the distal foot (Fig. 18–19*B*). This nerve supplies all of the plantar muscles of the foot, except for the four plantar muscles supplied by the medial plantar nerve. Cutaneous branches supply the skin of the lateral sole, the lateral side of the fifth toe, the skin between the fourth and fifth toes, and the ball of the fifth toe.

> **Injuries of the tibial nerve** are not common. When they occur, the nerve is typically damaged in the popliteal fossa, resulting in inability to plantarflex and push off with the affected foot. Patients compensate by shortening the stride length. The affected limb is moved forward by excessive flexion of the thigh.

The **inferior gluteal nerve** is a combination of fibers from spinal nerves L5, S1, and S2. It exits the pelvis via the greater sciatic foramen inferior to the piriformis muscle to innervate the gluteus maximus muscle (Figs. 18–19*A*, 18–20 and 18–21*A* and Table 18–5).

The **nerve to the obturator internus and gemellus superior muscles** is composed of fibers from spinal nerves L5, S1, and S2. It exits the pelvis via the greater sciatic foramen to innervate the posterior surface of the gemellus superior muscle. A branch crosses the ischial spine and reenters the pelvis via the lesser sciatic foramen to innervate the obturator internus muscle from its pelvic side (Figs. 18–19*A*, 18–20, and 18–21*B* and Table 18–5).

The **nerve to the piriformis muscle** originates from fibers of spinal nerves S1 and S2. It innervates the piriformis muscle via its anterior surface (Fig. 18–21*A* and Table 18–5).

The **posterior femoral cutaneous nerve** is a small nerve, which originates from spinal nerves S1 to S3. The posterior femoral cutaneous nerve exits the pelvis via the greater sciatic foramen inferior to the piriformis

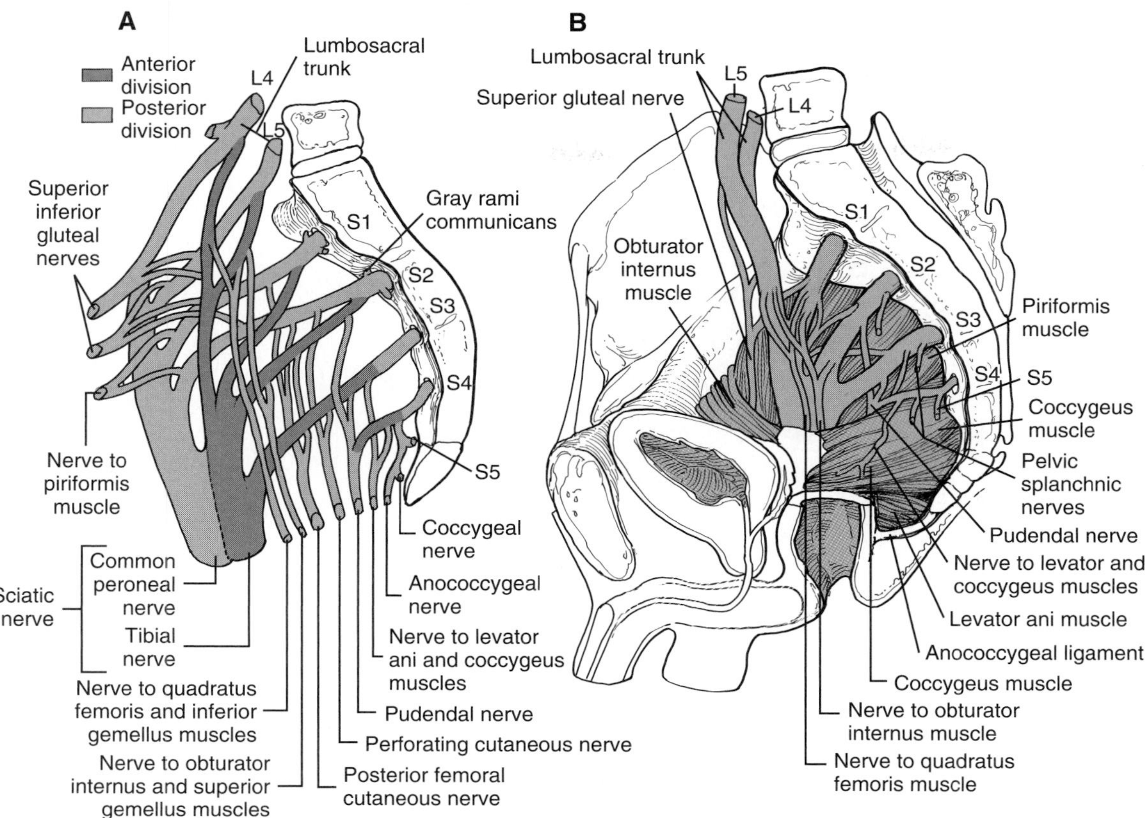

FIGURE 18–21
Sacral muscular branches and coccygeal plexus. **A.** Schematic drawing. **B.** Topographic view.

muscle and descends toward the posterior thigh under cover of the gluteus maximus muscle (Figs. 18–19*A*, 18–20, and 18–21*A*). Small cutaneous branches curl under the fold of the gluteus maximus muscle to innervate the skin covering the inferolateral border of the muscle. A **perineal branch** innervates the skin of the superomedial thigh and the labia majora or scrotum. The main trunk of the posterior femoral cutaneous nerve descends through the posterior compartment of the thigh just deep to the fascia lata. It gives off many cutaneous branches to the skin of the posterior thigh and pierces the fascia lata to enter the superficial fascia in the back of the knee where it joins the short saphenous vein. The posterior femoral cutaneous nerve continues to descend within the superficial fascia of the leg, giving off many cutaneous branches (Fig. 18–20 and Table 18–5).

The **perforating cutaneous nerve** typically arises from spinal nerves S2 and S3 (Figs. 18–19*A* and 18–21). It exits the pelvic cavity by piercing the sacrotuberous ligament and innervates the inferomedial skin of the buttock (Fig. 18–20 and Table 18–5).

The **pudendal nerve** is formed by fibers of spinal nerves S2 to S4. This nerve leaves the pelvis via the greater sciatic foramen between the coccygeus and piriformis muscles. It crosses the ischial spine and courses through the pudendal canal to the ischiorectal fossa. Its branches innervate the rectum, perianal region, and perineum (Figs. 18–21 and 18–22 and see Chapter 15).

The **pelvic splanchnic nerves** arise from visceral fibers of spinal nerves S2 to S4 (Fig. 18–21*B*). Their relationships and functions are described in Chapter 14.

Small **sacral muscular branches** composed of fibers from spinal nerve S4 innervate the coccygeus and levator ani muscles and external anal sphincter. Cutaneous branches escape the pelvis by piercing the coccygeus muscle. They supply the skin between the coccyx and anus (Fig. 18–21 and Table 18–5).

Nerves of the sacral plexus and their targets are summarized in Table 18–5.

Coccygeal Plexus. A branch of the ventral ramus of spinal nerve S4 and the ventral rami of spinal nerves S5 and Co1 make up the coccygeal plexus. **Muscular branches** innervate the coccygeus muscle. A **cutaneous branch** pierces the sacrotuberous ligament to supply the skin adjacent to it (Figs. 18–21*B* and 18–22 and Table 18–6).

Nerves of the coccygeal plexus and their targets are summarized in Table 18–6.

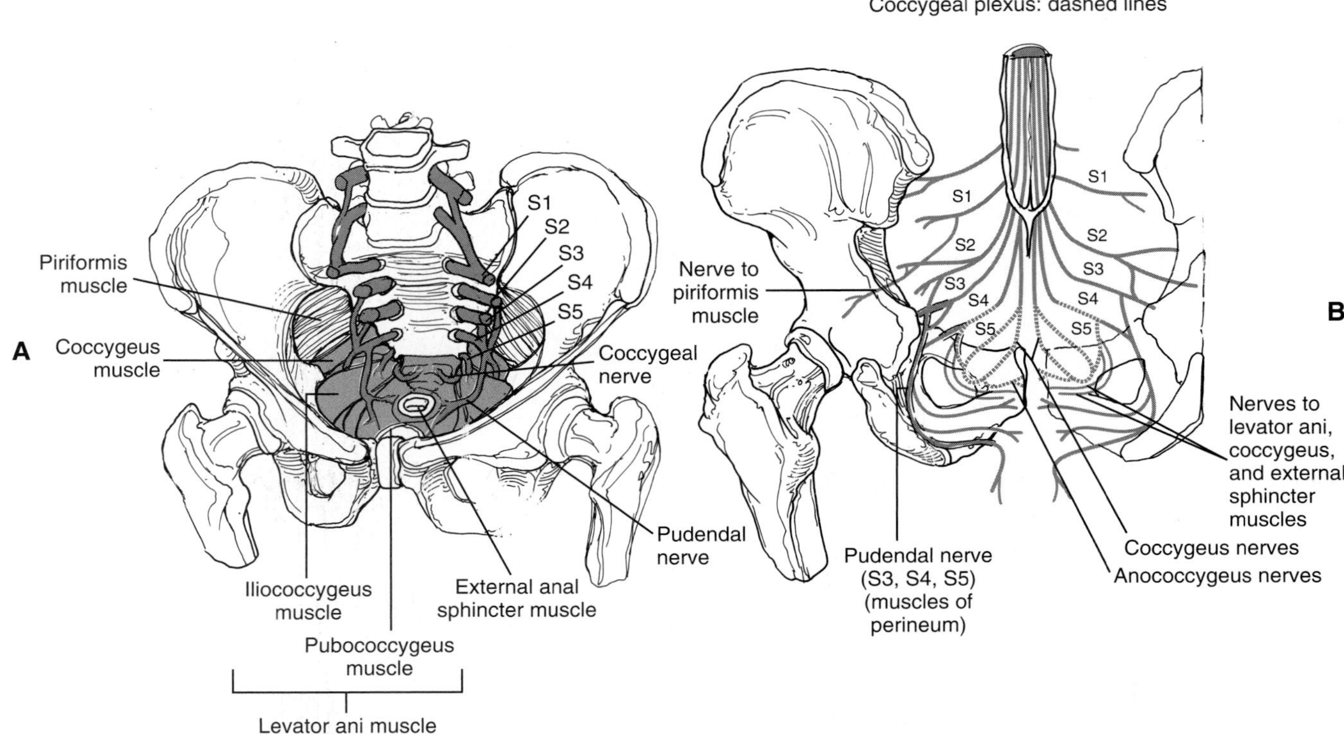

FIGURE 18–22
Nerves of the coccygeal plexus and the muscles they supply. **A.** Muscles innervated by the coccygeal nerves. **B.** Relationship of sacral nerves to coccygeal nerves.

TABLE 18–6
Nerves of the Coccygeal Plexus

Nerve	Origin	Structures Innervated
Coccygeal plexus	S4, S5, Co1	
Muscular branches		Coccygeus muscle
Cutaneous branches (anococcygeal nerves)		Skin over sacrotuberous ligament

19 Bones and Joints of the Upper Extremities

INTRODUCTION TO THE UPPER LIMB

Development of the Upper Extremity

The upper limbs arise from paddle-shaped buds of the lateral flank in the lower cervical and upper thoracic regions

Both the **upper** and **lower limb buds** arise from the lateral flank between weeks 4 and 8 of embryologic development (see Chapter 16). The upper limb buds form at the levels of somites C4 to T1 (Fig. 19–1*A*). Growth of the lateral plate mesoderm in these regions is initiated via signals from adjacent somites. Further proliferation of the **mesodermal core** of the limb bud is maintained by signals from a thickened craniocaudal ectodermal band at the distal edge of the hand plate called the **apical ectodermal ridge.** Development of the digits is organized in the craniocaudal axis with the thumb, or **pollex,** forming at the cranial edge of the hand plate and the little finger, the **digitus minimus,** at the caudal edge. The ventral side of the limb bud becomes the **palmar surface,** and the dorsal side becomes the **dorsum** of the hand (Fig. 19–1*B*). The development of both pairs of limb buds continues throughout the embryonic period, but the upper extremities begin to develop slightly earlier than the lower extremities.

As in the lower extremities, the **bones of the upper extremities** condense from elongated bars of mesenchyme, which form within the central axis of the limb bud. The bars arise from lateral plate mesoderm. Later, presumptive joints appear when fibroblastic **interzones** differentiate within these mesenchymal condensations. The interzones differentiate into ligaments, synovial membranes, and cartilage. The mesenchymal precursors of the appendicular skeleton **chondrify** during weeks 5 to 7 and **ossify** during weeks 6 to 12 in a proximal-to-distal sequence. However, the carpal bones do not ossify completely until early childhood. It should be noted that the **clavicle,** a bony segment unique to the upper extremity, ossifies directly from mesenchyme and, therefore, lacks a cartilaginous precursor.

Rotation of the Upper Extremities During Development

Upper limbs rotate only slightly during development

The upper extremities rotate slightly in a lateral direction during development (Fig. 19–2) in contrast to the 180-degree medial rotation of the lower extremities. As a consequence, the relative positions of the precursors of muscles, nerves, and vessels within the upper limb buds are not fundamentally altered during development. For example, the definitive flexor muscles of the upper limbs remain in the ventral location that their precursors occupied in the embryonic limb bud. Likewise, extensors remain located in posterior compartments of the arm, forearm, and hand (see Chapter 20). In addition, nerves of the brachial plexus that innervate upper extremity structures maintain their original craniocaudal and dorsoventral relationships within the definitive upper limbs. Thus, the ventral rami of spinal nerves C5 and C6 tend to innervate muscles and integument on the lateral (radial) side of the upper limb, while the ventral rami of spinal nerves C8 and T1 innervate muscles and integument on the medial (ulnar) side of the upper limb (see discussion of the brachial plexus in Chapter 21). Nerves that innervate muscle precursors on the dorsal side of the limb bud ultimately innervate extensors of the definitive upper limb. Nerves that innervate muscle precursors on the ventral side of the limb bud ultimately innervate flexors of the definitive limb (see Chapter 21).

Congenital Abnormalities of the Upper Limbs

Congenital malformations of the upper limbs are similar to those of the lower limbs

As in the lower limb, congenital malformations of the upper limb include **reduction defects,** ranging from total absence of the limb (amelia) to absence of part of the limb (meromelia). Meromelia of the upper limb is characterized by the absence of all of the proximal segments of the limb so that the hand is directly attached to the shoulder (phocomelia). Congenital anomalies of the upper limb also include **duplication defects,** such as duplication of the digits (polydactyly); **dysplasia,** such as fusion of the digits (syndactyly); and **gigantism,** or excessive growth of limb segments.

As has been noted in Chapter 16, congenital anomalies of the limb may be caused by specific mutations or chromosomal defects or may be a response to teratogenic substances. For example, homeotic transformation of limb seg-

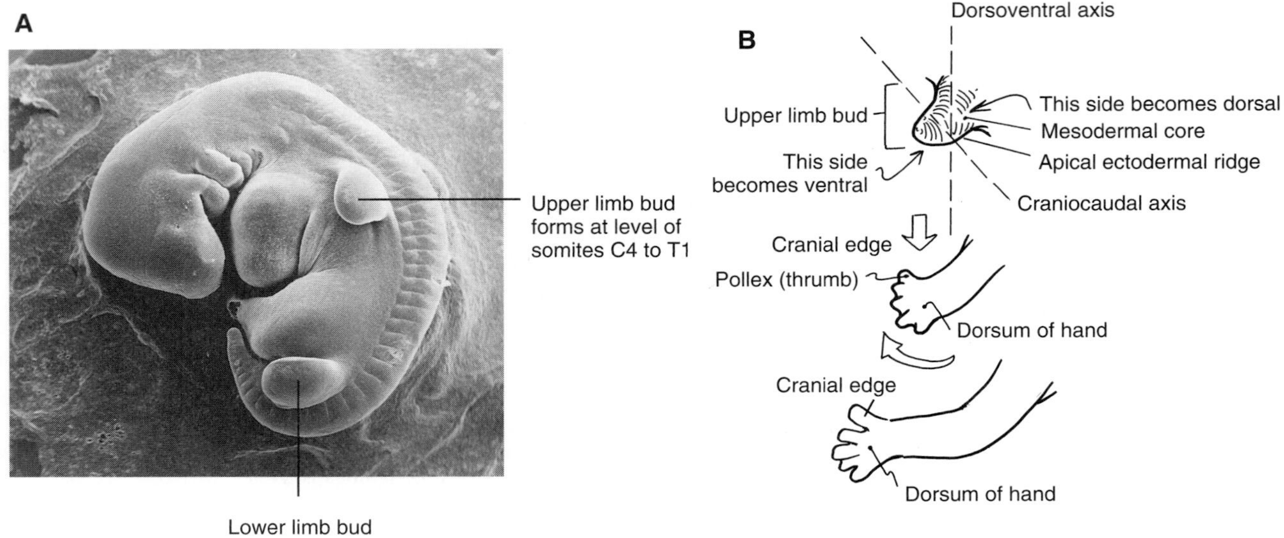

FIGURE 19–1
Development of the upper extremity. **A.** Upper limb bud in human embryo at approximately the fourth week of development. **B.** Craniocaudal and dorsolateral organization of developing upper limb.

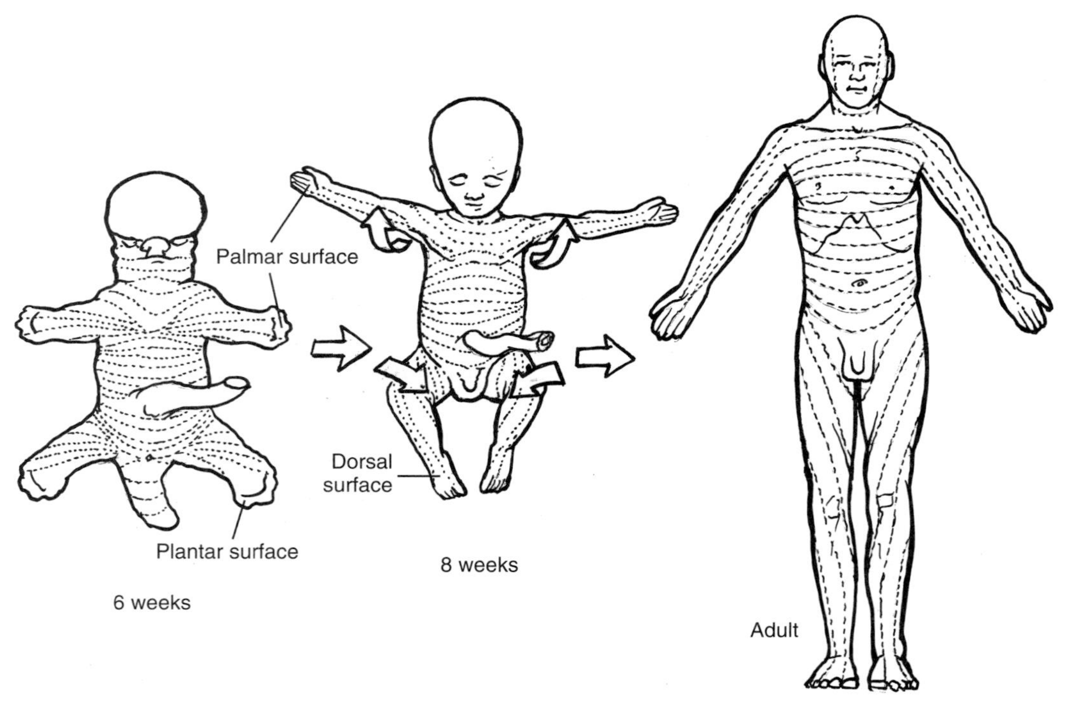

FIGURE 19–2
Rotation of the upper extremities during development.

ments may arise from the mutation of specific HOX genes, resulting in syndactyly and defects of the metacarpals or forearm. Some of the most hazardous teratogens are therapeutic drugs, including analogs of retinoic acid used for treatment of acne, phenytoin used for treatment of epilepsy, and thalidomide given as a sedative-hypnotic.

▲ Structure of the Definitive Upper Extremities

Surface Anatomy of the Upper Extremities

The integument of the upper extremity consists of the epidermis and dermis, which overlie the fatty hypodermis, or superficial fascia. The skin and superficial fascia of the upper extremity are organized in the same way

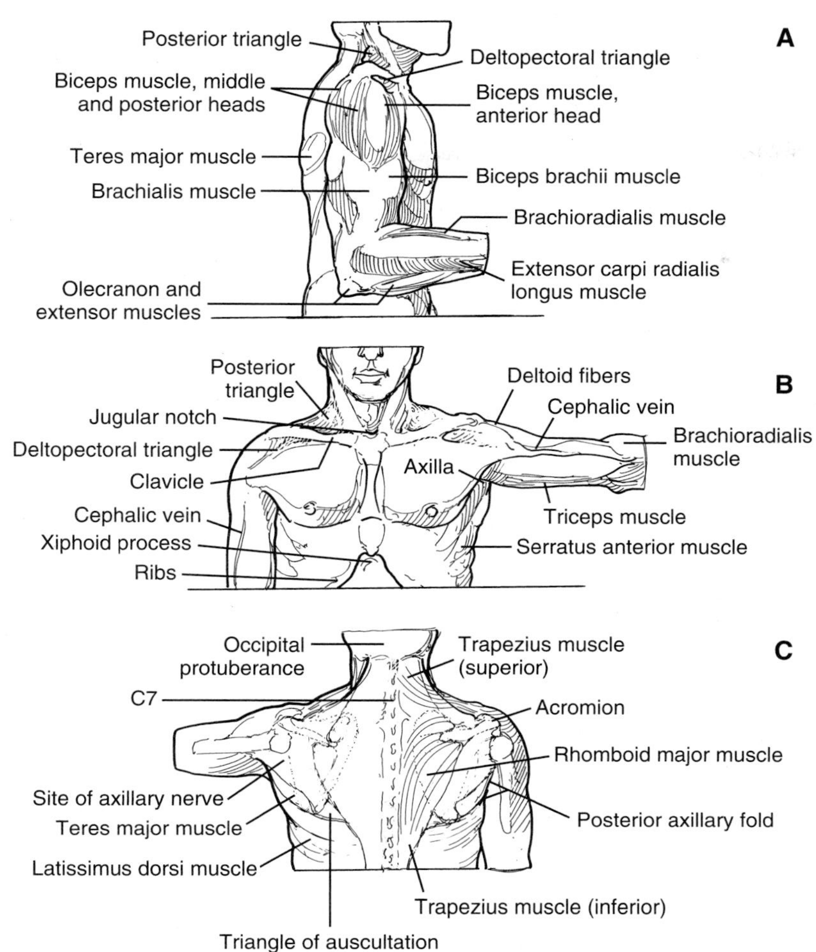

FIGURE 19–3
Muscles defining the surface anatomy of the upper extremities. **A.** Lateral view of features of the shoulders and upper arm. **B.** Anterior view showing axilla. **C.** Posterior view showing posterior axillary fold.

as integumentary elements elsewhere in the body. As in the lower extremity, their complete investment of the limb provides stability for muscles and joints. Deep to the superficial fascia, a layer of deep fascia invests the muscles, anchoring them, segregating them into functional compartments, and helping coordinate their actions within compartments (see Chapter 20).

The bulges of the **shoulders** are defined by the deltoid muscles, while the muscular bulge of the **pectoral region** reveals the underlying pectoralis major and minor muscles (Fig. 19–3*A*). The pectoralis major muscle forms the **anterior axillary fold** just anterior to the **axilla (armpit)** (Fig. 19–3*B*). The latissimus dorsi and teres major muscles form the **posterior axillary fold** just posterior to the axilla.

Contours of the **arm** (between the shoulder and the elbow joints) are defined by bulges of the flexor muscles ventrocranially and extensor muscles dorsocaudally. The **elbow joint,** between the arm and the forearm, is defined on its ventral side by a hollow called the **cubital fossa** (Fig. 19–4*A*) and on its dorsal side by a sharp extension of bone, the **olecranon process of the ulna** (Fig. 19–4*B*). The **forearm** (between the elbow and the wrist joints), or **antebrachial segment,** is defined by a **radial side** and an **ulnar side** based on the relative positions of the radius and ulna bones. In anatomic position (in which the upper limbs are supinated, or rotated outward), the thumb (digit 1) is on the radial side (in relation to the radius bone of the forearm). The fifth digit (little finger) is on the ulnar side (in relation to the ulnar bone of the forearm).

Other surface features of the upper extremities include prominent **flexure lines** of the wrists and hands (Fig. 19–4). For example, transverse creases are prominent on the dorsal surface in the regions of the radiocarpal, carpal, metacarpophalangeal, and interphalangeal joints (see below). These lines tend to disappear when the joints are flexed and tend to deepen when the

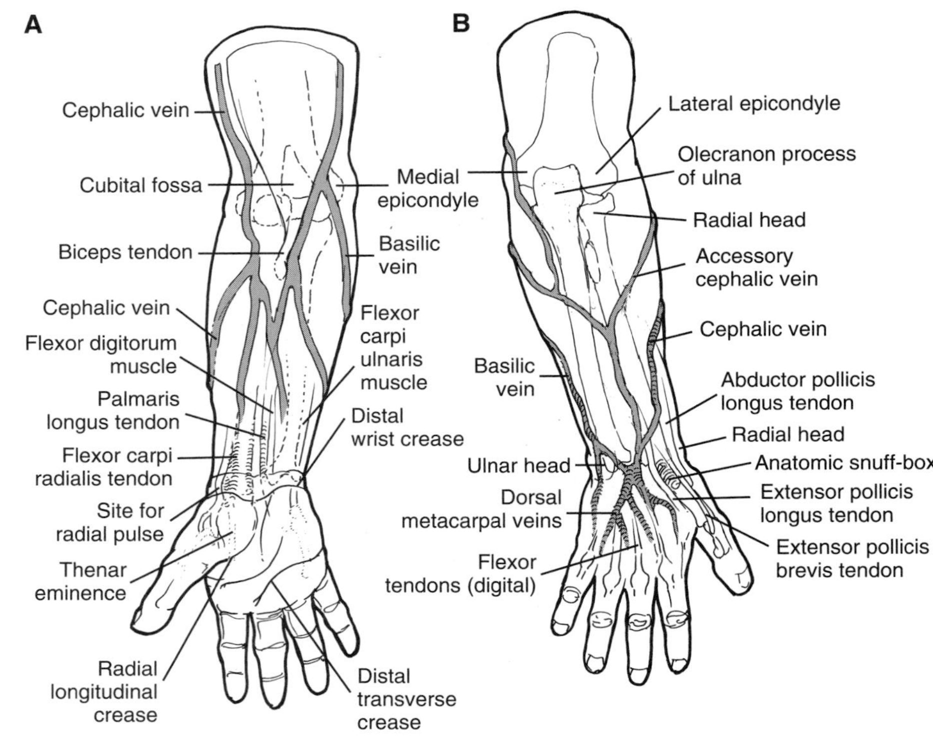

FIGURE 19–4
Surface anatomy of the forearm showing positions of bones, flexure lines, and superficial veins. **A.** Ventral side. **B.** Dorsal side.

joints are extended. Creases on the palmar side of the wrist and hand may serve as useful landmarks for deeper structures. For example, the most proximal of the three creases on the palmar side of the radiocarpal joint indicates the proximal limit of the flexor synovial sheaths; the intermediate crease lies over the radioulnar joint; and the most distal crease lies immediately superficial to the proximal boundary of the flexor retinaculum (see below). Creases of the palm include a radial longitudinal one outlining the **thenar eminence** (the bulge at the base of the thumb) and proximal and distal transverse lines (Fig. 19–4A). Transverse lines are also prominent on the palmar side of the bases of the digits and in the regions of all of the interphalangeal joints.

As in the lower extremity, **superficial veins** are prominent surface features of the upper extremity (see discussion of vasculature below).

Mobility of the Upper Extremities

The upper extremity is designed for mobility at the expense of stability

The function of the upper extremities is largely prehensile (i.e., they are used for grasping). Thus, control and smoothness of fine movement is particularly well developed in these appendages. If one views the upper limb as a proximodistal series of finely controlled skeletal platforms, each with specific, unique vectors of movement, one is able to see that, as the platforms work together from the shoulder to the hand, they enable the fingertips to be placed in infinitely varied ways so that the fingertips can grasp or touch objects in three-dimensional space (see discussion of prehensile function below). In contrast, the function of the lower extremities is largely to support the weight of the body while a person is standing or moving. In the upper extremities, stability is sacrificed so that mobility can be enhanced, and the anatomy and clinical vulnerabilities of the upper limbs reflect this fact (see discussion of injuries of the skeleton and joints below). For example, the bones of the shoulder joint, in contrast to the bones of the hip joint, are loosely bound and stabilized primarily by muscle attachments. Moreover, in the shoulder, the spheroidal humeral head sits upon a relatively flat glenoid fossa so that the humeral head has several degrees of freedom. Because of these arrangements, trauma to the shoulder tends to result in dislocation of the humerus from the glenoid fossa (see below).

Bones of the upper extremity are lighter and weaker than bones of the lower extremity

Bones of the upper extremity are smaller and lighter than those of the lower extremity. The femur and tibia, in keeping with their load-bearing functions, are massive compared with their counterparts, the humerus and ulna. Because the joints of the upper extremity facilitate prehensile function, they have a far greater range of motion than comparable joints of the lower extremity. Some of this mobility results from differences in skeletal anatomy, while some results from differences in the structure of the menisci, capsules, and ligaments.

Stabilizing elements of the upper limbs are less substantial and more lax than homologous elements of the lower limbs

As in the case of the lower extremity, several types of structural and stabilizing elements play pivotal roles in the function of the upper extremity. In the upper extremity, these elements must, to a far greater degree than in the lower extremity, provide for the increased mobility needed to carry out prehensile movements. Thus, in almost all cases, these structures are less substantial and more lax than similar structures in the lower extremity. They include skeletal elements; joints, including menisci, ligaments, and joint capsules (see below); retinacula and synovial tendon sheaths (see Chapter 20); the integument; and the deep fascia.

Relationships between structures of the upper extremity and their functions and the range of motion of specific joints are discussed below.

SKELETAL FRAMEWORK AND JOINTS OF THE UPPER EXTREMITY

Bones and joints of the upper extremity provide an unstable but mobile framework for intricate movements and prehensile function

An understanding of the skeletal structure of the upper extremity provides a framework for establishing the anatomic relationships of soft tissues, including muscles, vessels, and nerves. An understanding of joint structures provides a basis for learning muscle actions in the upper extremity.

The **appendicular skeleton of the upper extremity** is composed of the following bones, which are listed in a proximal-to-distal sequence:

- clavicle,
- scapula,
- humerus,
- ulna and radius,
- carpals (which make up the carpus, or wrist),
- metacarpals (which make up the metacarpus, or hand), and
- phalanges.

Joints of the upper extremity include the

- sternoclavicular joint;
- acromioclavicular joint;
- shoulder (glenohumeral, humeral) joint;
- elbow (cubital) joint;
- proximal, middle, and distal radioulnar joints;
- radiocarpal joint;
- intercarpal joints;
- carpometacarpal joints;
- intermetacarpal joints;
- metacarpophalangeal joints; and
- interphalangeal joints (Fig. 19–5).

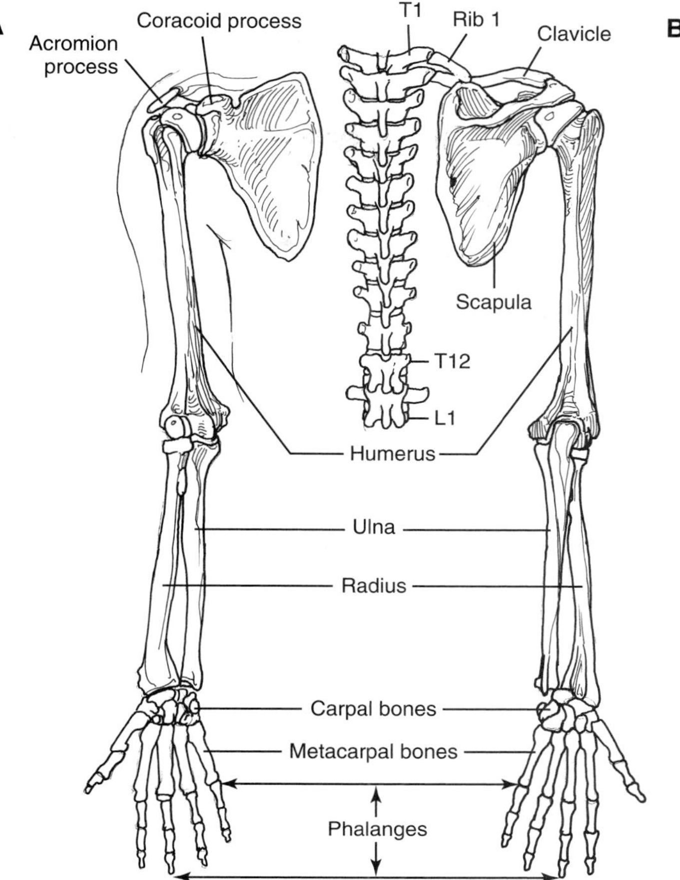

FIGURE 19–5
The appendicular skeleton of the upper extremity. **A.** Anterior view. **B.** Posterior view.

Upper extremity bones and joints are described in a proximal-to-distal order.

Skeletal Framework of the Upper Extremity

Shoulder Girdle

Clavicle. The sternoclavicular joint is the only bony connection between the upper appendicular skeleton and the axial skeleton. Muscles form all the other connections between the upper limb and the trunk (see Chapter 20).

The short, curved **clavicle** has no counterpart in the pelvic girdle (Fig. 19–6). The clavicle becomes bone mainly by dermal (intramembranous) ossification early in the second month of embryonic development. It is the first bone of the entire body to ossify. Its rounded **sternal head** articulates with the **clavicular notch of the manubrium,** and its flattened **acromial head** articulates with the **acromial process of the scapula** (Table 19–1). A short, tough **coracoclavicular ligament** further binds the lateral end of the clavicle to the coracoid process of

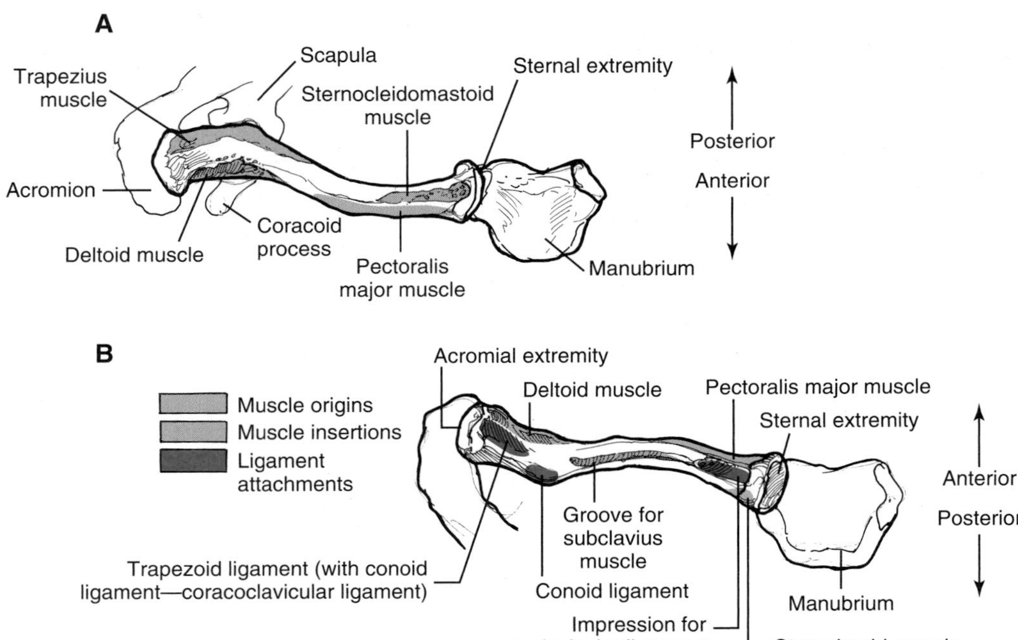

FIGURE 19–6
The clavicle bone, which is part of the shoulder girdle. The joint between this bone and the sternum is the only bony connection between the upper appendicular skeleton and the axial skeleton. **A.** Superior surface of the clavicle. **B.** Inferior surface of the clavicle.

the scapula. Several muscles also bind the clavicle to the axial skeleton, scapula, and humerus (see Chapter 20). Clavicular tubercles raised by these muscles are most obvious in males (Fig. 19–6).

Fracture of the Clavicle. Fractures of the clavicle are common for two reasons. First, the clavicle is the only bone of the upper extremity that is attached to the axial skeleton. Second, the sternoclavicular joint is so stable that it is difficult to dislocate. Thus, falling on an outstretched hand typically results in fracture of the clavicle as the force of the impact is transmitted from the hand (see the following display and Fig. 19–7).

Hand → Carpometacarpal joints → Carpus →
Radiocarpal joint → Radius →
Interosseous membrane and proximal and
distal radioulnar joints →
Ulna → Humeroulnar articulation (elbow joint) →
Humerus → Glenohumeral joint → Scapula →
Acromioclavicular joint → Clavicle

Fractures of the clavicle resulting from falls typically occur at the clavicle's weakest region, which is the boundary between its lateral one-third and its medial two-thirds (Fig. 19–7). This is an especially common fracture in children. The consequence of such fractures is that the medial two-thirds of the clavicle is elevated by the sternocleidomastoid muscle, while the lateral one-third is depressed by the weight of the upper extremity. Fortunately, this displacement spares the subclavian artery and vein as well as vulnerable elements of the brachial plexus (see below). Fracture of the clavicle at the boundary between its lateral two-thirds and its medial one-third is also common. This fracture most typically occurs as the consequence of a blow to the shoulder. In all bone fractures, it must be determined whether the fracture is the result of an underlying disorder such as osteoporosis or cancer (pathologic fracture) or a traumatic injury.

Scapula. The scapula is a triangular bone with medial, lateral, and superior borders (Fig. 19–8). The **superior border** is marked by a prominent **suprascapular notch,** which is bridged by a **suprascapular ligament.** The apices of the triangular scapula are the lateral, superior, and inferior angles. The **lateral angle** may also be characterized as the **head of the scapula,** which is attached to the scapular **body** by a slightly constricted **neck.** The **inferior angle** serves as a point of reference for rotational movements of the scapula. In **medial rotation,** the inferior angle moves medially, and in **lateral rotation,** it moves laterally (see below). The lateral surface of the scapular head forms a shallow fossa called the **glenoid fossa** (depression), which articulates with the proximal head of the humerus (see Table 19–1). The scapula has a flattened **costal (subscapular) surface,** which is slightly concave. This surface contains the subscapularis muscle. The scapula has a **dorsal surface** separated by a prominent **spine** into a **superior supra-**

TABLE 19–1
Specialized Skeletal Processes of Upper Extremity Bones and their Major Attachments and Articulations

Bone	Process	Attachments	Articulations
Clavicle	Sternal head		Clavicular notch of manubrium
	Acromial head		Acromial process of scapula
Scapula	Glenoid fossa		Head of humerus
	Supraglenoid tubercle	Long head of biceps brachii muscle	
	Infraglenoid tubercle	Long head of triceps brachii muscle	
	Scapular spine	Supraspinatus, infraspinatus, trapezius muscles	
	Acromial process		Acromial head of clavicle
	Coracoid process	Coracoclavicular ligament, pectoralis minor muscle	
Humerus	Head		Glenoid fossa of scapula
	Anatomic neck		Joins head and shaft of humerus
	Lesser tubercle	Subscapularis muscle	
	Greater tubercle	Supraspinatus, infraspinatus, teres minor muscles	
	Intertubercular sulcus		Occupied by tendon of long head of biceps muscle
	Surgical neck (just distal to greater and lesser tubercles)	Proximal shaft of humerus (common site of fracture)	
	Deltoid tuberosity	Deltoid, brachialis muscles	
	Lateral supracondylar ridge	Extensor carpi radialis longus muscle	
	Lateral epicondyle	Common tendon for superficial forearm extensors	
	Medial supracondylar ridge	Humeral head of pronator teres muscle	
	Medial epicondyle	Common tendon for superficial forearm flexors	
	Modified condyle (distal)		Ulna and radius
	Trochlea		Trochlear notch of ulna
	Capitulum		Radius
	Coronoid fossa		Coronoid process of ulna when forearm is fully flexed
	Radial fossa		Head of radius when forearm is fully flexed
	Olecranon fossa		Olecranon process of ulna when forearm is fully extended
Ulna	Trochlear notch		Trochlea of humerus
	Olecranon process		Olecranon fossa of humerus
	Coronoid process		Coronoid fossa of humerus
	Supinator crest (proximal extension of interosseous border)	Supinator muscle	
	Radial notch		Radius
	Styloid process	Ulnar collateral ligament	
Radius	Proximal head		Humerus and ulna
	Radial tuberosity	Distal tendon of biceps muscle	
	Distal head		Scaphoid and lunate bones
	Ulnar notch		Ulna
	Styloid process	Lateral ligament of wrist joint	
Hamate bone	Hamulus	Flexor retinaculum	
Trapezium bone	Trapezial tubercle	Opponens pollicis, flexor pollicis brevis muscles	

spinous fossa and an **inferior infraspinous fossa** (Fig. 19–8*B*). The **lateral border** of the scapular spine and the dorsal surface of the neck of the scapula contribute to the boundaries of the **greater scapular notch.** The supraspinous fossa houses the supraspinatus muscle, and the infraspinous fossa houses the infraspinatus muscle (see below).

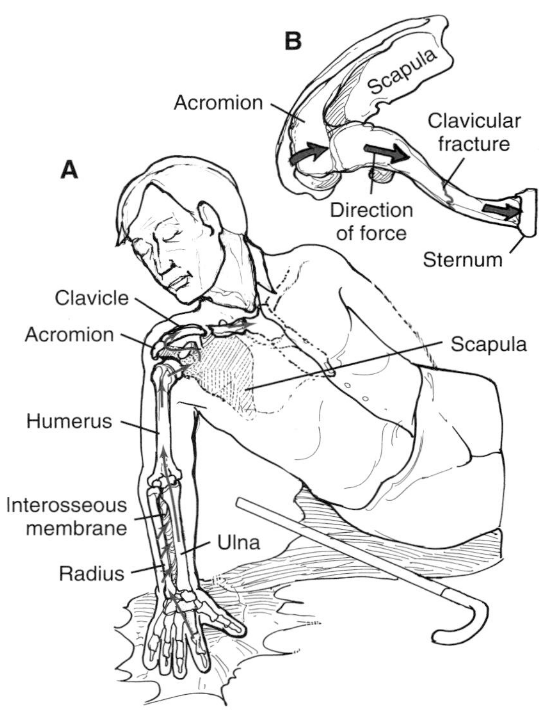

FIGURE 19–7
Fracture of the clavicle. **A.** Typical fall transmitting the force of impact to the clavicle. **B.** Common fracture point.

The scapula bears a posterolateral **acromial process** and an anterior **coracoid process.** The acromial process is a lateral extension of the scapular spine. It articulates with the acromial head of the clavicle (Fig. 19–8). The coracoid process provides an attachment site for the coracoclavicular ligament (see above) and for the origin of the pectoralis minor muscle. This process is an anterior projection of the scapular neck.

As has been noted, the scapula is bound to the clavicle at the acromioclavicular joint and to the humerus at the glenohumeral joint (Fig. 19–8). It is also bound to the trunk, clavicle, and humerus by many muscular attachments (see below).

Fracture of the Scapula. The scapula is seldom fractured. Fracture occurs only when the bone is subjected to direct trauma.

Upper Arm

Humerus. The long **shaft** of the humerus joins its two expanded ends: a proximal hemispheric head, which articulates with the scapula, and a distal modified condyle, which articulates with the ulna and radius of the forearm (Fig. 19–9 and see Table 19–1). Like many other long bones, the shaft of the humerus, which is triangular in cross section, has anterior, lateral, and medial borders and anterolateral, anteromedial, and posterior surfaces (Fig. 19–9).

The proximal **head** of the humerus is joined to the **shaft** by a constricted neck called the **anatomic neck** of the humerus, which is the site of attachment of the shoulder joint capsule (compare this structure with the **surgical neck** below).

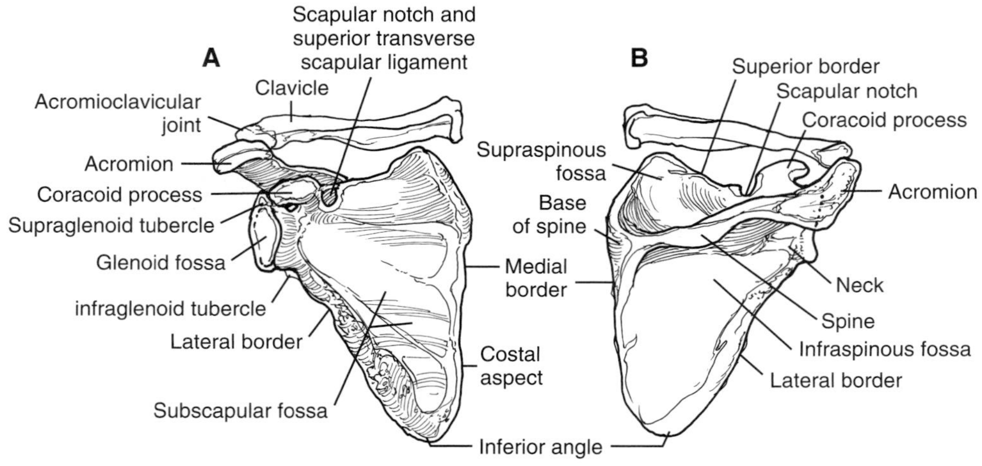

FIGURE 19–8
Anatomic features of the scapula, including its joints with the clavicle and humerus bones. **A.** Anterior view. **B.** Posterior view of dorsal surface.

Surface features of the proximal end of the shaft of the humerus include a medial **lesser tubercle** and lateral **greater tubercle** (see Table 19–1). Between these two tubercles lies the **intertubercular sulcus (bicipital groove),** which contains the long tendon of the biceps brachii muscle (Fig. 19–9). Just distal to the greater and lesser tubercles is the slightly constricted **surgical neck** of the humerus, so named because it is a common site of fracture (Fig. 19–9). The prominent **deltoid tuberosity** is apparent about halfway along the shaft at the lateral border of the humerus (Fig. 19–9). The other surfaces of the shaft are relatively smooth, providing sites for attachments of many muscles of the shoulder (proximal) and elbow (distal) joints (Fig. 19–9 and see below).

The expanded distal end of the humerus is characterized by a **lateral supracondylar ridge, lateral epicondyle, medial supracondylar ridge,** and **medial epicondyle** (Fig. 19–9). The intervening articular part of the condyle of the humerus consists of a pulley-shaped **trochlea,** which articulates with the ulna, and a hemispheric **capitulum,** which articulates with the proximal head of the radius (Fig. 19–9 and see Table 19–1). On the anterior surface, just proximal to the trochlea, a shallow **coronoid fossa** accommodates the coronoid process of the ulna when the forearm is fully flexed. Also on the anterior surface, a shallow **radial fossa** just proximal to the capitulum accommodates the margin of the head of the radius when the arm is fully flexed (Fig. 19–9 and see Table 19–1). On the posterior surface, a deep **olecranon fossa** accommodates the olecranon process of the ulna when the forearm is in full extension (Fig. 19–9 and see Table 19–1).

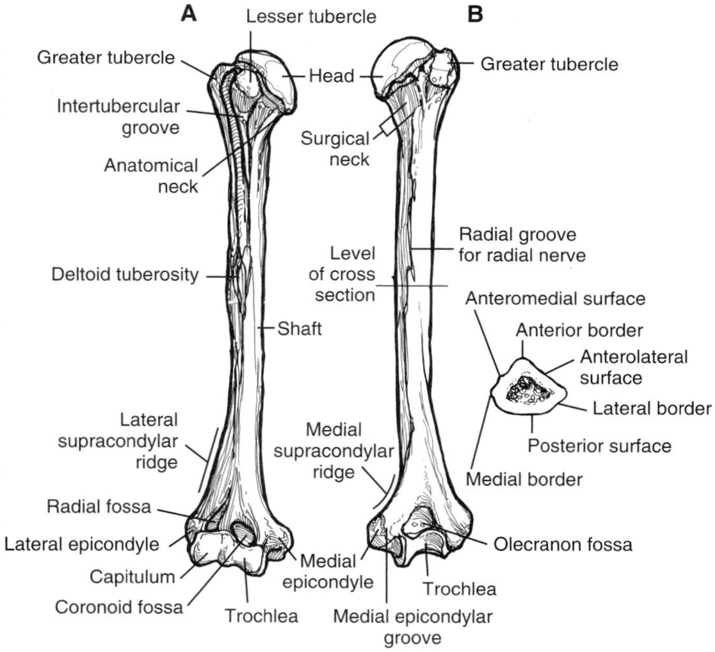

FIGURE 19–9
Surface features and articulating surfaces of the right humerus bone of the upper arm. **A.** Anterior view. **B.** Posterior view.

Fracture of the Humerus. The humerus is stronger than the clavicle or radius and is seldom fractured unless it is subjected to **direct trauma.** For example, trauma to the shoulder in an automobile accident may result in fracture of the humeral tuberosity or the surgical or anatomic neck of the humerus (Fig. 19–10*A* and see Fig. 19–9). The surgical neck is often fractured in elderly individuals as a consequence of a fall on the elbow. Direct trauma to the arm may result in fracture of the midshaft of the humerus (Fig. 19–10*B*). These fractures may also result in **injury to the radial nerve** (see Chapter 21). Trauma to the distal end of the humerus or forced abduction of the elbow may result in **avulsion of the medial epicondyle** (Fig. 19–10*C*). In this situation, **injury to the ulnar nerve** may also occur (see Chapter 21).

Forearm

Ulna. The ulna is medial to the radius within the supinated forearm (i.e., when the forearm is in anatomic position with the palms facing forward). When the forearm is pronated (i.e., when the palms are facing backward), the distal end of the radius twists anteriorly and

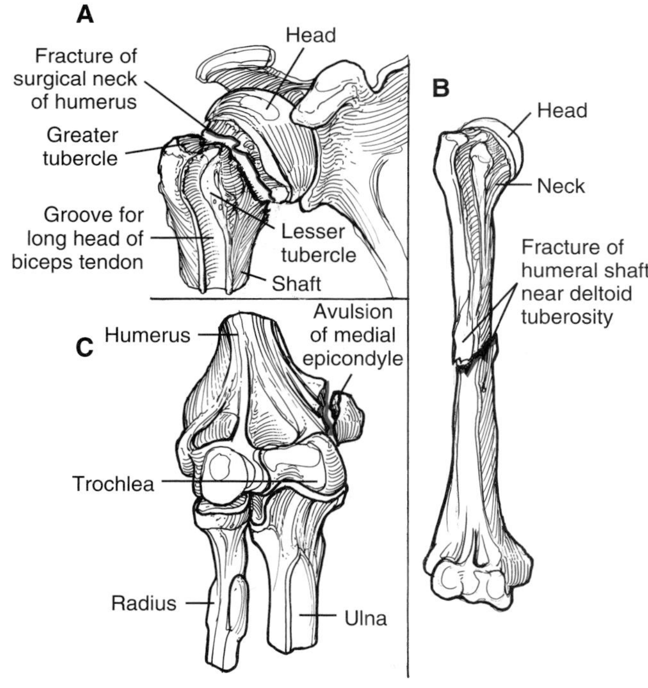

FIGURE 19–10
Fractures of the humerus. **A.** Fracture of the surgical neck may be caused by direct trauma to the shoulder. In elderly individuals, it is often caused by a fall on the elbow. **B.** Fracture of the midshaft by direct trauma to the arm. **C.** Avulsion of the medial epicondyle by trauma to the distal end of the humerus.

medially and the distal end of the ulna then lies lateral to the radius (see below). The ulna's proximal end articulates with the humerus and adjoining radius. The ulna's distal end articulates with a cartilaginous disc, which, in turn, articulates with the medial carpus (see below) and adjoining radius (Fig. 19–11*A* and *B*).

The anterior surface of the proximal end of the ulna has a smooth, concave **trochlear notch,** which articulates with the trochlea of the humerus (see Table 19–1 and above). The midregion of this articular surface is interrupted by a roughened nonarticular band and is divided into medial and lateral parts by a smooth longitudinal ridge. The beak-shaped **olecranon process** projects from the most proximal edge of the notch and the **coronoid process** from the most distal edge. An articulating surface for the radius, consisting of an oval **radial notch,** is located just lateral to the coronoid process (Fig. 19–11*A* and *B* and see Table 19–1).

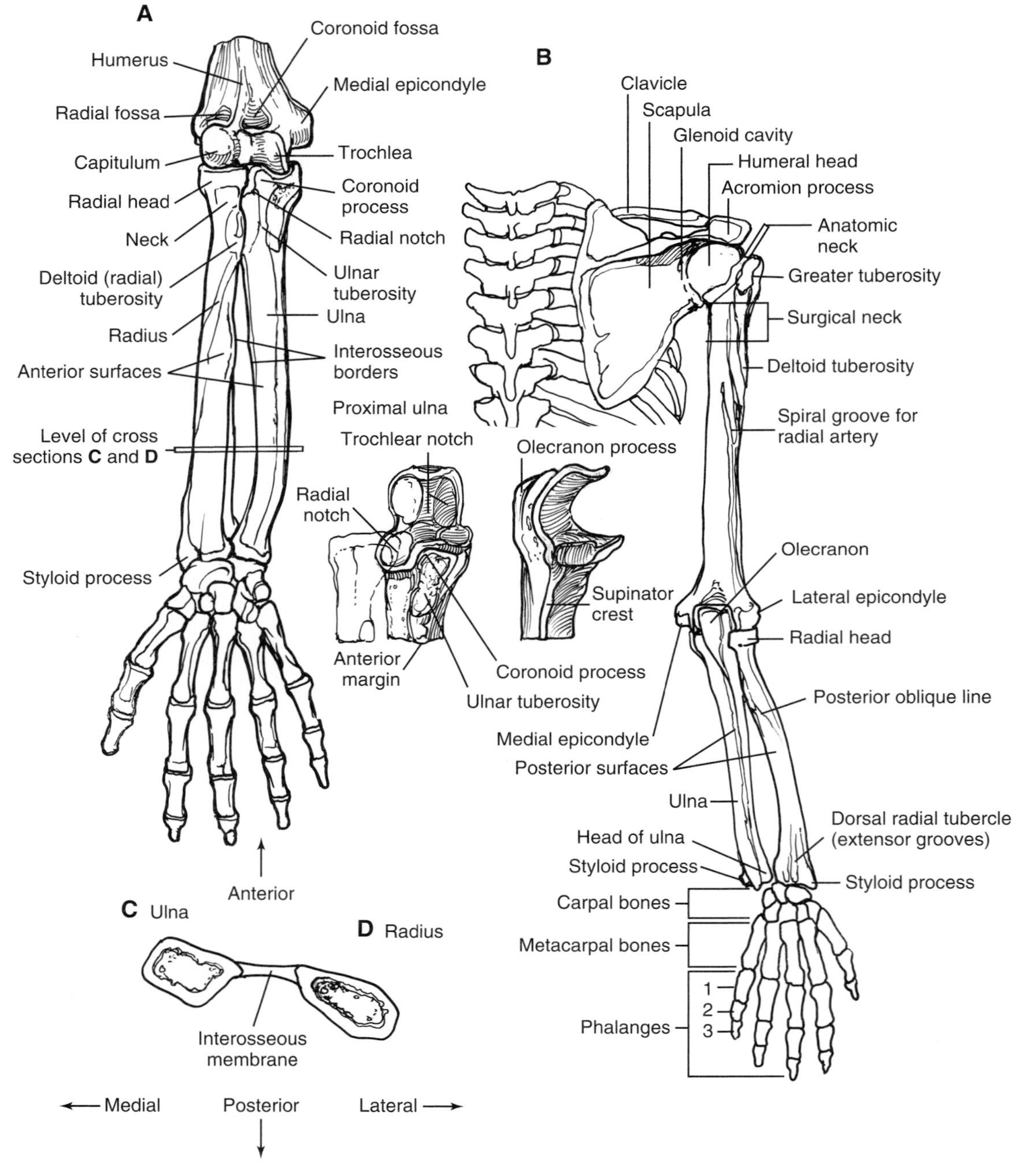

FIGURE 19–11
Bones of the forearm in anatomic position (supination) with surface features and articulation points of the ulna and radius bones. **A.** Anterior view of the right hand. **B.** Posterior view. **C.** Cross section of ulna. **D.** Cross section of radius.

The **shaft of the ulna** is triangular in cross section and has **anterior, posterior,** and **interosseous borders** and **anterior, posterior,** and **medial surfaces.** The lateral interosseous border is most apparent in the middle half of the shaft (Fig. 19–11*C*). The interosseous border is an attachment site for the interosseous membrane, which connects the ulna to the radius (Fig. 19–11*A* and *B* and see discussion of joints below). The proximal extension of the interosseous border is the **supinator crest** (see Table 19–1).

The **distal end of the ulna** has an expanded **head** and a **styloid process** (Fig. 19–11*A* and *B*). The distal surface of the head abuts a triangular articular disc, which articulates with the radius and abuts the medial part of the lunate bone and the triquetral bone of the medial carpus (Fig. 19–11*A* and *B*). The lateral convex surface of the ulnar head articulates with the **radial notch of the ulna** on the medial surface of the radius (see below). A posterolateral projection of the ulna's distal end is the **styloid process** (Fig. 19–11*A* and *B* and see Table 19–1). It is separated from the ulnar head by a deep longitudinal groove.

Fracture of the ulna is discussed with fracture of the radius, below.

Radius. The radius is the lateral bone of the forearm when the arm is in anatomic position (Fig. 19–11*A* and *B*). Its proximal end articulates (medially) with the ulna and (proximally) with the humerus. Its distal end articulates (medially) with the ulna and (distally) with the scaphoid and lunate bones of the lateral carpus.

The **proximal end of the radius** has a head, neck, and tuberosity (Fig. 19–11*A* and *B* and see Table 19–1). The superior surface of the proximal discoidal **head** has a shallow fossa, which articulates with the capitulum of the humerus. The constricted **neck** is just distal to the head. The anteromedial **radial tuberosity** is just distal to the neck of the radius. The radial tuberosity is an attachment site for the distal tendon of the biceps brachii muscle (see below).

The **shaft of the radius** is less obviously triangular in cross section than other long bones of the extremities. **Anterior, posterior,** and **interosseous (medial) borders** can be identified but only in certain regions (see Fig. 19–11*D*). The **anterior border** is best defined at the proximal and distal ends of the shaft. The shaft is rounded in between. The **posterior border** is deficient at both the proximal and distal ends of the shaft, and the **interosseous border** is deficient at the distal end (Fig. 19–11*A* and *B*). The **interosseous membrane** connects the distal three fourths of the interosseous (medial) border of the radius with the distal three fourths of the interosseous (lateral) border of the ulnar shaft (Fig. 19–11 and discussion of joints below). The radius has **anterior, posterior,** and **lateral surfaces,** but these are poorly defined by the incomplete radial borders just described (Fig. 19–11*A* and *B*).

The **distal head of the radius** has **anterior, posterior, medial,** and **lateral surfaces** and a **proximal (carpal) articular surface** (Fig. 19–11*A* and *B*). The carpal articular surface is divided into lateral triangular and medial quadrangular regions by a bony ridge. The lateral surface articulates with the scaphoid bone of the carpus and the medial surface with the lunate bone of the carpus (see Fig. 19–5). The medial surface has an **ulnar notch,** which articulates with the convex articulating surface on the lateral side of the distal head of the ulna (Fig. 19–11*A* and *B* and see below). A **styloid process** projects from the lateral surface of the distal radial head (Fig. 19–11*A* and *B*). A lateral **carpal ligament** is connected to the apex of the styloid process. Shallow grooves on the lateral and posterior surfaces of the styloid process carry tendons (see Table 19–1).

Fracture of the Radius and Ulna. **Fracture of the radius** may occur from a fall on an outstretched hand (Colles' fracture). The fracture typically occurs in the distal region of the radius (Fig. 19–12*A* and *B*). The distal segment of the broken radius is pulled proximally and superiorly. The styloid process of the ulna may also be fractured in such a fall. In a fall onto the back of the hand that results in a radial fracture, the distal fragment of the radius may be pulled proximally and anteriorly onto the proximal fragment (Smith's fracture). In children, the fracture more often occurs in the middle of the radial shaft (Fig. 19–12*B* and *D*). **Fracture of both the radius and ulna** may occur in a fall on an outstretched hand, particularly when twisting of the radius occurs. **Fractures of the ulna** are more commonly the consequence of direct trauma to the forearm. Repairs of forearm fractures are usually straightforward, although the swelling of muscles within forearm compartments may result in entrapment of the median nerve (see Chapter 21). Surgical cutting of the forearm fascia may relieve pressure on the nerve.

Wrist

Carpus. The carpus of the upper extremity consists of eight **carpal bones** organized in two rows: a proximal row of four and a distal row of four (see Fig. 19–11*A* and *B*). When the hand is supinated in anatomic position, the lateral-to-medial sequence of the proximal row is the **scaphoid, lunate, triquetral,** and **pisiform bones.** The lateral-to-medial sequence of the distal row is the **trapezium, trapezoid, capitate,** and **hamate bones.** All the carpal bones articulate with adjacent bones in the coronal plane except for the pisiform bone, which articulates only with the palmar aspect of the triquetral bone (see Fig. 19–11*A* and *B*).

Articulations of the carpal bones form a convex arch, which extends dorsally between the forearm and the metacarpals of the hand. The ventral concavity of

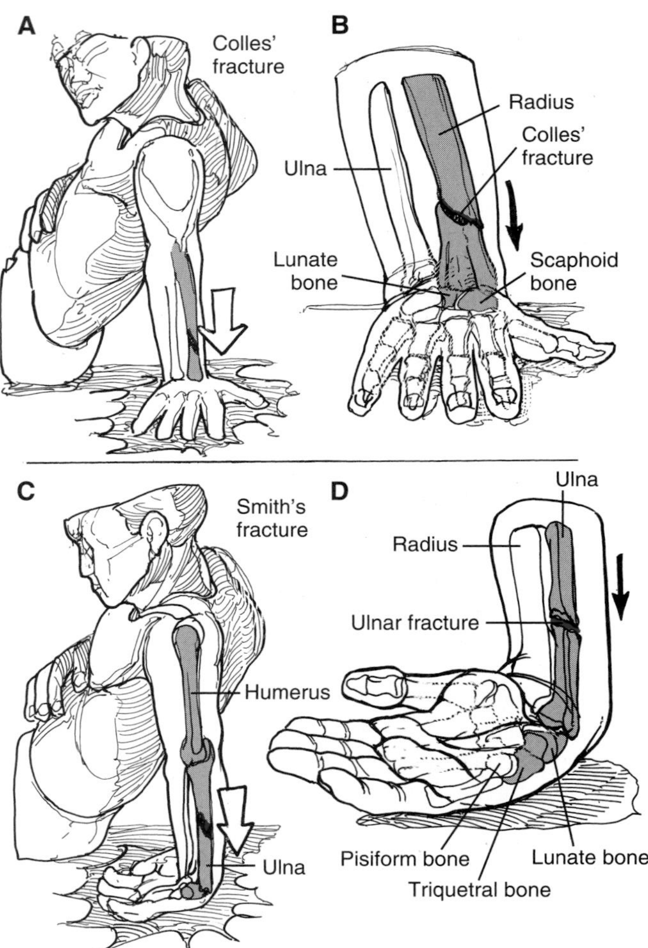

FIGURE 19–12
Fractures of the radius and ulna. **A** and **B.** Colles' fracture caused by a fall on an outstretched hand. Fracture of the radius is shown, but the ulna may also be fractured. **C** and **D.** Smith's fracture caused by a fall onto the back of the hand. Fracture of the ulna is shown. Fracture of the radius is more common, but both bones may be fractured, particularly if twisting occurs.

the arch is the **carpal groove.** This shallow groove is "roofed over" by a fibrous **flexor retinaculum** attached to its lateral and medial edges (including the hamulus of the hamate bone) to form a **carpal tunnel** (see discussion of connective tissue structures below).

The first bone at the lateral side of the most proximal row of carpal bones is the **scaphoid bone,** which is also the largest proximal carpal bone (Fig. 19–13). The rough dorsal and lateral surfaces of the scaphoid bone are its only nonarticular surfaces. The semilunar **lunate bone** just medial to the scaphoid bone has rough dorsal and palmar surfaces (Fig. 19–13). All of the other surfaces articulate with adjoining bones. The pyriform **triquetral bone** is roughened in the proximal part of its confluent dorsal and medial surfaces but articulates with adjacent bones in all other regions. The **pisiform bone** (shaped like a pea) has only one articular facet, which is at its dorsal surface and articulates with the triquetral bone (Fig. 19–13). It is classified as a sesamoid bone (see Chapter 16).

The first bone at the lateral side of the distal row of carpal bones is the **trapezium bone,** which has roughened dorsal, palmar, and lateral surfaces. All of its other surfaces articulate with adjacent bones. The most significant of these is the distolateral surface, which has a deep fossa that articulates with the base of the pollical (thumb) metacarpal. The trapezium bone also has a palmar tubercle and groove (Fig. 19–13). The **trapezoid bone** has roughened palmar and dorsal surfaces. All of its other smooth surfaces articulate with adjacent bones. Its distal end articulates with the second metacarpal. The distal end of the **capitate bone,** the largest bone of the carpus, articulates with the third metacarpal while its other surfaces articulate with adjacent carpal bones. Only the capitate's dorsal and palmar surfaces are roughened. The cuneiform (wedge-shaped) **hamate bone** defines the medial limit of the distal row of carpal bones. Its dorsal and palmar surfaces, along with a thin strip of its medial surface, are roughened. Its distal articular surface articulates with the fourth and fifth metacarpal bones. The distal region of its palmar surface bears a hooklike projection, called the **hamulus.** The hamulus contributes to the medial side of the carpal groove and serves as an attachment site for the flexor retinaculum, which forms the "roof" of the carpal tunnel (see above and Table 19–1).

Injuries of the Carpal Bones. The **scaphoid bone** is infrequently fractured as a consequence of a direct fall on an outstretched hand. These fractures are difficult to visualize in radiographs of the wrist.

Anterior dislocation of the **lunate bone** may occur when one falls forward on an outstretched hand. This may cause compression of the median nerve. Symptoms of this condition are similar to those of carpal tunnel syndrome.

Hand

Metacarpals. The **metacarpus** contains five **metacarpal bones,** which are numbered one to five in a lateral to medial sequence (i.e., from the thumb to the little finger). All of these bones have a head, shaft, and base (Fig. 19–13). The base of each metacarpal articulates with the distal row of carpal bones and adjacent metacarpals (see below). The shaft of each metacarpal radiates distally. Each head forms one of the knuckles. The second to fifth metacarpals are arched with convex dorsal and concave ventral surfaces. The convexity of the ventral side of the metacarpus houses the palmar muscles (see below). The original dorsoventral axis of the first (pollical) metacarpal bone is shifted 90 degrees so that its concave ventral surface faces medially and its convex dorsal sur-

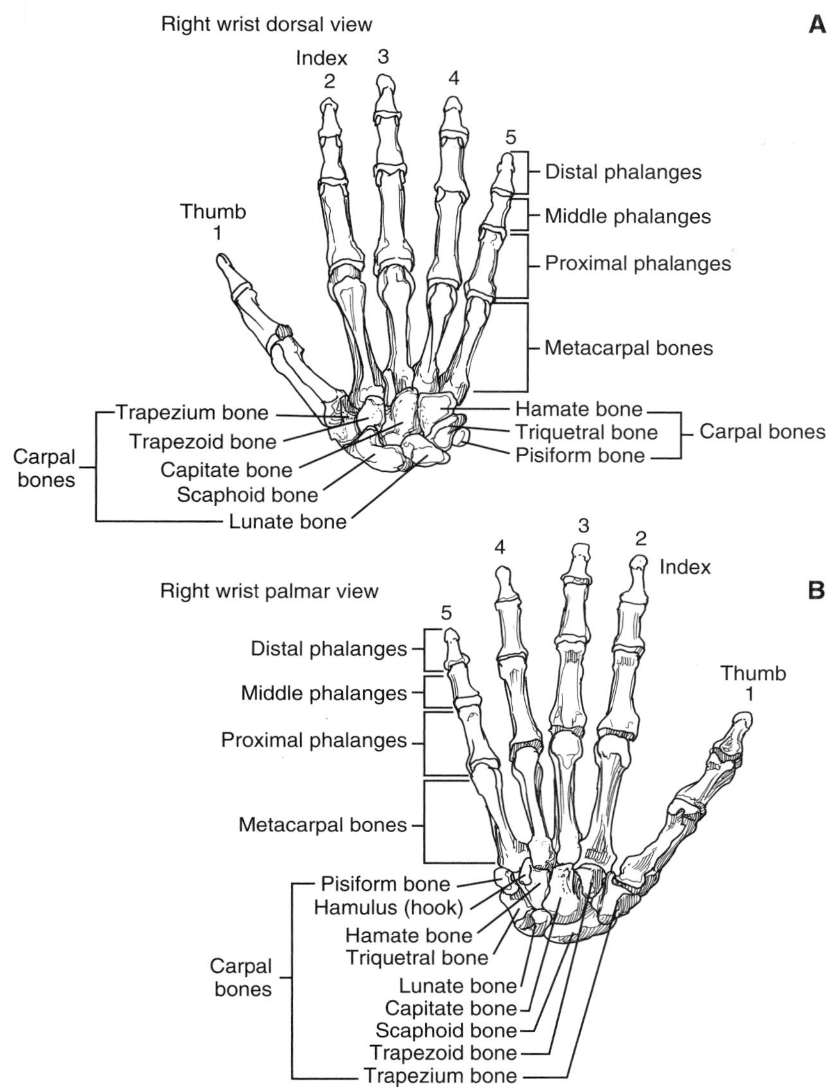

FIGURE 19–13
Carpal bones of the wrist and metacarpals and phalanges of the hand. **A.** Dorsal view of the right hand. **B.** Palmar view of the right hand.

face faces laterally (Fig. 19–13). This arrangement aids in the oppositional function of the thumb (see below).

Phalanges. Like the metacarpals, the 14 **phalangeal bones** (two in the thumb and three in the other fingers) have a proximal base, shaft, and distal head (Fig. 19–13). The rounded base of each proximal phalanx articulates with the concave facet of the corresponding metacarpal head. The bases of the middle and distal phalanges, however, have grooved articulations, which extend to the palmar surface of each bone. Heads of the proximal and middle phalanges have articulations that conform to the pulleylike articulations of the phalangeal bases. In contrast, the heads of the most distal phalanges provide roughened, nonarticular surfaces for the attachment of thickened connective tissues on the palmar sides of the fingertips (Fig. 19–13).

▲ Joints of the Upper Extremity

General Features of Upper Extremity Joints

As in the lower extremity, most of the joints of the upper extremity are **diarthroses (synovial joints).** These joints connect bone to bone via a cavitated connective tissue element in the following arrangement:

Bone ⟷ Articular hyaline cartilage ⟷ Cavity lined by synovial membrane containing synovial fluid ⟷ Articular hyaline cartilage ⟷ Bone

Synovial joints of the upper extremity may be **simple joints** with only two articulating surfaces; **compound joints** with more than two articulating surfaces; or **complex joints** with an intracapsular cartilaginous disc, the **meniscus,** between the articulating surfaces.

The first metacarpophalangeal joint is an example of a simple synovial joint with two articulating surfaces, the elbow (cubital) joint is an example of a compound joint (see Fig. 19–20), and the sternoclavicular joint is an example of a complex synovial joint (see Fig. 19–14).

Like some joints of the lower extremity, the shoulder and elbow joints have **extracapsular bursae** (see Figs. 19–17 and 19-20). The bursa is filled with synovial fluid in the shoulder joint, but it encloses fatty pads in the elbow joint. The cavities of the bursae may or may not be continuous with the synovial cavity of the joint.

The ulna and radius articulate by means of synovial joints at their proximal and distal ends. The shafts of the two bones are joined together by **syndesmoses** (fibrous synarthroses) along most of their lengths (see Fig. 19–22*D*). The connective tissue elements in these joints include an **interosseous membrane** (along the distal three fourths of the shafts) and an **oblique ligament** or **cord** (at the proximal ends of the shafts).

Like the lower extremity joints, joints of the upper extremity may degenerate as a consequence of **osteoarthritis** or **rheumatoid arthritis.**

Range of Motion of Upper Extremity Joints

Joints of the upper extremity are more mobile and less stable than joints of the lower extremity

As in the lower extremity, the range of motion of upper limb joints depends on the bony architecture, structure of capsules and ligaments, and encapsulation of skeletal elements by muscles, tendons, and the overlying integument. Many joints of the upper extremity are far more lax than comparable joints of the lower extremity. The hip and glenohumeral joints can be used for an interesting comparison. Differences in **bony structure** account primarily for the major differences in the mobility and stability of these joints. In lower extremity joints, **cartilaginous menisci** often help the bones fit snugly together. In upper extremity joints, this is less common. This can be seen when one compares the shoulder and hip joints or the knee and elbow joints (see Chapter 16). Perhaps one of the most functionally interesting differences in bony structure can be seen when one compares the first metacarpophalangeal joint with the first metatarsophalangeal joint. The skeletal anatomy of the first carpometacarpal joint is the basis for the thumb's ability to oppose the other digits of the hand. The anatomy of this joint allows flexion to begin in a coronal plane. Medial rotation of the first metacarpal occurs next. This sequence allows the pulp of the thumb to oppose the other four digits (see discussion of function of the digits below).

The **clavicle,** a skeletal segment unique to the upper extremity, provides additional mobility for the shoulder girdle, in part, through the function of its two unique joints: the sternoclavicular and acromioclavicular joints. Although the range of motion of each of these joints is slight, their combined range of motion allows for extensive, varied movements of the scapula, including rotation, protraction, retraction, elevation, and depression (see below). This arrangement provides a highly mobile platform (the glenoid fossa of the scapula), which supports more distal motions of the humerus and remaining upper extremity segments. Moreover, the scapulae, in keeping with their contribution to prehensile function, are small, separate, and mobile in contrast to their pelvic homologs in the lower extremity, which are massive, act as a single unit, and are stably bound to the vertebral column.

The **laxity of joint capsules and ligaments** also contributes to the enhanced mobility of the upper

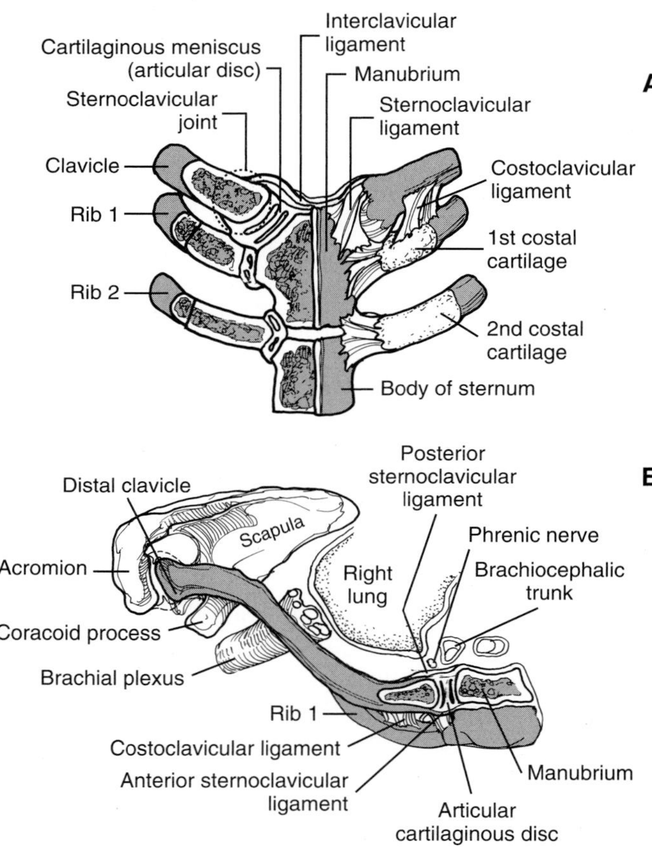

FIGURE 19–14
The sternoclavicular joint is a complex synovial joint. **A.** Sternoclavicular joint showing the area of the meniscus (intracapsular cartilaginous disc) between sternal and clavicular fibrocartilaginous surfaces, and articulation of this disk with the first costal cartilage of rib 1. **B.** Coronal section of the sternoclavicular joint region showing sternoclavicular and costoclavicular ligaments.

limbs. Although the shoulder joint is completely invested by a fibrous capsule (see below), this glenohumeral capsule and its associated ligaments are so loose that the humeral head can be pulled laterally 2 to 3 cm from the glenoid fossa. The tough interosseous membrane between the ulna and the radius provides significant stability of the forearm, but the anatomy of the proximal and distal radioulnar joints allows significant supination and pronation of the forearm in contrast to the leg, where such movements are negligible. The interosseous membrane of the forearm also readily twists or spirals to allow these movements. In addition, the **ligaments** enclosing the radial head do not directly bind the radius to the ulna but rather act as a sling, allowing rotation of the radial head adjacent to the ulna. The **skeletal anatomy** of the hemispheric humeral capitulum provides a pivot for radial rotation.

Anatomy of Specific Joints of the Upper Extremity

The joints of the upper extremity are described in a proximal-to-distal order.

Sternoclavicular and Acromioclavicular Joints. The **sternoclavicular joint** is a synovial diarthrosis of the complex type, with a circular cartilaginous meniscus interposed between the fibrocartilaginous surfaces of the sternoclavicular notch and the proximal, rounded end of the clavicle (Fig. 19–14). The proximal end of the clavicle also articulates just slightly with the superior surface of the proximal end of the first costal cartilage, so this joint may also be classified as a compound synovial joint (Fig. 19–14*A*).

The fibrous capsule of the sternoclavicular joint is reinforced by **anterior** and **posterior sternoclavicular ligaments;** by ligaments connecting the right and left sternoclavicular joints, the **interclavicular ligaments;** and by more laterally placed **costoclavicular ligaments** (Fig. 19–14*B*).

The **acromioclavicular joint** is a synovial diarthrosis providing articulation between the flattened acromial head of the clavicle and the medial surface of the medial rim of the acromial process of the scapula (Fig. 19–15). In some persons, it contains a cartilaginous articular disc, but the disc is rarely complete.

The fibrous capsule of the acromioclavicular joint is strengthened by the **acromioclavicular ligament** (Fig. 19–15*B* and *C*), which joins the upper surface of the clavicle's acromial head with the acromial process of the scapula. This joint is further reinforced by a separate

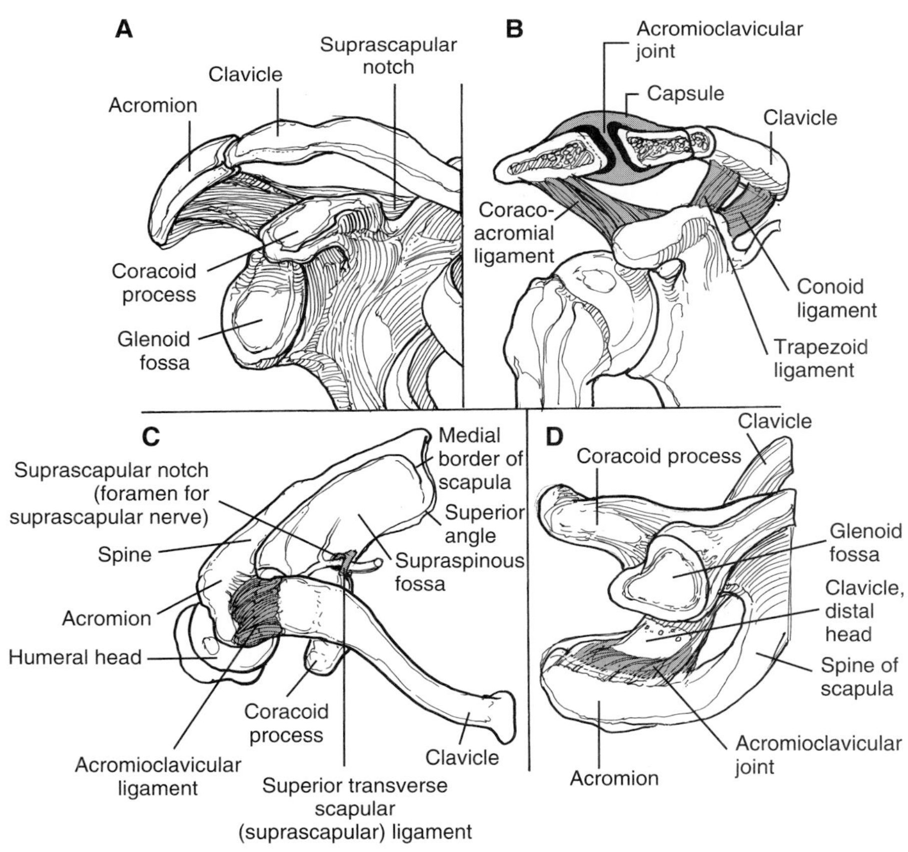

FIGURE 19–15
The acromioclavicular joint is a synovial diarthrosis. **A.** Bony anatomy of the joint area. **B.** Cross section (coronal view) of the joint. **C.** Superior view showing ligaments and suprascapular notch. **D.** Inferior view.

coracoclavicular ligament, which is not part of the acromioclavicular joint capsule. This ligament joins the clavicle to the coracoid process.

The scapula has two intrinsic ligaments that are not directly associated with joints: the coracoacromial ligament and the superior transverse scapular (suprascapular) ligament (Fig. 19–15*B* and *C*). The triangular **coracoacromial ligament** joins the coracoid process and acromium of the scapula above the humeral head. A flattened band called the **suprascapular ligament** joins the base of the coracoid process to the medial side of the suprascapular notch (see discussion of scapula above), forming a **suprascapular foramen** for transport of the suprascapular nerve (Fig. 19–15 and see below).

Movements of the Clavicular and Acromioclavicular Joints. Movements of the clavicle at the sternoclavicular joint are somewhat restricted but include finite elevation, depression, and forward and backward movement of the lateral end of the clavicle (Fig. 19–16 and Table 19–2). The clavicle is also capable of some rotation about its own axis. These movements are largely facilitated by the sliding of the medial clavicular head upon the articular disc. However, movements of the sternoclavicular joint are usually considered along with **movements of the scapula at the acromioclavicular joint.** Indeed, typically, movements of the clavicle occur in conjunction with movements of the scapula and, in some cases, with movements of the humerus. Thus, **elevation** of the clavicle and scapula is most often effected by the upper fibers of the trapezius muscle and the levator scapulae muscles as the sternal head of the clavicle slides down along the sternoclavicular articular disc (see Fig. 19–16*A*). Elevation of the clavicle is checked by opposing muscles (see discussion of depression below), the costoclavicular ligament, and the inferior part of the capsule of the sternoclavicular joint. **Depression** of the clavicle and scapula together is accomplished primarily by the forces of gravity but may be assisted by the serratus anterior and pectoralis minor muscles (Fig. 19–16*A*). During clavicular depression, the sternal head of the clavicle typically slides up upon the sternoclavicular articular disc. The subclavius muscle may participate in pulling the clavicle forward and stabilizing it against the thorax and the articular disc of the sternoclavicular joint. Depression of the clavicle at the sternoclavicular joint is checked by opposing muscles (see discussion of elevation, above): the interclavicular and sternoclavicular ligaments and the sternoclavicular articular disc. **Protraction** of the scapula is usually associated with forward movement of the acromial process over the lateral head of the clavicle (at the acromioclavicular joint) and with posterior translation (gliding) of the sternoclavicular head and its associated disc upon the sternal facet (Fig. 19–16*B*). Posterior translation of the sternal head of the clavicle is checked by opposing muscles (see discussion of retraction below) and anterior sternoclavicular and costoclavicular ligaments. These movements are typically effected by the serratus anterior and pectoralis minor muscles. Moreover, as the serratus anterior muscle pulls the scapula laterally and forward around the trunk, its action, along with the upper border of the latissimus dorsi muscle, presses the medial border of the scapula close to the thoracic wall. **Retraction** of the scapula is accompanied by backward movement of the scapular acromion upon the lateral clavicular head and by anterior translation of the sternal head of the clavicle and its associated disc within the sternal facet. This movement is affected by the rhomboid muscles and trapezius muscle (Fig. 19–16*B*). Retraction is checked by opposing muscles (see discussion of protraction above) and by posterior sternoclavicular and costoclavicular ligaments. **Lateral rotation** (defined by lateral movement of the inferior angle of the scapula; and sometimes called **forward rotation**) of the scapula is accompanied by elevation of the clavicle (at the sternoclavicular joint) and abduction of the scapula upon the lateral clavicular head at the acromioclavicular joint (Fig. 19–16*C*). This latter movement is checked by the coronoid ligament. These movements rotate the glenoid fossa upward most typically to assist in abduction of the arm (see below). Lateral rotation of the scapula is primarily affected by the upper part of the trapezius muscle and lower part of the serratus anterior muscles. **Medial rotation** (defined by medial movement of the inferior angle of the scapula and sometimes called **return rotation)** of the scapula is accompanied by downward rotation of the scapula at the acromioclavicular joint and depression of the clavicle (Fig. 19–16*D*). This movement is typically effected by gravity and controlled by the gradual relaxation of the trapezius and serratus anterior muscles. Medial rotation of the scapula may be assisted by the pectoralis minor, rhomboid major and minor, and levator scapulae muscles.

Clinical Disorders of the Sternoclavicular and Acromioclavicular Joints. The **sternoclavicular joint** is infrequently dislocated because it is relatively stable. Instead, falls upon the outstretched hand more often result in clavicular fracture (see above), while direct force upon the pectoral girdle often results in **rupture of the acromioclavicular capsule** and **dislocation of the acromioclavicular joint.** This latter injury is particularly serious when the coracoclavicular and acromioclavicular ligaments are torn. Dislocation of the acromioclavicular joint causes the weight of the arm to pull the arm away from the shoulder. **This dislocation is often incorrectly characterized as a shoulder separation** (see discussion of shoulder separation below).

Infection of the subacromial bursa (subacromial bursitis) results in pain that interferes with the action of the supraspinatus muscle and abduction of the humerus (see discussion of the supraspinatus muscle in Chapter 20).

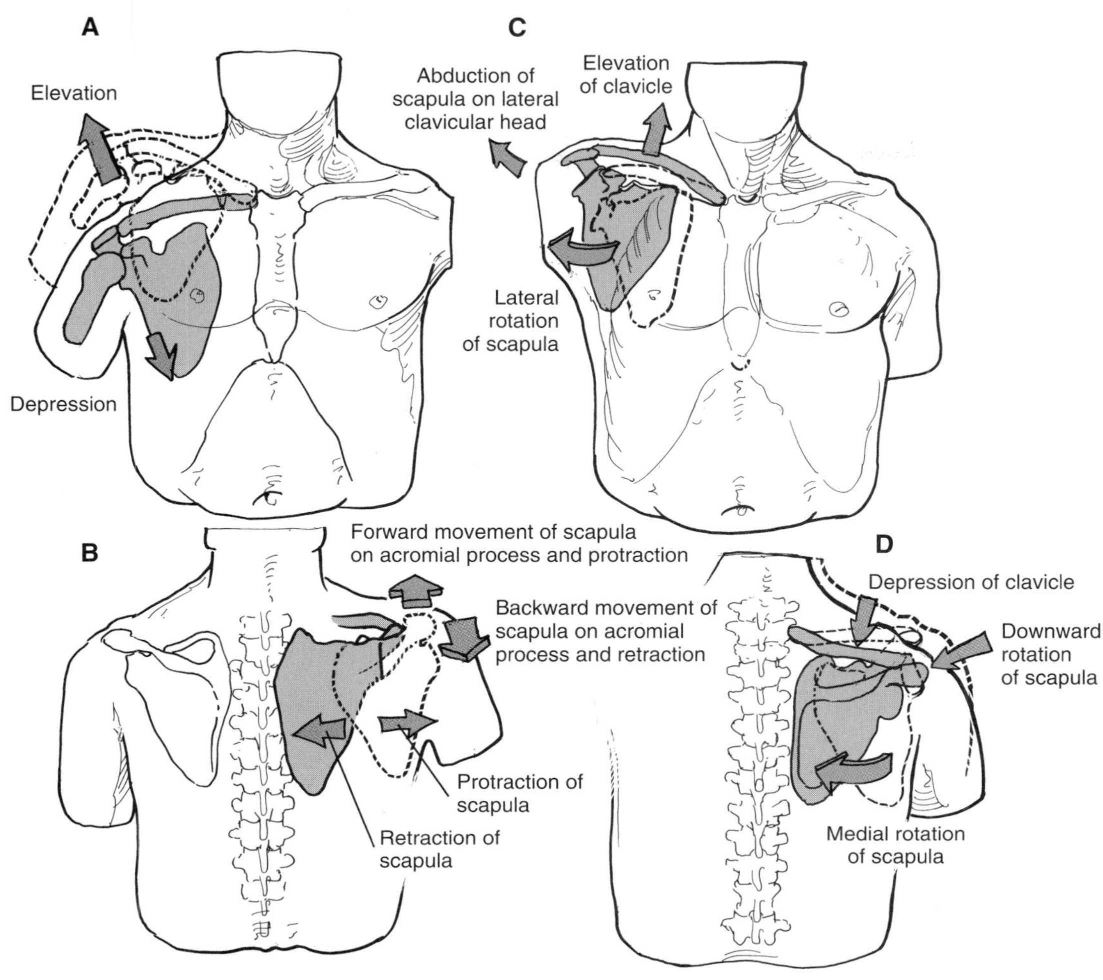

FIGURE 19–16

Movements of the clavicular and acromioclavicular joints. **A.** Elevation and depression. **B.** Protraction and retraction of the scapula. **C.** Lateral rotation (sometimes called *forward rotation*) of the scapula. **D.** Medial rotation (sometimes called *return rotation*) of the scapula.

Infection of the synovial cavity of the elbow joint results in excess accumulation of synovial fluid and consequent elevation of fat pads. Swelling may be particularly prominent in the region of the olecranon process, although some swelling may also occur around the head of the radius.

Constant rubbing and abrasion of the elbow may result in **infection of the subcutaneous olecranon bursa (student's elbow).** Less commonly, the subtendinous olecranon bursa may become infected as a consequence of repeated flexion and extension of the elbow, which causes friction between the distal triceps brachii tendon and the olecranon process.

Shoulder (Glenohumeral; or Humeral) Joint. The **glenohumeral joint** is a synovial diarthrosis of the simple type. This articulation joins the glenoid (shallow) fossa of the scapula and the head of the humerus. The glenoid fossa of the scapula is deepened slightly by a cartilaginous **glenoid lip,** a ring of fibrocartilage that is thick at its outer edge and deficient at its center (Fig. 19–17*A*).

A **fibrous capsule** encloses the entire joint through its proximal circumferential attachment to the edge of the glenoid fossa and its distal attachment to the neck of the humerus (Fig. 19–17*B*, *C*, and *D*). It thus encloses the entire glenoid lip of the scapula and articular surface of the head of the humerus. The capsule extends proximally onto the coracoid process to enclose the attachment of the tendon of the long head of the biceps brachii muscle (see below). The capsule extends distally along the medial side of the shaft of the humerus. However, the capsule is quite loose, allowing significant movement of the humeral head upon the glenoid fossa.

The capsule is reinforced by several ligaments, including three **glenohumeral ligaments** (superior, middle, and inferior ligaments) and the **coracohumeral** and **transverse humeral ligaments,** in addition to several tendons and muscles that span the joint (Fig. 19–17*B* and *C* and see below).

TABLE 19–2
Movements of Joints of the Upper Extremity

Joint	Movement	Forces of Gravity or Muscles Involved*
Sternoclavicular	Elevation of clavicle and scapula	Trapezius (upper fibers), levator scapulae muscles
	Depression of clavicle and scapula	Forces of gravity; serratus anterior, pectoralis minor muscles
Sternoclavicular and acromioclavicular	Protraction of scapula with forward gliding of acromial process on lateral clavicular head and posterior translation of sternal clavicular head in clavicular facet of sternum	Serratus anterior, pectoralis minor muscles; upper border of latissimus dorsi muscle holds scapula against trunk
	Retraction of scapula with backward gliding of acromial process on lateral clavicular head and anterior translation of sternal clavicular head in clavicular facet of sternum	Rhomboid major and minor, trapezius muscles
	Lateral rotation of scapula with elevation of clavicle and upward translation of acromial process on lateral clavicular head	Trapezius (upper fibers), serratus anterior (lower part) muscles
	Medial rotation of scapula with depression of clavicle and downward translation of acromial process on lateral clavicular head	Forces of gravity; pectoralis minor, rhomboid major and minor, levator scapulae muscles, **trapezius and serratus anterior muscles**
Glenohumeral	Flexion	Clavicular part of pectoralis major muscle; anterior fibers of deltoid muscle; coracobrachialis, biceps brachii muscles
	Extension	Posterior fibers of deltoid muscle; teres major, latissimus dorsi muscles; sternocostal head of pectoralis major muscle
	Abduction	Deltoid, supraspinatus muscles countered by subscapularis, infraspinatus, teres minor muscles to maintain position of humeral head
	Adduction	Forces of gravity; subscapularis, infraspinatus, teres minor muscles; adduction against resistance by pectoralis major, teres major, latissimus dorsi muscles
	Medial rotation	Pectoralis major muscle; anterior fibers of deltoid muscle; latissimus dorsi, teres major, subscapularis muscles
	Lateral rotation	Infraspinatus muscle; posterior fibers of deltoid muscle; teres minor muscle
Elbow	Flexion	Brachialis, biceps brachii, brachioradialis muscles assist in rapid flexion; pronator teres, flexor carpi radialis muscles assist against resistance
	Extension	Forces of gravity; triceps brachii, anconeus muscles
Proximal and distal radioulnar	Pronation	Pronator teres, pronator quadratus muscles assist against resistance
	Supination	Supinator, biceps brachii muscles in rapid supination and against resistance
Radiocarpal and intercarpal	Flexion	Flexor carpi radialis, flexor carpi ulnaris, palmaris longus, flexor digitorum superficialis, flexor digitorum profundus, flexor pollicis longus, abductor pollicis longus muscles
	Extension	Extensor carpi radialis longus, extensor carpi radialis brevis, extensor carpi ulnaris, extensor digitorum, extensor digiti minimi, extensor indicis, extensor pollicis longus muscles
	Adduction	Flexor carpi ulnaris, extensor carpi ulnaris muscles
	Abduction	Flexor carpi radialis, extensor carpi radialis longus, extensor carpi radialis brevis, abductor pollicis longus, extensor pollicis brevis muscles

*Muscles in boldfaced type produce the primary action. Muscles in regular type assist the primary muscles.

TABLE 19–2, cont'd
Movements of Joints of the Upper Extremity

Joint	Movement	Forces of Gravity or Muscles Involved
First carpometacarpal	Flexion with medial rotation	Flexor pollicis brevis, opponens pollicis muscles
	Extension with lateral rotation	Abductor pollicis longus, extensor pollicis brevis, extensor pollicis longus muscles
	Adduction	Adductor pollicis muscles
	Abduction	Abductor pollicis brevis, abductor pollicis longus muscles
	Opposition	Opponens pollicis, flexor pollicis brevis, adductor pollicis, flexor pollicis longus muscles to increase pressure between opposed digits
Lateral intermetacarpal	Slight gliding movements	Thenar, hypothenar muscles acting together, especially when thumb is opposed to digit 4 or 5
Metacarpophalangeal	Flexion	Flexor digitorum superficialis, flexor digitorum profundus muscles; lumbrical and interosseous muscles of digits 2 to 5 under certain conditions and assisted at digit 5 by flexor digiti minimi brevis muscle
	Extension	Digits 2 to 5 by extensor digitorum muscle; digit 1 by extensor pollicis brevis, extensor pollicis longus muscles; assisted at digit 5 by extensor digiti minimi muscle; assisted at digit 2 by extensor indicis muscle
	Adduction	Digit 1 by adductor pollicis, first palmar interosseous muscles; digit 2 by second palmar interosseous muscle; digit 3, none; digit 4 by third palmar interosseous muscle; digit 5 by adductor digiti minimi muscle
	Abduction	Digit 1 by abductor pollicis brevis muscle; digit 2 by first dorsal interosseous muscle; digit 3 by second and third dorsal interosseous muscles; digit 4 by fourth dorsal interosseous muscle; digit 5 by abductor digiti minimi muscle
Interphalangeal	Flexion	Proximal joints of digits 2 to 5 by flexor digitorum superficialis muscle, which may be assisted by interosseous and lumbrical muscles acting together, and by flexor digitorum profundus muscle, which also flexes distal joint; digit 1 by flexor pollicis longus muscle
	Extension	Proximal and distal joints of digits 2 to 5 by extensor digitorum muscle; assisted at digit 5 by extensor digiti minimi muscle; assisted at digits 2 to 5 by lumbricals when they are active in flexion of metacarpophalangeal joints; digit 1 by extensor pollicis brevis muscle assisted by abductor pollicis, extensor pollicis brevis muscles

The fibrous capsule of the shoulder joint is lined by a **synovial membrane.** This membrane also encloses a **synovial sheath,** which transports the tendon of the long head of the biceps brachii muscle. The synovial lining of the shoulder joint may extend into two of the many bursae associated with the shoulder joint, namely, the **bursae** between the subscapular tendon and neck of the scapula and between the infraspinatus tendon and capsule (Fig. 19–17*A* to *C*). Other associated bursae are lined by synovial membranes but do not communicate with the shoulder joint. These include the subacromial bursa, a bursa between the deltoid muscle and capsule, a bursa between the teres minor muscle and long head of the triceps brachii muscle, and bursae anterior to and posterior to the tendon of the latissimus dorsi muscle.

Movements of the Shoulder Joint. The shoulder joint is highly mobile. It is classified as a multiaxial spheroidal (ball and socket) joint with movement about three axes. Specific movements of the humerus at the shoulder joint thus include extension, flexion, abduction, adduction, medial rotation, and lateral rotation (Fig. 19–18

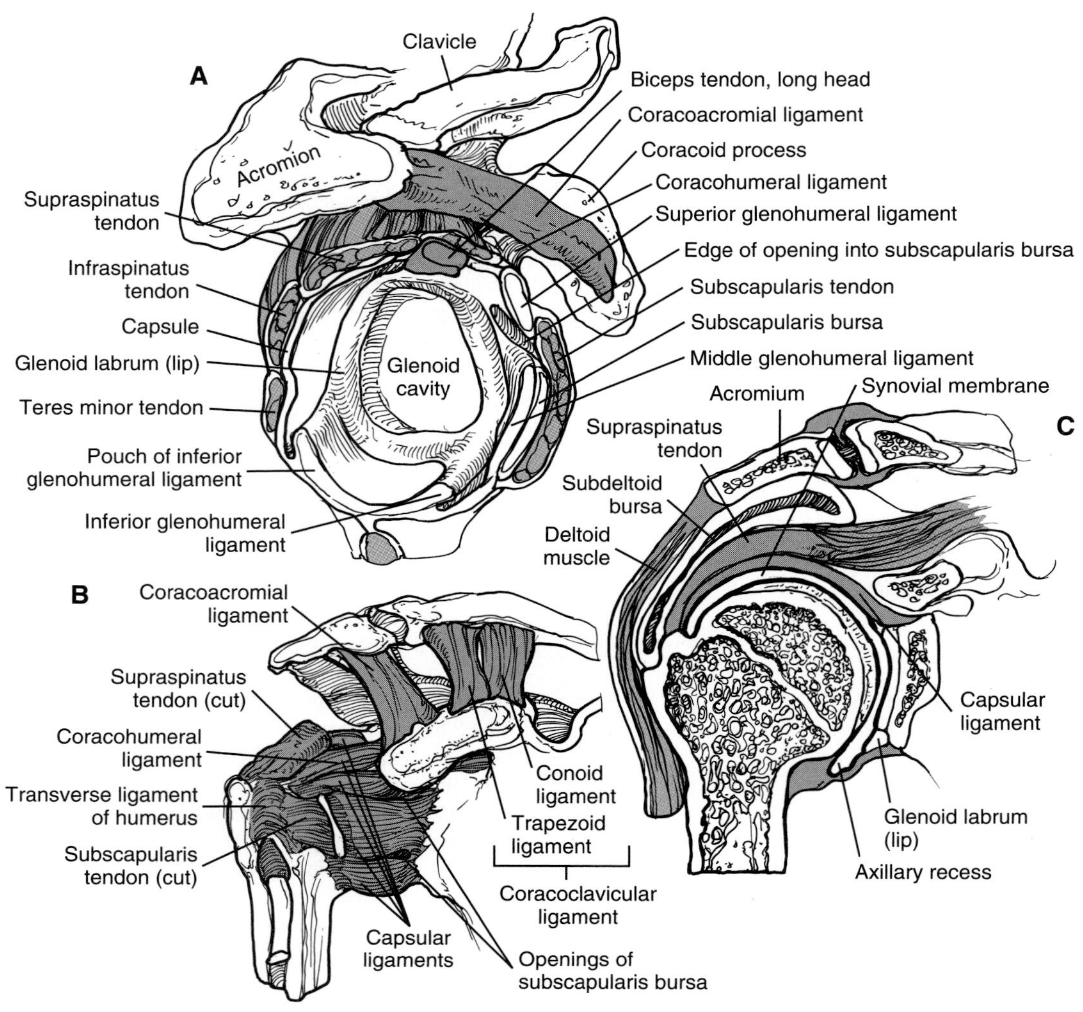

FIGURE 19–17
The shoulder joint (glenohumeral, or humeral, joint) is a synovial diarthrosis of the simple type. **A.** Anterosuperior view of the glenoid fossa and surrounding structures. **B.** Overview showing the fibrous capsule. **C.** Coronal section.

and see Table 19–2). In addition, by combining all of these movements in an appropriate sequence, the humerus may be circumducted at the glenohumeral joint. Because of the shoulder joint's remarkable mobility and inherent lack of stability, it is the most commonly dislocated joint of the body (see below). **Extension** occurs in a parasagittal plane (Fig. 19–18*B*) and is effected by posterior fibers of the deltoid muscle and the teres major muscle. These muscles are assisted by the latissimus dorsi muscle and the sternocostal head of the pectoralis major muscle if the humerus is extended against resistance. **Flexion** at the glenohumeral joint also occurs in a parasagittal plane (see Chapter 1) and is effected by the clavicular part of the pectoralis major muscle, the anterior fibers of the deltoid muscle, and the coracobrachialis muscles (Fig. 19–18*A*). The biceps brachii muscle assists in this movement. **Abduction** of the arm occurs within a coronal plane (Fig. 19–18*C*). It is effected largely by the deltoid muscle, which is assisted by the supraspinatus muscle in conjunction with resistance by the subscapularis, infraspinatus, and teres minor muscles. Actions of these latter three muscles ensure **upward rotation of the humeral head upon the glenoid fossa** and, at the same time, prevent the deltoid muscle from simply pulling the humeral head directly upward. In addition, the bicipital tendon checks the upward movement of the humeral head onto the lower surface of the acromial process. The arm may be abducted about 150 degrees through combined movements at the glenohumeral, acromioclavicular, and sternoclavicular joints. The first 30 degrees of abduction occurs wholly at the glenohumeral joint. The final 120 degrees occurs via simultaneous actions of the glenohumeral joint (60 degrees) and lateral rotation of the scapula (60 degrees). **Adduction** also occurs in a coronal plane and is largely a function of the forces of grav-

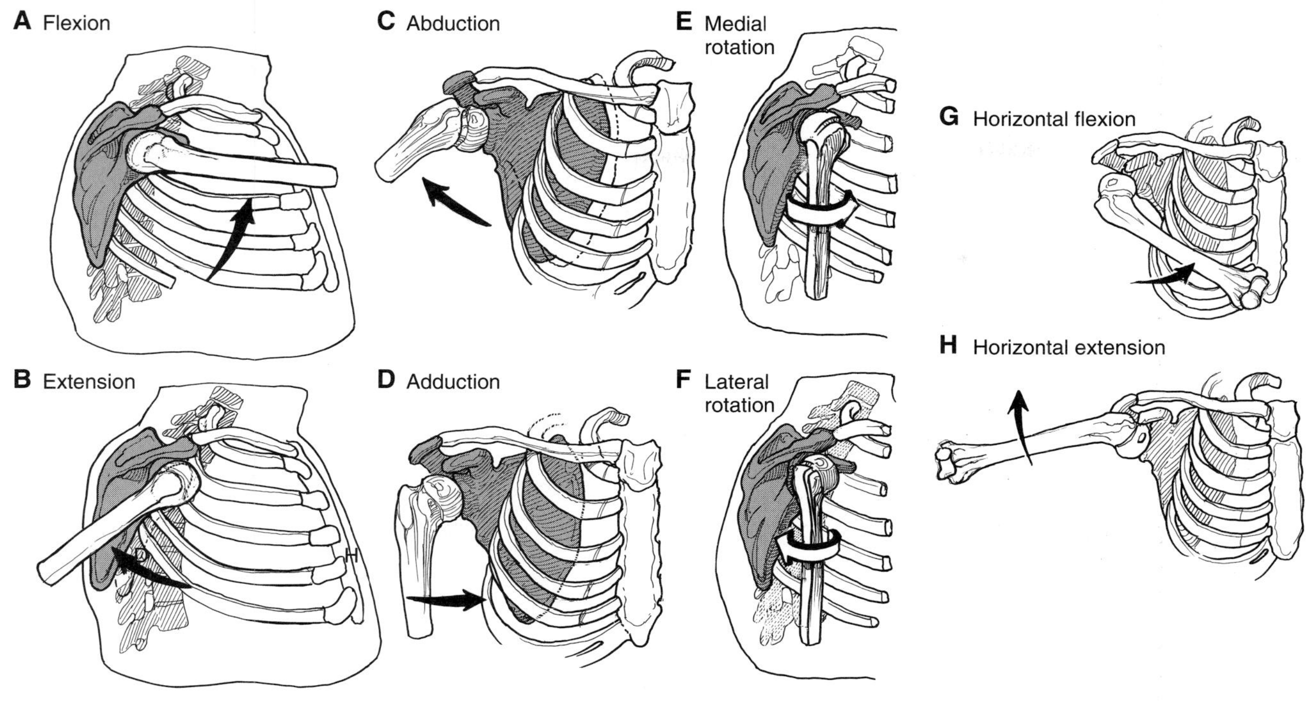

FIGURE 19–18
Movements of the shoulder joint. **A.** Flexion. **B.** Extension to hyperextension. **C.** Abduction. **D.** Adduction. **E.** Medial rotation. **F.** Lateral rotation. **G.** Horizontal flexion. **H.** Horizontal extension.

ity aided by resistance of muscles active in abduction (Fig. 19–18*D*). Adduction against resistance, however, is effected by the pectoralis major, teres major, and latissimus dorsi muscles. **Medial rotation** of the humerus is largely a function of the pectoralis major muscle, the anterior fibers of the deltoid muscle, the latissimus dorsi muscle, the teres major muscle, and the subscapularis muscle (Fig. 19–18*E*). **Lateral rotation** of the humerus is largely a function of the infraspinatus muscle, the posterior fibers of the deltoid muscle, and the teres minor muscle (Fig. 19–18*F*). **Horizontal flexion** is a function of the clavicular head of the pectoralis major muscle and the anterior fibers of the deltoid muscle (Fig. 19–18*G*). **Horizontal extension** is a function of the sternocostal head of the pectoralis major muscle and the posterior fibers of the deltoid muscle (Fig. 19–18*H* and Table 19–2).

Injuries of the Shoulder Joint. Shoulder separation is usually a consequence of direct trauma to the arm. Individuals under the age of 18 to 20 years are particularly prone to these injuries because the proximal epiphysis has not yet fused with the humeral shaft. Since the articular capsule is stronger than the epiphyseal plate, the **humeral shaft physically separates from the humeral head,** which is retained within the glenoid fossa.

Dislocation of the glenohumeral joint occurs more often than dislocation of any other joint of the body. Typically, the dislocation occurs in an **anteroinferior direction** where the capsule is thinnest. It often occurs during forced abduction of the humerus when it is extended and laterally rotated. As the humerus is forcefully abducted (often during a fall), the greater tuberosity is pushed against the underside of the acromial process so that the acromium acts as a fulcrum to lever the head of the humerus out of the glenoid cavity (Fig. 19–19). This often results in tearing or rupture of the glenoid labrum and capsule. Reduction of the dislocation is usually simple, and surgical repair is infrequently required. However, **rehabilitation of the rotator cuff muscles** is usually recommended, particularly when the shoulder is chronically dislocated. Posterior dislocations of the shoulder are relatively uncommon (about 2%). They may be caused by a fall on the outstretched limb, direct trauma to the anterior side of the joint, or severe muscle spasm.

Elbow (Cubital) Joint. The elbow joint includes two articulations and is, therefore, a **compound synovial diarthrosis.** The humerus articulates with the ulna (humeroulnar articulation) and radius (humeroradial articulation). The compound elbow joint shares some elements with the contiguous proximal radioulnar joint (see below). Thus, all three of these articulations together are defined as the **cubital complex.** However, the proximal radioulnar joint is defined as a separate joint (Fig. 19–20 and see below). The humeroulnar articulation of the elbow joint occurs between the humeral

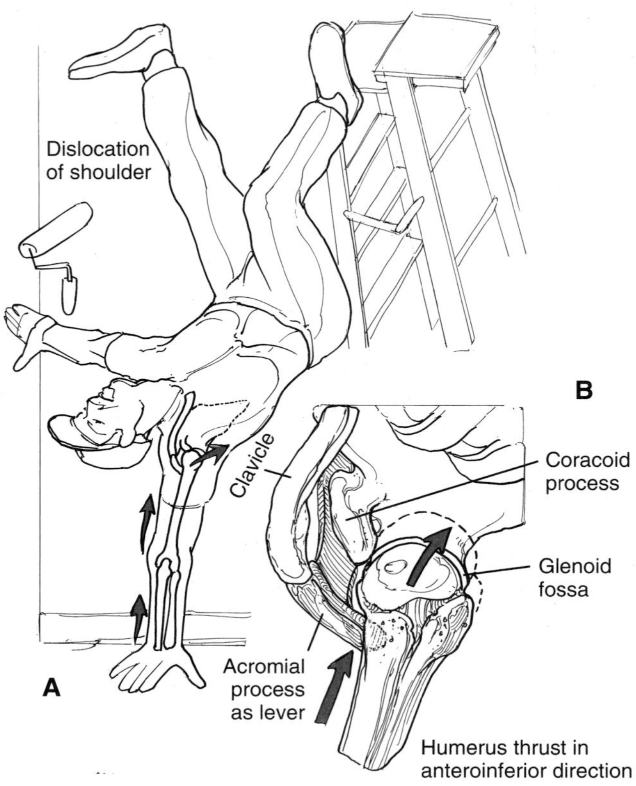

FIGURE 19–19
Dislocation of the glenohumeral joint. **A.** Forced abduction of the humerus caused by a fall. The drawing shows how the bone is extended and laterally rotated. **B.** Enlarged view of the area of dislocation.

trochlea and the ulnar trochlear notch, while the humeroradial articulation occurs between the humeral capitulum and the proximal radial head (Fig. 19–20 and see Figs. 19–9 and 19–11 and above).

The **fibrous capsule of the elbow joint** is thin both anteriorly and posteriorly. Anteriorly, its proximal attachment is to the medial epicondyle of the humerus and to the humeral shaft just superior to the coronoid and radial fossae (Fig. 19–20*A* to *C*). The distal attachment of the fibrous capsule at its anterior aspect is to the edge of the ulnar coronoid process and to the **annular ligament,** which binds the radius to the ulna at the proximal radioulnar joint (Fig. 19–20*A* to *C*). Posteriorly, the proximal attachment of the fibrous capsule is to the posterior surface of the medial epicondyle and to the posterior surface of the inferior end of the humeral shaft. The distal attachment of the fibrous capsule at its posterior aspect is to the superior edge of the olecranon process (Fig. 19–20*B* and *C*). Lateral and medial regions of the fibrous capsule of the elbow joint are reinforced by ligaments, which are thickened bands of the capsule (Fig. 19–20*B* and *C*). These include the **radial collateral ligament (lateral cubital ligament)** and **ulnar collateral ligament (medial cubital ligament).** The radial collateral ligament is a single triangular thickened band (Fig. 19–20*B*). The ulnar collateral ligament is formed by three discrete but contiguous bands (anterior, posterior, and oblique bands) (Fig. 19–20*C*).

Synovial membranes line the olecranon, radial, and coronoid fossae and the medial trochlear surface of the humerus. The membranes are reflected onto the inner surface of the investing joint capsule (Fig. 19–20*D* and *E*). The membranes are also reflected outward (between the distal end of the humerus and the proximal ends of the ulna and radius) to form **posterior** and **anterior fat-filled synovial bursae** (Fig. 19–20*F* and *G*). The posterior bursa is pushed into the olecranon fossa to cushion the ulna's olecranon process during extension. The anterior fat-filled bursa is forced into the coronoid and radial fossae during flexion. The subcutaneous and subtendinous olecranon bursae are small posterior bursae that lie just under the skin or deep to the triceps brachii tendon, as their names imply. A small radioulnar bursa lies between the radiohumeral joint and the overlying extensor digitorum and supinator muscles.

Movements of the Elbow Joint. The elbow joint is a complex joint consisting of both humeroradial and humeroulnar joints and is classified as a hinge joint or uniaxial joint. Major movements at the elbow joint are limited to flexion and extension of the ulna and radius with respect to the humerus (Fig. 19–21 and Table 19–2). The ulna articulates with the trochlea of the humerus, while the proximal radial head articulates with the capitulum of the humerus. Minor movements of the elbow joint include **slight medial rotation of the ulna** (with the ulna slightly pronated) during extension of the forearm and **slight lateral rotation** of the ulna (with the ulna slightly supinated) during flexion of the forearm. **Flexion** of the elbow joint is mainly effected by the brachialis and biceps brachii muscles, although the brachioradialis muscle may be enlisted in more rapid flexion. The pronator teres and flexor carpi radialis muscles may contribute when the forearm is flexed against resistance. **Extension** at the elbow joint is largely effected by the triceps brachii and anconeus muscles and by the forces of gravity.

Clinical Disorders of the Elbow Joint. Dislocation of the elbow joint is much less common than dislocation of the shoulder joint because the elbow joint has a more stable intrinsic skeletal architecture. Infrequently, however, a fall on an outstretched limb may dislocate the ulna and radius posteriorly as the distal humeral head breaks through the weak anterior wall of the capsule. In addition, direct trauma to the posterior side of the flexed elbow may dislocate the ulna and radius anteriorly. **Fractures** of the coronoid process, radial head, and medial epicondyle of the humerus may also occur.

Repetitive movements of the elbow joint, particularly pronation and supination, may result in premature degeneration and inflammation of the attachment of the superficial extensor tendons at the lateral epicondyle of the humerus. This painful condition is called **elbow tendinitis, tennis elbow,** or **lateral epicondylitis.**

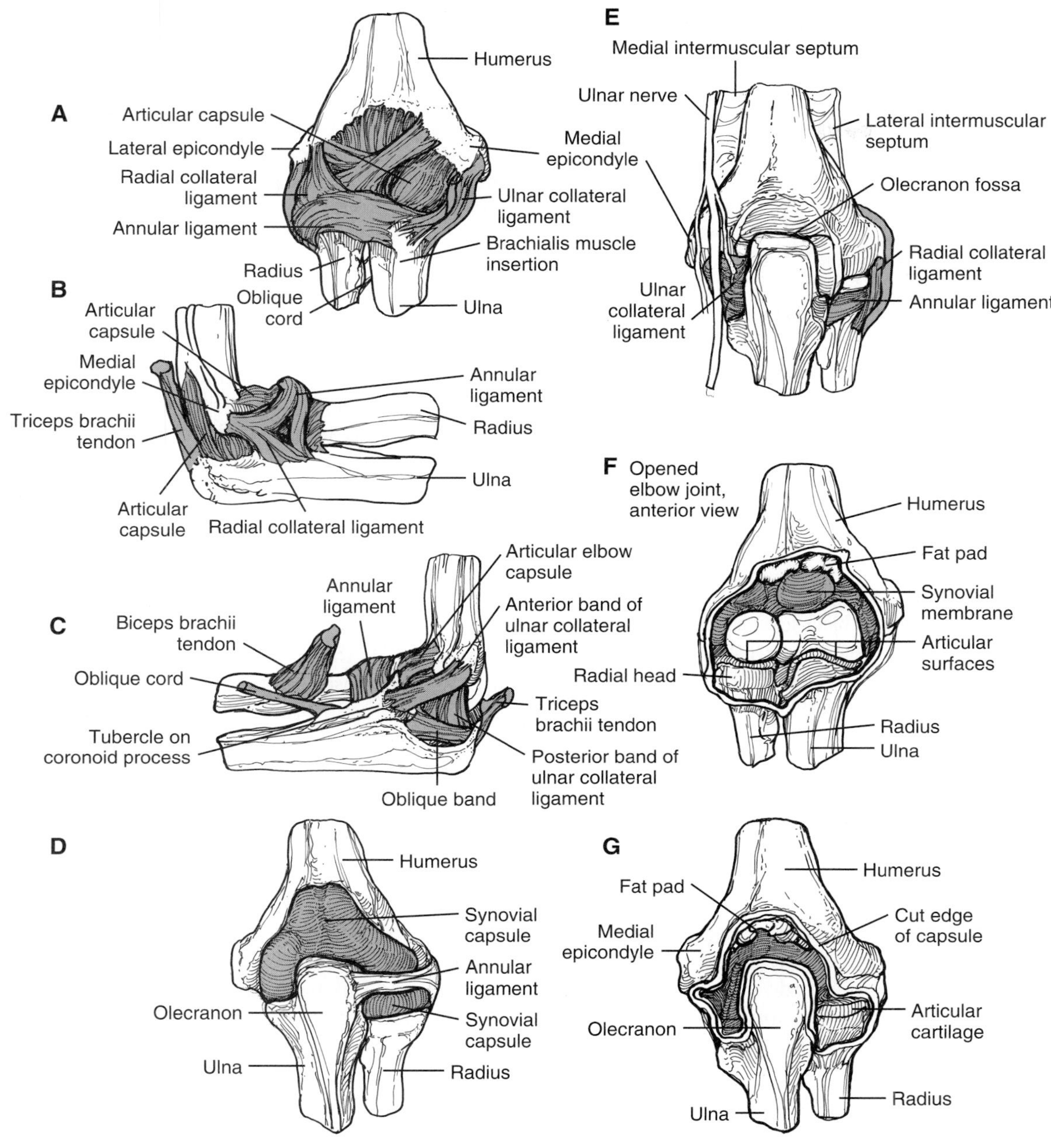

FIGURE 19–20
Cubital (elbow) joint is a compound synovial diarthrosis. **A** to **C** show the fibrous capsule of the right elbow joint and its ligaments. **A.** Anterior view. **B.** Lateral view. **C.** Medial view. **D, E,** and **G.** Synovial membranes, posterior views of joint. **F.** Opened anterior view of elbow joint showing fat pads and synovial membrane. **G.** Posterior view of joint with capsule cut showing fat pads.

Radioulnar Joint. The radius and ulna articulate through three distinct joints: **proximal, middle,** and **distal radioulnar joints** (Fig. 19–22*A, B,* and *C*). The proximal radioulnar joint is a simple diarthrosis. It provides a mechanism for the rotation of the disc-shaped head of the radius (upon a notch on the lateral side of the ulna). The middle radioulnar joint is made up of syndesmoses (i.e., a flexible interosseous membrane and a proximal ligament or cord), which loosely connect the radial and ulnar shafts. The distal radioulnar joint (a simple complex diarthrosis) provides a mechanism for the pivoting of the distal head of the radius about the distal head of the ulna.

In the **proximal radioulnar joint,** the proximal discoidal head of the radius is stabilized within the concave radial notch of the ulna by the radial ligament (see Figs. 19–20*A* to *C* and 19–22*A* and *B*). Posterior and lateral fibers of the radial ligament blend with the radial collat-

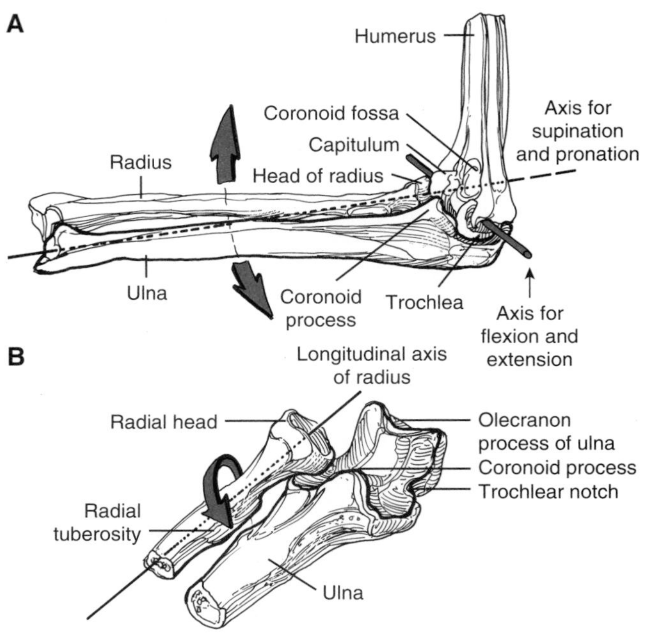

FIGURE 19–21
Movements of the elbow joint—a hinge joint that allows flexion and extension of the ulna and radius with respect to the humerus. **A.** Axis for supination and pronation and axis for flexion and extension. **B.** Medial and lateral rotation occur along a longitudinal axis.

eral ligament. A thin layer of cartilage lines the ligament and notch. Anterior and posterior regions of the annular ligament are also lined by a synovial membrane.

The **oblique cord of the middle radioulnar syndesmoses** connects the lateral side of the tuberosity of the ulna to the shaft of the radius just distal to the tuberosity of the radius (Fig. 19–22*A*, *D*, and *E*). The **interosseous membrane of the middle radioulnar joint** is a broad sheet of collagenous connective tissue composed of fibers, which descend in a distomedial orientation from the medial border of the radius to the lateral border of the ulna. The membrane is deficient in the upper third of the forearm, providing a gap for the transmission of vessels and nerves. A small foramen exists within the center of the membrane a few inches from its distal end. This small foramen transports the anterior interosseous artery and vein to the back of the forearm (Fig. 19–22*A* and *D*).

The **distal radioulnar joint** provides a mechanism for pronation and supination of the hand (Fig. 19–22*A*, *C*, and *E*). Articulating surfaces are the dome-shaped distal head of the ulna and distal ulnar notch of the radius (Fig. 19–22*C*). The capsule is thicker anteriorly than posteriorly. It is lined by a synovial membrane that forms a small sac that protrudes distally between the distal ends of the ulna and radius. Movements of the distal radioulnar joint are facilitated by an articular disc.

Movements of the Radioulnar Joints. Movements facilitated by the radioulnar joints are supination and pronation of the forearm (Fig. 19–22*D* and *E* and Table 19–2). In **supination,** the radius, with the attached hand, is twisted laterally (from a pronated position) over the anterior surface of the ulna (Fig. 19-22*D*). Thus, in complete supination, the palms face forward and the entire shaft of the radius lies parallel and lateral to the shaft of the ulna. In **pronation,** the radius, with the attached hand, is twisted medially (Fig. 19–22*E*). In **complete pronation,** the palms face backward and the distal end of the radius is medial to the distal end of the ulna (Fig. 19–22*E*). However, the proximal end of the radius remains lateral to the proximal end of the ulna. During pronation and supination, the proximal radial head rotates within the radial ligament and ulnar radial notch. In addition, the ulna glides slightly upon its humeral articulation (trochlea) in a posterolateral direction during pronation and in an anteromedial direction during supination. The ulnar notch on the medial surface of the distal head of the radius pivots about the convex lateral surface of the distal head of the ulna. In addition to this pivoting motion, the radial ulnar notch glides upon the distal head of the ulna. During the twisting motions of pronation and supination, the interosseous membrane of the middle radioulnar joint twists or spirals but does not check these movements (Fig. 19–22*D*). Indeed, the interosseous membrane is most relaxed in full pronation and supination and most taut between these two extreme positions. Pronation and supination at the radioulnar joints alone are limited to a range of approximately 150 degrees, but with contributions from the shoulder joint (and when the elbow joint is fully extended), the range may be increased to about 360 degrees. The major effector of pronation is the pronator teres muscle. It is assisted in rapid movements and in opposing resistance by the pronator quadratus muscle. The supinator muscle is the primary supinator of the forearm but is assisted by the biceps brachii muscle in rapid supination or in supination against resistance. The fact that supination is more forceful than pronation and the fact that most people are right handed are considerations in the design of screws and bolts.

Injuries of the Proximal Radioulnar Joint. Dislocation of the radial head is common in children under age 5 years when a sudden force on the pronated forearm pulls the radius anteriorly out of the annular ligament. This may occur when someone pulls the child away from danger, lifts the child off the ground, or swings the child by the arm.

Wrist (Radiocarpal) and Intercarpal Joints. The **wrist joint** is an articulation of the distal end of the radius (on the lateral side) and triangular articular disc (on the medial side) with the proximal articulating surfaces

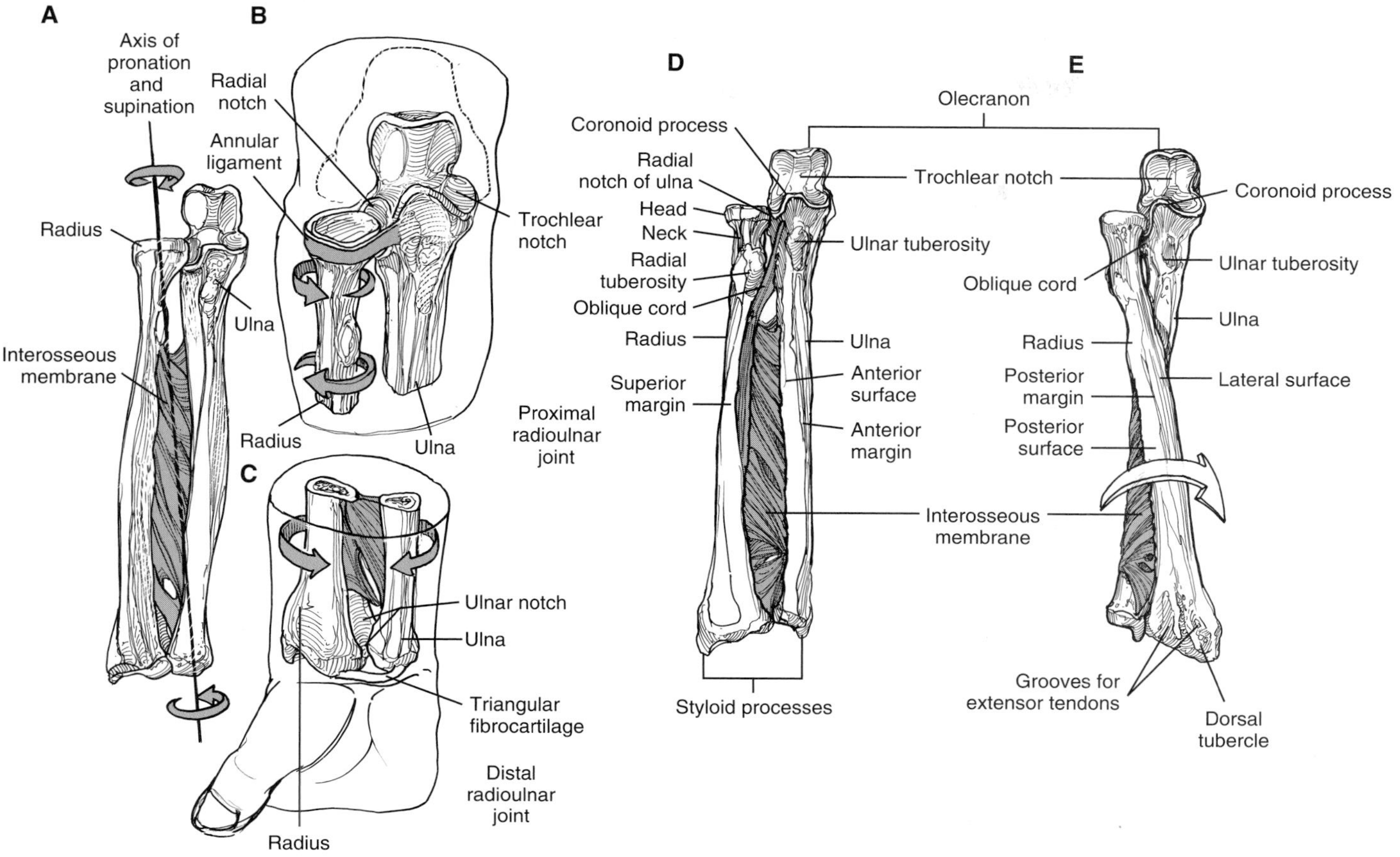

FIGURE 19–22
The three distinct joints articulating the radius and ulna. **A.** Relationship of the radius and ulna showing the axis of pronation and supination. **B.** Proximal radioulnar joint—a simple diarthrosis joint. **C.** Distal radioulnar joint—a simple complex diarthrosis joint—providing a mechanism for pronation and supination of the hand. **D.** Supinated position showing the oblique cord of the middle radioulnar syndesmoses and interosseous membrane. **E.** Radius and ulna in pronated position.

(from lateral to medial) of the scaphoid, lunate, and triquetral bones (Fig. 19–23*A* and *B*). In addition, a small triangular meniscus separates the distal tip of the ulnar styloid process from the proximal surface of the triquetral bone (Fig. 19–23*A* and *B*). The **fibrous capsule** is lined by a synovial membrane that encloses a synovial cavity. This synovial cavity is typically separated from the synovial cavity of the distal radioulnar joints and from synovial cavities within the carpus (Fig. 19–23*B*). The capsule is reinforced by several thickened ligaments. These include **ulnar** and **radial collateral ligaments** on the medial and lateral sides of the capsule (Fig. 19–23*C* and *D*). The ventral wall is reinforced by a broad **palmar radiocarpal ligament** (Fig. 19–23*C*) and the posterior wall by a broad triangular **dorsal radiocarpal ligament** (Fig. 19–23*D*).

Individual **intercarpal joints** can be classified in three categories: joints connecting carpal bones of the proximal row to each other, joints connecting carpal bones of the proximal row to those of the distal row **(midcarpal joints)**, and joints connecting carpal bones of the distal row to each other (Fig. 19–23*B*).

The synovial cavities of these three classes of joints are continuous. The scaphoid, lunate, and triquetral bones of the proximal row are connected by palmar, dorsal, and interosseous ligaments, as are the trapezium, trapezoid, capitate, and hamate bones of the distal row (Fig. 19–23*B*). The joint between the pisiform bone and the palmar surface of the triquetral bone is enclosed within a thin capsule but is more firmly connected to the hook of the hamate bone by a pisohamate ligament and to the base of the fifth metacarpal bone by the pisometacarpal ligament. The synovial cavity of the pisotriquetral joint is usually isolated from the synovial cavities of all other intercarpal joints (Fig. 19–23*B*).

Movements of the Radiocarpal and Intercarpal Joints. The radiocarpal and intercarpal joints act together. Their movements facilitate flexion, extension, adduction, abduction, and circumduction of the hand (see Table 19–2). However, circumduction is achieved through suc-

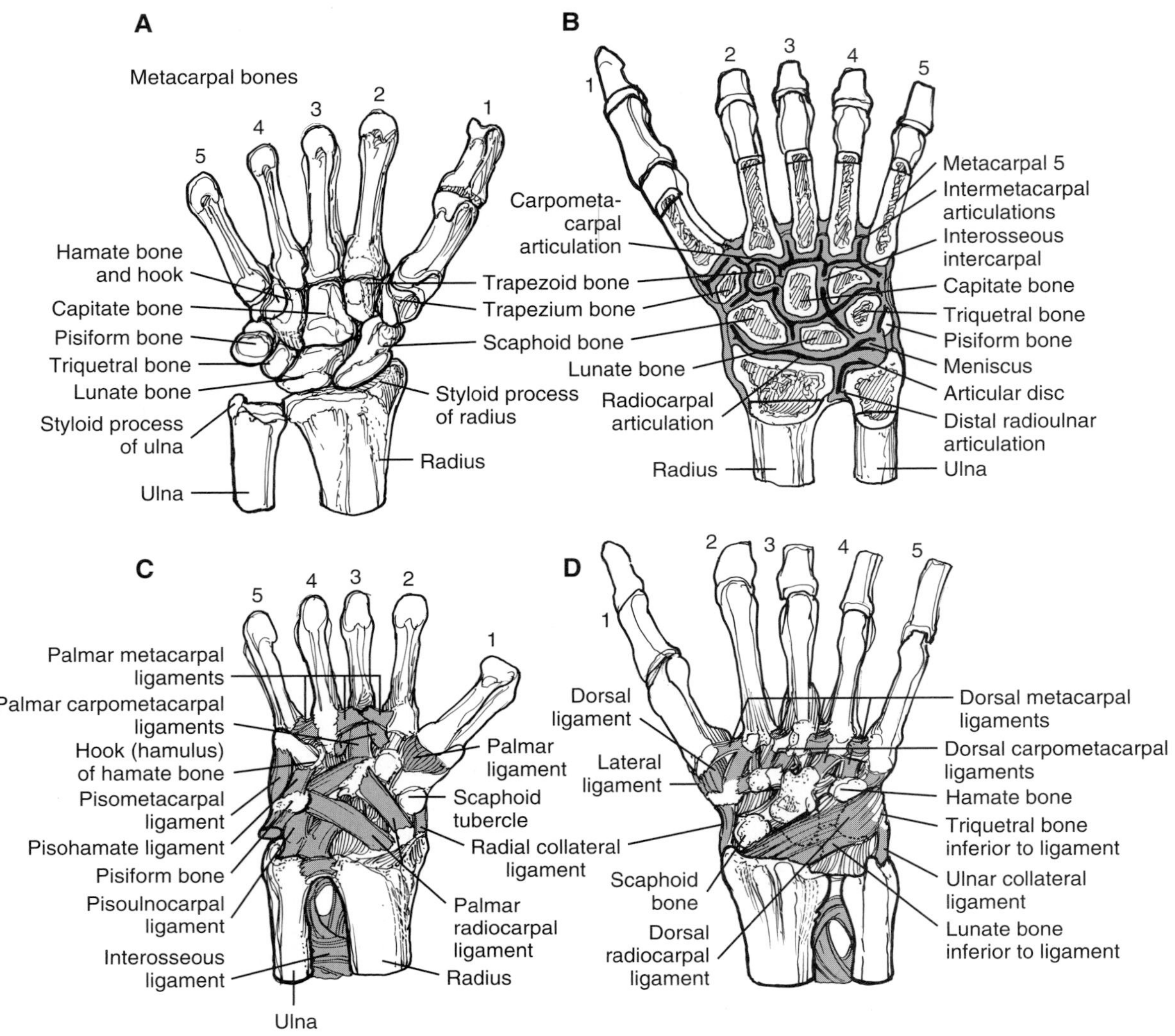

FIGURE 19–23
Radiocarpal (wrist) and intercarpal joints. **A.** Palmar view of carpal and metacarpal bones. **B.** Dorsal view of carpal and metacarpal bones showing area of meniscus and synovial cavity. **C.** Palmar view showing ligaments. **D.** Dorsal view showing ligaments.

cessive flexion, adduction, extension, and abduction of the wrist (Fig. 19–24). **Flexion** at these joints is achieved by the flexor carpi radialis, flexor carpi ulnaris, and palmaris longus muscles, assisted by the flexor digitorum superficialis, flexor digitorum profundus, flexor pollicis longus, and abductor pollicis longus muscles (Fig. 19–24*A*). Flexion is checked by opposing extensor muscles (see below) and dorsal carpal ligaments. **Extension** at the wrist is executed by the extensor carpi radialis longus, extensor carpi radialis brevis, and extensor carpi ulnaris muscles, assisted by the extensor digitorum, extensor digiti minimi, extensor indicis, and extensor pollicis longus muscles (Fig. 19–24*B*). Extension is checked by opposing flexor muscles (see above) and palmar carpal ligaments. **Adduction** is effected by the flexor carpi ulnaris and extensor carpi ulnaris muscles (Fig. 19–24*C*). Abduction is executed by the flexor carpi radialis, extensor carpi radialis longus, and extensor carpi radialis brevis muscles, assisted by the abductor pollicis longus and extensor pollicis brevis muscles (Fig. 19–24*D*).

Clinical Disorders of the Wrist Joint. Infections of the synovial sheaths of flexor tendons in the wrist result in swelling of the affected digit and pain with movement of the affected digit. Since the cavities within the synovial sheaths of digits 2 to 4 are independent of one another, infection is usually confined to a single digit. However, connections between the synovial sheaths of flexor tendons of digits 1 and 5 and the common flexor sheath provide an avenue for the spread of infection. Serious infection of the sheaths of the common flexor tendon may result in **swelling just proximal and distal to the flexor retinaculum.**

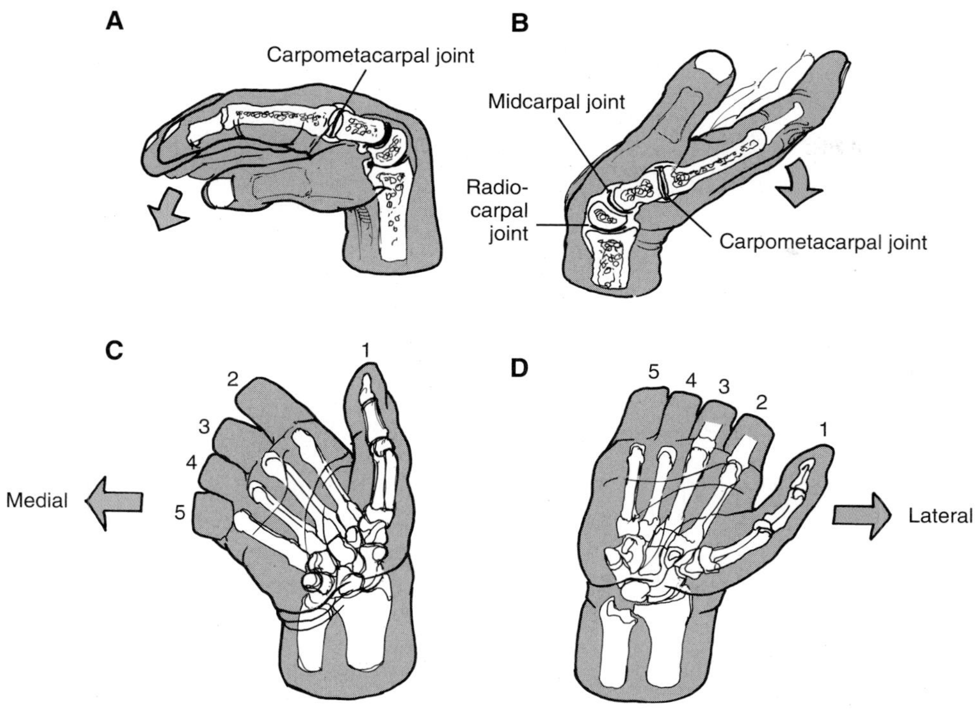

FIGURE 19–24
Movements of the radiocarpal and intercarpal joints. **A.** Flexion at these joints. **B.** Extension of the wrist. **C.** Adduction. **D.** Abduction.

Carpometacarpal Joints. The carpometacarpal joints can be considered in two groups: the joint between the first metacarpal (of the pollex) and the trapezium bone and the articulations between the bases of the second to fifth metacarpals and the carpus (Fig. 19–23*B* to *D*).

The **carpometacarpal joint of the thumb** is much more mobile than the carpometacarpal joints of the other digits because its articulating surfaces are more extensive. The joint is bound within a capsule lined by a synovial membrane and is stabilized by dorsal, palmar, and lateral ligaments (Fig. 19–23*C* and *D*). The dorsal and palmar ligaments unite the dorsal and palmar surfaces of the trapezium bone with the base of the first metacarpal. The lateral ligament unites the radial side of the trapezium bone with the radial side of the first metacarpal.

The **carpometacarpal joints of digits 2 to 5** have more limited movement. These joints are stabilized by capsules, which are lined by a synovial membrane and reinforced by dorsal, palmar, and interosseous ligaments (Fig. 19–23*C* and *D*). The second metacarpal is bound to the trapezium and trapezoid bones by two distinct dorsal ligaments and two distinct palmar ligaments; the third metacarpal is joined to the trapezoid and capitate bones by two distinct dorsal ligaments and three distinct palmar ligaments; the fourth metacarpal is joined to the capitate and hamate bones by two distinct dorsal ligaments and two distinct palmar ligaments; and the fifth metacarpal is joined to the hamate bone by a single dorsal ligament that is continuous with a single palmar ligament. There are only two interosseous ligaments, and these join the capitate and hamate bones with the third and fourth metacarpals.

Movements of the Carpometacarpal Joints. Movements of the first carpometacarpal joint include flexion, extension, adduction, abduction, rotation, circumduction, and opposition (see Table 19–2). The longitudinal axis of the first metacarpal (thumb), however, is rotated about 60 degrees with respect to the second, third, fourth, and fifth metacarpals. Adduction and abduction of the thumb thus occurs within an oblique plane with respect to the palm and dorsoventral axis (Fig. 19–25*B*). In **abduction,** for example, the thumb moves away from the palm and also somewhat laterally. In **adduction,** the thumb moves toward the palm and somewhat medially. Although flexion at the first carpometacarpal joint is initiated in a plane roughly 30 degrees from the plane of the palm (Fig. 19-25*C*), the thumb may rotate medially (at the carpometacarpal and metacarpophalangeal joints) so that its axis of flexion slowly turns to approximate the palmar plane and then moves toward the dorsoventral axis. Thus, the **combination of flexion and medial rotation of the first digit results in opposition of the thumb to the tips of digits two to five** (Fig. 19–25*D*). Conversely, extension of the first carpometacarpal joint may be accompanied by lateral rotation (Fig. 19–25*C*). **Flexion** (along with medial rotation) of the first metacarpal is thus effected by the flexor

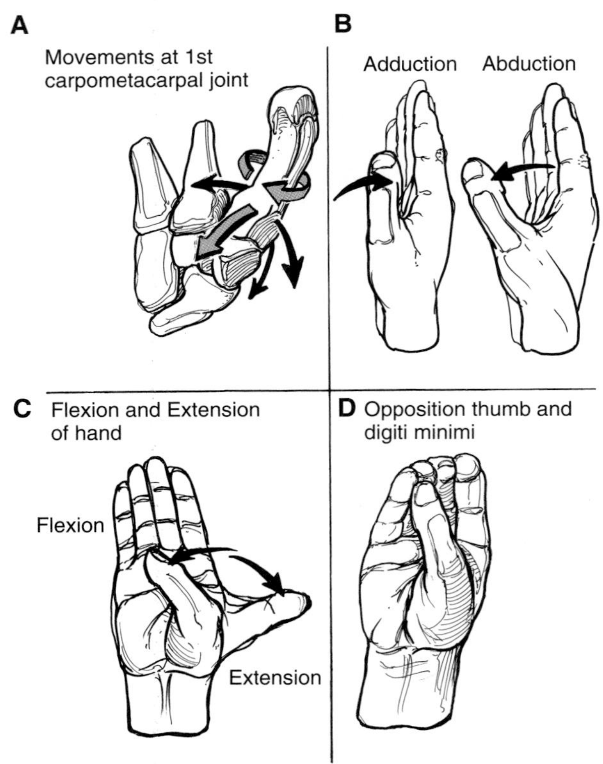

FIGURE 19–25
Movements of the first carpometacarpal joint (thumb). **A.** Planes of movement of the thumb. **B.** Adduction and abduction. **C.** Flexion and extension. **D.** Opposition of the thumb to the tips of digits 2 to 5—a combination of flexion and medial rotation.

pollicis brevis and opponens pollicis muscles. It is assisted by the flexor pollicis longus muscle when the metacarpophalangeal and interphalangeal joints are flexed at the same time. Conversely, **extension** of the first metacarpal (along with lateral rotation) is effected by the abductor pollicis longus, extensor pollicis brevis, and extensor pollicis longus muscles. Adduction is facilitated by the adductor pollicis muscle, and abduction occurs through the combined actions of the abductor pollicis brevis and abductor pollicis longus muscles. **Oppositional movements of the thumb** are executed by the opponens pollicis and flexor pollicis brevis muscles as they simultaneously flex and medially rotate the first metacarpal. Once the pulp of the first digit is in contact with the pulp of digit 2, 3, 4, or 5, however, the adductor pollicis and flexor pollicis longus muscles assist by contracting to increase the pressure between the opposed digits. There is **little flexion or extension at the carpometacarpal joints of digits 2 to 5,** but there may be slight gliding movements, which assist the lateral intermetacarpal joints in cupping the palm (see below). There is slightly more movement at the fifth carpometacarpal joint than at the second, third, and fourth carpometacarpal joints.

Intermetacarpal Joints. The intermetacarpal joints join the bases of the second to fifth metacarpal bones in the plane of the palm. The joints are stabilized by dorsal, palmar, and interosseous ligaments. Their synovial cavities tend to be continuous with those of the carpometacarpal joints described above (see Fig. 19–23*B*).

Movements of the Intermetacarpal Joints. Movements at the lateral intermetacarpal joints are slight gliding movements, which are most useful when the hand forms a "cup" shape as the thumb is opposed to the fourth or fifth digit. Thenar and hypothenar muscles acting together affect these movements.

Metacarpophalangeal Joints. The rounded bicondylar heads of all five metacarpal bones articulate with slight concavities within the bases of the proximal phalanges (see Fig. 19–13). They are stabilized by a single palmar ligament (plate) and two collateral ligaments, one on either side of each joint. In addition, the metacarpophalangeal joints of digits 2 to 5 are stabilized by deep transverse metacarpal ligaments, which unite the palmar ligaments of adjacent digits.

Movements of the Metacarpophalangeal Joints. Movements of the metacarpophalangeal joints include flexion, extension, adduction, abduction, and circumduction (see Table 19–2). Slight rotation may occur in conjunction with flexion and extension. This is especially evident in the first digit and essentially nonexistent in the third digit. All other movements are more restricted in the metacarpophalangeal joint of the first digit. **Flexion of digits 1 to 4** is produced by actions of the flexor digitorum superficialis and flexor digitorum profundus muscles and is assisted by the lumbrical and interosseous muscles (digits 2 to 5). **Flexion of the fifth digit** is assisted by the flexor digiti minimi brevis muscle and **flexion of the first digit** by the flexor pollicis longus and flexor pollicis brevis muscles. **Extension of the second to fifth digits** occurs through the action of the extensor digitorum muscle. However, **extension of the fifth digit** is assisted by the extensor digiti minimi muscle and **extension of the second digit** by the extensor indicis muscle. **Extension of the first digit** is effected by the extensor pollicis longus and extensor pollicis brevis muscles. Abduction and adduction occur with respect to an axial line drawn through the third digit (see Fig. 20–22). **Abduction of the digits** (only when they are extended) is produced by the following muscles: digit 1 by the abductor pollicis brevis muscle; digit 2 by the first dorsal interosseous muscle; digit 3 by the second and third dorsal interosseous muscles; digit 4 by the fourth dorsal interosseous muscle; and digit 5 by the abductor digiti minimi muscle. **Adduction of the digits** (only when they are extended) is accomplished as follows: digit 1 by the adductor pollicis and first palmar interosseous muscles, digit 2 by the second palmar interosseous muscle; digit 3 cannot be adducted and so has no adductors; digit 4 by the third palmar interosseous muscle; and digit 5 by the adductor digiti minimi muscle.

Interphalangeal Joints. The interphalangeal joints of all five digits (one within the first digit and two each within digits 2 to 5) are similar. They are hinge joints enclosed by a fibrous capsule, which is lined by a synovial membrane. Each joint is stabilized by one palmar and two collateral ligaments.

Movements of the Interphalangeal Joints. The interphalangeal joints are classified as uniaxial hinge joints. In addition to flexing and extending the digits, they also rotate them slightly (see Table 19–2). The range of rotation is greatest within the proximal and middle interphalangeal joints. Lateral rotation of phalanges 2 to 5 is associated with flexion of these joints, while medial rotation accompanies extension of these joints. The lateral rotation that accompanies flexion of these digits facilitates opposition of the fingers to the thumb and adaptation of the fingers to the various shapes of "grasped" objects. **Flexion at proximal interphalangeal joints of digits 2 to 5** is effected by the flexor digitorum superficialis and flexor digitorum profundus muscles. **Flexion of the distal interphalangeal joints of digits 2 to 5** is usually effected by the flexor digitorum profundus muscle only, but there may be assistance from the interosseous and lumbrical muscles acting together. **Flexion of the single interphalangeal joint of the first digit** is executed by the flexor pollicis longus muscle. **Extension at both interphalangeal joints of digits 2 to 5** is produced by the extensor digitorum muscle. **Extension at the single interphalangeal joint of digit 1** is produced by the extensor pollicis longus muscle. **Extension at digit five** is assisted by the extensor digiti minimi muscle and **extension at digit 1** by the abductor pollicis longus and extensor pollicis brevis muscles. In addition, it is thought that when the lumbricals are active in **flexion of the metacarpophalangeal joints of digits 2 to 5,** they are active in **extension at the interphalangeal joints of these digits** (see discussion of dorsal digital expansions and prehensile mechanisms in Chapter 20).

20 Muscles of the Upper Extremities

MUSCLES OF THE UPPER LIMB

Development of Upper Limb Muscles

The distribution of muscles and nerves is relatively unaltered during embryonic development

Upper limb muscles arise from somitic mesoderm as somitic myoblasts migrate into the upper limb buds to form dorsal and ventral muscle masses. Because the upper limb buds rotate only slightly in a lateral direction during development (in contrast to the lower extremity limb buds) (see Fig. 19–2), the embryonic dorsal and ventral muscle masses are displaced only slightly from their original positions. Thus, the ventral muscle mass directly forms the cranioventral muscles and the dorsal muscle mass forms the caudodorsal muscles of the definitive upper limb. Cranioventral muscles typically function as flexors and pronators, while caudodorsal muscles function as extensors and supinators.

Thus, muscles of the definitive upper limbs maintain their original cranial or caudal relationships. Cranial somitic mesoderm forms muscles within the radial side of the definitive upper extremity (i.e., the side of the forearm containing the radius). Caudal somitic mesoderm forms muscles within the ulnar side of the definitive upper extremity (i.e., the side of the forearm containing the ulna). As one would expect with this arrangement, radial muscles are innervated by nerves closer to the cranium (spinal nerves C5, C6, and C7) and ulnar muscles by nerves closer to the caudal region of the spinal cord (spinal nerves C7, C8, and T1) (see discussion of brachial plexus in Chapter 21).

It should be noted that many upper extremity muscles such as the serratus anterior, latissimus dorsi, levator scapulae, and rhomboid muscles migrate onto the wall of the trunk during embryonic development to intermingle with muscles of the trunk. The specific nerves of the brachial plexus (see below) that innervate each muscle elongate along behind each muscle as it migrates.

Organization of Definitive Upper Extremity Muscles

Deep fascia invests all of the muscles of the upper extremity. It plays much the same role as in the lower extremity. It assists in stabilizing the joints, anchoring specific muscles, and forming compartments for muscles with the same function (see below). In some cases, the functional compartments are divided into superficial and deep compartments.

The appendicular muscles of the shoulder are located in two major compartments: the **posterior (scapular)** and **anterior (pectoral) thoracic compartments** (Fig. 20–1). The appendicular muscles tend to move or stabilize (or both) the clavicle, scapula, and humerus. Muscles of the scapular compartment either connect the upper limb to the vertebral column or connect proximal segments of the upper limb to one another. Muscles of the pectoral compartment tend to connect the upper limb to the body wall.

As has been noted above, the upper extremity limb buds rotate laterally only slightly during development. Thus, when the upper limb is in anatomic position, the flexor compartments of the arm and forearm face anteriorly and the extensor compartments face posteriorly. The **upper arm (arm)** includes muscles of an anterocranial **flexor compartment** and a posterocaudal **extensor compartment** (Fig. 20–2), both of which act primarily to mobilize the arm and forearm. The forearm is characterized by an anterocranial **antebrachial (forearm) flexor compartment** (Fig. 20–3) and a posterocaudal **antebrachial (forearm) extensor compartment.** Unlike the flexor compartment of the arm, the flexor compartment of the forearm is divided into three distinct layers: the **superficial, intermediate,** and **deep layers.** The extensor compartment is divided into **superficial** and **deep layers.** The forearm muscles function in movements of the forearm, hand, and fingers.

Finally, there are three groups of small **intrinsic muscles of the hand:** the abductor, adductor, flexor, and opponens muscles of the thumb, the **thenar muscles;** the abductor, opponens, and flexor muscles of the little finger, the **hypothenar muscles;** and the lumbrical and interosseous muscles associated with the **central palm** and **intermetacarpal spaces** (Fig. 20–4).

As in the case of other skeletal muscles throughout the body, muscles of the upper extremity may serve both dynamic and postural functions as they mobilize segments of the upper limb or stabilize segments by re-

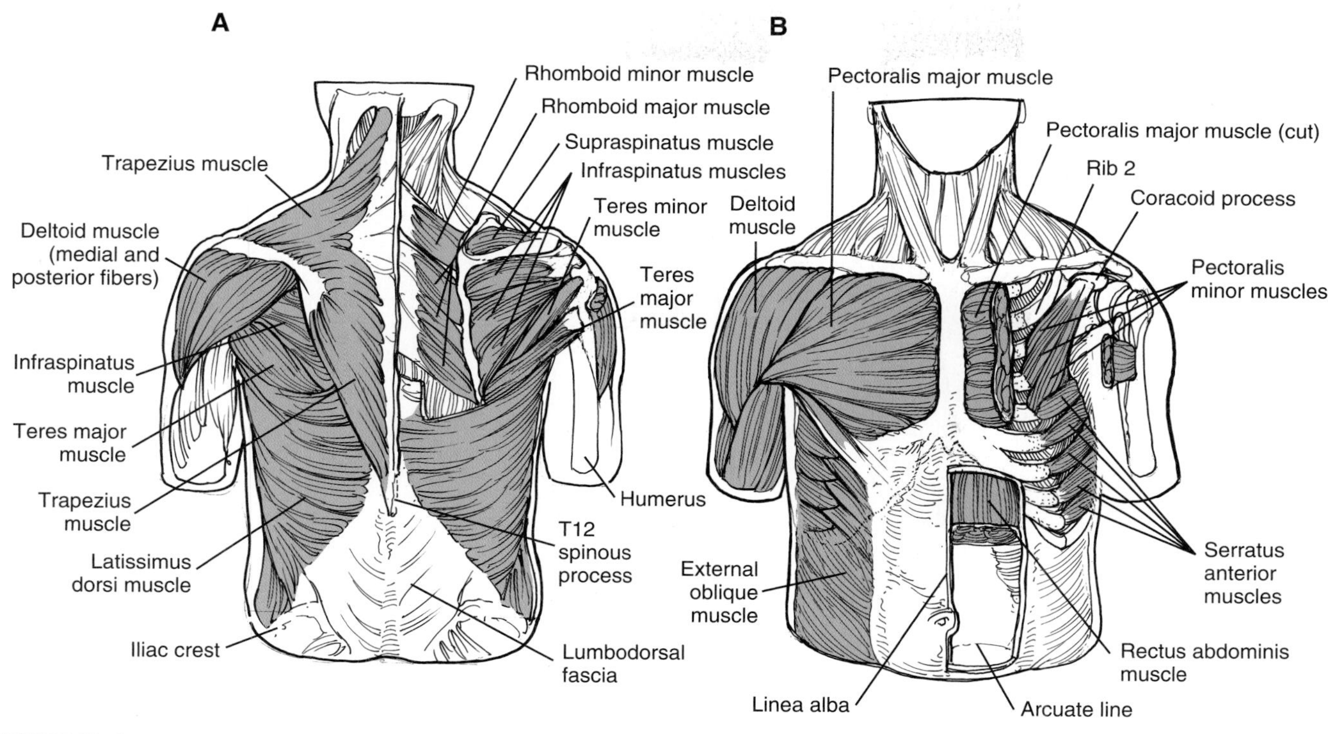

FIGURE 20–1
Appendicular muscles of the shoulder. **A.** Posterior (scapular) compartment. **B.** Anterior (pectoral) thoracic compartment.

sisting the actions of opposing muscles or outside forces, including gravity. The synergy of muscle actions is especially important in the upper limb because it allows the execution of the fine, smooth movements that characterize the limb's precise prehensile function.

The following descriptions of specific upper extremity muscles are organized from proximal to distal (i.e., from the shoulder to the fingers) and with respect to their locations within specific muscle compartments and layers.

▲ Specific Muscles of the Upper Extremity

Scapular Thoracic Muscles

Some scapular muscles connect the upper extremity to the vertebral column

Scapular muscles that connect the upper extremity to the vertebral column include the latissimus dorsi, trapezius, levator scapulae, and rhomboid major and minor muscles. The primary function of these muscles is to stabilize the shoulder or control movements of the scapula (elevation, depression, retraction, protraction, and medial and lateral rotation).

Latissimus Dorsi Muscle. Each latissimus dorsi muscle is triangular with its base lying along the vertebral axis that extends from the midthoracic to the sacral region (Fig. 20–5*A*). The muscle's superior fibers thus arise from the lower six thoracic vertebrae. Its inferior fibers originate from the posterior layer of the thoracolumbar fascia (see Chapter 5), supraspinous ligaments, posterior part of the iliac crest, and a region of the iliac crest just lateral to the erector spinae muscle within the lumbar and sacral regions. The upper fibers of the latissimus dorsi muscle are horizontal and overlap the inferior angle of the scapula. The middle fibers are oblique and the lower fibers almost vertical. All fibers of the latissimus dorsi muscle converge to form a single lateral tendon, which inserts into the intertubercular groove (sulcus) of the humerus (Fig. 20–5*A*). As the fibers converge to form the tendon, they spiral so that fibers arising from the lowest levels of the back insert more superiorly upon the humerus than fibers arising from the highest levels of the back. The insertion of the latissimus dorsi muscle is just anterior to the insertion of the teres major muscle (see below).

Actions of the latissimus dorsi muscle include adduction (against resistance) and extension of the humerus (see Fig. 19–18*B* and *D*). Adduction is particularly forceful when the humerus is abducted and slightly extended. The latissimus dorsi muscle adducts the humerus against resistance (with the sternocostal region of the pectoralis major muscle and with the teres major muscle). The latissimus dorsi muscle is a particularly strong medial rotator of the humerus (see Fig. 19–18*E* and Box 20–1). The latissimus dorsi muscle is typically active in backward swinging of the arm and is classically cited as a major promoter of the backward motion of

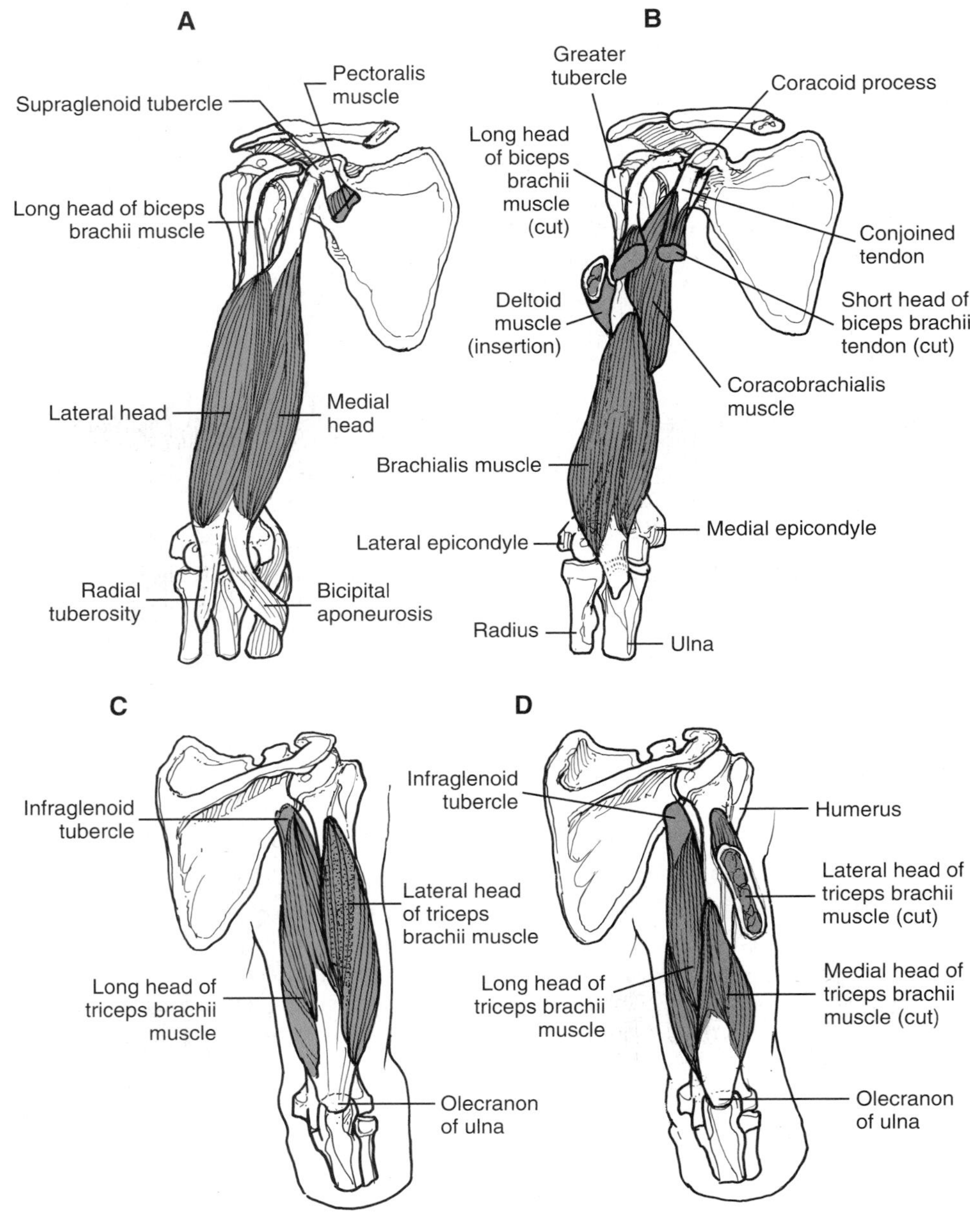

FIGURE 20–2

Flexor and extensor muscle compartments of the upper arm. **A** and **B**. Anterocranial flexor compartment. **A**. Superficial muscles. **B**. Intermediate muscles. **C** and **D**. Posterocaudal extensor compartment. **C**. Superficial muscles. **D**. Intermediate muscles.

the upper limb in the butterfly stroke in swimming. It is also activated as a respiratory muscle in forced expiration, coughing, and sneezing (see Chapter 6).

Trapezius Muscle. The trapezius muscle on each side of the body is triangular. The paired triangular trapezius muscles together assume the shape of a trapezoid (Fig. 20–6). The superior angle of each muscle is at the **occipital protuberance,** and the inferior angles converge at the spine of vertebra T12. The lateral angle of each muscle is at the shoulder. The base of the triangle is thus oriented along the midline from the occipital protuberance to the spine of vertebra T12, and all muscle fibers course from the base of the triangle to the lateral angle at the shoulder. However, fibers arising at the occipital protuberance course inferolaterally, while fibers arising at the twelfth vertebral spine course superolaterally. Fibers arising from the spine of vertebra T1 course horizontally.

Superior fibers of the trapezius muscle arise from the occipital protuberance, the medial one third of the superior nuchal line, and the superior extension of the interspinous ligament (ligamentum nuchae). These

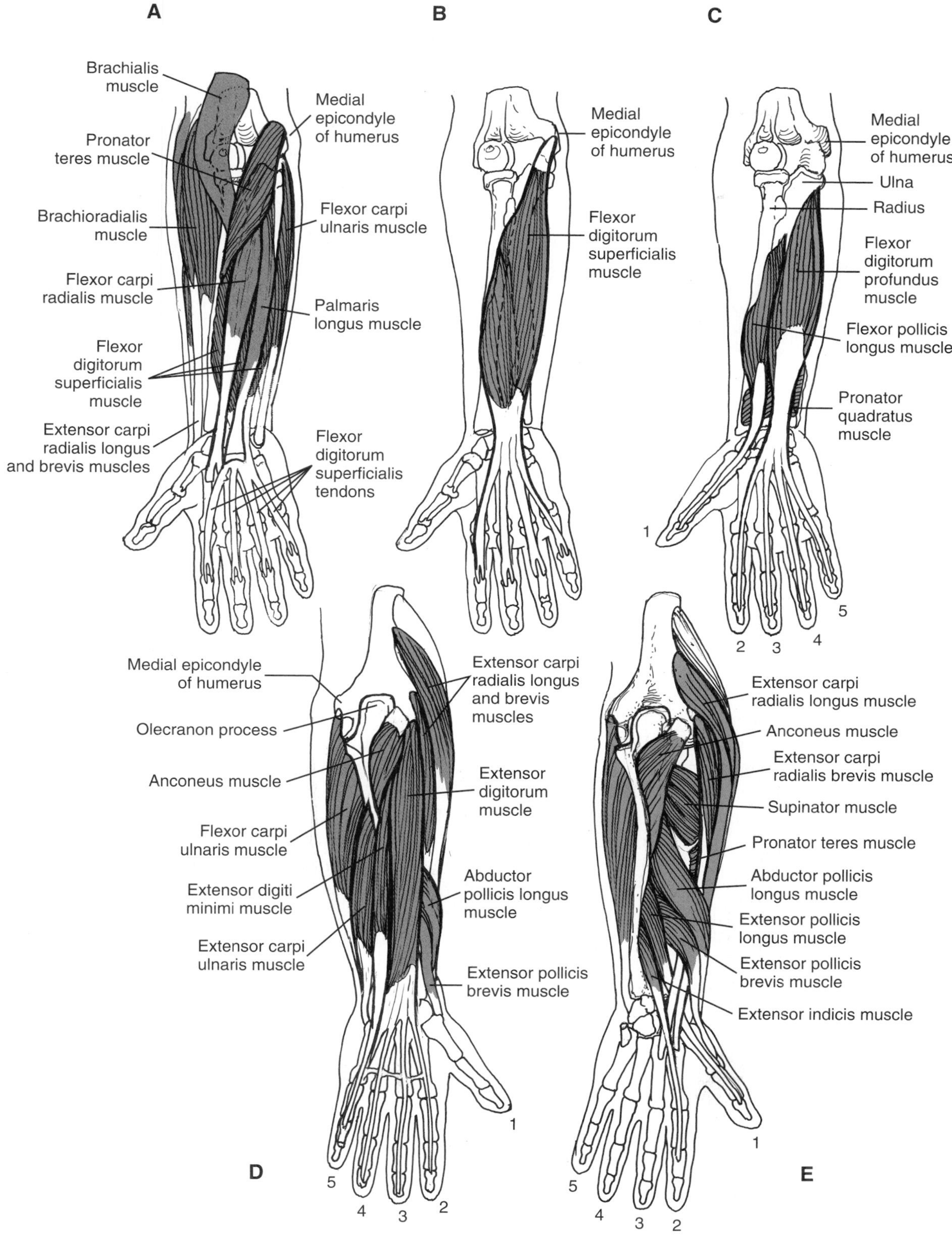

FIGURE 20–3

Flexor and extensor muscle compartments of the forearm. **A** to **C**. Antebrachial flexor compartment, palmar view. **A**. Superficial muscles. **B**. Intermediate muscles. **C**. Deep muscles. **D** and **E**. Antebrachial extensor compartment. **D**. Dorsal (volar) view of superficial muscles. **E**. Dorsal view of deep muscles.

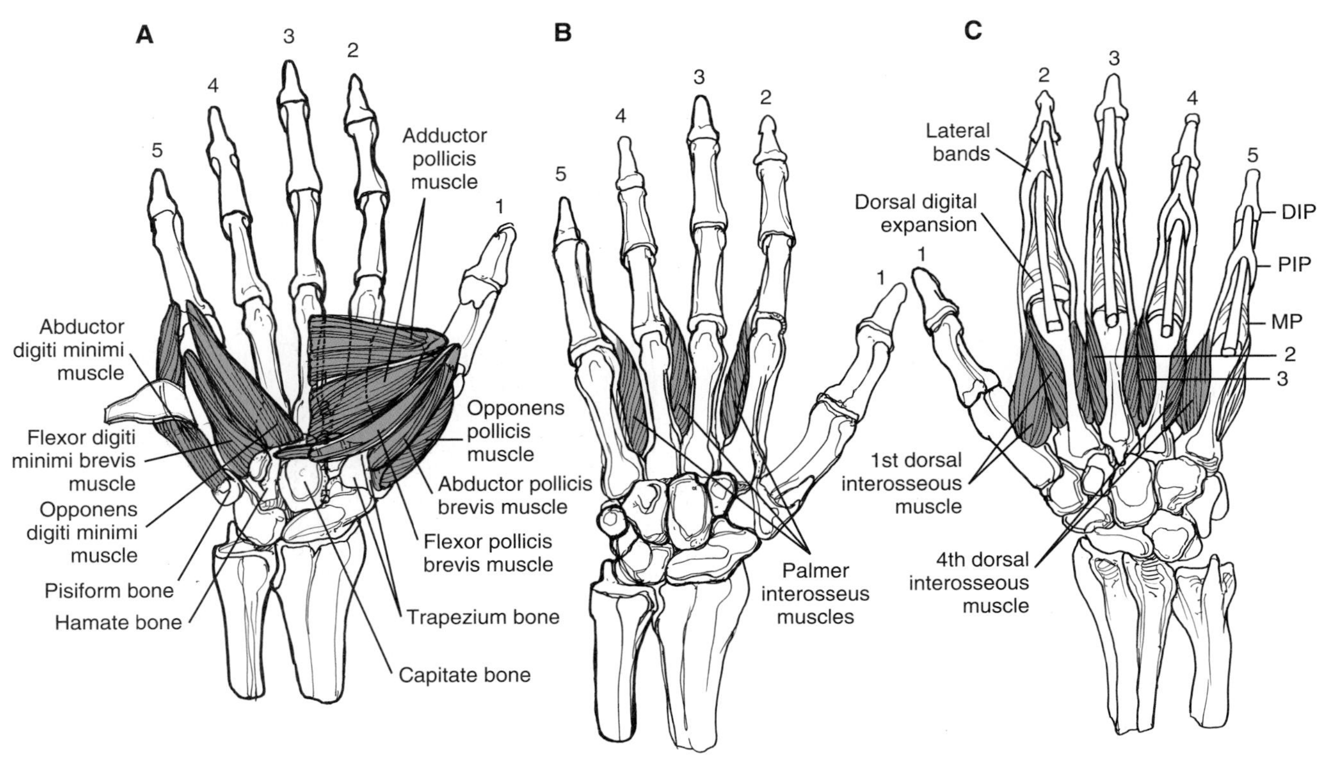

FIGURE 20–4
Intrinsic muscles of the hand. **A.** Thenar and hypothenar muscles. **B.** Palmar interosseous muscles. **C.** Dorsal interosseous muscles.

fibers course obliquely downward to insert upon the posterior border of the lateral third of the clavicle (Fig. 20–6*D*). The middle fibers arise from dense superficial connective tissue at the base of the skull and from an aponeurosis extending from the spines of vertebrae C6 to T3. These middle fibers course horizontally to insert upon the medial margin of the acromial process and all along the superior edge of the scapular spine. Inferior fibers of each trapezius muscle arise from vertebral spines T3 to T12 and course obliquely upward to insert upon the medial end of the scapular spine. Thus, the trapezius muscle connects the clavicle and scapula to the vertebral column and also connects the clavicle and scapula (see Fig. 20–5).

The varied orientations of its muscle fibers allow the trapezius muscle to perform many dynamic functions in addition to its main function of steadying the shoulder (maintenance of poise). Actions include elevation of the scapula (with the levator scapulae muscle); elevation of the clavicle; medial rotation of the scapula (i.e., the inferior angle is displaced medially); retraction of the scapula (i.e., the scapula is pulled toward the midline) (with the rhomboid major and minor, levator scapulae, and pectoralis minor muscles); and lateral rotation of the scapula (i.e., the inferior angle is displaced laterally) (with the serratus anterior muscle) (Fig. 19–16). With the shoulder fixed, the trapezius muscle may also bend the neck and head posteriorly or posterolaterally.

Levator Scapulae Muscle. Superior fibers of the levator scapulae muscle typically arise from the transverse processes of vertebrae C1 and C2 and the spines of vertebrae C3 and C4. From these points, muscle fibers course inferolaterally to attach to the superior angle of the scapula. Variations include separation of the muscle into two or more slips and origination of some fibers from the mastoid process, occipital bone, or adjacent muscles (see Fig. 20–5*C*).

Actions of the levator scapulae muscle (with the cervical vertebral column fixed) include elevation of the scapula (with the trapezius muscle) (Fig. 19–16*A*) and medial rotation of the scapula (with the trapezius, pectoralis minor, and rhomboid major and minor muscles) (see Fig. 19–16*D* and Table 20–1). With the scapula fixed, the levator scapulae muscle laterally flexes the neck.

Rhomboid Minor Muscle. The rhomboid minor muscle arises from the inferior part of the ligamentum nuchae and the spines and supraspinous ligaments of vertebrae C7 and T1 (Fig. 20–5*D*). Its fibers course inferolaterally to attach to the medial edge of the scapula near the medial end of the scapular spine (Fig. 20–6*D*).

Actions of the rhomboid minor muscle include retraction of the scapula (with the rhomboid major and trapezius muscles) and medial rotation of the scapula (with the trapezius, levator scapulae, rhomboid major, and pectoralis minor muscles) (Table 20–1 and see Fig. 20–5*D*).

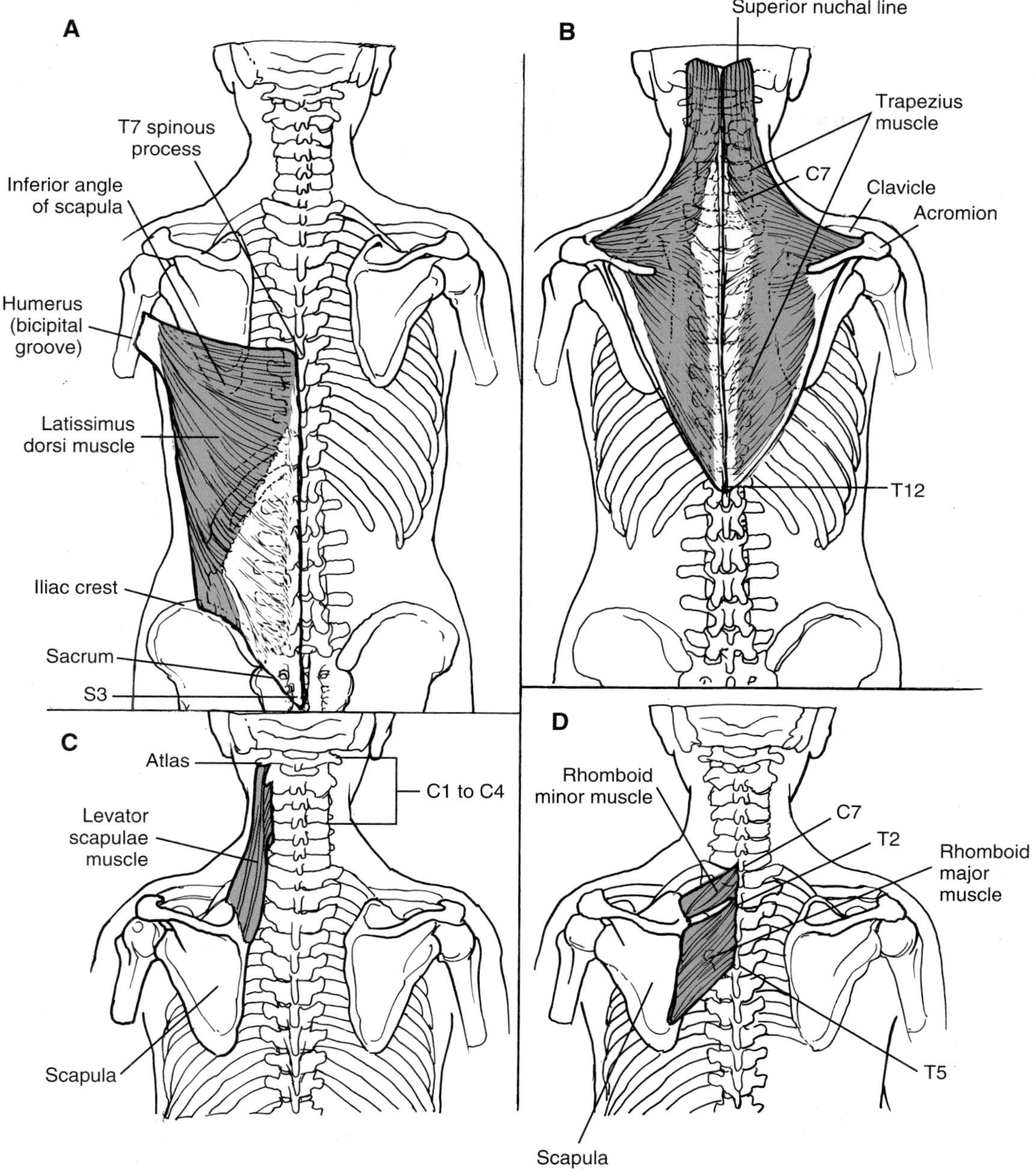

FIGURE 20–5

Scapular thoracic muscles that connect the upper extremity to the vertebral column. **A.** Latissimus dorsi muscle. **B.** Trapezius muscle. **C.** Levator scapulae muscle. **D.** Major and minor rhomboid muscles.

BOX 20–1

MUSCLES OF THE DORSAL AND VENTRAL MUSCLE MASSES IN THE UPPER EXTREMITY

Muscles of Dorsal Muscle Mass	Muscles of Ventral Muscle Mass
Levator scapulae; rhomboids; supraspinatus; infraspinatus; teres major and minor; latissimus dorsi; subscapularis; serratus anterior; posterior compartment muscles of arm and forearm; lateral compartment muscles of forearm and hand	Anterior compartment muscles of arm and forearm; all muscles of palmar side of hand

Rhomboid Major Muscle. The rhomboid major muscle arises from the spines of vertebrae T2 to T5 and their supraspinous ligaments. These fibers course inferolaterally to the medial border of the scapula (between the medial end of the scapular spine and the inferior angle) (Fig. 20–5*D*).

Actions of the rhomboid major muscle include retraction of the scapula (with the rhomboid minor and trapezius muscles) (see Fig. 19–16*B*) and medial rotation of the scapula (with the trapezius, rhomboid minor, levator scapulae, and pectoralis minor muscles) (see Fig. 19–16*D* and Table 20–1).

Scapular Muscles That Connect the Shoulder Girdle to the Arm

Some scapular muscles connect the shoulder girdle to the arm

Scapular muscles that connect the shoulder girdle (scapula and clavicle) to the humerus include the deltoid muscle, teres major muscle, and muscles of the ro-

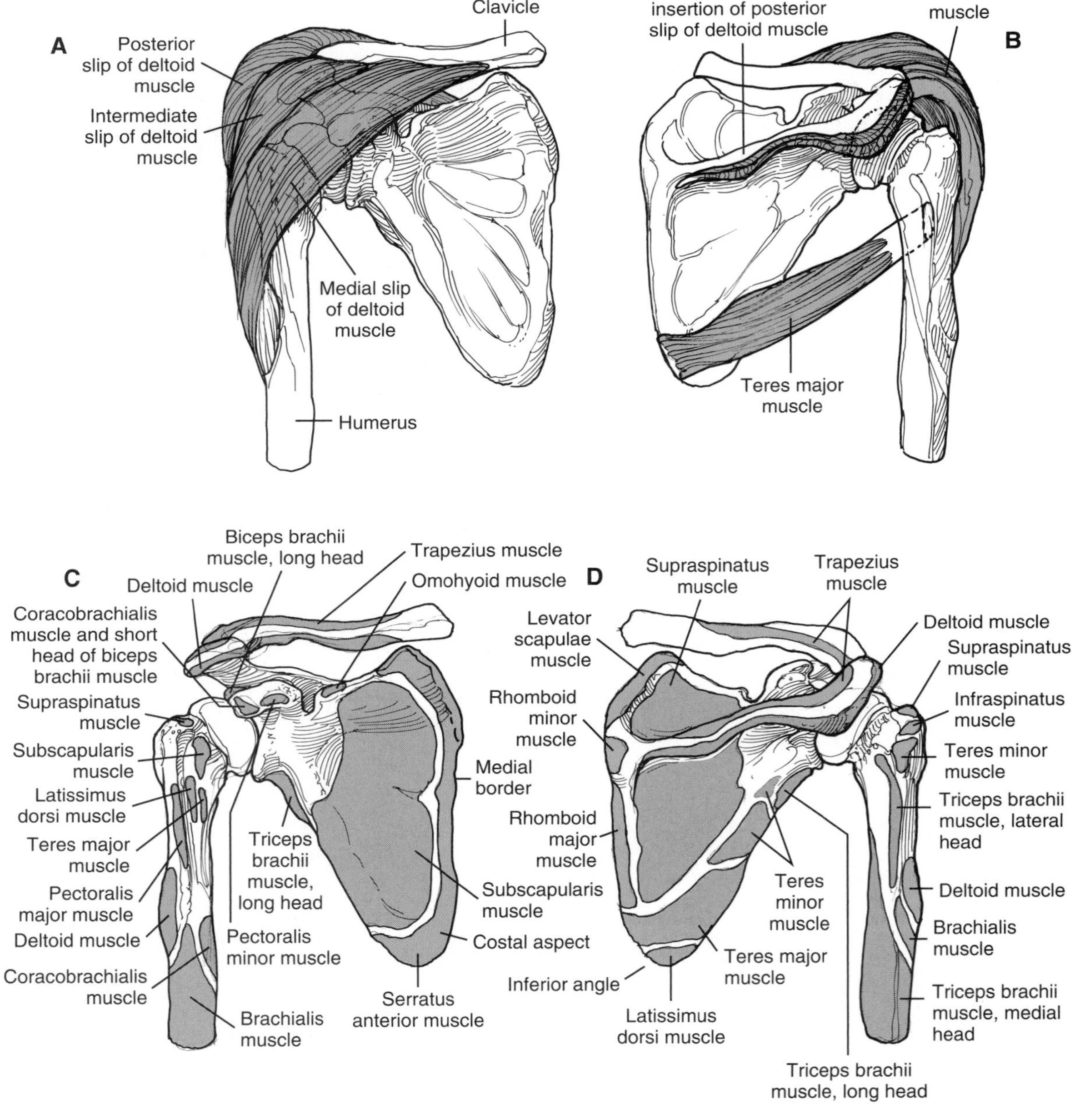

FIGURE 20–6
Scapular muscles that connect the shoulder girdle to the arm. **A.** Anterior view of deltoid muscle. **B.** Posterior view of deltoid and teres major muscles. **C.** and **D.** Origins and insertions for muscles of the shoulder girdle. Origins are gray, and insertions are red. **C.** Anterior view. **D.** Posterior view.

tator cuff (supraspinatus, infraspinatus, teres minor, and subscapularis muscles). These muscles primarily stabilize the humerus or control movements of the arm (extension, horizontal extension, flexion, horizontal flexion, adduction, and abduction).

Deltoid Muscle. The deltoid muscle can be seen as the rounded bulge of the shoulder (see surface anatomy; Fig. 20–6). The muscle consists of groups of anterior, intermediate, and posterior fibers, which enclose the shoulder joint, except for its inferior aspect. **Anterior fibers** arise from the lateral third of the clavicle, **intermediate fibers** from the superior surface and lateral margin of the acromium of the scapula, and **posterior fibers** from the lower edge of the crest of the scapular

TABLE 20–1
Attachments and Actions of Scapular Muscles

Muscle Group	Individual Muscle	Proximal Attachment	Distal Attachment	Muscle Action
Scapular thoracic muscles	Latissimus dorsi	Lower six thoracic vertebrae, lumbar fascia, lumbar supraspinous ligaments, iliac crest	Intertubercular groove of humerus	Adducts humerus against resistance, extends humerus, adducts humerus against resistance, medially rotates humerus
	Trapezius	Occipital protuberance, medial one third of superior nuchal line, ligamentum nuchae, aponeurosis from vertebra C6 to spine of vertebra T3, spines of vertebrae T3 to T12	Lateral third of clavicle, medial margin of acromial process and superior edge of scapular spine, medial end of scapular spine	Elevates scapula and clavicle, retracts scapula, laterally rotates scapula, hyperextends neck
	Levator scapulae	Transverse processes of vertebrae C1 and C2, spines of vertebrae C3 and C4	Superior angle of scapula	Elevates and medially rotates scapula, laterally flexes neck when scapula is fixed
	Rhomboid minor	Inferior part of ligamentum nuchae, spines and supraspinous ligaments of vertebrae C7 to T1	Medial edge of scapula	Retracts scapula, medially rotates scapula
	Rhomboid major	Spines and supraspinous ligaments of vertebrae T2 to T5	Medial edge of scapula	Retracts scapula, medially rotates scapula
Scapular muscles that connect the shoulder girdle to the arm	Deltoid	Lateral third of clavicle, acromial process of scapula, scapular spine	Deltoid tuberosity of humerus	Initially abducts humerus; *anterior fibers* flex, horizontally flex, medially rotate humerus; *posterior fibers* extend, horizontally extend, laterally rotate humerus
	Teres major	Inferior angle of scapula	Medial lip of intertubercular sulcus of humerus	Extends and medially rotates humerus, maintains posture of humerus and scapula
	Supraspinatus	Medial two thirds of supraspinous fossa of scapula	Glenohumeral joint capsule, superior edge of greater tubercle of humerus	Abducts humerus, stabilizes glenohumeral joint with other muscles of rotator cuff
	Infraspinatus	Medial two thirds of infraspinous fossa of scapula	Greater tubercle of humerus	Medially rotates humerus, stabilizes glenohumeral joint with other muscles of rotator cuff
	Teres minor	Dorsal surface of lateral border of scapula	Lower part of greater tubercle of humerus	Medially rotates humerus, stabilizes glenohumeral joint with other muscles of rotator cuff
	Subscapularis	Medial two thirds of subscapular fossa of scapula	Lesser tubercle of humerus	Laterally rotates humerus, stabilizes glenohumeral joint with other muscles of rotator cuff

spine. All three groups of fibers course laterally and then inferiorly. They converge to form a short, strong tendon, which is connected to the deltoid tuberosity. The **deltoid tuberosity** is a lateral tubercle on the midpart of the humeral shaft.

Actions of all of the fibers together (with the supraspinatus, infraspinatus, subscapularis, and teres minor muscles) abduct the arm (see Fig. 19–18*C*). The **intermediate fibers** of the deltoid muscle (with the supraspinatus muscle) play the most important role in initial abduction of the arm. Further abduction, which is needed to raise the arm over the head, requires lateral rotation of the scapula (see Fig. 19–16*C* and Table 20–1). Contraction of the **anterior** and **posterior fibers** of the deltoid muscle mainly steadies the arm during abduction. However, anterior fibers may also contract (with the pectoralis major muscle) to play a more active role in flexion, horizontal flexion, and medial rotation of the arm. Posterior fibers may contract (with the latissimus dorsi and teres major muscles) to extend, horizontally extend, and laterally rotate the arm.

Teres Major Muscle. The origin of the broad, flat teres major muscle is the inferior angle of the scapula. Fibers course superolaterally, passing anterior to the tendon of the long head of the triceps brachii muscle and posterior to the tendon of the latissimus dorsi muscle (Fig. 20–6). The distal regions of the teres major and latissimus dorsi muscles form the posterior axillary fold. The distal tendon of the teres major muscle inserts upon the medial lip of the intertubercular sulcus.

Actions of the teres major muscle include extension and medial rotation of the arm, particularly in arm swinging (Fig. 20–6 and Table 20–1). The muscle also plays a static role in maintaining the posture of the arm and scapula.

Muscles of the Rotator Cuff. The rotator cuff is a group of four muscles: the supraspinatus, infraspinatus, teres minor, and subscapularis muscles (Fig. 20–7). Together, they bind the humerus to the scapula. Their distal tendons invest and strengthen the shoulder joint.

The belly of the **supraspinatus muscle** arises from the medial two thirds of the supraspinous fossa of the scapula. As the muscle's fibers course laterally, they converge under the acromial process of the scapula, forming a tendon that courses over the superior lip of the glenohumeral joint where it attaches to the joint capsule. The tendon then continues inferiorly to attach to the most superior region of the greater tubercle of the humerus (Fig. 20–7).

The belly of the **infraspinatus muscle** arises from the medial two thirds of the infraspinous fossa of the scapula. As its fibers course laterally, they converge to form a tendon that passes over the posterior lip of the glenohumeral joint to attach to the greater tubercle of the humerus. A bursa, which may or may not communicate with the synovial cavity of the shoulder joint, typically separates the tendon from the glenohumeral capsule (Fig. 20–7).

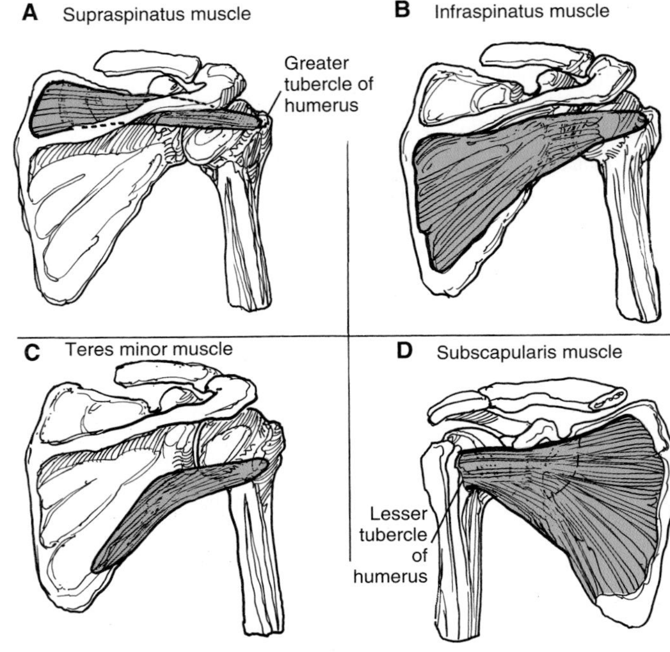

FIGURE 20–7
Rotator cuff muscles that bind the humerus to the scapula. **A.** Supraspinatus muscle. **B.** Infraspinatus muscle. **C.** Teres minor muscle. **D.** Subscapularis muscle.

The **teres minor muscle** arises from the dorsal surface of the lateral border of the scapula between the infraspinatus and teres major muscles (see above). As the fibers of the teres minor muscle course superolaterally, they converge to form a tendon that passes over the inferoposterior lip of the glenohumeral joint. The tendon then inserts upon the lowest region of the greater tubercle of the humerus (Fig. 20–7*C*).

The **subscapularis muscle** arises from the medial two thirds of the subscapular fossa on the anterior surface of the scapula. As the muscle's fibers course laterally, they converge to form a tendon that passes over the anterior surface of the scapular neck. Here, the tendon is separated from the scapular neck by a bursa, which communicates with the synovial cavity of the glenohumeral joint. The tendon then courses over the anterior lip of the glenohumeral joint and inserts upon the lesser tubercle of the humerus (Fig. 20–7*D*).

Tendons of the Rotator Cuff. The tendons of the rotator cuff play a critical role in stabilizing and mobilizing the glenohumeral joint, primarily by preventing excessive downward, anterior, or posterior sliding of the humeral head upon the glenoid fossa. The tendon of the subscapularis muscle tends to prevent forward sliding of the humeral head, while tendons of the infraspinatus and teres minor muscles prevent backward sliding. The tendon of the supraspinatus muscle, espe-

TABLE 20–2
Attachments and Actions of Pectoral Muscles

Muscle	Proximal Attachment	Distal Attachment	Muscle Action
Pectoralis major	Anterior surface of sternum and costal cartilages of ribs 1 to 7, anterior surface of sternal end of clavicle	Lateral lip of intertubercular sulcus	Adducts, medially rotates, horizontally flexes, extends humerus; forced inspiration
Pectoralis minor	Ribs 3 to 5 and fascia covering intervening intercostal spaces	Coracoid process of scapula	Depresses clavicle, pulls scapula forward; forced inspiration
Subclavius	Medial part of rib 1 and its costal cartilage	Underside of middle part of clavicle	Depresses clavicle, stabilizes clavicle
Serratus anterior	Ribs 1 to 9 and fascia covering intervening intercostal spaces	Anteromedial scapular border near its superior angle	Protracts scapula, stabilizes scapula, initially abducts humerus; lower fibers assist in lateral rotation of scapula

cially, tends to prevent subluxation (downward dislocation) of the humeral head by suspending the humerus from above (see below). The tendon of the long head of the biceps brachii muscle prevents excessive upward movement of the humeral head onto the lower surface of the acromium and also contributes to stabilization of the glenohumeral joint during movements of the arm (see below).

Function of the Rotator Cuff. The rotator cuff acts to steady or stabilize the humeral head within the flat glenoid fossa of the shoulder joint (see below). Dynamic actions of the muscles of the rotator cuff are varied. The subscapularis muscle is active in lateral rotation of the humerus (see Fig. 19–18*F*), while the infraspinatus and teres minor muscles are active in medial rotation of the humerus. The supraspinatus muscle is active in abduction of the humerus (with the deltoid muscle) (see Fig. 19–18C).

Injury to the Rotator Cuff. Injury to the rotator cuff from trauma or disease typically results in instability of the shoulder joint. **Trauma** to the rotator cuff is frequently experienced by baseball pitchers and football quarterbacks. **Degenerative tendinitis** of rotator cuff muscles is more common with aging.

Pectoral Thoracic Muscles

Pectoral (anterior) thoracic muscles connect the upper limb to the anterior thoracic wall

Muscles of the pectoral region include the pectoralis major, pectoralis minor, subclavius, and serratus anterior muscles (Table 20–2). In addition to stabilizing the upper extremity, these muscles control movements of the clavicle (elevation, depression, and circumduction) and raise the ribs.

Pectoralis Major Muscle. The broad, triangular pectoralis major muscle has two parts: a **sternocostal part** and a **clavicular part.** Fibers of the sternocostal head of each pectoralis major muscle arise from half of the anterior surface of the sternum and from the costal cartilages of ribs 1 to 7 (Fig. 20–8). Fibers of the superior sternal head of the pectoralis major muscle arise from the anterior surface of the sternal end of the clavicle. The larger sternocostal and smaller clavicular heads of the pectoralis major muscle are typically separated from each other by a deep groove. As fibers from both parts of the muscle course laterally, they converge to form a broad tendon. However, they also spiral in a medial direction (about 90 degrees) so that fibers of the clavicular head become inferior to fibers of the sternocostal head at their attachments to the humerus. The tendon is attached to the upper third of the humeral shaft in a long insertion upon the lateral lip of the intertubercular sulcus (bicipital groove) (Fig. 20–8).

A fascial specialization arises from the lower edge of the pectoralis major muscle and spans the axilla to invest the latissimus dorsi muscle. The region of axillary fascia that spans the lower boundary of the axilla is connected to the skin of the axilla. This part of the axillary fascia is called the **suspensory ligament of the axilla** (Fig. 20–9).

Actions of the pectoralis major muscle are adduction, medial rotation, horizontal flexion, and horizontal extension of the humerus. Both heads of the muscle are active in adduction and medial rotation. The clavicular part is active in horizontal flexion (with anterior fibers of the deltoid muscle and the coracobrachialis muscle) (see Fig. 19–18*G*). The sternocostal part is active in horizontal extension (with the latissimus dorsi and teres major muscles and posterior fibers of the deltoid muscle) (see Fig. 19–18*H*). Both heads of the pectoralis major muscle are active in climbing movements, as when one is holding onto a rocky ledge and pulls the trunk upward toward the hands, and in forced inspiration (see Chapter 8).

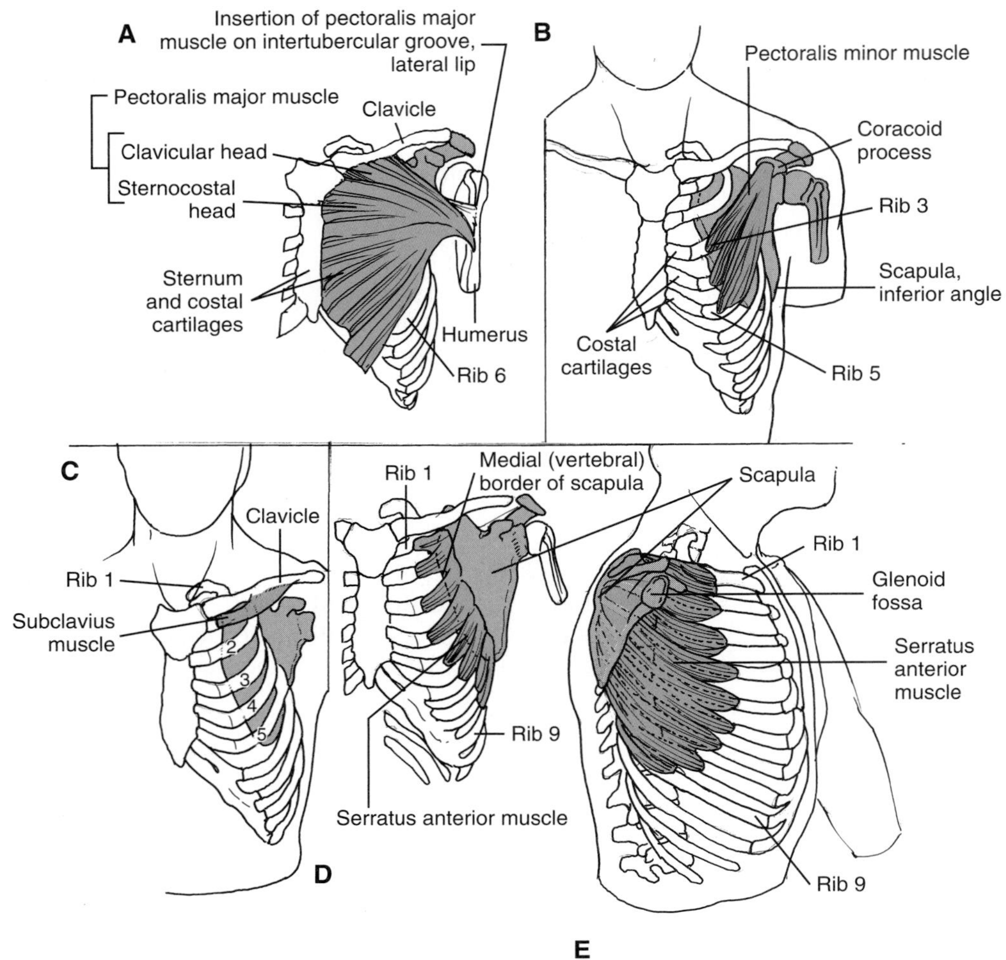

FIGURE 20–8

Pectoral thoracic muscles that connect the upper limb to the anterior thoracic wall. **A.** Pectoralis major muscle. **B.** Pectoralis minor muscle. **C.** Subclavius muscle. **D.** Anterior view of serratus anterior muscle. **E.** Lateral view of serratus anterior muscle.

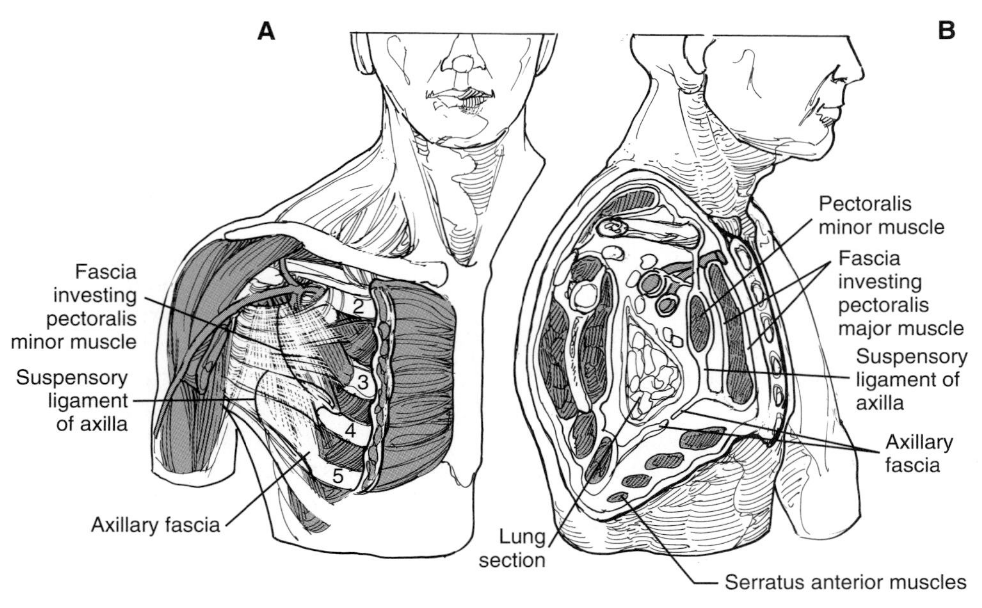

FIGURE 20–9

Suspensory ligament of the axilla and clavipectoral fascia. **A.** Anterior view. **B.** Lateral cut-away view.

Pectoralis Minor Muscle. Fibers of the thin, triangular pectoralis minor muscle arise from ribs 3 to 5 and from the deep fascia covering the intervening external intercostal muscles of the anterior chest wall between these ribs (see Fig. 20–8). As fibers of the pectoralis minor muscle course superolaterally, they converge to form a tendon, which may attach to the coracoid process of the scapula or to the coracoacromial and coracohumeral ligaments (or to both bone and ligaments).

Actions of the pectoralis minor muscle include depressing the clavicle (see Fig. 19–16*A*) and pulling the scapula forward (with the serratus anterior muscle). The pectoralis minor muscle also depresses the shoulder by depressing the clavicle (see Fig. 20–16*A*) (with the levator scapulae and rhomboid muscles as they medially rotate the scapula) (see Fig. 19–16*D*). With the scapula fixed, contraction of the pectoralis minor muscle may raise the ribs (e.g., in forced inspiration).

Subclavius Muscle. Fibers of the small, triangular subclavius muscle arise from the medial part of the first rib and its costal cartilage (see Fig. 20–8*C*). The fibers course superolaterally to attach to the undersurface of the middle part of the clavicle.

The primary action of the subclavius muscle is to depress the clavicle (see Fig. 19–16*A*). It may also stabilize the clavicle, particularly when one is climbing or hanging by one's hands.

Serratus Anterior Muscle. Fibers of the serratus anterior muscle arise as "fingers," or digitations, from the anterior surfaces of ribs 1 to 9 and from the deep fascia covering the intervening external intercostal muscles (see Fig. 20–8*D* and *E*). The line of attachment of these digitations is oblique. Superior digitations are more medial and inferior digitations more lateral. This flat sheet of muscle then courses around the lateral side of the thorax to the back as its fibers converge to form a wide tendon, which inserts upon the medial border of the scapula. Fibers arising from superior digitations of the muscle insert upon the anteromedial scapular border near its superior angle. Fibers of the inferior digitations insert upon the anteromedial border of the scapula near its inferior angle (i.e., there is no spiralization of these fibers).

Actions of the serratus anterior muscle include protraction (away from the midline) of the scapula (with the pectoralis minor muscle) (see Fig. 19–16*B*). All of the fibers of the serratus anterior muscle assist the trapezius muscle in stabilizing the scapula during the initial stages of abduction of the humerus. However, only the inferior fibers actively assist the trapezius muscle in lateral rotation of the scapula, which allows the arm to be raised above the head. The serratus anterior muscle may also assist in stabilizing the scapula against the trunk when one is carrying heavy objects or using the upper extremity to hold the body close to a fixed object.

Deep Fascia of Scapular and Pectoral Appendicular Muscles. In the scapular region, the deep fascia provides a strong anchor for the underlying trapezius muscle by connecting it directly to the nuchal lines of the skull, ligamentum nuchae, spine and acromial process of the scapula, and vertebral spines. In the lumbar region, the deep fascia anchors the latissimus dorsi muscle to the vertebral spines. This deep fascia is continuous with the **thoracolumbar fascia** of the back and the deep fascia of the axilla, anterior thorax, and abdomen. Inferiorly, it is connected to the iliac crests (see Chapter 5).

A specialization of deep fascia in the thorax is the **clavipectoral fascia.** This fascia arises from an inferior region of the posterior fascia of the pectoralis major muscle (see Chapter 6). It ascends as a single sheet, which splits into anterior and posterior sheets to invest the pectoralis minor muscle. These anterior and posterior layers recombine at the superior edge of the pectoralis minor muscle. They form a single sheet, which connects the muscle to the lower edge of the subclavius muscle. Here the sheet again splits into two sheets to invest the subclavius muscle. This fascia is pierced by pectoral branches of the thoracoacromial trunk, the medial and lateral pectoral nerves, and the cephalic vein (see Chapter 6).

Infections of the clavipectoral fascia may be superficial or deep. **Superficial infections** may occur between the pectoralis major and pectoralis minor muscles. An abscess may appear at the edge of the anterior axillary fold or in the groove between the pectoralis major and deltoid muscles on the anterior thoracic wall. **Deep infections** occur posterior to the pectoralis minor muscle and may enter the axilla to surround vessels and nerves. Pus may spread superiorly into the neck or inferiorly along brachial vessels into the arm. Access to this compartment for drainage of pus is through the inferior boundary of the axilla. This also provides a route for administering medications or, in the case of surgery of the upper extremity, for administering anesthesia for an **axillary nerve block.**

Muscles of the Arm

Muscles of the arm are separated by thickened **lateral** and **medial intermuscular septa** into an anterior flexor group and a posterior extensor group (Fig. 20–10). The flexor group includes the biceps brachii, brachialis, and coracobrachialis muscles; the extensor group consists mainly of the long, lateral, and medial heads of the triceps brachii muscle but also includes the diminutive subanconeus (articularis cubiti) muscle (Table 20–3).

The **lateral intermuscular septum** of the arm originates superiorly from the deep fascia of the deltoid muscle and is anchored to the lateral lip of the intertubercular sulcus. More inferiorly, it is anchored to the lateral surface of the humeral shaft and to the lateral supracondylar ridge and lateral epicondyle of the humerus (Fig. 20–10). The lateral intermuscular septum

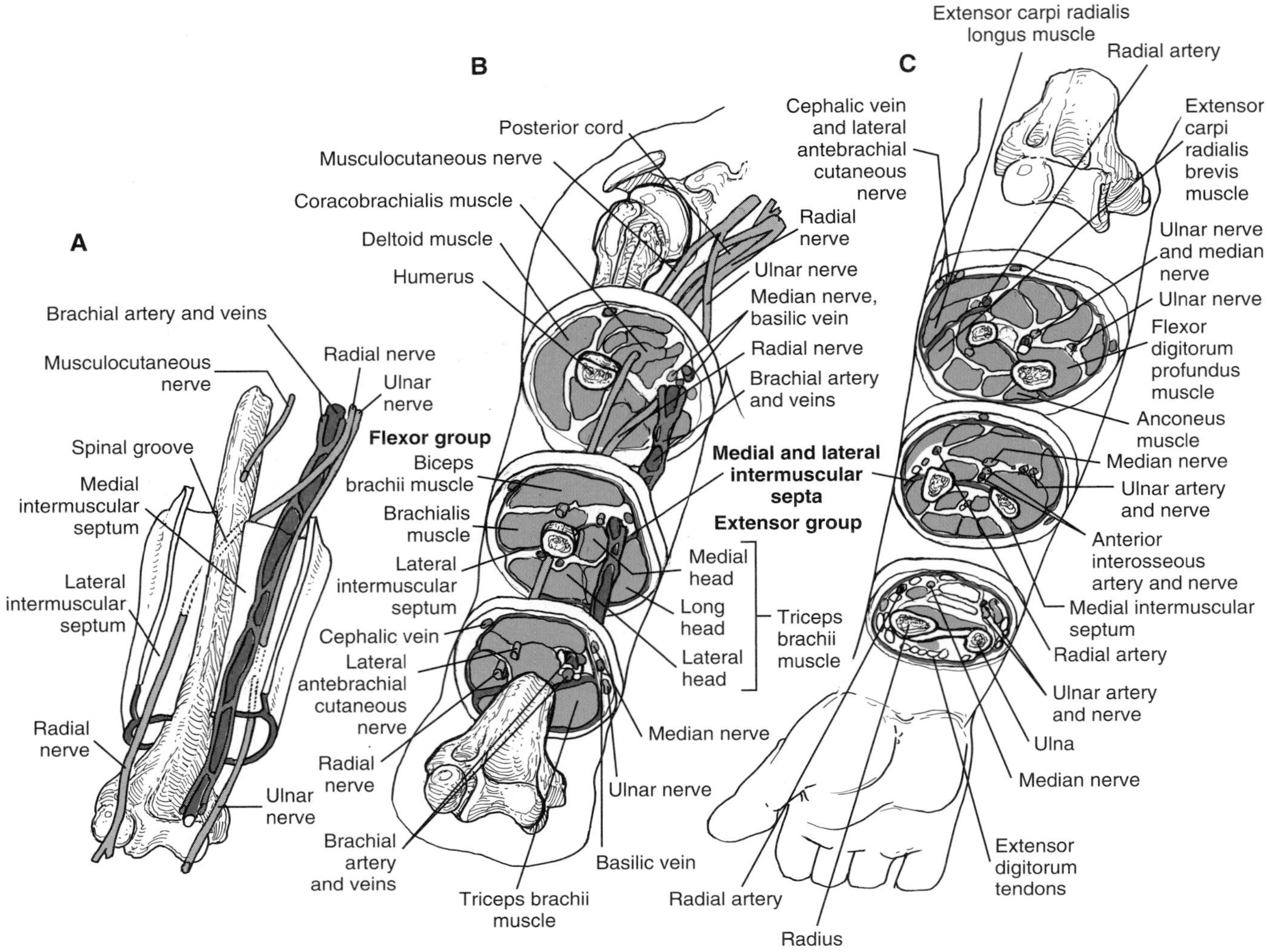

FIGURE 20–10
The lateral and medial intermuscular septa divide the arm muscles into anterior flexor and posterior extensor groups. **A.** Schematic drawing of intermuscular septa. **B.** Cross sectional view of the upper arm, showing intermuscular septa. **C.** Cross sectional view of the forearm, showing intermuscular septa.

serves as an anchoring site for the triceps brachii muscle posteriorly and the brachialis, brachioradialis, and extensor carpi radialis longus muscles anteriorly.

The thicker **medial intermuscular septum** of the arm arises from deep fascia of the teres major muscle and is anchored superiorly to the medial lip of the intertubercular sulcus. It is anchored more distally to the medial surface of the humeral shaft and to the medial supracondylar ridge and epicondyle of the humerus. In this region, it is also firmly attached to the tendon of the coracobrachialis muscle and to the olecranon process of the elbow (Fig. 20–10). The medial intermuscular septum provides an anchoring site for the triceps brachii muscle posteriorly and the brachialis muscle anteriorly. Deep fascia of the arm is continuous with deep fascia of the forearm.

Muscles of the Anterior (Flexor) Compartment. Muscles of the anterior compartment of the arm flex the arm horizontally and flex and supinate the forearm. Thus, the **coracobrachialis muscle** crosses the shoulder joint (Fig. 20–11*A*); the **biceps brachii muscle** crosses the glenohumeral and elbow joints (Fig. 20–11*B*); and the **brachialis muscle** crosses the elbow joint only (Fig. 20–11C). Both heads of the biceps brachii muscle and its tendons are superficial to the coracobrachialis and brachialis muscles.

The proximal tendon of the **coracobrachialis muscle** arises from the coracoid process of the scapula, along with the proximal tendon of the short head of the biceps brachii muscle (Fig. 20–11*A*). Its fibers course inferolaterally to insert upon the medial surface of the humeral shaft.

The main action of the coracobrachialis muscle is horizontal flexion of the humerus (see Fig. 19–18G). The muscle also stabilizes the humerus during abduction of the arm.

TABLE 20–3
Attachments and Actions of Muscles of the Arm

Muscle Group	Individual Muscle	Proximal Attachment	Distal Attachment	Muscle Action
Anterior (flexor) compartment of arm	Coracobrachialis	Coracoid process of scapula	Medial surface of humeral shaft	Horizontally flexes humerus, stabilizes humerus during abduction
	Biceps brachii	Short head from coracoid process of scapula, long head from supraglenoid tubercle of scapula	Radial tuberosity of radius	Flexes forearm, supinates forearm
	Brachialis	Anterior surface of inferior half of humerus, deltoid tuberosity	Coronoid process of ulna	Flexes forearm
Posterior (extensor) compartment of arm	Triceps brachii	Long head from infraglenoid tubercle of scapula, lateral head from posterior surface of inferior third of humerus, medial head from posterior surface of lower three fourths of humerus	Olecranon process of ulna, deep fascia of ventral forearm	Abducts arm; horizontally extends upper arm, extends arm, extends forearm
	Subanconeus	Distal deep medial head of triceps	Cubital capsule of elbow	Retracts capsule of elbow joint during extension

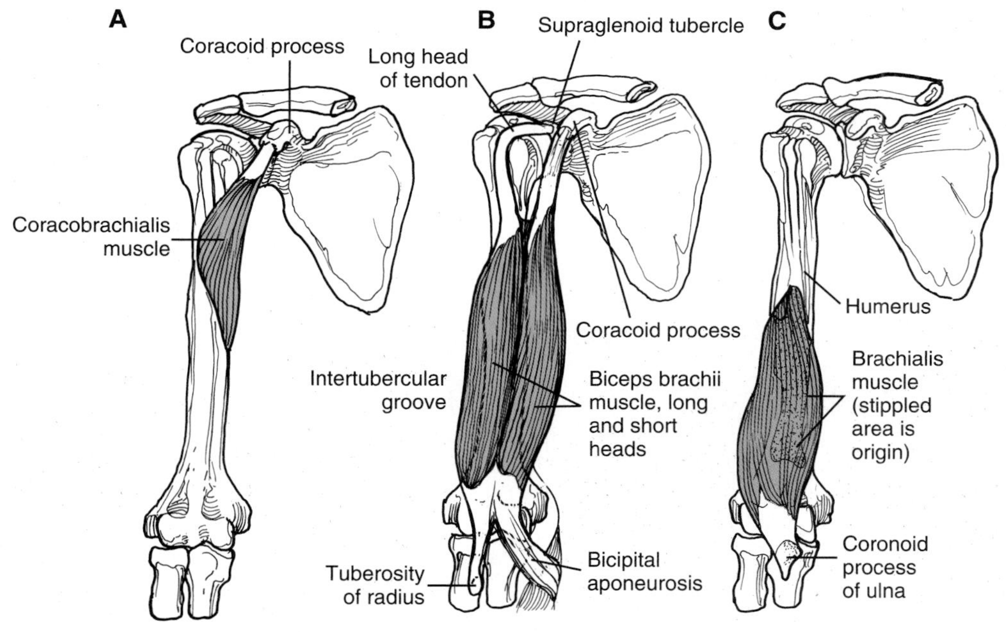

FIGURE 20–11
Muscles of the anterior (flexor) compartment of the arm. **A.** Coracobrachialis muscle. **B.** Biceps brachii muscle. **C.** Brachialis muscle.

The **biceps brachii muscle** has two expanded heads. The **short head** arises from a proximal tendon attached to the coracoid process of the scapula, and the **long head** arises from a proximal tendon attached to the **supraglenoid tubercle** of the scapula. The proximal tendon of the long head of the biceps brachii muscle courses over the humeral head through the **bicipital groove** (between the greater and lesser tubercles of the humerus) (Fig. 20–11*B*). Distal fibers of both heads converge to form a single distal tendon, which inserts upon the **radial tuberosity** of the radius. The tendon also has an expansion called the **bicipital aponeurosis,** which is attached to deep fascia covering the superficial flexors of the forearm. When the hand is supinated in anatomic position, the radial tuberosity is an elevated tubercle on the anterior surface of the radial shaft just distal to the proximal head and neck of the radius (Fig. 20–11*B*). With the hand and radius pronated, the radial tuberosity faces in a medial direction.

The main actions of the biceps brachii muscle are flexion and supination of the forearm. Supination (from a pronated position) occurs as the distal tendon of the muscle pulls the radial tuberosity anteriorly (see Fig. 19–22*D*). This action is strongest when the elbow is fixed in a flexed position. Indeed, the biceps brachii muscle is such a strong supinator of the radius that bolts and nuts are threaded so that they can be tightened by right-handed supination. The biceps brachii muscle also functions in flexion of the arm.

The **brachialis muscle** arises from a broad proximal tendon, which is attached to the anterior surface of the inferior half of the humerus and from the deltoid tuberosity (Fig. 20–11C). The muscle descends to cross the elbow joint and attaches to the medial and anterior aspects of the coronoid process of the ulna.

The main action of the brachialis muscle is to flex the elbow joint (see Fig. 19–21).

Muscles of the Posterior (Extensor) Compartment. The main muscle of the extensor compartment of the arm is the triceps brachii muscle. As its name implies, the muscle has three heads (Fig. 20–12). A diminutive second muscle in the extensor compartment is the subanconeus muscle.

The **long head** arise from the infraglenoid tubercle, and the **lateral head** from an oblique crest on the posterior surface of the upper third of the humeral shaft (Fig. 20–12*A*). The **medial head** arises from the lower three fourths of the posterior humeral surface (Fig. 20–12*B*). These heads are distinct throughout most of the extensor compartment, but as their fibers descend, they converge to form superficial and deep tendons about half as long as the humeral shaft. As these two flat tendons approach the olecranon process of the ulna, they fuse together, attach to the olecranon process, and then course distally to fuse with the deep fascia of the ventral forearm (Fig. 20–12*B*). The long head of the triceps brachii muscle descends between the teres minor and teres major muscles, dividing the lenticular-shaped space between them into a lateral **quadrangular space** and a medial **triangular space** (Fig. 20–12*C*). The boundaries of the quadrangular space are, therefore, the subscapularis and teres minor muscles superiorly, teres major muscle inferiorly, long head of the triceps brachii muscle medially, and humerus muscle laterally. The triangular space is bounded above by the teres minor muscle, below by the teres major muscle, and laterally by the long head of the triceps brachii muscle. The quadrangular space transmits the posterior humeral circumflex vessels and axillary nerve, while the triangular space encloses the circumflex scapular vessels (see below).

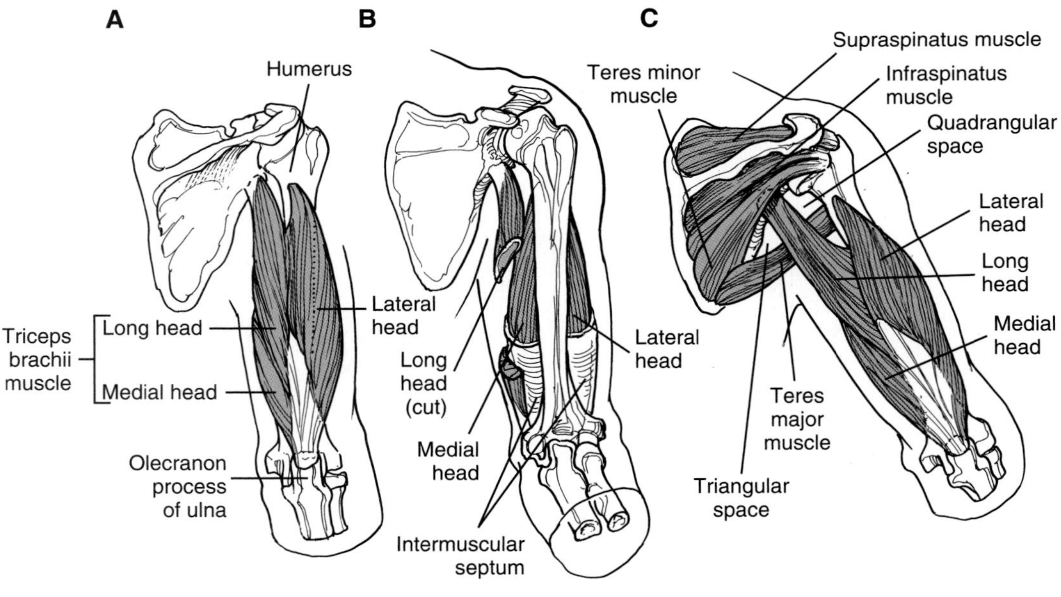

FIGURE 20–12
Muscles of the posterior (extensor) compartment. **A.** Posterior view of the triceps brachii muscle of the right arm. **B.** Anterior view of the medial head of the triceps brachii muscle of the left arm. **C.** Posterior view of the quadrangular and triangular spaces of the right arm.

The triceps brachii muscle acts to abduct and horizontally extend the upper arm and to extend the arm and forearm. It is the most important extensor of the elbow. The medial head of the triceps brachii muscle is active in all forms of extension, but the lateral and long heads are especially active in resisted extension (as when one is doing pushups). The long head, which crosses the inferior part of the shoulder joint, helps support the joint when the arm is raised.

The **subanconeus muscle,** sometimes called the **articularis cubiti muscle,** arises from fibers of the distal deep surface of the medial head of the triceps brachii muscle and inserts within the cubital capsule of the elbow. It *acts* to retract the capsule of the elbow joint during extension.

Muscles of the Forearm

Deep fascia of the forearm arises at the olecranon process and posterior border of the ulna. In this region, it gives rise to **lateral** and **medial intermuscular septa,** which, with the ulna, radius, and interosseous membrane, separate 19 forearm muscles into anterior (flexor) and posterior (extensor) groups (Table 20–4). Two additional **transverse septa** further separate muscles of the anterior and posterior antebrachial groups into the superficial and deep layers described below. As in the arm, these intermuscular septa provide attachment sites for muscles.

The anterior flexor compartment contains eight muscles, five in the superficial compartment and three in the deep compartment. One of the superficial flexors, the flexor digitorum superficialis muscle, is located between the other four superficial muscles and the three muscles of the deep compartment. It is, therefore, often classified as belonging to an intermediate layer of forearm flexors. The posterior extensor compartment contains 11 muscles—6 in the superficial compartment and 5 in the deep compartment. Superficial muscles in both the anterior and posterior compartments tend to originate from the humerus, while deep muscles in both compartments tend to originate from the ulna, radius, or interosseous membrane. Muscles of the forearm are usually named for their actions, locations, or shapes. Muscles named for their **actions** include the pronator teres muscle, which pronates the radius; the flexor carpi ulnaris muscle, which flexes the wrist; and the extensor digitorum muscle, which extends the digits. Muscles named for their **locations** include the brachioradialis muscle, which courses from the brachium (arm) to the radius of the forearm; the flexor digitorum superficialis muscle, which is in the superficial flexor compartment; and the anconeus muscle, which is near the elbow (ancon). A muscle named for its **shape** is the pronator quadratus muscle, which has a quadrilateral shape.

Several muscles of the flexor compartment could not function without the mechanism of the **flexor retinaculum.** In the lower extremity, the retinacula and enclosed synovial sheaths of the ankles serve as pulleys for muscles of the legs that must act on the feet and toes (see Chapter 17). In the same way, retinacula in the wrist facilitate the actions of forearm muscles serving the hands and fingers.

Anterior Antebrachial Flexors. Although the anterior compartment of the forearm is named the "flexor" compartment, it also includes two "pronators": the pronator teres muscle in the superficial compartment and pronator quadratus muscle in the deep compartment. All of the superficial flexors act on the elbow, wrist, hand, or finger joints. The deep flexors act only on the wrist, hand, or finger joints. The actions of some of these muscles are facilitated by a fibrous band—the **flexor retinaculum.** The flexor retinaculum is connected to the pisiform bone and hook of the hamate bone medially (i.e., on the ulnar side of the wrist). On the lateral (radial side) of the wrist, the flexor retinaculum splits into superficial and deep laminae. The superficial lamina attaches to the scaphoid and trapezium bones, while the deep lamina dives deep to attach to a deeper medial projection of the trapezium bone, forming a small tunnel that encloses the synovial sheath and tendon of the flexor carpi radialis muscle. The more median region deep to the flexor retinaculum encloses the median nerve and two synovial sheaths. The lateral sheath invests the flexor pollicis longus tendon only. The medial sheath invests tendons of the flexor digitorum superficialis muscles (superficial group) and flexor digitorum profundus (deep group) (Fig. 20–13*B*). This restricted space between the flexor retinaculum and the carpal bones that encloses tendons and the medial nerve is called the **carpal tunnel.** Any condition that causes inflammation within the carpal tunnel may result in pain (see Chapter 21).

The ulnar nerve, cutaneous branches of the ulnar and median nerves, ulnar vessels, and tendons of the palmaris longus and flexor carpi ulnaris muscles are superficial to the flexor retinaculum (Fig. 20–13*B*). Transverse fibers of the palmar aponeurosis (sometimes called the **palmar carpal ligament**) and the tendon of the palmaris longus muscle pass over the superficial palmar branch of the radial artery on the radial side of the wrist and the ulnar vessels and nerves on the ulnar side of the wrist (Fig. 20–15*A*). This layer of fascia is distinct from the superficial lamina of the carpal tunnel.

Superficial Compartment. The five muscles of the superficial flexor compartment of the forearm, called the **superficial anterior antebrachial flexors,** are the pronator teres, flexor carpi radialis, palmaris longus, flexor carpi ulnaris, and flexor digitorum superficialis muscles (Fig. 20–14).

The **pronator teres muscle** has two heads. The large **humeral head** arises from the humerus just proximal to the medial epicondyle and common flexor ten-

TABLE 20–4
Attachments and Actions of Muscles of the Forearm

Muscle Group	Individual Muscle	Proximal Attachment	Distal Attachment	Muscle Action
Superficial anterior antebrachial flexors	Pronator teres	Humerus just proximal to medial epicondyle, common flexor tendon attached to medial epicondyle of humerus, medial side of coronoid process of ulna	Lateral surface of midregion of radius	Pronates forearm and hand
	Flexor carpi radialis	Common flexor tendon attached to medial epicondyle of humerus	Base of second metacarpal	Flexes wrist, abducts hand
	Palmaris longus	Common flexor tendon attached to medial epicondyle of humerus	Palmar aponeurosis	Weakly flexes wrist, tenses connective tissue of palm
	Flexor carpi ulnaris	Common flexor tendon attached to medial epicondyle of humerus, medial edge of olecranon process and proximal two thirds of posterior ulnar surface	Pisiform, hamate, fifth metacarpal	Flexes wrist, adducts hand
	Flexor digitorum superficialis	Common flexor tendon attached to medial epicondyle of humerus, ulnar collateral ligament, medial side of coronoid process of ulna, anterior border of radius just distal to radial tuberosity	Superficial tendon splits to serve digits 3 and 4, deep tendon splits to serve digits 2 and 5 by attaching to sides of middle phalanx in each case	Flexes wrist and proximal and middle phalanges of digits 2 to 5
Deep anterior antebrachial flexors	Flexor digitorum profundus	Posterior border of ulna, anterior surface of upper third of ulna, upper third of ulnar half of interosseous membrane	Bases of distal phalanges of digits 2 to 5	Flexes distal phalanges of digits 2 to 5
	Flexor pollicis longus	Anterior surface of radius distal to radial tuberosity	Palmar surface of base of most distal phalanx of thumb	Flexes both phalanges of thumb
	Pronator quadratus	Oblique ridge on anterior surface of distal ulna	Lower fourth of anterior surface of radius	Pronates forearm and hand
Superficial posterior antebrachial extensors	Brachioradialis	Upper two thirds of supracondylar ridge on lateral side of humerus	Lateral surface of radius near midpoint or to styloid process, or both	Flexes elbow, although muscle is innervated by radial nerve (see text)
	Extensor carpi radialis longus	Distal third of supracondylar ridge on lateral side of humerus, common extensor tendon attached to lateral epicondyle of humerus	Dorsal side of base of second metacarpal	Extends wrist, abducts wrist
	Extensor carpi radialis brevis	Common extensor tendon attached to lateral epicondyle of humerus	Radial side of base of third metacarpal	Extends wrist, abducts wrist
	Extensor digitorum	Common extensor tendon attached to lateral epicondyle of humerus	Dorsal digital expansions and bases of proximal phalanges of digits 2 to 5	Extends wrist, extends all phalanges of digits 2 to 5
	Extensor digiti minimi	Common extensor tendon attached to lateral epicondyle of humerus	Dorsal digital expansion of digit 5	Extends wrist, extends all phalanges of digit 5
	Extensor carpi ulnaris	Common extensor tendon attached to lateral epicondyle of humerus	Base of fifth metacarpal	Extends wrist, adducts hand
	Anconeus	Independent tendon attached to lateral epicondyle of humerus	Lateral surface of olecranon process and posterior surface of proximal end of ulna	Extends forearm

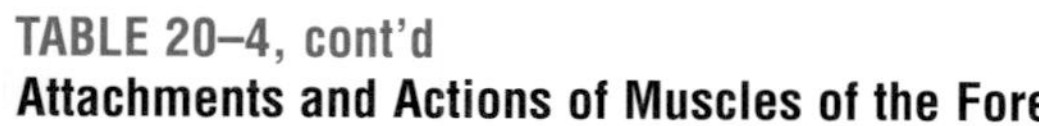

TABLE 20–4, cont'd
Attachments and Actions of Muscles of the Forearm

Muscle Group	Individual Muscle	Proximal Attachment	Distal Attachment	Muscle Action
Deep posterior antebrachial extensors	Supinator	Lateral epicondyle, radial collateral ligament, annular ligament, supinator crest	Lateral surface of proximal end of radial shaft	Supinates forearm and hand
	Abductor pollicis longus	Posterior surface of ulna, posterior surface of interosseous membrane, middle third of posterior surface of radial shaft	Radial side of base of first metacarpal, trapezium	Abducts thumb, assists in extension of thumb
	Extensor pollicis brevis	Posterior surface of radius and posterior surface of interosseous membrane	Posterolateral surface of base of first metacarpal	Extends thumb
	Extensor pollicis longus	Posterior surface of middle third of ulna, posterior surface of adjacent region of interosseous membrane	Base of distal phalanx of thumb	Extends thumb
	Extensor indicis	Posterior surface of ulna; posterior surface of adjacent region of interosseous membrane	Dorsal surface of base of proximal phalanx of digit 2	Extends digit 2

don in this region. The smaller **ulnar head** arises from the medial side of the coronoid process of the ulna. Its fibers descend laterally to attach to the lateral surface of the radius in its midregion (Fig. 20–14*A*).

As its name implies, the pronator teres muscle acts as a pronator. With the pronator quadratus muscle, it pulls on the supinated radius to pronate the palm (i.e., to turn the palm medially and posteriorly).

The **flexor carpi radialis muscle** is located just medial to the pronator teres muscle. This radial flexor of the wrist arises from the common flexor tendon attached to the medial epicondyle of the humerus (Fig. 20–14*B*). Its fibers course distally and somewhat laterally, quickly tapering to form a long tendon. This tendon slips into the palm through a canal formed by fibers of the flexor retinaculum within a synovial sheath cradled in a groove in the trapezium bone (see above). The tendon then inserts upon the base of the second metacarpal.

The action of the flexor carpi radialis muscle is to flex the wrist (with the flexor carpi ulnaris, flexor digitorum superficialis, and palmaris muscles) and abduct the hand (with the extensors on the radial side of the posterior extensor compartment) (see Fig. 19–24).

The **palmaris longus muscle** is a slender muscle, which lies just medial to the flexor carpi radialis muscle. Like the pronator teres and flexor carpi radialis muscles, its proximal tendon arises from the common flexor tendon attached to the medial epicondyle of the humerus (Fig. 20–14*C*). Fibers within the short belly of this muscle descend and quickly taper to form a long distal tendon, which passes over the flexor retinaculum of the wrist (see above). This tendon inserts into a tough aponeurosis of superficial connective tissue in the proximal region of the palm (Fig. 20–14*C*). Indeed, lateral, central, and medial parts of the **palmar aponeurosis** cover the entire palm (Fig. 20–15). The thin lateral and medial parts cover the thenar and hypothenar muscles. The tendon of the palmaris longus muscle splays into the thickened triangular central region, which covers the digital flexor tendons and superficial palmar arch. Digital extensions emanate from the distal edge of this central region of the palmar aponeurosis. Transverse fibers at the proximal end of the palmar aponeurosis are sometimes called the *palmar carpal ligament.*

Infections of the palmar aponeurosis may occur in response to repeated injury and infection and may eventually result in the progressive, disabling **Dupuytren's contracture** of the aponeurosis. Tightening of the palmar fascia may also result in forced flexion of the fourth digit. Infection may spread to the pulp of the fingers and flexor synovial sheaths, particularly the common flexor sheath and sheaths of the first and fifth digits (see above).

The palmaris longus muscle acts to weakly flex the wrist and tense the connective tissue of the palm.

A
Palmaris longus tendon
Hamate hook
Flexor retinaculum
Pisiform bone
Ulnar artery
Ulnar nerve
Flexor carpi ulnaris tendon
Thenar muscles
Trapezium bone
Radial artery
Flexor carpi radialis tendon
Flexor retinaculum
Median nerve
Flexor digitorum superficialis tendon

C
(2) Extensor carpi radialis brevis and longus tendons
(3) Extensor pollicis longus synovial sheath
Extensor retinaculum
(1) Abductor pollicis longus muscle
(4) Extensor indicis and extensor digitorum tendons
(5) Extensor digiti minimi tendon
(6) Extensor carpi ulnaris tendon
(1) Extensor pollicis brevis tendon

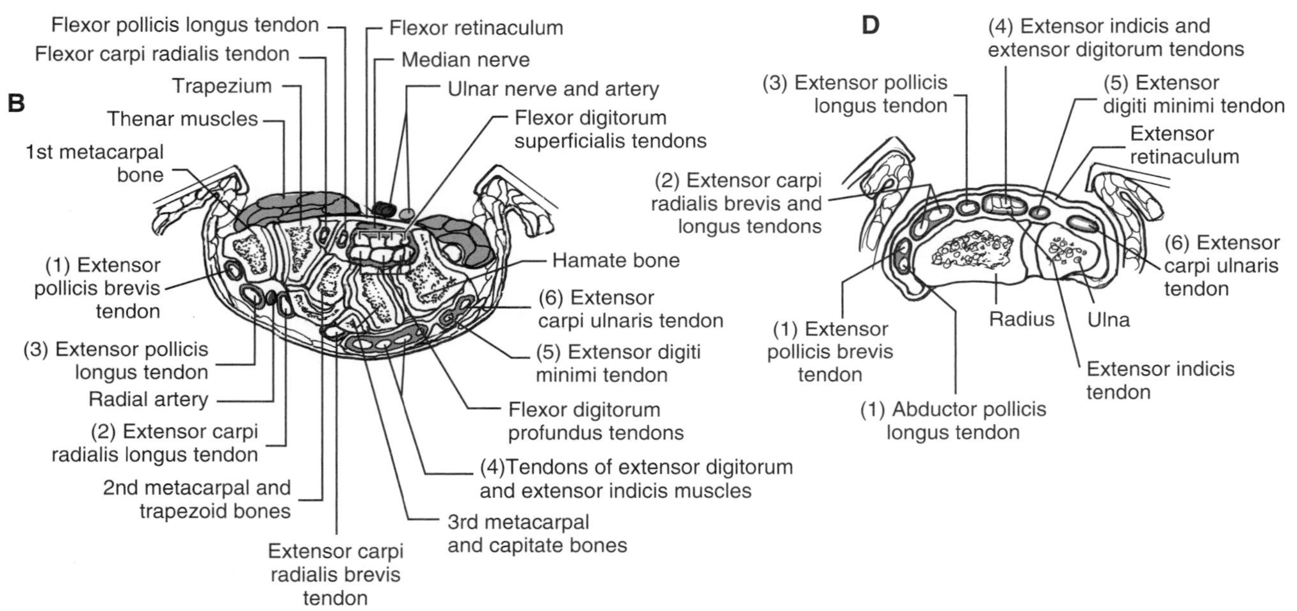

FIGURE 20–13

Relationship of retinacula within the wrist to anterior antebrachial flexors and posterior antebrachial extensors acting at the level of the wrist. The figure shows the retinacula, synovial sheaths, tendons, and area of the carpal tunnel. **A.** Palmar view of "flexor" compartment. **B.** Cross section through the wrist at the level of the flexor retinaculum. **C.** Dorsal view of extensor compartment, showing extensor retinaculum, tendons, and synovial sheaths. **D.** Cross section proximal to wrist, showing extensor retinaculum.

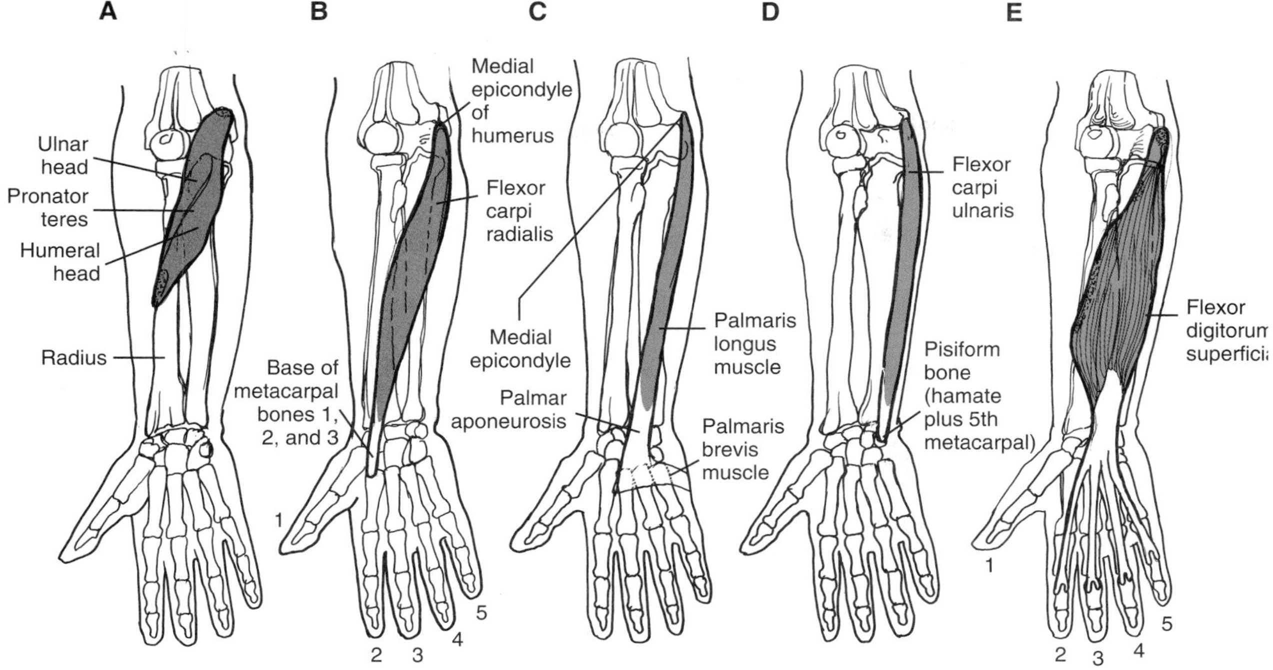

FIGURE 20–14
Muscles of the superficial flexor compartment of the forearm. **A.** Pronator teres muscle. **B.** Flexor carpi radialis muscle. **C.** Palmaris longus muscle. **D.** Flexor carpi ulnaris muscle. **E.** Flexor digitorum superficialis muscle.

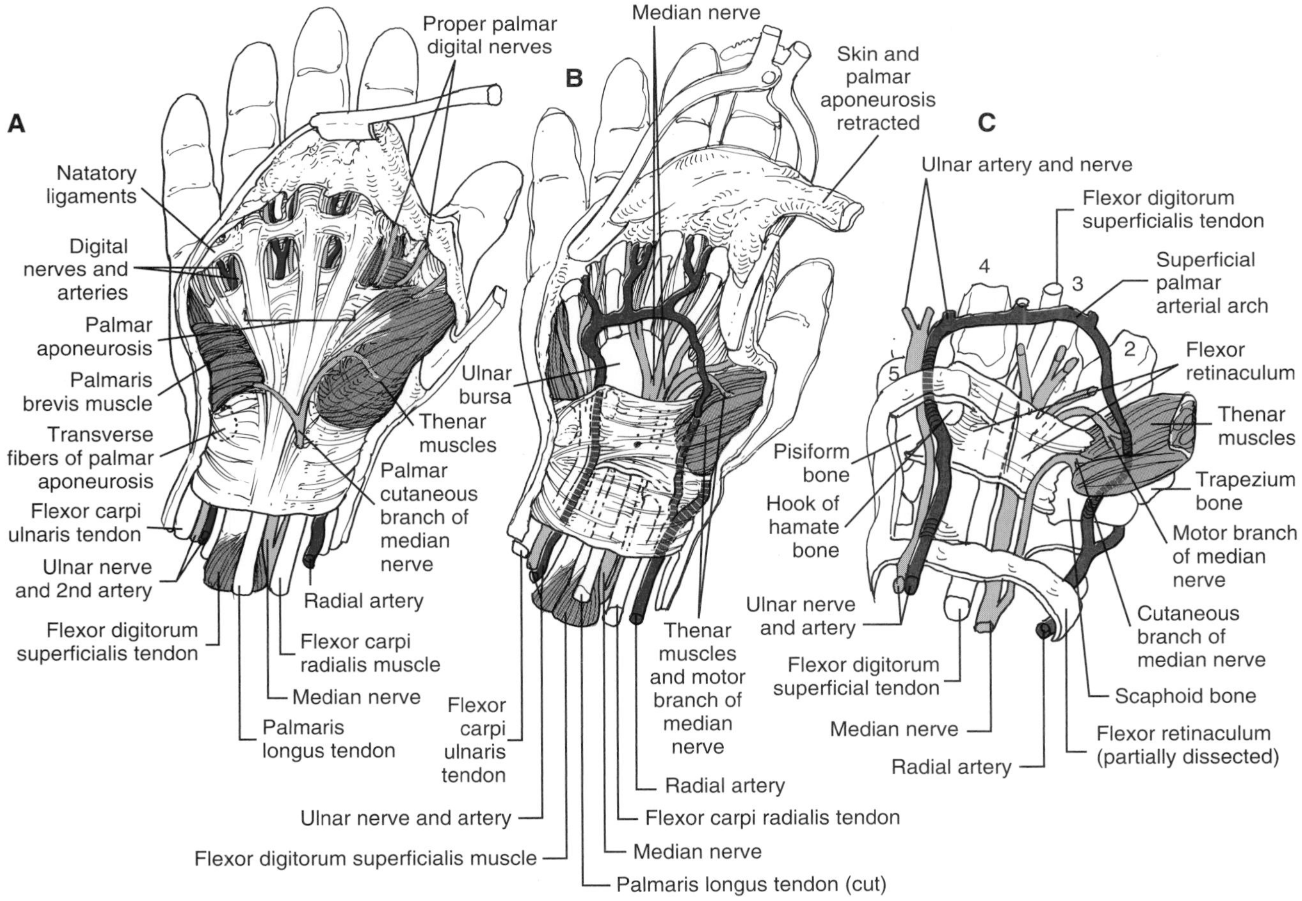

FIGURE 20–15
Palmar aponeurosis. **A.** Superficial palmar view. **B.** Palmar aponeurosis retracted. **C.** Schematic drawing of area of carpal ligament. Dotted red lines indicate possible surgical incision lines through flexor retinaculum for relieving symptoms of carpal tunnel syndrome.

The **flexor carpi ulnaris muscle** is the most medial flexor of the superficial anterior forearm. It has two heads. The small **humeral head** arises from the common flexor tendon attached to the medial epicondyle of the humerus. The **ulnar head** arises from the medial edge of the olecranon process of the ulna and from the proximal two thirds of the posterior ulnar surface. Fibers from the two heads converge and course distally along the medial edge of the forearm, tapering to form a distal tendon, which inserts upon the pisiform, hamate, and fifth metacarpal bones (Fig. 20–14*D*).

Actions of the flexor carpi ulnaris muscle include flexion of the wrist (with the flexor carpi radialis, flexor digitorum superficialis, and palmaris longus muscles) and adduction of the hand (with the extensor carpi ulnaris muscle) (see Fig. 19–24).

The **flexor digitorum superficialis muscle** flexes the fingers. It lies just deep to the four muscles described above and superficial to deep antebrachial flexors in an "intermediate" layer (see Fig. 20–3*B*). It arises from two heads. The distal tendon of its **humeroulnar head** arises from the common flexor tendon associated with the medial epicondyle of the humerus, from the ulnar collateral ligament, and from the medial side of the coronoid process of the ulna. The distal tendon of its **radial head** is attached to the anterior border of the radius, just distal to the radial tuberosity. Muscle fibers of both heads descend, converging to form superficial and deep tendons. The superficial tendon divides into two parts to serve digits 3 and 4, while the deep tendon splits into two parts to serve digits 2 and 5 (see Fig. 20–14*E*). All four tendons pass deep to the flexor retinaculum (see above) and diverge in the palm to course to the digits they serve. At the base of each proximal phalanx, each tendon splits. The split fibers of the tendon reunite to surround a deeper tendon from the flexor digitorum profundus muscle, which is a muscle of the deep forearm flexor group. The tendon splits again to attach to both sides of the shaft of the middle phalanx (see Figs. 20–17 and 20–24).

The flexor digitorum superficialis muscle acts to flex the wrist and the proximal and middle phalanges.

Deep Compartment. The three muscles of the deep flexor compartment of the forearm, the **deep anterior antebrachial flexors,** are the flexor digitorum profundus, flexor pollicis longus, and pronator quadratus muscles (Fig. 20–16).

The **flexor digitorum profundus muscle** is the most medial muscle of the deep flexor compartment. Its distal tendon arises from the posterior border of the ulna (with the flexor carpi ulnaris muscle), the anterior surface of the upper third of the ulna, and the upper third of the ulnar half of the interosseous membrane (Fig. 20–16*A*). Its fibers descend within the forearm deep to the flexor digitorum superficialis muscle and then within the midregion of the forearm. The fibers split into two tendons, one serving digit 2 and the other serving digits 3 to 5. The latter tendon splits into three separate tendons in the distal third of the forearm. All four tendons course under the flexor retinaculum (see above), deep to the tendons of the flexor digitorum superficialis muscle. Each of these deep flexor tendons

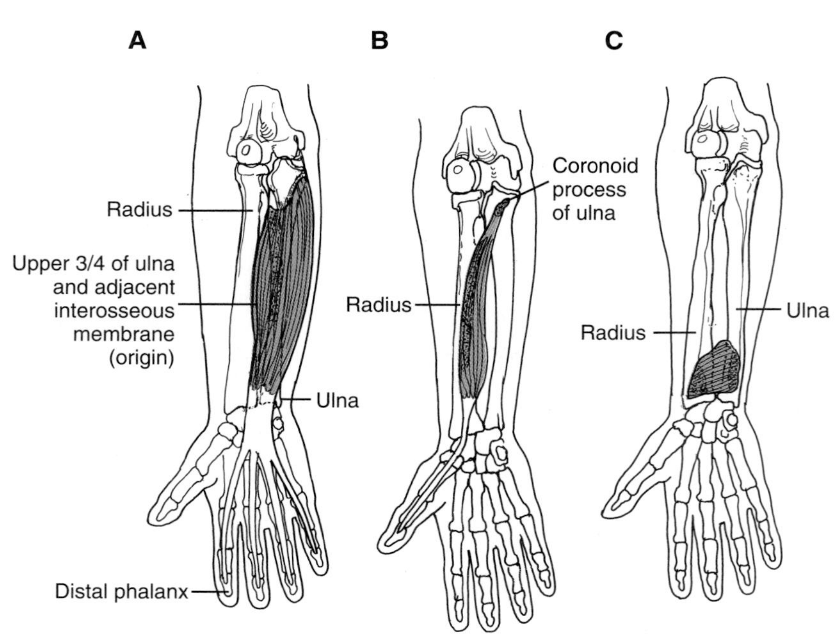

FIGURE 20–16
Deep flexor compartment of the forearm. **A.** Flexor digitorum profundus muscle. **B.** Flexor pollicis longus muscle. **C.** Pronator quadratus muscle.

courses to the base of each proximal phalanx where each tendon enters the channel created by the splitting of tendons of the flexor digitorum superficialis muscle (see above). After emerging from these tendinous canals, each profundus tendon inserts upon the palmar surface of the base of the distal phalanx that it serves (Fig. 20–17*A*). The split tendons of the flexor digitorum superficialis muscles (along with **digital fibrous flexor sheaths** and their enclosed **synovial sheaths**) serve as pulleys for the flexor digitorum profundus muscle (Fig. 20–17).

The action of the flexor digitorum profundus muscle is to flex the distal phalanx as the flexor digitorum superficialis muscle flexes the middle and proximal phalanges (Fig. 20–17 and see Fig. 20–24*B*). The actions of the flexor digitorum profundus muscle are also modified by resistance from the dorsal extensors (typically when only one digit is flexed) and by the interosseous and lumbrical muscles (Fig. 20–17). It should also be noted that weak flexion of the hand and digits is accomplished by contraction of the flexor digitorum superficialis muscle alone, whereas strong flexion (which includes flexion of the distal phalanges) requires the additional action of the flexor digitorum profundus muscle.

The **flexor pollicis longus muscle** is located adjacent and lateral to the flexor digitorum profundus muscle (see Fig. 20–16*B*). Its distal tendon arises from the anterior surface of the radius between the radial tuberosity and the attachment of the pronator quadratus muscle in the lower third of the forearm and the radial half of the interosseous membrane. Its fibers descend within the forearm, converging to form a single flat proximal tendon just anterior to the pronator quadratus muscle. This tendon narrows as it slips into the palm under the flexor retinaculum (see above). It then

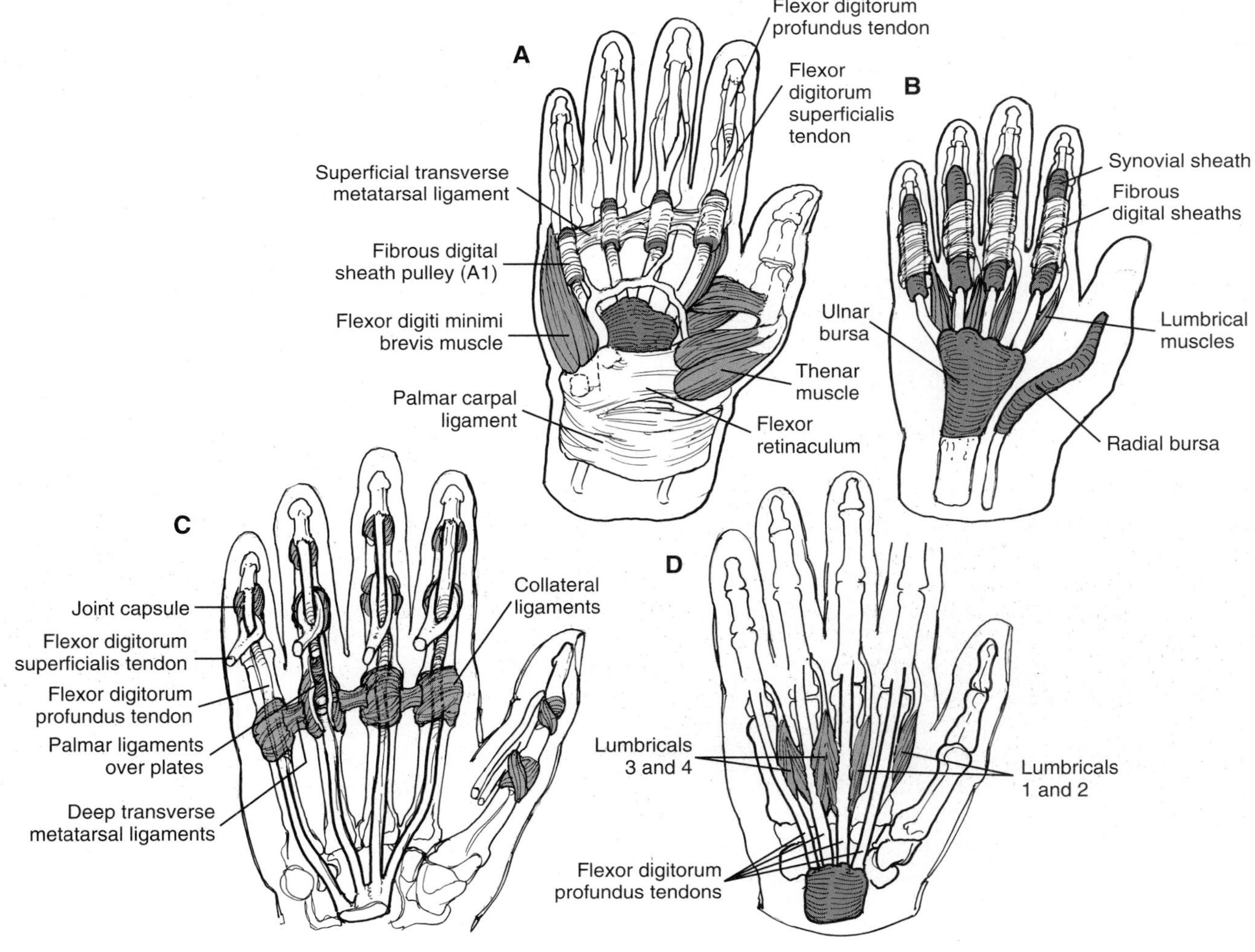

FIGURE 20–17
Split tendons, along with digital fibrous flexor sheaths and synovial sheaths, serve as pulleys for the flexor digitorum profundus muscle. **A.** View showing split tendons of flexor digitorum superficialis muscle. **B.** Synovial sheath, fibrous digital sheaths, and bursa. **C.** Joint capsules and collateral ligaments. **D.** Lumbrical muscles in relation to the flexor digitorum profundus tendons.

inserts upon the palmar surface of the base of the most distal phalanx of the thumb. Because the tendon is not split, it does not form a canal as do the tendons for digits 2 to 5 (see Fig. 20–16*B*).

The primary action of the flexor pollicis longus muscle is to flex both phalanges of the thumb.

The quadrilateral **pronator quadratus muscle** arises from the oblique ridge on the anterior surface of the ulna. It then courses laterally (and somewhat distally) to insert upon the lower fourth of the anterior surface of the radius (see Fig. 20–16*C*).

The action of the pronator quadratus muscle is to pronate the radius (with the more proximal pronator teres muscle), moving the palm medially so that it faces posteriorly. The pronator quadratus muscle also assists the interosseous membrane in preventing forceful separation of the ulna and radius.

Posterior Antebrachial Extensors. Muscles of the posterior compartment of the forearm function mainly as extensors. The only exception is the brachioradialis muscle, which is a flexor and which also assists the biceps brachii muscle in supination. All of the muscles within the posterior compartment of the forearm act upon a proximodistal series of joints (from the elbow or wrist to the wrist or phalanges), except for the brachioradialis and anconeus muscles (which act upon the elbow joint only) and the supinator muscle (which acts upon the radioulnar joint). The actions of several posterior antebrachial muscles that act on the hand and fingers are facilitated by an extensor retinaculum. The **extensor retinaculum** is attached to the anterior border of the radius (laterally) and to the triquetral and pisiform bones (medially). It contains six synovial sheaths that enclose tendons of the following nine muscles (listed from lateral to medial):

1. extensor pollicis brevis and abductor pollicis longus muscles,
2. extensor carpi radialis longus and extensor carpi radialis brevis muscles,
3. extensor pollicis longus muscle,
4. extensor digitorum and extensor indicis muscles,
5. extensor digiti minimi muscle, and
6. extensor carpi ulnaris muscles (Fig. 20–13*C* and *D*).

The superficial branches of the ulnar and radial nerves course over the extensor retinaculum.

Superficial Compartment. Muscles of the superficial extensor (posterior) compartment of the forearm—the **superficial posterior antebrachial extensors**—are the brachioradialis, extensor carpi radialis longus, extensor carpi radialis brevis, extensor digitorum, extensor digiti minimi, extensor carpi ulnaris, and anconeus muscles.

The proximal tendon of the **brachioradialis muscle** originates from the upper two-thirds of the supracondylar ridge on the lateral side of the humerus (Fig. 20–18*A*). Its muscle fibers cross (and may even fuse with) the lower fibers of the brachialis muscle (see above). The fibers descend to form a distal tendon, which usually inserts upon the lateral surface of the radius near its midpoint but may extend as far as the styloid process.

The brachioradialis muscle acts to flex the elbow (especially against resistance). The muscle is innervated by the radial nerve, which, however, mainly innervates the extensor muscles.

The **extensor carpi radialis longus muscle** is adjacent to and just medial to the brachioradialis muscle (Fig. 20–18*B*). Its proximal tendon arises from the distal third of the supracondylar ridge on the lateral surface of the humerus and from the common extensor tendon. Its muscle fibers then sweep distally along the lateral forearm, converging to form a distal tendon at the lower boundary of the middle third of the forearm. This flat tendon descends under the abductor pollicis muscle (see below) and extensor pollicis brevis muscle within a dorsal groove on the radius. The tendon then slips into the dorsum of the hand by passing deep to the extensor retinaculum. The tendon inserts on the dorsal side of the base of the second metacarpal.

Actions of the extensor carpi radialis longus muscle are extension of the wrist (with the extensor carpi radialis brevis and extensor carpi ulnaris muscles) and abduction (with the extensor carpi radialis brevis and flexor carpi radialis muscles).

The **extensor carpi radialis brevis muscle** is located just medial and deep to the extensor carpi radialis longus muscle (Fig. 20–18*C*). It arises from the lateral epicondyle of the humerus via the common extensor tendon and radial collateral ligament. Its fibers descend within the forearm, converging to form a tendon in its midregion. This flat tendon passes deep to the abductor pollicis longus and extensor pollicis brevis muscles. It then passes under the extensor retinaculum to insert upon the radial side of the base of the third metacarpal.

Actions of the extensor carpi radialis brevis muscle are extension of the wrist (with the extensor carpi radialis longus and extensor carpi ulnaris muscles) and abduction of the wrist (with the extensor carpi radialis longus and flexor carpi radialis muscles).

The **extensor digitorum muscle** arises from the lateral epicondyle of the humerus via the common extensor tendon (Fig. 20–18*D*). Its fibers descend within the forearm just adjacent and medial to the belly of the extensor carpi radialis longus muscle. In the midregion of the forearm, the extensor digitorum muscle splits into four tendons, which pass deep to the extensor retinaculum within a synovial sheath. This synovial sheath also carries the tendon of the extensor indicis muscle (Fig. 20–18*D*). Each tendon courses distally to form a **dorsal digital expansion** on phalanges 2 to 5. "Wings" of the dorsal digital expansion are attached to the lateral sides of the base of each proximal phalanx through their connections to interosseous tendons (see below). Prox-

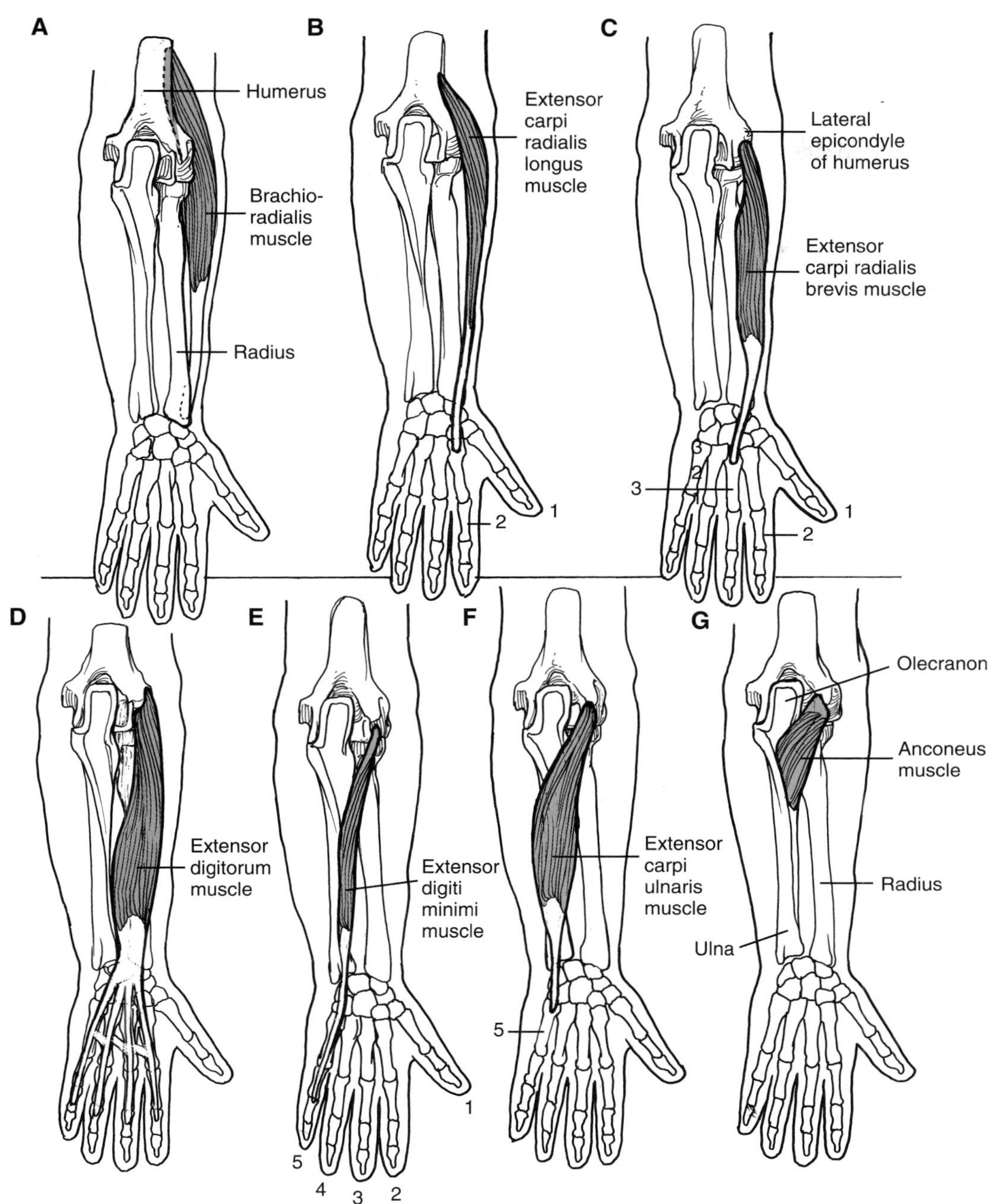

FIGURE 20–18

Superficial posterior extensor compartment of the forearm. **A.** Brachioradialis muscle. **B.** Extensor carpi radialis longus muscle. **C.** Extensor carpi radialis brevis muscle. **D.** Extensor digitorum muscle. **E.** Extensor digiti minimi muscle. **F.** Extensor carpi ulnaris muscle. **G.** Anconeus muscle.

imal continuations of these dorsal digital expansions are also attached to the dorsal surfaces of the bases of the middle and distal phalanges.

The extensor digitorum muscle acts to extend the wrist and the metacarpophalangeal and interphalangeal joints of digits 2 to 5.

The **extensor digiti minimi muscle,** which lies just medial to the extensor digitorum muscle, arises from the common extensor tendon attached to the lateral epicondyle of the humerus (Fig. 20–18*E*). Its fibers descend within the forearm, converging to form a tendon at its midpoint. This flat tendon passes under the extensor retinaculum (within its own synovial sheath) and onto the dorsum of the fifth digit. Here, the distal tendon splits into two slips, which are joined by the tendon of the extensor digitorum muscle to the fifth digit.

All three of these tendons are, together, attached to the dorsal digital expansion of the fifth digit, which is attached to the proximal, middle, and distal phalanges in the manner described above (Fig. 20–18*E*). The extensor digiti minimi muscle acts to extend the wrist and the metacarpophalangeal and interphalangeal joints of the fifth digit (with the extensor digitorum muscle).

The **extensor carpi ulnaris muscle** is the most medial muscle of the superficial posterior (extensor) compartment of the forearm (Fig. 20–18*F*). Its proximal tendon arises from the common extensor tendon attached to the lateral epicondyle of the humerus. Its fibers course medially as they descend within the forearm and then converge in its midregion to form a tendon that passes under the most medial region of the extensor retinaculum within its own compartment. This tendon slips within a groove between the distal ulnar head and ulnar styloid process and inserts upon the medial tubercle at the base of the fifth metacarpal.

The extensor carpi ulnaris muscle acts to extend the wrist (with the extensor carpi radialis longus and extensor carpi radialis brevis muscles). It adducts the hand (with the flexor carpi ulnaris muscle).

The **anconeus muscle** is a short muscle associated with the posterior side of the elbow joint. It arises from an independent proximal tendon from the lateral epicondyle of the humerus (Fig. 20–18*G*). Its fibers sweep medially over the annular ligament to form a tendon that inserts upon the lateral surface of the olecranon process and posterior surface of the proximal end of the ulna (Fig. 20–18*G*).

The action of the anconeus muscle is to extend the elbow joint (with the triceps brachii muscle).

Deep Compartment. Muscles of the deep extensor (posterior) compartment of the forearm, the **deep posterior antebrachial extensors,** are the supinator, abductor pollicis longus, extensor pollicis brevis, extensor pollicis longus, and extensor indicis muscles.

The proximal tendon of the **supinator muscle** arises from the lateral epicondyle, radial collateral ligament, annular ligament, and supinator crest (i.e., the proximal extension of the interosseous border) of the ulna (Fig. 20–19*A* and *B*). Its fibers course medially and inferiorly, converging to form a broad proximal tendon, which inserts upon the lateral surface of the proximal end of the radial shaft.

The supinator muscle acts to supinate the hand, turning the palm to face anteriorly from a pronated position. The supinator muscle acts with the biceps brachii muscle, particularly when the forearm is flexed or is in the process of being flexed.

The proximal tendon of the **abductor pollicis longus muscle** originates from the posterior surface of the ulna (just distal to the anconeus muscle), the posterior surface of the interosseous membrane, and the middle third of the posterior surface of the radial shaft (just distal to the insertion of the supinator muscle) (Fig. 20–19*C*). The abductor pollicis longus muscle descends obliquely toward the thumb. Its fibers converge to form a distal tendon, which usually splits into two tendons. One of these tendons inserts onto the radial side of the base of the first metacarpal. The other tendon inserts onto the trapezium bone of the carpus.

As its name implies, the abductor pollicis longus muscle acts to abduct the thumb (with the abductor pollicis brevis muscle). It may also assist in extension of the thumb (with the extensor pollicis brevis and extensor pollicis longus muscles).

The proximal origin of the **extensor pollicis brevis muscle** is from the posterior surface of the radius and the interosseous membrane. Its muscle fibers descend obliquely along the posterior forearm just medial to the belly of the abductor pollicis longus muscle (Fig. 20–19*D*). Its fibers converge to form a tendon just proximal to the posterolateral carpus. This tendon courses within a groove on the lateral side of the radial head. (This groove also carries the distal tendon of the abductor pollicis longus muscle.) The tendon of the extensor pollicis brevis muscle inserts upon the posterolateral surface of the base of the first metacarpal.

The extensor pollicis brevis muscle acts to extend the thumb (with the extensor pollicis longus and abductor pollicis longus muscles).

The proximal tendon of the **extensor pollicis longus muscle** arises from the posterior surface of the middle third of the posterior surface of the ulna (just distal to the origin of the abductor pollicis longus muscle) and from the posterior surface of the adjacent interosseous membrane (Fig. 20–19*E*). Muscle fibers of the extensor pollicis longus muscle descend obliquely within the deep posterior compartment of the forearm, just medial to the abductor pollicis longus muscle and then to the extensor pollicis brevis muscle (Fig. 20–19*E*). The muscle forms a distal tendon just proximal to the carpus. This tendon passes under the extensor retinaculum and into a groove on the dorsal surface of the distal radial head to insert upon the base of the distal phalanx of the thumb. This tendon and the tendon of the extensor pollicis brevis muscle are readily apparent when the thumb is extended because there is a noticeable depression, known as the **anatomic snuffbox,** between them at the lateral border of the hand (Fig. 20–19*F*).

The action of the extensor pollicis longus muscle is to extend the thumb (with the extensor pollicis brevis and abductor pollicis longus muscles).

The **extensor indicis muscle** is the most medial of the deep muscles of the posterior compartment of the forearm. Its proximal origin is to the posterior side of the ulna and adjacent interosseous membrane just distal to the origin of the extensor pollicis longus muscle (Fig. 20–19*G*). Its narrow belly descends laterally just

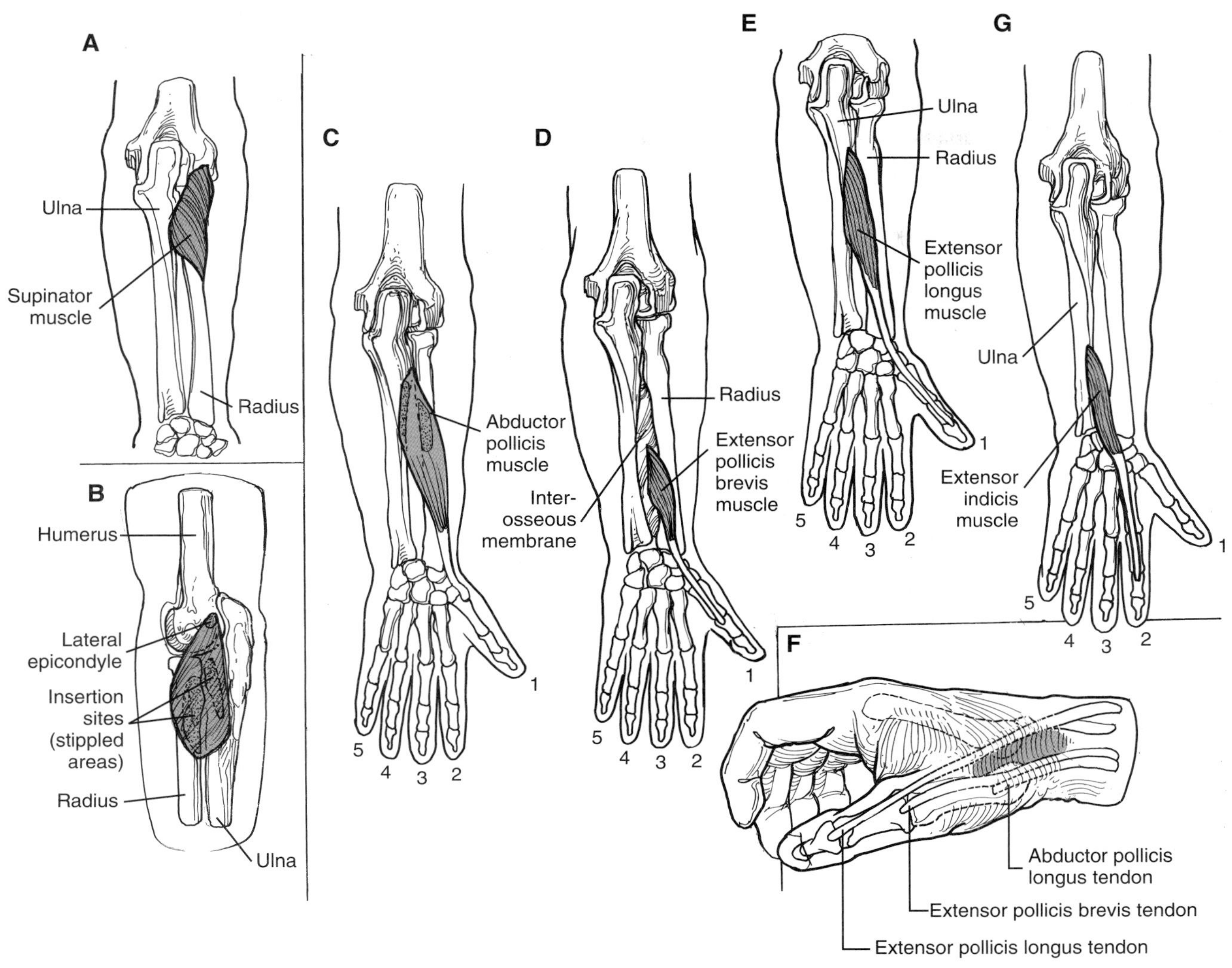

FIGURE 20–19
Muscles of the deep extensor posterior compartment of the forearm (deep posterior antebrachial extensors). **A.** Supinator muscle, posterior view. **B.** Supinator muscle, lateral view. **C.** Abductor pollicis longus muscle. **D.** Extensor pollicis brevis muscle. **E.** Extensor pollicis longus muscle. **F.** Anatomic "snuffbox." **G.** Extensor indicis muscle.

adjacent to the extensor pollicis longus muscle and forms a distal tendon just proximal to the carpus. This tendon courses under the extensor retinaculum with tendons of the extensor digitorum muscle of the superficial posterior compartment of the forearm. The distal tendon of the extensor indicis muscle fuses with the tendon of the extensor digitorum muscle that serves the second digit. This combined tendon inserts upon the dorsal surface of the base of the proximal phalanx of the second digit as is described above.

The extensor indicis muscle acts to extend the second digit (with the extensor digitorum muscle).

Comparison of Flexion and Extension in the Upper and Lower Extremities. The anatomy of **tendons of the phalangeal extensors (extensor sheath or dorsal digital expansion)** accounts for significant differences in the ranges of motion of upper and lower extremity segments. For example, metacarpophalangeal joints can readily flex, while flexion is far more limited at metatarsophalangeal joints. Conversely, these latter joints of the lower extremity are capable of significant hyperextension in contrast to their counterparts in the upper extremity.

Intrinsic Muscles of the Hand

There are three main groups of intrinsic muscles of the hand: 4 **thenar muscles** associated with the thumb; 4 **hypothenar muscles** associated with the little finger; and 11 muscles of the central palm and intermetacarpal spaces, namely, 4 **lumbrical** and 7 **interosseous muscles** (Table 20–5). Thus, there are 19 intrinsic muscles of the hand (see Fig. 20–4). The lumbricals have no counterpart in the foot.

Five of the intrinsic muscles of the hand can be classified as flexors. The four lumbricals extend the mid-

TABLE 20–5
Attachments and Actions of Intrinsic Muscles of the Hand

Muscle Group	Individual Muscle	Proximal Attachment	Distal Attachment	Muscle Action
Thenar muscles	Abductor pollicis brevis	Flexor retinaculum, scaphoid, trapezius	Radial side of base of proximal phalanx of thumb, dorsal digital expansion of thumb	Abducts thumb
	Opponens pollicis	Flexor retinaculum, tubercle of trapezium	Lateral border and dorsal surface of first metacarpal	Medially flexes thumb to effect opposition
	Flexor pollicis brevis	Flexor retinaculum, tubercle of trapezium	Lateral surface of base of proximal phalanx of digit 1	Flexes proximal phalanx of thumb; in extreme flexion it flexes and medially rotates first metacarpal to assist in opposition
	Adductor pollicis brevis	Capitate and bases of second and third metacarpals, palmar surface of distal half of third metacarpal	Base of proximal phalanx of thumb	Adducts thumb
Hypothenar muscles	Palmaris brevis	Ulnar side of flexor retinaculum	Dermis of ulnar border of palm	Wrinkles skin over hypothenar eminence
	Abductor digiti minimi	Pisiform, tendon of flexor carpi ulnaris	Ulnar side of base of proximal phalanx of digit 5, dorsal digital expansion of digit 5	Abducts digit 5
	Flexor digiti minimi brevis	Hook of hamate, flexor retinaculum	Medial side of phalanx of digit 5	Flexes digit 5, assists in opposition by laterally rotating digit 5
	Opponens digiti minimi	Hook of hamate, flexor retinaculum	Medial surface of fifth metacarpal	Flexes digit 5, laterally rotates digit 5 to oppose thumb
Lumbrical muscles of the palm and intermetacarpal spaces	First lumbrical	Lateral side of profundus tendon of digit 2	Dorsal digital (extensor) expansion of digit 2	Extends middle and distal phalanges of digit 2, assists in flexion of proximal phalanx of digit 2
	Second lumbrical	Medial side of profundus tendon of digit 2, lateral side of profundus tendon of digit 3	Dorsal digital expansion of digit 3	Extends middle and distal phalanges of digit 3, assists in flexion of proximal phalanx of digit 3
	Third lumbrical	Medial side of profundus tendon of digit 3, lateral side of profundus tendon of digit 4	Dorsal digital expansion of digit 4	Extends middle and distal phalanges of digit 4, assists in flexion of proximal phalanx of digit 4
	Fourth lumbrical	Medial side of profundus tendon of digit 4, lateral side of profundus tendon of digit 5	Dorsal digital expansion of digit 5	Extends middle and distal phalanges of digit 5, assists in flexion of proximal phalanx of digit 5
Interosseous muscles of palm and intermetacarpal spaces	Adductor of digit 2	Lateral side of second metacarpal	Lateral side of dorsal digital expansion of digit 2	Adducts digit 2
	Adductor of digit 4	Medial side of fourth metacarpal	Medial side of dorsal digital expansion of digit 4	Adducts digit 4
	Adductor of digit 5	Medial side of fifth metacarpal	Medial side of dorsal digital expansion of digit 5	Adducts digit 5
	Abductor of digit 2	Lateral side of second metacarpal	Lateral side of dorsal digital expansion of digit 2	Abducts digit 2
	Abductor of digit 3 (medial)	Lateral side of fourth metacarpal, medial side of third metacarpal	Lateral side of dorsal digital expansion of digit 3	Abducts digit 3
	Abductor of digit 3 (lateral)	Medial side of second metacarpal, lateral side of third metacarpal	Lateral side of dorsal digital expansion of digit 3	Abducts digit 3
	Abductor of digit 4	Lateral side of fifth metacarpal, medial side of fourth metacarpal	Medial side of dorsal digital expansion of digit 4	Abducts digit 4

dle phalanges of digits 2 to 4. Six of the intrinsic muscles of the hand are abductors and four are adductors (as in the toes; see Chapter 16). These muscles are distributed so that one pair of flexors acts on the thumb and another pair on the little finger, although one muscle of each pair is called an "opponens" muscle (see below). The fifth flexor, which is also classified as a hypothenar muscle, acts on the skin of the palm. Four of the intrinsic abductors are interosseous muscles and two are specialized abductors, one of the thumb and one of the little finger. Three of the adductors are interosseous muscles, and one is a special adductor (of the thumb). Unlike in the foot where the axis of abduction and adduction is the second digit, the axis of abduction and adduction in the hand is the third digit (see below).

Thenar Muscles. The **thenar prominence** of the palm is the bulge just proximal to the thumb. The bulge is produced by four thenar muscles. These are, from lateral to medial, the abductor pollicis brevis, flexor pollicis brevis, opponens pollicis, and adductor pollicis muscles (Fig. 20–20). There are no lumbricals that act upon the thumb (see below).

The **abductor pollicis brevis muscle** is a small muscle, which arises from the flexor retinaculum and scaphoid and trapezium bones of the carpus. Its thin belly lies on the lateral aspect of the thenar eminence. Its distal tendon inserts upon the lateral (radial) side of the base of the proximal phalanx of the thumb and into its dorsal digital expansion (Fig. 20–20*A*).

The abductor pollicis brevis muscle acts to pull the phalanges of the thumb laterally in the plane of the palm (abduction).

The **opponens pollicis muscle** lies deep to the abductor pollicis brevis and flexor pollicis brevis muscles. Its proximal tendon arises from the lateral side of the distal edge of the flexor retinaculum and from the trapezial tubercle of the carpus (Fig. 20–20*B*). Its fibers descend laterally to insert upon the lateral border and adjacent dorsal surface of the first metacarpal.

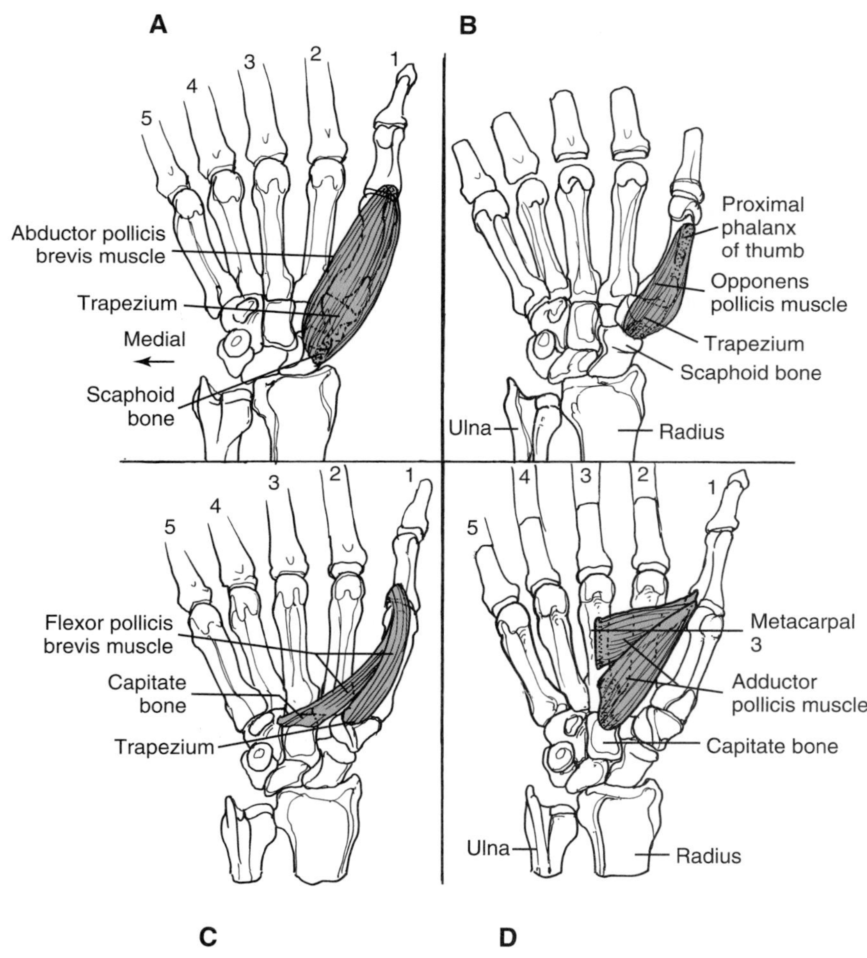

FIGURE 20–20
Thenar muscles. **A.** Abductor pollicis brevis muscle. **B.** Opponens pollicis muscle. **C.** Flexor pollicis brevis muscle. **D.** Adductor pollicis brevis muscle.

The opponens pollicis muscle acts as a flexor of the thumb. However, because the first metacarpal is rotated 90 degrees, the first metacarpal bone flexes medially, across the palm, allowing the thumb to oppose the ventral surfaces of the tips of digits 2 to 5.

The **flexor pollicis brevis muscle** is superficial to the abductor pollicis brevis and opponens pollicis muscles. Its belly lies slightly medial to the abductor muscle (Fig. 20–20*C*). Like the opponens pollicis muscle, the flexor pollicis brevis muscle arises from the flexor retinaculum and trapezial tubercle. However, it inserts upon the lateral (radial) surface of the base of the proximal phalanx of the first digit.

The flexor pollicis brevis muscle acts to flex the proximal phalanx of the thumb. In extreme flexion, however, it also flexes and medially rotates the first metacarpal, assisting the opponens pollicis muscle in allowing the thumb to oppose digits 2 to 5.

The **adductor pollicis brevis muscle** has two parts: a proximal oblique part and a distal transverse part (Fig. 20–20*D*). The oblique part arises from the capitate bone of the carpus and the bases of the second and third metacarpals. The transverse part arises from the palmar surface of the distal half of the third metacarpal. The fibers of both parts converge to insert at the base of the proximal phalanx of the first digit.

The action of the adductor pollicis brevis muscle is to pull the thumb toward the palm (adduction).

Hypothenar Muscles. The **hypothenar prominence** of the palm is the swelling just proximal to the fifth digit. It is created by fibers of four muscles: the palmaris brevis, abductor digiti minimi, flexor digiti minimi brevis, and opponens digiti minimi muscles (Fig. 20–21). The palmaris brevis muscle is superficial to the other three muscles, which are described below in medial to lateral order.

The **palmaris brevis muscle** is a thin hypothenar muscle lying superficial to other muscles of the hypothenar prominence. It arises from the ulnar side of the flexor retinaculum and inserts into the dermis of the ulnar border of the palm (Fig. 20–21*A*).

The palmaris brevis muscle acts to wrinkle the skin that lies over the hypothenar eminence.

The proximal tendon of the **abductor digiti minimi muscle** arises from the pisiform bone and the tendon of the flexor carpi ulnaris muscle. Its fibers course distally and converge to form two distal tendons: one that inserts upon the medial (ulnar) side of the base of the proximal phalanx of the fifth digit and one that inserts upon the dorsal digital expansion of the extensor digiti minimi muscle (Fig. 20–21*B*).

The action of the abductor digiti minimi muscle is to pull the fifth digit medially in the plane of the palm (abduction).

The **flexor digiti minimi brevis muscle** lies lateral to the abductor digiti minimi muscle. The proximal tendon of the flexor digiti minimi brevis muscle arises

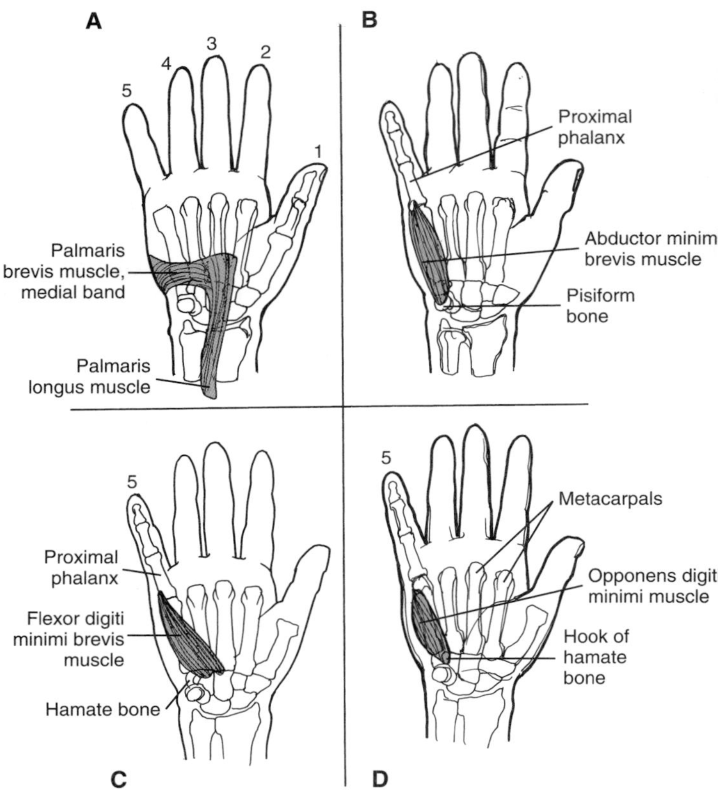

FIGURE 20–21
Hypothenar muscles. **A.** Palmaris brevis muscle. **B.** Abductor minimi brevis muscle. **C.** Flexor digiti minimi brevis muscle. **D.** Opponens digiti minimi muscle.

from the hook of the hamate bone and from the ulnar side of the flexor retinaculum. Its fibers course distally, converging to form a distal tendon, which inserts upon the medial (ulnar) side of the base of the proximal phalanx of the fifth digit (along with the tendon of the abductor digiti minimi muscle) (Fig. 20–21*C*). According to the rules of anatomic nomenclature, a flexor digiti minimi *longus* muscle should also exist, but this is not the case. The term *brevis* simply characterizes this muscle as a short flexor of the little finger.

The flexor digiti minimi brevis muscle acts to flex the fifth digit at the metacarpophalangeal joint. It also assists the opponens digiti minimi muscle in lateral rotation and opposition of the fifth digit to the thumb.

The **opponens digiti minimi muscle** lies lateral to the flexor digiti minimi brevis muscle. The proximal tendon of the opponens digiti minimi muscle arises from the ulnar side of the flexor retinaculum and from the hook of the hamate bone (Fig. 20–21*D*). Its fibers descend medially to insert upon the entire medial (ulnar) surface of the fifth metacarpal.

The opponens digiti minimi muscle acts to flex the fifth metacarpal. It also rotates the fifth metacarpal laterally (with the flexor digiti minimi brevis muscle) to oppose the thumb.

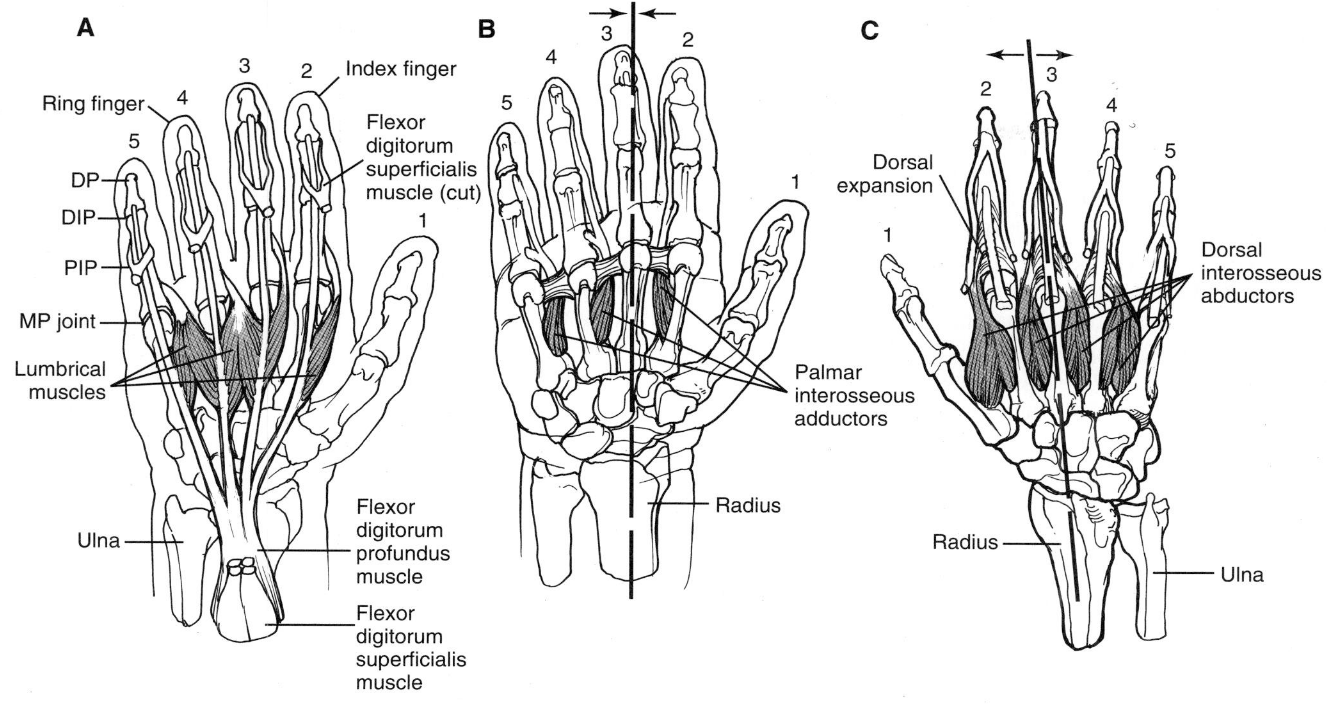

FIGURE 20–22

Lumbrical and interosseous muscles of the palm and intermetacarpal spaces. **A.** Palmar lumbrical muscles. **B.** Palmar interosseous adductors. The action plane of adduction is shown. **C.** Dorsal interosseous abductors, including action plane of abduction.

Muscles of the Palm and Intermetacarpal Spaces. Muscles of the palm and intermetacarpal spaces include the four lumbrical muscles and seven interosseous muscles (Fig. 20–22). The lumbricals are active in extension of the middle phalanges of digits 2 to 4 and the interosseous muscles in abduction and adduction of the digits as described below.

Lumbrical Muscles. The four lumbrical muscles (from the Latin, meaning *earthworm*) act upon digits 2 to 4. They arise in similar ways from the distal tendons of the flexor digitorum profundus muscle and insert upon the extensor expansions of digits 2 to 4 (Fig. 20–22*A*).

The **first lumbrical muscle** arises from the lateral (radial) side of the profundus tendon to the index finger (second digit). Its distal tendon courses around the same side of the second metacarpophalangeal joint to insert upon the extensor expansion of the second digit (Fig. 20–22*A*).

The **second lumbrical muscle** arises from the medial (ulnar) side of the profundus tendon to digit 2 and the lateral (radial) side of the profundus tendon to digit 3. It courses around the radial side of the third metacarpophalangeal joint to insert upon the extensor expansion of the third digit (Fig. 20–22*A*).

The **third lumbrical muscle** arises from the ulnar surface of the profundus tendon to digit 3 and from the radial surface of the profundus tendon to digit 4. It courses around the radial side of the fourth metacarpophalangeal joint to insert upon the extensor expansion of the fourth digit (Fig. 20–22*A*).

The **fourth lumbrical muscle** originates from the ulnar surface of the profundus tendon to digit 4 and from the radial side of the profundus tendon to digit 5. It courses around the radial side of the fifth metacarpophalangeal joint to insert upon the extensor expansion of the fifth digit (Fig. 20–22*A*).

Because the lumbricals to digits 2 to 4 are inserted into the extensor expansions, one of their actions is to extend the interphalangeal joints of these three digits. However, unlike the lumbricals of the toes, the lumbricals of the fingers probably do not play a role in flexion of the metacarpophalangeal joints of digits 2 to 4 (see Chapter 16). It has been argued that they may assist the interosseous muscles in flexing the proximal phalanges of digits 2 to 4.

Interosseous Muscles. Like the foot, the hand contains seven interosseous muscles: three palmar adductors and four dorsal abductors (Fig. 20–22*B* and *C*). The main actions of these muscles are characterized with respect to a longitudinal axis running through the middle digit. Palmar adductors pull digits toward the extended axis of the third digit, while dorsal abductors pull digits away from this axis.

Thus, the **palmar interosseous adductor muscle** acting on digit 5 arises from the medial (ulnar) side of the fifth metacarpal, courses around the ulnar side of the fifth metacarpophalangeal joint, and inserts upon the ulnar side of the dorsal digital expansion of digit 5 (Fig. 20–22*B*). Likewise, the palmar adductor muscle acting on digit 4 arises from the ulnar side of the fourth metacarpal, courses around the ulnar side of the fourth metacarpophalangeal joint, and inserts upon the ulnar side of the dorsal digital expansion of digit 4. In contrast, the palmar adductor muscle acting upon digit 2 arises from the lateral (radial) side of the second metacarpal, courses around the radial side of the second metacarpophalangeal joint, and inserts on the radial side of the dorsal digital expansion of digit 2. Obviously, the middle digit (digit 3) is not acted upon by palmar adductors. The interosseous muscles serving digit 3 are two dorsal abductors (Fig. 20–22*C*).

The **dorsal interosseous abductor muscle** acting on digit 4 arises from the fourth and fifth metacarpals, courses around the ulnar side of the fourth metacarpophalangeal joint, and inserts upon the ulnar side of the dorsal digital expansion of digit 4 (Fig. 20–22*C*). The third digit has two dorsal interosseous abductors. They arise from the radial side of the fourth metacarpal and the ulnar side of the third metacarpal (the abductor muscle on the ulnar side of the digit) and from the radial side of the third metacarpal and ulnar side of the second metacarpal (the abductor muscle on the radial side of the digit). The dorsal abductor muscle on the ulnar side of digit 3 inserts upon the ulnar side of the dorsal digital expansion of digit 3 while the radial abductor inserts on the radial side of the dorsal digital expansion. Finally, the dorsal abductor acting on digit 2 arises from the radial side of the second metacarpal and ulnar side of the first metacarpal. Its fibers course around the radial side of the metacarpophalangeal joint of digit 2 and insert on the radial edge of the dorsal digital expansion of digit 2.

An easy way to remember the attachments and actions of the interosseous muscles is to know that the 5 fingers have a total of 10 abductors and adductors. There must be six abductors and four adductors because digit 3, which is the axis of these actions, can only be abducted. Since digit 5 has a specific hypothenar abductor muscle (the abductor digiti minimi muscle), only its adductor is one of the palmar interosseous muscles. Digits 4 and 2, however, have both a dorsal interosseous abductor and a palmar interosseous adductor. Digit 3, as noted, has two dorsal interosseous abductors. Finally, the thumb has a specific thenar adductor (the adductor pollicis muscle) and a specific thenar abductor (the abductor pollicis brevis muscle). It should be noted that some anatomists suggest that the thumb also has a palmar interosseous adductor.

Finally, it should be noted that the adductor (palmar) interosseous muscles are active in preventing uncontrolled abduction during extension of the digits. Conversely, the abductor (dorsal) interosseous muscles prevent uncontrolled adduction during flexion of the digits. These preventive functions are important in the playing of musical instruments, such as the violin, guitar, or piano.

Mechanism of the Dorsal Digital Expansions. *Intrinsic muscles of the hand modify or balance actions of the long flexor and extensor muscles.* Flexion and extension of digits 2 to 5 are more complicated than has just been implied. For example, although it is true that the metacarpophalangeal joint and all of the interphalangeal joints may be flexed or extended together (Fig. 20–23*A*), it is also true that all of the interphalangeal joints may be flexed while the metacarpophalangeal joint remains extended (Fig. 20–23*B*). In addition, the interphalangeal joints may be extended while the metacarpophalangeal joint remains flexed (Fig. 20–23*C*). Moreover, the proximal and distal interphalangeal joints may be extended individually (Fig. 20–23*D* and see below). Finally, many of these movements may be carried out by single digits acting independently. In order to understand these complex movements, one must learn the anatomy of the extrinsic flexor and extensor muscle tendons and the attachments and functions of intrinsic muscles within the hands.

Actions of intrinsic muscles depend on their attachments to the dorsal (extensor) digital expansion

In addition to their functions in adduction and abduction, the **interosseous muscles assist the lumbrical muscles in flexion and extension of the metacarpophalangeal and interphalangeal joints.** These synergistic interactions are particularly important because they allow the joints to flex and extend independently of each other. Thus, the interphalangeal joints may be flexed or extended no matter what the state of the metacarpophalangeal joints (Fig. 20–23).

The intrinsic muscles accomplish this function, in part, through their effects upon the action and shape of the dorsal digital expansions to which they are connected. The **dorsal (extensor) digital expansions** are elaborations of the long extensor tendons. They are diamond-shaped structures. Each has a proximal and a distal "wing." These wings provide insertions for the dorsal interosseous and lumbrical muscles and, in conjunction with other bony insertion sites of these muscles, play a critical role in the dissociation of movements at different joints (Fig. 20–24). For example, the dorsal interosseous muscles (which arise from the shafts of the metacarpal bones) have a pair of distal tendons that insert into the **proximal wings of the dorsal digital expansions** on each side of the digit. The proximal wings of the dorsal digital expansions, in turn, course distally along both sides of the distal interphalangeal joint to insert upon the dorsal central band of the long extensor tendon (Fig. 20–24*A* and *B*). This central band then inserts upon

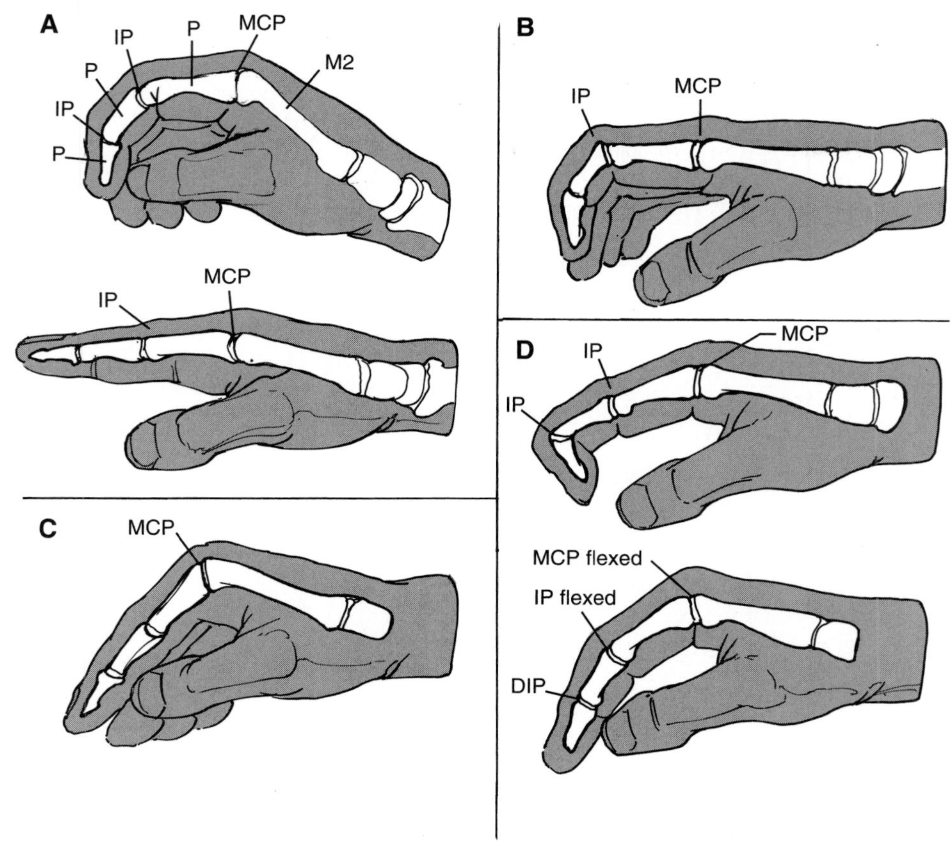

FIGURE 20–23
Complex mechanisms of dorsal digital expansions: Intrinsic muscles of the hand balance actions of the flexor and extensor muscles. **A.** The metacarpophalangeal joint and all the interphalangeal joints are flexed or extended together. **B.** All interphalangeal joints are flexed, and the metacarpophalangeal joint is extended. **C.** The interphalangeal are joints extended, and the metacarpophalangeal joint is flexed. **D.** Proximal and distal interphalangeal joints may be extended individually.

the dorsal surface of the base of the middle phalanx (Fig. 20–24*B*). A second pair of distal tendons of these muscles attaches to the lateral and medial surfaces of the bases of the proximal phalanges (Fig. 20–24*A* to *C*). Because of the double insertion of the dorsal interosseous muscles (one pair at the lateral and medial surface of the base of the proximal phalanx, and the other on the proximal wings of the distal expansion), the contraction of these muscles results in flexion of the metacarpophalangeal joint and extension of the proximal interphalangeal joint (Fig. 20–24*B* to *D*).

On the other hand, the combined distal tendons of the lumbrical and palmar interosseous muscles insert into the **distal wings of the dorsal digital expansions** (Fig. 20–24*B*). From the point at which these combined tendons become confluent with the distal wings of the dorsal digital expansions, the tendons course distally along the base of the shaft of the middle phalanx and then dorsally to insert upon the dorsal surface of the base of the distal phalanx (Fig. 20–24*B* to *D*). The palmar interosseous muscles originate from the sides of the shafts of the metacarpal bones, and the lumbricals arise from the long digital flexor tendons within the palm. Thus, the palmar interosseous and lumbrical muscles work together to extend the distal interphalangeal joint while they assist in flexion of the metacarpophalangeal joint (Figs. 20–23*C* and 20–24*D*).

It should also be noted that the interosseous and lumbrical muscles, acting together, increase the efficiency of the extensor digitorum muscle in extending the distal interphalangeal joint. They do this by pulling the dorsal digital expansion down upon the dorsum of the digit, preventing hyperextension at the proximal interphalangeal joint.

Finally, contraction of the lumbricals and palmar interosseous muscles changes the shape of the dorsal digital expansion because the muscles pull upon the expansion's distal wings. This action provides more slack within the long extensor tendon proximal to the distal wings, allowing the interphalangeal joints to be flexed or extended as the metacarpophalangeal joint is flexed.

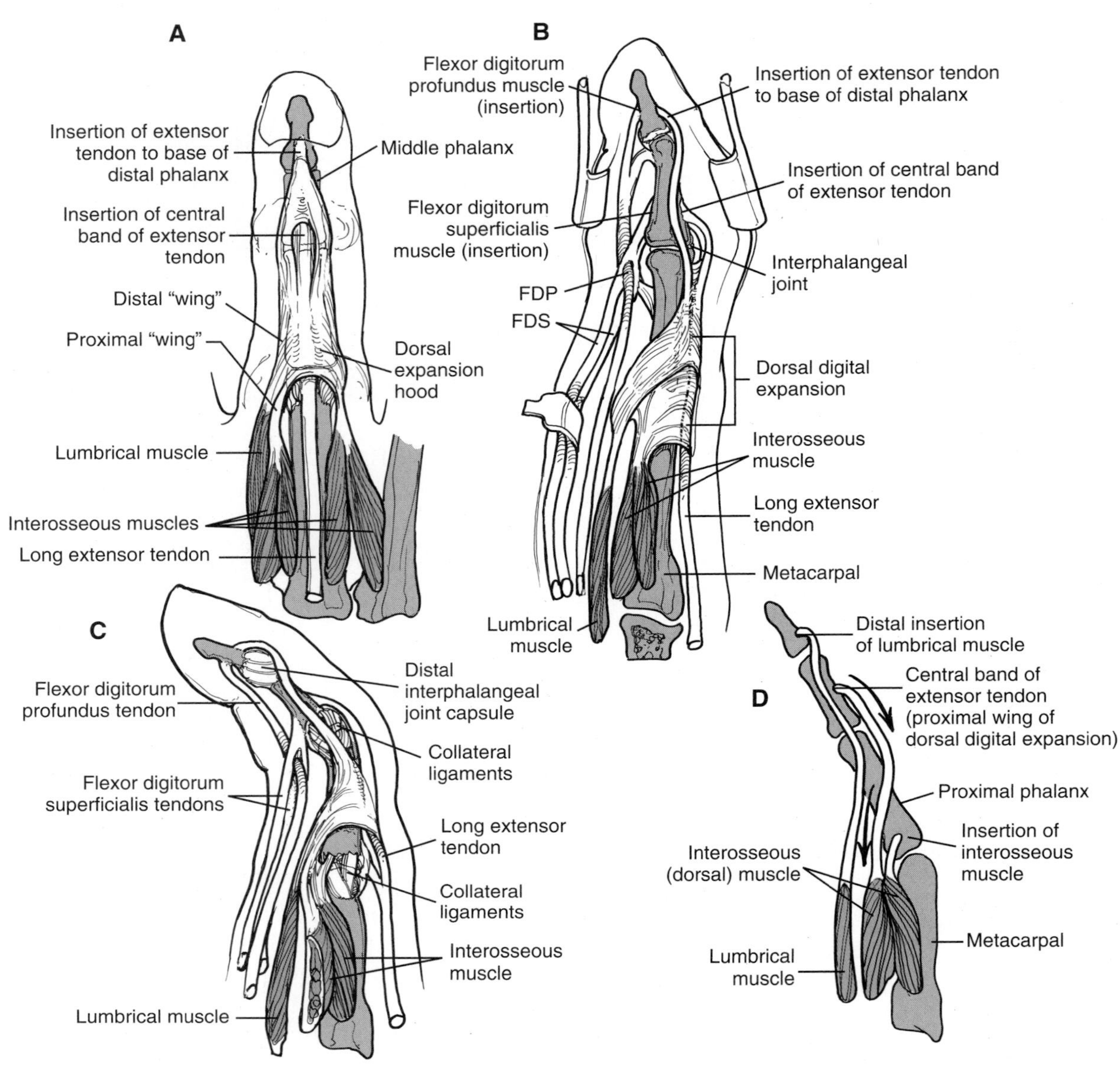

FIGURE 20–24

The ability of joints to flex and extend independently of each other depends on attachments of the dorsal extensor digital expansions (long extensor tendons) coupled with the interaction of lumbrical and interosseus muscles. **A.** Relationship of tendon insertions and interosseus and lumbrical muscles in the middle phalanx (dorsal view). **B.** Lateral view of dorsal digital expansion in relation to the above structures. **C.** Flexion of phalanx. **D.** Schematic drawing showing flexion of the metacarpophalangeal joint and extension of the proximal interphalangeal joint. Note insertion of lumbrical and interosseous muscles.

▲ Prehensile Function of the Upper Extremity

The upper extremity can be described as a series of movable platforms, which position the hands for grasping, pushing, hitting, or supporting the weight of the body (see Chapter 16 and above). The clavicle and scapula (shoulder girdle) provide a movable base for extension, flexion, abduction, and adduction of the arm (at the glenohumeral joints) and extension and flexion of the forearm (at the elbow joint). These movements pull the hand toward or push the hand away from the body. In addition, pronation and supination of the forearm and flexion, extension, adduction, and abduction of the wrist allow even more refined placement of the hand.

The human hand is a flexor-extensor mechanism

Movements of individual segments of the hand are relatively limited, but, as has already been discussed, the range of motion and degree of freedom of movement are increased by synergistic additive or cumulative

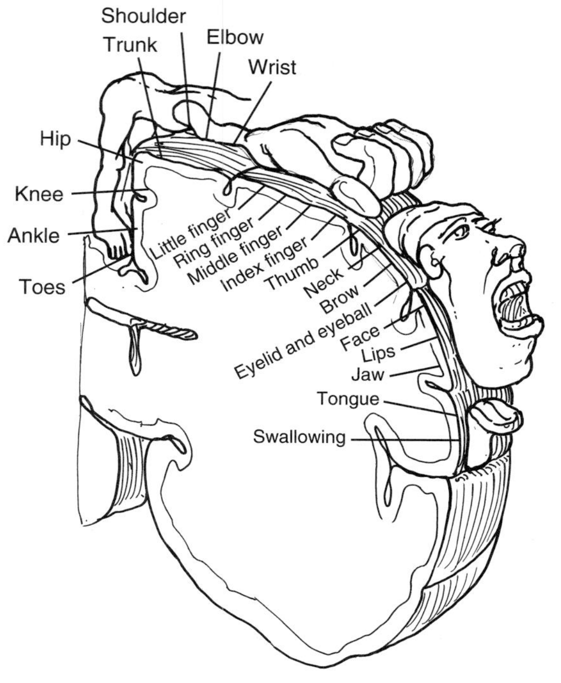

FIGURE 20–25
Motor homunculus. Motor area of the cerebral cortex devoted to controlling the hand.

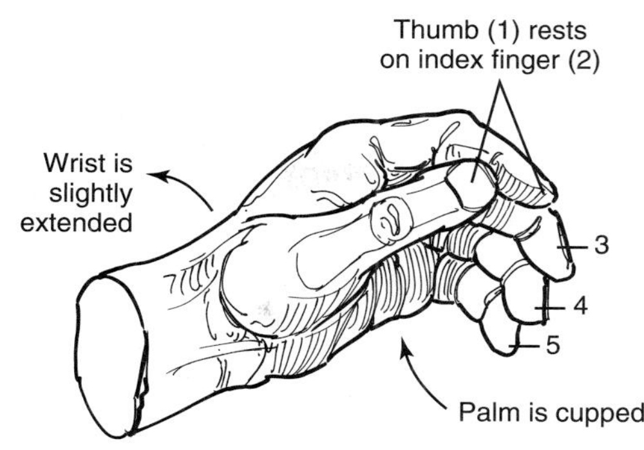

FIGURE 20–26
The hand in the position of rest.

actions of muscles. In addition, movements of the hand are so effective because they can be finely controlled. This control is the consequence of the basic anatomy of bones, joints, and tendons of the hand and of the functional balance between actions of extrinsic and intrinsic muscles of the hand. In addition to flexion and extension, the digits may be adducted and abducted and the thumb may be opposed to digits 2 to 5, in part, through rotational movements of the metacarpals and phalanges (see below).

As has been described above, the metacarpophalangeal and interphalangeal joints are essentially uniaxial and their primary motions are flexion and extension. Flexion and extension at these joints results from the action of extrinsic and intrinsic flexors and extensors of the digits. Thus, the primary function of these muscles is to close and open the hand. As was described in Chapter 5 and elsewhere, however, muscles may function either dynamically or in a postural capacity to maintain tension against an opposing force. This is true of the flexors and extensors of the digits. Thus, dynamic activity of the flexors of the digits (the flexor digitorum superficialis, flexor digitorum profundus, flexor digiti minimi longus, flexor digiti minimi brevis, flexor pollicis longus, and flexor pollicis brevis muscles) is countered by the graded postural activities of the extensors (the extensor digitorum, extensor indicis, extensor digiti minimi, and extensor pollicis muscles). Conversely, the dynamic activity of extensor muscles is countered by the graded postural activities of flexors of the hand.

The movements of the hand are so complex and so important to human survival and development that a larger area of the motor portion of the cerebral cortex is devoted to controlling the hand than the entire lower extremity. Incredibly, about half of this area is devoted to the thumb (Fig. 20–25 and see below).

A major function of the hand is prehensile

The normal attitude of the hand is its **position of rest** in which the wrist is slightly extended, the metacarpophalangeal and interphalangeal joints are slightly flexed, the thumb rests against the index and middle fingers, and the transverse metacarpal arch is quite pronounced (i.e., the palm is cupped) (Fig. 20–26).

One major function of the hand is **grasping,** which occurs through a power grip, precision grip, or hook grip. Use of only the thumb and index finger is a **pliers (pincer) grip** (Fig. 20–27*A*). In the **power grip,** some or all of digits 2 to 5 are opposed by the thumb as when one firmly grasps an object such as a book (Fig. 20–27*B*). Use of the thumb and two or more digits is a **chuck grip.** The major muscles used in the power grip are extrinsic muscles of the hand, particularly those on the ulnar side.

Grasping an object for fine manipulation is facilitated by the **precision grip** (Fig. 20–27*C*). This is the grip one uses when writing with a pen or pencil or performing other fine manipulative movements. Here, the actions of extrinsic muscles are significantly modified by the actions of intrinsic muscles of the hand (see below).

Finally, the **hook grip** primarily uses digits 2 to 5. The thumb is usually not involved. This grip is used for carrying a briefcase by its handle or for pulling the body toward an object as when one climbs a tree or goes rock climbing (Fig. 20–27*D*).

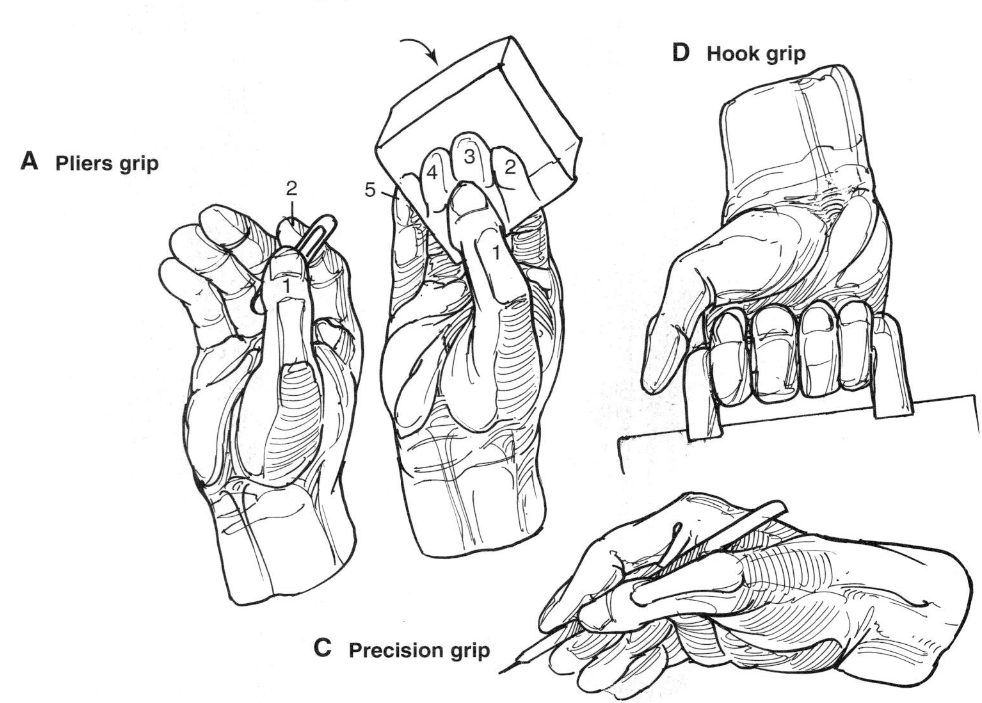

FIGURE 20–27
Functional movements of the hand. **A.** Pliers (pincher) grip, using only the thumb and index finger. **B.** Power grip (chuck grip), using the thumb opposed to two or more digits. **C.** Precision grip for fine manipulation. **D.** Hook grip, using primarily digits 2 to 5.

More than one type of grip may be used at the same time by the same hand. For example, a pen may be held by its base in a power grip while the cap is twisted off by the thumb and forefinger in a precision grip. A baseball pitcher or football quarterback may grasp a ball tightly in a power grip, but as the ball is released, it is manipulated to spin with a precision grip by the thumb and some of the other digits.

The prehensile activities of the hand are not unique to humans. They are shared by chimpanzees, gorillas, and some monkeys. Gibbons have lost oppositional capability in the hands. Their hands have instead become specialized to perform strong hook grips so that they can suspend their bodies from tree branches.

The action of the thumb is integral to the prehensile function of the hand

In the description of movements of the first carpometacarpal joint, above, it is clear that the natural movement of the thumb is **opposition.** The opponens pollicis and flexor pollicis brevis muscles cause the thumb to gently oppose the index and middle fingers. In order for the thumb to oppose digits 4 and 5, digits 4 and 5 must be moved by both hypothenar and thenar muscles. As has been noted, oppositional movements are accompanied by medial rotation of digit 1 and lateral rotation of digit 2, 3, 4, or 5. In oppositional grasping (power grip), the abductor pollicis brevis and flexor pollicis longus muscles are also engaged to increase the strength of the grip once the pulp of the thumb touches the pulp of the digit. Finally, hypothenar muscles may become more active in firm opposition of the thumb to digits 2 and 3 because these muscles affect the exaggeration of the transverse metacarpal arch.

▲ Pushing and Supportive Functions of the Upper Extremity

The upper limbs may be used to push objects away from the body or to support the weight of the body

The upper limbs are used to push objects away from the body or to fend off moving objects. They may also be used to support the body or prevent collisions of the body with other objects (e.g., as may occur in falls or sports activities). The upper limbs may even support a weight exceeding the weight of the body. In such a situation, the bones of the joints are typically packed closely together to provide strength for the limb as it resists the object or the forces of gravity. As a consequence, the long bones are often broken in falls when the outstretched limb is not able to flex or recoil in a controlled manner. The clavicle and radius are particularly prone to such trauma (see Chapter 19).

21 Vessels and Nerves of the Upper Extremities

SYSTEMS THAT INTEGRATE THE ANATOMY OF THE UPPER EXTREMITY

This chapter describes the vasculature and innervation of the bones, joints, and muscles of the upper extremity. Like the review of these frameworks for the lower limbs in Chapter 18, the review in this chapter helps to integrate the skeletal and muscular systems of the upper limbs. Also, this chapter discusses the compartmentalization of upper extremity muscles by substantial deep fascial septa. The foramina in these barriers allow vessels and nerves to pass from one compartment to another. Major examples of these foramina include the following:

- **fenestrae** (windowlike openings) of the clavipectoral fascia,
- the **hiatus** deep to the bicipital aponeurosis,
- a superior hiatus of the interosseous membrane,
- multiple **perforations** of the interosseous membrane,
- the lowest perforation of the interosseous membrane, and
- **apertures** in the deep fascial intermuscular septa of the arm and forearm.

All of these mechanisms are described in greater detail where appropriate.

Vasculature of the Upper Extremity

The upper extremity is vascularized by brachial arteries and their accompanying deep veins and by a system of superficial veins

During embryogenesis, the seventh cervical intersegmental arteries give rise to the **subclavian arteries** and their extensions (the **axillary** and **brachial arteries).** These vessels provide the chief arterial supply of the upper extremity. Deep veins of the same names accompany these major arteries. Deoxygenated blood is drained from the upper limb via the smaller tributaries (the **venae comitantes)** of the deep veins. As in the lower extremity, **superficial veins** also develop to drain the upper extremities (see below).

Arteries of the Upper Extremity

The right and left subclavian arteries have different embryonic origins

The right subclavian artery and its axillary continuation are derived from a small part of the aortic sac (i.e., the distal end of the truncus arteriosus), the right fourth aortic arch, a small segment of the right dorsal aorta, and the right seventh cervical intersegmental artery. The left subclavian and axillary arteries are derived wholly from the left seventh cervical intersegmental artery. On both the right and left sides, however, the seventh cervical intersegmental artery grows into the limb bud as a primary axial (axis) artery, which directly or indirectly (by sprouting), gives rise to all of the arteries in the definitive limb. The brachial and anterior interosseous arteries and a portion of the deep palmar arch are all derived directly from the embryonic axis (primary axial) artery. All other arteries of the upper extremities arise as sprouts of this main axial trunk (Figs. 21–1 and 21–2 and Table 21–1).

Subclavian Artery and Its Branches

Before entering the limb, the subclavian artery gives rise to branches that supply thoracic structures and the shoulder

Branches of the subclavian artery are most often described in relation to their first, second, and third parts. The anterior scalene muscle serves as a pivotal landmark in defining these three segments. This muscle arises from the anterior tubercles of vertebrae C2 to C6 (see Chapters 3 and 26). Its fibers descend behind the sternocleidomastoid muscle to attach to the first rib (Fig. 21–3*A*). The first part of each subclavian artery courses from its origin at the arch of the aorta to the medial border of the anterior scalene muscle. The second part courses directly behind the anterior scalene muscle. The third part courses from the lateral border of the anterior scalene muscle to the lateral boundary of the first rib (Fig. 21–3*A*). Branches that supply muscles or other structures of the upper extremity are emphasized in the following description (Table 21–1).

The **first part of the left subclavian artery** gives rise to the following branches:

- the vertebral artery,
- internal thoracic artery,
- thyrocervical trunk, and
- costocervical trunk (Fig. 21–3*A*).

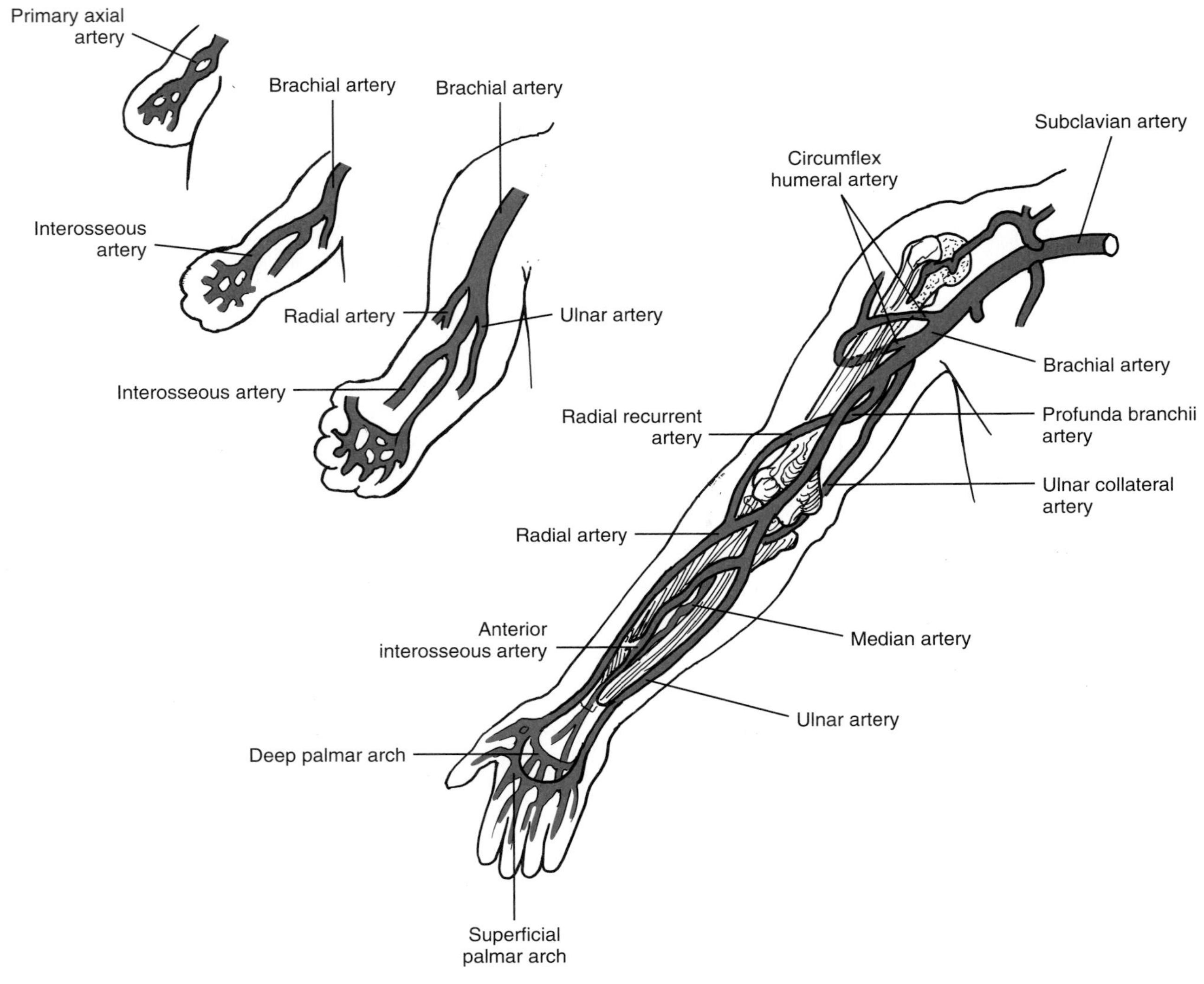

FIGURE 21–1
Development of the arterial system of the upper limb.

The **first part of the right subclavian artery** gives rise to the following branches:

- the vertebral artery,
- internal thoracic artery, and
- thyrocervical trunk (Figs. 21–3*A* and 21–4*A*).

The **vertebral artery** is introduced in Chapter 5 and described fully in Chapter 27, along with vessels of the head and neck. A brief description of the artery is given here. This first branch of the subclavian artery arises from the superior side of the first part of the subclavian artery and ascends through the transverse foramina of vertebrae C6 to C1. It enters the foramen magnum to supply the meninges and brainstem (Figs. 21–3*A* and 21–4*A* and Table 21–1). Before entering the skull, the vertebral artery gives rise to branches that supply the spinal cord (see Chapter 4) and suboccipital muscles (see Chapter 5).

The **internal thoracic artery** is the second branch of the first part of the subclavian artery (Figs. 21–3*A* and 21–4*A* and see Chapter 6). It arises from the inferior side of the subclavian artery and descends behind the sternum and costal cartilages, giving rise to anterior intercostal, pericardial, pericardiacophrenic, and mediastinal branches (Table 21–1 and see Chapter 6). In the region of the seventh to ninth costal cartilages, the internal thoracic artery branches to form a musculophrenic artery (see Chapter 13) and then continues as the superior epigastric artery (see Chapter 10).

As the internal thoracic artery descends in the region of the upper five or six intercostal spaces, it gives rise to **perforating branches,** which supply the pectoralis major muscle and overlying skin. In females, these branches also supply the mammary glands (see Table 21–1 and Chapter 6).

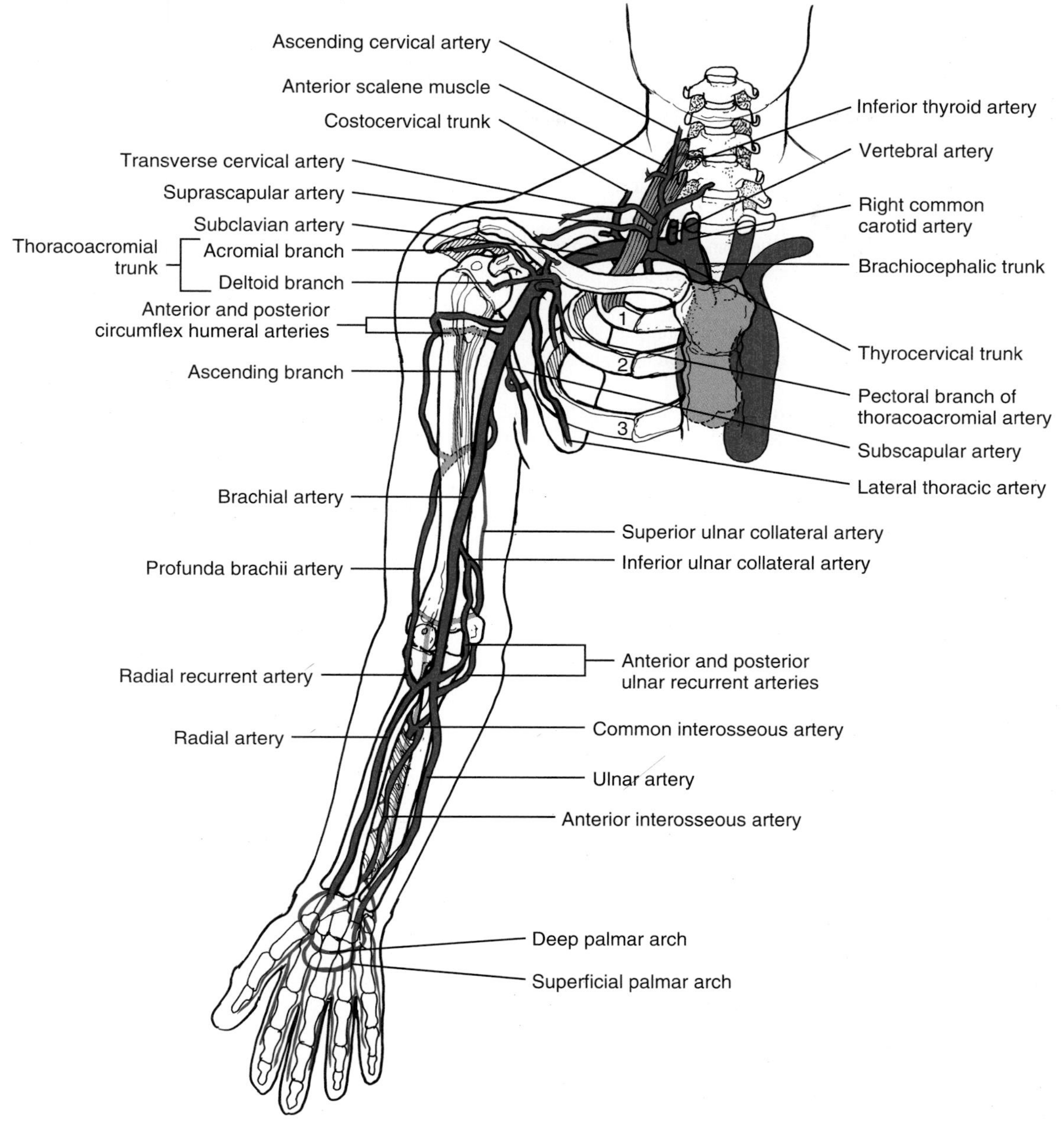

FIGURE 21–2
Arteries of the upper extremities.

The **thyrocervical trunk** branches from the anterior side of the first part of the subclavian artery just at the medial border of the anterior scalene muscle (Figs. 21–3*A* and 21–4). This short, fat artery immediately branches into the inferior thyroid, transverse cervical, and suprascapular arteries.

The **inferior thyroid artery** supplies muscles of the neck and the thyroid gland (Fig. 21–4*A* and Table 21–1 and see Chapter 24).

The **transverse cervical artery** crosses in front of the anterior scalene muscle and crosses the floor of the posterior triangle of the neck (Figs. 21–3*B* and 21–4 and see Chapter 27). It splits into a **superficial branch,** which supplies the trapezius muscle, and a **deep branch,** which supplies the levator scapulae and rhomboid muscles (Figs. 21–3*B* and 21–4*B* and Table 21–1). In some persons, the deep branch of the transverse cervical artery branches directly from the subclavian artery and is then called the **dorsal (descending) scapular artery** (Fig. 21–3*C*). The superficial branch, which then branches directly from the thyrocervical trunk, is called the **superficial cervical artery** (Fig. 21–3*C*).

Another branch of the thyrocervical trunk, the **suprascapular artery,** at first, courses laterally over the

TABLE 21–1
Muscles and other Structures Supplied by Branches of the Subclavian Artery

Artery	Muscles Supplied	Other Regions or Structures Supplied
FIRST PART OF SUBCLAVIAN ARTERY		
Vertebral artery	Suboccipital muscles	Cervical vertebrae, spinal cord, and meninges; skull; brain; cranial meninges (see Chapter 27)
Internal thoracic artery	Intercostal muscles, diaphragm, pectoralis major, abdominal muscles	Sternum, skin of anterior thorax, mammary glands
Branches of thyrocervical trunk		
Inferior thyroid artery	Infrahyoid, longus colli, inferior scalene, inferior constrictor, longus capitis, laryngeal muscles	Cervical vertebrae, cervical spinal cord, and meninges; larynx, esophagus, thyroid and parathyroid glands
Transverse cervical artery	Trapezius muscle (superficial branch or superficial cervical artery if there is no deep branch), levator scapulae, rhomboid major and minor, teres major and minor muscles (deep branch)	
Suprascapular artery	Subclavius, sternocleidomastoid, subscapularis, supraspinatus, infraspinatus muscles	Clavicle, scapula, skin of upper thorax and shoulder, acromioclavicular and glenohumeral joints
Left costocervical trunk	Muscles of first two intercostal spaces; semispinalis capitis, semispinalis cervicis muscles	Cervical vertebrae, spinal cord, meninges
SECOND PART OF SUBCLAVIAN ARTERY		
Right costocervical trunk	Muscles of first two intercostal spaces; semispinalis capitis, semispinalis cervicis muscles	Cervical vertebrae, spinal cord, meninges
THIRD PART OF SUBCLAVIAN ARTERY		
Dorsal (descending) scapular artery (if there is no deep branch of the transverse cervical artery)	Levator scapulae, rhomboid major and minor, teres major and minor muscles	Scapula

anterior surface of the anterior scalene muscle. It passes posterior to the clavicle and subclavius muscle (which it supplies, along with the sternocleidomastoid muscle) and splits into two major branches. One of these descends anteriorly to supply the subscapularis muscle within the subscapular fossa. The other courses over the superior border of the scapula in the region of the suprascapular ligament to enter the supraspinous fossa of the scapula next to the bone (Fig. 21–4*A*). Here it supplies the supraspinatus muscle before it continues around the greater scapular notch (see Fig. 21–2 and above) to enter the infraspinous fossa. It remains close to the bone within the infraspinous fossa and supplies the infraspinatus muscle (see Fig. 21–5*A* and *B*). Other branches anastomose with the deep branch of the transverse cervical artery (or dorsal scapular artery) and the circumflex scapular artery, which is a branch of the subscapular artery (Fig. 21–4*B* and Table 21–1 and see discussion of collateral circulation below).

The suprascapular artery also has branches that supply the clavicle, scapula, and acromioclavicular and glenohumeral joints (see Table 21–1).

The **left costocervical trunk** is a short artery, which arises from the posterior side of the first part of the left subclavian artery. It has two branches: the superior intercostal artery and deep cervical artery. The **deep cervical artery** ascends to supply muscles of the neck. It is described in Chapter 27. The **left superior intercostal artery** descends within the subserous fascia of the pleura, posterior to the first two ribs, where it branches to form the first and second posterior intercostal arteries.

The **second part of the left subclavian artery** has no branches (see Fig. 21–3*A*). The **second part of the right subclavian artery** gives rise to the right costocervical trunk (see Fig. 21–3*A*).

Like the left costocervical trunk, the **right costocervical trunk** splits into a deep cervical artery (described

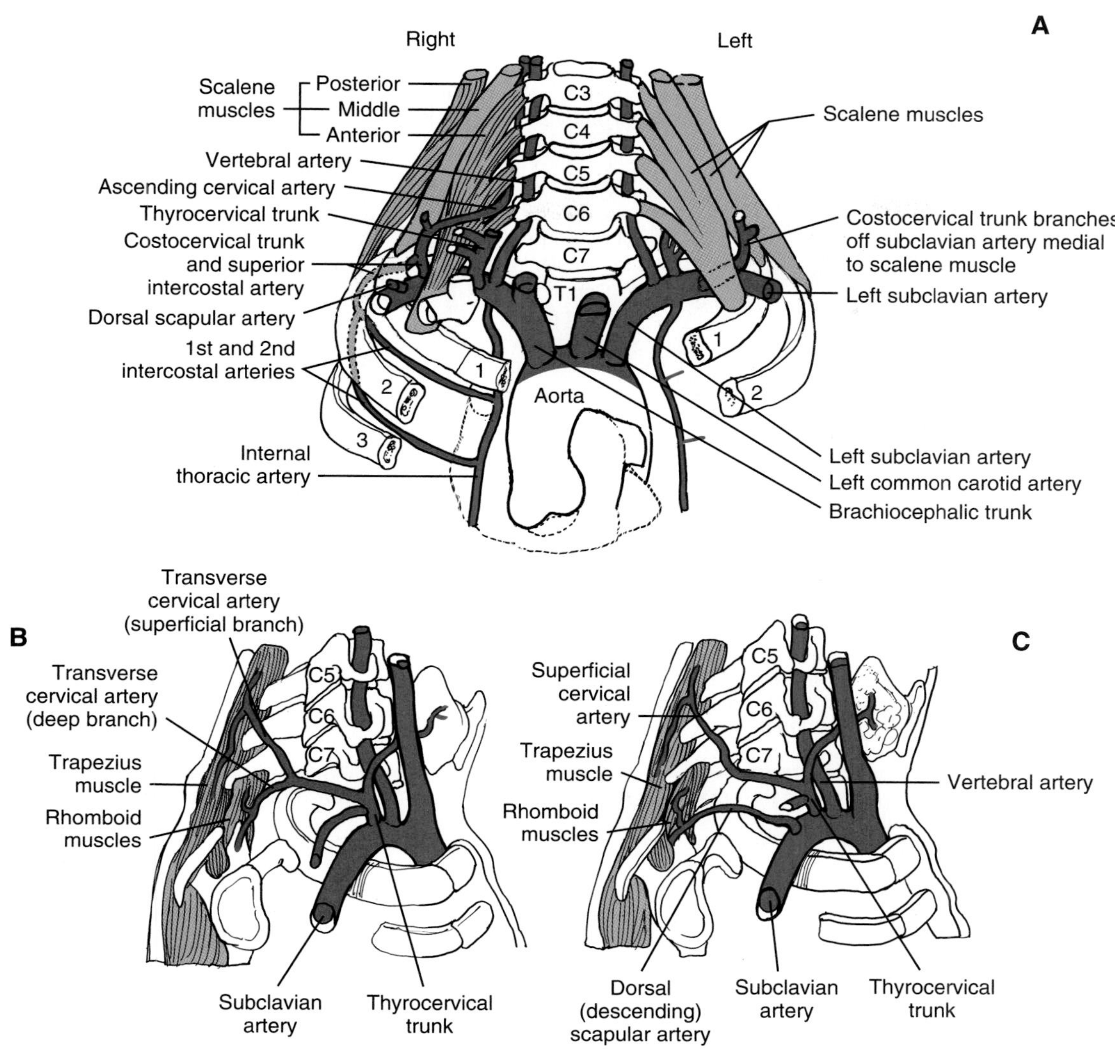

FIGURE 21–3
Subclavian artery and its branches. **A.** Anterior view. **B.** Subclavian artery branches of the right side. **C.** Variation showing dorsal descending scapular artery branching directly from the subclavian artery.

in Chapter 27) and a **right superior intercostal artery.** This artery branches to form the first and second right posterior intercostal arteries (Fig. 21–4*A*).

If the deep branch of the transverse cervical artery is absent, the **third parts of the left** and **right subclavian arteries** may each give rise to a descending (dorsal) scapular artery (see Fig. 21–3*C*). Thus, if the dorsal scapular artery exists, it courses laterally and posteriorly to supply the levator scapulae and rhomboid major and minor muscles (see Fig. 21–3*C*).

Axillary Artery and Its Branches

Before entering the limb, the axillary artery gives rise to branches that supply thoracic structures and the shoulder

The axillary artery is an extension of the subclavian artery. The axillary artery starts at the lateral border of the first rib and ends at the inferior border of the teres major muscle (Fig. 21–4*B*). Here, it enters the limb as the brachial artery. As is the case for branches of the subclavian artery, branches of the axillary artery are often described in relation to the three parts of the artery. The three parts are defined by the pectoralis minor muscle, which crosses the artery in its middle third. Thus, the first part is proximal (and medial) to the medial edge of the pectoralis minor muscle; the second part is posterior to the muscle; and the third part is distal (and lateral) to the muscle (Fig. 21–5*A*).

The **first part of the axillary artery** gives rise to one major branch, the **superior (supreme) thoracic artery** (Fig. 21–5*A*). This small branch arises from the axillary artery just under the lower border of the subclavius muscles and medial to the medial border of the pectoralis mi-

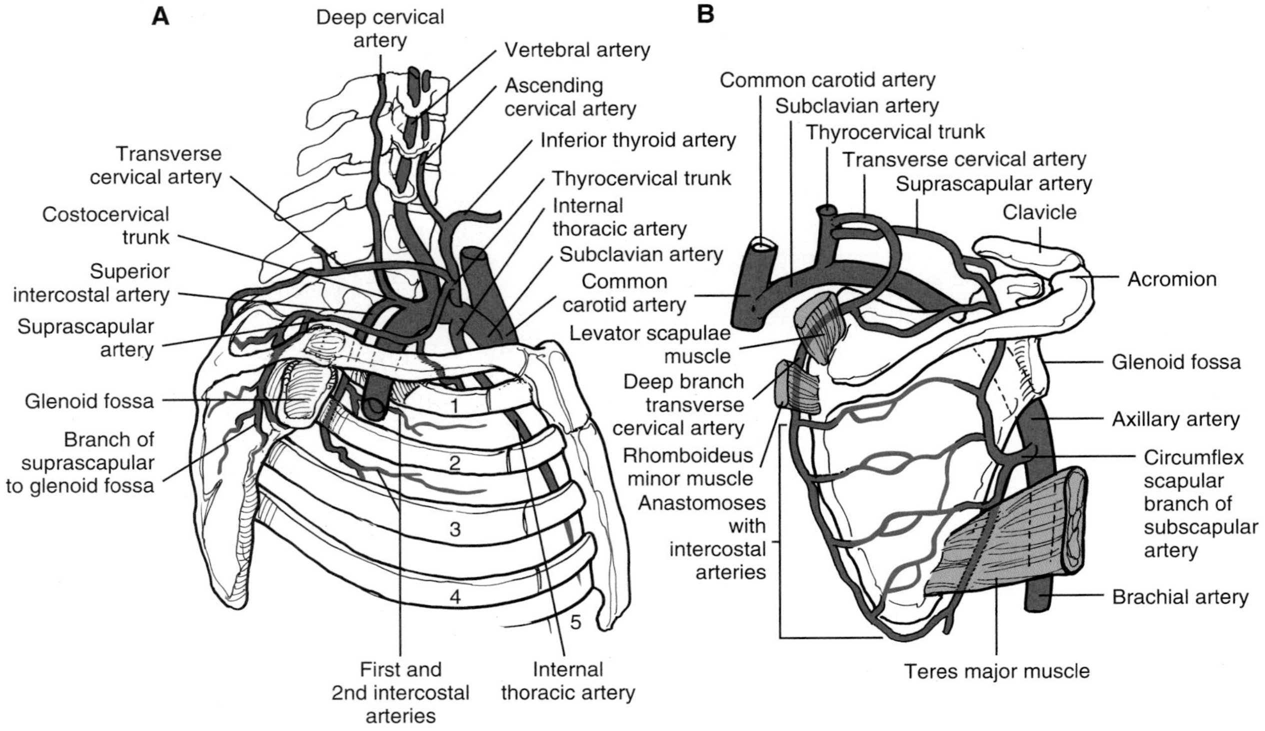

FIGURE 21–4
Thyrocervical trunk and costocervical trunk and their branches. **A.** Lateral view. **B.** Posterior view showing branch of suprascapular artery passing around the scapula.

nor muscle (Fig. 21–5*A*). It passes between the pectoralis minor muscle and the pectoralis major muscle to reach the thoracic wall. It supplies the subclavius and pectoralis minor and major muscles and anastomoses with the internal thoracic and anterior intercostal arteries.

The **second part of the axillary artery** gives rise to two branches, the thoracoacromial trunk and lateral thoracic artery (Fig. 21–5*A*). In some persons, the thoracoacromial artery arises from the first part of the axillary artery.

Typically, the **thoracoacromial artery** arises from the second part of the axillary artery just at the medial edge of the pectoralis minor muscle. It courses around the medial border of the pectoralis minor muscle and pierces the clavipectoral fascia as it splits into four branches (Fig. 21–5*A*). These branches include the **pectoral branch,** which supplies the pectoralis major and minor muscles; the **acromial branch,** which courses under the acromial process to supply the deltoid muscle; the **deltoid branch,** which crosses the pectoralis minor muscle (and accompanies the cephalic vein) to supply the deltoid and pectoralis major muscles; and the **clavicular branch,** which rises to supply the sternoclavicular joint and subclavius muscle (Fig. 21–5*A* and Table 21–2).

The **lateral thoracic artery** descends along the lateral border of the pectoralis minor muscle and over the anterior surface of the serratus anterior muscle (Fig. 21–5*A*). It supplies the pectoralis major and minor, serratus anterior, and subscapularis muscles (Table 21–2). Branches anastomose with the anterior intercostal arteries, subscapular artery, and pectoral branch of the thoracoacromial trunk (Fig. 21–5*A* and see Fig. 21–9). In females, the lateral thoracic artery supplies the lateral part of the mammary gland (see Chapter 6). Clinicians often refer to the lateral thoracic artery as the mammary artery.

The **third part of the axillary artery** has three branches: the subscapular artery, which is the largest branch of the axillary artery, and the anterior and posterior humeral circumflex arteries (see Fig. 21–5*A*).

The **subscapular artery** branches from the axillary artery near the inferior border of the subscapularis muscle (see Fig. 21–5*A*). Small branches anastomose with the lateral thoracic artery and adjacent intercostal arteries (see Fig. 21–9).

Within a few centimeters of the origin of the subscapular artery, a branch called the **scapular circumflex artery** arises from the main trunk. This vessel curves around the lateral border of the scapula, courses through the triangular space (see Fig. 21–12*C*), and follows the inferior border of the subscapularis muscle (which it supplies) to the inferior angle of the scapula. Here it splits into two branches. One branch supplies the infraspinatus and subscapularis muscles. It gives rise to other

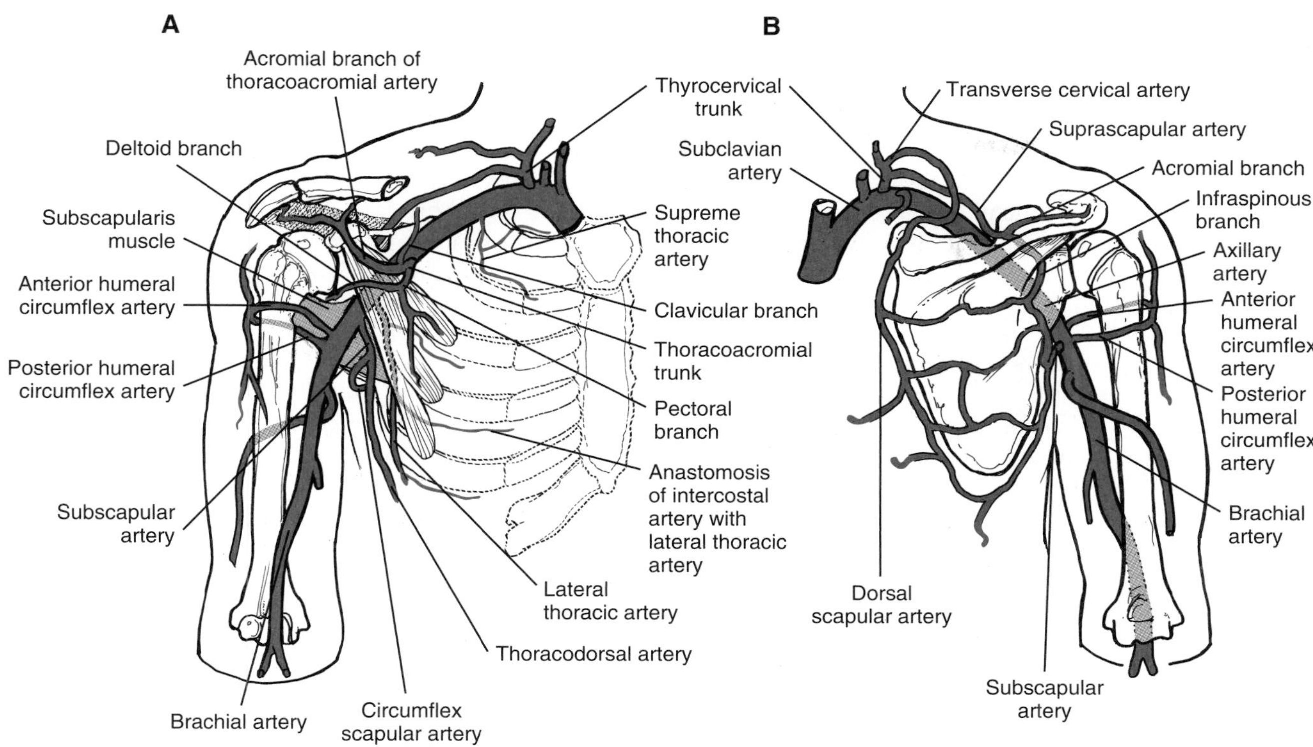

FIGURE 21–5
Axillary artery and its branches. **A.** Anterior view. **B.** Posterior view.

TABLE 21–2
Muscles and Other Structures Supplied by Branches of the Axillary Artery

Artery	Muscles Supplied	Other Regions or Structures Supplied
FIRST PART OF AXILLARY ARTERY		
Superior (supreme) thoracic artery	Subclavius, pectoralis major and minor muscles	
SECOND PART OF AXILLARY ARTERY		
Branches of thoracoacromial trunk		
Pectoral artery	Pectoralis major and minor, intercostal muscles	Mammary glands
Acromial artery	Deltoid muscle	
Deltoid artery	Deltoid, pectoralis major muscles	
Clavicular artery	Subclavius muscle	Sternoclavicular joint
Lateral thoracic artery	Serratus anterior, pectoralis major and minor, subscapularis muscles	Mammary glands
THIRD PART OF AXILLARY ARTERY		
Subscapular artery	Subscapularis, infraspinatus, intercostal, latissimus dorsi, deltoid muscles; long head of triceps brachii muscle	Scapula
Anterior humeral circumflex artery		Head of humerus, glenohumeral joint
Posterior humeral circumflex artery	Teres major and minor, deltoid muscles; long and lateral heads of triceps brachii muscle	Glenohumeral joint

branches that anastomose with the suprascapular artery and dorsal scapular artery (or deep branch of the transverse cervical artery). The other branch continues along the lateral scapular border and anastomoses with the dorsal scapular artery (see Fig. 21–9). Small branches supply the posterior part of the deltoid muscle and the long head of the triceps brachii muscle.

After giving off the scapular circumflex artery, the main trunk of the subscapular artery descends to supply the latissimus dorsi muscle as the **thoracodorsal artery** (Fig. 21–5A).

As the third part of the axillary artery turns downward to descend within the axilla, the **anterior humeral circumflex artery** arises from its lateral side (Fig. 21–5). It passes laterally between the surgical head of the humerus, short head of the biceps brachii muscle, and coracobrachialis muscle. It sends branches to the humerus and glenohumeral joint and circles the humerus under the deltoid muscle and the long head of the biceps brachii muscle to anastomose with the posterior humeral circumflex artery (see below).

The **posterior humeral circumflex artery** branches from the lateral side of the third part of the axillary artery just distal to the origin of the anterior humeral circumflex artery (Fig. 21–5). The posterior humeral circumflex artery, however, passes posteriorly through the quadrangular space (see above) with the axillary nerve. It circles posteriorly around the surgical neck of the humerus between the humerus and the long head of the triceps brachii muscle. It gives rise to branches that supply the teres major and minor muscles, deltoid muscle, long and lateral heads of the triceps brachii muscle, and glenohumeral joint. A **descending branch** may anastomose with the arteria profunda brachii (deep brachial artery), while the main trunk anastomoses with the anterior humeral circumflex artery (see Fig. 21–9).

Brachial Artery and Its Branches

The brachial artery (an extension of the axillary artery) and its branches supply blood to all compartments of the arm

The brachial artery is an extension of the axillary artery (Fig. 21–6). It originates at the inferior border of the tendon of the teres major muscle. It is a superficial artery, which courses just beneath the skin along the medial side of the arm. Within the arm, it gives rise to several branches, which serve the coracobrachialis, brachialis, and biceps brachii muscles, and to the arteria profunda brachii (deep brachial artery), nutrient artery of the humerus, superior ulnar collateral artery, and inferior ulnar collateral artery (Table 21–3). The brachial

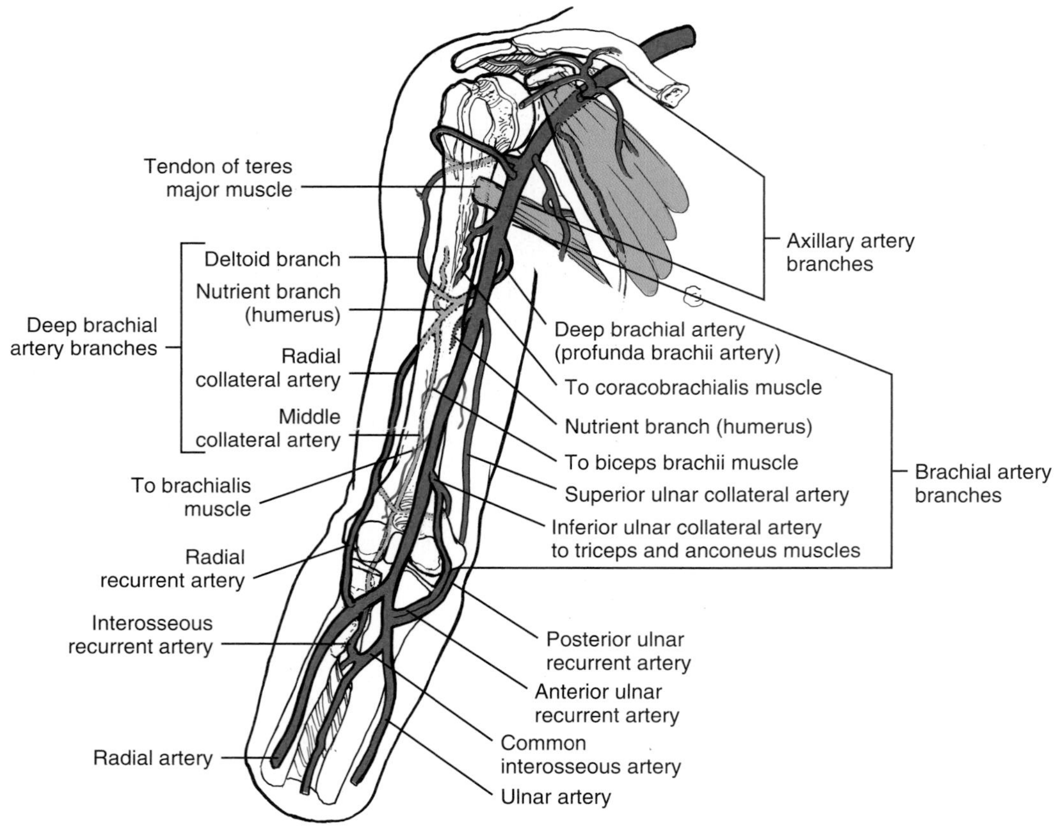

FIGURE 21–6
Brachial artery and its branches.

TABLE 21–3
Muscles and other Structures Supplied by Branches of the Brachial Artery

Artery	Muscles Supplied	Other Regions or Structures Supplied
BRANCHES OF ARTERIA PROFUNDA BRACHII (DEEP BRACHIAL ARTERY)		
Muscular branches	Lateral and medial heads of triceps brachii muscle	
Nutrient artery		Humerus
Deltoid artery		Anastomoses with posterior humeral circumflex artery (see text)
Middle collateral branch	Medial head of triceps brachii muscle, anconeus muscle	Anastomoses with recurrent interosseous and inferior ulnar collateral arteries
Radial collateral branch	Brachialis, brachioradialis muscles; lateral head of triceps brachii muscle	
MUSCULAR BRANCHES	Coracobrachialis, brachialis, biceps brachii, pronator teres muscles	
NUTRIENT BRANCHES		Humerus
SUPERIOR ULNAR COLLATERAL BRANCHES		Anastomose with posterior ulnar recurrent and inferior ulnar collateral arteries
INFERIOR ULNAR COLLATERAL BRANCHES		Anastomose with middle collateral branch of arteria profunda brachii
BRANCHES OF RADIAL ARTERY		
Muscular branches	Pronator teres, flexor carpi radialis, flexor digitorum superficialis, flexor pollicis longus, abductor pollicis longus muscles	
Radial recurrent artery	Brachioradialis, brachialis, supinator muscles	
Palmar carpal artery		Anastomoses with palmar carpal branch of ulnar artery, anterior interosseous artery, and recurrent branch of deep palmar arch to form cruciate palmar arch of wrist
Superficial palmar artery		Anastomoses with superficial palmar branch of ulnar artery to form superficial palmar arch
Dorsal carpal artery		Anastomoses with dorsal carpal branch of ulnar artery to form dorsal carpal arch
First dorsal metacarpal artery		Ulnar side of thumb, radial side of index finger
Princeps pollicis artery		Ulnar and radial sides of thumb; nutrient branch to first metacarpal; deep palmar branch anastomoses with deep palmar branch of ulnar artery to form deep palmar arch
Radialis indicis artery		Radial side of digit 2
BRANCHES OF ULNAR ARTERY		
Anterior recurrent ulnar artery	Brachialis, pronator teres muscles	Anastomoses with inferior ulnar collateral branch of brachial artery
Common interosseous artery		
Branches of anterior interosseous artery		
Muscular branches	Flexor digitorum profundus, flexor pollicis longus, extensor pollicis longus, abductor pollicis longus, pronator quadratus muscles	

Continued

TABLE 21–3, cont'd
Muscles and other Structures Supplied by Branches of the Brachial Artery

Artery	Muscles Supplied	Other Regions or Structures Supplied
BRANCHES OF ULNAR ARTERY—CONT'D		
Median branch		Median nerve
Nutrient branch		Ulna, radius
Branches of posterior interosseous artery		
Muscular branches	Supinator, abductor pollicis longus, extensor carpi ulnaris, extensor digitorum, extensor pollicis longus muscles	
Recurrent interosseous artery		Anastomoses with middle collateral branch of arteria profunda brachii
Muscular branches	Flexor carpi ulnaris, flexor digitorum superficialis, flexor digitorum profundus muscles	
Branches to ulnar nerve		Ulnar nerve
Dorsal carpal artery		Anastomoses with dorsal carpal branch of radial artery to form dorsal carpal arch (see text)
Deep palmar artery		Anastomoses with deep palmar branch of radial artery to form deep palmar arch (see text)

artery terminates just distal to the elbow joint at the level of the proximal radial head, where it splits into the ulnar and radial arteries (Fig. 21–6).

The **arteria profunda brachii (deep brachial artery)** is a large, deep vessel, which originates from the posteromedial surface of the brachial artery and courses posteriorly between the long and medial heads of the triceps brachii muscle to join the radial nerve (see below). Together, the arteria profunda brachii and radial nerve spiral around the posterior aspect of the humerus to its lateral side just deep to the lateral head of the triceps brachii muscle (Fig. 21–6 and Table 21–3). Here, after giving off muscular branches, the arteria profunda brachii splits into its four main terminal branches: the nutrient branch, deltoid branch, middle collateral branch, and radial collateral artery (Fig. 21–6).

Muscular branches of the arteria profunda brachii supply the lateral and medial heads of the triceps brachii muscle.

The **nutrient artery of the arteria profunda brachii** is not always present. If it is present, it enters the humerus just posterior to the deltoid tuberosity (Fig. 21–6).

The ascending **deltoid branch of the arteria profunda brachii** courses superiorly between the long and lateral heads of the triceps brachii muscle to anastomose with a descending branch of the posterior humeral circumflex artery (Fig. 21–6 and see Fig. 21–9).

The **middle collateral branch of the arteria profunda brachii** originates just posterior to the humerus. It descends within the substance of the medial head of the triceps brachii muscle and finally anastomoses with the recurrent interosseous and inferior ulnar collateral arteries (from the ulnar artery) (see below) just posterior to the lateral epicondyle (Fig. 21–6 and see Fig. 21–10). The middle collateral branch is the largest terminal branch of the arteria profunda brachii. It supplies the medial head of the triceps brachii muscle and the anconeus muscle (Table 21–3).

The **radial collateral branch** is the continuation of the **arteria profunda brachii.** Therefore, it pierces the lateral intermuscular septum (see below), along with the radial nerve, and descends between the brachialis and brachioradialis muscles just anterior to the lateral epicondyle (Fig. 21–6). Finally, it anastomoses with the radial recurrent artery, which is a branch of the radial artery (Fig. 21–6).

The **nutrient branch of the brachial artery** arises from the medial aspect of the artery. It dives deep between the coracobrachialis muscle and short head of the biceps brachii muscle to enter the nutrient canal of the humerus near the attachment of the coracobrachialis muscle (Fig. 21–6).

The **superior ulnar collateral artery** branches from the medial aspect of the brachial artery just distal to the midpoint of the humeral shaft (Fig. 21–6 and see Fig. 21–10). It pierces the medial intermuscular septum along with the ulnar nerve and courses inferiorly between the olecranon process and medial epicondyle of the humerus.

Then it anastomoses with the posterior ulnar recurrent artery (a branch of the ulnar artery) and the inferior ulnar collateral artery (see immediately below) behind the flexor carpi ulnaris muscle (Fig. 21–6 and see Fig. 21–10).

The **inferior ulnar collateral artery** branches from the medial aspect of the brachial artery just above the medial epicondyle of the humerus (Fig. 21–6 and see Fig. 21–10). It pierces the medial intermuscular septum and spirals posterolaterally around the humeral shaft to anastomose with the middle collateral branch of the arteria profunda brachii (Fig. 21–6 and see Fig. 21–10).

Direct **muscular branches of the brachial artery** supply the coracobrachialis, brachialis, and biceps brachii muscles (Fig. 21–6).

Radial Artery and Its Branches

The radial artery is a terminal branch of the brachial artery

The radial artery originates at the level of the proximal head of the radius within the anterior compartment of the forearm (Fig. 21–7 and Table 21–4). From its origin just medial to the radial neck, it passes under the belly of the brachioradialis muscle and courses distally, just deep to the skin, along the lateral side of the anterior forearm to the wrist. Here, it passes anterior to the radial styloid process and posterolaterally around the carpus to enter the hand (Figs. 21–7 and 21–8 and see Fig. 21–7). In the wrist and hand, with contributions from the ulnar artery, the radial artery forms the superficial palmar arch, deep palmar arch, and dorsal carpal arch (see Fig. 21–8). Thus, the radial artery and its branches course within three regions of the upper extremity: the forearm, wrist, and hand.

The most proximal branch of the radial artery is the **radial recurrent artery.** It arises from the lateral aspect of the radial artery at its origin. It then passes deep to the brachioradialis muscle to supply the brachioradialis, supinator, and brachialis muscles and the elbow joint. The radial recurrent artery anastomoses with the radial collateral branch of the arteria profunda brachii (Fig. 21–7 and see Fig. 21–10).

The radial artery gives off several direct **muscular branches** as it courses distally within the radial side of the forearm. In the forearm, these branches supply the pronator teres, flexor carpi radialis, flexor digitorum superficialis, flexor pollicis longus, and abductor pollicis longus muscles (Fig. 21–7).

The **palmar carpal branch** originates from the medial aspect of the radial artery just at the distal border of the pronator teres muscle (Fig. 21–7). It courses over the anterior aspect of the distal radial head and then courses in a medial direction deep to the long flexor tendons. It anastomoses with the palmar carpal branch of the ulnar artery, the anterior interosseous artery (a branch of the ulnar artery), and a recurrent branch from the deep palmar arch to form the **cruciate palmar carpal arch** (Figs. 21–7 and 21–8 and Table 21–4). These vessels supply the carpal bones and joints.

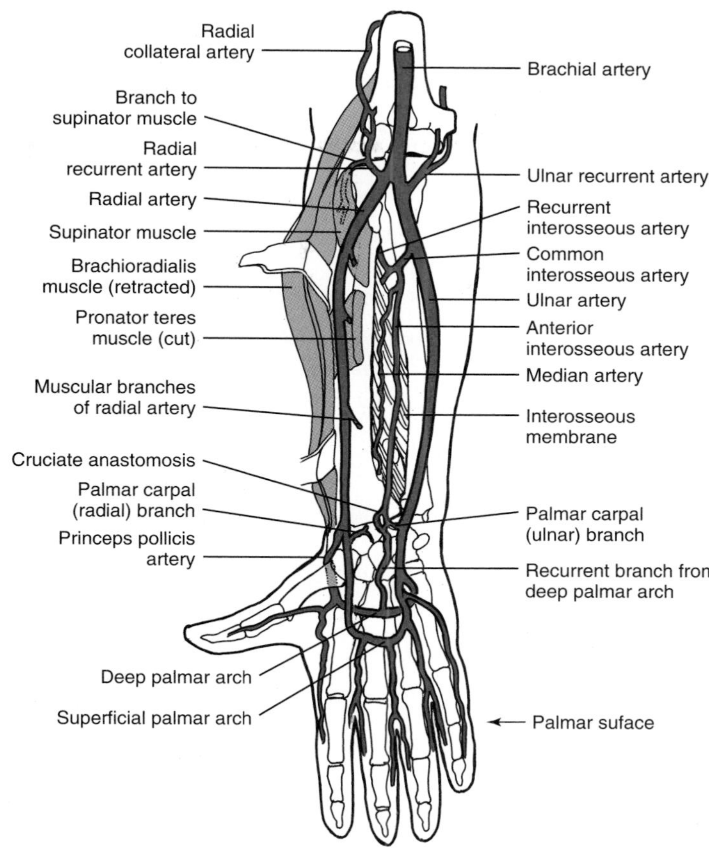

FIGURE 21–7
The radial and ulnar arteries and their branches of the right hand.

The **superficial palmar branch** of the radial artery originates just at the point where the palmar carpal branch arises from the radial artery and just proximal to the point at which the radial artery courses posteriorly around the lateral side of the carpus (Figs. 21–7 and 21–8). It anastomoses with a superficial palmar branch of the ulnar artery to form the **superficial palmar arch** (Fig. 21–8 and Table 21–4). The distal limit of the superficial palmar arch is at the midpoint of the shaft of the third metacarpal. The superficial palmar arch is described more completely below (see Arches Formed by the Ulnar and Radial Arteries).

The **dorsal carpal branch** of the radial artery branches from the radial artery at the lateral side of the carpus. It courses medially over the dorsal surface of the carpus and anastomoses with branches of the anterior and posterior interosseous arteries to form a **dorsal carpal arch** (Fig. 21–8 and Table 21–4). Branches of the dorsal carpal arch supply the carpal bones and their articulations and the epiphyseal regions of the distal ulna and radius (see below).

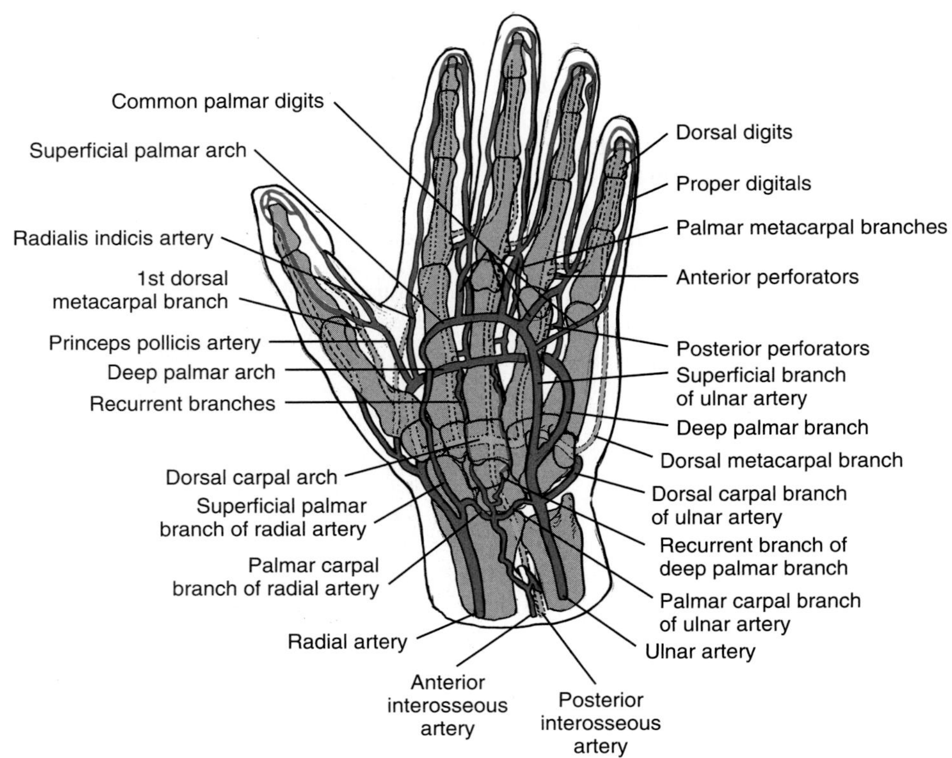

FIGURE 21–8
Palmar view of the arteries of the left hand.

TABLE 21–4
Terminal Branches of Radial or Ulnar Arteries: Palmar Arches

Palmar Arch	Terminal Branch of Radial or Ulnar Artery	Muscles Supplied	Other Regions or Structures Supplied
Dorsal carpal arch	Nutrient branch		Distal epiphyseal regions of ulna and radius
	Carpal artery		Bones and joints of carpus
	Dorsal digital artery	Lumbrical, interosseous muscles	Adjacent skin of digits 2 and 3, 3 and 4, 4 and 5; phalanges and nail beds of digits 2 to 5
Cruciate palmar arch of wrist	Carpal artery		Bones and joints of carpus
Superficial palmar arch	One proper palmar digital artery	Hypothenar muscles	Skin on ulnar side of digit 5; phalanges and nail bed of digit 5
	Three common palmar digital arteries split to form six proper palmar digital arteries	Lumbrical, interosseous muscles	Adjacent skin of digits 2 and 3, 3 and 4, 4 and 5; phalanges and nail beds of digits 2 to 5
Deep palmar arch	Three common palmar metacarpal arteries	Lumbrical, interosseous muscles	Anastomose with proper palmar digital arteries of superficial palmar arch, metacarpal bones
	Recurrent branch		Anastomoses with cruciate palmar arch of wrist

The **first dorsal metacarpal artery** branches from the radial artery just distal to the bases of the first and second metacarpals as the continuation of the radial artery (princeps pollicis artery) dives between the two heads of the first dorsal interosseous muscle (Fig. 21–8). The artery then immediately branches to supply the radial side of the index finger and ulnar side of the thumb. The radial side of the thumb is supplied by a separate twig of the radial artery that branches from the radial artery just at the level of the first carpometacarpal joint.

The **princeps pollicis artery** is a continuation of the radial artery. It returns to the palmar side of the hand as it dives between the first and second metacarpals (Figs. 21–7 and 21–8). At the base of the proximal phalanx of digit 2, it splits into a branch that supplies both sides of the thumb **(proper digital arteries of the thumb)** and a **deep palmar branch,** which anastomoses with the deep palmar branch of the ulnar artery to form a **deep palmar arch.** Branches of the deep palmar arch are described below (Table 21–4). The princeps pollicis artery provides a **nutrient branch** to the first metacarpal.

The **radialis indicis artery** is typically a branch of the princeps pollicis artery (Figs. 21–7 and 21–8). It courses along the radial side of digit 2.

Ulnar Artery and Its Branches

The ulnar artery is the larger terminal branch of the brachial artery

The ulnar artery branches from the brachial artery, along with the radial artery, between the lower edge of the brachialis muscle and upper edge of the pronator teres muscle (see Fig. 21–7). In addition to several named branches (see below), it gives rise to branches that supply muscles on the ulnar side of the medial side of the forearm and hand, the common synovial sheath of the long flexors, and the ulnar nerve. With branches of the radial artery, the ulnar artery also contributes to the superficial palmar arch, deep palmar arch, and dorsal carpal arch. Thus, the ulnar artery and its branches course within three regions of the upper limb: the forearm, wrist, and hand.

The first branch of the ulnar artery is the **anterior ulnar recurrent artery.** This artery courses proximally between the brachialis and pronator teres muscles and anastomoses with the inferior ulnar collateral branch of the brachial artery just anterior to the medial epicondyle of the humerus (see Fig. 21–7). The anterior ulnar recurrent artery supplies the brachialis and pronator teres muscles.

As the ulnar artery dives under the pronator teres muscle, it gives rise to the **posterior ulnar recurrent artery** (see Figs. 21–7 and 21–10). This branch courses proximally behind the medial epicondyle of the humerus to anastomose with the superior ulnar collateral artery. It supplies the flexor carpi ulnaris, pronator teres, and anconeus muscles; ulnar nerve; and elbow joint.

Distal to the origin of the posterior recurrent artery and anterior to the shaft of the ulna, the ulnar artery gives rise to the **common interosseous artery** (see Fig. 21–7 and 21–10). Almost immediately, at the proximal border of the interosseous membrane, this artery branches into the anterior and posterior interosseous arteries.

Just at its origin, the **anterior interosseous artery** gives rise to a long **median artery,** which supplies the median nerve (see Fig. 21–7). Then, as the anterior interosseous artery descends along the anterior surface of the interosseous membrane, several **muscular branches** supply deep flexors of the forearm, including the flexor digitorum profundus and flexor pollicis longus muscles (see Fig. 21–7). In addition, its **nutrient branches** supply the ulna and radius.

As it continues to course distally upon the interosseous membrane, small **muscular branches** pierce the membrane to supply muscles of the deep extensor compartment of the forearm. The most distal of these branches penetrates the interosseous membrane just proximal to the proximal boundary of the pronator quadratus muscle. This terminal branch anastomoses with the posterior interosseous artery (see below).

As has been described above, the anterior interosseous artery terminates by anastomosing with palmar carpal branches of the radial and ulnar arteries and a deep recurrent branch of the deep palmar arch to form the **cruciate palmar arch of the wrist** (see Figs. 21–7 and 21–8 and Table 21–4).

The **posterior interosseous artery** splits from the common interosseous artery to pass posterior to the interosseous membrane and between the supinator and abductor pollicis longus muscles. It first gives rise to a **recurrent interosseous branch,** which ascends between the lateral epicondyle and olecranon process to anastomose with the middle collateral branch of the arteria profunda brachii (see Fig. 21–7 and above). It then descends within the forearm between the superficial and deep extensor compartments, supplying (with **muscular branches**) the superficial extensor muscles (see Fig. 21–7). As has been noted above, its terminus anastomoses just proximal to the wrist with the terminus of the anterior interosseous artery and palmar carpal branch of the radial artery to form the **cruciate palmar arch of the wrist** (see Figs. 21–7 and 21–8 and Table 21–4).

Just after giving off anterior and posterior ulnar recurrent and common interosseous arteries, the main trunk of the ulnar artery descends within the ulnar side of the forearm between the deep and superficial flexor compartments. Here, it provides direct branches to the flexor carpi ulnaris, flexor digitorum profundus, and flexor digitorum superficialis muscles.

The **palmar carpal branch** of the ulnar artery arises from the radial side of the ulnar artery to course over the ventral aspect of the ulna and onto the ventral surface of the carpus where it anastomoses with the palmar carpal branch of the radial artery (see Figs. 21–7 and 21–8 and Table 21–4).

The **dorsal carpal branch** of the ulnar artery originates just proximal to the pisiform bone at the palmar aspect of the carpus. It then courses around the ulnar side of the wrist and onto the dorsal aspect of the carpus where it anastomoses with the dorsal carpal branch of the radial artery to form the **dorsal carpal arch.** It also gives rise to a **dorsal metacarpal branch,** which serves the ulnar side of digit 5 (see below).

The **deep palmar branch** of the ulnar artery arises from the ulnar side of the ulnar artery just distal to the pisiform bone. It passes between the flexor digiti minimi and abductor digiti minimi muscles and deep to the opponens digiti minimi muscle to anastomose with the deep palmar branch of the radial artery, forming a **deep palmar arch** (see Figs. 21–7 and 21–8 and Table 21–4).

Arches Formed by the Ulnar and Radial Arteries

Arches formed by terminal branches of the ulnar and radial arteries emit branches that serve the wrist, palm, and digits

The **dorsal carpal arch** is formed by dorsal carpal branches of the radial and ulnar arteries (see above). The dorsal carpal arch also receives contributions from the anterior and posterior interosseous arteries. The arch lies close to the dorsal surface of the carpus and gives rise to three dorsal metacarpal arteries and branches, which supply the distal epiphyseal regions of the ulna and radius, carpal bones, and intercarpal joints (see Fig. 21–8).

The three digital arteries that emanate from the dorsal carpal arch course between metacarpals 2 and 3, 3 and 4, and 4 and 5. In the regions of the metacarpophalangeal joints, each artery splits into two dorsal digital arteries, which supply the ulnar side of digit 2 and radial side of digit 3, the ulnar side of digit 3 and radial side of digit 4, and the ulnar side of digit 4 and radial side of digit 5 (see Fig. 21–8). To complete the arterial supply to the digits, a dorsal metacarpal branch of the radial artery gives rise to digital branches supplying the ulnar side of the thumb and radial side of digit 2 (see Fig. 21–8). The dorsal metacarpal artery serving the ulnar side of digit 5 arises from the dorsal carpal branch of the ulnar artery (see above).

The **cruciate palmar arch of the wrist** is an anastomosis of the palmar carpal branch of the radial artery, the palmar carpal branch of the ulnar artery, the anterior interosseous artery (a branch of the ulnar artery), and a recurrent branch of the deep palmar arch. It is located deep to flexor tendons in the wrist and supplies the carpal bones and their joints (see Fig. 21–8).

The **superficial palmar arch,** typically formed by superficial palmar branches of the radial and ulnar arteries, lies between the palmaris brevis muscle, palmar aponeurosis, flexor digiti minimi muscle, long flexor tendons, and lumbrical muscles. Alternatively, it is occasionally supplied only by a superficial palmar branch of the ulnar artery. Branches of the superficial palmar arch include a **proper palmar digital artery,** which supplies the ulnar side of digit 5, and three **common palmar digital arteries,** which split to form six proper palmar digital arteries. These supply the palmar and radial sides of digit 5; the palmar, ulnar, and radial sides of digits 4 and 3; and the palmar and ulnar sides of digit 2 (see Fig. 21–8). The radial side of digit 2 is supplied by the arteria radialis indicis. Both sides of the thumb are supplied by branches of the princeps pollicis artery. Both of these latter arteries are branches of the radial artery.

The **deep palmar arch** is formed by deep palmar branches of the radial and ulnar arteries and gives rise to three **palmar metacarpal branches,** each of which anastomoses with one of the three common digital branches of the superficial palmar arch (see Fig. 21–8). The deep palmar arch also gives rise to a **recurrent branch,** which anastomoses with palmar carpal branches of the radial and ulnar arteries (see Fig. 21–8).

Collateral Arterial Circulatory System. *As in the lower extremity, there is an extensive collateral circulatory system in the vicinity of the joints of the upper extremity.* A collateral circulatory system of arteries is extensive around the shoulder, glenohumeral, and elbow joints; proximal and distal radioulnar joints; and joints of the wrist, hand, and digits. Anastomoses of vessels within the wrist, hand, and digits are largely described by the **arterial arches** illustrated immediately above.

Collateral Arteries of the Scapula. *Three main arterial trunks of the subclavian and axillary arteries anastomose around the scapula.* The extensive collateral circulatory system around the scapula is provided by branches of the **suprascapular** and **deep cervical branches of the thyrocervical trunk** (a branch of the **subclavian artery**) and the **subscapular branch of the axillary artery** (Fig. 21–9). All of these major vessels provide significant contributions to an extensive anastomotic network of vessels within the supraspinous and infraspinous fossae of the scapula (Fig. 21–9). In addition, the **lateral thoracic artery** may contribute to the collateral circulation of the scapula through branches connected to the subscapular artery.

Collateral Arteries of the Glenohumeral Joint. *The anterior and posterior humeral circumflex arteries anastomose in the vicinity of the glenohumeral joint.* As has been described above, the **anterior** and **posterior humeral circumflex arteries** course around the neck of the humerus to form an anastomosis on the lateral surface of the neck (Fig. 21–9). In addition, a **descending branch** of the posterior humeral circumflex artery anastomoses with an ascending **deltoid branch** of the arteria profunda brachii (Fig. 21–9).

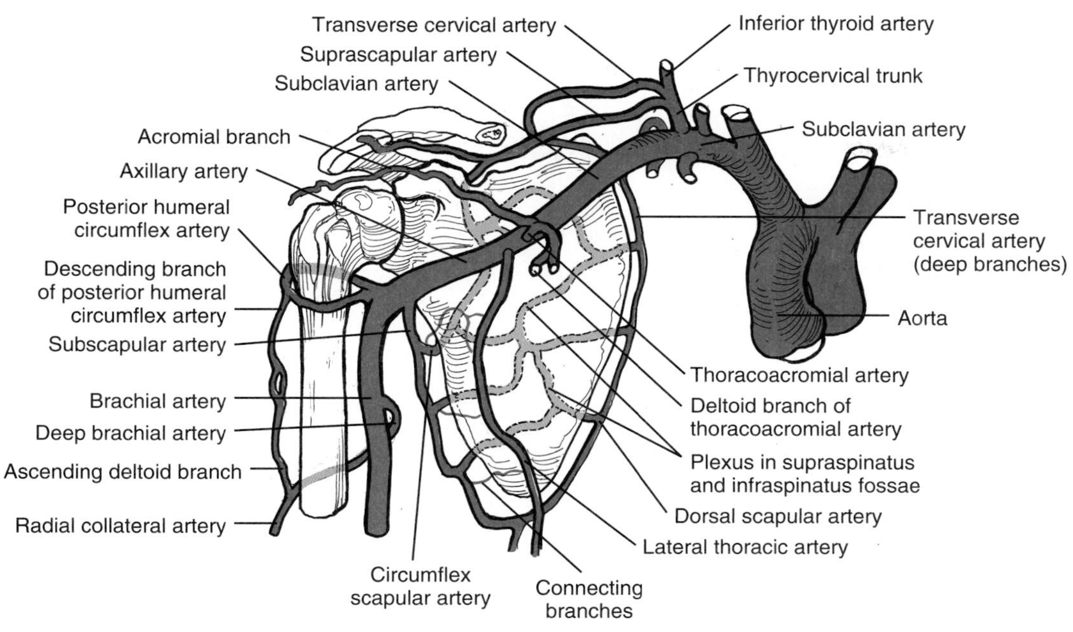

FIGURE 21–9
Collateral arteries of the scapula and glenohumeral joint.

Collateral Arteries of the Elbow Joint. *A network of collateral branches invests the elbow joint.* As has been described above, the brachial artery and arteria profunda brachii give rise to branches above the elbow joint. These branches anastomose with branches of the ulnar, radial, and posterior interosseous arteries that arise from these vessels below the elbow joint. On the ulnar side of the joint, the brachial artery gives rise to a very high branch **(superior ulnar collateral artery),** which descends within the medial arm and behind the medial epicondyle of the humerus to anastomose with the **posterior ulnar recurrent branch** of the ulnar artery (Fig. 21–10). An **inferior ulnar collateral branch** arises from the brachial artery just above the cubital fossa and descends anterior to the elbow joint to anastomose with the **anterior ulnar recurrent branch** of the ulnar artery (Fig. 21–10). Anastomoses may also form between the superior and inferior ulnar collateral branches. On the radial side of the elbow joint, the arteria profunda brachii splits to form two branches: an anterior descending branch and a middle collateral (posterior descending) branch. The **anterior descending branch** passes anterior to the lateral epicondyle of the humerus to anastomose with a **radial recurrent branch** of the radial artery. The **middle collateral (posterior descending) branch** passes behind the elbow joint to anastomose with a **recurrent interosseous branch,** which arises from the posterior interosseous artery on the anterior side of the interosseous membrane (Fig. 21–10). This recurrent interosseous branch gains access to the posterior region of the elbow joint by passing between the ulna and radius and over the superior edge of the interosseous membrane (Fig. 21–10). The ulnar and radial collaterals just described may anastomose with each other through a connection between the inferior ulnar collateral branch of the brachial artery and the middle collateral branch of the arteria profunda brachii in the distal region of the posterior arm (Fig. 21–10).

Collateral Arteries of the Wrist and Hand. *An extensive collateral circulatory system in the wrist and hand is provided by branches that connect the dorsal carpal arch, cruciate palmar arch of the wrist, and deep and superficial palmar arches of the hand.* Direct anastomoses between the dorsal carpal arch and cruciate palmar arch of the wrist are formed on both the ulnar and radial sides of the wrist via branches of the ulnar and radial arteries (see Fig. 21–8). In addition, an anterior ascending branch of the cruciate palmar arch of the wrist is connected to the dorsal carpal arch via the anterior and posterior interosseous arteries (see Fig. 21–8). The cruciate palmar arch of the wrist also anastomoses with the deep palmar arch via **ascending branches** of the deep palmar arch. The deep palmar arch, in turn, connects to **common palmar digital branches** of the superficial palmar arch via **palmar metacarpal arteries.** The common palmar digital arteries connect to the **dorsal metacarpal branches** of the dorsal carpal arch via **ante-**

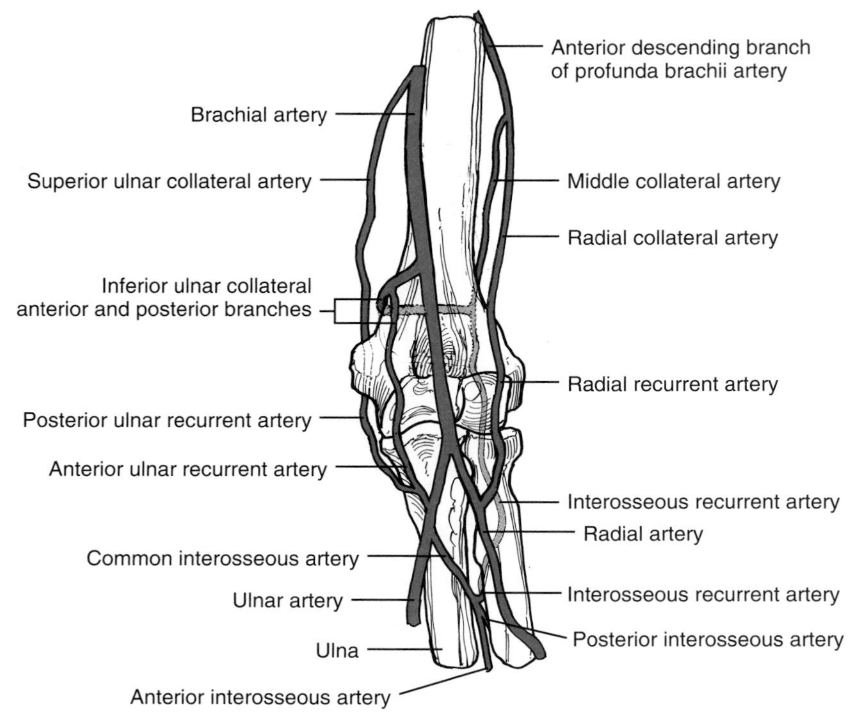

FIGURE 21–10
Collateral arteries of the elbow joint. Anterior view of left elbow.

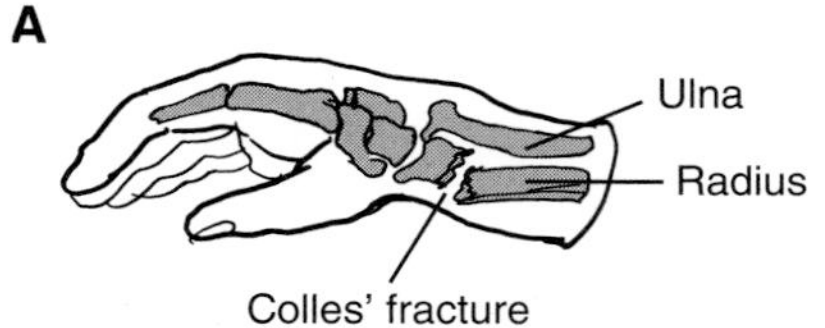

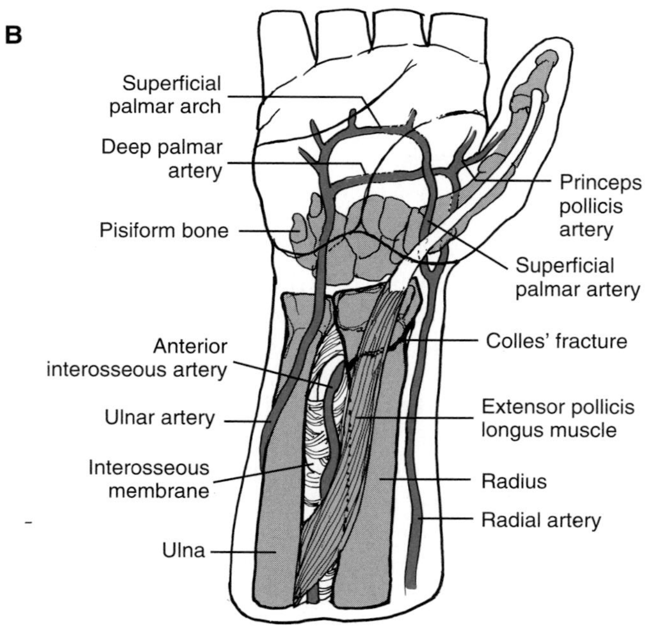

FIGURE 21–11
Colles' fracture may include rupture of a tendon as well as damage to arteries.

rior perforating branches, which course between the bases of the proximal phalanges. Similarly, the palmar metacarpal branches of the deep palmar arch are connected to **dorsal metacarpal branches** of the dorsal carpal arch via **posterior perforating branches,** which course between the metacarpal bones (see Fig. 21–8).

Arterial Injuries. The **axillary artery** is one of the most commonly injured vessels of the body. It is particularly prone to injury if it is diseased. Typically, it may be lacerated during reduction of shoulder dislocations.

In addition, injury to an artery may lead to disorders of surrounding structures. For example, compromise of the **anterior interosseous, radial,** or **pollical artery** as a consequence of **Colles' fracture** may result in avascular necrosis and rupture of the tendon of the extensor pollicis longus muscle (Fig. 21–11).

Because the collateral circulatory system of the **palmar arches** is so extensive, the ligature of any single vessel contributing to any of the arches will be insufficient to stop the bleeding following injury of an arch. Even the ligature of both the ulnar and radial arteries may be ineffective because carpal branches of the interosseous arteries also supply the injured arteries (see Fig. 21–8).

Raynaud's Disease and Raynaud's Phenomenon. Raynaud's disease and Raynaud's phenomenon result in the constriction of digital arteries. This first causes blanching (reduced blood flow), then cyanosis (stagnation of poorly oxygenated blood), and then redness (return of oxygenated

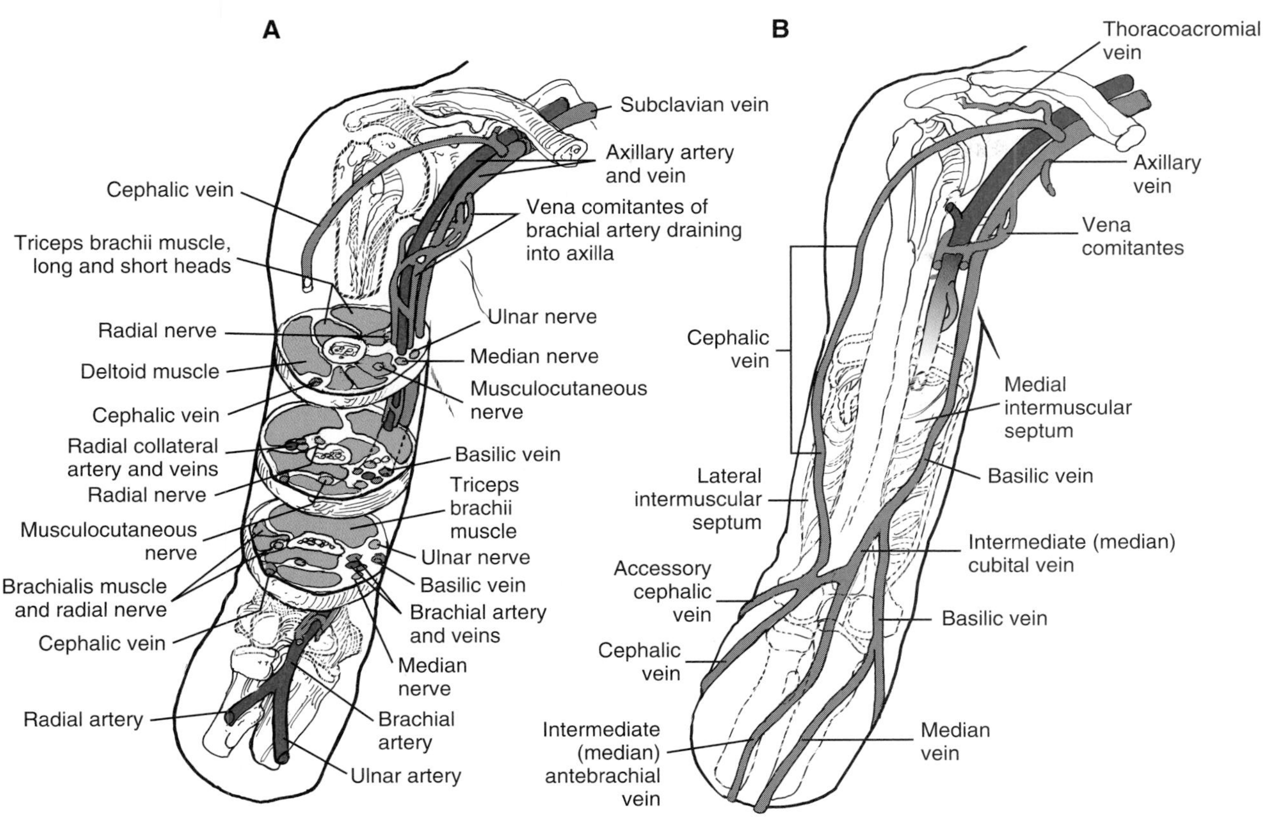

FIGURE 21–12
Veins of the upper extremity. **A.** Deep veins. **B.** Superficial veins.

blood) of the involved digits. Raynaud's disease often accompanies **systemic sclerosis,** an autoimmune disease characterized by the progressive degeneration of epithelia throughout the body. Constrictions of digital vessels may occur in both the upper and lower extremities. Raynaud's phenomenon is typically restricted to the upper limbs. It results from compression of the brachial plexus or upper extremity vasculature.

▲ Veins of the Upper Extremity

The venous system of the upper extremity is composed of deep and superficial vessels

Deep veins with the same names as the arteries described above accompany the arteries. These **venae comitantes** are often small but paired (Fig. 21–12*A*). Digital veins drain into deep and superficial venous arches. The deep venous arches are drained by **radial veins** and the superficial venous arches by **ulnar veins.** The radial and ulnar veins combine at the level of the cubital fossa to form two small **brachial veins,** which course within the arm to drain into the **axillary vein** (Fig. 21–12*A*).

The axillary vein also receives blood from the **basilic vein,** a **superficial vein** (Fig. 21–12). The large basilic vein originates on the ulnar side of the dorsal surface of the hand and then ascends along the dorsal side of the forearm to its midpoint, where it courses around the ulnar side of the forearm to its ventral surface. At the elbow, the basilic vein is joined by a **median (intermediate) cubital vein,** which drains the cephalic and median (intermediate) antebrachial veins (Fig. 21–13 and see below). The basilic vein continues its superior course along the ulnar side of the arm and pierces the deep fascia until it reaches a position just medial to the brachial artery. It terminates at the lower border of the teres major muscle where it drains directly into the axillary vein (Fig. 21–12*B*). At the lower border of the clavicle, the axillary vein becomes the **subclavian vein,** which is joined by the common jugular vein (from the head and neck; see Chapter 27) to form a **brachiocephalic vein** (on both sides). Both of the brachiocephalic veins drain into the superior vena cava, which drains into the right atrium of the heart (Fig. 21–14).

As has been noted, in addition to the basilic vein, other major superficial veins of the upper limb include the median, cubital, and cephalic veins. The **median vein** courses from the palmar surface of the hand (draining the palmar digital veins and palmar venous plexus) to the ventral surface of the wrist and forearm to drain into the cubital vein or basilic vein, or both (Fig. 21–15). The **cephalic vein** courses from the radial side of the dorsal surface of the hand and fingers and then ascends to the midpoint of the forearm where it curves

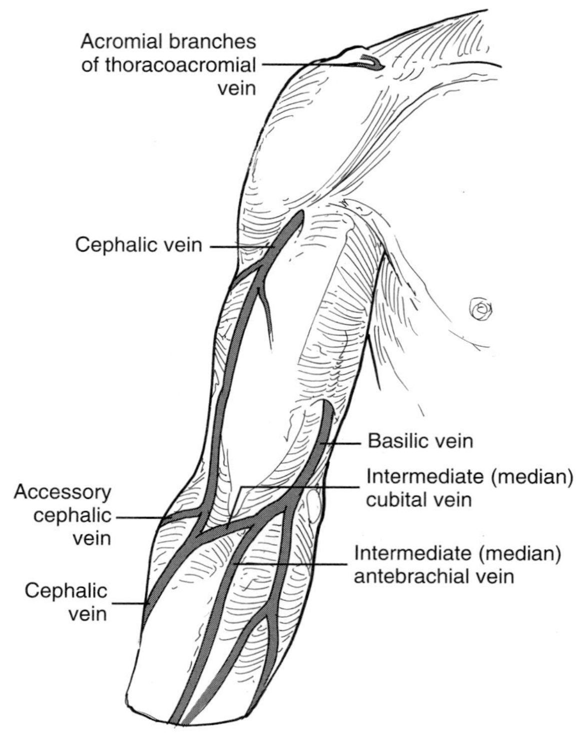

FIGURE 21–13
Superficial veins of the arm in relation to surface anatomy.

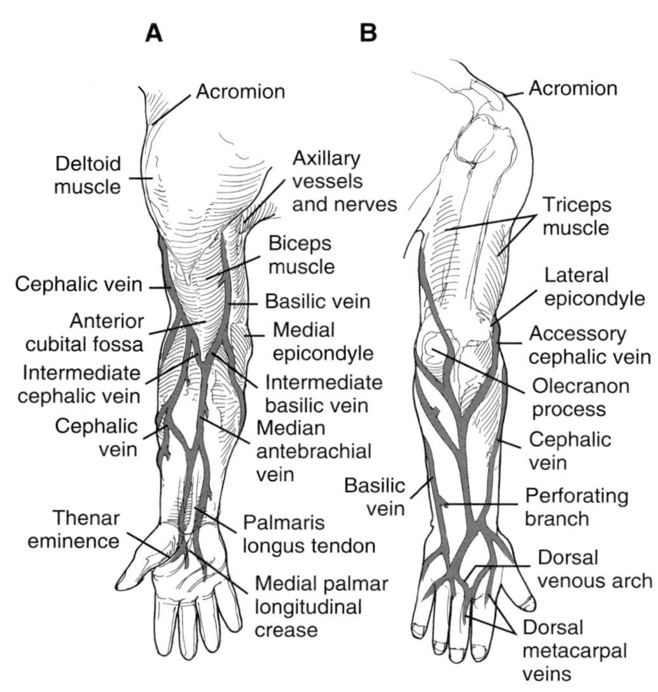

FIGURE 21–15
Venous system of the arm. **A.** Palmar view. **B.** Dorsal view.

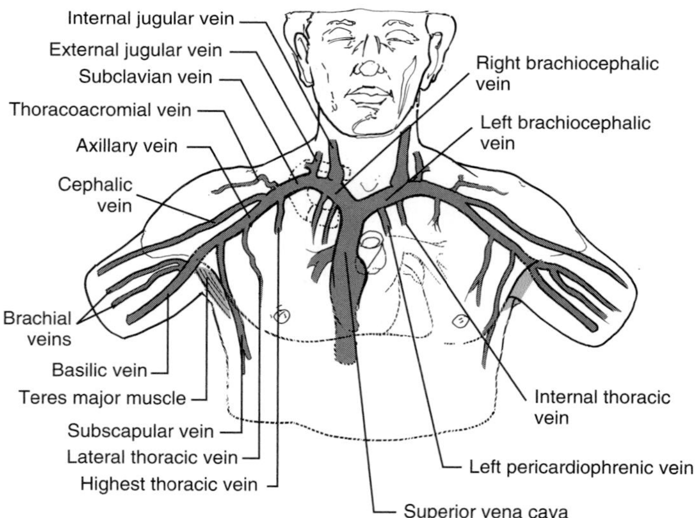

FIGURE 21–14
System of veins draining the upper portion of the body. Anterior view of brachiocephalic veins leading to the superior vena cava, which drains into the right atrium of the heart.

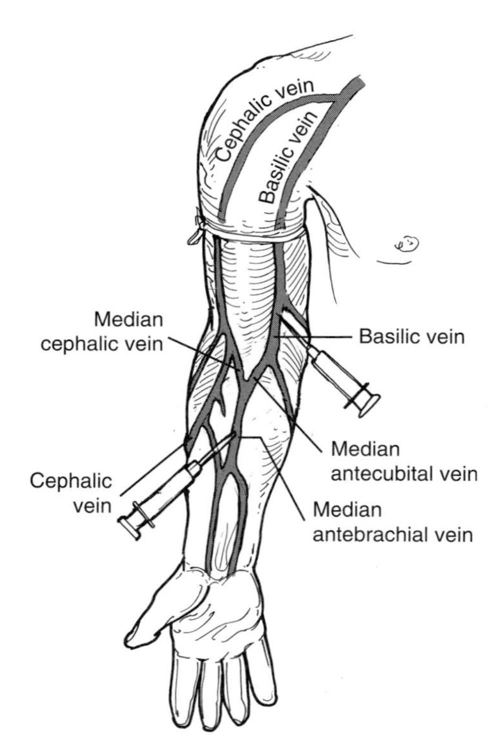

FIGURE 21–16
Points for venipuncture of median antecubital or basilic vein for drawing blood or administering medication.

around to the radial side of the ventral surface of the forearm (Fig. 21–15). At the elbow, the cephalic vein may give rise to the **cubital vein,** or, in cases where the cubital vein arises from the median vein (see above), the cephalic vein may be joined by a median cephalic branch of the median vein (Fig. 21–15). At this point, the main trunk of the cephalic vein continues to ascend on the radial side of the arm between the biceps brachii and brachioradialis muscles (Fig. 21–15). At the boundary defined by the anterior axillary fold, the cephalic vein continues to ascend (toward the head; hence its name) between the deltoid and pectoralis major muscles (Figs. 21–12*B* and 21–14). It then pierces the clavipectoral fascia to pass behind the clavicular head of the pectoralis major muscle and joins the axillary artery just inferior to the clavicle (Figs. 21–12*B* and 21–14).

Perforating Veins of the Collateral Circulation

The deep and superficial veins of the upper extremity are connected by many perforating veins

Many perforating veins connect deep veins to superficial veins throughout the upper extremity (see Fig. 21–15). The actions of muscle contraction and relaxation and the structure of valves within the perforating veins cause blood to flow from superficial veins into deep veins. However, most of the blood in the superficial basilic vessels drains directly into the brachial veins and most of the blood in the cephalic vessels drains directly into the axillary veins.

Diagnostic Procedures that Use Upper Extremity Arteries and Veins

Venipuncture. Superficial veins of the upper limbs are typically used for drawing blood or administering medication (venipuncture). Typically, the **median cubital** or the **basilic vein** is used for these purposes (Fig. 21–16). Identifying a superficial vein and penetrating it by a hypodermic needle or a catheter are facilitated by tying a tourniquet around the arm to impede the return of blood flow. This causes the vein to swell. A danger of venipuncture in this region is accidental injection into an anomalous, superficial brachial artery. This may have serious clinical consequences.

Measurement of Blood Pressure. The blood pressure is usually measured in an upper limb. A **sphygmometer,** which consists of a pressure cuff and manometer, is usually used (Fig. 21–17). The pressure cuff is fastened around the arm to compress the brachial artery against the humerus, completely blocking blood flow to the ulnar and radial arteries (Fig. 21–17*A*). The pressure is released, allowing blood to flow into the forearm. The pressure recorded on the manometer when

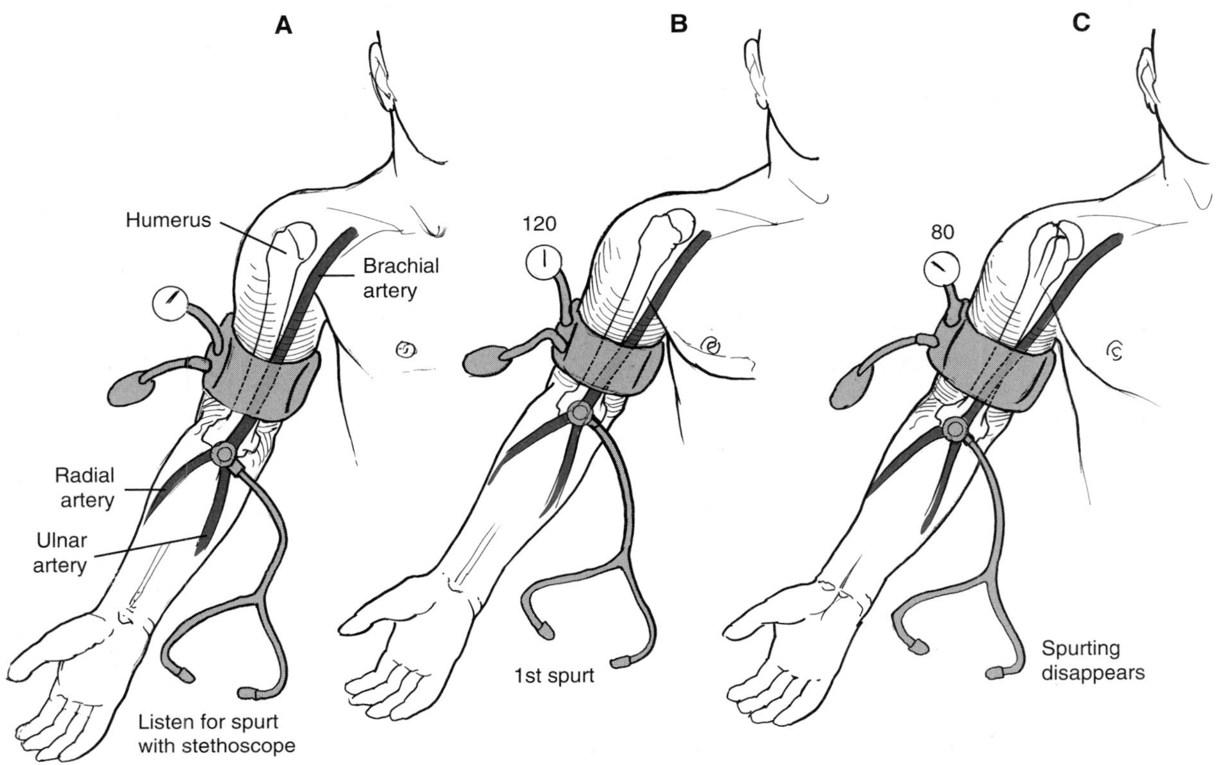

FIGURE 21–17
Measurement of blood pressure. **A.** Blood pressure cuff squeezes the brachial artery against the humerus to stop the blood flow. **B.** Pressure in the cuff is released until the first spurt of blood flows into the radial and ulnar arteries (systolic pressure). **C.** Pressure in the cuff is released further until the spurting stops (diastolic pressure).

blood flow is first detected below the cuff is the **systolic pressure** (Fig. 21–17*B*). This initial flow of blood may be detected by a stethoscope pressed against the cubital fossa, so that the physician can hear blood spurting into the underlying artery. Alternatively, the initial blood flow can be detected distal to the cuff by palpation of a pulse within the ulnar or radial artery (see below). As pressure is released further, the sound of spurting blood distal to the cuff disappears. This occurs at a pressure equal to the **diastolic pressure** (Fig. 21–17*C*).

Measurement of Pulse Rate. Arteries of the upper limbs are often used in measurements of the pulse rate. The **brachial artery** pulse may be taken with a stethoscope where the artery lies upon the distal end of the humerus (Fig. 21–18*A*). The **ulnar artery** may be palpated upon the surface of the pisiform bone (Fig. 21–18*A*). The **radial artery,** which lies upon the anterior surface of the distal radial head (between the tendons of the flexor carpi radialis and abductor pollicis longus muscles), is particularly useful (Fig. 21–18*A*). The "anatomic snuff-box" is also a useful site for measurement of the radial pulse rate (Fig. 21–18*B*).

Cardiac Catheterization. The **subclavian** and **axillary veins** are often used for **cardiac catheterization.** Fine catheters may be threaded through these veins to place pressure sensors or to deliver contrast medium to cardiac chambers for diagnosis before surgery (Fig. 21–19).

Lymphatics of the Upper Extremity

All of the lymphatic fluid from tissues of the upper extremity drains into the **axillary nodes.** These nodes can be classified as lateral, pectoral, subscapular, central, and apical (Fig. 21–20 and see Chapter 6). Other groups of upper extremity nodes include the **cubital (supratrochlear) nodes** (near the medial epicondyle of the humerus) and the **infraclavicular nodes** (associated with the cephalic vein just under the clavicle). Lymphatic vessels follow both deep and superficial veins.

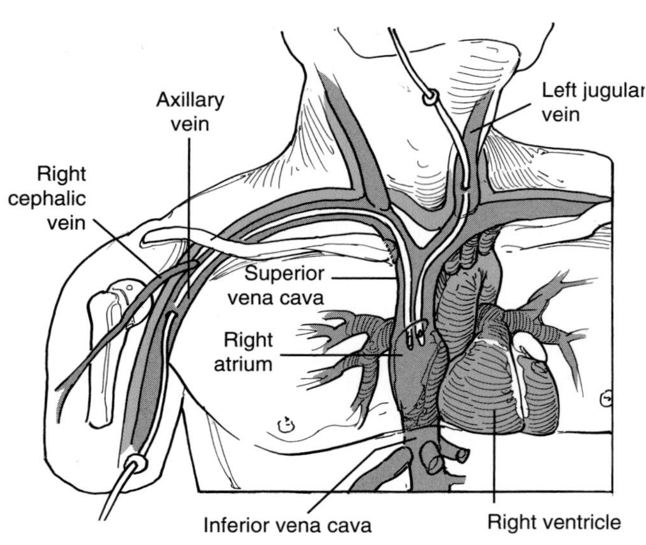

FIGURE 21–19
Subclavian or axillary veins are often used for cardiac catheterization.

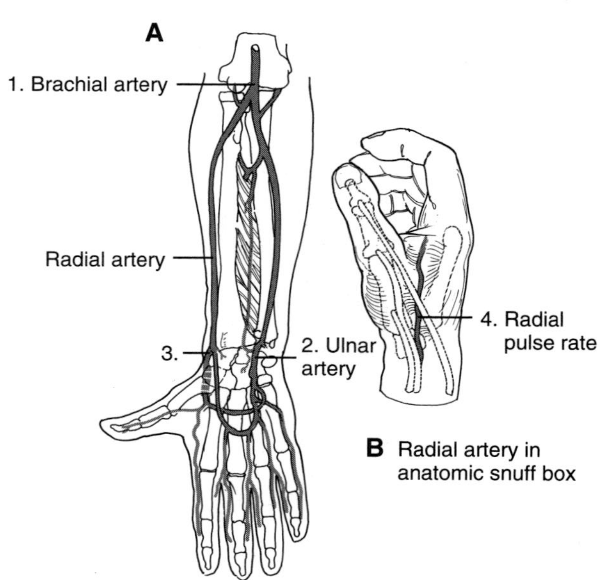

FIGURE 21–18
Measurement of pulse rate. **A.** *1,* The point at which the brachial artery may be palpated. *2,* The point at which the ulnar artery may be palpated. *3,* The radial pulse rate can be obtained from the radial artery. **B.** The radial artery in the anatomic snuffbox showing the point at which the pulse can be measured.

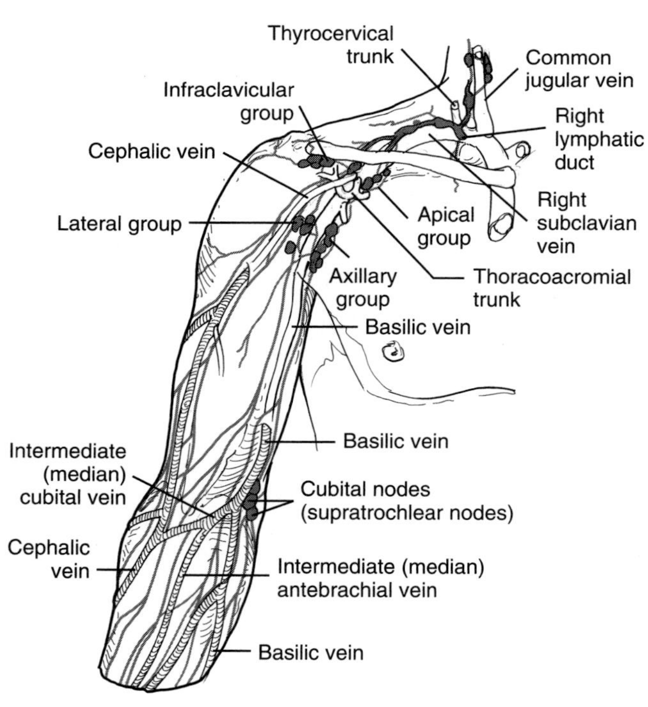

FIGURE 21–20
Lymphatics of the upper extremity.

Those associated with the superficial veins are larger and more numerous. Ultimately, lymph drained from the upper extremities empties into the systemic circulation near the junction of the common jugular and subclavian arteries (Fig. 21–20).

▲ Innervation of the Upper Extremity

The upper extremity is innervated and organized by the brachial plexus

Upper extremity muscles and sensory organs are innervated by nerves formed by different combinations of ventral rami from spinal nerves C5 to T1 (with variable contributions from spinal nerves C4 and T2). These nerves include somatic motor and sensory fibers as well as postganglionic sympathetic fibers. As the growth cones of these **ventral rami (nerve roots)** grow toward the limb bud during development, they mix to form a **brachial plexus.**

Roots, Trunks, Divisions, and Cords of the Brachial Plexus

The brachial plexus is comprised of roots, trunks, divisions, and cords

The typical brachial plexus is formed as the **nerve roots** (ventral primary rami) of spinal nerves C5 to T1 combine to form three trunks: the **superior (upper) trunk** (ventral rami of spinal nerves C5 and C6), **middle trunk** (ventral ramus of spinal nerve C7), and **inferior (lower) trunk** (ventral rami of spinal nerves C8 and T1) (Fig. 21–21*A*). On occasion, the superior trunk may contain a contribution from the ventral ramus of spinal nerve C4 (prefixed plexus). The inferior trunk may sometimes contain a contribution from the ventral ramus of spinal nerve T2 (postfixed plexus). In any case, each trunk splits to form an **anterior** and a **posterior division.** The divisions combine to form the cords of the brachial plexus. The anterior divisions of the superior and middle trunks form the **lateral cord;** the posterior divisions of the superior, middle, and inferior trunks form the **posterior cord;** and the anterior division of the inferior trunk forms the **medial cord.** The roots and trunks give rise to the **supraclavicular nerves** of the upper extremity, which are above the clavicle within the posterior triangle of the neck. The cords give rise to the **infraclavicular nerves,** which are below the clavicle (Fig. 21–21*A* and Table 21–5 and see below).

The intermixing of the spinal nerve root fibers that contribute to the plexus is important anatomically and functionally for two reasons:

1. The plexus distributes fibers from all of the spinal nerve ventral rami contributing to it (spinal nerves

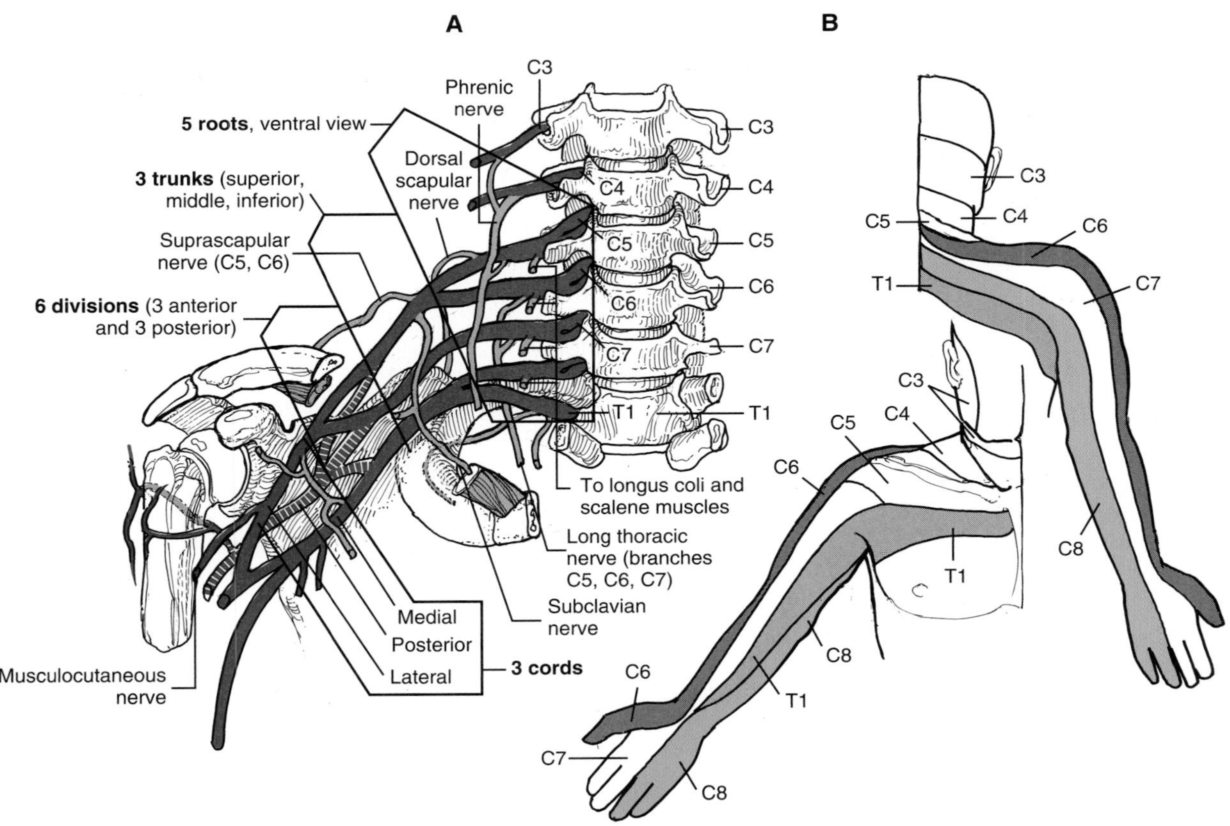

FIGURE 21–21
Roots, trunks, divisions, and cords of the brachial plexus. **A.** Overview of the brachial plexus. **B.** Dermatomes (areas) served by nerves of the brachial plexus.

TABLE 21–5
Nerves of the Brachial Plexus and Structures that They Innervate

Nerve	Contributing Ventral Rami	Structures Innervated
SUPRACLAVICULAR NERVES		
Contribution to phrenic nerve	C5	With C3 and C4, form nerves that innervate diaphragm
Dorsal scapular nerve	C5	Levator scapulae, rhomboid major and minor muscles
Unnamed muscular branch	C5, C6	Longus colli muscle
Suprascapular nerve	C5, C6	Supraspinatus, infraspinatus muscles; glenohumeral, coracoacromial joints
Nerve to subclavius muscle	C5, C6	Subclavius muscle
Long thoracic nerve	C5, C6, C7	Serratus anterior muscle
Unnamed muscular branches	C5, C6, C7, C8	Anterior, middle, and posterior scalene muscles
INFRACLAVICULAR NERVES		
Nerves of lateral cord		
Lateral pectoral nerve	C5, C6, C7	Clavicular head of pectoralis major muscle
Musculocutaneous nerve	C5, C6, C7	Long and short heads of biceps brachii muscle, brachialis muscle, elbow joint
Lateral cutaneous nerve of forearm		Skin of lateral forearm, wrist, and thenar region of hand
Lateral rami of median nerve	C5, C6, C7	Skin and muscles of radial forearm (see text)
Nerves of medial cord		
Medial rami of median nerve	C7, C8, T1	Medial skin and muscles of forearm (see text)
Medial pectoral nerve	C8, T1	Pectoralis minor muscle and sternocostal head of pectoralis major muscle
Medial cutaneous nerve of arm	C8, T1	Skin of medial arm from midpoint to elbow (with intercostobrachial nerve; T1, T2)
Medial cutaneous nerve of forearm	C8, T1	
Unnamed cutaneous branches		Skin over biceps brachii muscle in arm
Anterior branch		Skin over ulnar side of cubital fossa, flexor region of forearm
Posterior branch		Skin over ulnar side of extensor region of forearm
Ulnar nerve	C8, T1	
Articular branch		Elbow joint
Unnamed muscular branches		Flexor carpi ulnaris muscle, medial side of flexor digitorum profundus muscle
Palmar cutaneous dorsal branch		Skin of palm
Three dorsal digital nerves		Nerve 1: ulnar half of digit 5; Nerve 2: radial half of skin of digit 5; Nerve 3: ulnar half of skin of digit 4
Superficial terminal branch		
Cutaneous branch		Medial palmar skin
Unnamed muscular branch		Palmaris brevis muscle
Palmar digital nerves		Ulnar side of digits 4 and 5 and radial side of digit 5
Deep terminal branch		Flexor digiti minimi brevis, abductor digiti minimi, opponens digiti minimi muscles; all interosseous muscles; third and fourth lumbricals
Combined nerve of lateral and medial cords		
Median nerve	Lateral root: C5, C6, C7; Medial root: C7, C8, T1	
Vasomotor branch		Brachial artery
Unnamed muscular branch		Pronator teres muscle
Anterior interosseous branch		Flexor pollicis longus, flexor digitorum profundus, pronator quadratus muscles; distal radioulnar, radiocarpal, intercarpal joints
Palmar cutaneous branch		Skin of radial side of wrist and palm, skin covering thenar eminence
Unnamed muscular branches		Flexor pollicis brevis, abductor pollicis brevis, opponens pollicis muscles

TABLE 21–5, cont'd
Nerves of the Brachial Plexus and Structures that They Innervate

Nerve	Contributing Ventral Rami	Structures Innervated
Median nerve branch		
Three common palmar digital nerves (which give rise to 7 proper palmar digital branches)		Nerve 1: palmar, radial, ulnar skin of thumb and dorsal skin of distal phalanx of thumb, first lumbrical and first dorsal interosseous muscles, radial half of skin of palmar side and radial side of skin of digit 2, radial half of dorsal skin of distal phalanx of digit 2; Nerve 2: 2nd lumbrical, palmer skin and dorsal surface of distal phalanx of digit 2; Nerve 3: palmar skin and dorsal surface of distal phalanx of digit 3, radial half of palmar skin and of dorsal surface of distal phalanx of digit 4
Nerves of posterior cord		
Upper (superior) subscapular nerve	C5, C6	Subscapularis muscle
Lower subscapular nerve	C5, C6	Subscapularis, teres major muscles
Axillary (humeral circumflex) nerve	C5, C6	
Articular branch		Glenohumeral joint
Anterior branch		Deltoid muscle
Posterior branch		Teres minor muscle, posterior head of deltoid muscle
Cutaneous branch		Skin over deltoid muscle and superior part of long head of triceps brachii muscle
Thoracodorsal nerve	C6, C7, C8	Latissimus dorsi muscle
Radial nerve	C5, C6, C7, C8, T1	
Posterior cutaneous nerve of arm		Skin of dorsal surface of arm
Unnamed muscular branches		Medial, long, lateral heads of triceps brachii muscle; anconeus muscle; lateral part of brachialis muscle; brachioradialis, extensor carpi radialis longus muscles
Lower lateral cutaneous nerve of arm		Skin on lower lateral part of arm
Posterior cutaneous nerve of forearm		Posterior skin of forearm from elbow to wrist
Articular branch		Elbow joint
Superficial terminal branch		
Four dorsal digital nerves		Nerve 1: skin on radial side of thenar eminence and thumb; Nerve 2: skin on ulnar side of thumb and radial side of second digit; Nerve 3: skin on ulnar side of second digit and radial side of third digit; Nerve 4: skin on radial side of fourth digit. Nerves 1 to 4 usually supply dorsal surfaces of digits 1 to 3 and radial half of digit 4 up to most distal interphalangeal joints. Midpoint between ulnar and radial innervation may vary—can be middle of digit 3
Deep terminal branch (posterior interosseous nerve)		
Unnamed muscular branches		Extensor carpi radialis brevis, supinator, extensor digitorum, extensor digiti minimi, extensor carpi ulnaris, extensor pollicis longus, extensor indicis, abductor pollicis longus, extensor pollicis brevis muscles
Articular branches		Distal radioulnar, intercarpal, carpometacarpal, metacarpophalangeal, interphalangeal joints

C5 to T1) to the flexor (anterior) and extensor (posterior) compartments of the upper limb.

2. Although the fibers of the ventral rami (nerve roots) that enter the plexus are combined and mixed within the trunks, separated into anterior and posterior divisions, and recombined within the various cords and nerves of the plexus, the fibers are in the same order (from superior to inferior) at the end of this process as they were at the beginning of it. That is, nerves that contain fibers from spinal nerves C5 and C6 are the most superior (radial) nerves in the arm, while nerves that contain fibers from spinal nerves C8 and T1 are the most inferior (ulnar) nerves in the arm (Fig. 21–21*B*). This arrangement and redistribu-

tion of nerve fibers within the brachial plexus is described in more detail below.

Location of the Brachial Plexus

The brachial plexus is located within the posterior triangle of the neck and axilla

The proximal part of the brachial plexus is located within the **posterior triangle of the neck.** This triangle is defined by a superolateral border (anterior edge of the trapezius muscle), a medial border (lateral edge of the sternocleidomastoid muscle), and an inferior border (superior surface of the clavicle). Within this triangle, the roots of the brachial plexus course laterally between the anterior scalene and medial scalene muscles. The roots then combine to form the trunks of the plexus (Fig. 21–22). The trunks are, therefore, covered by skin, superficial fascia, the diminutive omohyoid muscle, a thin platysma muscle, and thin fascia. The triangle is easily palpated in this region. It is susceptible to traumatic injury (see below).

The trunks of the brachial plexus split within the posterior triangle. Just behind the clavicle and subclavian artery, the divisions of the trunks form the lateral, posterior, and medial cords (Fig. 21–22). As the cords course inferolaterally from behind the clavicle, they follow the axillary artery into the axilla. The cords surround the second part of the axillary artery in a manner described by their names (i.e., medial, lateral, and posterior). Finally, just in front of the medial border of the latissimus dorsi muscle (in the distal region of the axilla), the cords form the musculocutaneous, axillary, radial, median, and ulnar nerves (Fig. 21–22).

Muscles Innervated by Fibers of the Brachial Plexus

Nerves of the posterior cord tend to innervate extensor muscles, while nerves of the medial and lateral cords tend to innervate flexor muscles

It is important to realize that the highly evolved human upper limb and nerves of the brachial plexus maintain the fundamental, primitive, anterior and posterior relationships that developed in the first vertebrates with appendages (i.e., the fish). With few exceptions, **extensor (posterior) muscles** are innervated by nerves of the **posterior cord,** while **flexor (anterior) muscles** are innervated by nerves of the more anterior **medial** and **lateral cords** of the brachial plexus (Fig. 21–23). Thus, spinal nerve fibers from all spinal cord levels within the plexus (i.e., spinal nerves C5 to T1) are integrated and then distributed to the extensor and flexor compartments of the upper limb (Fig. 21–23 and see below).

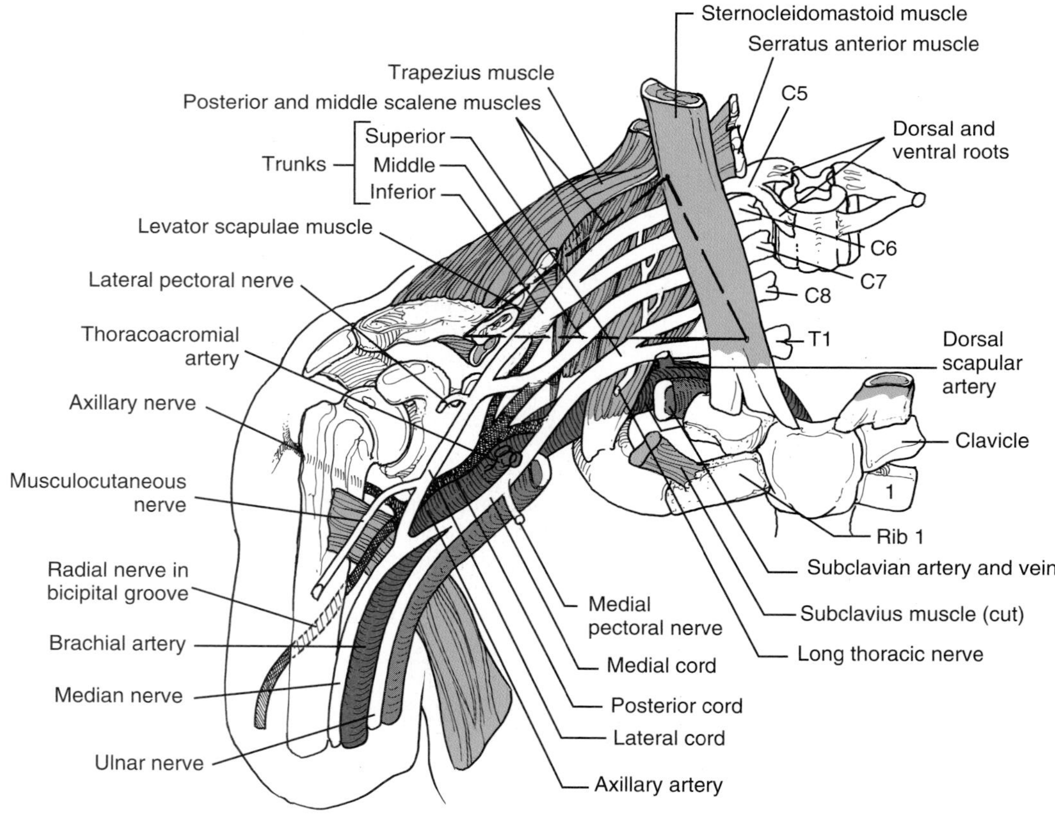

FIGURE 21–22
Location of the brachial plexus within the posterior triangle of the neck. The borders of the triangle are the anterior edge of the trapezius muscle, lateral edge of the sternocleidomastoid muscle, and superior surface of the clavicle.

Position of Nerve Fibers within the Brachial Plexus

Fibers of distal nerves maintain the same order from superior to inferior as the proximal nerve roots that contribute to the plexus

In spite of the apparently complex mixing and separating of ventral rami within the brachial plexus, the **general pattern of innervation of the upper limb** can be understood by studying the development and organization of the brachial plexus within the embryonic upper limb bud. First, as has been noted above, nerves of the posterior cord innervate muscles of the posterior compartments of the limb. These extensors and supinators are derived from the dorsal muscle mass of the limb bud (Fig. 21–24). In contrast, nerves of the lateral and medial cords innervate anterior flexor and pronator muscles derived from the ventral muscle mass of the limb bud (Fig. 21–24). In both the anterior and posterior compartments of the upper extremities, however, the ventral rami of more superior spinal nerves tend to innervate muscles and skin that form within the superior region of the limb bud, while spinal nerves at lower levels tend to innervate muscles and skin that form within more caudal regions of the limb bud. Because the upper extremity limb buds rotate very little during development, the muscles and skin on the **radial side**

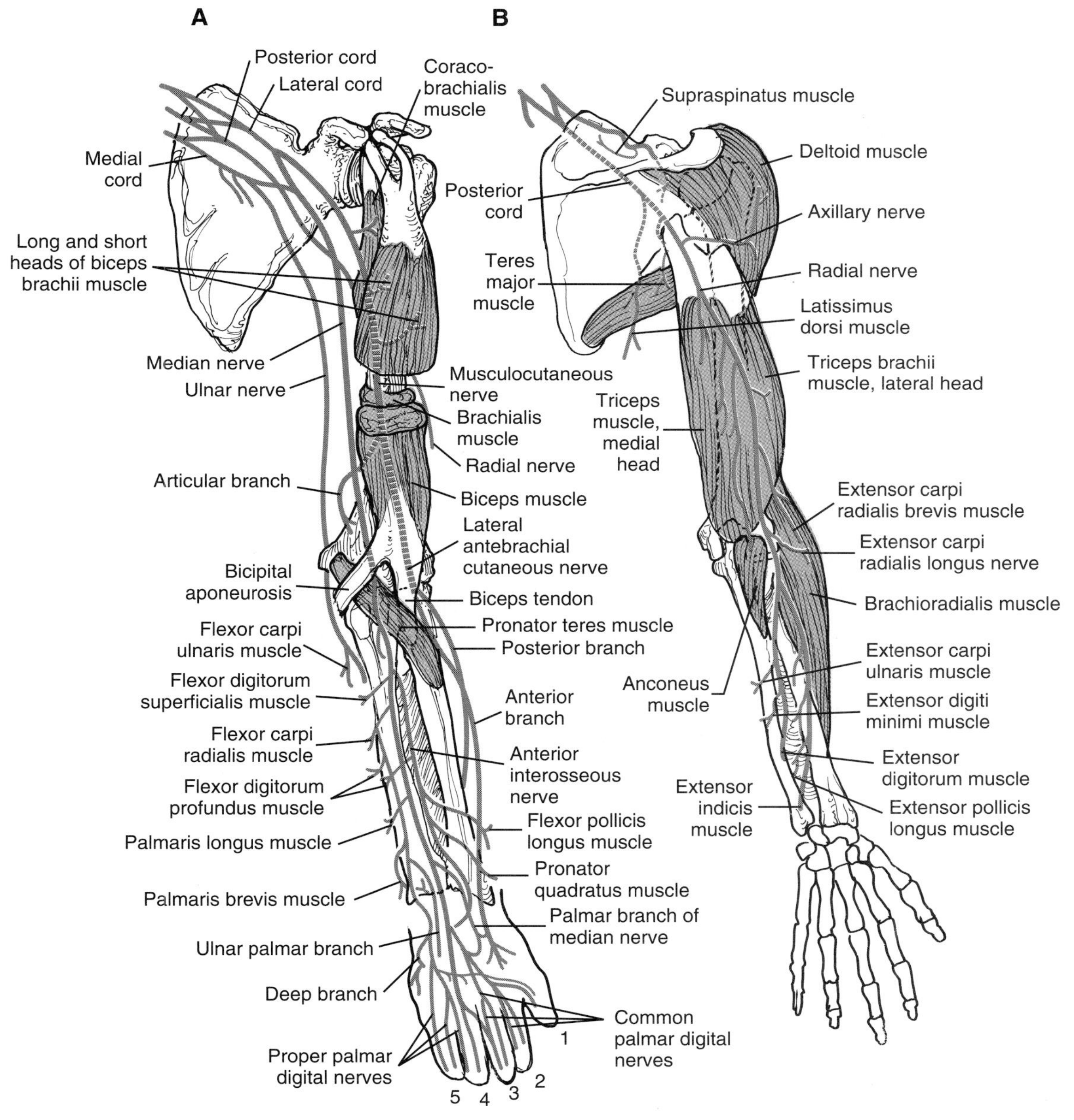

FIGURE 21–23

Muscles innervated by fibers of the brachial plexus. Extensor (posterior) muscles are innervated by nerves of the posterior cord, and flexor (anterior) muscles are innervated by nerves of the more anterior medial and lateral cords. **A.** Anterior view of left arm. **B.** Posterior view of right arm.

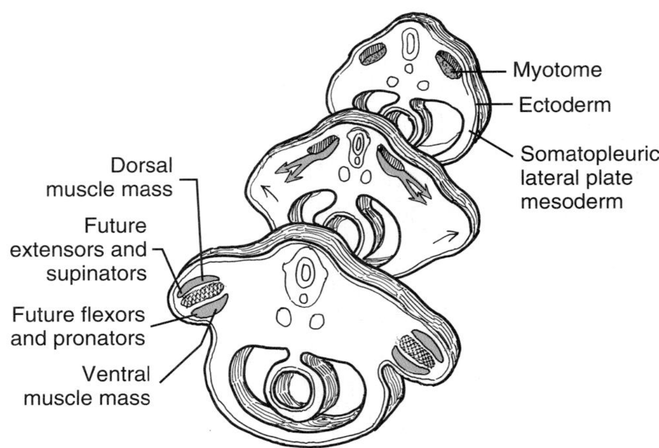

FIGURE 21–24

The general pattern of innervation of the upper limb follows the development and organization of the embryonic upper limb bud. Extensors and supinators from the dorsal muscle mass tend to be innervated by ventral rami of more *superior* spinal nerves C5, C6, and C7. Flexors and pronators from the ventral muscle mass tend to be innervated by combinations of ventral rami of *lower* spinal nerves C7, C8, and T1.

(formerly the superior edge) of the upper extremity tend to be innervated by nerves formed by ventral rami of spinal nerves C5, C6, and C7. Muscles and skin on the **ulnar side** (formerly the caudal edge) of the upper extremity tend to be innervated by nerves formed by combinations of ventral rami of spinal nerves C7, C8, and T1 (see Fig. 21–21*B*). Thus, the superior-to-inferior order of nerve roots of the brachial plexus is reflected within the more distal trunks, divisions, cords, and nerves of the plexus (see Fig. 21–21*B*). Indeed, as has just been noted, the posterior cord, which serves the posterior (extensor) compartments of all segments of the upper limb, from its radial side to its ulnar side, typically contains fibers from all levels (i.e., spinal nerves C5 to T1).

This simple pattern of innervation of the upper extremity may be complicated somewhat by the **migration of some appendicular muscles onto the trunk.** For example, the serratus anterior muscle, which migrates onto the anteroinferior thoracic wall, is innervated by cranially derived fibers of the long thoracic nerve (spinal nerves C5, C6, and C7). The pectoralis major and minor muscles migrate together onto the superior thorax. The pectoralis major muscle is innervated by both the lateral pectoral nerve (spinal nerves C5, C6, and C7) and the medial pectoral nerve (spinal nerves C7, C8, and T1). The pectoralis minor muscle is innervated by the medial pectoral nerve only.

Injuries to Nerves of the Brachial Plexus. Disabilities that ensue from damage to **upper roots of the brachial plexus** (in contrast to lower roots) reflect the basic cranial-to-caudal distribution of nerve fibers within the extremity.

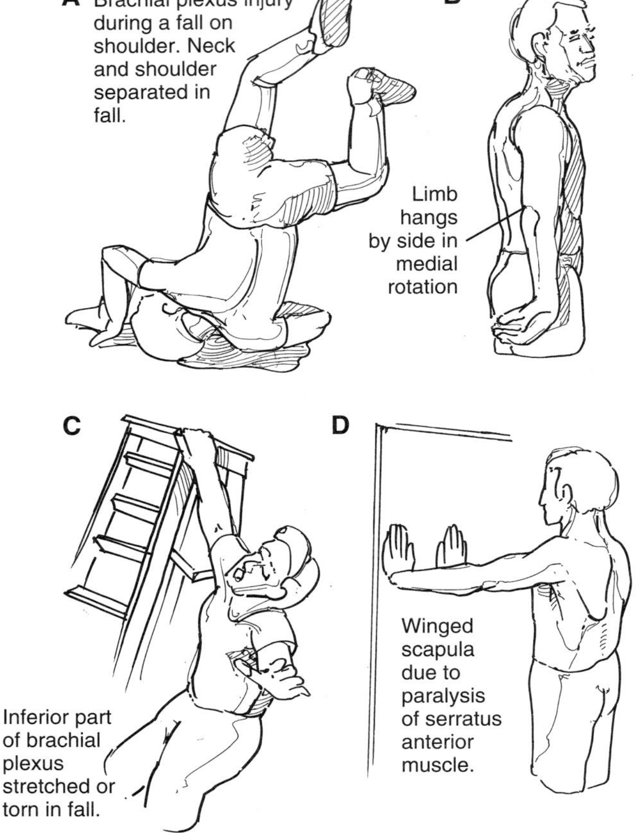

FIGURE 21–25

Injuries to nerves of the brachial plexus. **A.** Damage to the upper roots of the brachial plexus as a consequence of extreme downward displacement of the shoulder. The neck and shoulder are separated during the fall. **B.** Erb-Duchenne paralysis, one consequence of the fall shown in **A.** The limb hangs by the side in medial rotation. **C.** Damage to the lower roots of the brachial plexus caused by upward displacement of the shoulder. **D.** Winged scapula resulting from paralysis of the serratus anterior muscle.

For example, upper roots of the brachial plexus (spinal nerves C5 and C6) may be stretched or even pulled out of the spinal cord. This is often a consequence of severe downward displacement of the shoulder, as might occur when one falls on the shoulder (Fig. 21–25*A*). This injury may result in **Erb-Duchenne paralysis,** which is characterized by inability to flex and supinate the forearm. The elbow is extended, and the wrist is flexed and pronated in the "tip-taker's position" (Fig. 21–25*B*). A **"stinger,"** or **"burner,"** is a less severe sports-related injury to the upper roots of the plexus. This injury results in transient weakness of forearm flexors and supinators.

In contrast, **lower roots of the brachial plexus** (spinal nerves C8 and T1) may be injured by upward displacement of the shoulder, as might occur when one attempts to break a fall from a great height (Fig. 21–25*C*). This may result in

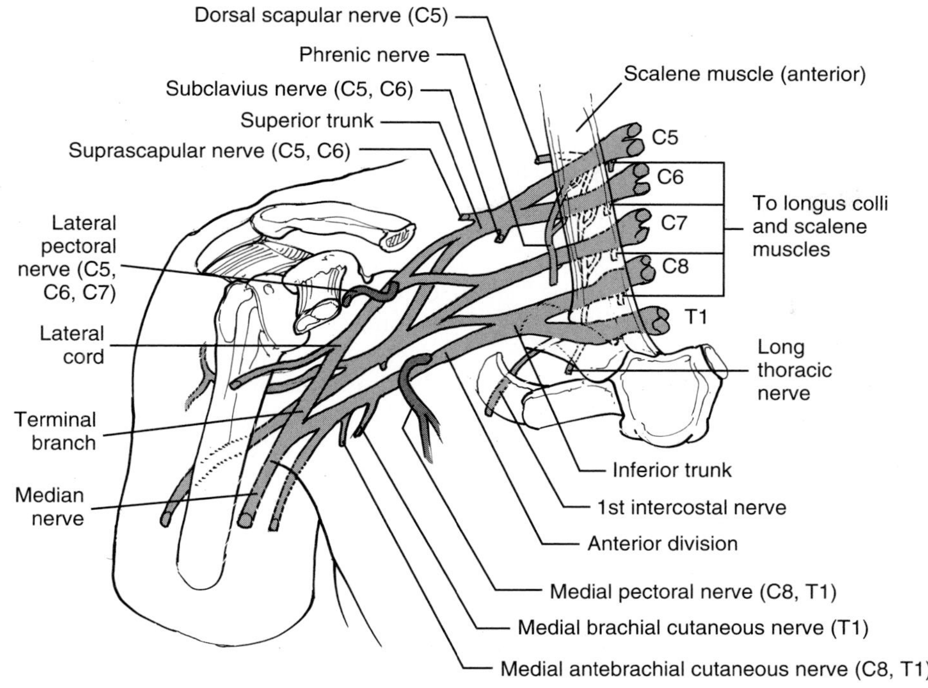

FIGURE 21–26
Supraclavicular branches of the brachial plexus arise from cervical roots and trunks. Infraclavicular branches arise from lateral, medial, and posterior cords.

Klumpke's palsy. Symptoms are similar to those of a median ulnar nerve injury affecting the intrinsic muscles of the hand. Over time, these muscles atrophy and shorten, causing flexion of the fingers **(clawhand).**

Specific Branches of the Brachial Plexus

Supraclavicular Branches. *Supraclavicular branches of the brachial plexus arise from cervical roots and trunks of the plexus.* The roots and trunks of nerves that combine to form the brachial plexus give rise to seven major nerves located superior to the clavicle but within the posterior triangle of the neck. **Supraclavicular nerves** of the brachial plexus include:

- ♦ a nerve to the scalene and longus colli muscles,
- ♦ a contribution to the phrenic nerve,
- ♦ the first intercostal nerve (spinal nerve T1),
- ♦ the dorsal scapular nerve,
- ♦ the long thoracic nerve,
- ♦ the nerve to the subclavius muscle, and
- ♦ the suprascapular nerve.

The first five nerves arise from cervical and thoracic roots of the brachial plexus, while the last two arise from the superior trunk of the plexus (Fig. 21–26 and see Fig. 21–21).

Nerves to the scalene and **longus colli muscles** arise from spinal nerve roots C5 to C8. Indeed, they branch from these four roots just after these spinal nerves exit the intervertebral foramina (Fig. 21–26 and see Fig. 21–21). Thus, in a sense, these nerves are simply spinal nerve branches rather than intrinsic nerves of the brachial plexus. Branches of more superior ventral rami also contribute to the innervation of these longitudinal muscles. For example, the longus colli muscles are innervated by branches of spinal nerves C2 to C6; the anterior scalene muscles by branches of spinal nerves C4 to C6; the middle scalene muscles by branches of spinal nerves C3 to C8; and the posterior scalene muscles by branches of spinal nerves C6 to C8 (see Chapter 24).

A **contribution to the phrenic nerve** branches from the inferior surface of the fifth cervical root of the brachial plexus just distal to the nerve to the scalene and longus colli muscles. This branch from spinal nerve C5 is joined by branches from spinal nerves C3 and C4 to form the phrenic nerve. In a sense, this nerve is also not an intrinsic nerve of the brachial plexus (Fig. 21–26 and see Fig. 21–21*A*).

The **first intercostal nerve** is merely a branch of the ventral root of spinal nerve T1, which innervates intercostal muscles within the first intercostal space (see Fig. 21–21*A* and Chapter 6).

The **dorsal scapular nerve** is a branch of the cervical ventral ramus of spinal nerve C5. It courses posteriorly, piercing the middle scalene muscle to supply the rhomboid major and rhomboid minor muscles. It may also supply the levator scapulae muscle (Fig. 21–26 and see Fig. 21–21).

The **long thoracic nerve** (from spinal nerve roots C5, C6, and C7) descends posterior to the brachial plexus and first part of the axillary artery. It continues its descent along the lateral surface of the serratus anterior muscle, which it supplies (Fig. 21–26 and see Fig. 21–21).

The long thoracic nerve is especially prone to injury because of its vulnerable location within the posterior triangle of the neck. Injury of this nerve weakens the serratus anterior muscle to the degree that it can no longer hold the scapula against the posterior body wall. This results in **winged scapula** (see Fig. 21–25*D*). Abduction of the humerus is also more limited because the scapula is unable to rotate laterally. Thus, the patient cannot raise the arm fully or effectively push objects away from the body.

The **nerve to the subclavius muscle** (spinal nerves C5 and C6) arises from the anterior aspect of the superior trunk just at the junction of the ventral rami from spinal nerves C5 and C6. It courses anterior to the third part of the subclavian artery and the subclavian vein to supply the subclavius muscle (Fig. 21–26 and see Fig. 21–21).

The **suprascapular nerve** arises from the superior aspect of the superior trunk of the brachial plexus at the junction of the fifth and sixth cervical ventral rami. It is comprised of fibers from spinal nerves C5 and C6. It courses lateral to the trapezius muscle, entering the supraspinous fossa through the supraspinous notch (and it passes under the supraspinous ligament; see above). As the suprascapular nerve courses around the lateral side of the scapular spine, it gives rise to branches that supply the supraspinatus and infraspinatus muscles as well as the glenohumeral and acromioclavicular joints (Fig. 21–26 and see Fig. 21–21).

Infraclavicular Branches. *Infraclavicular nerves of the brachial plexus arise from lateral, medial, and posterior cords.* The brachial plexus gives rise to 12 major nerves of the upper extremity. **Nerves arising from the lateral cord** include the:

- lateral pectoral nerve,
- musculocutaneous nerve, and
- lateral root of the median nerve (see Figs. 21–21*A* and 21–23*A*).

Nerves arising from the medial cord include the:

- medial pectoral nerve,
- medial cutaneous nerve of the arm,
- medial cutaneous nerve of the forearm,
- ulnar nerve, and
- medial root of the median nerve (see Figs. 21–21 and 21–23*A*).

Nerves arising from the posterior cord include the:

- upper subscapular nerve,
- thoracodorsal nerve,
- lower subscapular nerve,
- axillary nerve, and
- radial nerve (see Figs. 21–21 and 21–23*B*).

Note that one of these nerves, the **median nerve,** is composed of fibers from both the lateral and medial cords.

The nerves emanating from each cord are listed and described below in order from proximal to distal.

Nerves of the Lateral Cord. The **lateral pectoral nerve** (spinal nerves C5, C6, and C7) arises from the lateral cord of the brachial plexus. It descends in front of the second part of the axillary artery. It then pierces the clavipectoral fascia along with the pectoral branch of the thoracoacromial trunk to supply the clavicular head of the pectoralis major muscle (see Fig. 21–26). The sternocostal head of the muscle is supplied by the medial pectoral nerve (spinal nerves C7, C8, and T1; see below).

The **musculocutaneous nerve** (spinal nerves C5, C6, and C7) branches from the lateral cord near the lateral border of the pectoralis minor muscle. It innervates flexors in the arm and the skin of the forearm, wrist, and thenar region of the hand. Before entering the coracobrachialis muscle, the musculocutaneous nerve emits a branch that supplies this muscle (Fig. 21–27). Then the musculocutaneous nerve emerges from the coracobrachialis muscle and courses distally along the lateral side of the arm between the brachialis and biceps brachii muscles. Here, it emits branches that supply both heads of the biceps brachii muscle, the brachialis muscle, and the elbow joint. The musculocutaneous nerve descends to the lateral side of the arm and elbow where it pierces the deep fascia lateral to the biceps brachii tendon. It emerges into the superficial fascia where it continues its descent as the lateral cutaneous nerve of the forearm. Once it is within the superficial fascia of the radial side of the forearm, the **lateral cutaneous nerve of the forearm** courses deep to the cephalic vein to the carpus. It terminates in cutaneous branches that innervate the skin covering the radial side of the wrist and the thenar eminence (Fig. 21–27).

The **lateral root of the median nerve** (spinal nerves C5, C6, and C7) arises from the lateral cord just superior to the third part of the axillary artery. The lateral root of the median nerve sweeps around the axillary artery. It merges with the medial root of the median nerve (spinal nerves C8 and T1 from the medial cord) on its anterior side to form the median nerve (see discussion of nerves of the medial cord below).

The **median nerve** supplies the pronator teres muscle of the arm and all of the superficial and deep flexor muscles of the forearm, except the flexor carpi ulnaris muscle. The median nerve also supplies thenar muscles, some radial lumbricals, an interosseous muscle, and the skin of digits 1 to 4 (Fig. 21–27 and see Table 21–5). The median nerve typically enters the arm just lateral to the brachial artery. It crosses the artery and descends

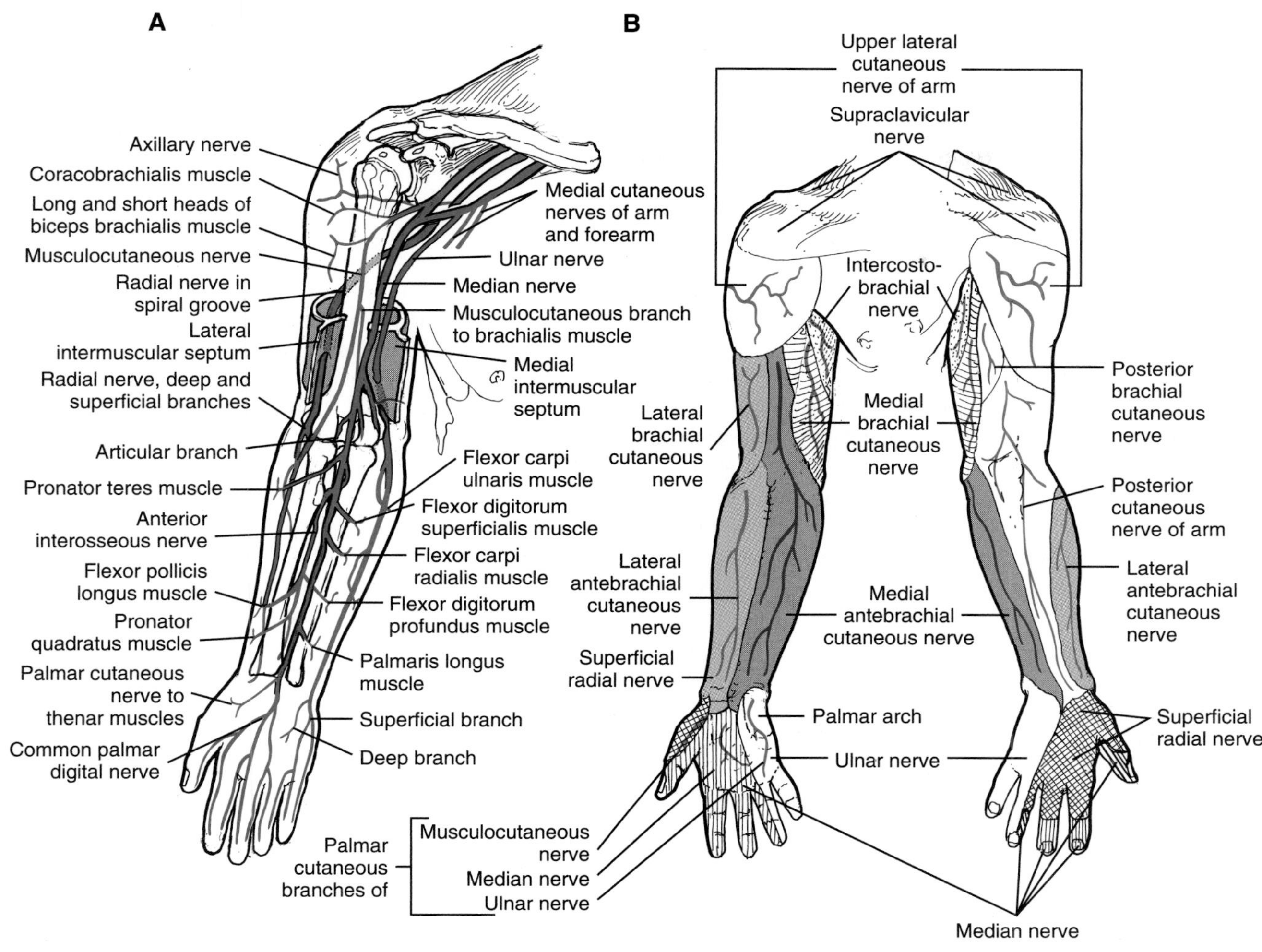

FIGURE 21–27
Nerves of the lateral cord, including the lateral pectoral nerve, musculocutaneous nerve, and lateral root of the median nerve. **A.** Motor branches. **B.** Cutaneous distribution.

medial to it within the arm. It supplies the brachial artery with vasomotor fibers. The median nerve courses under the bicipital aponeurosis in the cubital fossa and enters the forearm between the heads of the pronator teres muscle, which it supplies (Fig. 21–27*A*). It also gives off an **anterior interosseous branch** as it courses between the two heads of the pronator teres muscle. The anterior interosseous nerve descends within the forearm just anterior to the interosseous membrane and deep to the flexor pollicis longus muscle and lateral side of the flexor digitorum profundus muscle, which it supplies (Fig. 21–27). It then innervates the pronator quadratus muscle as it passes under it. Terminal **articular branches of the anterior interosseous nerve** supply the distal radioulnar, radiocarpal, and intercarpal joints (Fig. 21–27).

After giving off the anterior interosseous branch in the proximal forearm, the median nerve descends within the forearm between the flexor digitorum superficialis and flexor digitorum profundus muscles, usually with the medial branch of the anterior interosseous artery. As the median nerve descends, it supplies only three superficial flexors: the flexor digitorum superficialis, flexor carpi radialis, and palmaris longus muscles (Fig. 21–27*A*).

The median nerve emerges into the superficial fascia of the lower forearm after coursing around the lateral edge of the flexor digitorum superficialis muscle. It gives off a **palmar cutaneous branch,** which supplies the skin of the radial side of the wrist and palm and the skin covering the thenar eminence (Fig. 21–27). The continuation of the median nerve dives deep to pass under the flexor retinaculum (Fig. 21–27 and see below).

After passing under the flexor retinaculum, branches of the median nerve within the palm first supply the flexor pollicis brevis, abductor pollicis brevis, and opponens pollicis muscles (Fig. 21–27*A*). More distal **palmar digital branches** supply the palmar skin of digits 2 and 3 and the radial palmar skin of digit 4 (Fig. 21–27*B*). Dorsal branches of these nerves also supply the nails of digits 1, 2, and 3 and the radial half of the nail bed of digit 4 (Fig. 21–27*B*). Muscular branches supply the first and second lumbricals. Vasomotor branches supply vessels in the radial side of the hand and digits.

Entrapment of the median nerve may result from repetitive flexion and extension of the wrist as when one is typing or using a computer. Such entrapment may also result from arthritic changes to carpal bones or even infection. Adhesions may form within the carpal tunnel (see above) or in the more medial region of the wrist between the carpus and flexor retinaculum. This condition creates pressure against the median nerve and a tingling or prickling sensation in the hand **(paresthesia),** reduced sensation **(hypesthesia),** or complete cessation of feeling **(anesthesia).** This is **carpal tunnel syndrome.** In the absence of treatment, muscles of the thenar eminence may become paralyzed and atrophy. In addition, the two radial lumbrical muscles may become paralyzed. Relief of pressure is typically obtained by incision of the flexor retinaculum **(carpal tunnel release)** (see Fig. 20–15*C*).

Nerves of the Medial Cord. The **medial pectoral nerve** is formed by fibers from spinal nerves C8 and T1. It arises from the medial cord just inferior to the thoracoacromial trunk of the second part of the axillary artery and deep to the tendon of the pectoralis minor muscle (see Fig. 21–26). It immediately crosses under the lateral pectoral nerve and courses lateral to it under the belly of the pectoralis minor muscle. The medial pectoral nerve pierces and supplies the pectoralis minor muscle in the muscle's midregion. The nerve emerges from the anterior surface of the pectoralis minor muscle to penetrate the sternocostal head of the pectoralis major muscle, which it also supplies. It should be noted that the medial and lateral pectoral nerves are named for their origins from the medial and lateral cords of the brachial plexus, not for their positions at their distal ends (see Chapter 6).

The **medial cutaneous nerve of the arm (medial brachial cutaneous nerve)** branches from the inferior surface of the medial cord of the brachial plexus just distal to the origin of the medial pectoral nerve. At its origin, the medial cutaneous nerve of the arm contains fibers from the ventral rami of spinal nerves C8 and T1 (Fig. 21–28). The medial cutaneous nerve courses medially into the axilla. At the lateral edge of the latissimus dorsi muscle, it is joined by the **intercostobrachial nerve,** a branch of the second (thoracic) intercostal nerve (see Chapter 6). The medial cutaneous nerve of the arm, which now consists of fibers from spinal nerves C8, T1, and T2, courses medial to the brachial artery and vein, emerging to innervate the skin of the medial arm from the midpoint of the arm to the elbow.

The **medial cutaneous nerve of the forearm (medial antebrachial cutaneous nerve)** consists of fibers from spinal nerves C8 and T1. It arises from the inferior surface of the medial cord of the brachial plexus just distal to the origin of the medial cutaneous nerve of the arm (Fig. 21–28). The medial cutaneous nerve of the forearm courses medially through the axilla and descends along the medial aspect of the arm between the brachial artery and brachial vein. At the midpoint of the arm, the nerve emits a branch that innervates the skin covering the biceps brachii muscle (Fig. 21–28). The main trunk of the nerve continues to descend toward the elbow, medial to the brachial artery. Just proximal to the medial epicondyle of the humerus, the trunk splits into anterior and posterior branches (Fig. 21–28). The **anterior branch** passes anterior to the medial epicondyle and descends within the superficial fascia of the medial side of the flexor region of the forearm to supply the skin of the medial cubital fossa and forearm to the wrist (Fig. 21–28). The **posterior branch** also passes anterior to the medial epicondyle of the humerus but then sweeps around to the posterior side of the forearm to innervate the posteromedial skin of the extensor side of the forearm to the wrist (Fig. 21–28).

The **ulnar nerve** is an extension of the medial cord of the brachial plexus. Thus, it typically consists of fibers of ventral rami from spinal nerves C8 to T1 (Fig. 21–28). It commonly also receives contributions from the ventral ramus of spinal nerve C7. The ulnar nerve courses through the axilla and into the medial region of the arm just deep to the brachial artery and vein (Fig. 21–28). In the midregion of the arm, the ulnar nerve perforates the medial intermuscular septum. It continues to descend just anterior to the medial head of the triceps brachii muscle (Fig. 21–28).

At the elbow, the ulnar nerve passes between the olecranon process and medial epicondyle of the humerus and then into a groove on the dorsal surface of the epicondyle. An **articular branch** innervates the elbow joint. Finally, the ulnar nerve enters the medial side of the flexor compartment of the forearm between the two heads of the flexor carpi ulnaris muscle. It descends anterior to the flexor digitorum profundus muscle and lateral to the flexor carpi ulnaris muscle. It supplies the flexor carpi ulnaris muscle and the medial side of the flexor digitorum profundus muscle (Fig. 21–28). (The lateral side of the flexor digitorum profundus muscle is innervated by the median nerve; see above). The ulnar nerve is separated from the ulnar artery in the upper third of the forearm, but the nerve and artery become closely related in the lower third.

In the midregion of the forearm, the ulnar nerve gives off a **palmar cutaneous branch,** which descends to innervate the skin over the palm of the hand. Just proximal to the wrist, a **dorsal branch** arises from the ulnar nerve and sweeps around the dorsal side of the carpus. It divides into two or three **dorsal digital nerves,** which innervate the dorsal skin covering digits 4 and 5 (Fig. 21–28). The ulnar nerve and artery pass under the flexor retinaculum to enter the palmar compartment of the

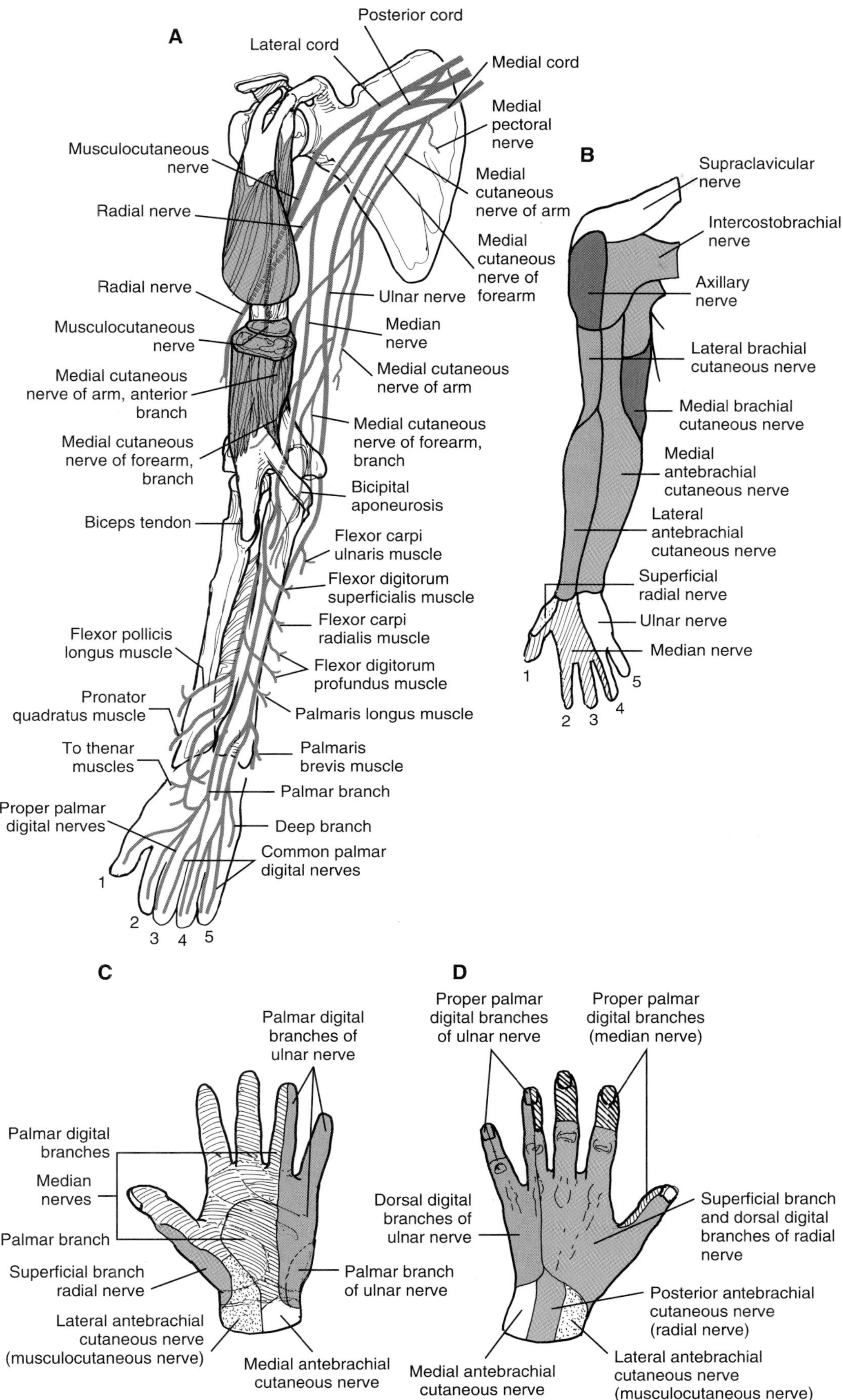

FIGURE 21–28

Nerves of the medial cord, including the medial pectoral nerve, medial cutaneous nerve of the arm, medial cutaneous nerves of the forearm, and ulnar nerve. **A.** Overview of nerves of the medial cord. **B.** Cutaneous innervation by sensory nerves. **C.** Palmar view of cutaneous nerve areas of the wrist and hand. **D.** Dorsal view of cutaneous nerve areas of the wrist and hand.

hand. At this point, the ulnar nerve divides into superficial and deep terminal branches (Fig. 21–28). The **superficial terminal branch** innervates the medial palmar skin and palmaris brevis muscle. The branch splits to form two **palmar digital nerves.** The more medial palmar digital nerve innervates the medial side of digit 5. The other palmar digital nerve splits into two proper digital nerves. One innervates the lateral side of digit 5 and one the medial side of digit 4 (Fig. 21–28). The **deep terminal branch** of the ulnar nerve courses between the short flexor muscle and abductor muscle of the little finger and penetrates the opponens digiti minimi muscle. It innervates all three of these short muscles. The main trunk dives deep to reach the deep palmar arch. Here it splits into branches that innervate all of the interosseous muscles and the third and fourth lumbrical muscles. The terminal muscular branches of the median nerve innervate the first dorsal interosseous muscle and the first, second, and third lumbrical muscles (see Fig. 21–27).

Damage to the ulnar nerve may occur with fracture of the medial epicondyle of the humerus. This injury results in atrophy and shortening of intrinsic muscles of the ulnar side of the hand and **clawing** of digits 4 and 5. **Entrapment of the ulnar nerve** may occur following injury and healing of the medial epicondyle of the humerus. Callus formation may entrap the nerve just posterior to the medial epicondyle, resulting in weakness of the ulnar intrinsic muscles and numbness in the medial region of the hand.

The **medial root of the median nerve** arises from the medial cord of the brachial plexus just inferior to the third part of the axillary artery (Fig. 21–28*A*). The medial root sweeps upward around the artery and joins with the lateral root of the median nerve to form the median nerve (Fig. 21–28*A* and see discussion of the median nerve above).

Nerves of the Posterior Cord. The **upper (superior) subscapular nerve** branches from the inferior side of the posterior cord of the brachial plexus and immediately innervates the anterior surface of the subscapularis muscle. The nerve is composed of fibers from spinal nerves C5 and C6 (Fig. 21–29*A* and *B* and see Fig. 21–21*A*).

The **thoracodorsal nerve** branches from the posterior cord just distal to the origin of the upper subscapular nerve and descends to innervate the latissimus dorsi muscle. It is composed of fibers from spinal nerves C6, C7, and C8 (see Figs. 21–21*A* and 21–29*A* and *B*).

The **lower (inferior) subscapular nerve** branches from the posterior cord just distal to the thoracodorsal nerve. It is composed of fibers from spinal nerves C5 and C6. It descends to the lower part of the subscapularis muscle, which it innervates (Fig. 21–29). Its terminus innervates the teres major muscle (Fig. 21–29*B*).

The **axillary (circumflex humeral) nerve** is comprised of fibers from ventral rami of spinal nerves C5 and C6. It branches from the superior side of the posterior cord, distal to the lower subscapular nerve. It courses laterally and traverses the quadrangular space (see above), along with the posterior humeral circumflex vessels (Fig. 21–29*A* to *C*). After giving off an **articular branch** to the glenohumeral joint, the axillary nerve splits into anterior and posterior branches. The **anterior branch** sweeps around the humeral neck with the posterior humeral circumflex vessels to supply the deltoid muscle. The **posterior branch** supplies the teres minor muscle and posterior head of the deltoid muscle. A **cutaneous branch** supplies the skin over the lower part of the deltoid muscle and the superior part of the long head of the triceps brachii muscle (Fig. 21–29*C*).

The **axillary nerve** may be injured in fracture of the surgical neck of the humerus or dislocation of the shoulder. The nerve injury will impair one's ability to abduct the arm and may result in flattening of the shoulder because of progressive atrophy of the deltoid muscle. Thus, this condition may simulate dislocation of the shoulder joint. Under these circumstances, it may be possible to insert the finger between the acromial process and the head of the humerus.

The **radial nerve** (the largest branch of the brachial plexus) is the continuation of the posterior cord. It contains fibers from the ventral rami of spinal nerves C5 to C8 and T1 (Fig. 21–29*D* and see Fig. 21–21*A*). The radial nerve passes through the axilla behind the axillary artery and gives rise to the **posterior cutaneous nerve of the arm** (Fig. 21–29*D*). This nerve sweeps out from under the inferior edge of the teres major muscle and around the medial surface of the long head of the triceps brachii muscle to innervate the skin of the dorsal surface of the arm. The main trunk of the radial nerve continues into the arm, posterior to the brachial artery (Fig. 21–29*D*).

The radial nerve passes into the posterior compartment of the arm with the arteria profunda brachii just under the inferior border of the teres major muscle and then between the long and medial heads of the triceps brachii muscle. It sweeps posteriorly around the shaft of the humerus at the junction of the upper and middle thirds of the shaft and descends obliquely (from medial to lateral) between the medial and lateral heads of the triceps brachii muscle (Fig. 21–29*D*). As the radial nerve descends, it innervates muscles in medial, posterior, and lateral groups. **Medial muscular branches** innervate the medial and long heads of the triceps brachii muscle. **Posterior muscular branches** supply the medial and lateral heads of the triceps brachii muscle and the anconeus muscle. Two cutaneous branches of the radial nerve pierce the lateral head of the triceps brachii muscle at the midpoint of the arm. One of these, the **lower lateral cutaneous nerve of the arm,** descends toward the lateral epicondyle of the humerus to innervate the skin on the lateral lower part of the arm (Fig. 21–29*D* and *E*). The other, the **posterior cutaneous nerve of the forearm,** follows much the same course at first but then moves onto

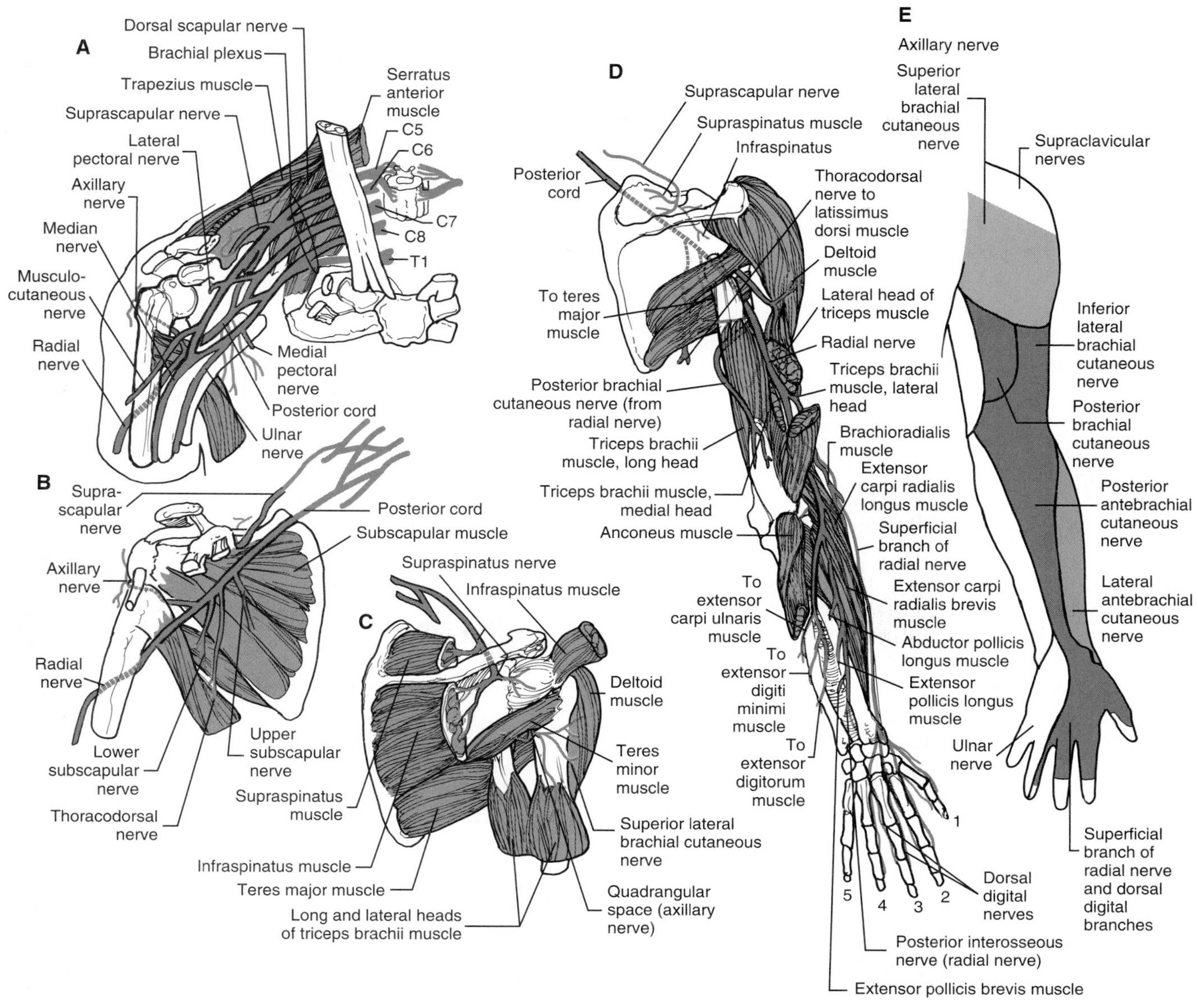

FIGURE 21–29

Nerves of the posterior cord, including the subscapular, thoracodorsal, axillary, and radial nerves. **A.** Anterior overview, showing posterior cord in relation to surrounding structures of the chest. **B.** Posterior cord branches. **C.** Posterior view of posterior cord. **D.** Branches of the radial nerve. **E.** Patterns of cutaneous innervation.

the dorsal surface of the forearm where it innervates the skin of the forearm from the elbow to the wrist (Fig. 21–29*D* and *E*). As the main trunk of the radial nerve continues to descend toward the elbow, it pierces the lateral intermuscular septum just below the midpoint of the arm. The main trunk first descends between the lateral edge of the biceps brachii muscle and medial edge of the brachioradialis muscle and then between the biceps brachii muscle and extensor carpi radialis longus muscle. Here, **lateral muscular branches** of the radial nerve innervate the lateral part of the brachialis muscle, the brachioradialis muscle, and the extensor carpi radialis longus muscle. Finally, just anterior to the lateral epicondyle of the humerus, the radial nerve gives off an **articular branch** to the elbow joint and splits into superficial and deep terminal branches (Fig. 21–29*D*). It is interesting to note that, although the brachialis and brachioradialis muscles are flexors of the elbow (see above), they are innervated by this "extensor nerve."

The **superficial terminal branch of the radial nerve** first descends within the radial edge of the forearm between the supinator and brachioradialis muscles. Then, just below the elbow, the superficial terminal branch of the radial nerve joins the radial artery. The nerve and artery course together, first between the pronator teres and brachioradialis muscles and then, more distally, between the flexor digitorum superficialis and brachioradialis muscles (Fig. 21–29*D*).

Just above the wrist, the superficial terminal branch of the radial nerve leaves the company of the radial artery to sweep around the radial side of the radius, over the extensor retinaculum, and onto the dorsum of the carpus where it branches into four **dorsal digital nerves** (Fig. 21–29*D*). The first dorsal digital nerve supplies the skin on the radial side of the thenar eminence and thumb; the second, the ulnar side of the thumb; the third, the ulnar side of digit 4; and the fourth, the adjoining skin on the ulnar side of digit 3 and the radial side of digit 4 (Fig. 21–29*D* and *E*). These dorsal digital nerves also supply the dorsal surfaces of digits 1 to 4 but only as far distally as the interphalangeal joint of the thumb, the most distal interphalangeal joint of digit 1, and the radial half of the dorsum (to the most distal interphalangeal joint) of digit 2. All of the skin at the tips of digits 1 to 3 (including the nail beds) is supplied by digital branches of the median nerve (see Fig. 21–29*E*).

The **deep terminal branch of the radial nerve** is also called the **posterior interosseous nerve.** The anterior interosseous nerve is a branch of the median nerve (see above). The deep terminal branch of the radial nerve first diverges medially from the superficial terminal branch but immediately gives rise to branches that innervate the extensor carpi radialis brevis and supinator muscles. Its main trunk pierces the supinator muscle (providing it with additional branches) and gains access to the plane between the superficial and deep extensor compartments (Fig. 21–29*D*). As the main trunk emerges, it gives rise to three short branches, which supply the extensor digitorum, extensor digiti minimi, and extensor carpi ulnaris muscles (Fig. 21–29*D*). It then gives rise to a long medial branch, which supplies the extensor pollicis longus and extensor indicis muscles, and a long lateral branch, which supplies the abductor pollicis longus and extensor pollicis brevis muscles (see Fig. 21–29*D*). The main trunk at first continues between the superficial and deep extensors, but at the lower border of the extensor pollicis brevis muscle, it lies upon the interosseous membrane.

The main trunk enters the wrist after passing deep to the extensor retinaculum and then courses upon the dorsum of the carpus. Here, it ramifies to form **articular branches,** which supply the distal radioulnar joint, intercarpal joints, and carpometacarpal joints. Distal digital branches supply the metacarpophalangeal and interphalangeal joints.

Injury to the radial nerve may be a consequence of midshaft fractures of the humerus because the nerve lies within the radial groove. This injury results in **wristdrop,** which is characterized by impaired ability to extend the elbow and wrist and grasp objects tightly.

Entrapment of the radial nerve may result from compression of the nerve against the humerus by an external force or swelling within the posterior compartment of the arm. This often occurs when the arm rests in an awkward position when a person is sleeping. Entrapment usually has no effect on the function of the triceps brachii muscle. This disorder also results in **wristdrop** (see above).

Communicating Branches of the Brachial Plexus

Nerves of the brachial plexus may interact through communicating branches

The discrete nerves described above may interact through communicating branches in some cases, sharing in the innervation of muscles or cutaneous targets in the upper limbs. For example, a communicating branch is typically found connecting the medial and lateral pectoral nerves in the vicinity of the brachial plexus (see Fig. 21–21*A*). This connection contains fibers of the lateral pectoral nerve. It provides limited innervation to the pectoralis minor muscle via the medial pectoral nerve.

While the following list is not exhaustive, it provides some other examples of communication between nerves of the brachial plexus:

- The lateral cutaneous nerve of the forearm (a branch of the musculocutaneous nerve) communicates with the posterior cutaneous branch of the forearm (a branch of the radial nerve) and superficial terminal branch of the radial nerve (on the dorsum of the hand).
- The posterior branch of the medial cutaneous nerve of the forearm (a branch of the medial cord) may emit branches that communicate with the medial cutaneous nerve of the arm (a branch of the medial cord), posterior cutaneous nerve of the forearm (a branch of the radial nerve), and dorsal branch of the ulnar nerve.
- The medial cutaneous nerve of the arm (a branch of the medial cord) may communicate with the intercostobrachial nerve (a branch of the second [thoracic] intercostal nerve). In some cases, the intercostobrachial nerve may entirely replace the medial cutaneous branch of the brachial plexus.
- The posterior cutaneous nerve of the arm (a branch of the radial nerve) may also communicate with the intercostobrachial nerve.
- The median nerve may emit one or more communicating branches within the axilla, arm, or forearm, which provide some fibers to the ulnar nerve. Thus, even though the thenar muscles are typically said to be innervated by the median nerve (see above), individual thenar muscles may alternatively receive their innervation from the ulnar nerve or from both the ulnar and median nerves.

SECTION 3

THE HEAD AND NECK

22 The Skull

INTRODUCTION TO THE HEAD AND NECK

Chapters 22 to 27 describe the development, anatomy, and functional and clinical significance of the head and neck. Chapter 22 describes the development and structure of the skull, which provides a skeletal framework for soft tissues of the head and neck. The foramina are also discussed. Foramina provide conduits for cranial nerves, vessels, and other structures so they can pass from the interior to the exterior of the skull.

Chapter 24 describes muscles, vessels, and nerves of the face, neck, and scalp. This discussion includes cranial nerves V and VII and their origins from the brain.

Chapter 25 focuses on the eyes and the ears and accompanying musculature, vasculature and cranial nerves II and VIII.

Chapters 26 and 27 describe the anatomy, vascularization, and innervation of the nasal cavity, oral cavity, pharynx, and larynx, as well as special sensory mechanisms, including olfactory and gustatory (taste) structures. Cranial nerves I, IX, X and XI will be described.

Evolutionary and Embryonic Origins of the Head and Neck

Different elements of the human head have diverse evolutionary origins

The head is a specialized structure designed to serve several important functions in humans.

1. The head has special sensory devices, such as the nose, ears, and eyes.
2. The head has a large, thick cranium that encloses, supports, and protects the brain, which is the most advanced and complex part of the central nervous system.
3. The head contains openings of well-developed mechanisms for eating, breathing, and vocalizing.

This diversity of structure and function is reflected in the complex origins and evolution of skeletal elements that support cranial structures. For example, some elements of the human head, such as the **chondrocranium, sensory capsules,** and **facial skeleton,** have been acquired from very primitive piscine (fish) relatives. Other features such as the **cranial vault, temporomandibular joint,** and **larynx** have evolved from more recent predecessors.

Chondrocranium

The base of the human brain case and sensory capsules develop from three pairs of cartilaginous precursors and the primitive sensory capsules of the earliest vertebrates

The **skull base,** or chondrocranium, in humans is derived from the prechordal, hypophyseal, and parachordal cartilages of early fishes. The **prechordal cartilages** formed the most anterior region of the medial skull base, the **ethmoid bone.** The primitive **hypophyseal cartilages** gave rise to the **body of the human sphenoid bone** in the region of the pituitary gland. The **parachordal cartilages** gave rise to part of the human **occipital bone** just anterior to the foramen magnum (Fig. 22–1). In addition, primitive capsules that developed around the sensory structures of primitive fishes have also contributed to the development of the more elaborate bony capsules that protect the olfactory (smell), ocular (sight), and auditory-vestibular (hearing and balance) mechanisms of humans. For example, the **primitive olfactory capsules** have given rise to the **turbinate** and **nasal bones** of the human olfactory capsule. The **greater** and **lesser wings of the sphenoid bone,** which are part of the human bony orbit, are derived from the **primitive ocular capsule** of early fishes (Fig. 22–1). Finally, the **periotic (petromastoid) bones** enclosing the human auditory-vestibular apparatus are derived from a **primitive otic capsule** (Fig. 22–1). All of these bony structures arise from cranial somitomeres or occipital and cervical somites. Because precursors of the bones of the skull base and the bony capsules surrounding olfactory, ocular, and auditory-vestibular areas in the skull are all initially formed in cartilage, they are converted to bone by the process of **endochondral ossification.**

Facial Skeleton

The facial skeleton of the human head is descended from the branchial (gill) apparatus of the jawless fishes

The facial skeleton and associated structures of the human face and anterior neck are descendants of the

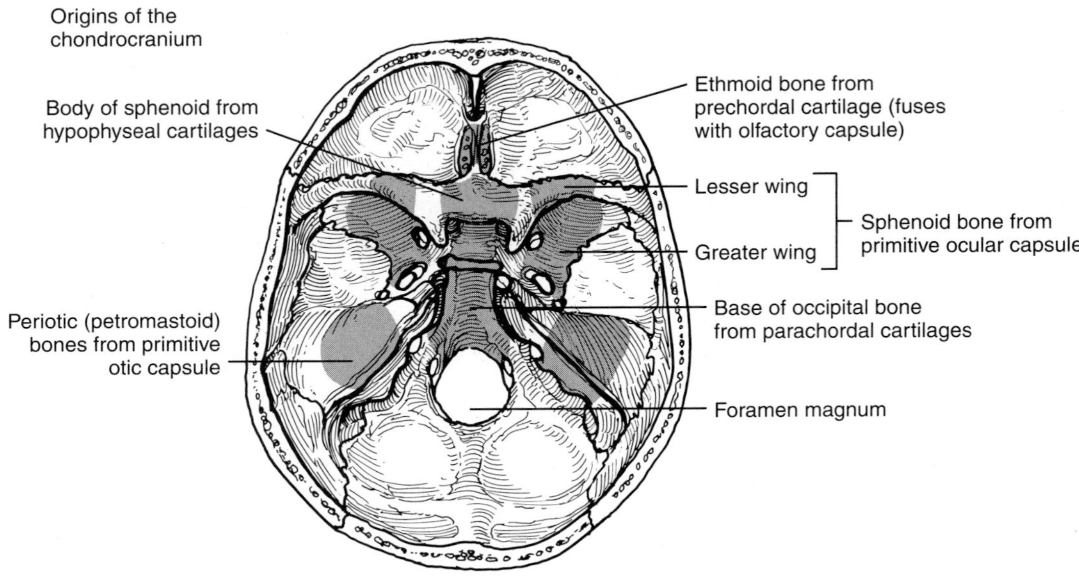

FIGURE 22–1
Origins of the chondrocranium. Ethmoid bone, occipital bone, and body of sphenoid bone develop from cartilaginous precursors. Greater and lesser wings of sphenoid bone, periotic bones, and turbinate and nasal bones (not shown) develop from primitive sensory capsules.

branchial arches that made up the feeding and respiratory apparatuses of jawless fishes. These were later modified in fishes with jaws and reptiles on the evolutionary line that led to humans to form the **pharyngeal arches** of the human embryo (Fig. 22–2*A* and *B*).

Typically, the branchial apparatus of the earliest fishes consisted of repeating, identical pairs of **gill bars,** or **branchial arches,** separated by paired openings, or **gill slits.** The gill bars contained an artery (of the aortic arch system) and were supported by small cartilaginous elements or bones. Each of these branchial arches also contained muscles that pulled water into the fish's mouth and then ejected it through the gill slits. During this process, the branchial apparatus filtered food particles from the water, directing them into the pharynx (throat), while capillaries within each branchial arch extracted oxygen for respiration. The number of gill bars and gill slits of ancestral fishes varied widely. The fish that gave rise to humans had six pairs of gill arches, but humans retain derivatives of only five pairs. They correspond to the first, second, third, fourth, and sixth pair of gill arches in the ancestral fish.

Obviously, the primitive branchial arches of the ancestral fishes have been markedly altered to serve much different functions in humans. For example, the respiratory function of the branchial arches has been lost in humans as lungs evolved for life on land. In some cases, the arches of humans have assumed completely novel functions. For example, arches 4 and 6 have been highly modified for vocalization (larynx). In one of the most striking transformations, supportive elements of the first branchial arch of the primitive jawless fishes were first transformed into the jaw joint of jawed fishes. As mammals arose from their reptilian ancestors, these jaw joint elements, the malleus and incus, migrated into the middle ear to join the stapes bone as two additional auditory ossicles (see below). On the other hand, many of the tissues derived from human arches 1, 2, and 3 continue to be used in eating (jaw and tongue) (Fig. 22–2*A* to *C*). Because structures derived from gill arches do not function as gills in humans (they are, instead, related to the pharynx), it is appropriate to refer to these embryologic arches as pharyngeal arches rather than branchial arches.

Although the pharyngeal arches have given rise to diverse structures of the head and neck, their initial embryonic anatomy is very similar both in form and content (Fig. 22–2*A* and *B*). Like the branchial arches of ancestral fishes, each embryonic human pharyngeal arch consists of a bar of mesenchyme covered on the outside by surface ectoderm and on the inside by endoderm. The ectomesenchymal (neural crest) component of the mesenchyme, however, forms cartilaginous or bony elements of the human facial skeleton, tendons, neurons, smooth muscles, and several other tissues. The mesenchyme of each human pharyngeal arch also includes paraxial mesoderm, which forms the striated muscle of the head and anterior neck and bones of the skull base. Each human pharyngeal arch also includes a specific cranial nerve and a single aortic arch artery. Each cranial nerve innervates a specific functional subset of muscles of the face or jaw (or both), and the aortic arches con-

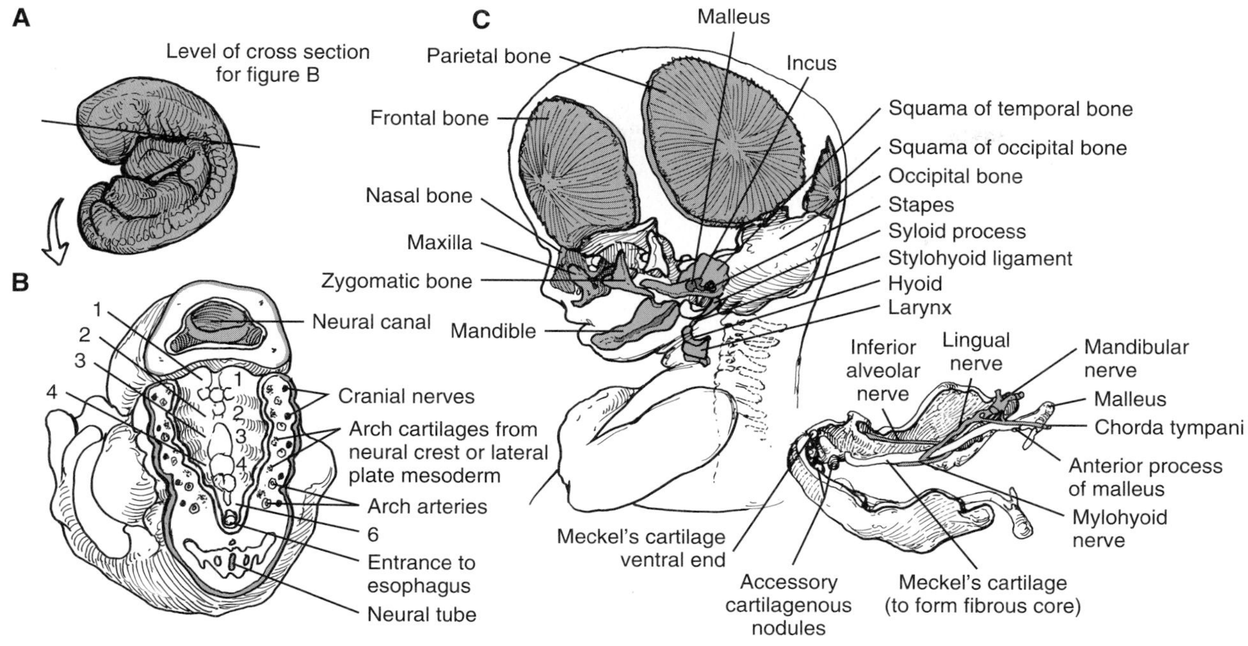

FIGURE 22–2

Prenatal development of the skull. Derivation of the facial skeleton from pharyngeal arches. **A.** Human embryo. **B.** Cross section indicated in **A** showing pharyngeal arches. **C.** Endochondrial facial skeletal elements, including structures from pharyngeal arch precursors, shown in red. Dermal bones of the cranial vault and facial skeleton shown in gray.

tribute to the development of the great arteries such as the aorta and common and internal carotid arteries. The pharyngeal arch nerves, muscles, and arteries are described in detail in Chapter 23.

As in the case of the somitomeres and somites of the trunk, the specific development and identity of the pharyngeal arches are regulated by a **combinatorial code of HOX genes** (and other regulatory genes).

Indeed, certain craniofacial defects in humans may arise through disruption of HOX gene expression in the embryonic head, either as a consequence of mutation or because of a response to teratogens such as retinoic acid (see Chapters 2 and 3 and the discussion of craniofacial defects below).

Derivation of the Facial Skeleton From Pharyngeal Arches. *The human facial skeleton is derived from neural crest or lateral plate mesoderm of the pharyngeal arches.* Neural crest cells within the first three arches and lateral plate mesoderm within arches 4 and 6 form specific arch-related structures of the facial skeleton. For example, the neural crest in the maxillary swellings (upper lip and cheeks) of the first arch gives rise to **part of the sphenoid bone** and the **incus bone** of the middle ear (an auditory ossicle) (Fig. 22–2C). The neural crest of the mandibular swellings (lower jaw) of the first arch gives rise to a **fibrous core within the mandible bone** and to the **malleus bone** of the middle ear. The neural crest of the second arch forms the **stapes bone** of the middle ear, **styloid process** of the temporal bone, **stylohyoid ligament,** and **upper rim** and **lesser horns of the hyoid bone.** The neural crest of the third arch forms the **lower rim** and **greater horns of the hyoid bone.** The lateral plate mesoderm of the fourth and sixth arches together forms the **laryngeal cartilages** (Fig. 22–2C).

Congenital Malformations of the Facial Skeleton.

A spectrum of anomalies called **holoprosencephaly** may affect the development of the skeleton of the midfacial region. In this syndrome, the induction of the forebrain by the prechordal mesoderm and notochord is disrupted during the third week of development, resulting in reduction of midventral parts of the central nervous system and consequent development of a single cerebral vesicle rather than two cerebral hemispheres. This results, in turn, in the reduction of midfacial structures, including skeletal and soft tissues. The affected infant may have a narrow forehead or hypotelorism (close-set eyes) and may be lacking a nose or philtrum (middle part of the upper lip). In extreme cases, the face may be so narrow that only a single eye is formed (cyclopia). This syndrome may result from disrupted expression (either through mutation or translocation) of the gene encoding the signal molecule that normally induces the midventral region of the central nervous system (sonic hedgehog). It may also result from mutations that occur in the absence of endogenous cholesterol production (Smith-Lemli-Opitz syndrome) or from excessive intake of alcohol by the mother during the third week of gestation (fetal alcohol syndrome).

During normal development, a midventral structure called the *intermaxillary process* fuses with the lateral maxillary swellings to form the maxilla bones of the upper jaw. Disruption of fusion on one side of the face may result in **unilateral cleft lip** and on both sides, **bilateral cleft lip.** This disruption is thought to result from reduced production of mesoderm within the maxillary swellings or the intermaxillary process (or both). Alternatively, the horizontal palatine shelves of the maxilla may also fail to fuse, resulting in a **cleft palate.** However, this anomaly is thought to arise by a mechanism distinct from the one that causes cleft lip.

Disrupted development of specific pharyngeal arches may result in specific arch-related defects. Usually, the malformation is attributed to inadequate proliferation of neural crest cells within the first and second pharyngeal arches, which leads to underdevelopment of the lower face and mandible. This class of malformations is called **mandibulofacial dysostosis.** Specific inherited examples of mandibulofacial dysostosis include Treacher-Collins syndrome and Hallermann-Streiff syndrome. Other syndromes may be caused by the mother's use of the oral antiacne medication, isotretinoin, during pregnancy.

Disruption of development of the third and fourth pharyngeal arches may result in a spectrum of malformations called **DiGeorge syndrome.** This syndrome includes defects of the ear, palate, and jaw; agenesis of the thyroid and thymus glands; and cardiovascular anomalies. DiGeorge syndrome may be caused by monosomy of chromosome 21 or by alcohol intake by the mother.

Dermal Bones of the Cranial Vault

The flat bones of the cranial vault arise from mesenchyme derived from the neural crest; this mesenchyme originally developed as protective armor in a line of bony fishes

Another innovation leading to the development of the human head is the **cranial vault.** The cranial vault has its origin in a line of bony fishes that was distinguished by a secondary bony armor covering the brain and head. This armor developed directly within the dermis of the integument from neural crest cells by a process of **membranous ossification** (Fig. 22–2C). The **dermal bones** of the cranial vault of humans include the **frontal bones, parietal bones,** and **flat (squamous) parts of the temporal** and **occipital bones.** More recently, in evolution, dermal bone has also replaced elements of the **facial skeleton** derived from the pharyngeal arches. These include most of the bones of the upper jaw and cheek such as the **maxilla** and **zygomatic bones** (Fig. 22–2C). In addition, the **jaw joint (temporomandibular joint)** of mammals is a novel dermal structure that has replaced the more primitive joint of reptiles, which was originally formed by the incus and malleus bones of the first arch (see above).

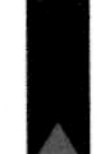

DEVELOPMENT AND ORGANIZATION OF THE DEFINITIVE SKULL

Prenatal Development of the Skull

The skull forms by endochondral ossification of the chondrocranium and facial skeletal elements and by membranous ossification of the cranial vault

The skull is the most complex bone of the **axial skeleton** (see Chapter 1). In part, this is because it originates from diverse precursors and because it must serve several diverse functions. As has been noted above, the bones of the base of the skull are formed by the ossification of cartilaginous precursors. These include the ethmoid and sphenoid bones, the petrous part of the temporal bone, and the occipital bone, with the exception of its squama. Likewise, bones of the facial skeleton, specifically the auditory ossicles, styloid process, and hyoid bone, also form by **endochondral ossification** of cartilaginous precursors within the pharyngeal arches. The skeletons of the epiglottis and larynx also form as cartilage but remain cartilaginous throughout adult life. In all of these cases, the skeletal elements first develop as condensed mesenchymal masses during the first and second months of embryonic life. Chondrification begins with the presumptive occipital bone in the second month and continues in an anterior direction within the base of the skull. Chondrification of elements of the facial skeleton also occurs within the second month. Ossification of most of the cartilaginous elements of the head is initiated before the completion of chondrification and continues even after birth (Figs. 22–2C and 22–3).

In contrast, bones of the cranial vault form through the direct condensation and ossification of mesenchyme within the dermis of the head, the **membranous ossification.** These mesenchymal precursors first appear at the beginning of the second month of embryonic development, and their ossification is initiated shortly thereafter (Fig. 22–2C). Complete ossification of the cranial vault, however, does not occur until early childhood (Fig. 22–3).

▲ Postnatal Development of the Skull

The length of the cranium increases after birth, largely through the accretion of new bone in the regions of the cartilaginous joints within the **chondrocranium** (between the ethmoid and sphenoid bones and between the sphenoid and occipital bones). This expansion continues until the late teens or early twenties.

By the ninth prenatal month, the individual bones of the **cranial vault** include the paired temporal and parietal bones, and the unpaired frontal bone and occipital squama (Fig. 22–3). These bones remain separated, however, by unossified **sutures** and six relatively large, unossified, membrane-covered **fonticuli (fontanelles).** The fontanelles are located at apposed angles of the individual calvarial plates (Fig. 22–3). There are two

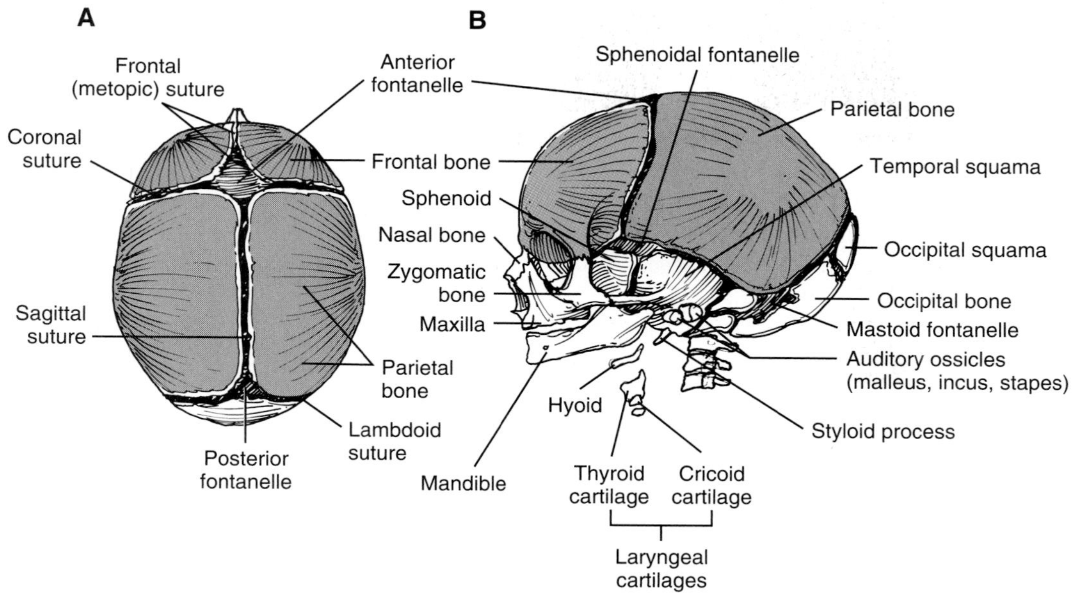

FIGURE 22–3
Postnatal development of the skull. **A.** Superior view of the human skull at birth, showing fontanelles. **B.** Lateral view of human skull at birth.

median fontanelles, the **anterior** and **posterior fontanelles.** There are also two pairs of **lateral fontanelles:** two anterolateral fontanelles (one on each side), called **sphenoidal fontanelles;** and two posterolateral fontanelles (one on each side) called **mastoid fontanelles** (Fig. 22–3*B*).

The unossified sutures and fontanelles between the bones of the cranial vault allow significant deformation of the proportionately large human head at birth. Indeed, individual bones may overlap during the birth process, allowing compression and compensatory elongation of the skull. These alterations in the shape of the skull may remain for as long as a week following birth. However, ossification of the sphenoidal and posterior fontanelles occurs by the second to third postnatal month, ossification of the mastoid fontanelles by the twelfth postnatal month, and ossification of the anterior fontanelle by the end of the second year of life. Although the sutures are not completely ossified until age 30 to 40 years (internally) or age 50 years (externally), they usually become stabilized through the complex interdigitation of apposed bones by the end of the second year of life.

The adult dimensions of the cranial vault are almost completely attained by age 7 years, although the vault may continue to grow a bit more until the person reaches the late teens. Growth of the cranial vault after birth occurs largely through the removal of bone (by absorption) from the internal side, the **inner table,** of the bone and through the concomitant addition or accretion of bone to the outside of the skull, the **external table.** Definitive bones of the skull typically have three layers: a compact **inner table,** a compact **outer table,** and a trabecular layer filled with red bone marrow called the **diploë,** which separates the inner and outer tables. In contrast, bones such as the vomer and medial and lateral pterygoid plates (see below) may be so thin that they have only a single compact layer.

In contrast to the cranial vault, the **facial skeleton** grows significantly during childhood and the early teens and even beyond puberty. Much of this growth in the mandible and maxilla results from eruption of the primary and secondary dentition. Growth of the upper face occurs as spaces within the diploë expand to form the air sinuses (see discussion of the paranasal sinuses below).

Development of Ridges and Processes of the Skull

The ridges and processes associated with the skull develop in response to the pull of attached muscles

The superciliary ridges, nuchal lines, occipital protuberance, and mastoid processes enlarge as the muscles attached to them increase in size and strength (see Table 22–2). It is, therefore, possible to estimate the age and sex of an individual by assessing the size and prominence of these structures. The structures are larger in males and older individuals. However, there are fewer differences between juvenile and adult human skulls and between male and female human skulls than is the case in other primates.

Craniosynostosis. In some fetuses, specific sutures of the skull fuse prior to birth. This restricts the growth of the brain and the cranial vault in the region of the suture. This phenomenon is called **craniosynostosis.** In order to compensate for the growth of the brain, other sutures remain open, resulting in abnormal expansion of surrounding regions of the skull. For example, when the coronal and lambdoid sutures fuse prematurely, the frontal suture widens, allowing excessive expansion of the forehead. The result is tower skull, called **acrocephaly,** which may be accompanied by hypertelorism (wide-set eyes) and cleft nose and upper lip. Rarely, the sagittal sutures fuse prenatally, forcing expansion of the skull both anteriorly (separation of the frontal and parietal bones by expansion of the frontal suture) and posteriorly (separation of the occipital and parietal bones by expansion of the lambdoid suture). This results in an elongated keel-shaped skull, **scaphocephaly.** This anomaly is sometimes accompanied by mental retardation. In these cases of craniosynostosis, reconstructive surgery may be attempted to restore the skull to its normal shape.

▲ General Features of the Definitive Skull

Composition of the Skull

Anatomically, the definitive skull is considered to consist of two main parts, the cranium and the facial skeleton

The **cranium,** or brainbox, is composed mainly of the bones of the skull base **(chondrocranium** or **neurocranium)** and the bones of the **cranial vault.** The upper domelike region of the cranial vault is called the **calvaria** or **calva.** Eight of the bones of the cranium enclose the brain. Seven other bones are more aptly described as bones that contribute to the structure of the nasal cavity or orbits (or both). The eight bones that enclose the brain are the unpaired occipital, sphenoid, frontal, and ethmoid bones and the paired parietal and temporal bones. The seven bones that contribute to the nasal cavities or orbits are the single vomer bone and the paired inferior nasal conchae, lacrimal, and nasal bones (Fig. 22–4).

The **facial skeleton (viscerocranium)** of the definitive skull is composed of seven bones: the single mandible and the paired maxilla, palatine, and zygomatic bones (Fig. 22–4). Other elements of the facial skeleton that have been defined developmentally above include the hyoid bone and the epiglottal and laryngeal cartilages. Specific details of the anatomy of these individual bones will be described where appropriate in Chapters 23 and 24. However, an understanding of the skull as a whole is of critical importance to a fundamental understanding of the soft tissues of the head and neck, so much of Chapter 22 is devoted to a more global description of the skull.

Joints of the Skull

Most bones of the skull are connected by sutures or synchondroses

All joints of the skull except for the temporomandibular joints are either immovable sutures or immovable synchondroses. **Sutures** are unique to the skull. They typically join bones of the cranial vault. They can be characterized by the following simple scheme:

Bone ⟷ Collagenous sutural ligament ⟷ Bone

On the other hand, **synchondroses of the skull** tend to join bones of the chondrocranium (e.g., they join the ethmoid bone to the sphenoid bone and the sphenoid bone to the occipital bones). They are similar in structure to the **epiphyses** of the long bones. The synchondroses are classified as joints in which apposed bones are joined by hyaline growth cartilage, as in the following scheme:

Bone ⟷ Hyaline growth cartilage ⟷ Bone

Like the epiphyses of long bones, the sutures and synchondroses of the cranium are **temporary joints** because the apposed bones eventually grow together, obliterating the intervening fibrous or cartilaginous junction between them. As has been noted, however, fusion of the skull sutures may not be complete until a person reaches 50 years of age.

One pair of movable **synovial joints** is also found in the skull. These are the **temporomandibular joints** of the jaw. They are described with the mandible at the end of this chapter.

▲ Anatomy of the Skull From Various Aspects

The anatomy of the definitive skull is described from various views or aspects (see Table 22–1)

The human skull is probably the most recognizable bone of the human body and has long held a fascination for painters, poets, playwrights, politicians, and spiritual leaders. Sadly, from time to time, measurements of various dimensions of the skull (craniometry) have been unjustifiably used as a basis for racial or religious discrimination. In recent times, however, craniometric measurements have proved useful in anthropologic studies and in forensic identification of skeletal remains, particularly when the skull can be compared with surviving photographic or radiographic records. General features of the definitive human skull can be readily seen when one observes the skull from **superior, anterior, posterior, inferior,** and **lateral aspects.**

Superior Aspect of the Skull (Norma Verticalis)

The parietal and frontal bones and a small superior part of the occipital bone are apparent in superior views of the skull

The cranium of a young adult has a modified ovoid (egg) shape when it is viewed from above. It is narrower from side to side anteriorly than posteriorly (Fig. 22–5). Running along the midline is the zigzag **sagittal suture,** which connects the paired **parietal bones.** A similarly elaborate interdigitation between the posterior edge of the single **frontal bone** and the anterior edges of the parietal bones demarcates the **coronal suture** (Fig.

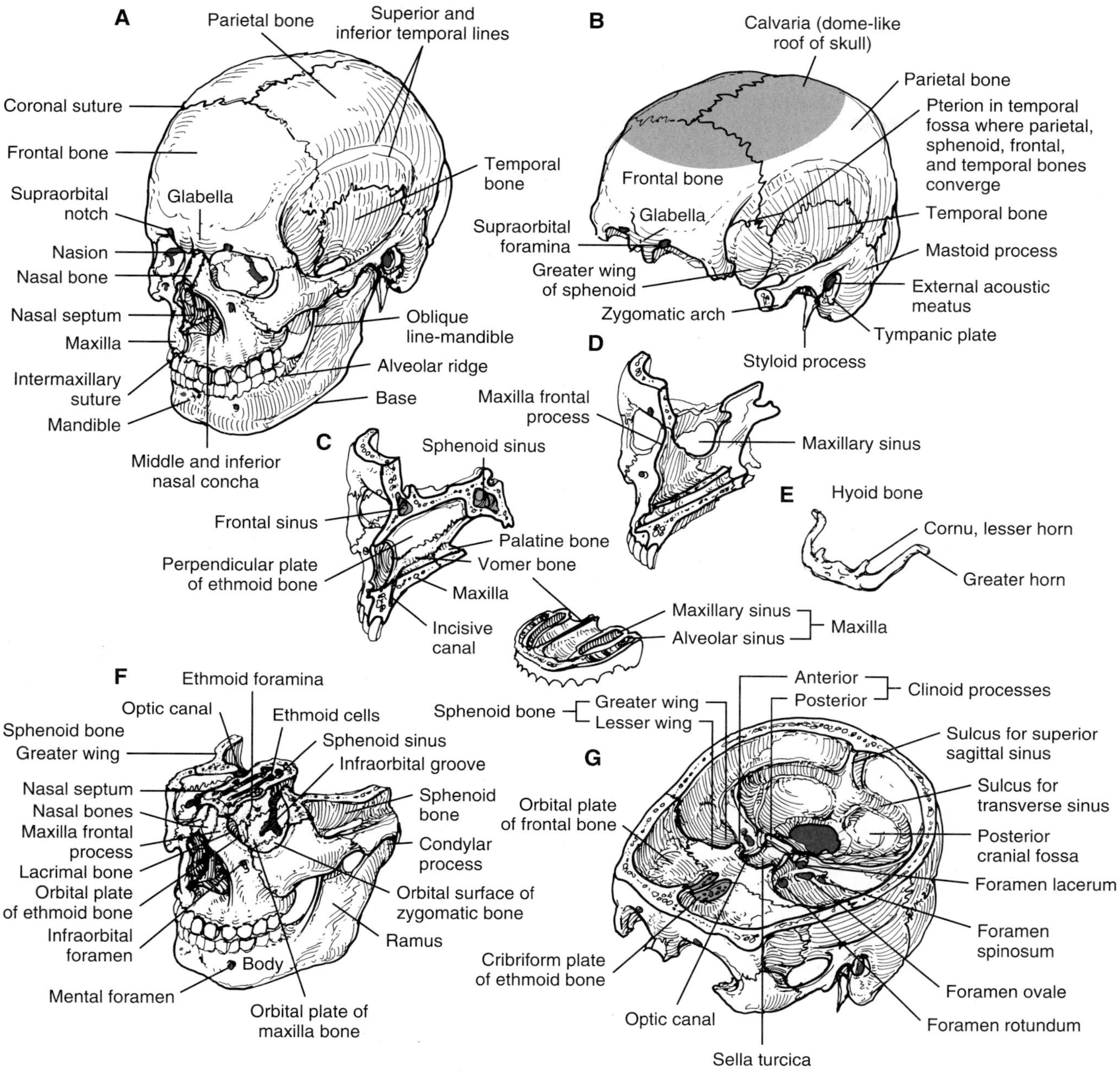

FIGURE 22–4
General features of the definitive skull, superior oblique views.

22–5). The point at which the frontal bone intersects with both parietal bones (junction of the sagittal and coronal sutures) is the **bregma.** This was the site of the original **anterior fontanelle.** Barely visible on the posterior surface of the skull is the **lambdoid suture,** which joins the inferoposterior edges of each parietal bone with the superoposterior edge of the **occipital bone** (Fig. 22–5). The point at which the two parietal bones and the occipital bone intersect (junction of the lambdoid and sagittal sutures) is the **lambda.** This is the site of the original **posterior fontanelle.** In about half of individuals, small, paired foramina are apparent just lateral to the lambda. These **parietal foramina** transport small **emissary veins,** which connect the superficial venous system of the scalp with the **superior sagittal sinus,** a part of the venous drainage system of the brain.

Posterior Aspect of the Skull (Norma Occipitalis)

The only bones apparent in posterior views of the skull are the paired parietal bones, occipital squama, and mandible

Prominent landmarks obvious in posterior views of the skull include a protuberance called the *external occipital protuberance* and three associated lines or ridges called (in superior to inferior order) the *highest, superior,* and *in-*

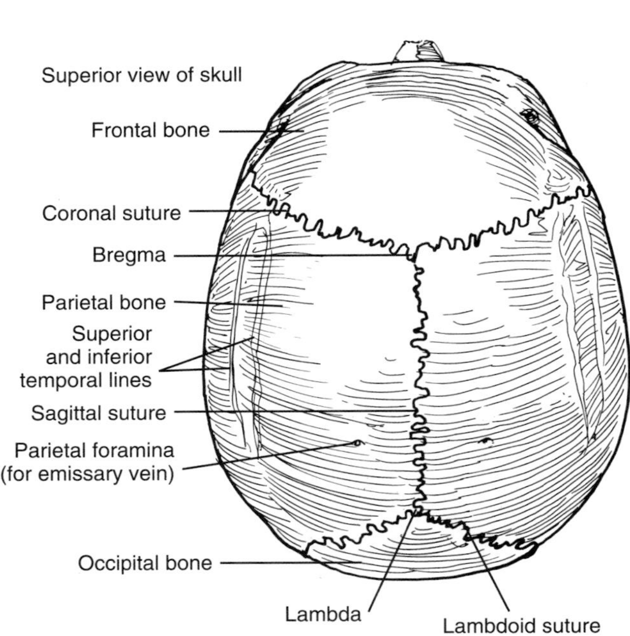

FIGURE 22–5
Superior view of the skull.

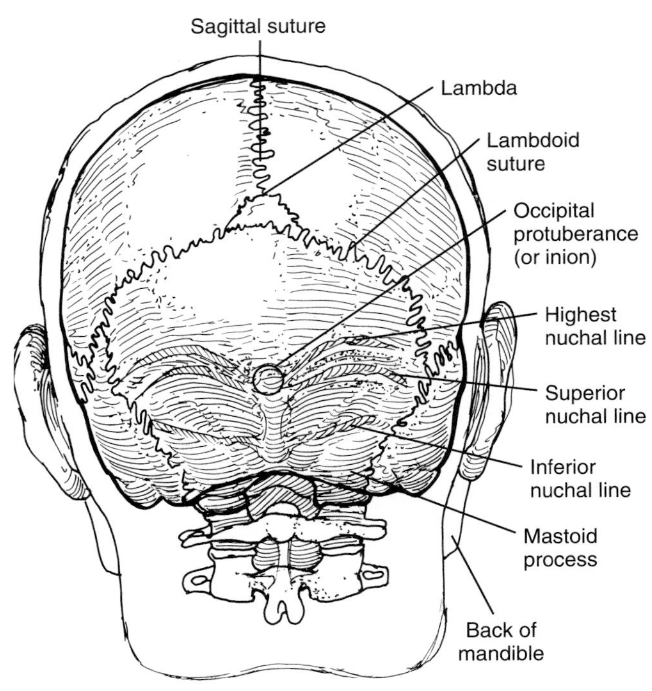

FIGURE 22–6
Posterior aspect of the skull.

ferior nuchal lines (Fig. 22–6). The apex of the **external occipital protuberance** is the **inion,** which is formed by the pull of the trapezius muscle at its most superior point and, more inferiorly, by the ligamentum nuchae (see Chapter 5). The superior attachment of the trapezius muscle also spreads laterally from the inion, forming the medial region of the **superior nuchal line.** The lateral region of the superior nuchal line is formed by the pull of medial fibers of the sternocleidomastoid muscle (see Fig. 24–21). The **highest nuchal line** is formed by the pull of the occipitofrontalis muscle. The **inferior nuchal line** is formed by the pull of the rectus capitis major muscle (laterally) and the rectus capitis minor muscle (medially). Two large processes just barely visible in this posterior view of the skull are the **mastoid processes.** They can be seen more clearly in lateral views of the skull (see below). Other prominent landmarks apparent in a posterior view of the skull include the **lambdoid suture** and the posterior extent of the **sagittal suture** (Fig. 22–6). Recall that the point of their intersection, the **lambda,** is the site of the former posterior fontanelle.

With the **mandible** in place, it is possible to view much of its internal surface from this posterior aspect (Fig. 22–6). This movable bone, however, is described in its entirety at the end of this chapter, along with the **temporomandibular joint.**

Anterior Aspect of the Skull (Norma Frontalis)

Bones of the forehead, cheek, and upper jaw are prominent features of the anterior skull

The perimeter of the anterior aspect of the skull is oval in shape. It is slightly wider above than below (Fig. 22–7). The **frontal bone** above is smooth, except for a median prominence called the **glabella,** which is bounded laterally by **superciliary arches** above the superior border of the orbits. The slight prominence above each superciliary arch is called a **frontal tuberosity.** The frontal bone also provides a superior border of the orbital cavity (orbit). This otherwise smooth **supraorbital margin,** however, may be broken by a **supraorbital notch,** which transmits the supraorbital nerve (a branch of the ophthalmic nerve) and supraorbital vessels to the forehead (see Chapter 24). Alternatively, the nerve and vessels may be transmitted to the forehead by distinct **supraorbital foramina.** In addition to contributing to the supraorbital margin of the orbit, the frontal bone also contributes to the superior parts of the **medial** and **lateral orbital margins.**

In contrast to the relatively simple forehead just described, the lower facial skeleton is quite irregular. It is broken by the paired orbits and the piriform (pear-shaped) opening to the nasal cavity. The paired, protruding **nasal bones** are joined in the midline by an **internasal suture.** The superior edge of each nasal bone is joined to the frontal bone by the **frontonasal suture.** The junction of the internasal and frontonasal suture is called the **nasion** (Fig. 22–7 and see Fig. 22–10).

One of the most prominent features of the lower part of the anterior face is the paired **maxilla bones.** Each of these bones is composed of three regions: a superomedial frontal process, a lateral zygomatic process, and an inferior alveolar process. The **frontal process**

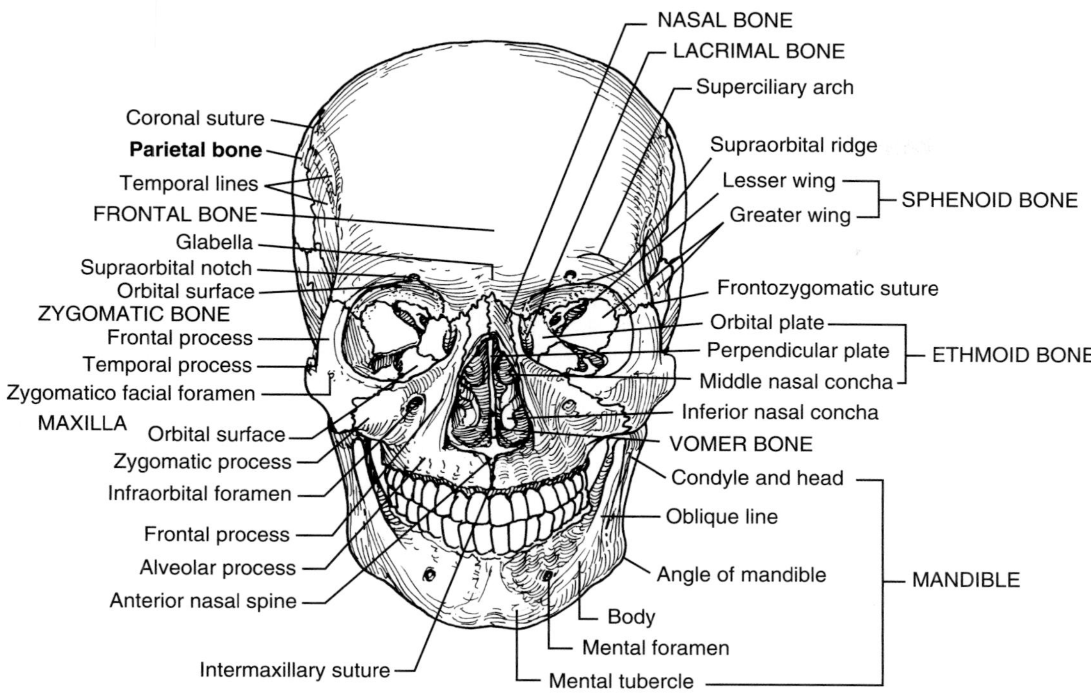

FIGURE 22–7
Anterior aspect of the skull.

joins the maxilla to the frontal bone by a frontomaxillary suture just inferior to the glabella. A **nasomaxillary suture** joins the medial edge of each frontal process with the more medial nasal bones (Fig. 22–7). The frontal process of the maxillary bone also contributes to the medial edge of the orbit. The **zygomatic process of the maxilla** is connected to the **maxillary process of the zygomatic bone** by a **zygomaticomaxillary suture** just inferior to the orbit. Together, the zygomatic process of the maxillary bone and the maxillary process of the zygomatic bone form the **infraorbital margin** of the orbit. **Infraorbital foramina** are apparent in the zygomatic process of the maxilla. They penetrate the maxilla about 1 cm below the infraorbital margin, in line with the supraorbital notch or supraorbital foramina above. They transmit the infraorbital nerve (from the ophthalmic nerve) and the infraorbital vessels. Finally, the **alveolar process** of each maxilla contains sockets (alveoli) for eight upper teeth (Fig. 22–7). These include two incisors, one canine tooth, two premolars, and three molars. The two alveolar processes are connected in the midline just under the nasal aperture by an **intermaxillary suture.** The superior part of this suture is marked by a protruding **nasal spine.**

Most of the **zygomatic bone** is apparent in a frontal or anterior view of the skull. As has been noted, its **maxillary process** joins the zygomatic process of the maxilla to form the infraorbital margin. In addition, its **frontal process** joins the frontal bone to form the lateral orbital margin. Its **temporal process** (more apparent in the lateral view; see below) is joined to the **zygomatic arch** of the **temporal bone.** A small **zygomaticofacial foramen** is usually apparent in the zygomatic bone near the inferior orbital margin (Fig. 22–7). This foramen carries the zygomaticofacial nerve and vessels.

The **mandible** of the skull is apparent immediately inferior to the alveolar processes of the maxilla bones. When it is in place, much of its external surface can be described from this anterior aspect. However, the mandible will be described in its entirety at the end of this chapter.

The skull is characterized as having five major cavities, which are the paired orbits, paired nasal passages, and cranial cavity. The orbits and nasal passages are apparent in anterior views of the skull. The cranial cavity is described below.

Fracture of Bones of the Anterior Face. Trauma to the anterior face is common when the head collides with a hard object, as may occur in automobile accidents or sports-related mishaps. In these cases, virtually any of the facial bones may be fractured, including the maxilla, nasal bones, and zygomatic bones. Three major types of facial fractures were described by Le Fort, a French surgeon in the early twentieth century, and these classifications remain useful to the present day. In a **type I fracture,** the alveolar process of the maxilla and the upper teeth and hard palate are separated from the more superior part of the skull (Fig. 22–8*A*). In a **type II fracture,** most of the maxilla, including the alveolar, zygomatic, and frontal processes and the nasal bones, is separated from the frontal and zygomatic bones (Fig. 22–8*B*). Fi-

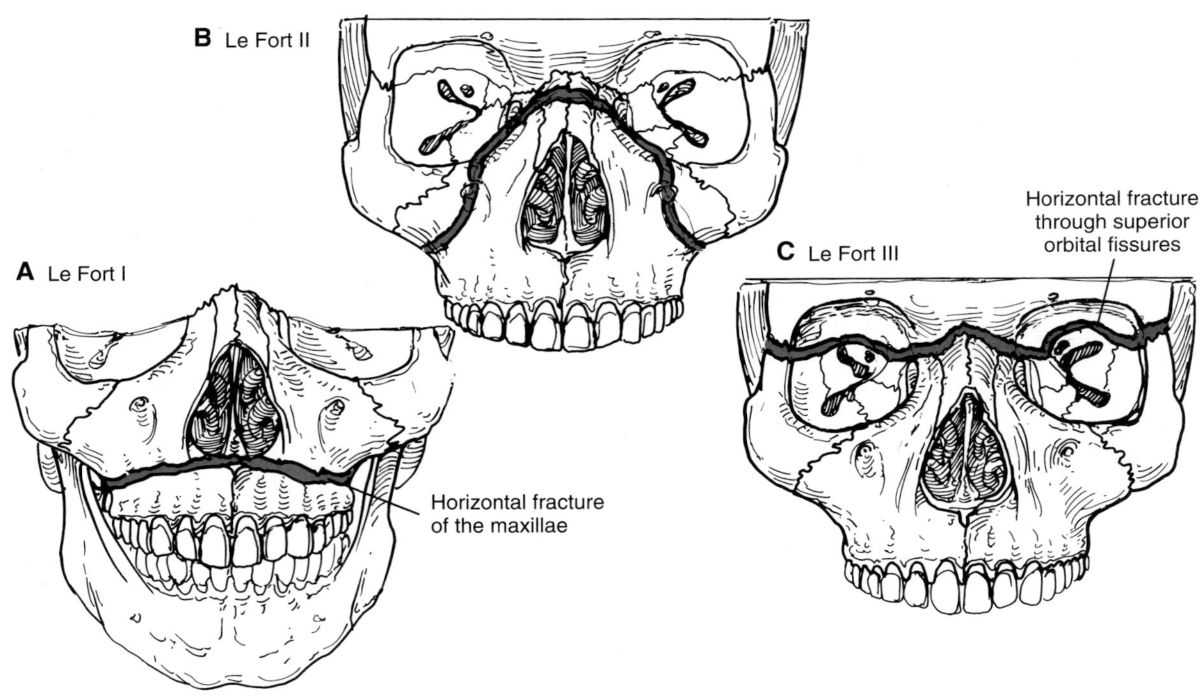

FIGURE 22–8
Fracture of bones of the anterior face. **A.** Type I fracture. **B.** Type II fracture. **C.** Type III fracture.

nally, in a **type III fracture,** virtually the entire facial skeleton, including the maxillae, nasal bones, and zygomatic bones, is separated from the frontal bone above it (Fig. 22–8*C*).

Orbits. *Bones of the orbital cavity are described with respect to their locations within the cavity's superior, inferior, medial, or lateral wall.* The cavity of the orbit is bounded by a superior "roof," an inferior "floor," and lateral and medial "walls." These boundaries may be considered as sides of a pyramid. The **base** of the pyramid is at the anterior opening of the orbit and the **apex** at the posterior end of the orbital cavity (Fig. 22–9*A* and *C*).

The **superior wall (roof)** of the orbital cavity is formed by two bones: the **frontal plate of the frontal bone** (main bone), and, posteriorly, by a small part of the **lesser wing of the sphenoid bone.** The thin frontal plate is the only barrier between the orbital cavity and the anterior fossa of the cranial cavity, which contains the frontal lobes of the brain (Fig. 22–9*A* and discussion of the interior of the cranium below). Anteromedially, the frontal plate elaborates a bony process, which serves as a pulley for the superior oblique muscle, an extrinsic muscle of the eyeball (see Chapter 25). Anterolaterally, the frontal plate is depressed to house the **orbital part** of **a tear gland, the lacrimal gland** (see Chapter 25).

The thin **medial wall** of the orbital cavity is formed by three bones: the **lacrimal bone** (anteriorly); the **orbital plate of the ethmoid bone,** which is just posterior to the lacrimal bone; and part of the **body of the sphenoid bone,** which is just behind the orbital plate of the ethmoid bone (Fig. 22–9*B*). This posterior sphenoidal part of the medial wall of the orbit is separated from the more superior frontal plate of the roof of the orbit by the **optic canal,** a foramen that transmits the **optic nerve** and **ophthalmic artery** from the **middle fossa** of the cranial cavity (see discussion of the interior of the cranium below). Anteriorly, the medial wall has a depression, the **lacrimal groove,** which houses the lacrimal sac. The lacrimal groove opens into a **nasolacrimal canal,** which drains tears into the inferior meatus of the nasal cavity (see below).

The thick **lateral wall** of the orbital cavity is formed by two bones: the **frontal process of the zygomatic bone** anteriorly and part of the **greater wing of the sphenoid bone** posteriorly (Fig. 22–9*C*). The frontal process of the zygomatic bone contains a small fissure for the zygomaticofacial nerve. A **superior orbital fissure** separates this part of the greater wing of the sphenoid bone from the part of the lesser wing of the sphenoid bone that forms the roof of the orbital cavity (Fig. 22–9*C*). The superior orbital fissure transmits the following structures between the middle cranial fossa of the cranial cavity and the orbital cavity:

- ♦ oculomotor nerve,
- ♦ trochlear nerve,
- ♦ abducens nerve,

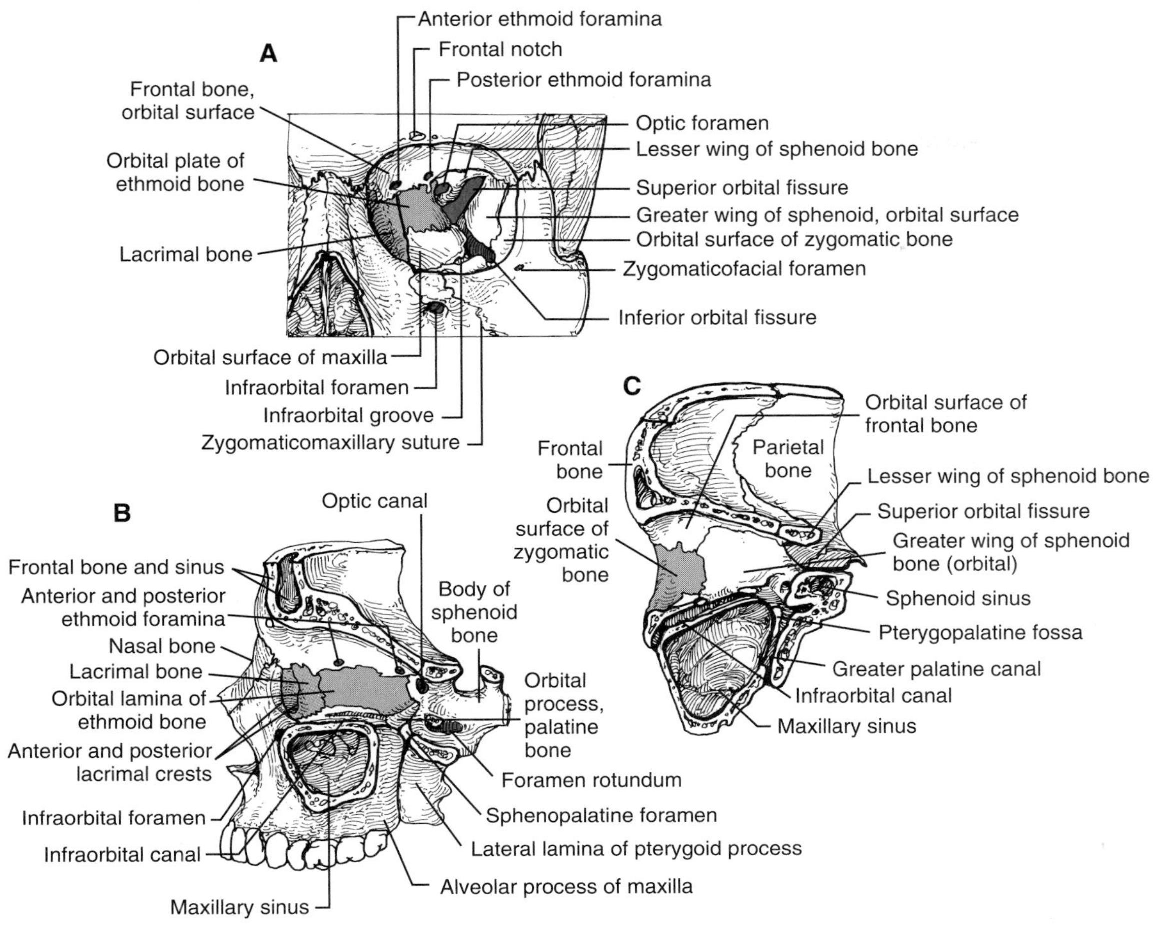

FIGURE 22–9

Bones of the orbital cavity. **A.** Anterior view. **B.** Parasagittal section showing medial wall of left orbit. **C.** Lateral wall of right orbit (viewed from medial side).

- branches of the ophthalmic nerve, and
- branches of the ophthalmic vein (see Chapter 23).

Separating the inferior boundary of the greater wing of the sphenoid bone from the floor of the orbital cavity is the **infraorbital fissure.** The infraorbital fissure transmits the following structures between the middle fossa of the cranial cavity and the orbital cavity:

- maxillary nerve,
- zygomatic nerve, and
- infraorbital vessels.

The **inferior wall (floor)** of the orbital cavity is comprised of three bones: the maxillary process of the zygomatic bone anteriorly, the zygomatic process of the maxilla, and part of the palatine process of the maxilla posteriorly (see discussion of the inferior aspect of the skull below).

Fractures of Bones of the Orbit. Fracture of the floor of the orbit (which is also the roof of the maxillary sinus; see below), may follow a blow to the eye. This fracture is called a **blowout fracture.** Pressure from the periorbital fat around the eyeball (globe) causes the eyeball to sag down into the maxillary sinus, resulting in **diplopia (double vision)** (see Chapter 23). Fractures of the medial and superior walls and apex of the orbit are also common, typically as a consequence of penetration by a sharp object. If penetration occurs in the anteromedial wall, the frontal sinus may be opened to the orbit. If the posteromedial wall is penetrated, ethmoidal sinuses may communicate with the orbit. An object that penetrates the apex of the orbit via the superior orbital fissure enters the middle cranial fossa and may damage the temporal lobe of the brain. Penetration of the roof of the orbit opens the anterior cranial fossa to the orbit, exposing the frontal lobe (see descriptions of the paranasal sinuses, below).

Nasal Cavity. The nasal cavity is a space bounded anteriorly by the pear-shaped **anterior nasal aperture** and posteriorly by paired **posterior nasal apertures (choanae),** which lead into the nasopharynx (Fig. 22–10*A* and *B* and see Chapter 26). Anteriorly, the **roof of the nasal cavity** is formed by the paired **nasal bones** (which specifically constitute the roof of the external

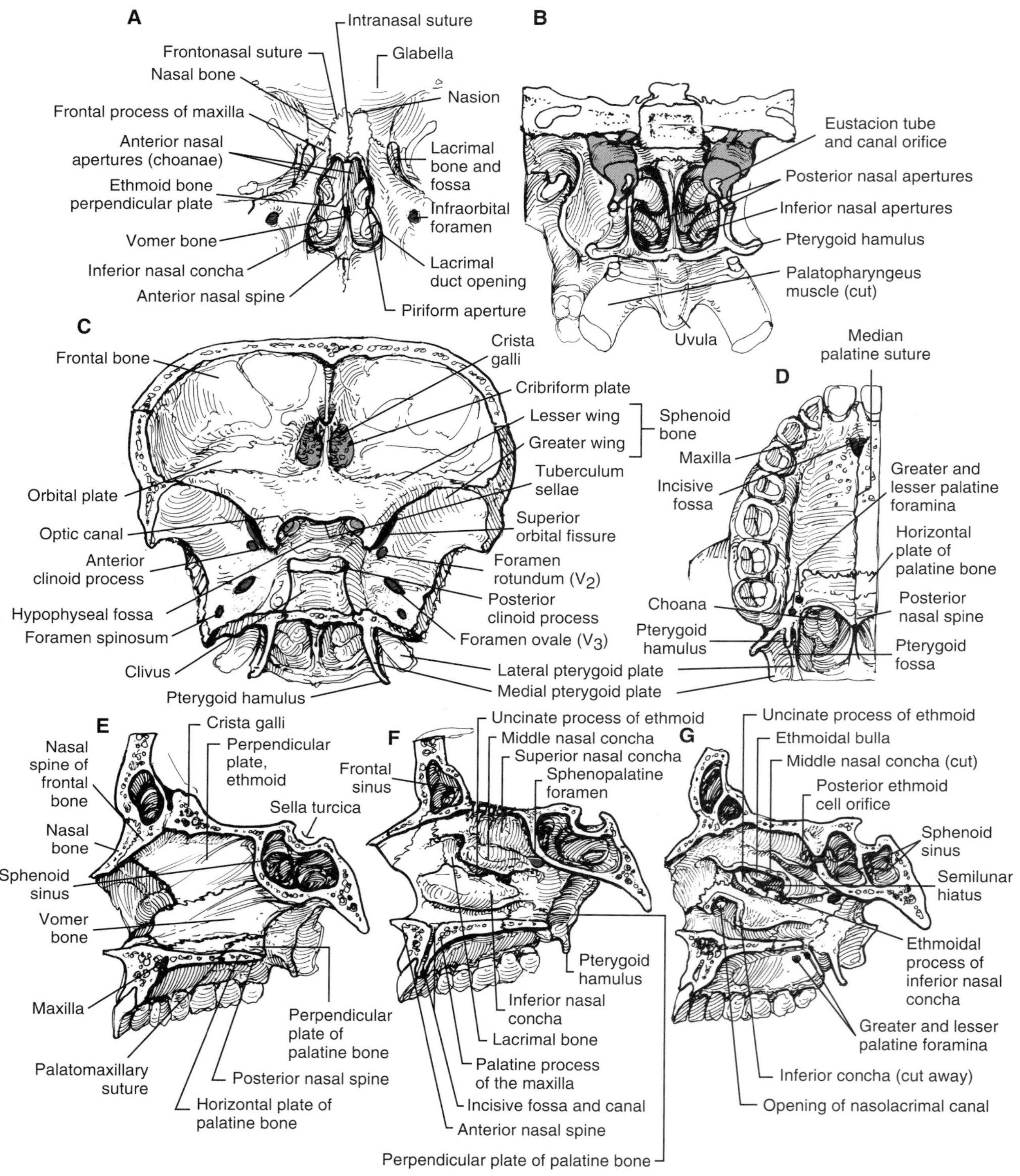

FIGURE 22–10

Bones of the nasal cavity. **A.** Anterior view. **B.** Posterior view. **C.** Roof of nasal cavity viewed from above. **D.** Floor of nasal cavity, inferior view. **E**, **F**, and **G**. Cross-sectional views. **E.** Median septum. **F.** Lateral wall of nasal cavity. **G.** Lateral wall with middle and inferior conchae partially cut away.

part of the nose) and the **nasal spine of the frontal bone** (Fig. 22–10*A* and *E*). Posteriorly, the roof of the nasal cavity is formed by part of the **body of the sphenoid bone.** The middle part of the roof, between the sphenoid bone and the nasal bones, is the **cribriform plate of the ethmoid bone** (Fig. 22–10*C* and *E*). The **floor of the nasal cavity** is composed of the bony palate, including the paired **palatine processes of the maxillary bones** and **horizontal processes of the palatine bones** (Fig. 22–10*D*). A palatomaxillary suture joins these bones at the junction between the middle third and posterior third of the nasal floor. In addition, two **incisive canals** connect the nasal cavity with the **incisive fossae** of the palatine bones in the anteromedial region of the nasal floor.

The nasal cavity is divided into two **nasal passages** by a single median septum formed primarily by a thin **vomer bone** and the **perpendicular plate of the ethmoid bone** (Fig. 22–10*A*, *B*, and *E*). Anteriorly, part of the septum is also formed by a **septal cartilage.** Minor contributions to the median septum include the **nasal bones, nasal spines of the frontal bones** anterosuperiorly, a short **rostrum** and **crest of the sphenoid bone** posterosuperiorly, and the **nasal crests of the maxilla** and **palatine bones** inferiorly. This median septum serves as a **medial wall for both nasal passages** (Fig. 22–10*E*). The **lateral walls** of the nasal cavity (and both nasal passages) are formed by part of the maxilla anteroinferiorly, the perpendicular plates of the palatine bones posteriorly, and the ethmoidal labyrinth superiorly (Fig. 22–10*F*). The ethmoidal labyrinth separates the nasal cavity from the orbit (see the orbital plate of the ethmoid bone in the discussion of orbits above). Minor contributions to the lateral wall of the nasal chamber are parts of the nasal bones, frontal processes of the maxillary bones, and the lacrimal bones.

The lateral walls of the nasal cavity also include three rounded projections: the **superior, middle,** and **inferior nasal conchae** (Fig. 22–10*F*). The superior and middle conchae are projections of the ethmoidal labyrinth, while the inferior concha is a separate bone. The posterior ends of the middle and inferior conchae articulate with the perpendicular plate of the palatine bone. In all cases, the thin conchae curve inferiorly to partially enclose intervening grooves. These are the **superior meatus** (under the superior concha), **middle meatus** (under the middle concha), and **inferior meatus** (under the inferior concha) (Fig. 22–10*F*). In addition, a narrow sphenoethmoidal recess separates the superior concha from the body of the sphenoid bone. A small foramen within the sphenoethmoidal recess opens into the sphenoidal air sinus (see Chapter 26). Likewise, small foramina in the superior meatus open into the posterior ethmoidal air cells of the ethmoid sinus and, posteriorly, a mucous-filled opening (sphenopalatine foramen) leads into the pterygopalatine fossa (see Chapter 26). The middle meatus can be viewed only by removing the middle concha. Once this is done, a rounded protrusion called the **ethmoidal bulla** is apparent (Fig. 22–10*G*). This projection contains middle ethmoidal air cells, which typically communicate with the nasal cavity by a foramen just superior to the bulla (see Chapter 26). Just inferior and anterior to the bulla is a bony projection called the **uncinate process** of the ethmoid bone, which crosses over a very large opening into the maxillary air sinus (see Chapter 26). In addition, an opening between the uncinate process and the bulla called the **hiatus semilunaris** is continuous with a short canal, the **ethmoidal infundibulum,** which provides an opening for anterior ethmoidal air cells (and frontal and maxillary sinuses) into the middle meatus. Alternatively, the frontal sinus may open independently into the middle meatus. The inferior meatus is the largest of the three. It has an opening near its anterior end, which is the inferior orifice of the nasolacrimal canal.

Inferior Aspect of the Skull (Norma Basalis)

The base of the skull may be divided into anterior, middle, and posterior parts

The base of the skull extends from the incisor teeth anteriorly to the superior nuchal line posteriorly. It is easier to describe, however, by dividing it into an **anterior part** (from the incisor teeth to the posterior limit of the hard palate), a **middle part** (from the posterior limit of the hard palate to a transverse line drawn through the most anterior boundary of the foramen magnum), and a **posterior part** (from the transverse line tangential to the anterior margin of the foramen magnum to the superior nuchal line) (Fig. 22–11). A significant feature of the base of the skull is the presence of numerous foramina, which transport nerves or vessels (or both) between the interior and exterior of the skull (see Table 22–3).

Anterior Part of the Base of the Skull. *The anterior part of the base of the skull consists mainly of the osseous palate.* The hard (osseous) palate and upper teeth are the main features of the anterior part of the base of the skull. The **hard palate** consists of four horizontally disposed bones: two **maxillary palatine processes** (horizontal extensions of the maxilla bones) and two **horizontal plates of the palatine bones.** The maxillary palatine bones meet at a midsagittal **intermaxillary suture** and the horizontal plates of the palatine bones at a midsagittal **interpalatine suture.** The transverse **palatomaxillary suture** marks the boundary between the maxillary palatine processes and the horizontal plates of the palatine bones (Fig. 22–11*A* and *D*). The intersection of the intermaxillary, interpalatine, and palatomaxillary sutures is called the **cruciate suture.** Medially, the posterior border of the hard palate projects as a **posterior nasal spine.** More laterally, small horizontal **palatine**

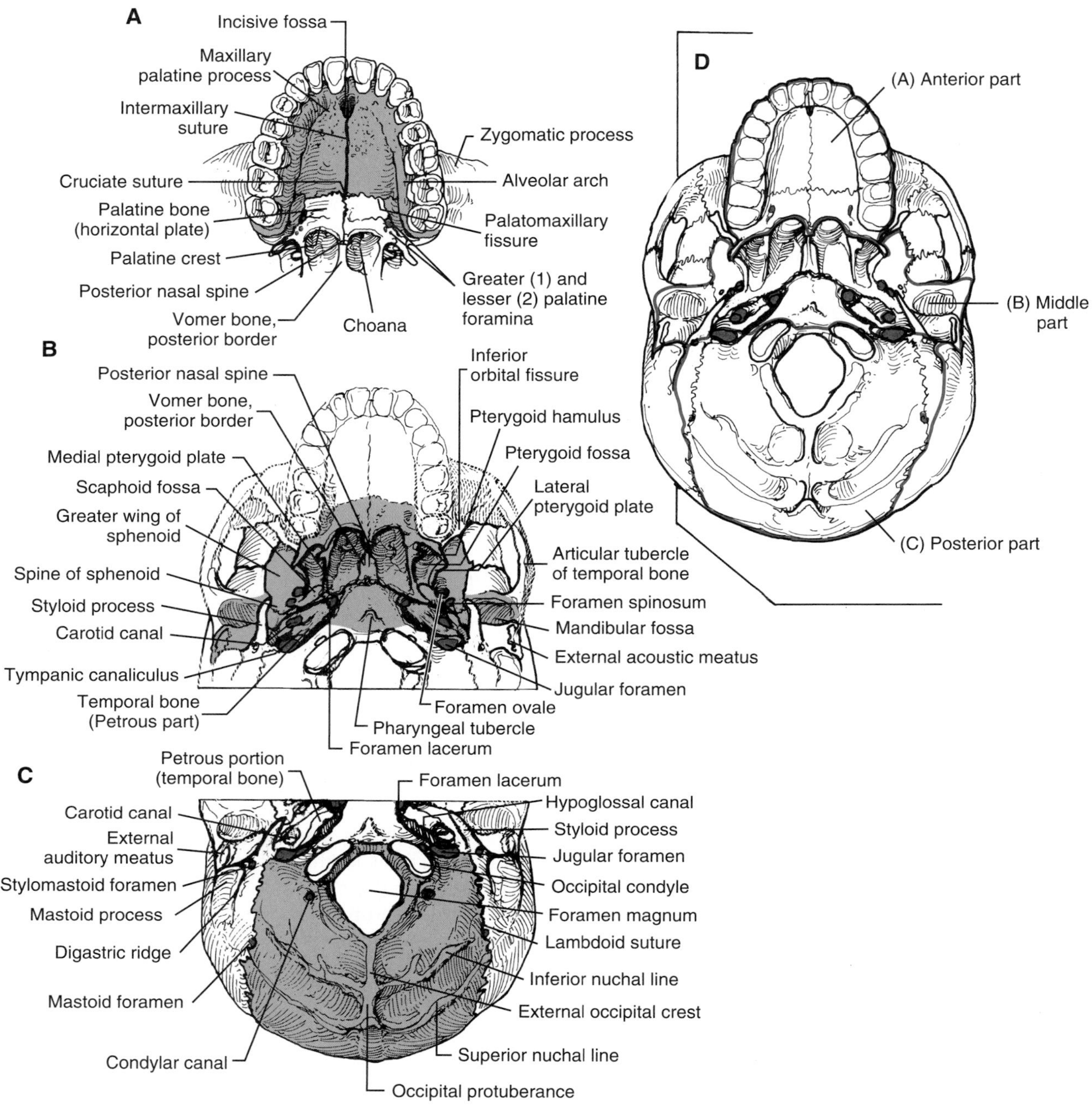

FIGURE 22–11
Inferior aspect of the skull. **A.** Anterior part, hard palate. **B** and **C.** Middle and posterior parts. **D.** Overview.

crests extend medially and posteriorly from the horizontal palatine plates. The prominent **alveolar arch** of the hard palate contains sockets (alveoli) for 16 upper teeth (see discussion of the anterior aspect of the skull above).

The hard palate displays a fossa and several foramina. An **incisive fossa** is located anteriorly and medially just behind the upper two incisor teeth. The fossa marks the point where the depressor septae muscle attaches to the upper surface of the hard palate (Fig. 22–11*A* and *D* and see discussion of the nasal cavity above). The depressor septa muscle is usually considered a part of the dilator nares muscle (see Fig. 24–23*E*). Two **lateral incisive foramina** are located within the lateral walls of the incisive fossa. These are openings for the two **lateral incisive canals,** which lead to the nasal cavity. Each incisive canal transports a greater palatine artery and a nasopalatine nerve (Chapter 24). A **greater palatine foramen** is located on each side of the palate, just posterior to the palatomaxillary suture. Two **lesser palatine foramina** are typically found behind each greater palatine foramen (Fig. 22–11*A* and *D*). The greater palatine foramina transport the greater palatine nerves and vessels, while the lesser palatine foramina transport the lesser palatine nerves and vessels.

Middle Part of the Base of the Skull. *The following discussion proceeds as if the anterior end of the skull is at the top, with the middle part of the base of the skull beginning at 12 o'clock position; the description proceeds in a clockwise direction.* The middle part of the base of the skull is bounded anteriorly by the posterior nasal apertures and posteriorly by the anterior border of the foramen magnum. Medially, the middle part of the base of the skull is composed of the inferior surfaces of the body of the sphenoid bone anteriorly and the basioccipital bone posteriorly. Although this region is mostly flat, it is marked by the posterior extension of the **vomer bone** (medially and anteriorly) and by a **pharyngeal tubercle** (Fig. 22–11*B* and *D*). The pharyngeal tubercle provides an attachment site for the superior constrictor muscle of the pharynx (see Chapter 26).

The **pterygoid bones,** which are rather complex, lie just lateral to this flat region of the skull base. Each pterygoid bone has a **medial** and a **lateral pterygoid plate** (Fig. 22–11*B* and *D*). These thin parasagittal plates are separated by a posterior-facing **pterygoid fossa.** The thinner medial pterygoid plate projects posteriorly, and a **pterygoid hamulus** projects inferiorly from its anterior edge. The pterygoid hamulus serves as a pulley for the tendon of the tensor veli palatini muscle (see Chapter 24). A shallow **scaphoid fossa** at the posterior base of the medial pterygoid plate provides an attachment site for the tensor veli palatini muscle. The thicker lateral pterygoid plate projects posterolaterally (Fig. 22–11*B* and *D* and below). The pterygoid plates and their intervening fossae thus lie between the medial nasal cavity and the lateral infratemporal fossa.

The **greater wings of the sphenoid bones** lie lateral to the pterygoid bones on each side of the middle part of the skull base (Fig. 22–11). They contribute to the roof of the infratemporal fossa and serve as an attachment site for part of the lateral pterygoid muscle (see Chapter 24). The **foramen rotundum** and **foramen spinosum** are also located here (Fig. 22–11*B* and *D* and see Fig. 22–10*C* and Table 22–3).

An inferior part of each **temporal squama** lies lateral to the greater wing of the sphenoid bone. The zygomatic arch projects anteriorly from the lateral side of the temporal squama. Other landmarks include an **articular tubercle,** which is continuous with the base of the zygomatic arch, and a **mandibular fossa,** which lies just posterior to the articular tubercle (Fig. 22–11*B* and *D*). The articular tubercle and mandibular fossa contribute to the articulation of the mandible (see below).

The **tympanic part (plate) of the temporal bone** lies just behind the mandibular fossa (Fig. 22–11*B* and *D*). It is separated from the temporal squama by a squamotympanic suture. This tympanic part of the temporal bone encloses the **external acoustic meatus** on its anterior, inferior, and posterior sides. Its superior side is bounded by the squamous part of the temporal bone. The external acoustic meatus is a canal of the external ear, which is bounded internally by the tympanic membrane (see Chapter 25). The temporal **styloid process** projects from the midregion of the posterior border of the temporal tympanic plate, and a large **carotid canal** is located in the most medial region of its posterior border. The carotid canal transports the internal carotid artery first into the foramen lacerum via its posterior wall. It then exits into the middle cranial fossa of the cranial cavity (see below) via the foramen lacerum.

The **petrous part of the temporal bone** lies just medial to the tympanic plate, posterior to the greater wing of the sphenoid bone, and lateral to the basioccipital bone (Fig. 22–11*B* and *D*). This rough region of the base of the skull houses the middle ear and inner ear (see Chapter 25) and a **facial canal,** which transports the facial nerve through the petrous bone to the stylomastoid foramen (see below). In this inferior view of the base of the skull, a large **foramen lacerum** can be seen at the apex of the petrous part of the temporal bone, adjacent to the posterolateral border of the body of the sphenoid bone (Fig. 22–11*B* and *D*). The inferior region of the foramen lacerum is filled with cartilage. The posterior wall of its superior region contains a small segment of the carotid artery (i.e., the segment that has left the carotid canal and is turning upward to enter the cranial cavity).

Posterior Part of the Base of the Skull. *The posterior part of the base of the skull is located between a line drawn through the anterior border of the foramen magnum and the superior nuchal line.* The most prominent feature of the posterior part of the base of the skull is the large foramen magnum, with its flanking occipital condyles (Fig. 22–11*C* and *D*). The **foramen magnum** is located at the petro-occipital suture. It contains the lower end of the brainstem, the medulla oblongata, the vertebral arteries (with accompanying sympathetic fibers), and the sensory spinal rami of the spinal accessory nerves (see Fig. 3–3). The **occipital condyles** articulate with superior articular facets on the lateral masses of the atlas (see Chapter 3 and Fig. 3–3). Their convex surfaces are smooth, but their medial aspects are roughened attachment sites for stabilizing ligaments of the atlanto-occipital joint (Fig. 22–11*C* and *D* and see Chapter 24). A **hypoglossal canal** is located within the occipital bone just anterior to each condyle. This foramen transports the hypoglossal nerve, a meningeal branch of the ascending pharyngeal artery and an emissary vein between the exterior of the skull and the posterior fossa of the cranial cavity (see Chapter 24). A **jugular canal (foramen)** is located just lateral and slightly posterior to the hypoglossal canal, within the posterior region of the petro-occipital suture. The jugular canal contains the glossopharyngeal, vagus, and spinal accessory nerves and the internal jugular vein (see Fig. 22–15*C*). A **stylomastoid foramen** at the posterior boundary of the base of the styloid process contains the facial nerve and a stylomastoid artery. Finally, a **condylar canal** posterior to each occipital condyle may carry a small emissary vein (Fig. 22–11*C* and *D*).

As has been described above, the **inferior nuchal lines** provide attachment sites for the rectus capitis posterior minor muscle (medially) and rectus capitis posterior major muscle (laterally). The region between the inferior and superior nuchal lines provides attachment sites for the semispinalis capitis muscle (medially) and the obliquus superior muscle (laterally). Medial to the superior nuchal line (at the **occipital protuberance** with the **inion** at its apex) is an attachment site for the trapezius muscle. The **superior nuchal line** provides attachment sites for the trapezius and sternocleidomastoid muscles. Anterior to these attachment sites, the superior nuchal lines provides attachment sites for the splenius capitis muscles (Fig. 22–11*C* and *D*).

Lateral Aspect of the Skull (Norma Lateralis)

A lateral view of the skull reveals bones of the chondrocranium, facial skeleton, and cranial vault; the mandible; the external auditory meatus; and the temporal, infratemporal, and pterygopalatine fossae

Bones apparent in lateral views of the skull include the **frontal, zygomatic,** and **parietal bones.** The **greater wing of the sphenoid bone,** the **nasal** and **lacrimal bones,** the **maxilla (particularly the alveolar and frontal processes),** and part of the **occipital squama** are also revealed in a lateral view of the skull (Fig. 22–12). In addition, most parts of the **temporal bone,** including the **squama, zygomatic arch,** and **styloid** and **mastoid processes,** are clearly visualized. Inferiorly, the **mandible** with its **condyloid** and **coronoid processes** is apparent. The mandible is described in detail below.

Prominent landmarks visible in lateral views of the skull include the superior and inferior temporal lines (Fig. 22–12). The **superior temporal line** is the site of attachment for fascia investing the temporalis muscle, while the **inferior temporal line** is an attachment site for the temporal muscle (see discussion of the temporal fossa below). Just posterior to the mandible, the **mastoid process of the temporal bone** protrudes inferiorly. This process is formed by the pull of the sternocleidomastoid muscle during childhood. A small mastoid foramen may be observed near the occipitomastoid suture. It transmits a small emissary vein from the sigmoid sinus (see below) within the cranium. Just anterior and medial to the mastoid process, the prominent **styloid process of the temporal bone** descends anteriorly and medially. A stylohyoid ligament and muscle suspend and elevate the hyoid bone via an attachment to its lesser horn (see Fig. 24–22*A*). Lateral views of the skull also reveal the bony opening to the **external auditory meatus,** which is located just inferior to the temporal squama, anterior to the mastoid process, and superior to the styloid process. An important clinical landmark observed in lateral views of the skull is the **pterion,** the region of fusion of the greater wing of the sphenoid bone, the temporal squama, and the frontal and parietal bones (Fig. 22–12 and Table 22–1). This region of the skull is especially prone to fracture.

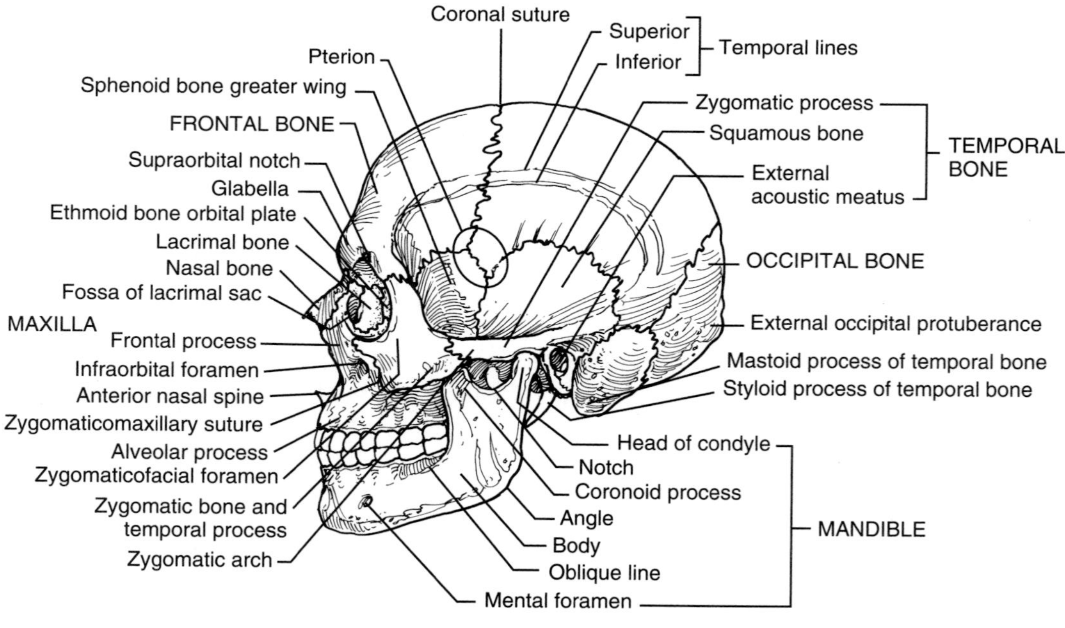

FIGURE 22–12
Lateral aspect of the skull.

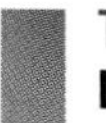

TABLE 22–1
Landmarks, Tubercles, and Processes of the Skull

Region of Skull	Landmark, Tubercle, or Process	Location, Attachments, or Articulations
Superior aspect	Bregma	Site of anterior fontanelle; intersection of posterior edge of frontal bone with both parietal bones (i.e., junction of frontal, coronal, and sagittal sutures)
	Vertex	Highest point of skull
Posterior aspect	Lambda	Site of posterior fontanelle; intersection of occipital bone with both parietal bones (i.e., junction of lambdoid and sagittal sutures)
	External occipital protuberance and crest	Median projection from occipital bone at level of superior nuchal line; attachment of trapezius muscle
	Inion	Apex of external occipital protuberance on posterior aspect of occipital bone; attachment of trapezius muscle
	Highest nuchal line	Posterior aspect of occipital bone medially and posterior aspect of parietal bone laterally; attachment of fronto-occipitalis muscle
	Superior nuchal line	Posterior aspect of occipital bone; attachment of trapezius muscle medially; attachment of sternocleidomastoid muscle laterally
	Inferior nuchal line	Posterior aspect of occipital bone; attachment of rectus capitis minor muscle medially; attachment of rectus capitis major muscle laterally
	Mastoid process	Mastoid part of temporal bone; attachment of sternocleidomastoid muscle
Anterior aspect	Glabella	Median prominence of frontal bone
	Superciliary arches	Above superior border of orbits (frontal bone); medially, attachment of corrugator supercilii muscle
	Anterior nasal spine	Small extension at superior end of intermaxillary suture
	Nasion	Junction of frontal and nasal bones
Inferior aspect	Alveolar process of maxilla	Alveolar arch at periphery of underside of maxilla; contains sockets for teeth (8 on each side)
	Incisive fossa of maxilla	At anterior end of intermaxillary fissure of hard palate; attachment of depressor septi muscle; contains lateral incisive canals, which transmit greater palatine artery and nasopalatine nerve
	Pterygoid process of sphenoid bone	Consists of perpendicular lateral and medial plates, which descend from junction of body and greater wing of sphenoid bone; attachments of lateral and medial pterygoid and tensor veli palatini muscles
	Posterior nasal spine	Medial posterior extension of palatines plates; attachment of musculus uvulae muscle
	Pterygoid hamulus	Projects from outer edge of medial pterygoid plate; serves as pulley for tensor veli palatini muscle
	Pharyngeal tubercle	Median prominence of basioccipital bone; attachment of superior constrictor muscle
	Scaphoid fossa	Posterior base of medial pterygoid plate; attachment of tensor veli palatini muscle
	Mandibular fossa of temporal squama	Part of articulation for temporomandibular joint
	Articular tubercle of temporal squama	Part of articulation for temporomandibular joint
	Spine of sphenoid bone	Attachment of sphenomandibular ligament
	Occipital condyles	Lateral to foramen magnum on lateral parts of occipital bone; articulate with atlas
Lateral aspect	Asterion	Junction of occipital, temporal, and parietal bones
	Pterion	Junction of greater wing of sphenoid bone plus temporal, frontal, and parietal bones
	Superior temporal line	Attachment of fascia of temporalis muscle
	Inferior temporal line	Attachment of temporalis muscle
	Mastoid process of temporal bone	Attachment of sternocleidomastoid muscle
	Maxillary tuberosity	Posteroinferior aspect of maxilla; attachment of medial pterygoid muscle
	Styloid process of temporal bone	Attachment of stylohyoid ligament and stylomandibular ligament

Continued

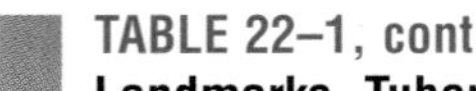

TABLE 22–1, cont'd
Landmarks, Tubercles, and Processes of the Skull

Region of Skull	Landmark, Tubercle, or Process	Location, Attachments, or Articulations
Lateral aspect—cont'd		
	Temporal tympanic plate	Anterior wall of external acoustic meatus
	External acoustic meatus	Bony investment of external auditory canal
	Zygomatic arch (zygoma)	Zygomatic process of temporal bone and temporal process of zygomatic bone form prominence of cheek; attachments of levator labis superiori, levator anguli oris, zygomaticus major, zygomaticus minor, and masseter muscles
	Temporal fossa	Shallow depression of lateral skull housing temporalis muscle (see Table 22–2)
	Infratemporal fossa	Depression of lateral skull housing several muscles, vessels, and nerves (see Table 22–2)
	Pterygopalatine fossa	Depression of lateral skull housing several vessels and nerves (see Table 22–2)

Fractures Near the Pterion. The thick convex dome of the cranial vault (calvaria) protects the brain and is resistant to fracture. In contrast, the thinner, flatter temporal region of the skull, particularly in the region of the pterion, is far more susceptible to injury. Here, lateral trauma to the head (often the consequence of automobile accidents in adults or bicycle accidents in children) may result in a **linear fracture,** which is a single line of fracture, or a **radiating fracture,** which may extend into the skull base, resulting in laceration of dural sinuses (including the cavernous sinus) and vessels that supply the brain (see Chapter 27). Ironically, the rigidity of the skull, typically cited as a protective feature, also predisposes an individual to life-threatening sequelae of such fractures. Edema or bleeding within the rigid brain case may result in increased intracranial pressure, leading to local brain damage or herniation of the brainstem through the foramen magnum, or both. Dislocation of the brainstem may lead to compromise of the respiratory center (see Chapter 8) and eventual respiratory failure.

Fractures of the Lateral Face. Fracture of the zygomatic bone is often described as "breaking the face." This type of injury, along with fractures of the calvaria or other facial bones, often occurs with severe trauma in automobile accidents.

Fossae of the Skull. Three major depressions, or fossae, may be identified in lateral views of the skull. They are the temporal, infratemporal, and pterygopalatine fossae. All three of these fossae and their anatomic landmarks may be useful frames of reference for locating soft tissues of the head (Fig. 22–13*A* and *B* and see Table 22–2).

Temporal Fossa. Boundaries of the temporal fossa are defined superiorly and posteriorly by the superior temporal line, inferiorly by the zygomatic arch of the temporal bone and the temporal and frontal processes of the zygomatic bone, and anteriorly by the zygomatic process of the frontal bone (Figs. 22–12 and 22–13*A* and Table 22–2).

Contents of the temporal fossa include the origin and upper part of the body of the temporalis muscle, which springs from the floor of the temporal fossa just inferior to the inferior temporal line (Table 22–2 and see Fig. 24–13*B*).

Infratemporal Fossa. Boundaries of the infratemporal fossa include a roof, which is provided by part of the temporal squama and the infratemporal surface of the greater wing of the sphenoid bone (Figs. 22–12 and 22–13*A*). The medial boundary of the infratemporal fossa is the lateral pterygoid plate. Its anterior wall is the posterior wall of the maxilla. The infratemporal fossa is open at its lateral, posterior, and inferior aspects (Fig. 22–13*A* and *B*). The anterior and medial walls of the infratemporal fossa are separated by a space called the **pterygomaxillary fissure.** This fissure allows communication between the medial region of the infratemporal fossa and the lateral part of the pterygopalatine fossa (see below). The pterygomaxillary fissure is also continuous with the posterior end of the infraorbital fissure (see above), allowing communication between the infratemporal fossa and the orbit. In addition, the infratemporal surface of the sphenoid bone forming part of the roof of the infratemporal fossa is pierced by the foramen ovale and foramen spinosum (see below). The **foramen ovale** transmits the mandibular nerve (which is a branch of the fifth cranial nerve, or the trigeminal nerve) from the middle cranial fossa, while the **foramen spinosum** transmits the middle meningeal artery and accompanying veins (see Tables 22–1 and 22–3).

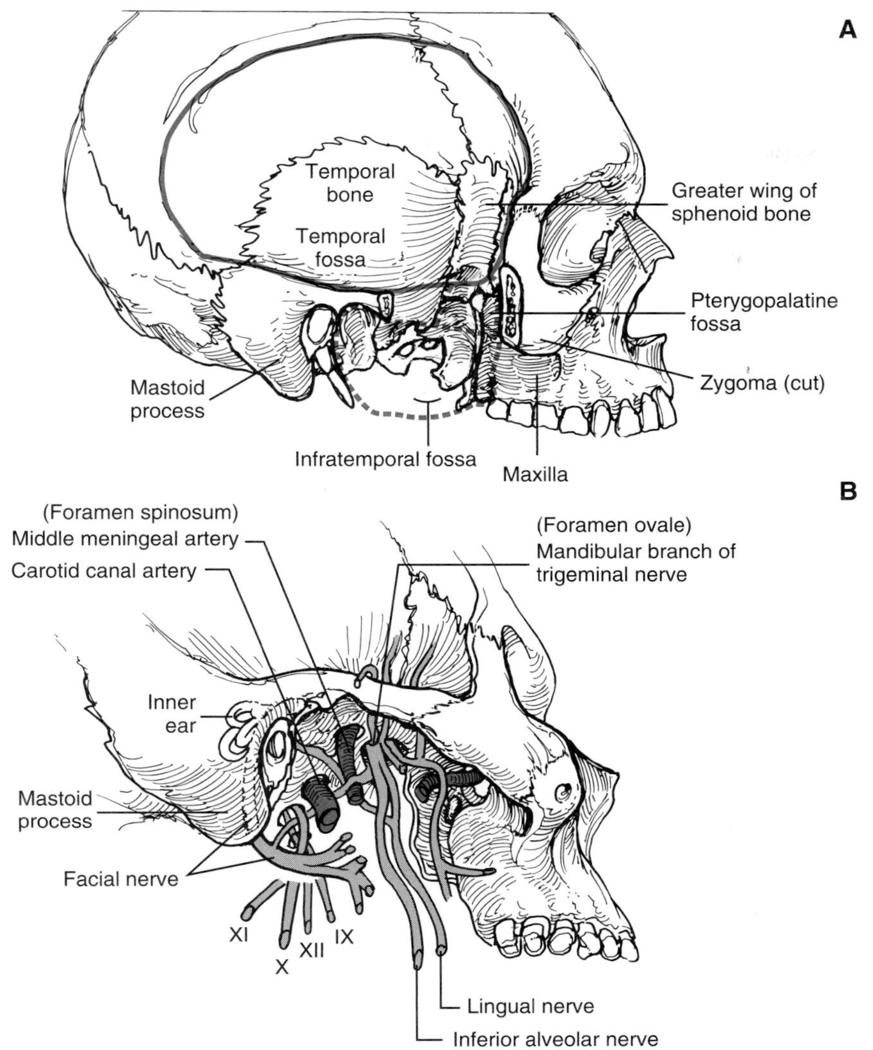

FIGURE 22–13

Temporal, infratemporal, and pterygopalatine fossae. **A.** Zygomatic arch and mandible removed to reveal fossae area. **B.** Schematic representation of nerves and vessles emerging from foramina within these fossae.

Contents of the infratemporal fossa include the lower part of the body of the temporalis muscle and the lateral and medial pterygoid muscles. The temporalis muscle is superficial. The maxillary artery and pterygoid venous plexus lie between the temporalis and lateral pterygoid muscles. The mandibular nerve and a specialized branch of the facial nerve, the chorda tympani, lie deep to the medial pterygoid muscle. The maxillary nerve may be found in the superior region of the infratemporal fossa near the infraorbital fissure (Fig. 22–13*B* and Tables 22–2 and 22–3 and see Chapter 24).

Pterygopalatine Fossa. The pterygopalatine fossa lies deep (medial) to the infratemporal fossa, communicating with it via the pterygomaxillary fissure (see bulleted list, below). Boundaries of the pterygopalatine fossa include an anterior wall, which is formed by the smooth posterior surface of the maxilla; a medial wall, which is formed by the maxillary surface of the palatine bone; and a posterior wall, which is composed of the root of the pterygoid process and anterior surface of the greater wing of the sphenoid bone. The superior boundary of the pterygopalatine fossa is the apex of the orbit .

Contents of the pterygopalatine fossa include the maxillary nerve, pterygopalatine ganglion, and terminus of the maxillary artery (see Table 22–2). In addition to the presence of these structures, the anatomic impor-

TABLE 22–2
Major Fossae of the Skull and Their Contents

Fossa	Boundaries	Contents
OUTSIDE SKULL		
Temporal fossa	*Superior:* superior temporal line; *inferior:* zygomatic arch of temporal bone; *anterior:* zygomatic process of frontal bone; *posterior:* superior temporal line; *medial:* greater wing of sphenoid bone, frontal bone, temporal squama, parietal bone; *lateral:* open	Origins and upper body of temporalis muscle
Infratemporal fossa	*Superior:* temporal squama, infratemporal surface of greater wing of sphenoid bone; *inferior:* pyramidal process of palatine bone; *anterior:* posterior wall of maxilla; *posterior:* pyramidal process of palatine bone; *lateral:* open	Lower part of body of temporalis muscle, lateral and medial pterygoid muscles, maxillary artery, pterygoid venous plexus, maxillary nerve
Pterygopalatine fossa	*Superior:* infraorbital fissure; *inferior:* perpendicular plate of palatine bone and medial surface of maxilla; *anterior:* posterior surface of maxilla; *posterior:* root of pterygoid process and anterior surface of greater wing of sphenoid bone; *medial:* maxillary surface of palatine bone; *lateral:* pterygomaxillary fissure	Maxillary nerve, terminus of maxillary artery, pterygopalatine ganglion, pterygoid nerve, pterygoid vessels, nasopalatine nerve and vessels, greater palatine artery and vein, lesser palatine artery and vein, and anterior, middle, and posterior palatine nerves
INSIDE CALVARIA		
Underside of calvaria	Both sides of sagittal suture	Granular foveolae for arachnoid granulations, grooves for middle meningeal arteries and veins, impressions for gyri of cerebrum
Anterior cranial fossa	*Anterior:* frontal bone; *posterior:* posterior edge of lesser wing of sphenoid bone, anterior clinoid processes, posterior edge of jugum of body of sphenoid bone; *lateral:* frontal bone; *floor:* orbital part of frontal bone, frontal crest, cribriform plate of ethmoid bone, crista galli of ethmoid bone, lesser wing of sphenoid bone, jugum of greater wing of sphenoid bone	Frontal lobes of cerebrum; olfactory bulbs
Middle cranial fossa	*Anterior:* posterior edge of lesser wing of sphenoid bone, anterior clinoid process, posterior edge of jugum of body of sphenoid bone; *posterior:* petrous part of temporal bone, dorsum sellae of sphenoid bone with posterior clinoid processes; *lateral:* temporal squama, parietal bones, greater wings of sphenoid bones; *floor:* parietal bones, temporal squama, greater wings of sphenoid bones with sella turcica (which includes tuberculum sellae, hypophyseal fossa, and dorsum sellae)	Temporal lobes of cerebrum, pituitary gland, optic nerves and optic chiasm, cavernous sinus, internal carotid artery, trigeminal ganglion and trigeminal nerves, superior petrosal sinus, inferior petrosal sinus, and oculomotor, trochlear, abducent, and ophthalmic nerves
Posterior cranial fossa	*Anterior:* dorsum sellae and posterior clinoid processes, body of sphenoid bone, basilar part of occipital bone; *posterior:* occipital squama; *lateral:* petrous part of temporal bones, mastoid part of temporal bones, mastoid angles of parietal bones; *floor:* basilar part of occipital bone, occipital squama, parietal bone	Cerebellum, pons, medulla oblongata, facial nerves, vestibulocochlear nerves, glossopharyngeal nerves, vagus nerves, accessory nerves, hypoglossal nerves, superior petrosal sinus, sagittal sinus, transverse sinus

tance of the pterygopalatine fossa is suggested by its strategic location between the infratemporal fossa, the orbit, the nasal cavity, and the pharynx and by the presence of several nerves and vessels that course within the fossa. Indeed, its function as a way station for the combination and distribution of nerves (see Chapter 24) is further emphasized by the large number of foramina within its walls (see Fig. 22–11*B* and Table 22–2).

Indeed, the pterygopalatine fossa communicates with other fossae or cavities of the skull by means of

TABLE 22–3
Foramina, Fissures, and Canals of the Skull from Outside of the Cranial Cavity

Region of Skull	Foramen, Fissure, or Canal	Specific Location	Structure Passing through Foramen, Fissure, or Canal
Calvaria (superior aspect of skull)	Parietal foramina	Lateral to sagittal suture and anterior to lambda in parietal bones	Emissary veins
Face	Supraorbital notches or foramina	Superior border of orbit	Supraorbital nerve and vessels
	Infraorbital notches or foramina	Inferior border of orbit	Infraorbital nerve and vessels
	Zygomaticofacial foramina	In zygoma at junction of inferior and lateral orbital margins	Zygomaticofacial nerve and artery
Anterior part of base of skull	Lateral incisive foramina and incisive canals	In lateral walls of incisive fossa of maxilla	Greater palatine artery and nasopalatine nerve
	Greater palatine foramina	Lateroposterior region of horizontal plates of palatine bones	Greater palatine nerves and vessels
	Lesser palatine foramina	Palatine pyramidal process between lateral and medial pterygoid plates	Lesser palatine nerves and vessels
Middle part of base of skull	Foramen rotundum	Infratemporal surface of greater wing of sphenoid bone	Maxillary division of trigeminal nerve
	Foramen ovale	Infratemporal surface of greater wing of sphenoid bone	Mandibular division of trigeminal nerve (V); accessory meningeal artery; lesser petrosal nerve
	Foramen spinosum	Infratemporal surface of sphenoid bone	Middle meningeal artery and vein; meningeal branch of mandibular nerve
	Foramen lacerum	Junction of basisphenoid bone; petrous part of temporal bone; basilar parts of occipital bone	Cartilage in inferior part; part of internal carotid artery and carotid plexus in posterior wall superiorly, along with greater petrosal nerve; meningeal branches of ascending pharyngeal artery and small veins traverse entire canal
	Pterygoid canal	At point of fusion between greater wing and body of sphenoid bone and pterygoid process	Pterygoid nerve and artery between anterior wall of foramen lacerum; pterygopalatine ganglion
	Carotid canal	At posteromedial border of tympanic plate	Carotid artery
	Palatovaginal canal	Between sphenoidal process of palatine bone and vaginal process of medial pterygoid plate	Pharyngeal branch of pterygopalatine ganglion; pharyngeal branch of maxillary artery (between pterygopalatine ganglion and pharynx)
	Pterygomaxillary fissure	Connects infratemporal and pterygopalatine fossa	Maxillary artery and nerve
Posterior part of base of skull	Foramen magnum	Between petrous part of temporal bone and occipital bone	Medulla oblongata
	Hypoglossal canal	Occipital bone anterior to occipital condyles	Hypoglossal nerve; meningeal branch of ascending pharyngeal artery; emissary vein
	Jugular foramen	Between petrous part of temporal bone and occiput	Inferior petrosal sinus in anterior part; glossopharyngeal, vagus, and accessory nerves in intermediate part; internal jugular vein in posterior part
	Stylomastoid foramen	Temporal squama at base of styloid process	Facial nerve; stylomastoid artery
	Facial canal	Within the petrous temporal bone	Facial nerve
	Mastoid foramen	Near or in occipitomastoid suture	Emissary vein
	External acoustic meatus	Below root of zygomatic bone	Meatus of external ear

Continued

TABLE 22–3, cont'd
Foramina, Fissures, and Canals of the Skull from Outside of the Cranial Cavity

Region of Skull	Foramen, Fissure, or Canal	Specific Location	Structure Passing through Foramen, Fissure, or Canal
Nasal cavity	Numerous small foramina	Cribriform plate of ethmoid bone	Olfactory nerves
	Anterior nasal apertures	Bounded superiorly by nasal bones and laterally and inferiorly by maxilla	Anterior openings to nasal passages
	Posterior nasal apertures	Bounded superiorly by sphenoid bone, inferiorly by horizontal plate of palatine bone, laterally by medial pterygoid plates. Medially, apertures are separated by vomer.	Opening between nasal cavity and nasopharynx
Orbit	Superior orbital fissure	Between roof and lateral wall of orbit, providing communication between orbit and middle cranial fossa	Oculomotor, trochlear, abducent nerves; branches of ophthalmic nerve; ophthalmic veins
	Inferior orbital fissure	Fissure in floor of orbit, providing communication between orbit and infratemporal and pterygopalatine fossae	Maxillary nerve, infraorbital vessels, zygomatic nerve; rami of pterygopalatine ganglion
	Optic canal	Between orbit and middle cranial fossa	Optic nerve and ophthalmic artery

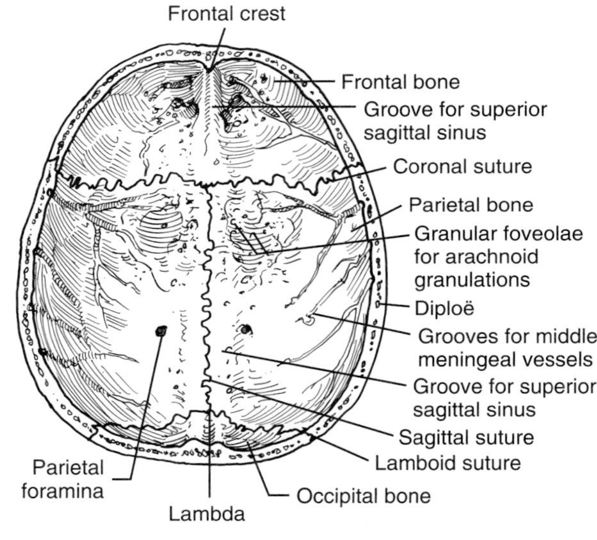

FIGURE 22–14
Inferior view of calvaria.

several fissures, foramina, and canals, including the following:

- The superior region of the pterygopalatine fossa communicates with the orbital cavity via the medial end of the **infraorbital fissure.** It transmits the maxillary nerve, infraorbital vessels, zygomatic nerve, and rami of the pterygopalatine ganglion.
- The lateral part of the pterygopalatine fossa communicates with the infratemporal fossa via the **pterygomaxillary fissure.** It transmits the maxillary artery and maxillary nerve.
- A small round hole in the posterior wall of the pterygopalatine fossa, the **foramen rotundum,** transmits the maxillary nerve from the cranial cavity to the face.
- Just inferomedial to the foramen rotundum, the **pterygoid canal** transmits the pterygoid nerve and pterygoid vessels from the anterior region of the **foramen lacerum** to the pterygoid ganglion.
- An inferomedial **palatovaginal canal** transmits the pharyngeal nerve from the pterygoid ganglion to the roof of the pharynx.
- A medial **sphenopalatine foramen (canal)** transmits the nasopalatine nerve and vessels into the nasal cavity.
- An inferior **greater palatine canal** transmits the anterior, middle, and posterior palatine nerves and greater and lesser palatine vessels to the bony palate.

Interior View of the Skull; Cranial Cavity

Once the calvaria (calva) is removed, the interior view of the skull reveals details of the cranial cavity (Fig. 22–14 and Table 22–4 and see Fig. 22–15). The bony surface within the cavity is lined by an outer layer of the dura mater, the **endocranium,** which penetrates all foramina of the skull to fuse with their more superficial periosteal lining, the **pericranium.** The pericranium and the endocranium blend with the sutural ligaments within the joints that bond individual bones of the skull.

Underside of the Calvaria. Viewing the underside of the calvaria from an inferior aspect (see Fig. 22–14), the lambdoid, sagittal, and frontal sutures may all be observed unless they have become obliterated (as in older skulls; see above). A **parietal foramen** for the transport of emissary veins is apparent on either side of the sagit-

TABLE 22–4
Foramina, Fissures, and Canals of the Skull from within the Cranial Cavity

Region of Skull	Foramen, Fissure, or Canal	Specific Location	Structure Passing through Foramen, Fissure, or Canal
Calvaria	Parietal foramina	Lateral to sagittal suture and anterior to lambda	Emissary veins
Anterior cranial fossa	Foramen cecum	Frontoethmoid suture	Vein connecting nasal veins and superior sagittal sinus when present
	Numerous small foramina	Cribriform plate of ethmoid bone	Olfactory nerves
	Anterior ethmoidal canal	Cribrifrontal suture	Anterior ethmoidal nerve and vessels
	Posterior ethmoidal canal	Posterolateral corners of cribriform plate	Posterior ethmoidal nerve and vessels
	Optic canal	Junction of body and lesser wing of sphenoid bone	Optic nerve; ophthalmic artery
Middle cranial fossa	Superior orbital fissure	Between middle fossa and orbit	Ophthalmic nerve and vein; oculomotor, trochlear, and abducent nerves
	Foramen rotundum	Within greater wing of sphenoid bone	Maxillary nerve
	Foramen ovale	Within greater wing of sphenoid bone	Mandibular nerve; accessory meningeal artery
	Foramen spinosum	Within greater wing of sphenoid bone	Middle meningeal artery and vein; meningeal branch of mandibular nerve
	Foramen lacerum	Junction of basisphenoid bone; petrous part of temporal bone; basilar part of occipital bone	Cartilage in inferior part; part of carotid artery with carotid plexus in posterior wall, superiorly, along with greater petrosal nerve. Meningeal branches of ascending pharyngeal artery and small veins traverse entire canal.
	Lesser petrosal sinus	Anterior wall of petrous part of temporal bone	Lesser petrosal nerve
	Greater petrosal canal	Anterior wall of petrous part of temporal bone	Greater petrosal nerve
Posterior cranial fossa	Internal acoustic meatus	Posterior wall of petrous part of temporal bone	Facial nerve (VII); vestibulocochlear nerve (VIII); labyrinthine artery
	Opening of vestibular aqueduct	Posterior wall of petrous part of temporal bone	Endolymphatic duct
	Mastoid foramen	Behind mastoid antrum within sigmoid sulcus	Emissary vein and meningeal branch of occipital artery
	Jugular foramen	In middle part of petro-occipital fissure	Internal jugular vein; spinal accessory, vagus, and pharyngeal nerves
	Hypoglossal canal	In lateral walls of foramen magnum	Hypoglossal nerve
	Foramen magnum	Junction between petrous part of temporal bone and occiput	Medulla oblongata and spinal cord

tal suture. In addition, a groove, or **sagittal sulcus,** along the midline of the calva reflects the location of a part of the venous system of the cranial cavity, the **superior sagittal sinus** (see Chapter 26). Projecting backward from the frontal bone toward the sagittal sulcus is a bony projection called the **frontal crest** (Fig. 22–14). The frontal crest provides an attachment site for a tough crescentic fold of dura mater called the **falx cerebri** (see Chapter 26). In life, the falx cerebri separates the cerebral hemispheres and encloses the superior sagittal sinus and other venous elements of the cranium (see Chapter 27). Deep depressions, or **granular foveolae,** may be seen on either side of the sagittal sulcus. In life, these depressions appose the **arachnoid granulations,** which transport cerebrospinal fluid from the subarachnoid space within the meninges investing the brain to

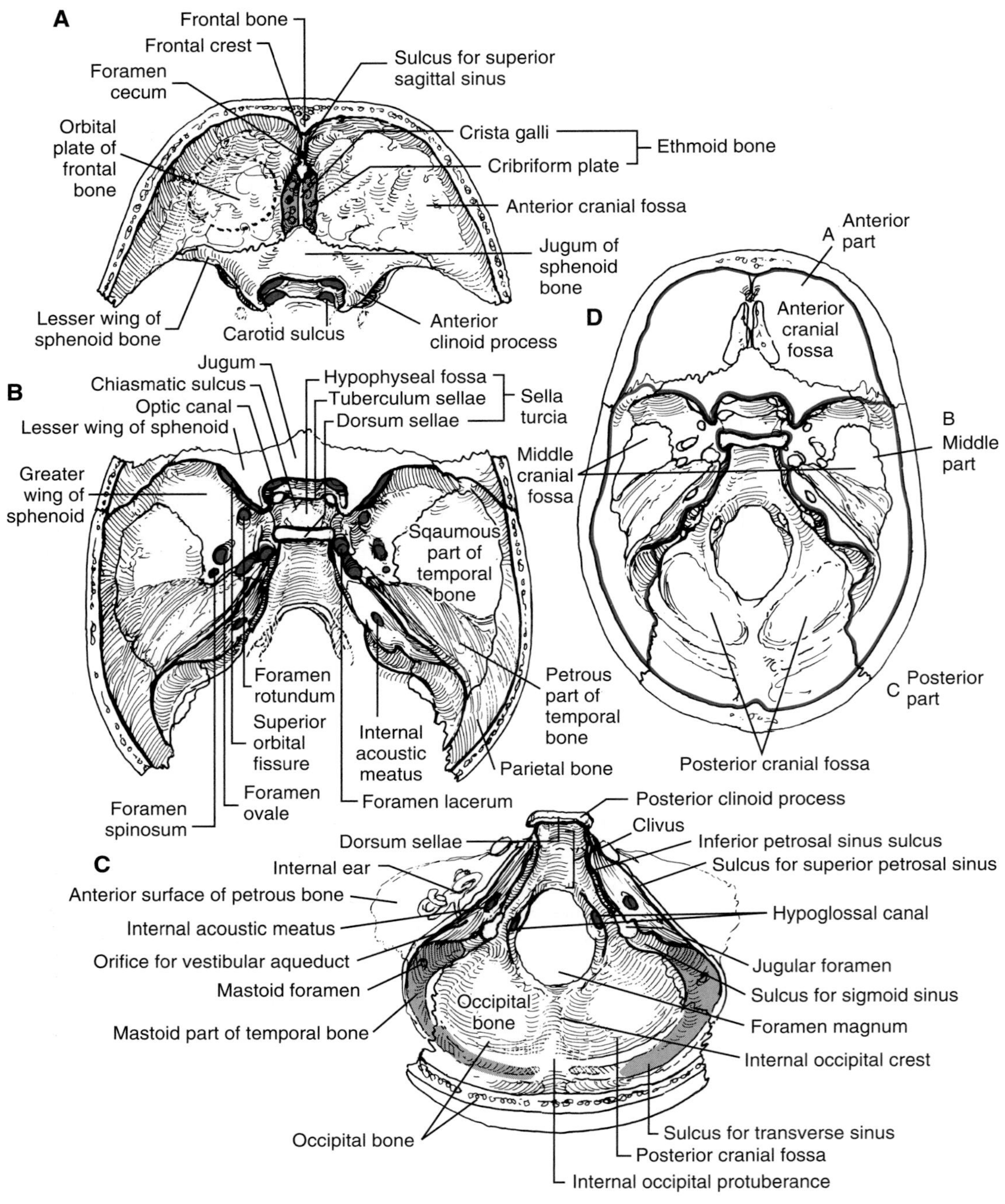

FIGURE 22–15
Fossae of cranial cavity. Superior view of the interior of the skull base. **A.** Anterior part. **B.** Middle part. **C.** Posterior part. **D.** Overview.

the venous sinuses (see Chapter 26). Finally, grooves for the **middle meningeal arteries** and their branches, as well as impressions for gyri of the brain, may be apparent in inferior views of the calvaria (Fig. 22–14 and Table 22–2).

Interior of the Skull Base. *The interior of the skull base may be divided into three fossae.* The interior of the skull base may be divided into anterior, middle, and posterior **cranial fossae** (Fig. 22–15 and see Table 22–2). All of these fossae are lined with endocranium, which blends with more superficial pericranium within the many foramina visible within the skull base. The irregular surfaces of the cranial fossae reflect the locations of cerebral gyri (see Chapter 26). The boundary between the anterior and middle cranial fossae is the posterior border of the lesser wing of the sphenoid bone (laterally) and the clinoid processes (medially). The boundary between the middle and posterior cranial fossae is the superior border of the petrous part of the temporal bone (laterally) and the dorsum sellae of the sphenoid bone (medially).

Anterior Cranial Fossa. The anterior cranial fossa is *bounded* anteriorly and laterally by the frontal bone. The lateral region of its posterior boundary is the posterior edge of the lesser wings of the sphenoid bone laterally with their anterior clinoid processes. (*Clinoid* is from the Greek, meaning shaped like a bed.) The medial part of the posterior boundary of the anterior cranial fossa is the jugum of the body of the sphenoid bone (Fig. 22–15*A* and *D* and see below). The anterior fossa contains the **frontal lobes of the cerebrum** and **olfactory bulbs** (see Table 22–2 and Chapter 26).

The "floor" of the anterior cranial fossa is comprised of the orbital plates of the frontal bone and their anterior connections, the cribriform plate of the ethmoid bone, and the lesser wings and body of the sphenoid bone (Fig. 22–15*A* and *D*). The **orbital plate of the frontal bone** separates the frontal lobes of the cerebrum from the orbit and, thus, constitutes most of the floor of the anterior cranial sulcus. A projection of the frontal bone called the **frontal crest** is located between the two orbits in the anteromedial region of the anterior fossa (Fig. 22–15*A*). The diploë of the frontal bone expands to form a **frontal sinus** (see discussion of the paranasal sinuses in Chapter 26) between the frontal crest in the cranial cavity and the glabella of the forehead (see Fig. 22–10 and Chapter 26). The medial side of each orbital plate is fused to a lateral side of the ethmoid cribriform plate (Fig. 22–15*A* and *D*). The posterior side of each orbital plate is connected to the anterior edge of the lesser wing of the sphenoid bone.

The **cribriform plate of the ethmoid bone** has a raised crest in the midline called the **crista galli** (Fig. 22–15*A* and *D*). (*"Cribriform"* is from the Latin, meaning *formed like a sieve. "Crista galli,"* also from the Latin, means *rooster's comb.*) Small **cribriform foramina** are located just lateral to the crista galli. These foramina transport olfactory nerves from the nasal cavity to the anterior fossa. The ethmoidal plate is joined to the frontal bone by a frontoethmoidal suture within a depression just anterior to the crista galli and posterior to the frontal crest. An aperture may also be observed in the posterior region of the crest. This is the **foramen caecum of the skull.** Infrequently, this foramen transports a small vein that connects nasal veins with the superior sagittal sinus (see Tables 22–1 and 22–3).

The surface of the body of the sphenoid bone, or **jugum** (from the Latin, meaning *yoke*), and **lesser wings of the sphenoid bone** cover the posterior part of the floor of the anterior fossa. Medially, the jugum is connected to the cribriform plate of the ethmoid bone, while laterally, the anterior edges of the lesser wings of the sphenoid bone are connected to the frontal bone. The posterior edge of the lesser wings overhang the middle cranial fossa. Medially, each forms a sloping **anterior clinoid process.**

The **optic canal** lies just anterior to the anterior clinoid process at the point where the sphenoidal body and lesser wings join together (both superior and inferior to the optic canal) (see Table 22–4).

Middle Cranial Fossa. The anterior boundary of the middle cranial fossa is the posterior edge of the lesser wing of the sphenoid bone (laterally) and the anterior clinoid process and chiasmatic groove (medially) (Fig. 22–15*B* and *D* and discussion of the optic chiasm in Chapter 25). The posterior boundary of the middle cranial fossa is the superior boundary of the petrous part of the temporal bone and the dorsum sellae and posterior clinoid processes of the sphenoid bone. The lateral boundary of the middle fossa is formed by the temporal squama, parietal bones, and greater wings of the sphenoid bone. Most of the middle fossa harbors the **temporal lobes of the cerebrum.** The hypophyseal fossa within the middle fossa contains the **pituitary gland** (see Table 22–2).

The **floor of the middle fossa** is composed of the body and greater wing of the sphenoid bone, part of the temporal squama, and the anterior wall of the petrous part of the temporal bone. Anteriorly, the body of the sphenoid bone elaborates the **chiasmatic groove.** Behind this is the saddlelike structure called the **sella turcica** (from the Latin, meaning *Turkish saddle*), which is composed of three parts: an anterior ridge called the **tuberculum sellae;** a central depression called the **hypophyseal fossa** (which contains the pituitary gland in a live person), and, posteriorly, a raised ridge called the **dorsum sellae.** The posterolateral edges of the dorsum sellae form small expansions called the **posterior clinoid processes** (Fig. 22–15*B* and *D*). The floor of the hypophyseal fossa also forms the roof of the sphenoidal air sinuses (see Table 22–2).

Prominent landmarks of the greater wing of the sphenoid bone include several large foramina such as the foramen rotundum, foramen ovale, and foramen lacerum (Fig. 22–15*B* and *D*). The **foramen rotundum** transports the second (maxillary) division of the fifth cranial (trigeminal) nerve. Posterolaterally, the **foramen ovale** transports the first (mandibular) division of the trigeminal nerve and the accessory meningeal artery. Still more posteriorly and laterally, the **foramen spinosum** transports the middle meningeal artery and vein and the meningeal branch of the mandibular nerve. Finally, the

foramen lacerum is located just medial to the foramen spinosum at the medial end of the petrous temporal bone where it joins the greater wing and body of the sphenoid bone and the basilar part of the occipital bone. The meningeal branches of the ascending pharyngeal artery and some small veins traverse the entire length of the foramen lacerum. The carotid artery traverses only the superior part of the foramen lacerum. The artery enters the foramen through its posterior wall as the artery exits the petrous canal. The greater petrosal nerve descends through the superior part of the foramen lacerum and exits through an opening in the foramen's anterior wall to enter the **pterygoid canal.** Here the greater petrosal nerve joins the deep petrosal nerve to form the pterygoid nerve (see Table 22–4 and Chapter 24).

Posterior Cranial Fossa. The posterior cranial fossa is bounded anteriorly by the dorsum sellae and posterior clinoid processes, the body of the sphenoid bone, and the basilar part of the occipital bone (Fig. 22–15*C* and *D*). Laterally, the fossa is bounded by the posteromedial wall of the petrous part of the temporal bone, the mastoid part of the temporal bone, and the mastoid angles of the parietal bones. Posteriorly, the fossa is bounded by the occipital squama. This most posterior of the cranial fossae is the deepest and largest fossa. It contains the **cerebellum, pons,** and **medulla oblongata** (see Table 22–2 and Chapter 26).

The floor of the posterior fossa consists largely of the basilar, lateral, and squamous parts of the occipital bone. Anteriorly, it includes some of the basilar part of the sphenoid bone, which, with the basilar part of the occipital bone, forms a sloping "ramp" called the **clivus** (from the Latin, meaning *slope*). The clivus is capped by the **posterior clinoid processes** laterally and the **dorsum sellae** medially (Fig. 22–15*C* and *D*). Just at the boundary of the middle fossa and posterior fossa (at the apex of the petrous part of the temporal bone), a small groove, or **sulcus,** marks the location of the **superior petrosal sinus.** Just medial to this in the anterolateral region of the floor of the posterior fossa, the medial wall of the petrous part of the temporal bone contains a **sulcus for the sigmoid sinus.** A small **mastoid emissary foramen** is apparent within the sigmoid sulcus. This foramen transmits an emissary vein and a meningeal branch of the occipital artery. Continuous with this groove is a more posterior groove in the occipital bone, which is the **sulcus for the transverse sinus** (Fig. 22–15*C* and *D*). The anterior part of the suture between the petrous part of the temporal bone and the basilar part of the occipital bone, the **petro-occipital fissure,** contains a **sulcus for the inferior petrosal sinus.** The sigmoid, transverse, and inferior petrosal sinuses constitute elements of the venous system within the skull (see Table 22–2 and Chapter 26).

Just posterior to the groove for the inferior petrosal sinus, the petro-occipital fissure widens into the **jugular foramen** (Fig. 22–15*C* and *D*). The jugular foramen transmits the spinal accessory nerve (cranial nerve XI), vagus nerve (cranial nerve X), glossopharyngeal nerve (cranial nerve IX), and internal jugular vein (Fig. 22–15*C* and *D* and see Chapter 26). Just lateral to the jugular foramen (within the medial wall of the petrous part of the temporal bone) is the **internal acoustic meatus.** The internal acoustic meatus transmits the facial nerve (cranial nerve VII) and vestibulocochlear nerve (cranial nerve VIII). Just posterior to the internal acoustic meatus, a small slitlike **opening for the vestibular aqueduct** transmits the endolymphatic duct, a part of the inner ear (Fig. 22–15*C* and *D* and see Chapter 25). A large egg-shaped **foramen magnum** is apparent in the central part of the posterior fossa, bounded anteriorly by the basilar part of the occipital bone, laterally by lateral parts of the occipital bone, and posteriorly by the squamous part of the occipital bone. The foramen magnum is located at the point where the spinal cord becomes continuous with the medulla oblongata of the hindbrain. Internal openings of the **hypoglossal canals** are located within the lateral walls of the foramen magnum. These canals transmit the hypoglossal nerves (cranial nerves XII) (Fig. 22–15*C* and *D* and see Table 22–4 and Chapter 26).

PARANASAL AIR SINUSES

The paranasal air sinuses are cavities within the trabecular parts of the maxillary, ethmoid, sphenoid, and frontal bones of the skull. While these enlargements of the diploë may first appear during fetal development, their most significant growth does not occur until late childhood, usually in conjunction with eruption of the secondary dentition (between ages 6 to 8 years) and continues until puberty.

The two large **maxillary sinuses** of the teenager or adult first appear as diminutive evaginations of the nasal sac during the third fetal month. These slowly expand into the maxilla on each side of the nasal cavity during childhood to form a large pyramidal cavity between the floor of the orbit and the alveolar process of the maxilla. By puberty, the maxillary sinuses may measure about an inch or more in height, depth, and width, with the superior apex extending into the zygomatic bone. Each sinus empties into the lower part of the hiatus semilunaris and then into the middle meatus of the nasal cavity (Fig. 22–16*A* and *B*). The roots of the first and second molars, first and second premolars, and canine teeth may protrude through the floors of the maxillary sinuses.

> Infections of the maxillary sinuses may spread from the teeth. Infections of any of the sinuses may spread from the nasal cavity.

Each **frontal sinus** lies just behind the superciliary arches within the frontal bones. The sinuses first appear

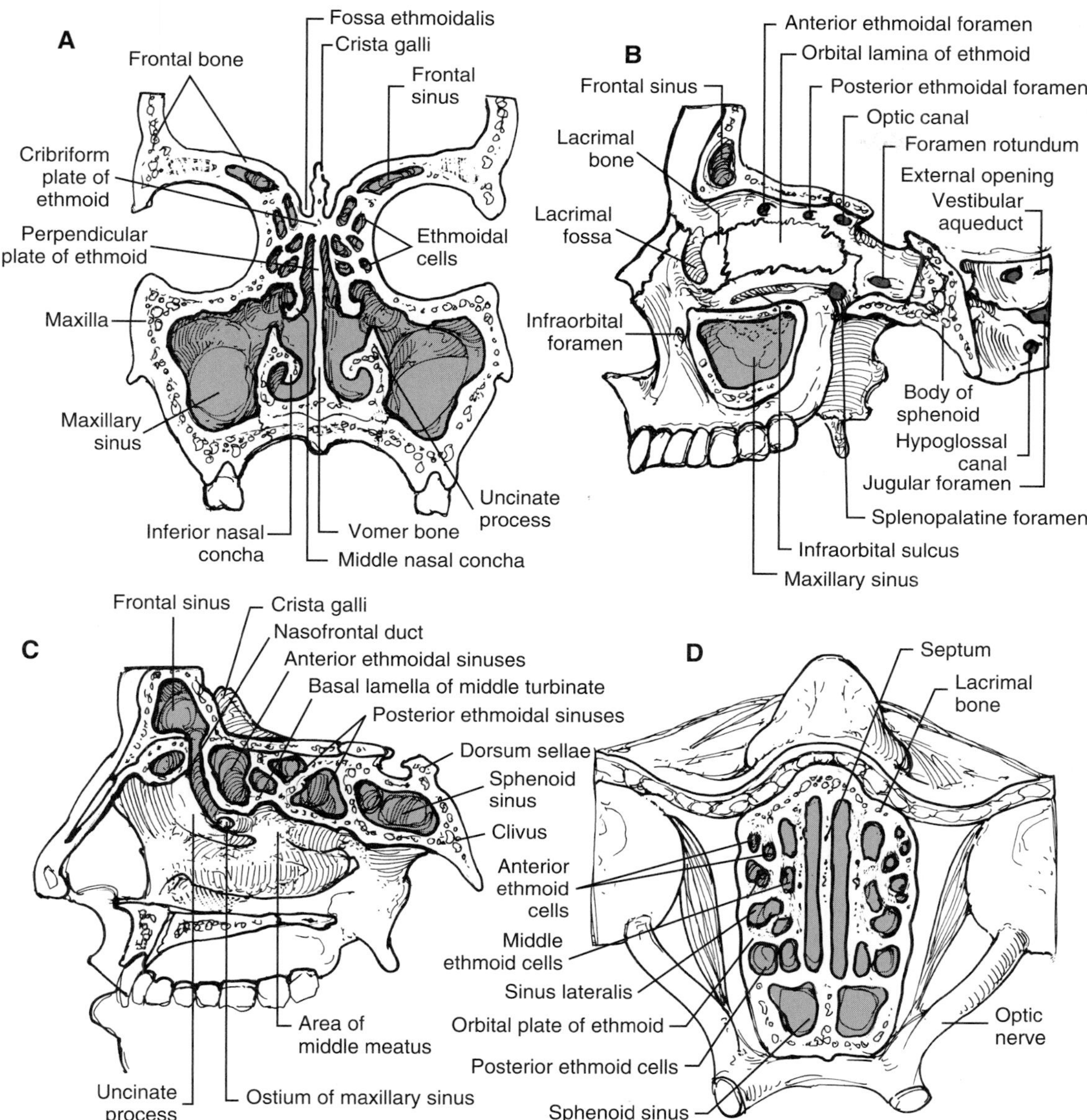

FIGURE 22–16

Paranasal air sinuses. **A.** Coronal section showing from superior to inferior: frontal, ethmoidal, and maxillary sinuses. **B.** Lateral view showing maxillary sinus in relation to medial wall of orbit. **C.** Ethmoid, frontal, and sphenoid sinuses in relation to lateral wall of nose. **D.** Horizontal section viewed from above.

during the fifth or sixth year of life and continue to grow throughout adolescence (Fig. 22–16*B* and *C*).

The **ethmoidal air cells (paranasal air sinuses)** first appear as evaginations of the middle meatus during the fifth fetal month. Their most expansive growth into the ethmoid bones, however, occurs from the age of 6 years through puberty and slightly beyond. Some anatomists characterize these air cells as belonging to one of three groups (i.e., anterior, middle, or posterior group), while others recognize only two groups (i.e., anterior and posterior groups). The anterior group of a few to as many as 18 partially separated cavities may open into the ethmoidal infundibulum (a canal that opens into the anterior ethmoidal, frontal, and maxillary air sinuses) into the middle meatus. Alternatively, this anterior group may open into the orifice of the frontonasal duct (the opening between the frontal air sinuses and the middle meatus; see below). The middle group of about three air cells is located within the ethmoidal bulla (see discussion of the nasal cavity above). These air cells open into the middle meatus via one to three openings. Finally, the posterior group of ethmoidal air cells (as many as seven) empty separately into the superior meatus just inferior to the superior concha (Fig. 22–16*C* and *D*).

The **sphenoidal air sinuses** form as cavities within the body of the sphenoid bone in the fifth fetal month. The two sinuses grow throughout infancy and childhood, expanding, in some cases, into the pterygoid processes and greater wings of the sphenoid bone and even into the basilar part of the occipital bone. In cases where the sinuses extend into the basiocciput, transphenoidal surgical approaches to the pituitary gland are possible. The sphenoidal sinuses open into the sphenoethmoidal recess of the nasal cavity (see above) just above the superior concha (Fig. 22–16*C* and *D*).

Functions and clinical problems of the paranasal sinuses are discussed in Chapter 26.

MANDIBLE AND TEMPOROMANDIBULAR JOINT

Anatomy of the Mandible

The mandible is the largest, strongest bone of the skull

The prominent lower jaw (mandible) is apparent below the alveolar process of the maxillary bone (Fig. 22–17*A*). It has a horseshoe-shaped **body,** which is composed of right and left **arms** and two posterior **rami.** The broad body of the adult mandible has an external surface, inferior border (base), superior border (alveolar part), and internal surface. The long axis of each **ramus** is oriented at a right angle to the long axis of each arm of the body. The **angles** are at the junctions of the arms of the body and each ramus. Superiorly, the rami exhibit two large processes: the posterior head (condylar process) and anterior coronoid process (Fig. 22–17*A* and Table 22–5). The **mandibular condyle** is the mandibular part of the temporomandibular joint (see discussion of the temporomandibular joint, below). It is attached to the ramus by a **neck.** The **coronoid process** provides an attachment site for the temporalis muscle.

The **external surface** of the body of the mandible is marked by the triangular **mental protuberance** in its inferior midline. A faint median line may course superiorly from the apex of the mental protuberance. This is the line of fusion (symphysis) between the two halves of the fetal mandible (Fig. 22–17*A*). A raised **mental tubercle** is apparent along each side of the mental protuberance. Near the apex of the mental protuberance, a shallow incisive fossa provides an attachment site for the mentalis muscle, which is used to push out the lower lip when one expresses doubt or disdain. A **mental foramen** is located lateral to each mental protuberance at the junction between the premolars and molars and about halfway between the superior border and inferior border of the mandibular body (Fig. 22–17*A*). The mental foramen transports the mental nerve and mental vessels. The base of the body of the mandible courses posterolaterally on each side of the jaw from the

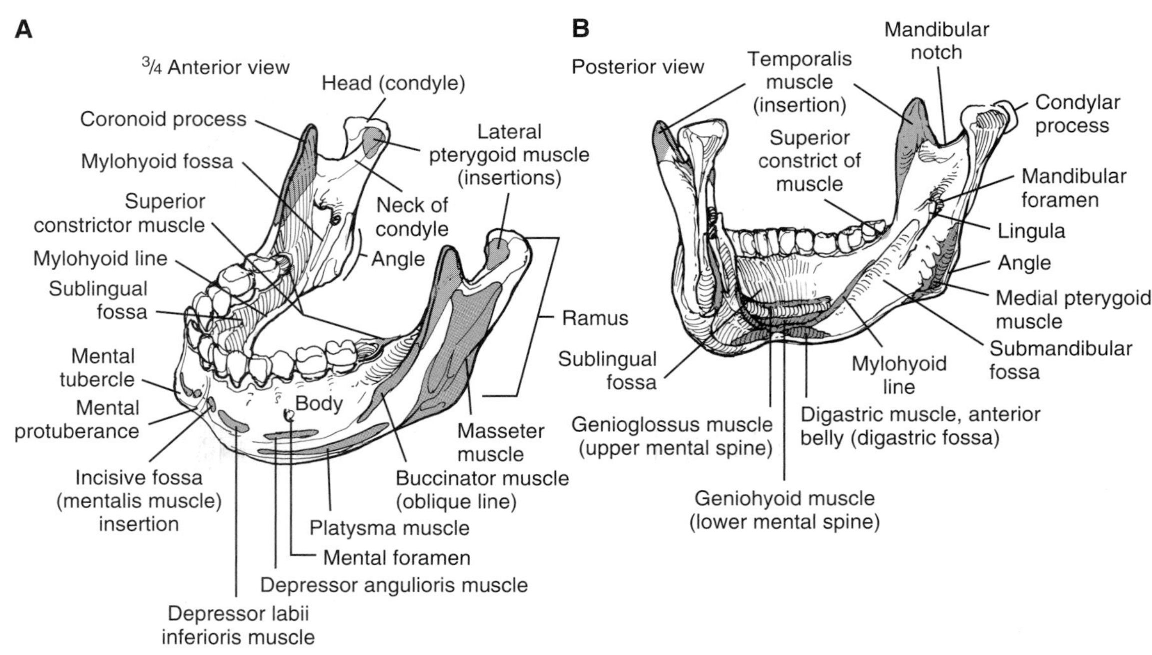

FIGURE 22–17
Anatomy of the mandible.

symphysis to blend with the base of the mandibular ramus at the level of the third molar (Fig. 22–17). The alveolar part of the body of the mandible contains alveoli (sockets) for 16 teeth (8 on each side). These include 4 incisors, 2 canines, 4 premolars, and 6 molars. The external surface of each ramus of the mandible is flat except in the inferior region, where oblique ridges form an attachment site for the masseter muscle (Fig. 22–17 and see Chapter 23).

The **internal surface** of the body of the mandible is divided by a distinct oblique **mylohyoid line** into two shallow fossae: the upper **sublingual fossa** and lower **mylohyoid fossa** (Fig. 22–17 and Table 22–5). The internal surface of each mandibular ramus possesses a prominent **mandibular foramen,** which is partially covered at its anteroinferior border by a small shelf of bone called the **lingula**. The lingula serves as an attachment site for the sphenomandibular ligament (Fig. 22–17 and discussion of the temporomandibular joint below). Inferiorly, a faint **mylohyoid groove** joins the mandibular foramen. The mandibular foramen transports the inferior alveolar nerves and vessels, while the mylohyoid groove transports the mylohyoid nerve and vessels.

Functions of the Mandible

Functions of the mandible in chewing and vocalization are discussed in Chapter 24.

Fracture of the Mandible. Mandibular fracture is usually caused by a blow to the ventral midline of the mandible. Fracture may occur at the point of impact within the mandibular body (usually in line with the second canine tooth) (Fig. 22–18*A*) or at the angles of the mandible (Fig. 22–18*B*). Fractures are often bilateral. Repair typically requires immobilization of the mandible with elastic bands and the wiring of separated fragments to prevent their displacement by the powerful masticatory muscles. Fractures may also occur at the base of the coronoid process (Fig. 22–18*C*) and through the neck of the mandibular ramus (Fig. 22–18*D*).

Lingula as a Guide to Anesthesia of the Inferior Alveolar Nerve. The sharp bony shelf at the anteroinferior border of the mandibular foramen (lingula) may be palpated to guide injections of anesthetic into the vicinity of the inferior alveolar nerve. This procedure is common in the dental office. Anesthetic is flooded into the region of the mandibular foramen, resulting in anesthesia of the lower teeth, gums, gingiva, and skin on the same side of the mandible (see Chapter 26).

▲ Anatomy of the Temporomandibular Joints

The skull has one pair of movable joints

The single pair of movable joints of the skull is the synovial temporomandibular joints. These are the condylar joints of the jaw, which join the mandible to

TABLE 22–5
Tubercles, Processes, and Fossae of the Mandible

Tubercle, Process, or Fossa	Location, Attachments, or Articulations
Coronoid process	Attachment of temporalis muscle
Oblique line of mandible	Attachment of buccinator muscle
Mandibular condyle	Articulates with temporal bone
Lingula	Attachment of sphenomandibular ligament
Mylohyoid line	Attachment of mylohyoid muscle
Upper mental spine	Attachment of genioglossus
Lower mental spine	Attachment of geniohyoid
Mylohyoid groove	Inside surface of mandibular ramus, extending anteroinferiorly from mandibular foramen; mylohyoid nerves and vessels
Mental protuberance	Triangular prominence on anterior surface of mandible
Mental tubercle	Ridges bordering lateral boundaries of mental tubercle
Incisive fossa (of mandible)	Attachment of mentalis muscle and part of orbicularis oris muscle
Digastric fossa	Attachment of anterior belly of digastric muscle
Submandibular fossa	Submandibular lymph nodes
Mandibular notch	Upper border of ramus between coronoid process and condyle. Transmits masseteric nerve and vessels from infratemporal fossa.

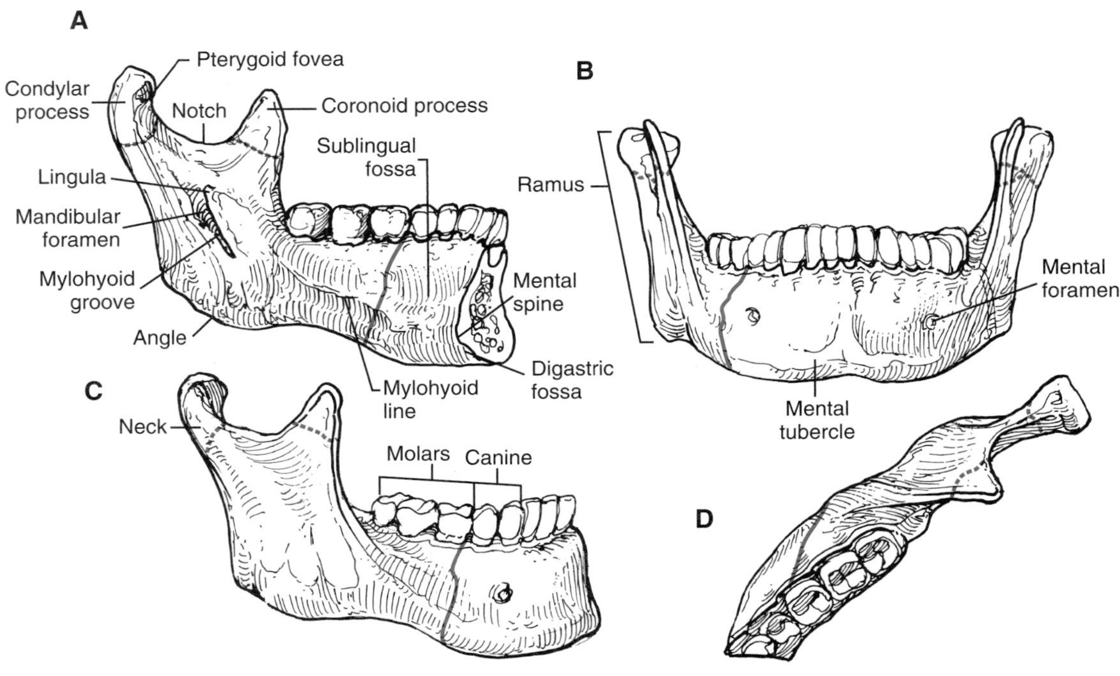

FIGURE 22–18
Fractures of the mandible. **A.** Interior view, left side. **B.** Anterior view. **C.** Exterior view, right side. **D.** Superior angle.

the temporal bone and may be characterized by the following scheme:

Bone ⟷ Articular hyaline cartilage ⟷ Cavity lined by synovial membrane containing synovial fluid and articular disc ⟷ Articular hyaline cartilage ⟷ Bone

As has been noted, this temporomandibular joint is novel in mammals, arising from the overgrowth of the temporal bones and mandible by dermal bone as the original incus and malleus are displaced into the middle ear where they serve as auditory ossicles along with the stapes. The human temporomandibular joint is thus formed by an articulation between the shallow **mandibular fossa** and **articular tubercle** of the temporal squama and the **mandibular condyle** of the mandible (Fig. 22–19). The mandibular fossa is located just posteromedially to the inferior side of the root of the zygomatic process. It is bounded anteriorly by the articular tubercle of the temporal squama and posteriorly by the anterior wall of the external acoustic meatus, the **temporal tympanic plate.**

Stability of the temporomandibular joint is maintained by a tough fibrous capsule and several ligaments. The **capsule** completely encloses the joint through its upper "temporal" connection to the articular tubercle (anteriorly), the squamotympanic fissure between the temporal bone and tympanic plate (posteriorly), and the periphery of the temporal fossa (laterally and medially). The capsule is connected all around the neck of the mandible below (Fig. 22–19A). A **lateral (temporomandibular) ligament** is attached to a tubercle of the zygomatic process of the temporal bone above and to the posterior and lateral surfaces of the neck of the mandible below. This ligament is closely apposed to the lateral surface of the fibrous capsule of the joint. The **sphenomandibular ligament** is attached above to the spine of the sphenoid bone and below to the lingula of the mandibular foramen (Fig. 22–19A). Some fibers of the sphenomandibular ligament cross the petrotympanic fissure to attach to the anterior process of the malleus bone. The **stylomandibular ligament** is attached above to the styloid process of the temporal bone and below to the angle and posterior border of the ramus of the mandible. Both the sphenomandibular and stylomandibular ligaments are clearly separated from the joint capsule, unlike the lateral ligament (see above).

The architecture of the mandibular fossa-articular tubercle and mandibular condyle appears at first glance to be a simple hinge joint. However, its movements, which open and close the jaw, are more complex than those of a simple hinge joint. The mandibular condyle has a "hinge" (or rotational) movement but also glides forward and backward and from side to side within the mandibular fossa. The mandible can, therefore, be elevated, depressed, protruded, retracted, and moved from side to side. These movements are facilitated by several

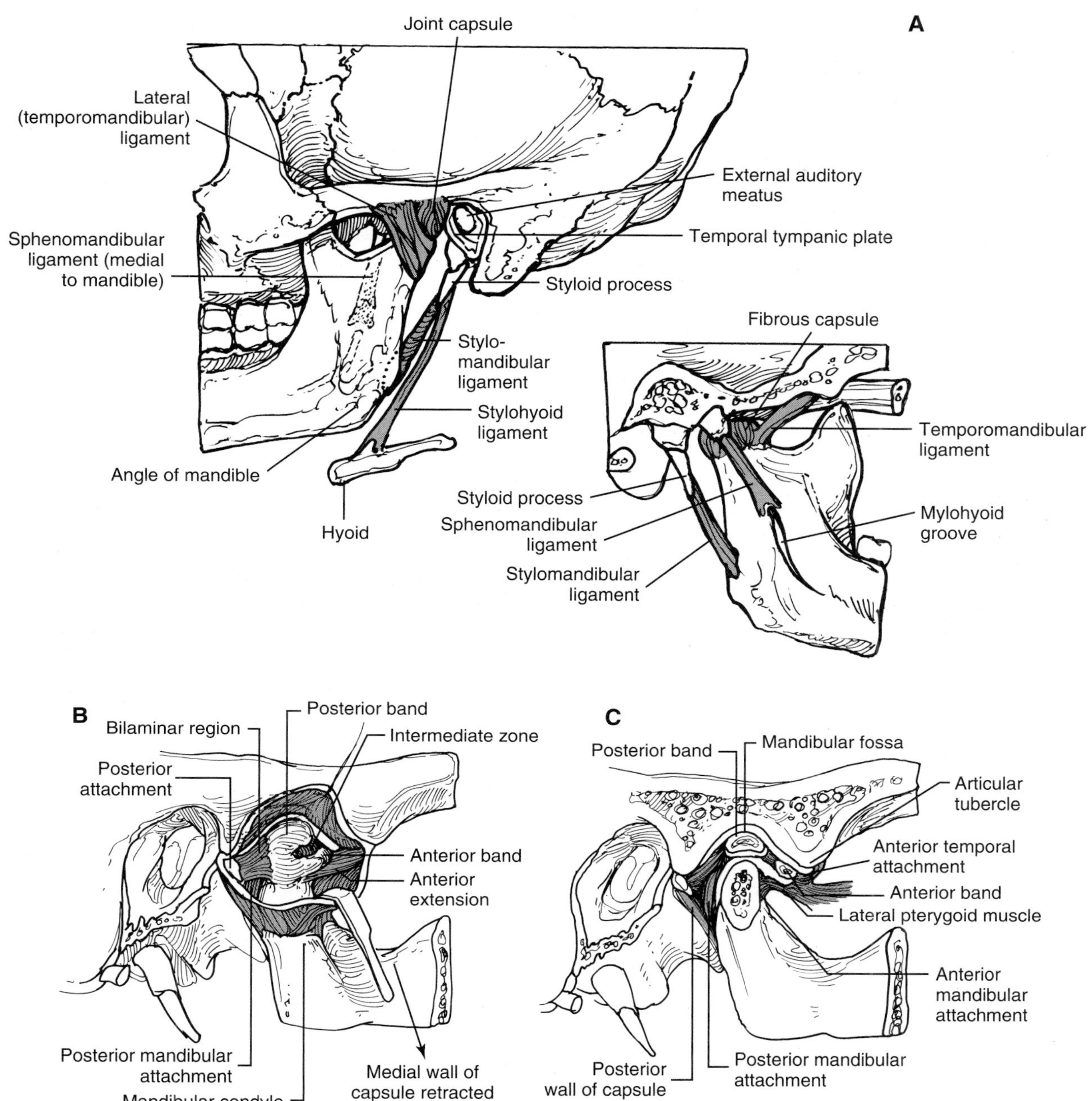

FIGURE 22–19
Temporomandibular joint. **A.** The lateral ligament completely encloses the lateral and posterior neck of the mandible. Stylomandibular and sphenomandibular ligaments (from styloid process of temporal bone and sphenoid bone, respectively) attach separately to the posterior ramus and medial lingula of the mandible. **B.** Exterior view of the unique articular disc. **C.** Cross-sectional view of the unique articular disc.

muscles, which act together on the mandible and articular disc of the temporomandibular joint (see below).

The complex movements of the mandible rely especially upon the complex architecture of a unique **articular disc,** which is intercalated between the mandibular fossa and mandibular condyle (Fig. 22–19*B* and *C*). The disc is attached to the apex of the articular tubercle anteriorly and to the anterior surface of the mandibular condyle by its **anterior extension.** The posterior edge of this anterior extension is attached to a thickened **anterior band,** which, in turn, is attached to a thicker **posterior band** by an intervening **intermediate zone.** In addition, anterior and posterior bands are attached to each other at their medial and lateral ends. Finally, the posterior surface of the posterior band is attached to both the tympanic plate and the posterior surface of the mandibular condyle by separate laminae at the posterior bilamellar region of the articular disc. The temporomandibular joint capsule completely encloses all of these elements of the disc (Fig. 22–19).

▲ Movements of the Temporomandibular Joints

Movements of the mandible require the actions of several muscles upon the mandible and also upon the articular disc of the temporomandibular joint.

Opening the Mouth

1. If the mouth is closed, the mandible is completely elevated. The initial depression of the mandible from this position requires bilateral actions of the digastric, geniohyoid, and mylohyoid muscles to **pull the mandible downward.**
2. The lateral pterygoid muscles pull the head of the mandible, with the articular disc, forward onto the articular tubercle. Indeed, this **protrusion** of the mandible (forward movement of the lower teeth over the upper teeth) requires only the forward gliding movements of the mandibular head and articular disc and, therefore, only bilateral actions of the lateral pterygoid muscles.
3. At this point, the mouth can be opened wider by **further depression of the mandible** by the digastric, geniohyoid, and mylohyoid muscles.

Closing the Mouth

1. Initial **elevation of the mandible** from a completely depressed position (i.e., the mouth is wide open) requires bilateral actions of the temporalis, masseter, and medial pterygoid muscles to pull the mandible upward.
2. Relaxation of the lateral pterygoid muscles allows the backward movement of the articular disc and backward gliding of the mandibular head into the

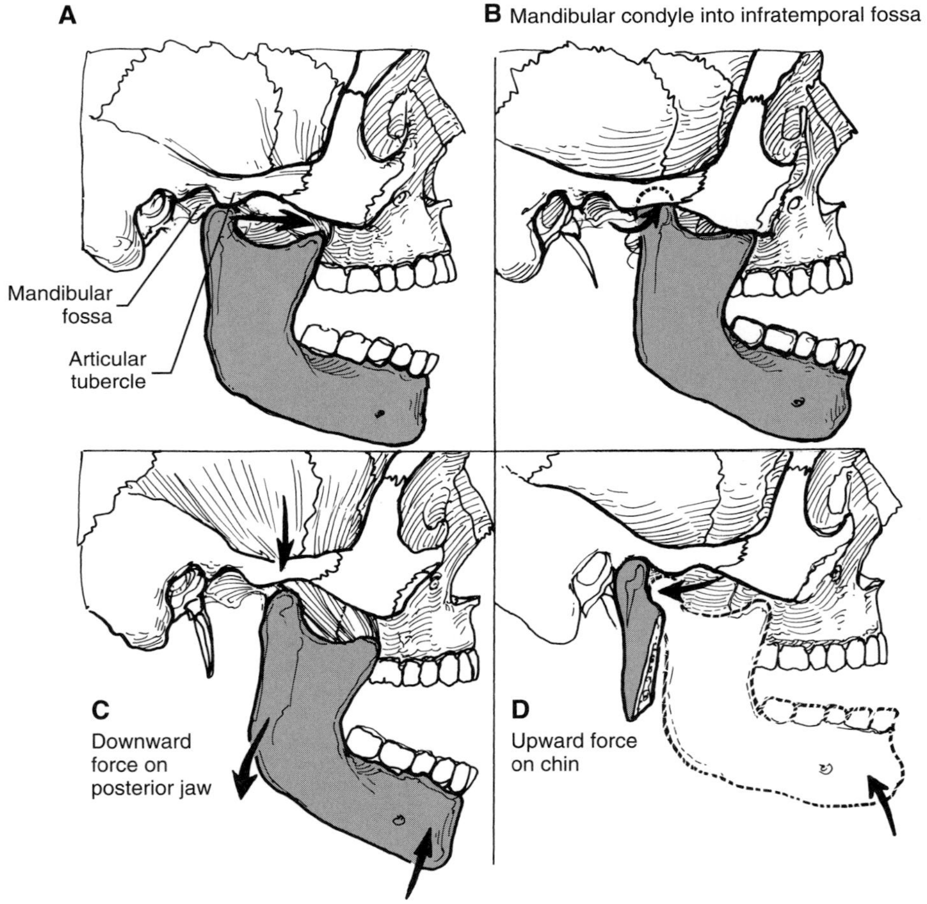

FIGURE 22–20

Dislocation of the temporomandibular joint. **A** and **B.** Head of mandible displaced anteriorly into infratemporal fossa. **C** and **D.** Downward pressure on posterior jaw and upward pressure on chin are required to overcome the actions of the temporalis, lateral pterygoid, and masseter muscles and to restore the jaw to its original position.

temporal fossa. This **retraction** of the mandible (backward movement of the lower teeth over the upper teeth) requires the action of the posterior fibers of the temporalis muscles (which may be assisted by the middle and deep parts of the masseter muscles and by the geniohyoid and digastric muscles).

3. Finally, complete elevation and closure of the jaw requires, once again, the actions of the temporalis, masseter, and medial pterygoid muscles.

Maintaining the Jaw in a Position of Rest. Maintaining the jaw in a position of rest (in which the upper and lower teeth are slightly separated) requires the action of the temporalis muscle only.

Dislocation of the Temporomandibular Joint

The temporomandibular joint may be dislocated (unilaterally or bilaterally) in an anterior direction, displacing the head of the mandible into the infratemporal fossa (Fig. 22–20*A* and *B*). This typically occurs when a person yawns suddenly and convulsively or when there is violent trauma to the chin while the mouth is open. Dislocations often accompany fractures of the mandible. In order to reduce the dislocation of the temporomandibular joint, the physician must place downward pressure on the posterior jaw (to overcome the actions of the temporalis, lateral pterygoid, and masseter muscles) while elevating the chin (to push the condyle posteriorly over the articular tubercle) (Fig. 22–20*C* and *D*). Dislocation may damage the articular disc, resulting in laxity, pain, and a clicking noise with movement.

HYOID BONE AND LARYNX

Although the hyoid bone and larynx are considered to be parts of the facial skeleton, their functions are more closely related to the oral cavity, pharynx, and neck. These skeletal elements will, therefore, be discussed in Chapter 27.

23 Development of the Head, Neck, and Cranial Nerves

EVOLUTIONARY ORIGINS OF THE HUMAN HEAD AND NECK AND THEIR FUNCTIONS

The vertebrate head evolved as vertebrate organisms developed organs of locomotion

During evolution, as certain protochordate larvae became mobile, a primitive "head" formed at the leading end of the larval organism. This line of protochordates was part of the evolutionary chain that eventually produced humans, and the primitive larval head was the precursor of the human head. As discussed in Chapter 22, the larval head housed and protected a small, concentrated group of neural elements, which formed the presumptive brain. These neural elements contained special structures that could sense the environment at the organism's leading end. A mouth also formed within the neural elements that could take in water for respiration and nourishment. As species developed along the evolutionary line that led to humans, these primitive structures changed extensively but their general functions have remained the same. Obviously, the human head

- houses and protects the brain;
- contains the eyes, nose, ears, and gustatory (taste) apparatuses, which sense the environment at the organism's leading end
- contains the nose and mouth, which serve as openings to the respiratory and digestive systems; and
- contains structures (especially the facial muscles and laryngeal apparatus) that allow a person to communicate in complex ways with other people or creatures.

EMBRYOLOGIC DEVELOPMENT OF THE HEAD AND NECK, INCLUDING THE CRANIAL NERVES

Most structures of the head and neck arise from five pairs of metameric units called **pharyngeal arches** (Fig. 23–1A). Pharyngeal arches are rudiments of the gill bars of ancestral fishes (see below). Most muscles of the face are formed within pharyngeal arches 1 and 2. Arches 1 and 2 also give rise to skeletal elements, including the auditory ossicles, styloid process, and upper part of the hyoid bone. Arches 3, 4, and 6 give rise to structures of the neck, including the lower part of the hyoid bone as well as the larynx and many of its associated muscles (see Chapter 22 and below).

Some structures of the head and neck arise from **tissues other than the pharyngeal arches.** For example, extrinsic ocular muscles and intrinsic muscles of the tongue arise from the paraxial mesoderm (see below). In addition, all dermal bones and the base of the skull are derived from tissues not associated with the arches (see Chapter 22).

Regardless of the specific origin of head structures, most are innervated by a special class of **cranial nerves,** which emanates mainly from the hindbrain (rhombencephalon). There are a total of 12 cranial nerves, 4 of which develop in association with the 5 pharyngeal arches. The other 8 nerves innervate structures that are not formed within the pharyngeal arches (Table 23–1). The 12 cranial nerves innervate virtually all structures of the head and some structures of the neck. Some sympathetic and somatic spinal nerves also innervate structures of the head and neck.

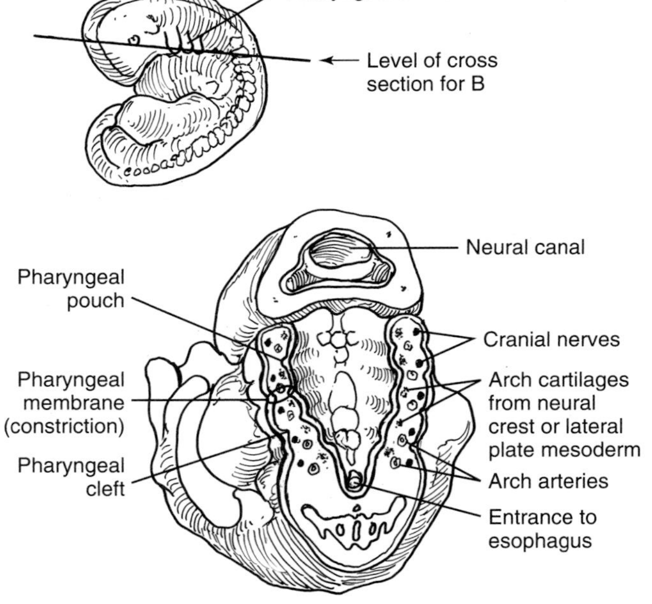

FIGURE 23–1
Embryonic development of the head and neck. **A.** Embryo at approximately 29 days. **B.** Common features of pharyngeal arches.

TABLE 23–1
Cranial Nerves: General Functions and Targets in the Head and Neck

Cranial Nerve	Functional Fibers	Targets
CRANIAL NERVES (OR BRANCHES) TO PHARYNGEAL ARCHES		
Trigeminal nerve (V); to arch 1	Branchial efferent (BE) fibers (special visceral efferent)	Muscles of mastication, including anterior belly of digastric and mylohyoid muscles; tensor muscle of tympanic membrane and tensor muscle of velum palatini
	General somatic afferent (GSA) fibers	Sensory receptors of face, scalp, eyeball, conjunctival sac, and lacrimal gland; external acoustic meatus and tragus and part of concha of pinna (external ear); mucosa of nasal cavity and paranasal sinuses; hard and soft palates; anterior two thirds of tongue and floor of mouth; gingiva and teeth; meninges of anterior and middle cranial fossae; temporomandibular joint; proprioceptors of muscles of mastication; proprioceptors of inferior oblique muscle, medial rectus muscle, and levator muscle of upper eyelid (oculomotor nerve [III]); proprioceptors of superior oblique muscle of eyeball (trochlear nerve [IV]); proprioceptors of lateral rectus muscle (abducens nerve [VI]).
Facial nerve (VII); to arch 2	BE fibers	Muscles of facial expression, stylohyoid muscle, posterior belly of digastric muscle, stapedius muscle
	GSA fibers	General sensory receptors around concha of pinna; proprioceptors of facial muscles
	Parasympathetic general visceral efferent (pGVE) fibers (pterygopalatine and submandibular ganglia)	Submandibular and sublingual salivary glands, lacrimal glands; mucous glands of nasal palatine and pharyngeal mucosa
	Special visceral afferent (SVA) fibers	Taste receptors in mucosa of palate and taste buds of anterior two thirds of tongue
Glossopharyngeal nerve (IX); to arch 3	BE fibers	Stylopharyngeal muscle
	GSA fibers	Sensory receptors of posterior third of tongue; epiglottis; palatine tonsils and pharynx; internal surface of tympanic membrane and skin of external ear; proprioceptors of stylopharyngeal muscle
	pGVE fibers (otic ganglion)	Parotid gland
	GVA fibers	Interoceptors of carotid sinus and carotid body
	SVA fibers	Taste receptors of posterior third of tongue
Superior laryngeal and pharyngeal branches of vagus nerve (X); to arch 4	BE fibers	Constrictors of pharynx, cricothyroid muscle, levator muscle of velum palatini
	GVA fibers	Sensory receptors of pharynx and larynx above vocal folds; proprioceptors of striated muscles innervated by superior laryngeal branch of vagus nerve
	pGVE fibers (several peripheral ganglia)	Mucous glands of pharynx and larynx above vocal folds
	GVA fibers	Interoceptors (chemoreceptors) of aortic body at arch of aorta; stretch receptors in aortic arch; visceral sensation from mucous membrane of epiglottis to most of larynx and vocal folds
	SVA fibers	Taste receptors in region of epiglottis
Recurrent laryngeal branch of vagus nerve (X); to arch 6	BE fibers	Intrinsic muscles of larynx
	GSA fibers	Sensory receptors of laryngeal lining below vocal cords (folds); proprioceptors of intrinsic laryngeal muscles
	pGVE fibers	Mucous glands of larynx below vocal folds
	GVA fibers	Visceral sensation from mucous membrane of larynx below vocal folds
Auricular branch of vagus nerve (X)	GSA fibers*	Skin of external ear, external auditory meatus, external surface of tympanic membrane
Meningeal branch of vagus nerve (X)	GSA fibers	Sensory receptors of meninges of posterior cranial fossa

*The trapezius and sternocleidomastoid muscles are also innervated by motor (GSE) fibers and sensory (proprioceptive, or GSA) fibers of spinal nerves C2 to C4.

Continued

TABLE 23–1, cont'd
Cranial Nerves: General Functions and Targets in the Head and Neck

Cranial Nerve	Functional Fibers	Targets
CRANIAL NERVES TO EXTRINSIC OCULAR MUSCLES		
Trochlear nerve (IV)	General somatic efferent (GSE) fibers	Superior oblique muscle
Abducens nerve (VI)	GSE fibers	Lateral rectus muscle
Oculomotor nerve (III)	GSE fibers (from ciliary ganglion)	Inferior oblique muscle, medial rectus muscle, levator muscle of upper eyelid
	pGVE fibers	Constrictor muscle of pupil and ciliary muscles of eye
OTHER CRANIAL NERVE TARGETS		
Optic nerve (II)	Special somatic afferent (SSA) fibers	Receptors of retina
Vestibulocochlear nerve (VIII)	SSA fibers	Auditory and balancing mechanisms
Olfactory nerve (I)	SSA fibers	Receptors of olfactory epithelium
Hypoglossal nerve (XII)	GSE fibers	Extrinsic and intrinsic muscles of tongue
Accessory nerve (XI)*		
Cranial root	BE fibers	Muscles of larynx, except for cricothyroid muscle after fibers join superior laryngeal branch of vagus nerve (X)
Spinal root (C1 to C5)	BE fibers	Trapezius and sternocleidomastoid fibers
Spinal nerve (C2 to C4)	GSE fibers	Trapezius and sternocleidomastoid muscles
Spinal nerve (C2 to C4)	GSA fibers	Proprioceptors of trapezius and sternocleidomastoid fibers

 The Pharyngeal Arches

Five pairs of pharyngeal arches give rise to most structures of the human face and some structures of the neck

Development of the Pharyngeal Arches

The human pharyngeal arches were introduced in Chapter 2 and were discussed in relation to the development of the facial skeleton in Chapter 22. As was noted, five pairs of pharyngeal arches develop in humans. These arches correspond to the first, second, third, fourth, and sixth pairs of branchial arches (gill bars) of ancestral fishes. In humans, the first pair of arches begins to develop on day 22 of embryologic life. The other pairs of arches then form in a craniocaudal sequence, until the sixth pair of arches is completed on day 29 (Fig. 23–1*A*).

Elements of the Pharyngeal Arches

Although the five pairs of human pharyngeal arches vary somewhat in shape and size, they are all composed of the same basic elements (see Fig. 23–1B)

Each pharyngeal arch is an expansion of mesoderm. There are intervening constrictions of mesoderm between the arches. Each arch is covered on the outside by a layer of surface ectoderm and on the inside by a layer of endoderm. The inner indentation of each intervening constriction is a **pharyngeal pouch;** the outer indentation is a **pharyngeal cleft.** The thin membrane of the constriction itself is the **pharyngeal membrane,** which has three layers: surface ectoderm, mesoderm, and endoderm. The elements within each pharyngeal arch include the following:

- an **aortic arch artery,**
- **paraxial mesoderm** (from somites or somitomeres),
- **neural crest cells (lateral plate mesoderm),** and
- a **cranial nerve.**

The **neural crest cells** of each arch primarily form skeletal structures of the head and neck and some of the dermis of the integument (see Chapter 22). The neural crest cells migrate into each arch from specific segments of the hindbrain called rhombomeres (Fig. 23–2). **Aortic arch arteries** give rise to parts of the great arteries or to parts of arteries that supply the face (see the discussion of vasculature of the head in Chapter 27). The **paraxial mesoderm** in each arch forms a specific functional group of striated muscles. These muscles arise from subsets of myoblasts, which develop in cranial somitomeres 4 to 6 and occipital somites. Finally, the **cranial nerve** that develops within a particular pharyngeal

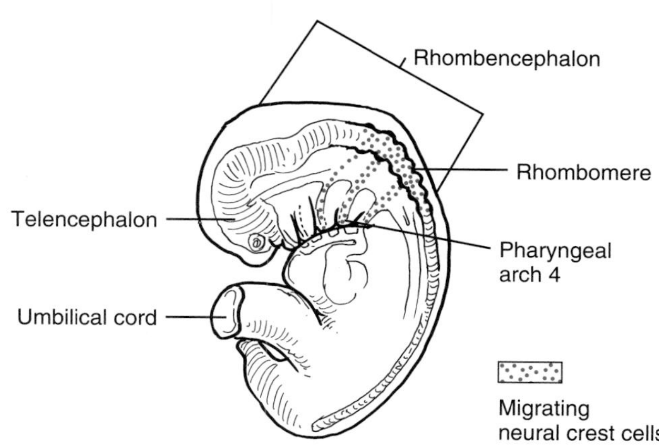

FIGURE 23–2
Migration of neural crest cells.

arch innervates structures also formed within that arch (see below).

Head and Neck Structures That Arise From the Pharyngeal Arches

Each of the pharyngeal arches forms a different part of the head or neck

The five pairs of pharyngeal arches form the skeleton and soft tissues of the face, oral cavity, pharynx, and anterior neck. As is the case for the somites of the trunk (see Chapter 2), the segmental identity and specific differentiation of each pharyngeal arch depends on the expression of a specific combinatorial code of HOX genes (Fig. 23–3). Indeed, mutations of HOX genes or environmental disruptions of HOX gene expression in the pharyngeal arches result in common craniofacial anomalies.

Pharyngeal arches 1 and 2 are involved particularly in the development of the middle and outer ears, auditory ossicles, styloid process, and hyoid bone. Arches 3, 4, and 6 form the larynx, muscles of mastication, and muscles of facial expression. Structures of the pharynx, including the mucosa of the tongue and the thyroid gland, are derived from pharyngeal arches 1, 3, and 4. The tonsils, thymus gland, and parathyroid glands are derived from the pharyngeal pouches.

Cranial Nerve Innervation of Structures That Arise From the Pharyngeal Arches

An understanding of the cranial nerve innervation of structures that arise from the pharyngeal arches is particularly useful because, as has been noted above, elements that develop within a particular pharyngeal arch are innervated by the specific cranial nerve or cranial nerve branch that develops within the same arch (Fig. 23–3). The pattern of development is as follows:

- The **first pair of pharyngeal arches** gives rise to the upper and lower jaws, muscles of mastication, two of the three auditory ossicles, and the mucosa of the most superior end of the oral cavity and tongue. The cranial nerve that innervates structures of the first pharyngeal arch is **cranial nerve V (trigeminal nerve).**
- The **second pair of pharyngeal arches** forms one of the auditory ossicles, the styloid process, the upper rim and lesser horns of the hyoid bone, the oral mucosa, and the muscles of facial expression, including the occipitofrontal muscle of the scalp. The cranial nerve that innervates structures formed in the second pharyngeal arch is **cranial nerve VII (facial nerve).**
- The **third pair of pharyngeal arches** forms the lower rim and greater horns of the hyoid bone in the neck, the mucosa of the oral cavity and posterior tongue, and the stylopharyngeal muscle. The cranial nerve that innervates structures formed within the third pharyngeal arch is **cranial nerve IX (glossopharyngeal nerve).**
- The **fourth pair of pharyngeal arches** forms cartilages and extrinsic muscles of the larynx, the most posterior mucosa of the tongue and pharynx, and the superior mucosa of the larynx. The cranial nerve that innervates structures formed in the fourth pharyngeal arch is the **superior laryngeal branch of cranial nerve X (vagus nerve).**
- The **sixth pair of pharyngeal arches** forms cartilages, intrinsic muscles, and inferior mucosa of the larynx. The cranial nerve that innervates tissues of the sixth pharyngeal arch is the **recurrent laryngeal branch of cranial nerve X (vagus nerve).**

Head and Neck Structures That Arise Directly From Tissues Not Associated with the Pharyngeal Arches

Some structures of the head and neck do not arise from the pharyngeal arches

Most structures of the head arise from tissues associated with the five pairs of pharyngeal arches just described. However, some structures arise directly from surface ectoderm, paraxial mesoderm, and neural crest cells not associated with the pharyngeal arches. Some structures, including the nose orbits and cranium, arise from the frontonasal prominence (see Fig. 22–2C). Other structures are evaginations of the brain or are formed from paraxial mesoderm that is not associated with any of the pharyngeal arches. Some examples are as follows:

- Seven pairs of cranial somitomeres and four pairs of occipital **somites** are arranged segmentally and in sequence, just like somites of the trunk. While much of this paraxial mesoderm is incorporated into the pharyngeal arches to give rise to muscles of the face and neck, some of it gives rise directly to the extrinsic ocular muscles, muscles of the tongue, and parachordal cartilages, which are precursors of the most caudal part of the chondrocranium.
- The **surface ectoderm of the frontonasal prominence** gives rise to the epidermis of the forehead, scalp, eyelids, and nose; lenses and conjunctivas of the eyes; and epithelium of the nasal cavities.

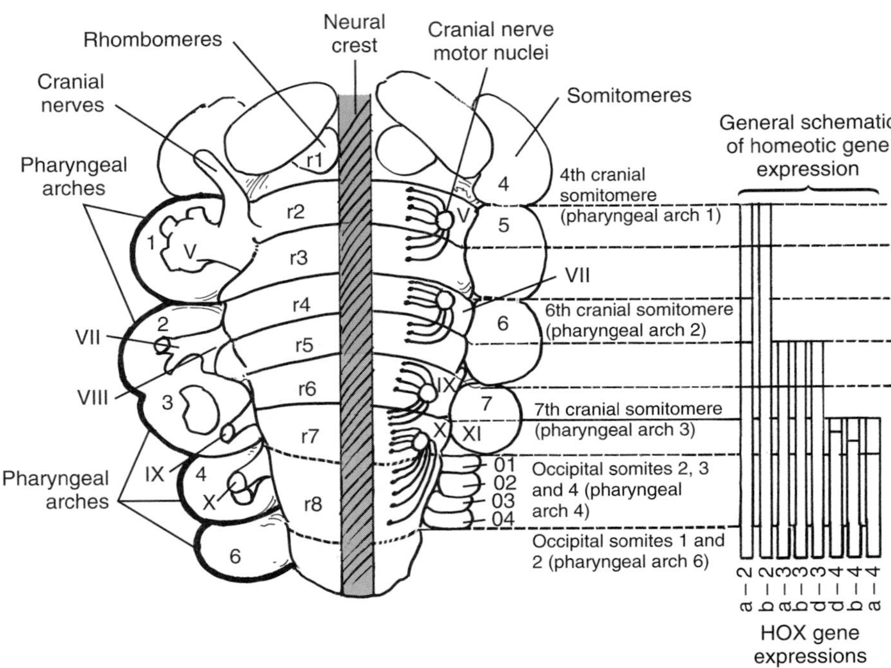

FIGURE 23–3
Stylized depiction of the brainstem showing spatial relationships of pharyngeal arches and cranial nerves and expressions of HOX genes.

- A subpopulation of neural crest cells, the **cranial neural crest cells,** arises mainly from the rhombencephalon (brainstem), although some may be formed by the mesencephalon and diencephalon. Much of this tissue invades the pharyngeal arches to form some of the bones and connective tissues of the face (see Chapter 22). Other cranial neural crest cells, however, give rise to the connective tissues and dermal bones of the cranial vault and to precursors of the prechordal and hypophyseal cartilages of the chondrocranium (see Chapter 22). Some cranial neural crest cells form the ciliary and dilator muscles of the eye, the sphincter muscle of the pupil, and the tendons of the extrinsic ocular muscles. Neural crest cells also give rise to odontoblasts of the teeth.
- Some structures of the human head arise as **evaginations of the forebrain (prosencephalon).** For example, the olfactory bulbs are direct outgrowths of the **telencephalon,** which is the most cranial region of the prosencephalon. The optic cups that form the pigment and neural retinas of the eyes are outgrowths of the **diencephalon,** which is the caudal part of the prosencephalon. See Table 23–2 for brain terminology.

Cranial Nerve Innervation of Head and Neck Structures Derived From Tissues Other Than the Pharyngeal Arches

Many parts of the head and neck formed from tissues not associated with pharyngeal arches are also innervated by cranial nerves

Structures that arise directly from somitomeres or somites, surface ectoderm of the frontonasal prominence, neural crest cells, or the brain itself are also innervated by specific cranial nerves. Examples are as follows:

- The skin and connective tissue of the scalp arises from the surface ectoderm and neural crest of the frontonasal prominence. While the **posterior region of the scalp** is innervated by **cervical nerves C2 and C3 (greater occipital nerve),** its anterior region is innervated by **cranial nerve V (trigeminal nerve).**
- The extrinsic muscles of the eyes arise from cranial somitomeres and are innervated by **cranial nerves III, IV,** and **VI (oculomotor, trochlear,** and **abducens nerves,** respectively).
- The sphincter muscle of the pupil and ciliary muscles of the eye arise independently from cranial neural crest cells and are innervated by **cranial nerve III (oculomotor nerve).**
- The neural retina arises from the diencephalon of the brain and is innervated by **cranial nerve II (optic nerve).**
- The olfactory epithelium arises from the ectoderm of the frontonasal prominence (nasal placode) and is innervated by **cranial nerve I (olfactory nerve).**
- The auditory and vestibular organs of the inner ear arise from the ectoderm of the frontonasal prominence (otic placode) and are innervated by **cranial nerve VIII (vestibulocochlear nerve).**
- Muscles of the tongue arise from occipital somites and are innervated by **cranial nerve XII (hypoglossal nerve).**

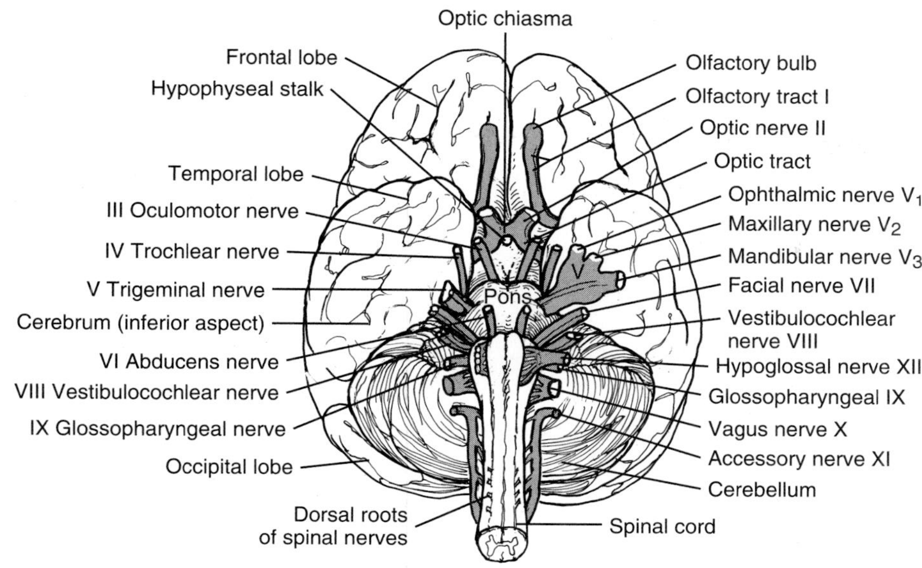

FIGURE 23–4
Emergence of the 12 cranial nerves from the brain (inferior view). Cranial nerves IX, X, and XI exit together through the jugular foramen while the hypoglossal nerve exits inferiorly through the hypoglossal canals in the lateral walls of the foramen magnum.

- Extrinsic muscles of the larynx (except for the cricothyroid muscle) are innervated by the cranial root of **cranial nerve XI (spinal accessory nerve).**

CRANIAL NERVE INNERVATION OF THE HEAD AND NECK

Numbering of the Cranial Nerves

Numbering of the cranial nerves from I to XII is based on the order of the nerves' origins along the base of the brain. Fig. 23–4 shows the relationship of each cranial nerve to the base of the brain, which determines its eventual route through the foramina of the skull to the exterior of the skull. Thus, the cranial nerves are arranged in the following order:

I (olfactory nerve) → II (optic nerve) → III (oculomotor nerve) →
IV (trochlear nerve) → V (trigeminal nerve → VI (abducens nerve) →
VII (facial nerve) → VIII (vestibulocochlear nerve) →
IX (glossopharyngeal nerve) → X (vagus nerve) →
XI (spinal accessory nerve) → XII (hypoglossal nerve)

▲ Using the Cranial Nerves as a Framework for Organizing Head and Neck Structures

The reader should recall that the framework of the peripheral nervous system was used to organize descriptions of the structure and function of the trunk. In the same way, the cranial nerves of the head and neck can be used as a framework to organize descriptions of head and neck structures, whether these structures arise from pharyngeal arches or from other tissues.

The discussion can be organized in two ways: (1) according to the sequence in which the cranial nerves originate from the base of the brain and (2) according to the specific anatomic targets and functions of the cranial nerves. The second method of organization (outlined in Table 23–1) is the most helpful and efficient.

Anatomic Targets of the Cranial Nerves

The specific functions of the cranial nerves depend on the nature of the nerves' anatomic targets. Cranial nerves V, VII, IX, and X innervate most of the head and neck structures (i.e., the skin, mucous membranes, striated and smooth muscles, and glands derived from the pharyngeal arches). Of these four nerves, cranial nerves V and VII innervate most of these structures. Cranial nerve IX innervates just a few structures of the head, oral cavity, pharynx, and neck. Most targets of cranial nerve X are in the trunk (see Chapters 4, 8, 9, and 11).

Each of the remaining eight cranial nerves innervates only a handful of end organs and has a more limited function. For example, cranial nerves III, IV, and VI innervate a few structures associated with the eye and orbit (mainly the extrinsic muscles of the eye). The three cranial nerves that innervate special sensory structures (I, II, and VIII) are each specialized to serve well-defined functions (i.e., smell, sight, balance, and hearing). Cranial nerve XII innervates muscles of the tongue. Finally, the cranial root of nerve XI innervates muscles of the larynx (except the cricothyroid muscle) after it joins the vagus nerve (X). The spinal roots of cranial nerve XI supply motor and sensory fibers to the trapezius and sternocleidomastoid muscles (see Table 23–1 and Chapter 27).

TABLE 23–2
General Terms Used in Discussion of Cranial Nerves

Terms	Brief Description	Example or Related Structures
Nucleus	Functionally related nerve cell bodies in the central nervous system (CNS)	Nucleus ambiguus
Ganglion	Nerve cell bodies located in a peripheral nerve usually visible as a "knot"	Trigeminal ganglion or geniculate ganglion
Tract	A bundle of parallel axons within the CNS	Optic tract
Nerve	Parallel axons and cells in the peripheral nervous system	Glossopharyngeal nerve
		Associated Cranial Nerve
BRAIN REGION		
Prosencephalon	The primary forebrain that develops into the cranial telencephalon and caudal diencephalon	
Rhombencephalon	The primary hindbrain that develops into the metencephalon and myelencephalon	
Telencephalon	Cranial region of forebrain	Olfactory bulb and tract (cranial nerve I)
Diencephalon	Ventral portion of the forebrain	Optic nerve II
Mesencephalon	Primary midbrain	Oculomotor nerve (III) and trochlear nerve (IV)
Metencephalon	Gives rise ventrally to the pons (the dorsal portion of the medulla); three cranial nerves exit the pons-medullar junction	Trigeminal nerve (V), abducens (VI) facial nerve (VII), vestibulocochlear nerve (VIII)
Myelencephalon	Caudal-most portion of the brain; gives rise to medulla oblongata (commonly called medulla)	Associated with cranial nerves IX–XII

Functions of the Cranial Nerves

As the targets listed above imply, the 12 cranial nerves of the human head may have motor, sensory, or autonomic functions

Like the spinal nerves of the trunk, the cranial nerves may innervate striated muscles or visceral structures or may carry impulses back to the central nervous system from sensory end organs. Moreover, the fundamental organization of all the cranial nerves, except for the olfactory (I) and optic (II) nerves, tends to include elements similar to those of spinal nerves of the trunk. Indeed, most of the 10 "spinal nerve-like cranial nerves" are associated with the brainstem (rhombencephalon; hindbrain), the part of the brain most like the spinal cord. While each cranial nerve may not contain all of the elements commonly found in a typical spinal nerve, when these elements are present, their anatomic relationships resemble the relationships of spinal nerve components and the spinal cord. Some examples follow:

- **Motor neurons** that innervate striated muscles of the head and neck are located in the ventral gray columns of the brainstem just as motor neurons that innervate striated muscles of the trunk are located in the ventral (basal) columns of the spinal cord (Figs. 23–5 and 23–6). Motor nuclei that arise from a pharyngeal arch and innervate striated muscle are classified as **branchial efferent (BE) neurons** (sometimes called special visceral efferent [SVE] neurons). Motor nuclei that arise from mesoderm not associated with the pharyngeal arches and innervate striated muscle are classified as **general somatic efferent (GSE) nuclei.** Axons emanating from both the BE and GSE motor nuclei leave the brainstem via a discrete **motor root** (see Figs. 23–5 and 23–6).
- **Central motor neurons of the cranial parasympathetic system** that innervate visceral structures of the head and neck (general visceral efferent [GVE] nuclei) are located near the medial sulcus of the midbrain or hindbrain just as central sympathetic neurons are located in intermediolateral cell columns of the spinal cord (Fig. 23–5).
- As in the case of the thoracolumbar sympathetic system, the **peripheral neurons of the cranial parasympathetic system** are located in peripheral ganglia. These are the ciliary ganglion of nerve III, the pterygopalatine and submandibular ganglia of nerve VII, the otic ganglion of nerve IX, and the many peripheral vagal ganglia of nerve X.
- Just as association neurons of the spinal cord are located in dorsal (alar) columns, **association neurons of cranial nerves** with general sensory functions are located in dorsal (alar) gray columns of the brainstem (Fig. 23–5).
- Like the dorsal root ganglia of the spinal nerves, cranial nerves with general somatic or visceral sensory

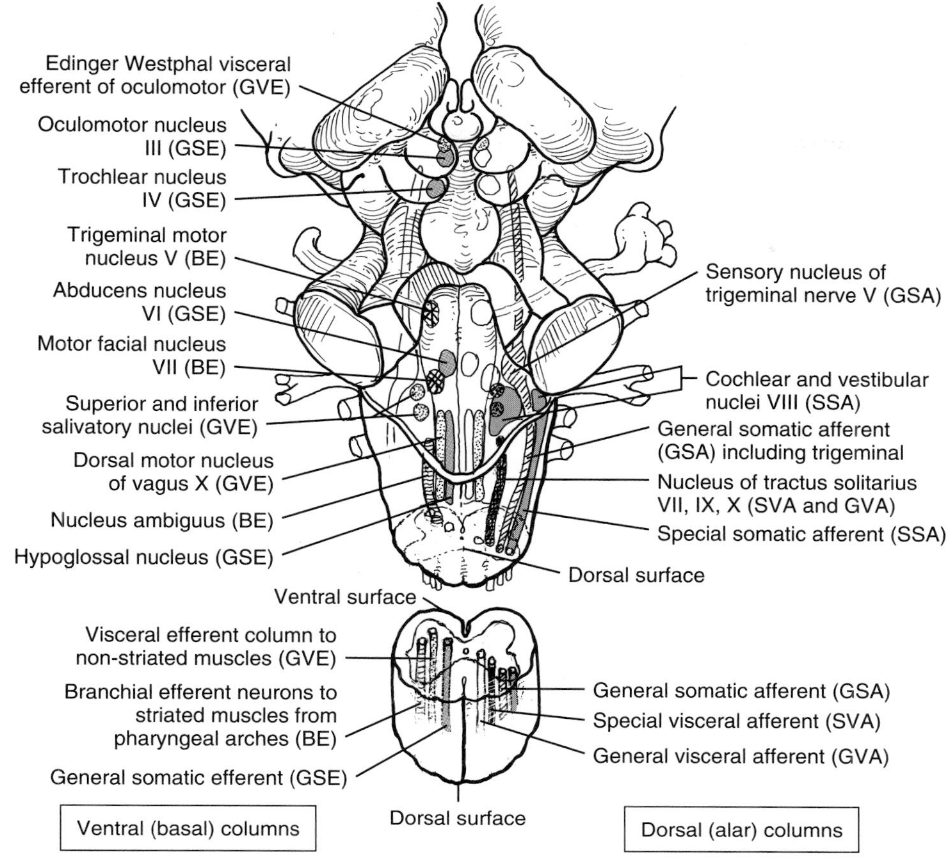

FIGURE 23–5
Anatomic relationships of cranial motor, sensory, and autonomic functions resemble the general organization of spinal nerve components in the spinal cord.

functions have sensory ganglia that contain **sensory neurons.** These are the trigeminal (semilunar) ganglion of nerve V, the combined superior ganglia of nerves IX and X, the inferior (petrosal) ganglion of nerve IX, the inferior (nodose) ganglion of nerve X, the combined superior ganglia of nerves VII and VIII, and the inferior (geniculate) ganglion of nerve VII. In addition, nerve VIII, which has a special sensory function, has a distal vestibular ganglion and a cochlear ganglion (Fig. 23–5). As in the case of the dorsal root ganglia, these cranial sensory ganglia contain unipolar axons, which innervate the association neurons related to the same nerve via an identifiable **sensory root.** These neurons also emit centrifugal axons, which innervate the sensory end organs that are related to the same nerve (Fig. 23–6).

The two cranial nerves whose organization deviates most significantly from this fundamental pattern are the olfactory nerve (I), which serves the function of smell, and the optic nerve (II), which serves the function of sight. These nerves are associated with the unique, more advanced part of the brain, the forebrain (see below).

Cranial Nerves With Sensory Function. *Individual cranial nerves may contain one, two, or three of the four different kinds of sensory fibers.* Many of the cranial nerves contain sensory fibers. The specific nature, functions, and importance of these fibers vary, with some being more important than others.

- Cranial nerves V (trigeminal nerve), VII (facial nerve), IX (glossopharyngeal nerve), and X (vagus nerve) contain **general somatic afferent (GSA) fibers.** These fibers carry general sensory impulses from receptors in the **skin** or **mucosa** of the nasal, oral, pharyngeal, or laryngeal cavities or from **proprioceptive endings** in striated muscles (Box 23–1).
- Cranial nerves IX and X have **general visceral afferent (GVA) fibers,** which innervate **interoceptors.** Interoceptors sense chemical and pressural changes of the blood in the **carotid sinus** and **carotid body** at the root of the internal carotid artery in the upper part of the neck or in the aortic body. Cranial nerves IX and X also carry GVA fibers from glands or smooth muscles of the head and neck.

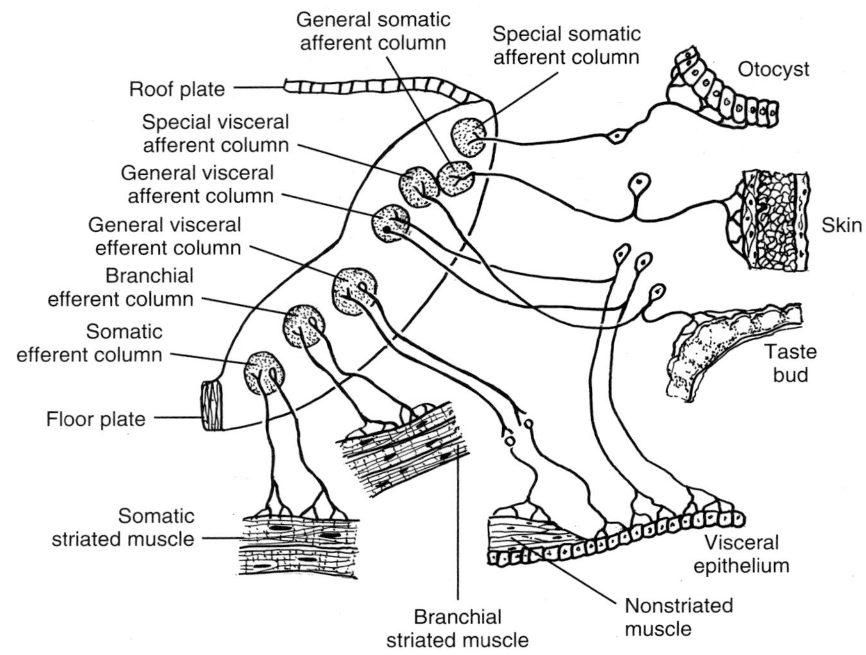

FIGURE 23–6
Idealized representation of organization of brainstem cranial nerve nuclei.

BOX 23–1
ANATOMIC ANNOTATION: CRANIAL NERVE FIBERS

GSA fibers, which carry proprioceptive (positional) information back to the brain from the striated muscles of the head and neck, are generally ignored when major functions of the cranial nerves are discussed. For example, note that nerves III, IV, VI, XI, and XII are not included in the list of nerves above that possess general sensory fibers. Nonetheless, the hypoglossal nerve (XII) does contain some general sensory fibers that carry proprioceptive impulses from muscles of the tongue back to the brainstem. Although the positional information of the tongue muscles is important for speech and deglutition, the proprioceptive fibers of nerve XII are simply ignored. The reason for this may be that there is no known clinical condition that affects only this component of the nerve. Nerves III, IV, and VI have also been omitted from this group because of the unusual proprioceptive innervation of the extrinsic ocular muscles. While the extrinsic ocular muscles contain proprioceptive end organs, the GSA fibers that innervate them are only present in distal regions of nerves III, IV, and VI. These distal fibers cross over to branches of the trigeminal nerve (V) to connect with cell bodies located in its semilunar (trigeminal) ganglion. Thus, even though these general sensory fibers innervate targets of nerves III, IV, and VI, they are more aptly considered to be components of cranial nerve V (see the detailed discussion of the cranial nerves in the text). Finally, the proprioceptive fibers that innervate the sternocleidomastoid and trapezius muscles are elements of spinal nerves C2 to C4 (see Table 23–1 and the discussion of cranial nerve XI in the text).

- In addition, cranial nerves VII, IX, and X contain **special visceral afferent (SVA) fibers,** which serve the function of **taste (gustation).**
- Finally, cranial nerves I, II, and VIII contain **special somatic afferent (SSA) fibers** (sometimes simply called *special sensory fibers*). The special sensory fibers of cranial nerve I (olfactory nerve) serve the function of **smell,** those of nerve II (optic nerve) the function of **sight,** and those of nerve VIII (vestibulocochlear nerve) the function of **balance** or **hearing,** or both.

Cranial Nerves With Motor Functions. *Individual cranial nerves may contain one or two of the three kinds of motor (efferent) fibers.* Nine of the twelve cranial nerves have motor fibers. In some cases, these efferent fibers innervate striated muscles derived from pharyngeal (branchial) arches and are called **BE fibers.** Cranial nerves with BE fibers include nerves V (trigeminal nerve), VII (facial nerve), IX (glossopharyngeal nerve), and X (vagus nerve) (Table 23–1). However, cranial nerve XI (accessory nerve) is also included in this group, not because the muscles it innervates are derived from a pharyngeal arch but because its neurons are located in the **nucleus ambiguus** (the same basal nucleus that serves nerves IX and X) or in basal columns closely related to the nucleus ambiguus (see Fig. 23–5).

As noted above, many other striated muscles of the head are derived from paraxial mesoderm that is not associated with a pharyngeal arch. These include the extrinsic muscles of the eye and muscles of the tongue. The cranial nerve motor fibers that innervate these muscles are called **general somatic efferent (GSE) fibers** as are the motor fibers in the spinal nerves that innervate striated muscles of the trunk and extremities. Cranial nerves with GSE fibers include nerves III (oculomotor nerve), IV (trochlear nerve), VI (abducens nerve), and XII (hypoglossal nerve) (see Table 23–1). GSE fibers arise from basal gray columns of the hindbrain located close to gray columns containing BE neurons (see Fig. 23–4).

Cranial Nerves With Autonomic Functions. Four cranial nerves that contain **general visceral efferent (GVE) fibers** (III, VII, IX, and X) carry out autonomic motor functions. Unlike the autonomic fibers of thoracic and lumbar spinal nerves, which have a sympathetic function, the autonomic fibers in these cranial nerves are **parasympathetic** in function. The organization of these parasympathetic mechanisms, however, is similar to that of the sympathetic nerves of the trunk. The central neurons of these parasympathetic pathways are located in intermediate gray columns near the medial sulci of the midbrain or hindbrain (Fig. 23–5). Their preganglionic fibers innervate neurons within one of four peripheral ganglia in the head: nerve III, the ciliary ganglion; nerve VII, the pterygopalatine and submandibular ganglia; nerve IX, the otic ganglion; and nerve X, a multitude of peripheral ganglia located in or near the walls of thoracic and abdominopelvic organs).

Autonomic nerves, whether parasympathetic or sympathetic, are considered to have a GVE function. In this textbook, sympathetic nerves will be designated as **sympathetic general visceral efferent (sGVE) nerves** and parasympathetic nerves as **parasympathetic general visceral efferent (pGVE) nerves.**

SPINAL NERVE INNERVATION OF THE HEAD AND NECK

Motor and Sensory Innervation of the Head and Neck by Spinal Nerves

Sensory fibers of spinal nerves C2 and C3 join to form the greater occipital nerve, which provides sensory innervation to the posterior part of the scalp (see Chapter 24). Spinal nerves C4 to C8 provide cutaneous innervation to the posterior skin of the neck. The lateral and anterior skin of the neck and inferior face is supplied by sensory branches of spinal nerves C2 to C4 via the cervical plexus (see Chapters 24 and 27). These include branches of the great auricular nerve (spinal nerves C2 and C3) and transverse cervical nerve (spinal nerves C2 and C3). Both motor and sensory fibers of spinal nerves C2 and C4 also assist the spinal roots of the spinal accessory nerve (C1 to C5) in the innervation of the trapezius and sternocleidomastoid muscles. Spinal nerves C1 to C8 provide motor innervation to many other muscles of the neck (see Chapters 5 and 27).

Sympathetic Innervation of the Head and Neck by Spinal Nerves

Sympathetic innervation of the head and neck is provided by thoracic spinal nerves

In addition to the parasympathetic innervation of head and neck structures by parasympathetic fibers from cranial nerves (see above), it should be noted that several structures of the head and neck are also innervated by sympathetic (sGVE) fibers from thoracic spinal nerves. Preganglionic fibers from central sympathetic neurons located within intermediolateral cell columns of the spinal cord at levels T1 to T3 or T4 rise within the upper thoracic and cervical sympathetic trunk to innervate peripheral sympathetic neurons housed within several pairs of cervical chain ganglia in the neck (Fig. 23–7 and see Chapters 4 and 27). There are usually three obvious pairs of these cervical sympathetic ganglia: a pair of **superior cervical ganglia** at vertebral levels C2 and C3, a pair of small **middle cervical ganglia** at vertebral level C6, and a pair of **cervicothoracic (stellate) ganglia.** Each superior cervical ganglion typically forms by fusion of the first four cervical sympathetic ganglia. The middle cervical ganglion represents the fifth and sixth cervical sympathetic ganglia. The cervical component of the stellate ganglion typically forms by fusion between the seventh and eighth cervical sympathetic ganglia. The entire stellate ganglion may include neurons from these two lowest cervical levels as well as thoracic ganglia from levels T1 to T4. A small **vertebral ganglion** is sometimes present between the middle cervical and stellate ganglia and is thought to represent a detached portion of one of these ganglia.

The cervical sympathetic ganglia do not possess white rami, since these ganglia obtain their innervation from the first three or four thoracic levels via the sympathetic trunk (Fig. 23–7). In order to innervate blood vessels and other smooth muscles of the neck, however, some of the postganglionic fibers emitted by the peripheral neurons in these ganglia travel to associated cervical spinal nerves via gray rami communicantes. On the other hand, in order to innervate various visceral

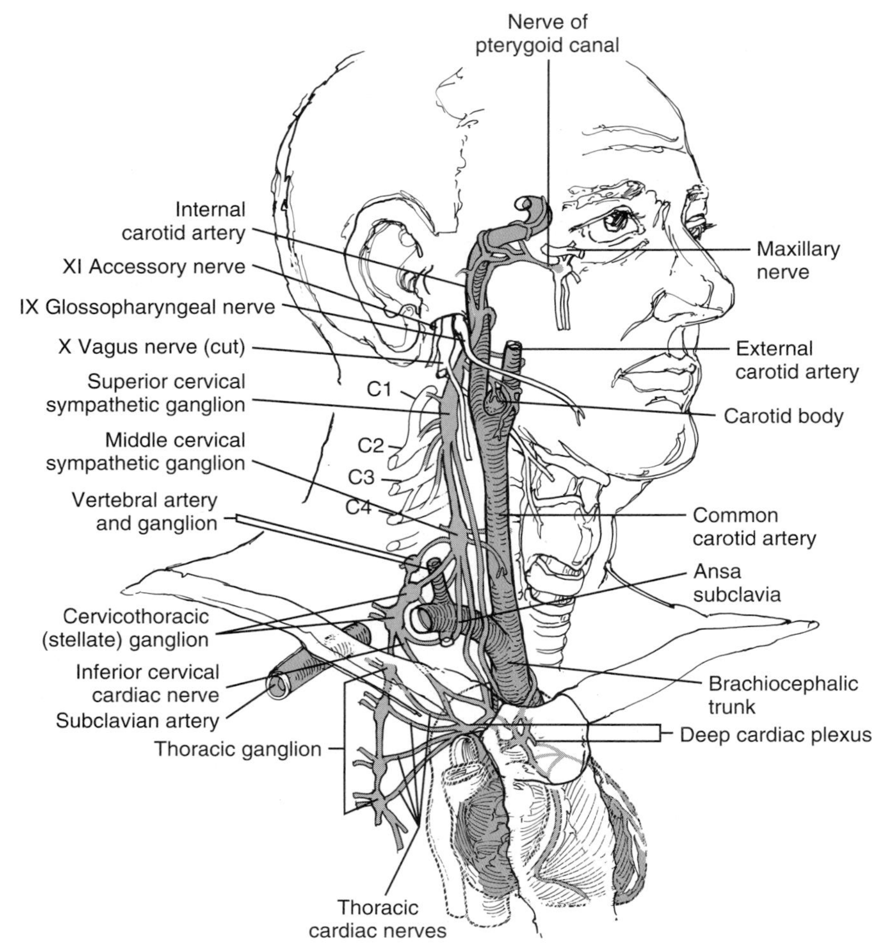

FIGURE 23–7
Sympathetic innervation of the head and neck.

structures of the head and neck, including glands and intrinsic ocular muscles, the peripheral neurons within the cervical chain ganglia emit postganglionic axons, which follow branches of the external or internal carotid arteries to their targets. In addition, some sympathetic postganglionic fibers may "hitch a ride" with various cranial nerve branches. They may even course through parasympathetic ganglia (without synapsing) to reach their targets. These various pathways are described in greater detail in Chapter 24.

24 The Scalp and Face

OVERVIEW OF THE HEAD AND NECK

This chapter describes the anatomy of the scalp and face. The orbit and ear are described in Chapter 25; the paranasal sinuses, nasal, oral, and pharyngeal cavities, and brain in Chapter 26; and the structures of the neck and vasculature of the head and neck in Chapter 27.

All of these chapters are organized according to the territories and targets of specific cranial nerves, spinal nerves, or related groups of cranial nerves.

This chapter on the scalp and face focuses on the territories and targets of cranial nerves V (trigeminal nerve) and VII (facial nerve).

In Chapter 25, on the orbit and ear, the first section describes the targets and functions of cranial nerves III (oculomotor nerve), IV (trochlear nerve), and VI (abducent nerve). These nerves innervate the extrinsic muscles of the eyeball. Discussions then focus on targets and functions of cranial nerves II (optic nerve) and VIII (vestibulocochlear nerve).

Chapter 26 begins with a discussion of the nasal cavity and cranial nerve I (olfactory nerve) and moves on to the oral cavity, pharynx, and cranial nerves IX (glossopharyngeal nerve), X (vagus nerve), and XII (hypoglossal nerve).

Cranial nerve XI (spinal accessory nerve) and its targets are discussed in Chapter 27.

The discussions of specific targets and territories of each nerve are accompanied by boxes describing the origin, structure, and pathway of the nerve. Although specific vessels are introduced in Chapters 24 to 26, the comprehensive discussion of the vasculature of the head and neck is presented in Chapter 27. This provides a framework for integrating and reviewing structures of the head and neck.

DEFINITIVE ANATOMY OF THE SCALP AND FACE

Anatomy of the Scalp and Face Based on Cranial Nerves V and VII and Spinal Nerves C2 and C3

Sensory territories and motor targets of cranial nerves V and VII and spinal nerves C2 and C3 can serve as a framework for most of the anatomy of the scalp, face, and nasal and oral cavities

It should be apparent from Table 23–1 that **cranial nerves V (trigeminal nerve)** and **VII (facial nerve)** are especially significant in the anatomy and function of structures of the scalp and face. These are the only two cranial nerves that serve moderately complex territories. It should also be clear that the other 10 cranial nerves serve quite specific structures and have limited functions (i.e., their territories are much less complicated than those of cranial nerves V and VII).

Sensory innervation of the scalp and face is mainly by branches of cranial nerve V with very small contributions made by cranial nerve VII and spinal nerves C2 and C3. **Motor innervation of facial muscles** is by cranial nerves V and VII. The first section of this chapter describes the sensory territory of the ophthalmic branch of the trigeminal nerve (i.e., the anterior scalp and superior face), gives a short introduction to branches of the facial nerve that innervate the occipitofrontal muscle of the scalp, and describes the sensory territories of the maxillary (midfacial) and mandibular (lower facial) divisions of the trigeminal nerve. The second part of the chapter describes the targets of motor branches of the mandibular branch of the trigeminal nerve (i.e., the muscles of mastication). The last part of the chapter focuses on targets of the facial nerve (i.e., general and special sensory territories, muscles of facial expression, and autonomic targets, including a variety of glands).

ANATOMY OF THE SCALP

The **scalp** is the soft tissue covering the superior region of the cranial vault and forehead between the highest nuchal line posteriorly and the supraorbital ridges (deep to the eyebrows) anteriorly. Its lateral boundaries are the temporal lines (Fig. 24–1).

Integument, Muscles, and Connective Tissues of the Scalp

The integument, muscles, and connective tissues of the scalp form five layers

The **integument of the scalp** consists of two layers: the **epidermis** and **dermis.** The skin from just above the supraorbital ridges anteriorly to the occipital protuberance and highest nuchal lines posteriorly is usually covered by a dense mat of hair. The skin of the scalp adheres firmly to an underlying **dense hypodermis,** much like the skin of the palms or soles (Fig. 24–2). The large, flat **oc-**

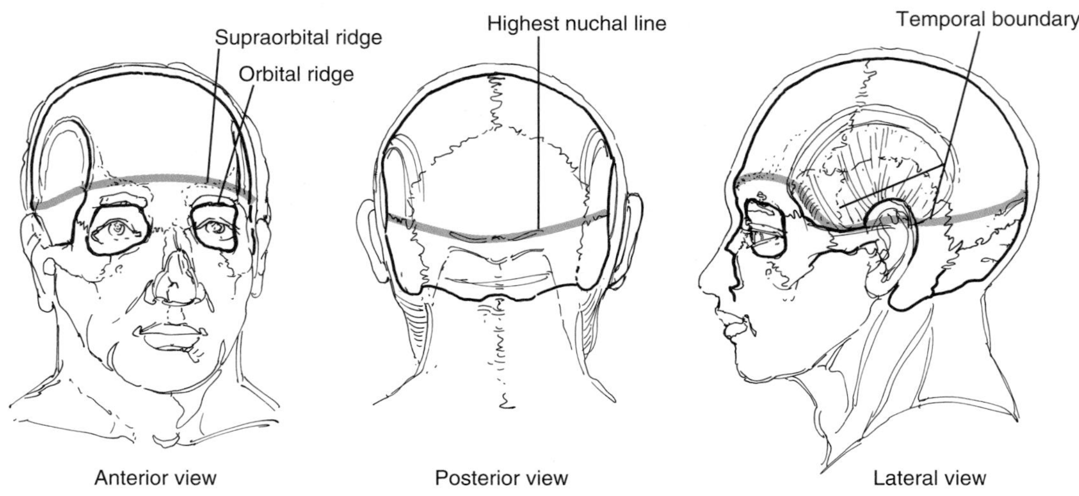

FIGURE 24-1
Boundaries of the scalp.

TABLE 24–1
Innervation of the Scalp

Definitive Structure	Nerve	Fibers
Integument of posterior scalp	Greater occipital nerve (C2, C3), dorsal rami	GSA
Integument of anteromedial forehead	Supratrochlear nerve of ophthalmic division of trigeminal nerve (V_1)	GSA
Integument of anterolateral forehead and most of anterior scalp	Supraorbital nerve of ophthalmic division of trigeminal nerve (V_1) Zygomaticotemporal nerve of maxillary division of trigeminal nerve (V_2)	GSA GSA
Frontal muscle	Temporal branch of facial nerve	BE
Occipital muscle	Posterior auricular branch of facial nerve	BE

GSA, General somatic afferent; *BE*, branchial efferent.

cipitofrontal (epicranial) muscle underlies the dense hypodermis and has four distinct bellies: a pair of anterior frontal muscles and a pair of posterior occipital muscles.

One of the anterior **frontal muscles** is on each side of the sagittal suture. These muscles are connected by an aponeurosis at their medial edges (Fig. 24–3). Their posterior edges are connected to the occipital muscles by an extensive flat aponeurosis called the **galea aponeurotica (epicranial aponeurosis).** Anteriorly, however, the frontal muscles simply blend with muscles and skin of the forehead in the region of the eyebrows. The frontal muscles thus have no direct connection to bone.

One of the paired posterior **occipital muscles** is also on each side of the sagittal suture. These muscles, however, are attached to the highest nuchal lines of the occipital bone posteriorly. They are connected across the midline by a fibrous aponeurosis (Fig. 24–3).

The frontal and occipital muscles and their aponeuroses adhere firmly to the more superficial, dense hypodermis but are only loosely connected to the deeper **loose areolar connective tissue.** This tissue covers the layer of **pericranium** that covers the calvaria of the skull (Fig. 24–2).

In summary, the five layers of the scalp, from superficial to deep, may be organized by the following acronym (Fig. 24–2):

S: Skin
C: Connective tissue (hypodermis)
A: Aponeurosis and muscle fibers of the occipitofrontal muscle
L: Loose areolar connective tissue
P: Pericranium (periosteum of the cranial vault)

It should be noted that, by convention, the **scalp proper** consists only of the three most superficial layers: the skin, dense hypodermis, and epicranial muscle and its aponeuroses.

▲ Vessels of the Scalp

The scalp's arterial supply is by branches of the carotid system (Fig. 24–4*A*). For example, the forehead and anterior scalp are vascularized by branches of the supraorbital artery (a branch of the internal carotid

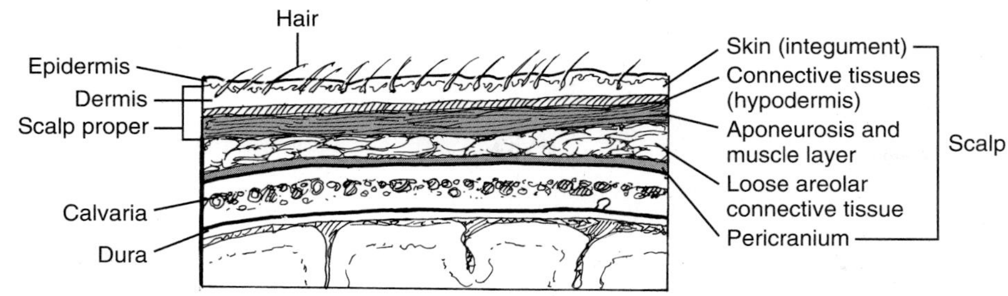

FIGURE 24-2
Layers of the scalp.

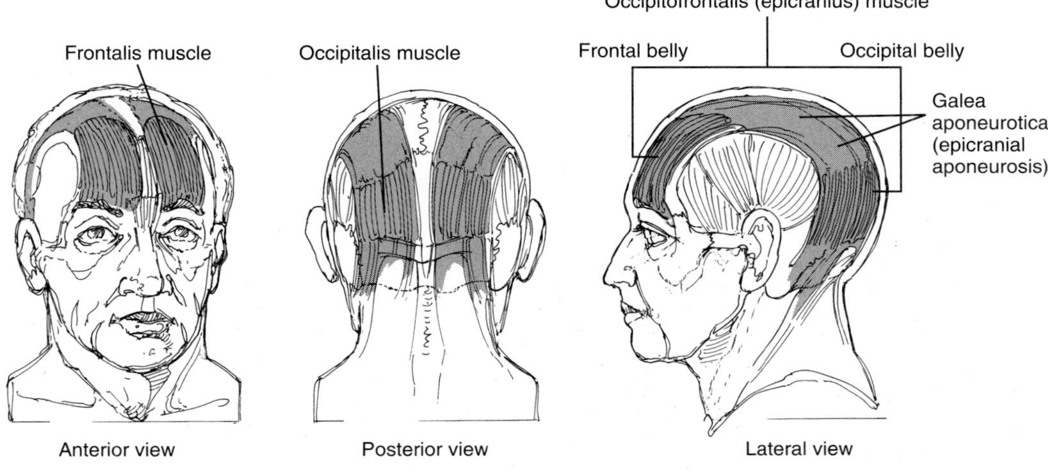

FIGURE 24-3
The occipitofrontalis muscle, its parts, and its connections.

artery); the temple and parietal part of the scalp by branches of the temporal artery (a branch of the external carotid artery); and the posterior scalp by the occipital artery (a branch of the external carotid artery).

Venous drainage of the scalp is by branches of the internal jugular system (supraorbital veins), by the external jugular system (facial, temporal, and posterior auricular veins), and by the vertebral system of veins (occipital veins) (Fig. 24–4).

Lymphatic fluids of the scalp drain ultimately into deep cervical lymph nodes and then into subclavian veins.

The vasculature of the entire head and neck is described in detail in Chapter 27.

▲ Developmental Origin of Tissues of the Scalp

The epidermis of the skin of the scalp, forehead, and nose is derived from surface ectoderm of the frontonasal prominence, while the dermis of the scalp is derived from cranial neural crest cells. These cranial neural crest cells form the hypodermis, loose areolar tissue, and pericranium (cranial periosteum) covering the calvaria. They also form bones of the cranial vault such as the frontal, parietal, temporal, and occipital squamae (see Chapter 22). The major muscle of the scalp, the occipitofrontal muscle, arises from paraxial mesoderm of the sixth cranial somitomeres associated with the second pharyngeal arches. Major blood vessels of the entire head and neck are derived from vessels of the pharyngeal arches (carotid arteries and jugular veins) and from intersegmental vessels of the neck (vertebral arteries and veins). The nerves of the scalp include branches of the cranial nerve to the first pharyngeal arch (trigeminal nerve), branches of the nerve to the second pharyngeal arch (facial nerve), and cervical spinal nerve branches (occipital nerves).

▲ Sensory Territories and Motor Targets in the Scalp

As has been noted, the scalp receives sensory fibers from both the C2 and C3 cervical spinal nerves and branches of cranial nerve V, the trigeminal nerve (Fig. 24–4*B* and *C* and Table 24–1). Motor innervation is provided solely by branches of cranial nerve VII. (Table 24–1).

Sensory Innervation of the Scalp by Cervical Spinal Nerves

Branches of spinal nerves C2 and C3 innervate the posterior scalp

Posteriorly, the skin of the scalp is innervated by general somatic afferent (GSA) fibers of the **greater occipital nerve.** This nerve is comprised of sensory

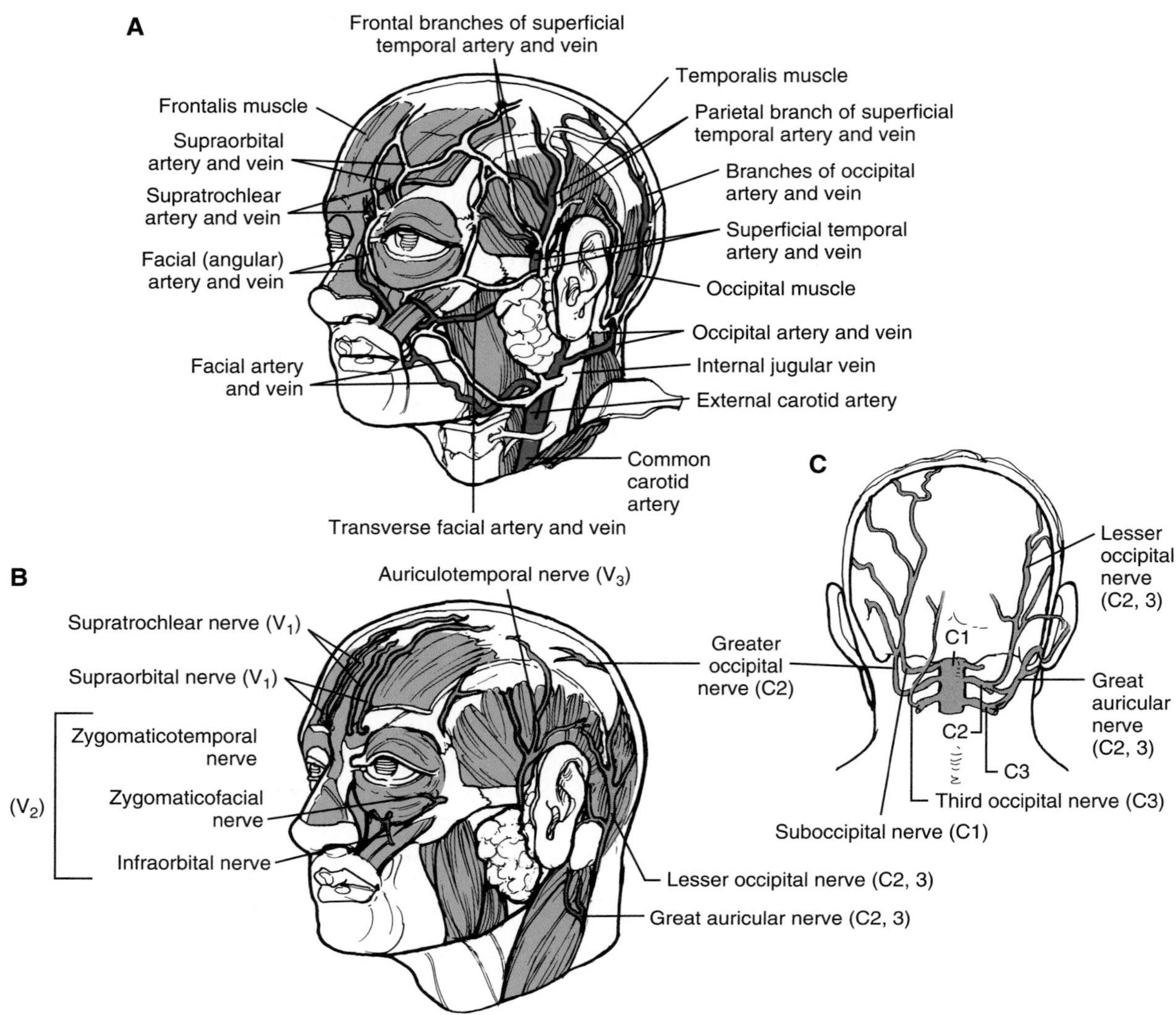

FIGURE 24-4
Nerves and vessels of the scalp. **A.** Arteries and veins of the scalp. **B.** Sensory innervation of the scalp by cervical spinal nerves and branches of cranial nerve V. **C.** Sensory cervical spinal nerve innervation of the scalp.

fibers from spinal nerves C2 and C3 (Fig. 24–4*B* and *C*, Table 24–1, and see Chapter 5). The reader may recall that spinal nerve C1 does not have sensory fibers and, therefore, is not involved in sensory innervation of the scalp.

Sensory Innervation of the Scalp by Cranial Nerves

Sensory innervation of the anterior scalp is by branches of the ophthalmic divisions of cranial nerve V

Sensory GSA innervation of the skin of the forehead and anterior scalp is provided by the supraorbital and supratrochlear branches of the **frontal nerve.** The frontal nerve is a branch of the ophthalmic division of cranial nerve V (trigeminal nerve) (Fig. 24–4*B*, Box 24–1, and see Table 24–1). The **supraorbital nerve** is lateral to the supratrochlear nerve. Its sensory territory includes much of the anterior scalp. However, the posterior boundary of its territory meets the anterior boundary of the sensory territory of the greater occipital nerve in the region of the **vertex** of the skull, which is the highest point of the cranial vault, or crown of the head (Fig. 24–4*B*). On the other hand, the **supratrochlear branch** of the frontal nerve provides sensory GSA innervation only to the anteromedial territory of the scalp, from the root of the nose to the hairline (Fig. 24–4*B* and see discussion of the relationships of ophthalmic branches of the trigeminal nerve below).

Cranial Nerve Motor Targets of the Scalp

The facial nerve innervates the occipitofrontal muscle

Because the occipitofrontal muscle arises from paraxial mesoderm of the second pharyngeal arch as a

BOX 24–1
INTRODUCTION TO CRANIAL NERVE V (TRIGEMINAL NERVE) AND ITS OPHTHALMIC DIVISION

The trigeminal nerve has sensory and motor functions

Because the trigeminal nerve has both sensory and motor functions, it possesses both sensory and motor roots. It is also associated with a large sensory trigeminal (semilunar) ganglion. Association neurons of the **sensory root** are located in three distinct nuclei: an elongated trigeminal nerve nucleus called the **mesencephalic nucleus,** the **principal sensory nucleus,** and the **nucleus of the spinal tract.** These nuclei are located in the alar columns of the mesencephalon (midbrain) and rhombencephalon (hindbrain) (Fig. 24–10).

The **sensory root** is larger than the motor root. It exits the ventrolateral surface of the pons near its upper border. The sensory root courses somewhat posterolaterally to the motor root, at first under the tentorium cerebelli and then under the superior petrosal sinus, to terminate on the posterior side of the trigeminal ganglion.

The **trigeminal (semilunar) ganglion** is located at the apex of the petrous temporal bone in a recess of the dura (trigeminal cave) covering the trigeminal recess. The posterior part of the cavernous sinus (see below) and the internal carotid artery lie just medial to each trigeminal ganglion. The trigeminal ganglion contains the unipolar general somatic sensory nerve cell bodies that serve all three divisions of the trigeminal nerve and that also give rise to the centripetal fibers that constitute the sensory root of the trigeminal nerve (Fig. 24–10). Some of these sensory neurons serve sensory receptors in the skin of the face, and others have proprioceptive functions.

Neurons that emit axons of the **motor root** are located in a small ovoid nucleus that lies just medial to the principal sensory nucleus at the cranial end of the hindbrain (Fig. 24–10). The motor root, like the sensory root, exits the brain from the ventrolateral surface of the pons near its superior border. It then courses under the tentorium cerebelli and superior petrosal sinus, terminating at the posterior side of the large trigeminal (semilunar) ganglion. These motor axons course through the semilunar ganglion without synapsing to provide motor fibers to the mandibular division of the trigeminal nerve. Three major nerves are emitted from the trigeminal ganglion: **ophthalmic nerve** (division 1 of the trigeminal nerve), **maxillary nerve** (division 2), and **mandibular nerve** (division 3).

All three divisions of the trigeminal nerve provide sensory innervation to the anterior scalp and most of the face; the third division also has motor fibers that innervate muscles of mastication

The **ophthalmic division** of the trigeminal nerve provides sensory innervation to the meninges, orbit, upper eyelid, side of the nose, paranasal air sinuses, forehead, and anterior scalp (see Table 24–2). The **maxillary division** sends sensory fibers to the meninges, lower eyelid***s,*** ala of the nose, cheeks, mucous membranes of the paranasal sinuses, nasal cavity, orbit***s,*** upper lip, upper teeth, and palate (see Table 24–3). The **mandibular division** provides sensory general somatic afferent (GSA) innervation to structures of the lower jaw, including the lower lip and lower teeth, external acoustic meatus, temporomandibular joint, and oral cavity and tongue (see Table 24–4). It also provides motor branchial efferent (BE) fibers to the muscles of mastication and associated muscles (see below).

The ophthalmic division of the trigeminal nerve contains only sensory (GSA) fibers, but some of its branches mix with fibers of other cranial nerves

Although the ophthalmic division of the trigeminal nerve is considered to be completely sensory, parasympathetic general visceral efferent (pGVE) fibers from the facial nerve and sympathetic fibers of the internal carotid plexus mix with distal segments of some ophthalmic nerve branches (see below). GSA fibers from the oculomotor, trochlear, and abducent nerves, which function in proprioception of extraocular muscles, also mix with branches of the trigeminal nerve. These associations are described immediately below and in discussions of the facial nerve.

The ophthalmic nerve branches from the semilunar ganglion

Once the **ophthalmic nerve** branches from the anteromedial side of the semilunar ganglion, it courses anteriorly along the lateral wall of the cavernous sinus, which is an expansion of the venous plexus just posterior to the superior orbital fissure and lateral to the body of the sphenoid bone (see below and Chapter 22). It is joined by sympathetic fibers from a plexus associated with the internal carotid artery and by fibers from the oculomotor, trochlear, and abducent nerves. These connections to nerves III, IV, and VI (which provide motor innervation to the extrinsic ocular muscle) are thought to be paths along which proprioceptive (GSA) fibers from extrinsic ocular muscles course back to the semilunar ganglion of cranial nerve V. Before it enters the orbit, the ophthalmic division usually ramifies into four branches: **recurrent tentorial nerve, lacrimal nerve, nasociliary nerve,** and **frontal nerve.**

1. The first branch that arises from the ophthalmic division is the **recurrent tentorial nerve.** This nerve innervates (with GSA fibers) the tentorium cerebelli, which is the large crescentic lamina of dura mater that covers the cerebellum and supports the overlying cerebral hemispheres (Fig. 24–10).

Continued

BOX 24–1, cont'd

INTRODUCTION TO CRANIAL NERVE V (TRIGEMINAL NERVE) AND ITS OPHTHALMIC DIVISION

2. Next, a small **lacrimal nerve** branches from the ophthalmic division. The lacrimal nerve enters the orbit along the lateral side of the superior orbital fissure to innervate the lacrimal gland (pGVE fibers) and associated epithelium of the conjunctival sac (GSA fibers). It then supplies the upper eyelid (GSA fibers) after joining with fibers of the facial nerve. The lacrimal nerve also receives fibers from the zygomaticotemporal branch of the maxillary nerve (intermediate division of the trigeminal nerve). It is thought that the zygomaticotemporal nerve provides the **secretomotor (pGVE) fibers** that innervate serous cells of the lacrimal gland. However, these secretomotor fibers ultimately originate from the facial nerve. They join the zygomaticofacial branch of the trigeminal nerve only after they pass through the pterygopalatine ganglion (Fig. 24–10).
3. A **nasociliary nerve** branches from the ophthalmic division and enters the orbit through the medial part of the supraorbital fissure. It crosses cranial nerve II (optic nerve), giving off several long ciliary nerves, the posterior ethmoidal nerve, and the infratrochlear nerve (Fig. 24–10). It then courses along the medial orbital wall where it becomes the **anterior ethmoidal nerve.** The anterior ethmoidal nerve then enters the cranial cavity via the anterior ethmoidal foramen and canal to course within a groove on the crista galli. It then penetrates the floor of the anterior fossa to enter the nasal cavity and splits into the following branches:
    - ♦ Two **internal nasal branches** supply the septal and lateral mucosa of the nasal wall
    - ♦ One **external nasal branch** exits the lower border of the nasal bone to supply the dorsum and apex of the nose
    - ♦ Two or three **long ciliary nerves** course anteriorly between the choroid and the sclera to supply the cornea and iris. The long ciliary nerves also supply sympathetic (sGVE) fibers from the internal carotid sympathetic plexus to the ciliary muscle and dilator pupillae muscles of the iris
    - ♦ One **infratrochlear nerve** branches in the vicinity of the anterior ethmoidal foramen courses between the medial wall of the orbit and the rectus medialis muscle (see Chapter 25). Along with fibers from the supratrochlear nerve, it supplies the medial upper eyelid, the lacrimal sac, caruncle, and skin of the lateral part of the root of the nose (Fig. 24–10).
    - ♦ One **posterior ethmoidal nerve** penetrates the medial orbital wall via the posterior ethmoidal foramen to supply the ethmoidal and sphenoidal air sinuses.
4. The fourth and final major branch of the ophthalmic division of the trigeminal nerve is the large **frontal nerve.** This nerve enters the orbit via the superior orbital fissure about halfway between the base and apex of the orbit and splits into the following:
    - ♦ a small **supratrochlear nerve** courses superiorly to the trochlea and exits the orbit to provide sensory (GSA) fibers to the conjunctive and skin of the upper eyelid. It continues to course superomedially (joining the infratrochlear nerve) to provide sensory (GSA) innervation to the skin of the lower forehead near the midline (Fig. 24–10).
    - ♦ **a larger** supraorbital nerve courses along the orbital roof and exits the orbit via the supraorbital notch (foramen) to provide sensory (GSA) innervation to the conjunctiva and upper eyelid. The nerve courses posteriorly in the scalp and splits into lateral and medial branches. The lateral supraorbital branch provides sensory innervation to the integument of the scalp as far posterior as the lambdoid suture (Fig. 24–10).

The nerves and targets of the ophthalmic division of the trigeminal nerve are summarized in Table 24–2.

muscle of facial expression, it is innervated by branches of cranial nerve VII (facial nerve). The frontal muscles (anterior bellies of the occipitofrontal muscle) are innervated by **temporal branches** (branchial efferent [BE] fibers) of the facial nerve. The occipital muscles (posterior bellies) are innervated by **posterior auricular branches** (BE fibers) of the facial nerve (see Fig. 24–24).

Function of the Scalp

The frontal muscles protract the scalp, raise the eyebrows, and wrinkle the forehead as in an expression of horror, surprise, or fear (Fig. 24–5). These muscles also produce wrinkles in the forehead when a person is frowning or angry. The occipital muscles retract the scalp. Thus, the frontal and occipital muscles working together pull the scalp back and forth (see also discussion of the facial nerve motor targets below). In general, blood vessels in the skin function to help regulate body heat. Because of the especially rich vasculature of the scalp (see Chapter 27), hair is important as an insulator to prevent excess loss of body heat.

Clinical Disorders of the Scalp

Injury to the Scalp. The three most superficial layers of the scalp (skin, subcutaneous connective tissue, and epicranial muscle and aponeuroses) are tightly fused, and so they often become detached as a unit when they are injured or when surgery is done. Indeed, if the epicranial muscle or galea aponeurotica remains undamaged by an incision or cut in the two most superficial layers, the muscle tends to hold the cut edges of the superficial layers together because it is so tightly fused to the overlying dense hypodermis.

The dense subcutaneous connective tissue tends to limit swelling of the scalp following injury. However, the presence of loose areolar tissue deep to the epicranial muscle allows blood, pus, or infection to spread within this layer. For this reason, it is called the **danger area of the scalp** (Fig. 24–6). Indeed, blood, pus, and infectious agents are not only able to spread through the region of the skull covered by loose areolar connective tissue, but may also gain access to the cranial cavity and meninges via emissary veins that penetrate the calvaria (see Chapter 27). Blood, pus, or infectious agents within the danger area of the scalp may also gain access to the eyelids and nose because the frontal muscles do not attach to bone anteriorly (Fig. 24–6). In contrast, infectious agents or fluids cannot spread to the back of the neck or lateral face inferior to the zygomatic arches because the epicranial connective tissue and its extensions are firmly fused to the occipital bone and zygomatic arches (Fig. 24–6).

Surgery of the Scalp. The scalp is vascularized and innervated by well-defined vessels and nerves from inferior sources (see Fig. 24–4 and Chapter 27). Therefore, when flaps of scalp tissue are detached to prepare the calvaria for a **craniotomy** to gain access to the cranial cavity, superior incisions are made so that the scalp may be reflected inferiorly from above to preserve its vascularization and innervation.

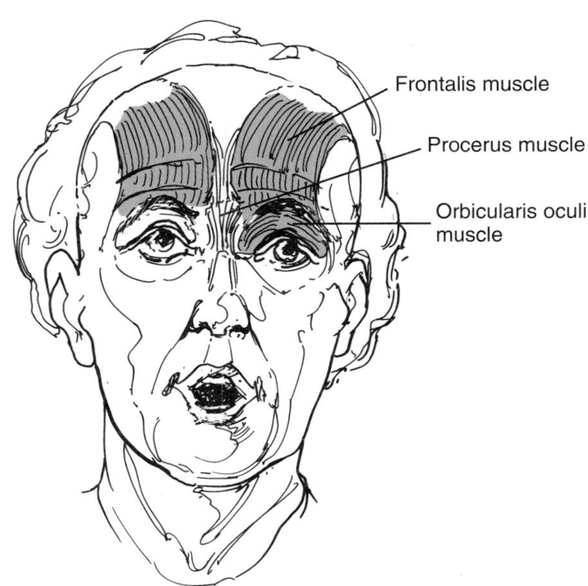

FIGURE 24-5
Frontalis and occipitalis muscles protract and retract the scalp, functioning in looks of surprise, horror, or fear. The frontalis muscle also produces wrinkles when a person is frowning.

ANATOMY OF THE FACE

Territory and Regions of the Face

The **territory of the face** extends from the forehead to the chin and from one ear to the other. The face arises from the embryonic **frontonasal prominence, two maxillary swellings,** and **two mandibular swellings.**

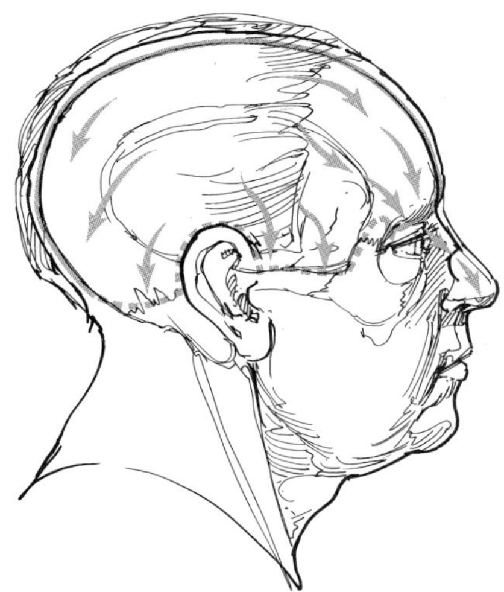

FIGURE 24-6
Danger area of the scalp: the area where blood or infection can be easily spread because of the presence of loose areolar tissue deep to the epicranius muscle.

The maxillary and mandibular swellings are structures of the first pharyngeal arch.

The **regions of the face** include the following (Fig. 24–7):

- **supraorbital region** (area directly above the orbit),
- **nasal region** (region of the nose),
- **orbital region** (region of the eye and eyelids),
- **infraorbital region** (area directly below the orbit),
- **zygomatic region** (bony prominence of the cheek),
- **buccal region** (soft part of the cheek),
- **oral region** (region surrounding the mouth),
- **mental region** (the chin),
- **masseteric region** (region where the mandibular ramus is covered by the masseter muscle; see below),
- **parotid region** (region of the parotid gland just anterior to the auricle), and
- **temporal region** (lateral face [temple]).

It should be understood that these regions blend with each other indistinctly. The face also has three deeper regions (fossae), which contain three important structures:

- **temporal fossa** (containing the upper part of the temporal muscle in the temporal region),
- **infratemporal fossa** (containing the lower part of the temporal muscle and the medial pterygoid muscle), and
- **pterygopalatine fossa** (containing the maxillary nerve, pterygopalatine ganglion, and terminus of the maxillary artery).

The temporal, infratemporal, and pterygopalatine fossae are described in Chapter 22 (see Fig. 22–13) in relation to muscles, nerves, and vessels, where appropriate.

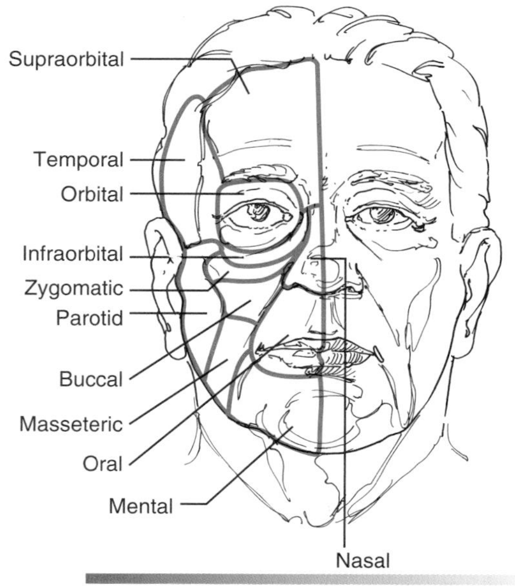

FIGURE 24-7
Regions of the face.

Surface Anatomy and Landmarks of the Face

The contours of the face are determined by the shapes of underlying bones and the mass and distribution of fat and muscles (Fig. 24–8). Notable landmarks of the face include the smooth **frontal tuberosities** of the frontal bone of the forehead and the prominence of the eyebrows, which covers underlying **superciliary arches.** The medial protrusion above the root of the nose is the **glabella** of the frontal bone (see below and Chapter 22). Below the superciliary arches are the **orbits** with their **globes (eyeballs), upper** and **lower eyelids,** and **medial** and **lateral canthi (angles).** Inferior to the glabella is the **nose** with its **root** (attachment to the forehead) and **apex** (tip of the nose), which are connected by an intervening **dorsum** (Fig. 24–8). The nasal openings (nostrils) are the **external nares,** each of which opens into a **nasal vestibule.** The external nares are separated by the **septum nasi.** Each nostril is bounded laterally by an **ala** (from the Latin for "wing"). Landmarks of the upper lip include the **philtrum,** a median groove bounded by **philtral ridges** laterally and a **philtral tubercle** inferiorly. The **nasolabial sulci** are grooves extending from each ala to the corner of the mouth. The **inferior buccolabial sulci** are grooves that extend inferiorly from each corner (angle) of the mouth. The **mentolabial sulcus** is a horizontal groove about halfway between the lower lip and the chin (Fig. 24–8). In addition, the cheeks, especially in infancy, are defined by protrusion of the **buccal fat pads,** which prevent the collapse of the cheeks when an infant is suckling. The opening of the mouth is the **oral fissure,** which is bounded at each side by an **oral angle.** Not technically considered parts of the face, the ears are characterized by prominent **auricles,** or **pinnae,** which are the projecting parts of the external ears. Each auricle encloses the external opening of the ear, the **external acoustic meatus** (Fig. 24–8). As discussed in Chapter 22, the shape of the face changes dramatically during infancy and early childhood as the paranasal sinuses and dentition develop and increase the size of the facial skeleton.

Structures of the Face

The tissues of the face include the integument and its appendages, associated fat, and connective tissue. Between the integument and the underlying skeleton are two groups of muscles: the muscles of mastication and muscles of facial expression. Interspersed with the connective tissue and muscles of the face are the nerves and vessels of the face (see below and Chapter 27).

Integument, Integumental Appendages, and Connective Tissues of the Face

The **integument of the face** varies in thickness. It is quite thin in the regions of the lips, auricle, and external acoustic meatus of the ears, eyelids, and nose. The skin of the face is connected to underlying bones by small, specialized ligaments called the **retinacula cutis.** In the regions of the external nares (nasal openings), lips, and eyelids, the skin is continuous with the mucous membrane lining the oral cavity, nasal chambers, and inner surfaces of the eyelids.

The skin of the face contains **specialized appendages,** including **hair follicles, sebaceous glands,** and **sweat glands.** The skin of the eyelids contains specialized sebaceous glands called **tarsal glands,** which secrete an oily substance that retains tears within the conjunctival sac. Modified sudoriferous (sweat) glands called **ciliary glands** of the eyelids open in the region of the roots of the eyelashes. The integument of the external acoustic meatus also contains modified sweat glands, the **ceruminous glands,** which secrete a waxy substance that protects the skin of the ear canal from water and may also discourage insects from entering the canal. Sebaceous glands are especially numerous and large in the skin of the nose. A large **parotid salivary gland** is located just anteroinferior to each auricle, thus overlying the mandibular ramus and posterior portion of the masseter muscle. A parotid duct issues from its anterior edge and courses over the anterior part of the masseter muscle. At the edge of the masseter muscle, the duct turns inward to penetrate the buccinator muscle. The **submandibular salivary glands** are located at the posterolateral edges of the mylohyoid muscles just inferomedial to the body of the mandible. The parotid and submandibular salivary glands are palpable, especially when inflamed. A third pair of salivary glands, the **sublingual salivary glands,** is located within the oral cavity just under and alongside the tongue. They extend to the **mandibular symphysis.** All three of these glands are discussed in detail below.

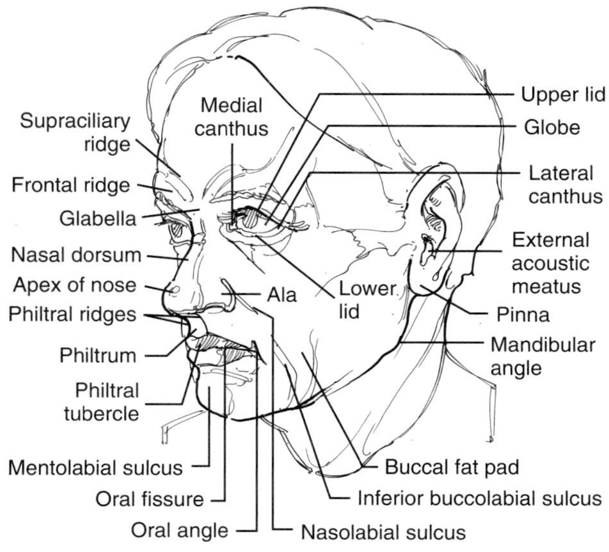

FIGURE 24-8
Surface anatomy of the face.

In most regions of the face, a relatively thin layer of **subcutaneous connective tissue** lies beneath the skin. In the buccal region, however, a thicker fat pad underlies the skin.

Clinical Disorders of the Palpebral Glands. Obstruction of the ciliary gland ducts may result in the formation of pus (suppuration). This may cause the eyelid to swell, and a **sty** may form on the eyelid. Inflammation of the tarsal gland may produce swelling that irritates the eyeball and causes extreme pain when a person blinks **(tarsal chalazion).** (*Chalazion* is from the Greek for "sty," "tubercle," or "cyst.")

Muscles of the Face

Several muscles of mastication and facial expression are sandwiched between the bones and the skin of the face. Most of these muscles are attached to underlying bone, but, in many cases, they are also intimately inserted into the overlying skin. It is thus quite difficult to dissect the facial skin free without damaging underlying muscles.

The **muscles of mastication** include the temporal, lateral, and medial pterygoid, masseter, and mylohyoid muscles (see Fig. 24–13). Associated muscles arising from the same source (see discussion of structures of the first pharyngeal arch below) are the anterior belly of the digastric muscle, tensor muscle of the tympanum, and tensor muscle of the velum palatini (see Fig. 24–14). All of these muscles are innervated by nerves of the mandibular division (the "third" division or V_3 of cranial nerve V [trigeminal nerve]).

The **muscles of facial expression** include the orbicular muscle of the eye; orbicular muscle of the mouth; and risorius, platysma, auricular, and occipitofrontal (epicranial) muscles, as well as many others (see Fig. 24–21). Associated muscles that arise from the same source include the buccinator muscle, posterior belly of the digastric muscle, stylohyoid muscle, and stapedius muscle (see Fig. 24–22). These muscles are innervated by branches of cranial nerve VII (facial nerve).

Although the muscles of mastication and muscles of facial expression originate from different sites, they migrate and intermix during development within the territory of the face. As the muscles migrate, however, individual branches of the trigeminal and facial nerves elongate to maintain connections to their original targets.

Vessels of the Face

The vasculature of the head and neck consists of branches of the internal and external carotid arteries, branches of the jugular system of veins, and a system of lymphatic vessels. These vascular systems are described as a unit in Chapter 27. Specific branches of these vessels, however, are described where appropriate in this and the following two chapters.

Developmental Origins of Tissues of the Face

The skin of the forehead, eyelids, nose, and philtrum is derived from surface ectoderm of the frontonasal prominence (see Chapter 23). The skin of the cheeks and lateral upper lip is derived from surface ectoderm of the maxillary swellings. The skin of the jaw arises from surface ectoderm of the mandibular swellings. The muscles of mastication arise from the paraxial mesoderm of the fourth somitomeres of the mandibular swellings of the first pharyngeal arch. The muscles of facial expression originate from the paraxial mesoderm of the sixth somitomeres of the second pharyngeal arch. The auricles of the ears are formed by the first and second pharyngeal arches. The dermis, hypodermis, and much of the bone of the facial skeleton arise from ectomesenchymal cells of the neural crest. Most of the vessels and nerves of the face are derived from precursors that develop in the first and second pharyngeal arches.

GENERAL INTRODUCTION TO SENSORY TERRITORIES AND MOTOR TARGETS OF THE FACE

Sensory innervation of the face is by branches of all three divisions of the trigeminal nerve (ophthalmic, maxillary, and mandibular divisions) and by branches of the greater auricular (C2 and C3) and transverse cervical (C2 and C3) spinal nerves (Fig. 24–9*B*). A very small amount of the cutaneous innervation of the ear is by GSA fibers of the facial nerve. In the following discussion, sensory innervation by branches of the ophthalmic, maxillary, and mandibular divisions of the trigeminal nerve and branches of the facial and cervical nerves are described by region. Comprehensive descriptions of the ophthalmic, maxillary, and mandibular divisions are provided in Boxes 24–1 to 24–4 and Tables 24–2 to 24–6. Facial nerve branches are described in Boxes 24–5 to 24–8 and Tables 24–7 and 24–8.

▲ Sensory Territories and Motor Targets of the Trigeminal Nerve

Ophthalmic (V_1) and maxillary (V_2) divisions carry only sensory fibers, while the mandibular division (V_3) has both sensory territories and motor targets.

Sensory territories of the trigeminal nerve are discussed first, followed by the motor innervation of the muscles of mastication by the mandibular division.

Motor targets of the face include the muscles of mastication and muscles of facial expression. The **muscles of mastication** are innervated by branches of the mandibular division of the trigeminal nerve (see Fig. 24–15). The **muscles of facial expression** are innervated by branches of the facial nerve (see Fig. 24–24).

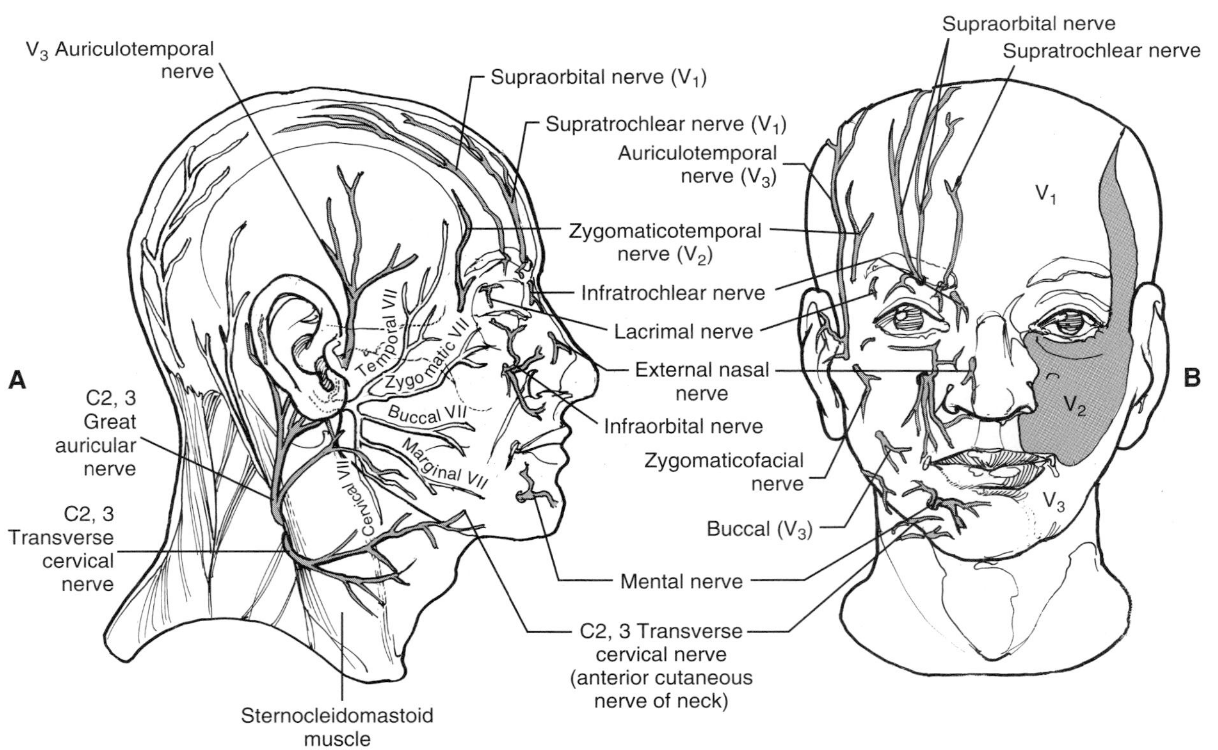

FIGURE 24-9

Sensory territories of the face served by ophthalmic V_1, maxillary V_2, and mandibular V_3 divisions of the trigeminal nerve. **A.** Lateral view (showing relative position of facial branches, VII). **B.** Frontal view showing branches of cranial nerve V only.

Cutaneous Innervation of the Supraorbital Region, Nasal Region, and Superior Part of the Orbital Region

The skin of the **supraorbital region** (forehead) is innervated by the **supraorbital** and **supratrochlear nerves** (GSA fibers). These are continuations of the frontal nerve (see Figs. 24–9 and 24–10 and discussion of the scalp above).

The skin of the **nasal region** is innervated by three major nerve branches (see Fig. 24–9). Two of these are branches of the ophthalmic division of the trigeminal nerve: the **infratrochlear branch** of the nasociliary nerve, which innervates the side of the root of the nose near the medial canthus (angle) of the eye, and the **external nasal branch** of the nasociliary nerve, which innervates the dorsum and apex of the nose (see Fig. 24–10 and Box 24–1). The third sensory nerve of the nose is a **nasal branch** of the infraorbital nerve of the trigeminal nerve's maxillary division (Box 24–2).

The skin of the superior part of the **orbital region** (encompassing the area of the upper eyelid) receives multiple branches of the ophthalmic division of the trigeminal nerve. For example, the upper eyelid and conjunctiva (inner epithelial lining of the eyelid) in the region of the medial canthus are innervated by the **infratrochlear branch** of the nasociliary nerve (GSA fibers) (see Figs. 24–9 and 24–10). More laterally, the

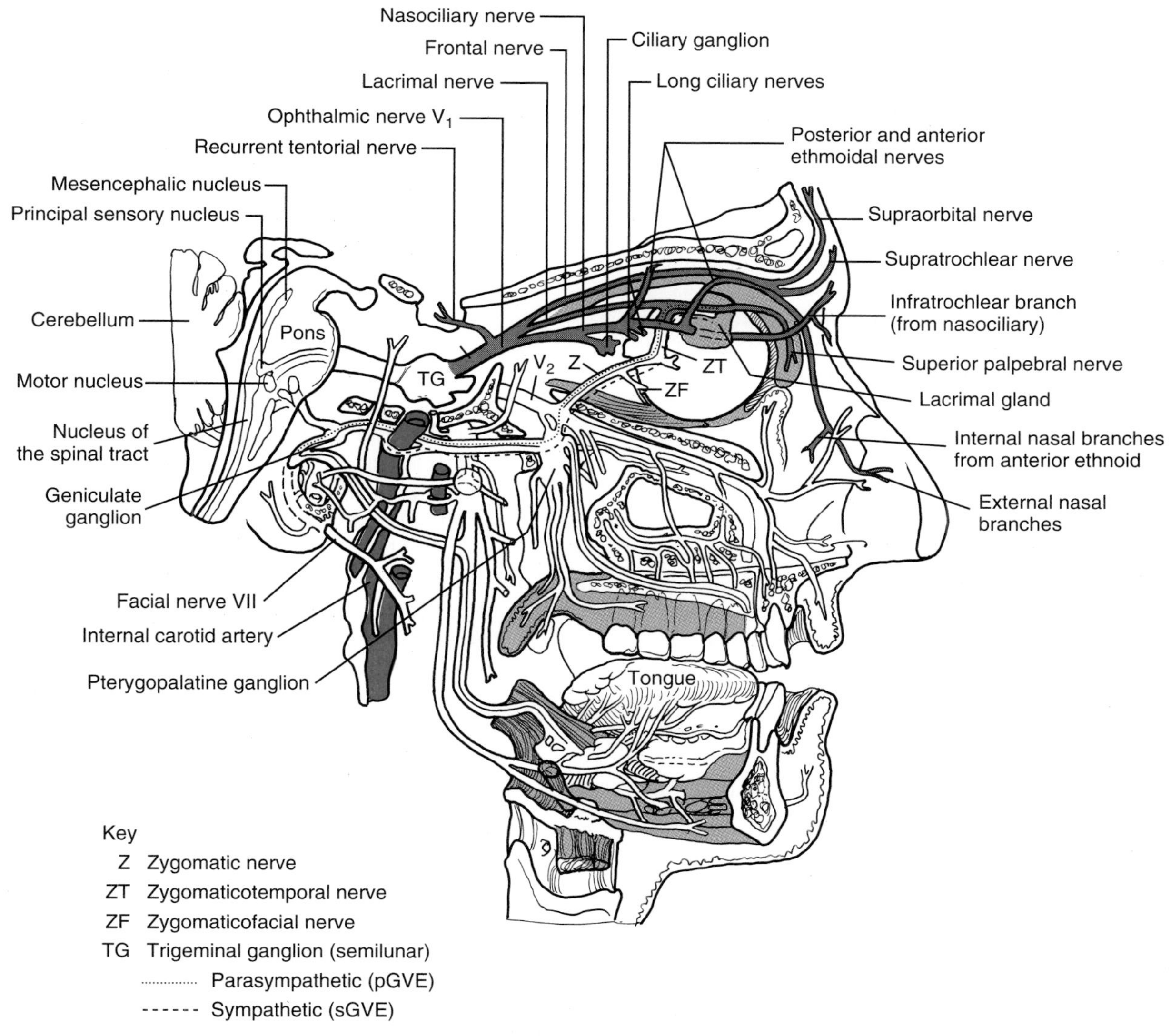

FIGURE 24-10

Sensory ophthalmic branch of the trigeminal nerve (shaded). Parasympathetic fibers from facial nerve VII and sympathetic fibers from the internal carotid plexus are carried by the zygomatic nerve to the lacrimal nerve.

BOX 24–2
MAXILLARY DIVISION OF THE TRIGEMINAL NERVE AND THE PTERYGOPALATINE GANGLION

The maxillary division of the trigeminal nerve contains only sensory fibers

Nerves that branch from the maxillary division of the trigeminal nerve, like those from the ophthalmic division, are sensory nerves only. However, some of these nerves may mix with sympathetic and parasympathetic motor fibers of the facial nerve in their peripheral regions (see below).

The maxillary nerve is a branch of the semilunar ganglion

The **maxillary division of the trigeminal nerve** branches from the semilunar ganglion just below the ophthalmic branch and courses anteriorly along the lateral wall of the cavernous sinus (see Fig. 24–11). It then exits the skull via the **foramen rotundum,** immediately passes through the superior region of the pterygopalatine fossa, and enters the orbit via the inferior orbital fissure (see Chapter 22).

The maxillary division of the trigeminal nerve ramifies into **three main branches** to the face: **zygomatic nerve, posterior superior alveolar (dental) nerve,** and **infraorbital nerve.** After passing through the pterygopalatine ganglion, it also produces branches called the *nerves of the pterygopalatine ganglion* (see Fig. 24–11).

1. Before entering the orbit, the maxillary nerve gives off a **zygomatic** *branch* within the pterygopalatine fossa. The zygomatic branch enters the orbit via the inferior orbital fissure. In the lateral wall of the orbit, it splits into two nerves: the **zygomaticotemporal nerve** and the **zygomaticofacial nerve** (see Fig. 24–11).
   - The **zygomaticotemporal nerve** exits the orbit via a foramen within the zygomatic bone. It then courses into the temporal fossa, piercing the temporal fascia and temporal muscle to provide general sensory innervation to the skin of the temple just laterosuperior to the eye. As it passes the lateral canthus of the eye, it gives off parasympathetic secretomotor fibers to the lacrimal nerve. These fibers innervate the lacrimal gland. However, the **parasympathetic (pGVE) fibers of the zygomaticotemporal nerve** originate from the facial nerve. They join the zygomaticotemporal nerve within the pterygopalatine ganglion (see Boxes 24–2 and 24–7). Parasympathetic fibers of the facial nerve also mix with other fibers of the maxillary division to form mixed nerves of the pterygopalatine ganglion (see Fig. 24–11).
   - The **zygomaticofacial nerve** exits the orbit via a foramen in the zygomatic bone to provide sensory innervation to the prominence of the cheek (zygomatic region) (see Fig. 24–11).
2. Below the zygomatic nerve, the maxillary nerve gives rise to a **posterior superior alveolar (dental) nerve.** This nerve branches from the maxillary nerve within the pterygopalatine fossa and gains entrance to the maxillary sinus, where it provides general sensory innervation to the mucosa of the maxillary sinus (see Fig. 24–11). The posterior superior alveolar nerve then splits into several branches to supply the molar teeth, associated gingivae, and adjacent cheek.
3. Below the point where the posterior superior alveolar nerve arises, the main trunk of the maxillary nerve enters the infraorbital groove. At this point, it is called the **infraorbital nerve** (see Fig. 24–11).
   - Within the infraorbital groove, the infraorbital nerve gives rise to a **middle superior alveolar branch.** This nerve enters the maxillary sinus where it supplies the lateral mucosal wall. It then splits into several branches, which supply the premolar teeth and their associated gingivae (see Fig. 24–11).
   - The infraorbital nerve next gives rise to an **anterior superior alveolar branch,** which gains entrance to the maxillary sinus to supply the mucosa of the anterior wall of the sinus and the incisor and canine teeth. It pierces the lateral wall of the inferior meatus of the nasal cavity to supply the mucous membrane in the floor and lateral wall of the nasal cavity (superior to the opening of the maxillary sinus). Its terminal branch supplies the nasal septum in the region of the anterior nasal spine (see Fig. 24–11).
   - After giving off the middle and anterior superior alveolar (dental) nerves, the infraorbital nerve continues to course anteriorly within the infraorbital canal. The infraorbital nerve then exits to the face via the infraorbital foramen of the maxilla (see Fig. 24–11). Once it has exited, it splits into a **nasal branch,** which supplies the ala of the nose, several **palpebral branches,** which innervate the lower eyelid, and the **superior labial branches** (see Fig. 24–11). These superior labial branches intermix with fibers from the facial nerve to form the **infraorbital plexus of nerves.** The branches then ramify to innervate (GSA fibers) the superior part of the buccal region (soft part of the cheek), upper lip (superior oral region), adjacent oral mucosa, and labial glands. The labial glands are small salivary glands that open into the vestibule of the oral cavity.
4. The maxillary division also produces several branches after it passes through the pterygopalatine ganglion in the pterygopalatine fossa. These branches may be referred to as **nerves of the pterygopalatine ganglion** (see below).

The **pterygopalatine ganglion** is a peripheral parasympathetic ganglion of cranial nerve VII (facial nerve) but is described here because of its intimate interactions with fibers of the maxillary division of cranial nerve V (trigeminal

BOX 24–2, cont'd
MAXILLARY DIVISION OF THE TRIGEMINAL NERVE AND THE PTERYGOPALATINE GANGLION

nerve). As has been noted, the maxillary nerve courses through the pterygopalatine fossa close to the pterygopalatine ganglion (see Fig. 24–11). Some of its fibers then enter the pterygopalatine ganglion but do not synapse there. Instead, they pass through, picking up postsynaptic parasympathetic fibers. These fibers are emitted by neurons within the ganglion that are innervated by presynaptic parasympathetic fibers arising from the parasympathetic central neurons of the facial nerve, which are located in a region of the hindbrain called the pons (part of the metencephalon of the hindbrain; see below). These facial parasympathetic presynaptic fibers from the pons emerge from the brain via the sensory root of the facial nerve **(nervus intermedius)** (see discussion of the facial nerve below), course through the sensory ganglion of the facial nerve **(geniculate ganglion)** (see below), and exit the geniculate ganglion with GSA fibers of the greater petrosal nerve (a sensory branch of the facial nerve carrying fibers that sense taste, mostly SVA fibers) (see Fig. 24–11).

The **greater petrosal nerve** joins with a collection of sympathetic fibers from the internal carotid plexus called the **deep petrosal nerve.** These two nerves enter the **pterygoid canal** together to form the **nerve of the pterygoid canal,** which contains GSA, SVA, pGVE, and sGVE fibers. The preganglionic parasympathetic fibers of the greater petrosal nerve synapse with neurons in the pterygoid ganglion. (All other fibers pass through the ganglion without synapsing to join with general sensory fibers from the maxillary division of the trigeminal nerve [see below]). Within the pterygopalatine ganglion, sensory (GSA) fibers of the maxillary nerve, postganglionic sympathetic (sGVE) fibers of the deep petrosal nerve, postganglionic parasympathetic (pGVE) fibers of the facial nerve, and special visceral afferent (SVA) fibers of the facial nerve intermix to form several **nerves of the pterygopalatine ganglion: orbital nerve, palatine nerve, nasal nerve,** and **pharyngeal nerve.**

- **Two or three tiny** orbital nerves enter the orbit via the infraorbital fissure to supply the orbital periosteum and orbital muscle (smooth muscle of unknown function spanning the inferior orbital fissure). Other fibers enter the ethmoidal foramen to innervate the mucosa of the ethmoidal and sphenoidal sinuses.
- The three **palatine nerves** are the one greater and two lesser (middle and posterior) palatine nerves (see Fig. 24–11). All three exit the inferior surface of the pterygopalatine ganglion to descend behind the perpendicular plate of the palatine bone. The **greater palatine nerve** gives off **posterior inferior nasal branches,** which penetrate the perpendicular plate of the palatine bone to gain access to the nasal cavity. These posterior inferior nasal nerves supply the inferior concha and middle and inferior meatuses. The greater palatine nerve continues downward to penetrate the hard palate via the greater palatine foramen. It courses forward on the underside of the hard palate to supply the mucosa and glands of the hard palate. It also communicates with branches of the nasopalatine nerve (see below). The **lesser palatine nerves** penetrate the hard palate via the lesser palatine foramina to supply the soft palate, uvula, and tonsils with GSA fibers. In addition, taste receptors of the palate are innervated by SVA fibers of the facial nerve that are carried by the greater and lesser palatine nerves, back through the pterygopalatine ganglion and greater petrosal nerve to the geniculate ganglion (see Box 24–6).
- Several **nasal branches** of the pterygopalatine ganglion are emitted from its anterior surface. These nerves enter the nasal cavity via the sphenopalatine foramen (see Fig. 24–11). Several **lateral posterior superior** and **medial posterior superior branches** innervate the mucosa of the roof of the nasal cavity, the posterior regions of the superior and middle nasal conchae and nasal septum, and the lining of the posterior ethmoidal air sinuses. A large **nasopalatine nerve** courses obliquely downward along the nasal septum, supplying the mucosa. It penetrates the hard palate via the nasopalatine foramen to supply the mucosa covering the most anterior region of the hard palate (see Fig. 24–11).
- Finally, a **pharyngeal nerve** is emitted from the posterior surface of the pterygopalatine ganglion. It gains entrance to the pharynx via the palatovaginal canal (see Chapter 22) to innervate the pharyngeal mucosa just posterior to the opening of the auditory tube (see Fig. 24–11).

upper eyelid and conjunctiva receive filaments from the **supratrochlear branch** of the frontal nerve. Laterally, the upper eyelid and conjunctiva receive sensory filaments from the **supraorbital branch** of the frontal nerve (see Fig. 24–9). In addition, a small branch of the **lacrimal nerve** supplies the skin and conjunctiva of the most lateral region of the upper eyelid (see Box 24–1).

Other Sensory Targets of the Ophthalmic Branch of the Trigeminal Nerve

Other sensory targets are the tentorium cerebelli, lacrimal sac, caruncle, associated conjunctiva of the upper eyelid, iris, cornea, and mucous membrane of the frontal, sphenoid, and ethmoid air sinuses

The **tentorium cerebelli** is a large crescentic lamina of dura mater that covers the cerebellum and serves as a supportive base for the cerebral hemispheres. It is provided with sensory innervation (GSA fibers) by the first nerve of the ophthalmic division of the trigeminal nerve, or recurrent tentorial nerve. The tentorium cerebelli also contains the **transverse sinuses** of the venous system, which drain structures of the cranial cavity and wall (see Chapter 27).

The **conjunctiva** is a mucous membrane that lines the inside of the eyelid (palpebral conjunctiva) and anterior aspect of the cornea of the eyeball (ocular, or bulbar, conjunctiva). The conjunctiva of the upper eyelid and all of the ocular conjunctiva are innervated by branches of the ophthalmic division (GSA fibers). The conjunctiva of the lower eyelid is innervated by branches of the maxillary division (GSA fibers) of the trigeminal nerve (Table 24–2 and see Box 24–1). The

TABLE 24–2
Ophthalmic Division of the Trigeminal Nerve and Its Branches and Territories

Nerve	Fibers	Target
Recurrent tentorial	GSA	Tentorium cerebelli
Lacrimal conjunctival	GSA	Lateral upper eyelid and its conjunctiva and associated lacrimal gland
	pGVE*	Lacrimal gland
	sGVE†	Lacrimal gland
Nasociliary		
Long ciliary	GSA	Iris, cornea (including all of ocular conjunctiva)
	sGVE†	Dilator pupillae muscle
Infratrochlear	GSA	Medial upper eyelid and its conjunctiva, lacrimal sac, caruncle, skin of lateral part of root of nose
Anterior ethmoidal	GSA	Mucous membrane of ethmoid air sinus
Internal nasal	GSA	Nasal septum and lateral wall of nasal chamber
	pGVE*	Mucous glands of nasal wall and septum, ethmoidal air sinus
	sGVE†	Mucous glands and blood vessels of nasal wall and septum, ethmoidal air sinus
External nasal	GSA	Dorsum, apex, vestibule of nose
	sGVE†	Blood vessels and sweat glands of dorsum, apex, vestibule of nose
Posterior ethmoidal	GSA	Ethmoidal and sphenoidal air sinuses
	pGVE*	Mucous glands of ethmoidal and sphenoidal air sinuses
	sGVE†	Mucous glands and blood vessels of ethmoidal, sphenoidal air sinuses
Frontal	GSA	Frontal air sinus, pericranium
	pGVE*	Mucous glands of frontal air sinus
	sGVE†	Mucous glands and blood vessels of frontal air sinus
Supraorbital	GSA	Anterolateral scalp to vertex, frontal air sinus, pericranium
	pGVE*	Mucous glands of frontal air sinus
	sGVE†	Mucous glands and blood vessels of frontal air sinus, blood vessels, arrector pili muscles and sweat glands of anterolateral scalp
Supratrochlear	GSA	Anteromedial scalp, frontal air sinus, pericranium
	pGVE*	Mucous glands of frontal air sinus
	sGVE†	Mucous glands and blood vessels of frontal air sinus and blood vessels, sweat glands, arrector pili muscles of hair of anteromedial scalp

GSA, General somatic afferent; *pGVE,* parasympathetic general visceral efferent; *sGVE,* sympathetic general visceral efferent.
*These pGVE fibers originate from cranial nerve VII (facial nerve) and are distributed to their targets by ophthalmic branches of the trigeminal nerve.
†These sGVE fibers originate from the internal carotid plexus and are distributed to their targets via branches of the ophthalmic division of the trigeminal nerve.

conjunctiva and conjunctival sac are more thoroughly described in Chapter 25.

The **lacrimal sac** is the superior opening of the nasolacrimal duct, which carries tears from the conjunctival sac (space between the inside surface of the eyelid and the anterior surface of the eyeball) to the nasal cavity (see Chapter 25). The **lacrimal caruncle** is an associated pinkish mass of tissue containing modified sweat and sebaceous glands. The lacrimal sac and caruncle are located within the medial canthus of the eye. Sensory innervation (GSA fibers) to the lacrimal sac and caruncle is provided by the infratrochlear nerve. The lacrimal gland is described in greater detail below as a parasympathetic target of the facial nerve and in the discussion of the orbit in Chapter 25.

The **iris** (from the Greek for "rainbow") is the delicate diaphragm that surrounds the pupil of the eye. The iris contracts and retracts to regulate the amount of light that strikes the retina (see Chapter 25). It is supplied with sensory innervation (GSA fibers) by the long ciliary nerve (see Fig. 24–10). The **cornea** is the anterior transparent covering of the eyeball (see Chapter 25) and is also supplied with sensory innervation (GSA fibers) by the long ciliary nerve. Its outer layer (ocular conjunctiva) is a mucous membrane, which is continuous with the conjunctival layer lining the inner eyelid. A rich sensory innervation to the cornea is necessary because of its extreme susceptibility to damage.

The **paranasal sinuses** are cavities within the bones of the face. They are virtually absent at birth but grow significantly during childhood. They include frontal, sphenoid, ethmoid, and maxillary sinuses. However, these cavities are of questionable function. The **mucous membrane** of the frontal, sphenoid, and ethmoid air sinuses is thinner and less vascular than the mucous membrane lining the nasal cavity (see below). Ciliary action propels the mucus formed within the sinuses into the nasal cavity (see Chapters 22 and 26 for more detailed discussions of the paranasal sinuses). The mucous membrane of the frontal sinus is provided with sensory innervation (GSA fibers) by a branch of the frontal nerve and by the supraorbital and supratrochlear nerves. The ethmoid sinus is provided with sensory innervation (GSA fibers) by the anterior and posterior ethmoidal branches of the nasociliary nerve and the sphenoid sinus by the posterior ethmoidal branch of the nasociliary nerve.

The **mucous membrane of the nasal septum** and **of the lateral walls of the nasal cavity** is highly vascularized and is provided with sensory innervation (GSA fibers) by the internal nasal branch of the nasociliary nerve (see Fig. 24–10). The function of this mucous membrane is to warm and moisten inspired air. This membrane is described more completely in discussions of maxillary nerve branches below. The nasal cavity is described in detail in Chapter 26.

While parasympathetic innervation of many structures (e.g., the lacrimal and mucous glands) is carried by distal segments of the trigeminal nerve, the source of these fibers is the facial nerve. These structures will be described at the end of this chapter.

Cutaneous Innervation of the Inferior Orbital, Zygomatic, Buccal, and Superior Oral Regions

The skin of the midregion of the anterior face (from the inferior orbital region to the superior oral region, including the cheek and ala of the nose) is innervated by branches of the **maxillary division** of the trigeminal nerve (Fig. 24–11 and see Fig. 24–9). These branches include zygomaticotemporal and zygomaticofacial nerves and palpebral, nasal, and superior labial branches. Their origins and relationships are described in Box 24–2. Specific sensory territories of these nerves include the following:

- The skin of the inferior part of the **orbital region** and the **infraorbital region** (encompassing the area of the lower eyelid and area just inferior to the lower eyelid) is innervated by **palpebral branches** (GSA fibers) of the infraorbital nerve of the maxillary division of the trigeminal nerve (Fig. 24–11 and see Box 24–2). The **infraorbital nerve** is a continuation of the maxillary division of the trigeminal nerve (see Box 24–2).
- The **zygomaticotemporal branch** of the zygomatic nerve (a branch of the maxillary nerve [see Box 24–2]) supplies a small ramus to the lacrimal nerve, which contains parasympathetic general visceral efferent (pGVE) fibers of the facial nerve (see above). The zygomaticotemporal nerve then enters the temporal fossa to supply general sensory afferent (GSA) fibers to the skin of the temple just laterosuperior to the eye (see Fig. 24–9 and Box 24–2).
- The skin of the **zygomatic region** (prominence of the cheek) is provided with sensory innervation (GSA fibers) by the **zygomaticofacial branch** of the zygomatic nerve (see Fig. 24–9*B*).
- The skin of the **ala of the nose** and the **vestibule** is innervated by **nasal branches** (GSA fibers) of the infraorbital nerve.
- Sensory innervation (GSA fibers) of the skin of the **superior labial region** (upper lip) is by the **superior labial branches** of the infraorbital nerve. Skin over the **buccal region** (soft part of the cheek) is innervated by the **buccal nerve** (joining buccal branches from the facial nerve) (see Fig. 24–9). A small patch of skin over the molar teeth is also innervated by the posterior superior alveolar dental nerve (GSA fibers).

Other Sensory Targets of the Maxillary Division of the Trigeminal Nerve. The **conjunctiva of the lower eyelid** is supplied by palpebral branches of the infraorbital nerve. The conjunctivas are described in detail in Chapter 25.

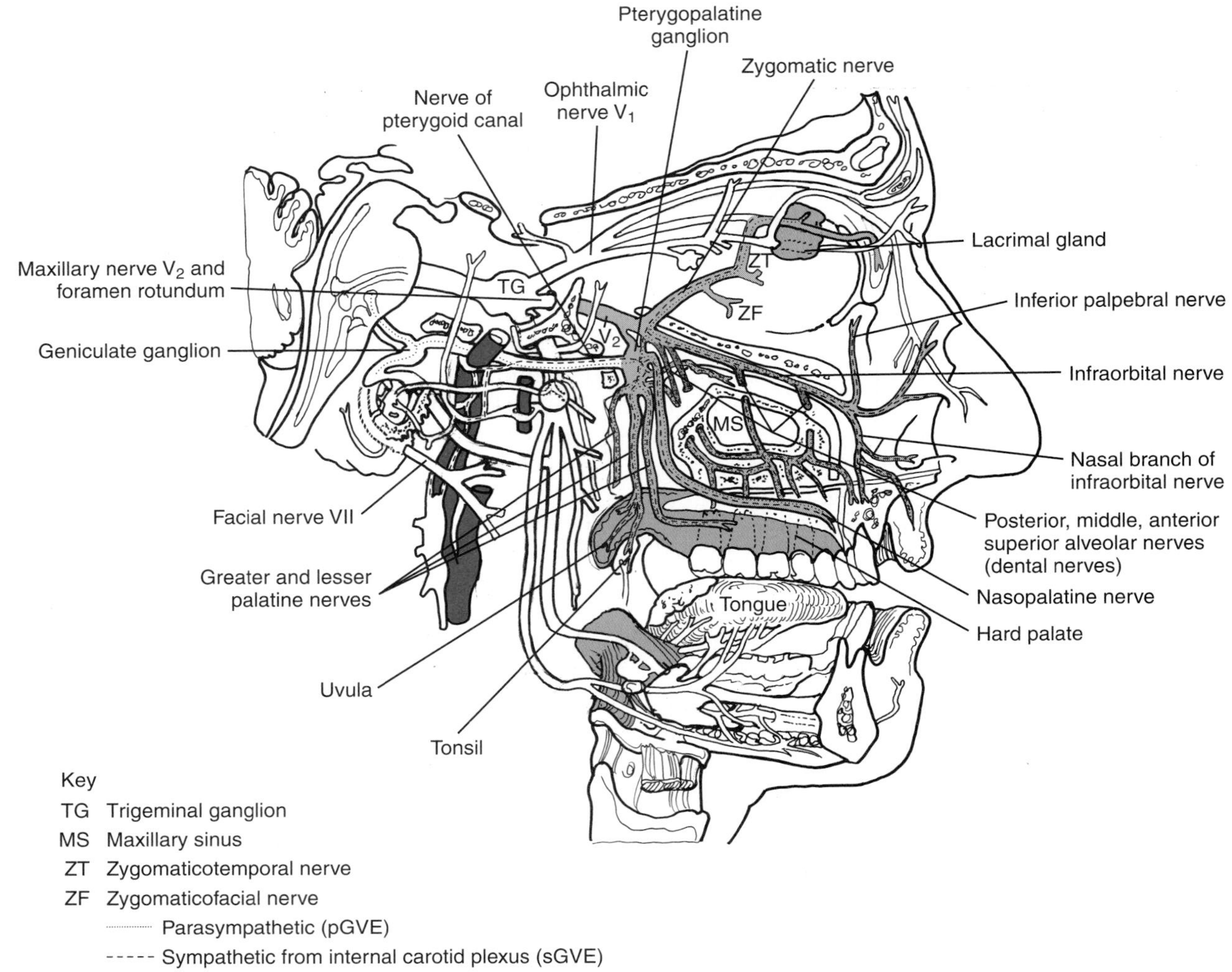

FIGURE 24-11
Sensory maxillary division of the trigeminal nerve (shaded). Branches pick up parasympathetic and sympathetic fibers as they pass through pterygopalatine ganglion.

The **mucosa of the maxillary sinus** is provided with sensory innervation (GSA fibers) by the posterior, middle, and anterior superior alveolar nerves (Fig. 24–11). The maxillary sinus is described in Chapters 22 and 26.

The **hard palate** consists of the bony primary palate (posterior extension of the intermaxillary process of the mid upper lip) and the bony part of the secondary palate, which is formed by medially growing palatine shelves of the maxillary processes. The hard palate (and soft palate) separate the upper nasal cavity from the lower oral cavity and pharynx. The mucous membrane of the hard palate is provided with sensory innervation (GSA fibers) by the greater (anterior) palatine and nasopalatine nerves. The **soft palate** is a posterior extension of the hard palate. It consists of muscle, lymphoid tissue, vessels, nerves, and mucous glands enclosed within a mucous membrane. The **uvula** is a small conical process that hangs from the middle of the lower border of the soft palate. GSA innervation of the soft palate and uvula is by the middle and posterior lesser palatine nerves (Fig. 24–11). The lesser palatine nerves also provide the **palatine tonsils** with GSA innervation. The palatine tonsils are concentrations of lymphoid tissue within the lateral walls of the oropharynx. (See Chapter 26 for further discussion of the hard palate, soft palate, and uvula.)

The **mucosa of most of the nasal cavity and nasal septum** is provided with GSA innervation mainly by branches of the maxillary division of the trigeminal nerve. A twig from the anterior superior alveolar nerve supplies the mucosa of the nasal septum in the region of the anterior nasal spine (Table 24–3).

A small region of the **mucous membrane of the pharynx** just posterior to the opening of the eustachian

TABLE 24–3
Nerves and Targets of the Maxillary Division of the Trigeminal Nerve

Nerve	Fibers	Target
ZYGOMATIC		
Zygomaticotemporal	GSA	Skin of temple just superolateral to eye
	sGVE*	Sweat glands, arrector pili muscles, blood vessels of skin just superolateral to eye
Ramus to lacrimal	pGVE†	Lacrimal gland
zygomaticofacial	GSA	Skin of zygomatic region
	sGVE*	Sweat glands, arrector pili muscles, blood vessels of skin of zygomatic region
SUPERIOR ALVEOLAR		
Posterior	GSA	Mucous membrane of maxillary sinus; maxillary molar teeth, associated gingiva, adjacent skin of buccal region
	pGVE†	Mucous glands of maxillary sinus and gingiva associated with maxillary molar teeth
	sGVE*	Mucous glands and blood vessels of maxillary sinus and sweat glands, arrector pili muscles, blood vessels of skin in region of maxillary molar teeth
Middle	GSA	Lateral mucosal wall of maxillary sinus, maxillary premolar teeth and associated gingiva
	pGVE†	Mucous glands of lateral wall of maxillary sinus and gingiva associated with maxillary premolar teeth
	sGVE*	Mucous glands and blood vessels of lateral wall of maxillary sinus and gingiva associated with maxillary premolar teeth
Anterior	GSA	Mucosa of anterior wall of maxillary sinus, maxillary incisor and canine teeth and associated gingiva, mucous membrane of nasal septum in region of anterior nasal spine
	pGVE†	Mucous glands of anterior wall of maxillary sinus; gingiva associated with maxillary canine teeth and nasal septum in region of anterior nasal spine
	sGVE*	Mucous glands and blood vessels of anterior wall of maxillary sinus, gingiva associated with canine teeth and anterior nasal septum
INFRAORBITAL		
Palpebral	GSA	Skin and conjunctiva of inferior orbital region (lower eyelid), skin of infraorbital region
	sGVE*	Sweat glands, arrector pili muscles, blood vessels of skin of inferior orbital region
Nasal	GSA	Skin of ala, vestibule of nose
	sGVE*	Sweat glands, arrector pili muscles, blood vessels of skin of ala and vestibule of nose
Superior labial	GSA	Skin of superior buccal region, skin of upper lip (superior oral region), adjacent oral mucosa
	pGVE†	Mucous and labial glands of oral mucosa
	sGVE*	Mucous and labial glands and blood vessels of oral mucosa, blood vessels, sweat glands, arrector pili muscles of superior buccal and superior oral regions
NERVES OF PTERYGOPALATINE GANGLION		
Orbital	GSA	Orbital periosteum, mucosa of ethmoidal and sphenoidal air sinuses
	pGVE†	Orbital muscle
	sGVE*	Orbital muscle
Palatine		
Greater (anterior)	GSA	Gums and mucous membrane of hard palate
palatine	pGVE†	Mucous glands of hard palate
	sGVE*	Mucous glands and blood vessels of hard palate
Posterior inferior	GSA	Mucosa of inferior concha and inferior and middle meatus
nasal branch	pGVE†	Mucous glands of inferior concha and inferior and middle meatus
	sGVE*	Mucous glands and blood vessels of inferior concha and inferior and middle meatus

GSA, General somatic afferent; *sGVE,* sympathetic general visceral efferent; *pGVE,* preganglionic general visceral efferent; *SVA,* special visceral afferent.

*sGVE fibers from the internal carotid plexus pass through the pterygopalatine ganglion and then "hitch a ride" with trigeminal nerve branches to innervate their targets.

†pGVE fibers from the facial nerve synapse in the pterygopalatine ganglion. Postganglionic fibers then "hitch a ride" with various trigeminal nerve branches to innervate their targets.

Continued

TABLE 24–3, cont'd
Nerves and Targets of the Maxillary Division of the Trigeminal Nerve

Nerve	Fibers	Target
NERVES OF PTERYGOPALATINE GANGLION—cont'd		
Lesser palatine (middle and posterior)	GSA	Mucosa of soft palate, uvula and tonsils
	SVA‡	Taste receptors of soft palate
	pGVE†	Mucous glands of soft palate, uvula, and tonsils
	sGVE*	Mucous glands and blood vessels of soft palate, uvula and tonsils
Nasal		
Lateral posterior superior and medial posterior superior	GSA	Mucosa of roof of nasal cavity, posterior regions of middle and posterior nasal conchae and of posterior ethmoidal air sinuses and nasal septum
	pGVE†	Mucous glands of posterior parts of superior and middle conchae, posterior ethmoidal air sinuses and posterior part of roof of nasal cavity and nasal septum
	sGVE*	Mucous glands and blood vessels of posterior parts of superior and middle conchae, posterior ethmoidal air sinuses and posterior part of roof of nasal cavity and nasal septum
Nasopalatine (long sphenopalatine)	GSA	Mucosa of nasal septum and anterior part of hard palate
	pGVE†	Mucous glands of nasal septum and anterior part of hard palate
	sGVE*	Mucous glands and blood vessels of nasal septum and anterior part of hard palate
Pharyngeal	GSA	Mucosa of pharynx just posterior to opening of auditory tube
	pGVE†	Mucous glands of pharynx just posterior to opening of auditory tube
	sGVE*	Mucous glands and blood vessels of pharynx just posterior to opening of auditory tube

‡SVA fibers of the facial nerve "hitch a ride" with greater and lesser palatine nerves, which carry them back to the pterygopalatine ganglion. These fibers course through the pterygopalatine ganglion without synapsing and then course to the geniculate ganglion of the facial nerve via the greater petrosal nerve. They then innervate taste receptors of the soft palate via the lesser palatine nerve and taste receptors of the hard palate via the posterior inferior nasal and nasopalatine nerves.

tube is provided with sensory innervation (GSA fibers) by a pharyngeal branch of the infraorbital nerve. The pharynx is discussed in detail in Chapter 26.

The **maxillary (upper) teeth** and associated **gingiva** are provided with GSA innervation by anterior, middle, and posterior superior alveolar nerves (Table 24–3). The teeth and gingiva are described in detail in Chapter 26.

Cutaneous Innervation of the Inferior Orbital Region by the Mandibular Division of the Trigeminal Nerve (V_3)

V_3 innervates the chin; masseteric, parotid, and temporal regions; auricle; external acoustic meatus; and tympanic membrane

The lower part of the face, chin, mandible, and temporal region are provided with sensory innervation by the third division of the trigeminal nerve, the **mandibular division** (see Fig. 24–9). Sensory nerves of the mandibular division include a meningeal branch and the buccal, auriculotemporal, lingual, and inferior alveolar (dental) nerves (Fig. 24–12, Box 24–3, and Table 24–4). The mandibular division of the trigeminal nerve also provides motor branches to the muscles of mastication, which are discussed in the following section (Box 24–4 and see Fig. 24–13 and Tables 24–5 and 24–6).

Innervation of most of the skin of the inferior part of the **oral region** (including the lower lip) and the **mental region** (chin) is by the **mental nerve** (GSA). The mental nerve is a branch of the inferior alveolar nerve. It penetrates the mandible via the mental foramen to gain access to the skin of the chin and inferior oral region (see below and Chapter 22). The most inferior skin of the mental region is innervated by spinal nerve branches of the anterior cutaneous nerve of the neck, which is a branch of the transverse cervical nerve (see Fig. 24–9 and Chapter 27).

The skin of the **masseteric region** of the face is innervated (GSA) by posterior branches of the mental nerve, anterior inferior branches of the buccal nerve, and spinal nerve branches (C2 and C3) of the great auricular nerve (see Fig. 24–9).

The skin of the inferior part of the **buccal region** of the face (over the soft part of the cheek) is supplied by the buccal nerve (see Fig. 24–9).

The buccal nerve also provides sensory innervation to the anterior part of the **parotid region.** The great auricular nerve supplies the posterior part of the parotid region (see Fig. 24–9).

Sensory innervation (GSA) to the skin of the **temporal region** is provided by superficial temporal branches of the auriculotemporal nerve (see Fig. 24–9).

Sensory innervation to the **skin of the auricle** and **external acoustic meatus** is provided by the mandibular division of the trigeminal nerve, the vagus nerve, and sensory branches of the great auricular and auriculotemporal nerves. Anterior auricular branches of the mandibular division of the trigeminal nerve in-

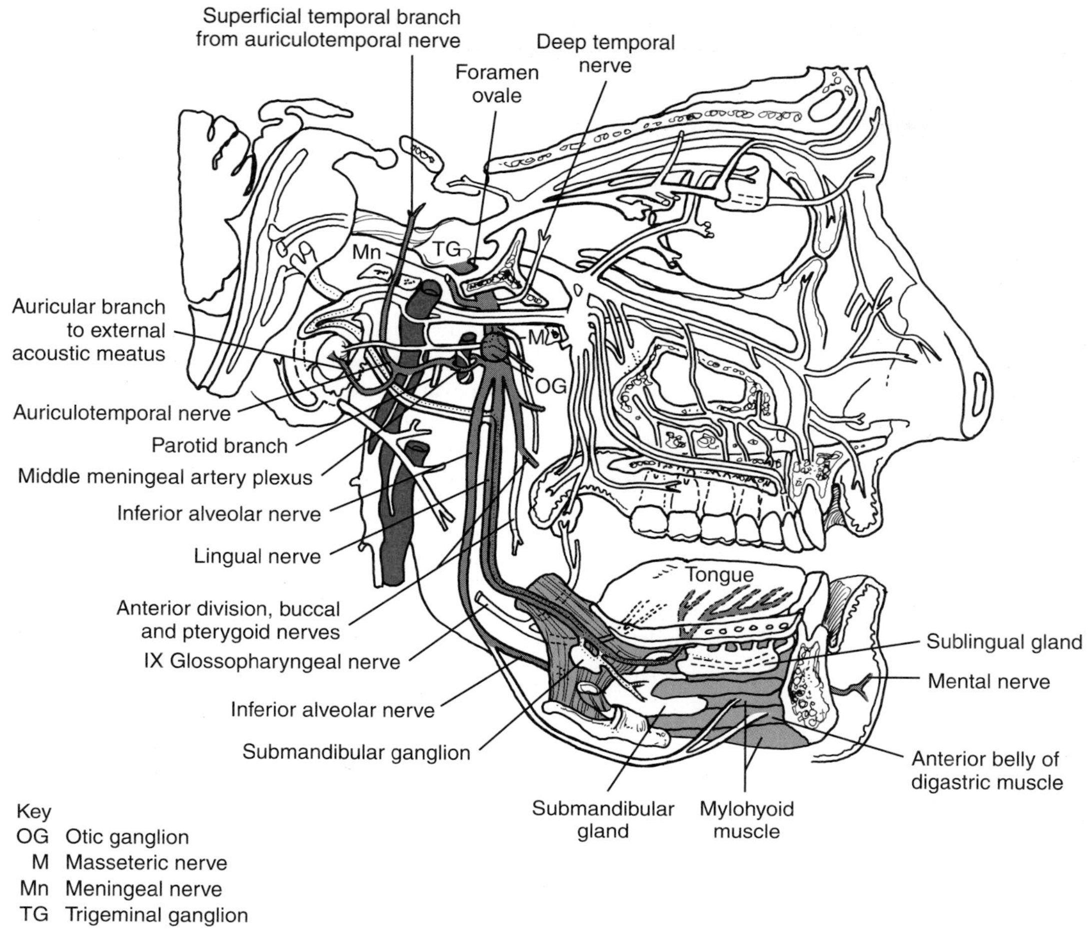

FIGURE 24-12
Sensory nerves of mandibular division of the trigeminal nerve (shaded). Both parasympathetic (pGVE) and sympathetic (sGVE) fibers are carried in the lingual and some branches of the auriculotemporal nerve. Buccal, mental, and meningeal nerves carry sympathetic fibers.

nervate the skin of the tragus and part of the helix of the auricle. The skin of the external acoustic meatus and the tympanic membrane is supplied by a V_3 (mandibular) branch to the external acoustic meatus. However, the skin on the cranial surface of the auricle, extending to the posterior wall of the external acoustic meatus and adjacent tympanic membrane, is supplied by an auricular branch of the vagus nerve (see below). Most of the skin of the anterior outer surface of the auricle, however, is innervated by spinal nerve branches of the great auricular nerve (C2 and C3), except for tiny areas of the conchal eminence and depression, which are innervated by facial nerve (GSA) sensory fibers that "hitch a ride" with the auricular branch of the vagus (see Fig. 24–19 and discussion of the facial nerve in Box 24–5).

Other Sensory Targets of the Mandibular Division of the Trigeminal Nerve

The meningeal branch of the mandibular nerve provides sensory innervation to the **dura of the middle cranial fossa** and some of the **anterior cranial fossa** and **calvaria.** The dura is a tough meningeal lining of the cranial cavity, which is formed from the periosteum and which encloses the brain. It also forms partitions that extend into the cranial cavity, the falx cerebri (which separate the cerebral hemispheres), and the falx cerebelli (which separate the cerebrum from the cerebellum). These structures also contain segments of the venous drainage system of the cranial cavity (see Chapter 27). The meningeal branch of the mandibular nerve also innervates the mucosa of the mastoid air sinuses. The **mucosa of the mastoid air cells** is also provided with sensory innervation by the meningeal branch of the mandibular nerve. The mastoid air cells are a group of intercommunicating cavities within the mastoid process. These cavities are continuous with cells in the petrous part of the temporal bone (mastoid antrum) and with the tympanic cavity (see Chapter 25).

The **gingiva** and **teeth of the mandible** are provided with general somatic afferent innervation by sev-

BOX 24–3

INTRODUCTION TO THE MANDIBULAR DIVISION OF THE TRIGEMINAL NERVE AND ITS SENSORY NERVES

The **mandibular division** of the trigeminal nerve has two roots: a **relatively large sensory root** and a **relatively small motor root.**

The **sensory root** courses from the lateral side of the semilunar ganglion and exits the skull immediately via the **foramen ovale.** The smaller **motor root** courses onto the anterolateral side of the semilunar ganglion and also exits the skull via the foramen ovale. The motor root then immediately joins the sensory root to form the **mandibular nerve** in the space between the medial pterygoid muscle and the tensor veli palatini muscle (see Fig. 24–12). Just beyond this point, the mandibular nerve gives rise to a **meningeal branch** (GSA and sympathetic fibers) and a **nerve to the medial pterygoid muscle** (branchial efferent fibers) (see discussion of motor nerves of the mandibular division in Box 24–4). Only the main sensory branches of the mandibular nerve are described here. They include the meningeal, buccal, auriculotemporal, lingual, and inferior alveolar nerves.

1. The **meningeal branch of the mandibular nerve** reenters the skull (with the middle meningeal artery) via the **foramen spinosum.** For this reason, it is also called the **nervus spinosum** (see Fig. 24–12). It then splits into anterior and posterior branches to supply the dura in the middle and anterior cranial fossae, the calvaria, and the mucous membrane of the mastoid air cells (see below and Chapter 22).

   After giving off the meningeal branch, the main trunk of the mandibular nerve immediately splits into **anterior** and **posterior trunks.** Both trunks contain sensory and motor fibers. However, the anterior division has mostly motor fibers and the posterior division mostly sensory fibers. The anterior division gives rise to a single sensory branch, the buccal nerve, and three motor branches (masseteric nerve, nerve to the lateral pterygoid muscle, and deep temporal branch). The posterior trunk gives rise to the auriculotemporal, lingual, and inferior alveolar (dental) nerves. These nerves are mainly sensory nerves, except that the inferior alveolar nerve gives rise to a small motor nerve to the mylohyoid muscle (and anterior belly of the digastric muscle; see below).
2. The **buccal branch of the mandibular nerve** arises from the **anterior trunk** of the mandibular nerve just inferior to the root of the nerve to the medial pterygoid muscle (see Fig. 24–12). It courses between the two heads of the lateral pterygoid muscle and descends deep to the temporal muscle and the ramus of the mandible (see below). It then emerges to provide sensory fibers to the skin of the inferior part of the buccal region, the mucous membrane that lines the inner surface of the buccal region, and the mucosa covering the adjacent buccal gingiva (fibrous connective tissue surrounding the roots of the teeth). Usually, these fibers join with buccal branches of the facial nerve (see below).
3. The **auriculotemporal branch of the mandibular nerve** usually arises from the **posterior trunk** of the mandibular nerve as two roots. Both roots course posteriorly, with the superior root passing over the middle meningeal artery and the inferior root passing under it. The two roots fuse just posterior to the artery to form the auriculotemporal nerve (see Fig. 24–12). The auriculotemporal nerve courses deep to the lateral pterygoid muscle, behind the temporomandibular joint, and just deep to the parotid gland (see Fig. 24–12). The nerve then courses upward, superficial to the posterior root of the zygomatic arch, and splits into several superficial temporal branches. Branches of the auriculotemporal nerve include anterior auricular branches, branches to the external acoustic meatus, articular branches, superficial temporal branches, and parotid branches.
   - Two **anterior auricular branches** provide sensory innervation to the tragus and part of the helix of the auricle (see Fig. 24–12).
   - Two **external acoustic meatal branches** supply the skin of the external acoustic meatus and the tympanic membrane (see Fig. 24–12).
   - One or two **articular branches** supply the temporomandibular joint (see Fig. 24–12 and discussion of clinical disorders of the temporomandibular joint below).
   - Several **superficial temporal branches** supply the skin of the temporal region (see above). The superficial temporal branches of the auriculotemporal nerve also communicate with the facial and zygomaticotemporal nerves (see Fig. 24–12).
   - The auriculotemporal nerve also communicates with the otic ganglion (picking up parasympathetic postganglionic fibers of the glossopharyngeal nerve to form **parotid branches** that provide secretomotor fibers to the parotid gland and sympathetic fibers to blood vessels of the parotid gland) (see Fig. 24–12).
4. The **lingual nerve** is another branch of the **posterior trunk** of the mandibular division of the trigeminal nerve. Just after branching from the posterior trunk, it courses between the tensor veli palatini and pterygoid muscles. At the inferior border of the lateral pterygoid muscle, the lingual nerve is joined by a branch of the inferior alveolar nerve and by a branch of the facial nerve, the chorda tympani. The chorda tympani carries fibers that function in taste (SVA fibers) and preganglionic parasympathetic (pGVE) fibers that innervate the submandibular ganglion (see discussion of facial

BOX 24–3, cont'd

INTRODUCTION TO THE MANDIBULAR DIVISION OF THE TRIGEMINAL NERVE AND ITS SENSORY NERVES

nerve below). The lingual nerve then courses anteriorly between the mandibular ramus and the medial pterygoid muscle along with, but slightly anterior to, the inferior alveolar nerve (see below). The lingual nerve passes inferiorly to the attachment of the superior constrictor of the pharynx (see Chapter 27) in the region of the third molar. From this point, it courses to the lateral surface of the tongue, running anteriorly. It first courses lateral to, then inferior to, and then medial to the submandibular salivary gland and its duct (see Figs. 24–12 and Fig. 24–26). Its terminal branches ramify to provide GSA innervation to the lingual mucosa of the presulcal part of the tongue (anterior two thirds, which is anterior to the sulcus terminalis), mucosa of the floor of the oral cavity, and mucous membrane covering the gingiva of the mandible. Terminal branches of the lingual nerve also supply the sublingual salivary gland with postsynaptic parasympathetic (pGVE) and sympathetic (sGVE) fibers.

5. The **inferior alveolar nerve** and lingual nerve split from the **posterior trunk** of the mandibular nerve together just superficial to the lateral pterygoid muscle. At the lower border of the muscle, the inferior alveolar nerve passes between the sphenomandibular ligament (see Chapter 22) and the mandible. It enters the ramus of the mandible via the mandibular foramen and travels inferior to the teeth within the mandibular canal. In most individuals, the nerve ramifies into several branches within multiple "mandibular canals," giving off **molar** and **premolar branches,** which innervate the molar and premolar teeth and their associated gingivae. The inferior alveolar nerve may also give off a **canine branch,** which innervates the canine tooth and its associated gingiva. The inferior alveolar nerve then splits into the **incisive nerve,** which innervates the incisor tooth (and sometimes the canine tooth), and the **mental nerve,** which exits the mandible via the mental foramen. The mental nerve splits into two ascending branches, which innervate the skin of the lower lip and its associated mucosa, and a descending branch, which innervates the skin of the chin. These nerves communicate with branches of the facial nerve (see Fig. 24–12 and below).

eral branches of the inferior alveolar nerve (see Chapter 26).

The **mucosa of the anterior two thirds of the tongue** is provided with sensory innervation by the lingual nerve. This is consistent with the origin of the mucosa of the presulcal part of the tongue from the first pharyngeal arch. Thus, the **mucosa of the floor of the oral cavity,** which is derived from the first arch, is also supplied with sensory innervation by the lingual nerve. The tongue and oral cavity are discussed in detail in Chapter 26.

Striated Muscles of the Face

There are three major groups of striated muscles of the face: muscles of mastication, muscles of facial expression, and extrinsic muscles of the eye.

The **muscles of mastication** (and associated muscles) are formed within the first pharyngeal arch. The muscles of mastication are all innervated by the mandibular division of cranial nerve V (trigeminal nerve) and are discussed immediately below. The **muscles of facial expression** (and associated muscles) are formed within the second pharyngeal arch. All of these muscles are innervated by cranial nerve VII (facial nerve). The **extrinsic muscles of the eye** are innervated by cranial nerves III (oculomotor nerve), IV (trochlear nerve), and VI (abducent nerve).

Motor Targets of the Mandibular Division of the Trigeminal Nerve: Muscles of the First Pharyngeal Arch

The muscles of mastication and some associated muscles all arise from the first pharyngeal arch and are innervated by branches of the mandibular division of the trigeminal nerve (V3)

The **muscles of mastication** include the masseter, temporal, lateral pterygoid, and medial pterygoid muscles (Fig. 24–13). **Other related muscles** that form from the fourth cranial somitomere within the first pharyngeal arch are the mylohyoid muscle, anterior belly of the digastric muscle, tensor veli palatini muscles, and tensor tympani muscles (Fig. 24–14). As has been noted, all of these muscles receive their innervation from the mandibular division of the trigeminal nerve (see Fig. 24–15 and Table 24–6). Most of these muscles function mainly in mastication and speech. The tensor tympani muscle functions in hearing.

Attachments, Innervations, and Specific Actions of Muscles of the First Pharyngeal Arch

The muscles of mastication are described in order, from the deepest (medial pterygoid muscle) to the most

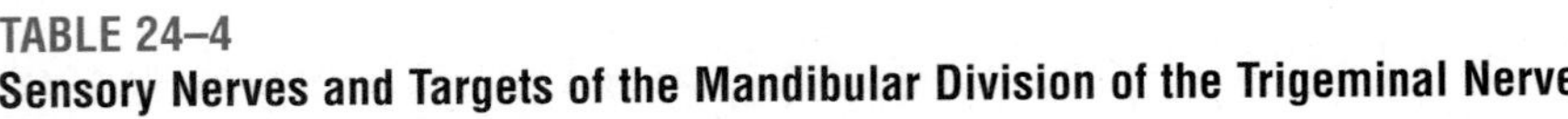

TABLE 24–4
Sensory Nerves and Targets of the Mandibular Division of the Trigeminal Nerve

Nerve	Fibers	Target
MENINGEAL	GSA	Dura mater of middle cranial fossa and some of anterior cranial fossa and calvaria, mucous lining of mastoid air cells
	sGVE[1]	From plexus on middle meningeal artery
ANTERIOR TRUNK OF MANDIBULAR DIVISION		
Buccal[2]	GSA	Skin covering anterior region of buccinator muscle, mucous membrane deep to buccinator muscle and associated gingiva
	sGVE[1]	Sweat glands, blood vessels, and arrector pili muscles of skin covering anterior region of buccinator muscle and mucous glands of gingiva in region of buccinator muscle
POSTERIOR TRUNK OF MANDIBULAR DIVISION		
Auriculotemporal		
Anterior auricular	GSA	Tragus and part of helix
	sGVE[1]	Sweat glands, blood vessels, and arrector pili muscles of tragus and helix
External acoustic meatus	GSA	External acoustic meatus and tympanic membrane
Articular	GSA	Temporomandibular joint
	sGVE[1]	Blood vessels of external acoustic meatus
Superficial temporal	GSA	Skin of temporal region
	sGVE[1]	Sweat glands, blood vessels, and arrector pili muscles of skin of temporal region
Parotid	GSA	Parotid gland
	pGVE[2]	Secretomotor fibers to parotid gland
	sGVE[1]	Blood vessels of parotid gland
Lingual	GSA	Mucosa of anterior two thirds of tongue, mucosa of floor of oral cavity, mucosa of mucous membrane covering gingiva of mandible, submandibular and sublingual salivary glands (see discussion of facial nerve below)
	SVA[3]	Taste receptors of anterior two thirds of tongue
	pGVE[4]	Secretomotor fibers to submandibular and sublingual salivary glands
	sGVE[5]	Submandibular and sublingual salivary glands
Inferior alveolar[6]		
Molar	GSA	Molar teeth and gingiva
Premolar	GSA	Premolar teeth and gingiva
Canine	GSA	Canine tooth and gingiva
Incisive	GSA	Incisor tooth and gingiva
Mental	GSA	Skin of inferior oral region, including chin and lower lip
	sGVE[7]	Sweat glands, blood vessels, and arrector pili muscles of skin of inferior oral region, including chin and lower lip

GSA, General somatic afferent; *sGVE,* sympathetic general visceral efferent; *pGVE,* parasympathetic general visceral efferent; *SVA,* special visceral afferent.

[1]sGVE fibers of the mandibular nerves are supplied by the nervous spinosus from a sympathetic plexus of the middle meningeal artery.

[2]pGVE fibers within parotid branches of the auriculotemporal nerve arise from cranial nerve IX (glossopharyngeal nerve) innervating the otic ganglion via the lesser petrosal nerve (see discussion of glossopharyngeal nerve in Chapter 26).

[3]SVA fibers of the chorda tympani branch of the facial nerve are carried by the lingual branch of the mandibular division of the trigeminal nerve to the taste buds (except the vallate papillae) of the tongue.

[4]Preganglionic pGVE fibers are conveyed to the submandibular ganglion via the facial nerve, chorda tympani, and lingual nerve. They synapse with peripheral neurons in the ganglion and then postganglionic pGVE fibers are carried to the submandibular and sublingual salivary glands by the lingual nerve.

[5]Postganglionic sGVE fibers from the facial nerve plexus are conveyed to the lingual nerve via the chorda tympani. After coursing through the submandibular ganglion without synapsing, a terminal branch of the lingual nerve conveys these fibers to the submandibular and sublingual salivary glands (see discussion of the facial nerve below).

[6]The inferior alveolar nerve also contains motor fibers that innervate the mylohyoid muscle and anterior belly of the digastric muscle (see Table 24–7).

[7]The buccal nerve also contains motor fibers that innervate the lateral pterygoid muscle.

BOX 24–4
MOTOR BRANCHES OF THE MANDIBULAR DIVISION OF THE TRIGEMINAL NERVE

The motor root of the mandibular nerve exits the skull via the foramen ovale, along with the much larger mandibular sensory root (see Fig. 24–12). The motor and sensory roots unite just outside the foramen ovale to form the **mandibular nerve.** As has been described above, the mandibular nerve almost immediately splits into an anterior and a posterior trunk. Before splitting, however, the mandibular nerve gives rise to a sensory meningeal branch and a motor branch to the medial pterygoid muscle. The **anterior trunk** forms the sensory buccal nerve (see Box 24–3) and the motor masseteric, deep temporal, and lateral pterygoid nerves, which are described below. The **posterior trunk** contains mostly sensory fibers but also some motor fibers. It gives rise to the sensory auriculotemporal, lingual, and inferior alveolar (dental) nerves. The inferior alveolar nerve, in turn, gives rise to motor nerves that innervate the mylohyoid muscle and anterior belly of the digastric muscle.

It should be noted that the so-called motor nerves just listed contain sensory proprioceptive fibers that innervate proprioceptive endings in these muscles of mastication. Thus, the motor nerves of the mandibular division of the trigeminal nerve include the following seven major branches:

1. The **nerve to the medial pterygoid muscle** arises from the mandibular nerve just after it emerges from the space between the lateral pterygoid muscle and the tensor veli palatini muscle (Fig. 24–15). It immediately gives rise to two small nerves:
   - ♦ The **nerve to the tensor tympani muscle** courses posteriorly to enter the canal containing the muscle (see above).
   - ♦ **The** nerve to the tensor veli palatini muscle courses anteriorly to innervate the muscle.

Both of these nerves pass through the **otic ganglion** of the glossopharyngeal nerve without synapsing before innervating their respective targets. The otic ganglion (see below) is just superficial to the point at which the anterior and posterior trunks of the mandibular nerve separate from each other (Fig. 24–15).

After giving rise to nerves to the tensor tympani and tensor veli palatini muscles, the **nerve to the medial pterygoid muscle** courses inferiorly to penetrate the lateral surface of the medial pterygoid muscle (Fig. 24–15).

1. The **masseteric nerve** arises from the anterior trunk and then courses laterally superior to the lateral pterygoid muscle, posterior to the temporal tendon, and anterior to the temporomandibular joint. It traverses the mandibular incisure (see Chapter 22), entering the deep surface of the masseter muscle, which it innervates (Fig. 24–15).
2. The anterior trunk of the mandibular nerve also gives rise to an **anterior temporal nerve** and a posterior deep temporal nerve.
3. The anterior temporal nerve and posterior deep temporal nerve course superiorly to the lateral pterygoid muscle and then enter the deep surface of the temporal muscle, which they innervate (Fig. 24–15).
4. The anterior trunk of the mandibular nerve gives rise to a **posterior deep temporal nerve.** This nerve also courses superiorly to the lateral pterygoid muscle and then enters the deep surface of the temporal muscle, which it innervates (Fig. 24–15).
5. The **nerve to the lateral pterygoid muscle** also arises from the anterior trunk of the mandibular nerve. Almost immediately, it enters the deep surface of the lateral pterygoid muscle, which it innervates (Fig. 24–15).

Variations of nerve branching include the origination of the anterior temporal nerve and nerve to the lateral pterygoid muscle from the buccal nerve.

The posterior trunk of the mandibular nerve gives rise to motor branches, which innervate the mylohyoid muscle and anterior belly of the digastric muscle.

6. The **nerve to the mylohyoid muscle** branches from the inferior alveolar nerve just before the nerve enters the mandibular foramen. The nerve to the mylohyoid muscle then penetrates and passes through the sphenomandibular ligament. It courses inferiorly along the medial surface of the ramus of the mandible and anteriorly just inferior to the mylohyoid line before it enters the inferior surface of the mylohyoid muscle, which it innervates (Fig. 24–15).
7. Just before entering the inferior surface of the mylohyoid muscle, the mylohyoid nerve gives rise to a **nerve to the anterior belly of the digastric muscle** (Fig. 24–15).

superficial (masseter muscle). Other muscles of the first pharyngeal arch are then discussed. The attachments and actions of all of these muscles are summarized in Table 24–5, and their innervation is summarized in Table 24–6 and Box 24–4.

The anterosuperior attachments of the **medial pterygoid muscle** include the medial surface of the lateral pterygoid plate, the pyramidal process of the palatine bone, and the lateral surfaces of the pyramidal process and tuberosity of the maxilla. The posteroinferior attachment to the mandible is to the medial surfaces of the ramus and angle (see Fig. 24–13). The me-

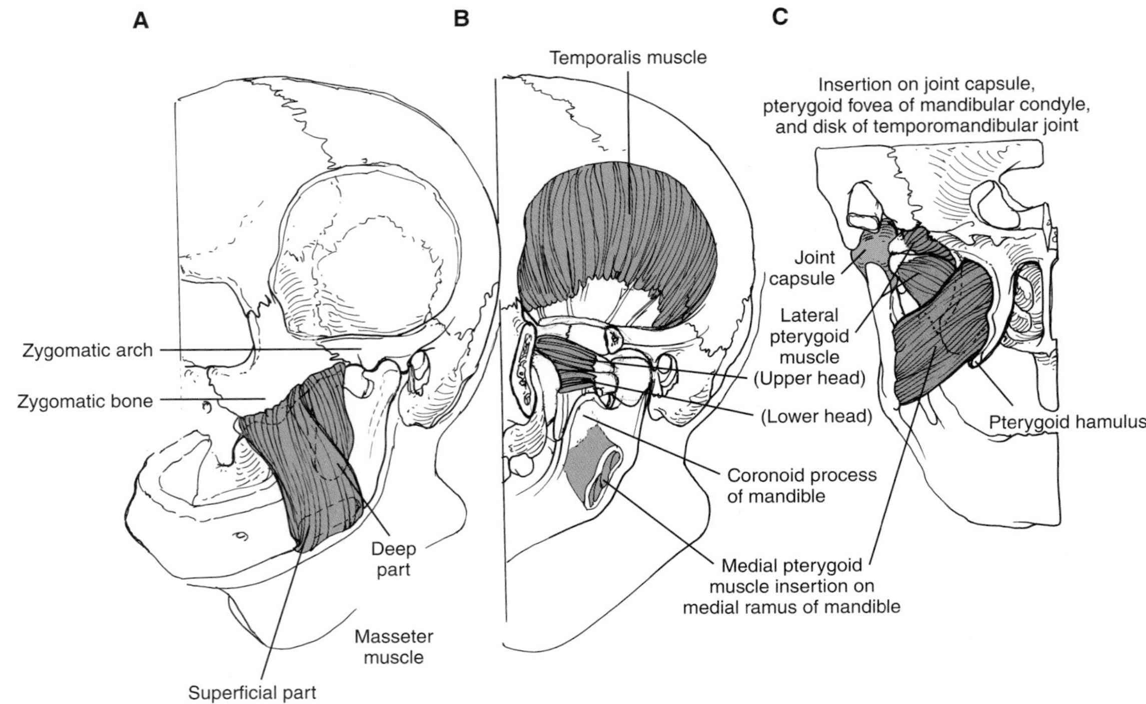

FIGURE 24-13
Muscles of mastication from the first pharyngeal arch, including the temporalis, the lateral and medial pterygoid, and the main division of the masseter muscle. **A.** Superficial front angle view of the masseter muscle. **B.** Intermediate front angle view of the lateral pterygoid and temporal muscles. **C.** Posterior view of the medial and lateral pterygoid muscles in relation to the pterygoid plate, temporomandibular joint and mandible.

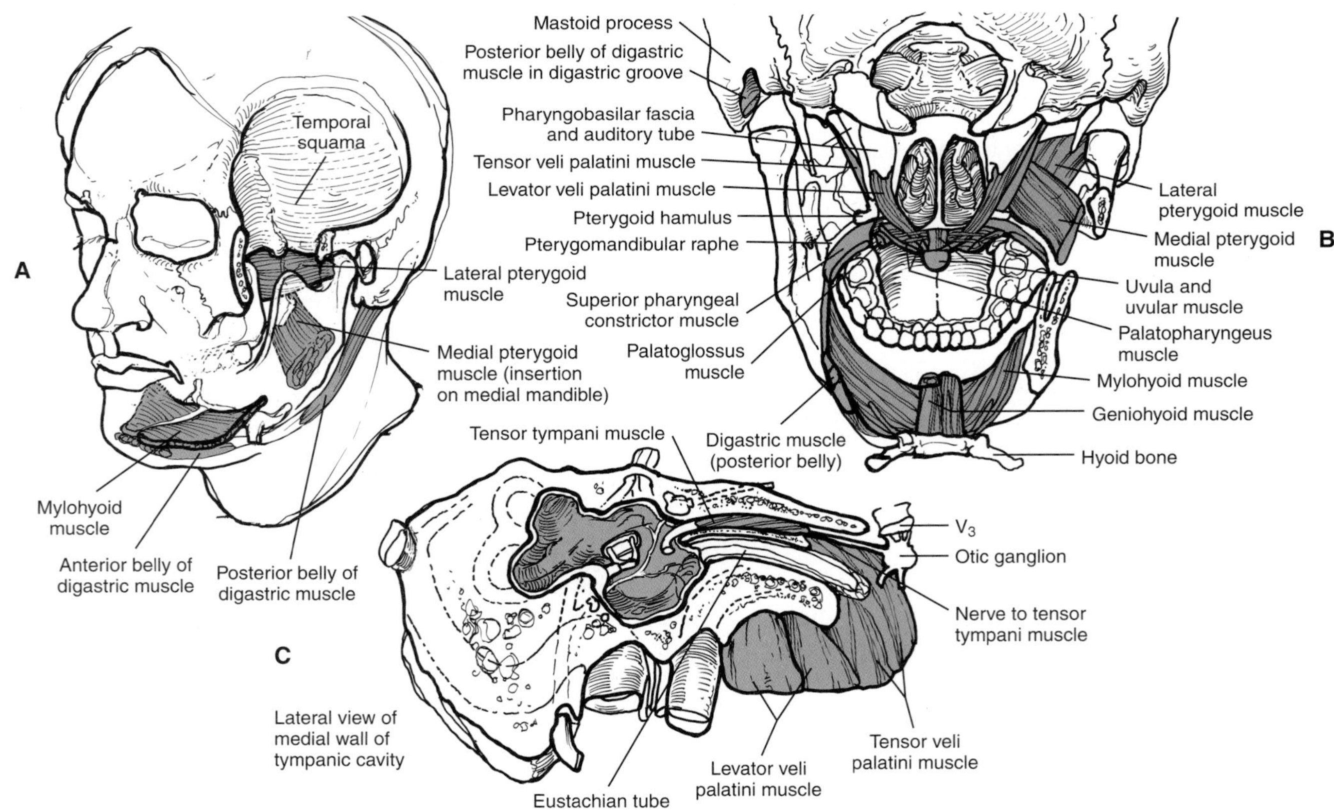

FIGURE 24-14
Other muscles associated with the first pharyngeal arch. **A.** The mylohyoid muscle and anterior belly of the digastric muscle. (The posterior digastric belly shown is from the second arch.) **B.** Posterior view showing geniohyoid muscles deep to the mylohyoid and tensor veli palatini muscle. **C.** Tensor tympani muscle above the auditory tube. (Attachment to the handle of the malleus is out of the plane of this view).

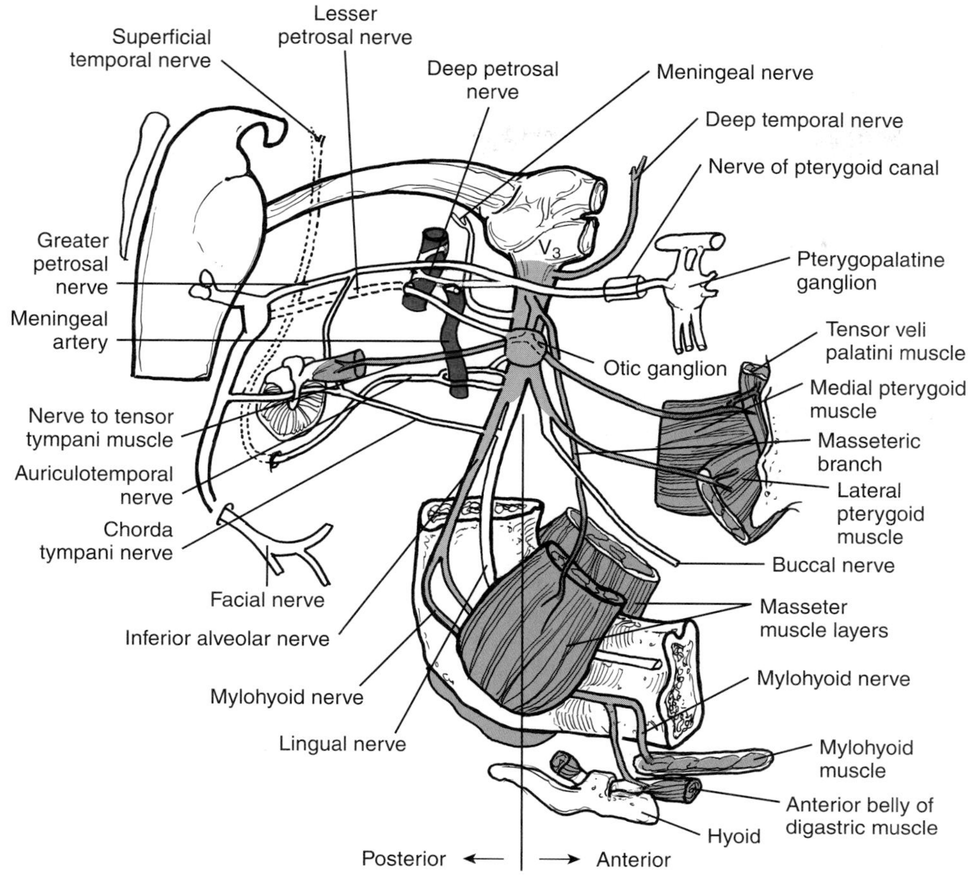

FIGURE 24-15
Schematic drawing of the motor nerves of the mandibular division. Motor branches (shaded) and nerves to the medial and lateral pterygoid, tensor veli palatini, tensor tympani, masseter, mylohyoid, and anterior digastric muscles. Note that inferior alveolar nerve is sensory but carries motor fibers.

dial pterygoid muscle, however, is separated from the ramus of the mandible by slips of the lateral pterygoid muscle and by the maxillary artery and inferior alveolar vessels, inferior alveolar and lingual nerves, sphenomandibular ligament, and part of the parotid gland. The tensor veli palatini muscle is deep to the medial pterygoid muscles. The medial pterygoid muscles are innervated by a branch of the mandibular nerve (nerve of the medial pterygoid muscle; see below). The actions of the medial pterygoid muscles include elevation and protrusion (with the lateral pterygoids) of the mandible. The two medial pterygoid muscles are also employed in mastication (see discussion of mastication below).

The **lateral pterygoid muscle** has two heads. The upper head is attached to the infratemporal surface and crest of the greater wing of the sphenoid bone. The lower head is attached to the lateral surface of the lateral pterygoid plate (see Fig. 24–13). The combined tendon of the upper and lower heads is attached to the mandibular neck, articular disc, and capsule of the temporomandibular joint. The medial pterygoid muscle lies medial to the lateral pterygoid muscle, and the masseter muscle lies lateral to it. The maxillary artery may course deep or superficial to the lateral pterygoid muscle. The lateral pterygoid muscle is innervated by a branch from the anterior trunk of the mandibular nerve (nerve to the lateral pterygoid muscle; see below). The lower head of the lateral pterygoid muscle acts with the medial pterygoid muscle to protrude the mandible. The upper head is used in mastication (see discussion of mastication below).

The **temporal muscle** is attached to the floor of the temporal fossa and deep temporal fascia superiorly. It descends to attach to the coronoid process and anterior border of the mandibular ramus inferiorly (see Fig. 24–13). The temporal fascia, in turn, is attached to the superior temporal line above and to the upper boundary of the zygomatic arch below. The fibers of the temporal muscle thus course between the cranium and the zygomatic arch. The temporal muscle is, therefore, deep

TABLE 24–5
Attachments and Actions of Muscles of the First Pharyngeal Arch: Muscles of Mastication and Associated Muscles

Muscle	Immovable Attachment	Movable Attachment	Action
Medial pterygoid	Medial surface of lateral pterygoid plate,pyramidal process of palatine bone, pyramidal process and tuberosity of maxilla	Medial surface of ramus and angle of mandible	Elevation and protrusion of mandible, mastication (with lateral pterygoid muscle)
Lateral pterygoid	Upper head: infratemporal surface of greater wing of sphenoid bone	Neck of mandible, articular disc and capsule of temporomandibular joint	Protrusion of mandible and mastication with medial pterygoid muscle (see discussion of mastication below), pulling of articular disc of temporomandibular joint anteriorly
	Lower head: lateral surface of lateral pterygoid plate	Neck of mandible, articular disc and capsule of temporomandibular joint	See action of upper head
Temporal	Bony surface of temporal fossa and temporal fascia connected to superior temporal line	Anterior border of mandibular ramus	Elevation of mandible
Masseter	Deep layer: deep surface of zygomatic arch	Upper part of mandibular ramus	Occlusion of teeth, side-to-side movement of mandible, protraction and retraction
	Middle layer: zygomatic arch	Middle part of mandibular ramus	See action of deep and middle layers
	Superficial layer: maxillary process of zygomatic bone and anterior two thirds of zygomatic arch	Lower posterior half of mandibular ramus	See action of deep and middle layers
Anterior belly of digastric muscle		Digastric fossa of mandible, tendon of posterior belly attached to hyoid bone	Depression of mandible, elevation of hyoid bone
Mylohyoid		Mylohyoid line of mandible, median tendinous raphe, body and greater cornu of hyoid bone	Depression of mandible, elevation of floor of oral cavity, elevation of hyoid bone
Tensor tympani	Auditory tube, greater wing of sphenoid bone, bony elements of its own canal	Handle of malleus	Tension in eardrum
Tensor veli palatini	Scaphoid fossa of pterygoid process, medial surface of spine of sphenoid bone, lateral lamina of cartilage of auditory tube	Palatine aponeurosis, horizontal plate of palatine bone	Unilateral pulling of soft palate to one side, bilateral tension of soft palate

TABLE 24–6
Motor Nerves and Targets of the Mandibular Division of the Trigeminal Nerve: Muscles of Mastication and Associated Muscles

Nerve	Fibers	Target
ANTERIOR TRUNK OF MANDIBULAR NERVE		
Nerve to medial pterygoid muscle	BE	Medial pterygoid muscle
Nerve to tensor tympani muscle	BE	Tensor tympani muscle
Nerve to tensor veli palatini muscle	BE	Tensor veli palatini muscle
Masseteric nerve	BE	Masseter muscle
Deep temporal nerves	BE	Temporal muscle
Buccal nerve*		
Nerve to lateral pterygoid muscle	BE	Lateral pterygoid muscle
POSTERIOR TRUNK OF MANDIBULAR NERVE		
Inferior alveolar nerve*		
Nerve to mylohyoid muscle	BE	Mylohyoid muscle
Nerve to anterior belly of digastric muscle	BE	Anterior belly of digastric muscle

BE, Branchial efferent.

*The buccal and inferior alveolar nerves are mainly sensory and are comprised of general somatic afferent fibers; they carry motor (BE) fibers that innervate the muscles indicated (see Table 24–4).

to most structures of the lateral face, including the masseter muscle, parotid gland, and various nerves and vessels. The temporal muscles are innervated by deep temporal branches of the anterior trunk of the mandibular nerve (see below). The temporal muscle *acts* to elevate the mandible while closing the mouth. This requires the synergistic activity of anterior and posterior fibers of the muscle, which simultaneously retract the jaw (posterior fibers) and elevate the mandible (anterior fibers; see the discussion of mandibular function, below).

The **masseter muscle** is a quadrilateral muscle with three layers. The deepest layer connects the deep surface of the zygomatic arch to the upper part of the mandibular ramus and the coracoid process. The middle layer connects the inferior edge of the zygomatic arch to the middle part of the mandibular ramus. The superficial layer connects the maxillary process of the zygomatic bone and anterior two thirds of the zygomatic arch to the angle and lateral surface of the lower posterior half of the mandibular ramus (see Fig. 24–13). The masseter muscle is also attached to an overlying layer of cervical fascia called the **parotid fascia.** The masseter muscles are innervated by a branch of the anterior trunk of the mandibular nerve (see below). The *actions* of the masseter muscle include occlusion of the teeth (the maxillary and mandibular teeth make contact). It is also involved in some side-to-side movement and in retraction and protraction of the lower jaw.

The **anterior belly of the digastric muscle** arises from the first pharyngeal arch, but its posterior belly is formed within the second arch. Thus, this muscle has dual innervation. Since both bellies always act together, they are both described here. The anterior belly is attached to the digastric fossa of the mandible near the midline (see Fig. 24–14*A*). It courses inferiorly and posteriorly, ending in a tendon that attaches to the posterior belly of the digastric muscle within a perforation of the stylohyoid muscle. This tendon is secured to the hyoid bone by a fibrous loop. The posterior belly of the digastric muscle arises from the temporal mastoid notch and courses anteroinferiorly to the tendon within the perforation of the stylohyoid muscle (see Fig. 24–14*B*). The anterior belly of the digastric muscle is superficial to the mylohyoid muscle (see below). The posterior belly is superficial (lateral) to the superior oblique and rectus capitis muscles of the suboccipital triangle (see Chapter 5) and several associated nerves and vessels of the lateral neck (see below and Chapter 27). The digastric muscle is deep to the platysma muscle (see muscles of facial expression below); splenius, longissimus capitis, stylohyoid, and sternocleidomastoid muscles; and mastoid process. The anterior belly of the digastric muscle is innervated by a branch of the inferior alveolar nerve (see below). The posterior belly of the digastric muscle is innervated by a branch of the facial nerve. The *actions* of the digastric muscle include depression of the mandible and elevation of the hyoid bone.

The **mylohyoid muscles** (one on each side) are suprahyoid muscles, which arise from the mylohyoid line of the mandible to form a muscular floor for the oral cavity. Their medial edges are attached to each other through decussation of their fibers in the midline. The fibers form a raphe, which extends from the chin to the hyoid bone (see Fig. 24–14*B*). The posterior edge of each mylohyoid muscle is attached to the anterior surface of the body of the hyoid bone (see Chapter 24). The mylohyoid muscle is deep and superior to the anterior belly of the digastric muscle to which it is sometimes fused. It is also deep to the platysma muscle; part of the submandibular salivary gland; the mylohyoid, submental, and facial vessels; and the nerve to the mylohyoid muscle (see below). It is superficial to the geniohyoid and styloglossus muscles and the hypoglossal and lingual nerves (see Fig. 24–14). The mylohyoid muscles are innervated by mylohyoid branches of the inferior alveolar nerve (see below). Actions of the mylohyoid muscles include elevation of the hyoid bone, depression of the mandible, and elevation of the floor of the oral cavity during swallowing (see Chapter 26).

The **tensor tympani muscle** arises from the cartilaginous part of the auditory (eustachian) tube, the greater wing of the sphenoid bone, and bony elements of the canal it occupies just above the osseous part of the auditory tube (see below). Its tendon courses posteriorly to curve around the trochleariformis muscle (from the Latin, meaning *pulley-shaped*) and then enters the tympanic cavity to attach to the handle of the malleus (see Fig. 24–14*C*). The tensor tympani muscle is innervated by a branch of the nerve to the medial pterygoid muscle, which, in turn, is a branch of the mandibular nerve (see below). The tensor tympani muscle *acts* to tighten the eardrum to dampen the effects of high-intensity sound and protect the inner ear (see discussions of the stapedius muscle and ear below).

The **tensor veli palatini muscle** is just medial to the medial pterygoid muscle. It arises from the scaphoid fossa of the pterygoid process, medial surface of the spine of the sphenoid bone, and lateral lamina of the cartilage of the auditory tube. It courses inferiorly, forming a tendon that curves around the hamulus of the pterygoid bone and penetrates the origin of the buccinator muscle (see below) to insert into the palatine aponeurosis and onto the horizontal plate of the palatine bone (Fig. 24–14*B*). The tensor veli palatini muscle is innervated by a branch of the nerve to the medial pterygoid muscle (see below). Each tensor veli palatini muscle *acts* alone to pull the soft palate to the right or left side. The muscles act together to tense the soft palate.

Functions of the Muscles of Mastication: Movements of the Mandible. Movements of the mandible require the actions of several muscles of mastication (and other muscles). The muscles act upon the mandible itself and upon the articular disc of the temporomandibular joint (see Fig. 24–16 and see Fig. 22–19).

Opening the Mouth. When the mandible is completely elevated (i.e., the mouth is closed), the bilateral actions of the digastric, geniohyoid (see below), and mylohyoid muscles are required to **pull the mandible downward** (Fig. 24–16*A*).

The lower heads of the lateral pterygoid muscles then pull the head of the mandible with the articular disc forward onto the articular tubercle (Fig. 24–16*B*). Indeed, this **protrusion of the mandible** (forward movement of the lower teeth over the upper teeth) requires only the forward gliding movements of the head of the mandible and the articular disc and, therefore, requires only the bilateral actions of the lateral pterygoid muscles.

At this point, the mouth can be opened even wider by **further depression of the mandible** by the digastric, geniohyoid (see below), and mylohyoid muscles (Fig. 24–16*C* and *D*).

Closing the Mouth. When the mandible is completely depressed (i.e., the mouth is wide open), the bilateral actions of the temporal, masseter, and medial pterygoid muscles are required to **pull the mandible upward** (Fig. 24–16*E*).

Relaxation of the lateral pterygoid muscles allows the articular disc to move backward and the head of the mandible to glide backward into the temporal fossa (Fig. 24–16*F*). This **retraction of the mandible** (backward movement of the lower teeth over the upper teeth) requires the action of the posterior fibers of the temporal muscles (which may be assisted by the middle and deep parts of the masseter muscles and by the geniohyoid [see below] and digastric muscles).

Finally, complete **elevation and closure of the jaw** requires action of the temporal, masseter, and medial pterygoid muscles (Fig. 24–16*G* and *H*).

Maintaining the Jaw in Its Position of Rest. Maintaining the jaw in its **position of rest** (in which the upper and lower teeth are slightly separated), requires the action of the temporal muscle only.

Function of the Mandible in Mastication. Alternating actions of the pterygoid muscles advance the condyle of the mandible on one side as they rotate the mandible on the vertical axis of the temporomandibular joint on the other side. This aids in **trituration** (i.e., reducing food to small pieces). Specifically, the lateral pterygoid muscle on one side acts with the ipsilateral medial pterygoid muscle on the same side to advance the condyle on that side and to rotate the mandibular head (in the vertical axis) at the temporomandibular joint on the side with the active muscles (Fig. 24–17). These muscles then relax, and the pterygoid muscles on the opposite side contract. In addition, side-to-side movements of the mandible are effected by alternating actions of the masseter muscles.

The crushing of food between the teeth is facilitated by the temporal, medial pterygoid, and masseter muscles on both sides acting together.

Nerve Damage in the Vicinity of the Temporomandibular Joint. **Dislocation** of the temporomandibular joint is described in Chapter 22. The articular branches of the auriculotemporal nerve that supply the joint and its capsule and lateral ligament may be injured in such dislocations or in fractures of the temporomandibular joint. This may cause weakness of the joint.

Surgery to or **injuries** of the region of the temporomandibular joint may also result in damage to the closely associated facial and auriculotemporal nerves (see below).

Other Clinical Disorders of the Trigeminal Nerve and Its Targets

Loss of Sensory and Motor Function. Functions of the trigeminal nerve may be disrupted by tumors, injury, infection, or vascular damage. Trigeminal nerve damage may also result from poliomyelitis and multiple sclerosis. If the function of the entire trigeminal nerve on one side is completely disrupted, there is loss of sensation in the anterior scalp and face, tragus, and part of the helix of the auricle on the affected side. The only unaffected areas are in the posterior parotid region, which is innervated by the posterior auricular nerve (C2 and C3), and the conchal eminence and depression, which are innervated by fibers of the facial nerve (see below). Sensation is also lost in the cornea and lining of the conjunctival sac, mucous membranes of the nose and paranasal air sinuses, floor of the oral cavity and anterior two thirds of the tongue, all of the teeth, and mucosa covering the gingiva of the upper and lower jaws. The muscles of mastication and other muscles formed within the first pharyngeal arch are first paralyzed and then atrophy. Because the lateral pterygoid muscle on the affected side is inactive, the mandible on that side protrudes (especially when the mouth is opened).

Loss of Sensory Innervation Only. Because the sensory and motor innervation of the face is provided by different nerves, sensory deficits may occur without accompanying motor deficits. **Trigeminal neuralgia (tic douloureux)** is an extremely painful condition involving the sensory nerves only of the maxillary or mandibular divisions of the trigeminal nerve on one side of the face. The pain is confined to the specific region innervated by the involved nerve branch. The pain is so intense that patients often attribute it to activities they were engaged in at the time of the attack, although there is no causal relationship. As more attacks occur, the patient often retreats from more and more activities until he or she becomes a "prisoner" of fear of an attack. "Trigger zones" on the face may be so sensitive that even a light breeze or gentle touch may trigger the stabbing pain.

The cause of trigeminal neuralgia is unknown, but it is believed that vascular compression of the relevant nerve roots or the presence of microneuromas (small neoplasms of cells of the nervous system) may be responsible.

There is no effective cure for this condition. The patient may elect to have the affected nerve surgically severed, preferring the ensuing numbness to the pain. Typically, the sensory root is transected just posterior to the semilunar gan-

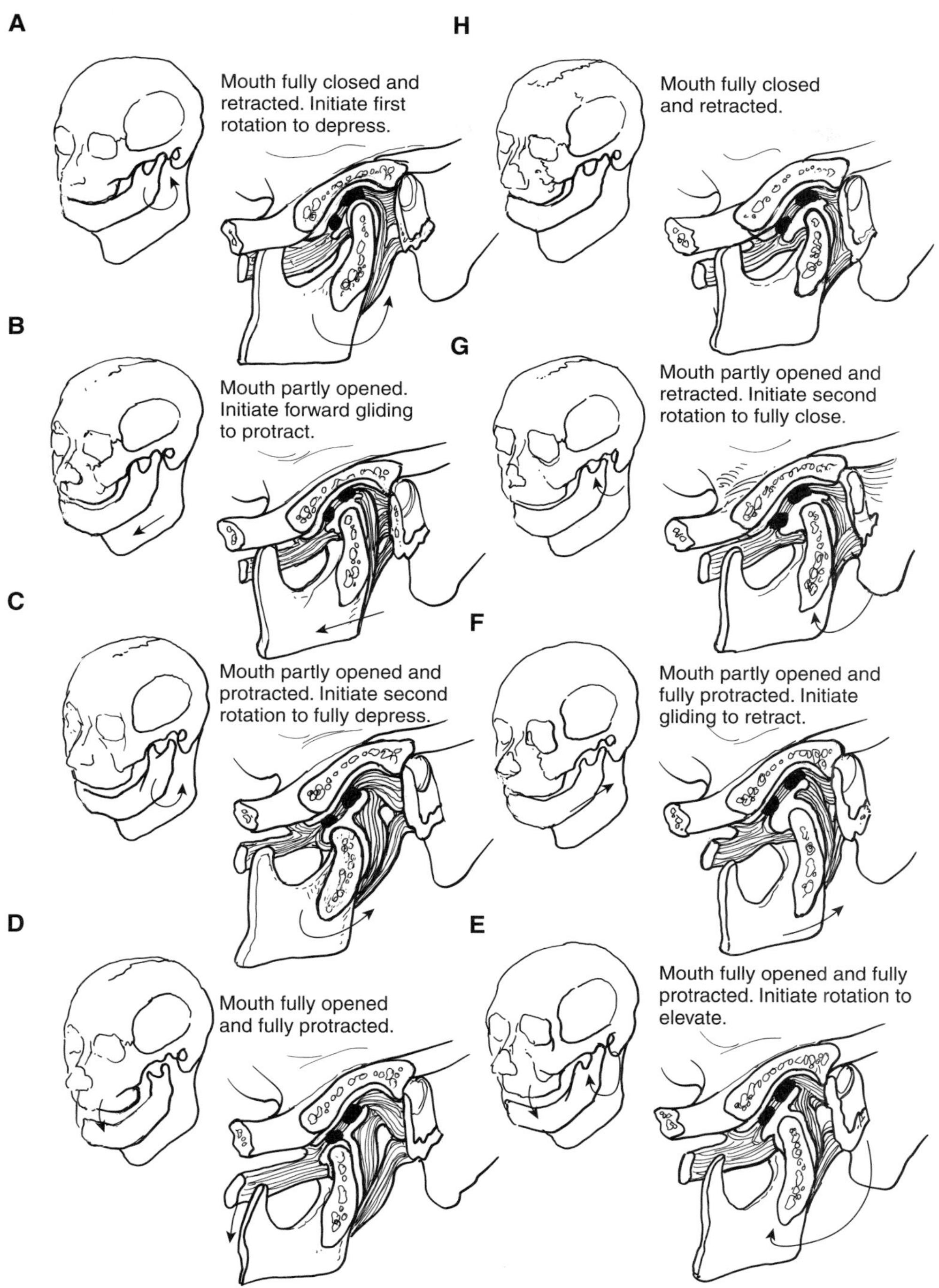

FIGURE 24-16

Movements of the mandible when opening the mouth **(A** to **D) A.** From a closed, retracted position, the mandible is pulled downward by bilateral actions of digastric, geniohyoid, and mylohyoid muscles. **B.** Protrusion of the mandible allows further opening by bilateral actions of the lateral pterygoid muscles. **C.** and **D.** Further depression of the mandible allows one to open the mouth even wider using the digastric, geniohyoid, and mylohyoid muscles. Closing the mouth **(E** to **H) E.** Elevation of the mandible in the depressed position by bilateral actions of the temporalis, masseter, and medial pterygoid muscles. **F.** Retraction of the mandible by relaxation of the lateral pterygoid muscles for backward gliding and assisted action of posterior fibers of the temporalis muscles. **G** and **H.** Complete elevation and closure of the jaw by actions of the temporalis, masseter, and medial pterygoid muscles.

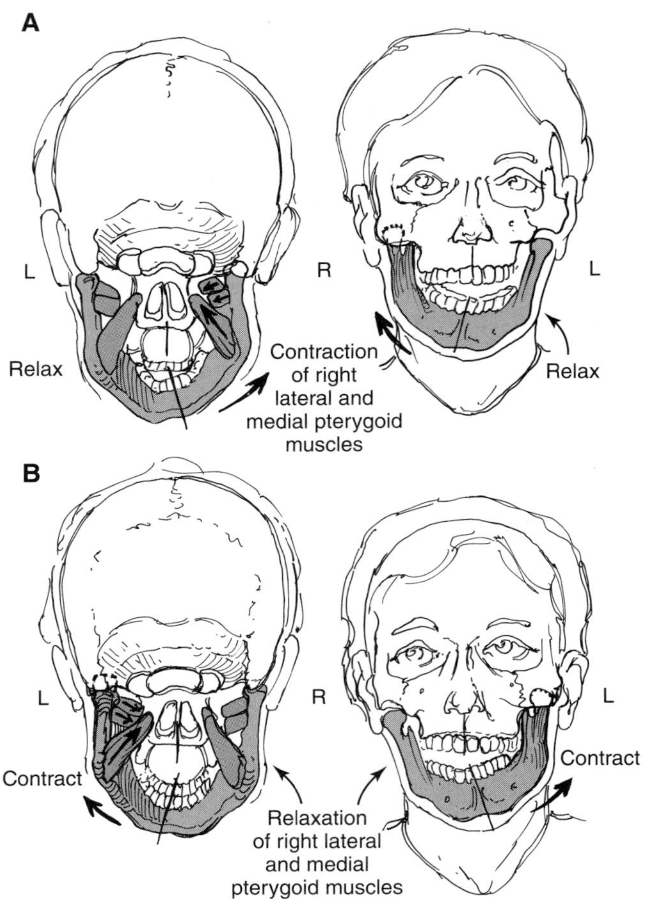

FIGURE 24-17

Function of the mandible in mastication. Alternate action of the lateral and medial pterygoid muscles coupled with alternate activity of the masseter muscles. Crushing of food between the teeth is facilitated by the temporalis, medial pterygoid, and masseter muscles on both sides acting together.

glion. Unfortunately, this operation results in denervation of the cornea, loss of the corneal reflex, and neuropathic keratitis of the cornea. Transection of the sensory root may thus be carried out to avoid damage to ophthalmic fibers, which are confined to the superomedial part of the root.

Referred Pain in Branches of the Trigeminal Nerve. Pain may be referred throughout the territories of nerves of the ophthalmic, maxillary, or mandibular divisions of the trigeminal nerve. The most common cause is dental caries. Referred pain may also indicate the presence of other, more severe clinical problems.

Pain may be referred throughout the area innervated by the **ophthalmic nerve,** particularly the supraorbital region, in sinusitis of the frontal or ethmoidal air sinuses or in glaucoma. **Maxillary neuralgia** (from the Greek root "neur," meaning *nerve,* and "algos," meaning *pain*) may result from dental caries of the maxillary teeth, from malignant growths or empyema (suppuration or formation of pus) in the maxillary sinus, or from disease of the inferior concha or nasal septum of the nose.

The most common cause of **mandibular neuralgia** is dental caries of the mandibular teeth. Pain radiates throughout the area of distribution of the auriculotemporal nerve, typically to the ear and temporal fossa. The pain is alleviated with treatment of the affected tooth or teeth. Pain referred throughout the distribution of the auriculotemporal nerve may also result from ulcers, cancers of the tongue, or diseases of the parotid salivary gland. The parotid salivary gland receives sensory innervation from the auriculotemporal nerve, also.

Clinical Anesthesia of Trigeminal Nerves. Local anesthesia of various regions of the face or oral cavity is often used in the repair of cuts or lacerations of the face, in facial surgery, or in dental repairs or extractions. Anesthesia of individual trigeminal nerve branches is guided by an understanding of their anatomic courses, particularly in relation to associated bony landmarks (Fig. 24–18).

In **anesthesia of the greater palatine nerve,** the second and third molar teeth are used as a reference point for injection of the anesthetic because this nerve emerges from the greater palatine foramen of the hard palate between these two teeth (Fig. 24–18A and see Chapter 22). An injection in this region anesthetizes the palatal mucosa and the bone and gingiva posterior to the upper canine teeth.

In **anesthesia of the nasopalatine nerve,** anesthetic is injected into the incisive fossa of the hard palate (Fig. 24–18B). This numbs the bone and mucosa of the hard palate and the gingiva and alveolar bone of the upper teeth.

In **anesthesia of the infraorbital nerve,** pressure is exerted upon the nerve in the region of the infraorbital foramen, resulting in development of pain (Fig. 24–18C and see Chapter 22). Care must be taken when one floods the region with anesthetic to avoid injecting it into associated blood vessels. Aspiration of blood prior to injection indicates penetration of a vessel. Care must also be exercised to avoid injecting anesthetic into the closely related orbit because this may cause paralysis of extraocular muscles. Anesthesia of the infraorbital nerve is typically used in repair of lacerations of the upper lip or cheek or in dental work on the upper incisors.

In **anesthesia of the mandibular nerve,** a needle may be passed from the outside through the mandibular notch of the ramus of the mandible to enter the infratemporal fossa (Fig. 24–18*D*). Flooding of anesthetic into this region will usually numb the inferior alveolar, auriculotemporal, lingual, and buccal nerves.

In **anesthesia of the inferior alveolar nerve,** the sharp, bony shelf at the anteroinferior border of the mandibular foramen **(lingula)** may be palpated to guide injections near it (Fig. 24–18*E* and see Fig. 22–18*A*). In this procedure, which is commonly used in the dental office to anesthetize all of the mandibular teeth and associated gingiva, anesthetic is flooded into the region of the mandibular foramen to numb the lower teeth, gums, gingiva, and skin on that side of the mandible.

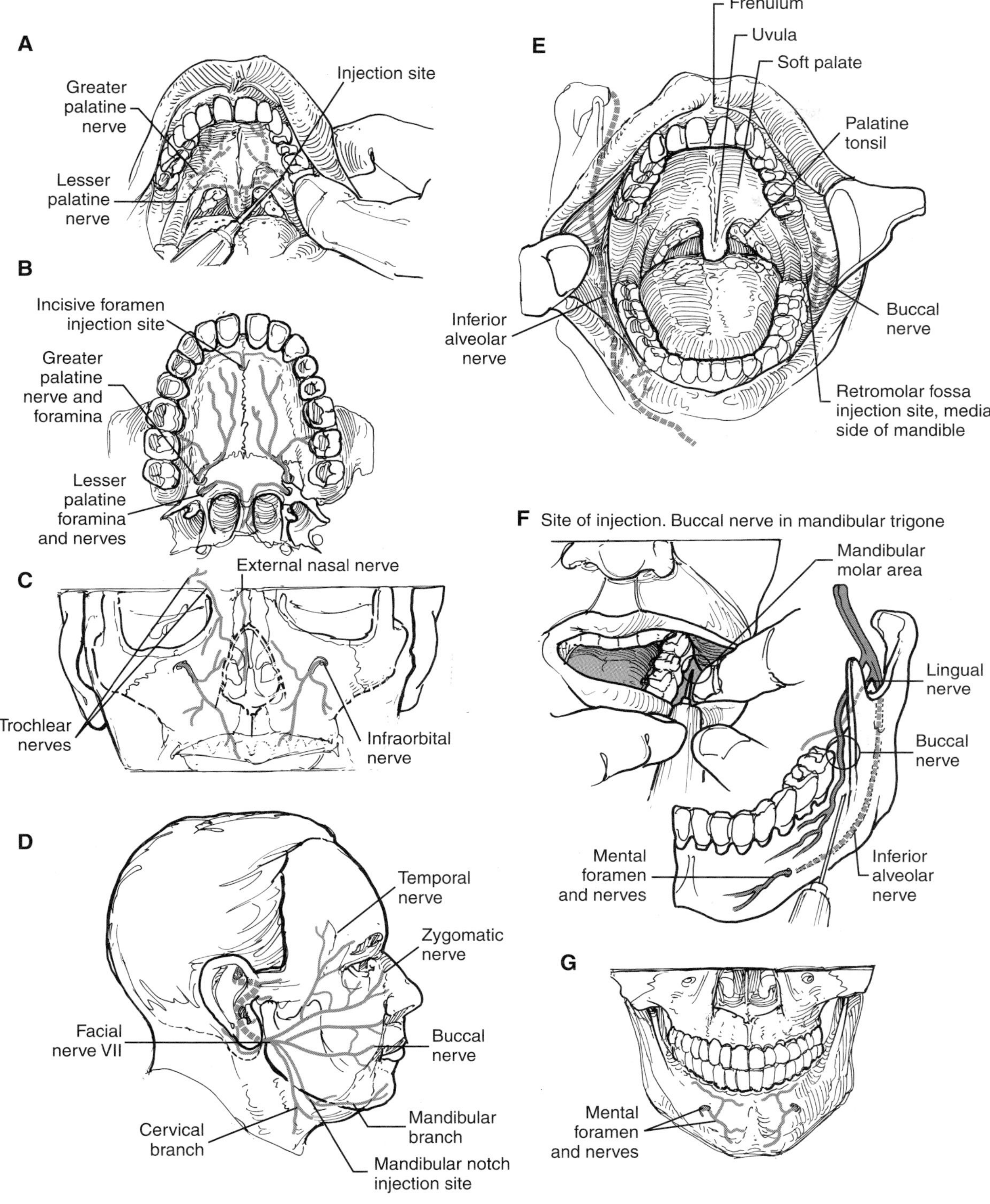

FIGURE 24-18

Landmarks for anesthesia of the trigeminal nerves. **A.** Anesthesia of the greater palatine nerve between the second and third molars. **B.** Anesthesia of the nasopalatine nerve in the incisive fossa of the hard palate. **C.** Anesthesia of the infraorbital nerve. **D.** Anesthesia of the mandibular nerve through the mandibular notch. **E.** Anesthesia of the inferior alveolar nerve. **F.** Anesthesia of the buccal nerve. **G.** Anesthesia of the mental nerve.

Anesthesia of the buccal nerve may be undertaken by locating and injecting the mucosa of the retromolar fossa just posterior to the molar of the mandible (Fig. 24–18*F*).

In **anesthesia of the mental nerve,** the mental foramen (Fig. 24–18*G* and see Chapter 22) may be palpated to anesthetize the skin and mucous membrane of the medial region of the lower lip, and bicuspid and cuspid teeth.

▲ Afferent Territories and Motor Targets of the Facial Nerve: Structures of the Second Pharyngeal Arch

A primary function of the facial nerve is to control the highly evolved muscles of facial expression (BE fibers), although the facial nerve also carries GSA, SVA, and pGVE fibers

Unlike the trigeminal nerve, the facial nerve carries a very small number of general somatic afferent (GSA) sensory fibers. These fibers innervate only a small part of the skin of the ear. However, the facial nerve also carries special taste, or gustatory, (SVA) fibers, which innervate taste buds of the tongue and palate. The primary function of the facial nerve, however, is the innervation of muscles that have developed within the second pharyngeal arch. These are mainly the muscles of facial expression, which arise from the sixth cranial somitomeres (BE fibers).

Although the second pharyngeal arch is a large, distinct entity of the embryo (see Chapter 23), most of the enclosed muscle precursors migrate away from the region of the second arch to occupy the definitive territories of cranial nerve V, which are the maxillary and mandibular swellings of the first pharyngeal arch. Thus, the second arch muscle precursors intermix with the muscles of mastication from the first pharyngeal arch as they come to lie under the skin of the scalp and face. Overlap of innervation of the facial and trigeminal nerves also occurs because the facial nerve carries parasympathetic pGVE fibers that tend to "hitch rides" to their targets with branches of the trigeminal nerve to innervate the lacrimal glands, mucous glands of the nasal cavity and palate, and submandibular and sublingual salivary glands. The trigeminal nerve branches (which do not carry parasympathetic fibers) provide GSA fibers to these same targets, resulting in considerable intermixing of facial nerve pGVE and trigeminal nerve GSA fibers.

The following paragraphs first describe general somatic and special visceral sensory territories of the facial nerve and then its motor targets (muscles of facial expression) and parasympathetic targets, along with all relevant facial nerve branches.

GSA Territories of the Facial Nerve

GSA fibers of the facial nerve innervate both sides of the auricular concha and proprioceptive endings in the facial muscles

The conchal eminence and depression are provided with sensory innervation by a small number of cutaneous GSA fibers of the facial nerve. However, distal segments of these fibers reach this final destination only by "hitching a ride" with the auricular branch of the vagus nerve (Fig. 24–19). Other facial nerve sensory fibers may assist the anterior auricular branch of the auriculotemporal nerve (mandibular division of the trigeminal nerve) in innervating the external acoustic meatus and outer surface of the tympanic membrane. Although GSA fibers are not typically described as traveling with the facial nerve, sensory fibers do accompany all motor branches of the facial nerve to relay proprioceptive impulses from the muscles of facial expression back to the brain (see Box 23–1). Some of these fibers may be responsible for the sensation of "deep facial pain," although this is controversial.

Structures Innervated by Special Visceral Afferent (SVA) Fibers of the Facial Nerve. The taste buds of the palate, tongue, epiglottis, and pharynx are innervated by the afferent nerve endings of centripetal axons of unipolar neurons housed in the sensory nucleus of the facial nerve (geniculate ganglion), by the glossopharyngeal nerve via its inferior ganglion, and by the vagus nerve via its inferior ganglion (Fig. 24–20 and see Chapter 26). **Taste buds** are specialized structures formed by modified epithelial cells. They are present in the anterior and posterior regions of the tongue and on the soft palate, epiglottis, and pharynx. They are most abundant on the posterior one third of the tongue. However, taste buds at the most posterior border of the tongue atrophy and disappear as a person ages. While taste buds of the vallate papillae at the posterior border of the anterior two thirds of the tongue are innervated by the glossopharyngeal nerve, all other taste buds of this presulcal (oral) part of the tongue are innervated by the chorda tympani branch of the facial nerve via the lingual nerve. (The **presulcal region of the tongue** is anterior to a groove **[sulcus terminalis]** that separates the anterior two thirds from the posterior one third of the tongue.) SVA fibers of cranial nerve VII also innervate taste buds of the inferior part of the soft palate via palatine branches (see Box 24–6).

It had long been presumed that taste buds in different regions of the tongue vary in their sensitivity to different substances, but this seems to be an oversimplification of the sensory process for the following reasons:

- Taste buds are found throughout the tongue and extend into the soft palate.
- Although peripheral and central neurons within taste buds may respond most strongly to one type of stimulus, they typically respond to more than one kind.
- Taste discrimination may depend one a pattern of activity across neurons or even a combination of information (similar to the photoreceptor responses in vision). Concentration of gustatory stimuli also plays a role.
- Some researchers even suggest the presence of a fifth "taste" for glutamate.

The anatomy of the tongue, including its mucosa and musculature, is described in greater detail in Chapter 26.

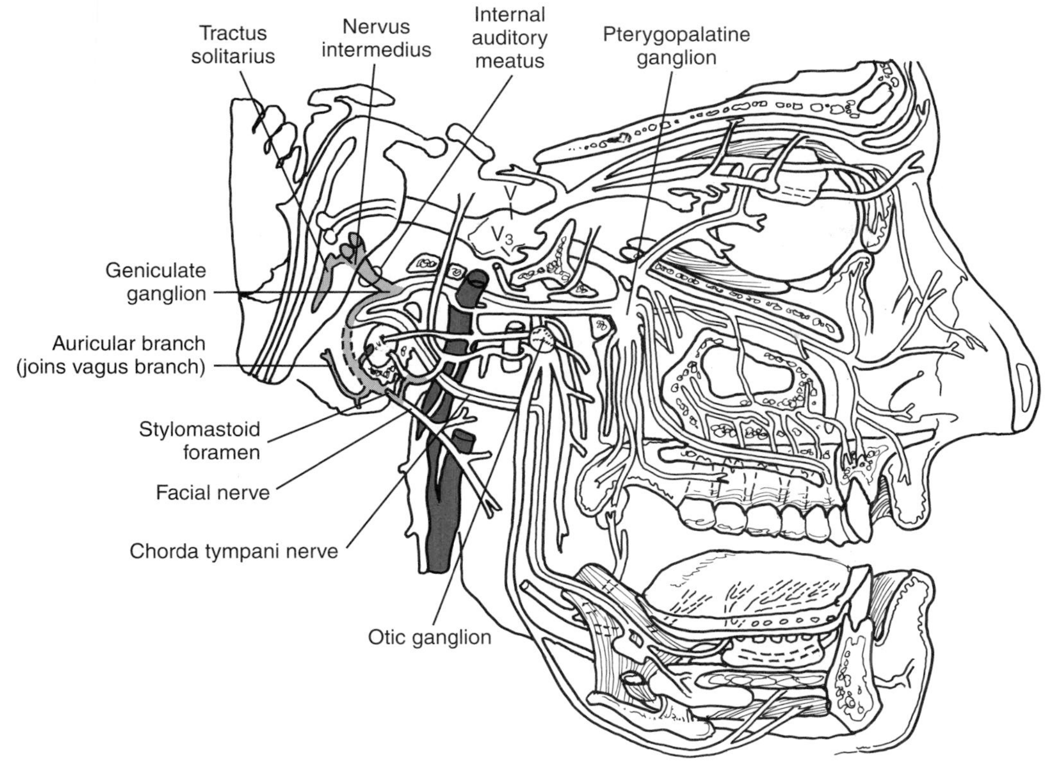

FIGURE 24-19

Facial nerve general somatic afferent (GSA) fibers join with the auricular branch of vagus to innervate the auricular concha region, communicating with branches of the great auricular and lesser occipital cervical nerves and the auriculotemporal nerve (V_3). Although not indicated here, motor branches also carry some proprioceptive GSA fibers.

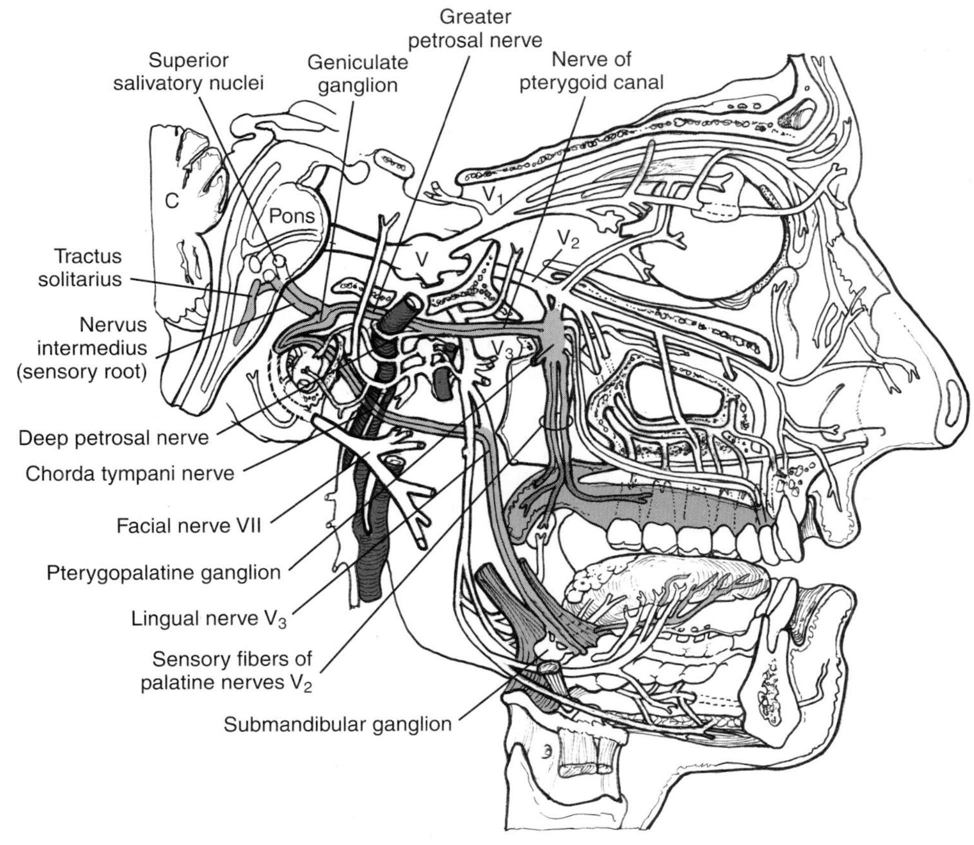

FIGURE 24-20

Special sensory taste (SVA) fibers from the sensory root of the facial nerve (with unipolar neurons in the geniculate ganglion) ultimately travel with cranial nerve V branches. The chorda tympani nerve joins the lingual nerve (V_3). Greater petrosal fibers travel through the pterygopalatine ganglion to palatine nerves (V_2). Taste information is conveyed to the cranial end of the tractus solitarius in the medulla.

Branchial Motor Targets of the Facial Nerve. *Branchial Efferent (BE) fibers of the facial nerve innervate muscles of facial expression.* As has been noted above, the striated muscles of facial expression and related muscles that arise from the second pharyngeal arch are innervated by motor (BE) fibers of the facial nerve. The muscles of facial expression include the occipitofrontal (see discussion of scalp above), corrugator supercilii, orbicularis oculi, zygomaticus major and minor, procerus, levator labii superioris, levator labii superioris alaeque nasi, levator anguli oris, nasalis, depressor septi nasi, orbicularis oris, depressor anguli oris, depressor labii inferioris, mentalis, risorius, buccinator, platysma, and auricular muscles (Fig. 24–21 and see below).

Other muscles that arise from the second pharyngeal arch include the stapedius and stylohyoid muscles and posterior belly of the digastric muscle (Fig. 24–22).

The stapedius muscle opposes the action of the tensor tympani muscle (see discussion of the mandibular division of the trigeminal nerve above). In this way, the stapedius muscle protects the inner ear by muting the effects of high-intensity sound. The stylohyoid muscle probably functions in mastication and vocalization, while the posterior belly of the digastric muscle functions in mastication and deglutition (swallowing).

Attachments, Innervation, and Specific Actions of Striated Muscles of the Second Pharyngeal Arch. Muscles of facial expression are described from the most superior (occipitofrontal muscle) to the most inferior (platysma muscle). By and large, this format organizes the muscles into groups that are innervated by specific branches of the facial nerve. Other muscles of the second pharyngeal arch are then discussed. The attachments, actions, and innervation of muscles of the second pharyngeal arch are summarized in Table 24–7. Branches of the facial nerve that innervate muscles of facial expression and other muscles arising from the second pharyngeal arch include the temporal, zygomatic, buccal, marginal mandibular, cervical, posterior auricular, digastric, stapedial, and stylohyoid branches. See also the discussion of the facial nerve BE branches in Box 24–7.

Muscles Innervated by Branches of the Temporal Nerve. The anterior **frontal bellies** of the occipitofrontal muscles (see Fig. 24–21) are described above (see discussion of the scalp). The frontal muscles are innervated by anterior branches of the temporal nerve. As has been noted, the anterior attachment of each frontal muscle is to the skin in the region of the eyebrow, and so these muscles act to protract the scalp (pull it forward) and to wrinkle the forehead in an expression of anger, concern, or frustration (Fig. 24–23*A*).

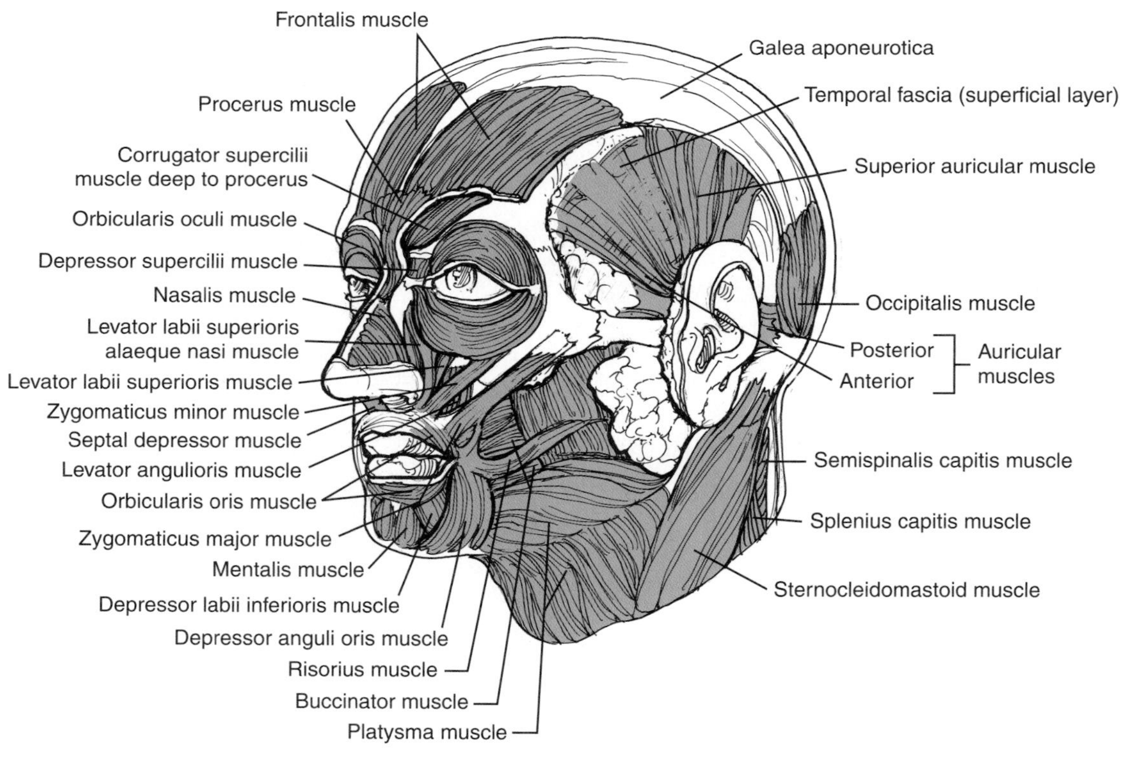

FIGURE 24-21
Muscles of facial expression from the second pharyngeal arch. Branchial efferent (BE) motor targets of the facial nerve.

The **corrugator supercilii muscles** are attached to bone at the medial ends of the superciliary arches. The muscle fibers course superolaterally to attach to the anterior edge of the frontal muscle and the superomedial edge of the orbicularis oculi muscle encircling each eye (see Fig. 24–21). The corrugator supercilii muscles are innervated by anterior branches of the temporal nerve. Their action pulls the skin above the eyes inferiorly, producing major and minor vertical wrinkles. This action shields the eyes from the sun and expresses disapproval or unhappiness when frowning (Fig. 24–23*B*).

Each of the flat, elliptical **orbicularis oculi muscles** encircles an eye (see Fig. 24–21). Fibers at the periphery of each muscle are attached to the nasal part of the frontal bone and procerus muscle (medially) and to the frontal part of the maxilla (inferomedially). These peripheral fibers sweep laterally (both superiorly and inferiorly around the eye) to blend with and attach to the levator labii superioris, alaeque nasi, and zygomaticus minor muscles inferiorly and to the frontal and corrugator supercilii muscles, skin, and associated hypodermis superiorly. These outer superior and inferior fibers meet and interdigitate at the lateral angle of the eye. Inner (more central) medial fibers of the orbicularis oculi muscle are attached to the medial palpebral ligament, which is a short ligament attached to the frontal process of the maxilla just anterior to the nasolacrimal groove (see Chapter 22). Other medial fibers originate from fascia posterior to the lacrimal sac. These inner fibers sweep laterally from their medial attachments into the upper and lower eyelids. The fibers meet again at the lateral canthi in a lateral palpebral raphe (a region where superior and inferior fibers interdigitate). The orbicularis oculi muscles are innervated by both temporal branches (superiorly) and zygomatic branches (inferiorly) of the facial nerve. The orbicularis oculi muscles act to close the eyes in sleep or to quickly and reflexively close them during blinking. Tension on the lacrimal fascia may help to dilate the lacrimal sac, aiding in the release and spreading of tears onto the surface of the cornea and promoting the secretions of the tarsal and ciliary glands. Closing the eyes produces horizontal wrinkles of the skin at the lateral angles and vertical wrinkles above the medial angles of the eyes (Fig. 24–23C). These wrinkles may become permanent as a person ages. The orbicularis oculi muscles are also involved in the squinting of the eyes when a person is closely inspecting an object or is expressing doubt or anger (Fig. 24–23C).

The **superior auricular muscle** arises from the lateral edge of the aponeurosis of the epicranial muscle and inserts into the superior edge of the auricle (see Fig.

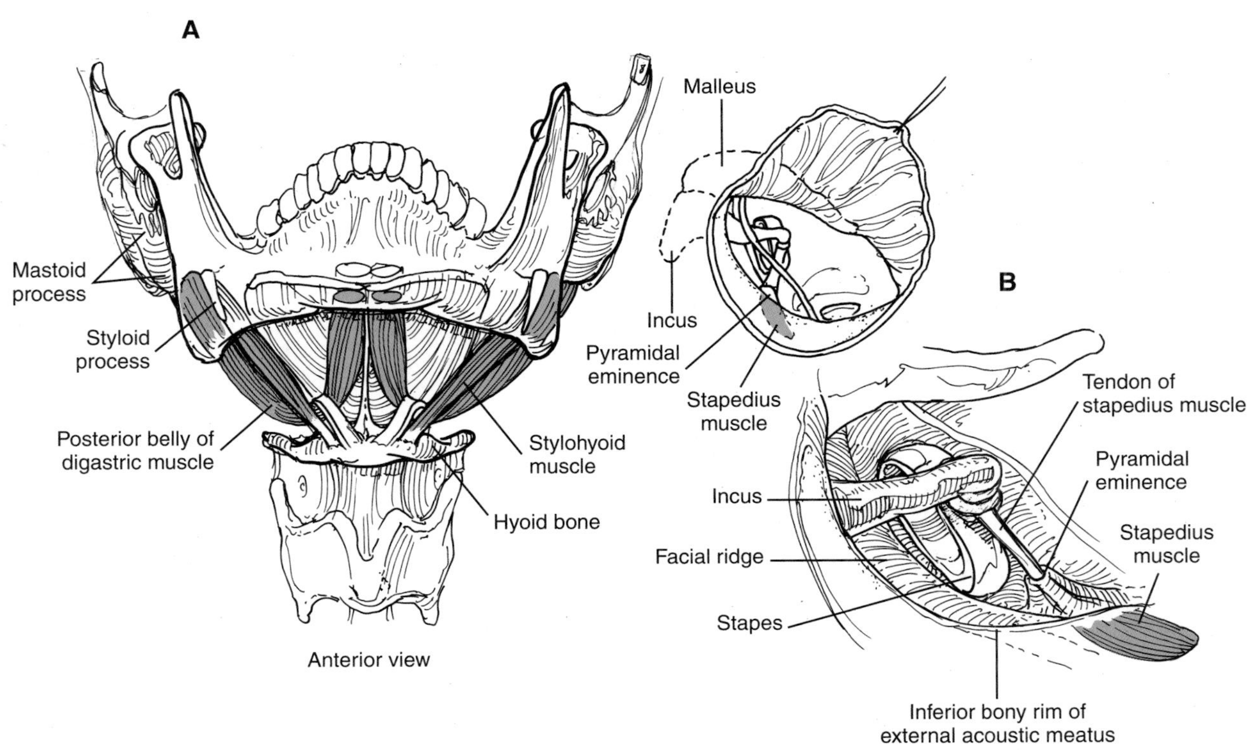

FIGURE 24-22
Other muscles that arise from the second pharyngeal arch. **A.** Stylohyoid muscle and posterior belly of the digastric muscle. **B.** Stapedius muscle.

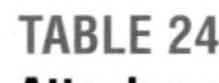

TABLE 24–7
Attachments and Actions of Muscles of the Second Pharyngeal Arch: Muscles of Facial Expression and Associated Muscles

Muscle	Immovable Attachment	Movable Attachment	Action
MUSCLES INNERVATED BY TEMPORAL NERVE			
Frontal		Epicranial aponeurosis, skin and connective tissue of eyebrows	Protraction of scalp, wrinkling of skin of forehead
Corrugator supercilii	Bone at medial end of superciliary arch	Anterior edge of frontal and superomedial edge of orbicularis oculi muscle	Pulling of skin above eye inferiorly
Orbicularis oculi	Nasal part of frontal bone, medial palpebral ligament	Levator labii superioris, levator labii superioris alaeque nasi, zygomaticus minor lateral fibers interdigitate, frontal and corrugator supercilii	Closing of the eyes, dilation of lacrimal sac, squinting
Anterior auricular	Lateral edge of epicranial aponeurosis	Anterior edge of auricle	Pulling of auricle forward
Intrinsic auricular muscles	Within auricles	Within auricles	Rudimentary
MUSCLES INNERVATED BY ZYGOMATIC NERVE			
Procerus nasalis	Fascia covering nasal bone	Skin of medial forehead	Pulling of medial eyebrows inferiorly to shield eyes from sunlight
Transverse slip	Maxilla	Transverse slip of contralateral side and procerus	Compression of nasal aperture at junction with vestibule
Alar slip	Maxilla	Alar cartilage	Dilation of outer edge of nasal aperture
Depressor septae	Maxilla	Mobile region of nasal septum	Assistance in dilation of nasal aperture
Zygomaticus major	Zygomatic bone	Modiolus	Pulling of angle of mouth superolaterally
Zygomaticus minor	Zygomatic bone	Muscles of upper lip	Elevation of upper lip
Levator labii superioris	Junction of maxilla and zygomatic bones	Muscles of upper lip	Elevation and eversion of upper lip
Levator labii superioris alaeque nasi	Frontal process of maxilla	Muscles of upper lip	Lateral slip elevates and everts upper lip; medial slip flares nostril
Levator anguli oris	Canine fossa of maxilla	Modiolus	Elevation of angle of mouth, exposing teeth
MUSCLE INNERVATED BY ZYGOMATIC AND BUCCAL NERVES			
Superior part of orbicularis oris			
Pars marginalis superioris		Skin of upper lip with mucous membrane	Formation of embrasure
Pars peripheralis superioris	Floor of incisive fossa of maxilla	Modiolus; contributing muscles	Assistance in closing mouth and pressing lips against teeth
MUSCLE INNERVATED BY BUCCAL NERVE			
Buccinator	Superior edge to alveolar process of maxilla; inferior edge to alveolar process of mandible; posterior edge of pterygomandibular raphe	Modiolus and into orbicularis oris	Compression of cheeks against teeth in mastication

TABLE 24–7, cont'd
Attachments and Actions of Muscles of the Second Pharyngeal Arch: Muscles of Facial Expression and Associated Muscles

Muscle	Immovable Attachment	Movable Attachment	Action
MUSCLES INNERVATED BY BUCCAL AND MARGINAL MANDIBULAR NERVES			
Inferior part of orbicularis oris			
Pars marginalis inferioris		Skin of lower lip and mucous membrane	Formation of embrasure
Pars peripheralis inferioris	Floor of incisive fossa of mandible	Modiolus; contributing muscles	Assistance in closing mouth and pressing lips against teeth
Risorius	Zygomatic arch; fascia of parotid gland, masseter, or platysma	Modiolus	Pulling of angles of mouth laterally
Depressor anguli oris	Mental tubercle and oblique line of mandible	Modiolus	Depression of modiolus and angles of mouth
MUSCLE INNERVATED BY MARGINAL MANDIBULAR NERVE			
Depressor labii inferioris	Oblique line of mandible	Skin and mucous membrane of lower lip	Depression and eversion of lower lip
MUSCLE INNERVATED BY MARGINAL MANDIBULAR AND CERVICAL NERVES			
Mental	Incisive fossa of mandible	Mental skin	Raising of skin of chin and depression of base of lower lip to assist in eversion of lower lip
MUSCLE INNERVATED BY CERVICAL NERVE			
Platysma	Fascia of deltoid and pectoralis major muscles	Inferior surface of mandible; lateral regions of lower lip; skin and subcutaneous connective tissue of lower face; modiolus	Tightening skin of anterior neck
MUSCLES INNERVATED BY POSTERIOR AURICULAR NERVE			
Occipital	Highest nuchal line of occipital bone	Epicranial aponeurosis	Retraction of scalp
Posterior auricular	Mastoid process of temporal bone	Posterior edge of auricle	Pulling of auricle posteriorly
MUSCLE INNERVATED BY DIGASTRIC NERVE			
Posterior belly of digastric	Mastoid notch of temporal mastoid process	Tendon of anterior belly of digastric	Depression of mandible, elevation of hyoid bone
MUSCLE INNERVATED BY STYLOHYOID NERVE			
Stylohyoid	Posterior surface of styloid process	Hyoid bone	Pulling of hyoid muscle posterosuperiorly, elongating floor of oral cavity
MUSCLE INNERVATED BY STAPEDIAL NERVE			
Stapedius	Cavity of pyramidal eminence	Neck of stapes	Pulling of stapes and tympanic membrane outward

BOX 24–5

INTRODUCTION TO THE FACIAL NERVE AND ITS GENERAL SOMATIC AFFERENT BRANCHES

The facial nerve has multiple functions

As has been noted in the text, **cranial nerve VII (facial nerve)** innervates structures derived from the second pharyngeal arch, mainly the muscles of facial expression (branchial efferent [BE] fibers). As has also been noted, however, the facial nerve contains a small number of general somatic afferent (GSA) fibers; some special visceral afferent (SVA) fibers, which innervate taste buds of the tongue and palate; and some autonomic preganglionic general visceral efferent (pGVE) fibers, which innervate the lacrimal gland, submandibular and sublingual salivary glands, and mucous glands of the nasal cavity and palate. The motor and sensory functions of the facial nerve arise from its motor and sensory roots. The facial nerve is also associated with a sensory ganglion, the **geniculate ganglion.** Because the facial nerve carries autonomic fibers, it is associated with autonomic ganglia, the **pterygopalatine** and **submandibular ganglia** (see Fig. 24–28).

The **sensory nucleus** of the facial nerve is located in the medulla at the cranial end of the tractus solitarius (see below). Its **motor nucleus** is part of the BE column located deep within the pons. The facial nerve is associated with two autonomic ganglia, which contain the peripheral neurons of the nerve's parasympathetic pathways. These are the **pterygopalatine** and **submandibular ganglia** (see Fig. 24–28). Central neurons of the facial parasympathetic (pGVE) fibers are located in a small nucleus within the pons called the **superior salivatory nucleus** (see Fig. 24–19).

Much of the facial nerve is encased in bone at the base of the skull

The sensory root **nervus intermedius** and the motor root of the facial nerve emanate from the caudal boundary of the pons and course anterolaterally within the posterior fossa of the cranial cavity (see Fig. 24–19). The sensory root is medial, and the motor root is lateral. Together, the roots enter the petrous part of the temporal bone through the medial end of the internal acoustic meatus (see Chapter 22), along with cranial nerve VIII (vestibulocochlear nerve). However, in the lateral region of the internal acoustic meatus, the roots diverge from the vestibulocochlear nerve and proceed anterolaterally into a horizontal part of the **facial canal.** Both roots terminate at the **geniculate ganglion,** which lies at the lateral end of the horizontal part of the facial canal (see Fig. 24–19).

The two major facial nerve branches of the geniculate ganglion are the greater petrosal nerve and the facial nerve

Two major facial nerve branches emanate from the geniculate ganglion: the **greater petrosal nerve** and the **facial nerve.**

1. The **greater petrosal nerve** contains mainly SVA fibers and presynaptic parasympathetic (pGVE) fibers. It issues from the anteromedial surface of the geniculate ganglion and passes anteromedially into the middle fossa of the cranial cavity via a small hiatus on the anterior surface of the petrous part of the temporal bone. It then passes under the semilunar (trigeminal) ganglion to reach the area of the foramen lacerum (see Chapter 22). Here the greater petrosal nerve penetrates the cartilage within the foramen lacerum. At this point, it is joined by the deep petrosal nerve. (The deep petrosal nerve originates as a plexus of sympathetic [sGVE] fibers associated with the internal carotid artery.) The greater petrosal and deep petrosal nerves course anteriorly together within the pterygoid canal as the **nerve of the pterygoid canal.** This nerve terminates at the pterygopalatine ganglion in the pterygopalatine fossa. Here the presynaptic parasympathetic fibers of the nerve of the pterygoid canal synapse with peripheral parasympathetic neurons, which emit postsynaptic axons. These postsynaptic fibers, along with SVA fibers of the facial nerve (which simply pass through the pterygopalatine ganglion without synapsing), are distributed to their targets by various trigeminal nerve branches (Boxes 24–6 and 24–7 and see Figs. 24–11 and Fig. 24–28).
2. The other major nerve that branches from the geniculate ganglion is the **facial nerve.** The facial nerve emanates from the inferior surface of the geniculate ganglion to enter the vertical part of the **facial canal,** descends through the vertical part, and exits onto the face via the **stylomastoid foramen.** Before it exits, however, it gives rise to a motor nerve (BE fibers), which innervates the stapedius muscle; a branch containing SVA fibers, which innervates taste buds in the anterior two thirds of the tongue **(chorda tympani);** and a ramus containing GSA fibers, which innervates the auricular branch of the vagus nerve (see Fig. 24–19). These GSA fibers of the facial nerve thus innervate the conchal eminence and depression via the auricular nerve. Once the facial nerve exits the stylomastoid foramen, its more distal part carries BE and presynaptic parasympathetic (pGVE) fibers onto the face. At first the facial nerve penetrates the parotid gland, and then, under cover of the parotid gland, it branches to innervate the muscles of facial expression and the submandibular ganglion (see Box 24–8).

GSA fibers of the facial nerve travel via the geniculate ganglion

GSA fibers within the sensory root of the facial nerve are centripetal fibers of unipolar GSA neurons located in the geniculate ganglion. It should be noted, however, that this sensory

BOX 24–5, cont'd

INTRODUCTION TO THE FACIAL NERVE AND ITS GENERAL SOMATIC AFFERENT BRANCHES

root also contains **SVA** fibers, which provide the sense of taste (Box 24–6), and presynaptic parasympathetic (pGVE) fibers, which innervate a variety of glands (see below and Box 24–8). As has been noted above, this "multifunctional" sensory root is the nervus intermedius.

The GSA fibers of the **nervus intermedius** originate in the pons from their synapses with association neurons of the superior end of the tractus solitarius (see Fig. 24–19 and discussions of the glossopharyngeal and vagus nerves in Chapter 26). These axons leave the brain near the inferior border of the pons. They course to the geniculate ganglion via the nervus intermedius to a unipolar cell body, which emits a centrifugal axon that courses into the facial nerve (see Fig. 24–19). These centrifugal GSA fibers cross over to the auricular branch of the vagus nerve via a small ramus that branches from the facial nerve in the vertical part of the facial canal (see above). The auricular nerve then distributes these "hitchhiking" facial nerve sensory fibers to the conchal eminence and depression of the auricle. The proximodistal route of cutaneous GSA fibers of the facial nerve can, therefore, be summarized as follows:

Centripetal fibers originate from
their synapses within the nucleus solitarius, →
course within the nervus intermedius →
to unipolar neurons of the geniculate ganglion. →
These unipolar neurons emit centrifugal fibers
that exit the geniculate ganglion, →
course within the facial nerve, →
and then course within a special ramus →
to auricular branches of the vagus nerve →
receptors in the skin of conchal eminence and depression.

24–21). It is innervated by a branch of the temporal nerve. It acts to raise the auricle slightly.

The **anterior auricular muscle** also arises from the lateral edge of the epicranial aponeurosis. It inserts into the anterior edge of the auricle (see Fig. 24–21). The anterior auricular muscles are innervated by a branch of the temporal nerve and act to pull the auricle forward.

The **intrinsic (lateral) auricular muscles** include several small fascicles of insignificant function. They are innervated by branches of the temporal nerve.

Muscles Innervated by Zygomatic Branches of the Facial Nerve. Inferior fibers of the **orbicularis oculi muscle** are innervated by zygomatic branches of the facial nerve. The attachments and actions of this muscle are described above (see Fig. 24–21).

The **procerus muscle** originates from fascia covering the nasal bone and inserts into the skin of the medial forehead (see Fig. 24–21). It is innervated by branches of the zygomatic nerve. By pulling the medial end of the eyebrow inferiorly, it acts to shield the eye from bright sunlight (Fig. 24–23*D*). This action also produces horizontal wrinkles at the root of the nose.

The **nasalis muscle** has a transverse and an alar slip (see Fig. 24–21). The transverse slip (compressor naris) has an inferolateral attachment to the maxilla. Its fibers then course superomedially to interdigitate with fibers of the transverse slip from the opposite side of the nose and with fibers of the procerus muscle. The alar slip originates on the maxilla just inferomedial to the attachment of the transverse slip. Its fibers then course inferomedially to attach to the alar cartilages. Both slips of the nasalis muscle are innervated by branches of the zygomatic nerve. The transverse slip acts to compress the nasal aperture at its junction with the vestibule, and the alar slip acts to depress the alar cartilage in dilation of the outer edge of the nasal aperture (Fig. 24–23*E*). These slips are very active during physical exertion and during the course of an emotional eruption.

The **depressor septi muscle** has an inferior attachment to the maxilla just superior to the medial incisor tooth. Its fibers then course superiorly to insert into the anterior mobile region of the nasal septum (see Fig. 24–21). The depressor septi muscle is innervated by zygomatic branches of the facial nerve. It acts to assist the alar slip of the nasalis muscle in dilating the nasal aperture (Fig. 24–23*E*).

The superior attachment of the **zygomaticus major muscle** is to the zygomatic bone (see Fig. 24–21). From this point, its fibers course inferomedially toward the angles of the mouth where its fibers interdigitate with fibers of the levator anguli oris, orbicularis oris, risorius, buccinator, and depressor anguli oris muscles and some fibers of the platysma muscle. The region of intersection and interdigitation of these muscles is called the **modiolus.** This dense fibromuscular mass is not fixed, and, therefore, its movements and fixation are synergistically regulated by the actions of all of the muscles that connect to it. The zygomaticus major muscle is innervated by branches of the zygomatic nerve. The muscle acts to

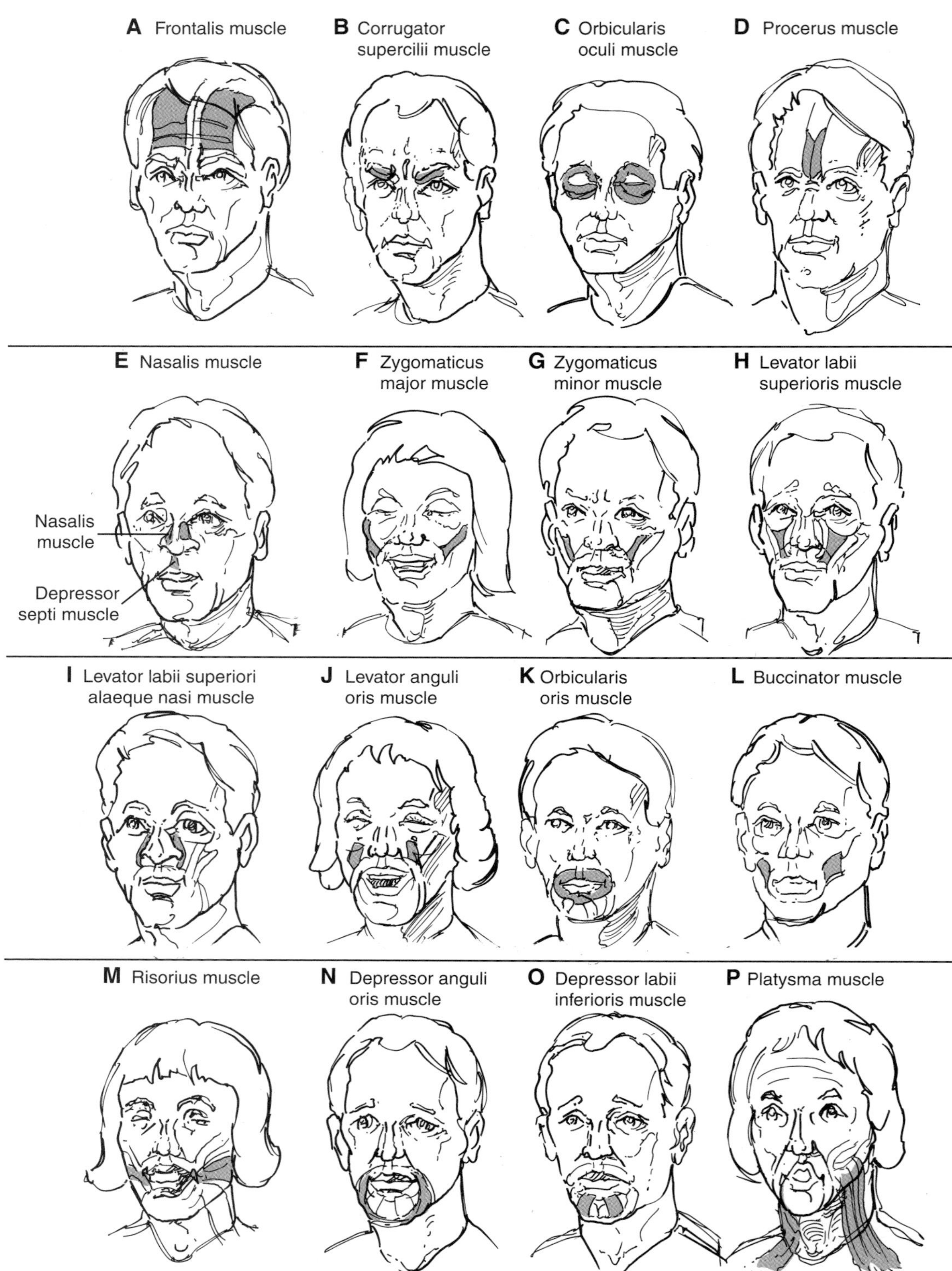

FIGURE 24-23

Specific muscles of facial expression. **A.** Frontalis muscle. **B.** Corrugator supercilii muscle. **C.** Orbicularis oculi muscle. **D.** Procerus muscle. **E.** Nasalis muscle. **F.** Zygomaticus major muscle. **G.** Zygomaticus minor muscle. **H.** Levator labii superioris muscle. **I.** Levator labii superioris alaeque nasi muscle. **J.** Levator anguli oris muscle. **K.** Orbicularis oris muscle. **L.** Buccinator muscle. **M.** Risorius muscle. **N.** Depressor anguli oris muscle. **O.** Depressor labii inferioris muscle. **P.** Platysma muscle.

pull the modiolus and, thus, the angle of the mouth laterosuperiorly when a person is laughing (Fig. 24–23*F*).

The superior attachment of the **zygomaticus minor muscle** is also to the zygomatic bone, just medial to the attachment of the zygomaticus major muscle (see Fig. 24–21). Its fibers course downward and medially to blend with muscle fibers of the upper lip, including those of the levator labii superioris alaeque nasi, levator labii superioris, and orbicularis oris muscles. The zygomaticus minor muscle is innervated by branches of the zygomatic nerve and acts to elevate the upper lip. It is used with the levator labii superioris alaeque nasi and levator labii superioris muscles to express contempt (see Fig. 24–23*G*).

The **levator labii superioris muscle** is attached superiorly to the region of the junction of the maxilla and zygomatic bones just above the infraorbital foramen (see Fig. 24–21 and Chapter 22). Its fibers course inferomedially to blend with fibers of the orbicularis oris muscle between the inferior attachments of the zygomaticus minor muscle (see above) and levator labii superioris alaeque nasi muscle (see below). The muscle is innervated by a branch of the zygomatic nerve and acts to elevate and evert the upper lip. In conjunction with the levator labii superioris alaeque nasi muscle, the levator labii superioris muscle accentuates the nasolabial sulcus (furrow) in expressions of sadness or remorse (Fig. 24–23*H*).

Each of the **levator labii superioris alaeque nasi muscles** is attached superiorly to the frontal process of the maxilla (see Fig. 24–21). A lateral slip courses inferolaterally to blend with fibers of the orbicularis oris muscle just medial to the inferior attachment of the levator labii superioris and zygomaticus minor muscles (see above). The medial slip courses inferomedially to attach to the alar cartilage of the nose. This muscle is innervated by branches of the zygomatic nerve. Its lateral slip acts to elevate and evert the upper lip, while its medial slip causes the nostril to flare (Fig. 24–23*I*). Because superior fibers of the levator labii superioris alaeque nasi muscle are also attached to the nasolabial ridge (superficially) and to the ventral surface of the levator labii superioris muscle (deeply), this muscle, in conjunction with the levator nasi superioris muscle, deepens the superior region of the nasolabial sulcus in expressions of sadness or remorse (Fig. 24–23*H*).

The **levator anguli oris muscle** is attached superiorly to the canine fossa just inferior to the infraorbital foramen of the maxilla. It courses inferomedially to attach to the modiolus (see Fig. 24–21). It is innervated by branches of the zygomatic nerve and acts to elevate the angle of the mouth and to expose the teeth when a person is smiling (Fig. 24–23*J*).

Muscle Innervated by Zygomatic and Buccal Branches of the Facial Nerve. The **orbicularis oris muscle** completely encircles the mouth (see Fig. 24–21). The **upper half of the orbicularis oris muscle** underlies the skin of the superior buccal region. The part of the upper half of the orbicularis oris muscle intrinsic to the lips is the **pars marginalis superioris muscle.** Oblique fibers of the pars marginalis superioris muscle connect the deep surface of the skin of the lips to the underlying mucous membrane of the oral cavity. The more peripheral part of the upper half of the orbicularis oris muscle is the **pars peripheralis superioris muscle.** Specialized slips of the pars peripheralis superioris muscle called the **incisivus labii superioris muscles** arise from the floor of the incisive fossa of the maxilla bone. These slips then course laterally to blend with other fibers of the pars peripheralis superioris and levator anguli oris muscles, which, in turn, insert into the modiolus. Some fibers of the orbicularis oris muscle, particularly those in the more superficial layers, are formed by muscle tissue of the orbicularis oris muscle proper. Fibers within the deep layer of the orbicularis oris muscle, however, are contributed by adjacent muscles such as the buccinator, levator labii superioris, zygomaticus major, zygomaticus minor, depressor anguli oris, and depressor labii inferioris muscles (see Fig. 24–21). The lateral attachment of the orbicularis oris muscle (including fibers of some of the contributing muscles such as the buccinator, zygomaticus major, and depressor anguli oris muscles) is to the fibromuscular modiolus at the angle of the mouth (see Fig. 24–21). The upper half of the orbicularis oris muscle is innervated by branches of the zygomatic and buccal nerves. The upper half of the orbicularis oris muscle acts with the lower half to close the lips and compress them against the teeth (Fig. 24–23*K*). The pars marginalis superior and inferior muscles play a particularly important role in the articulation of speech. This complex of muscles and the lips form an embrasure when a person plays a brass instrument (Fig. 24–23*K*).

Muscle Innervated by Buccal Branches of the Facial Nerve. The **buccinator muscle** is a quadrilateral muscle. It is attached along its superior and inferior edges to the alveolar processes of the maxilla and the mandible in the region of the molar teeth (see Fig. 24–21). The posterior end of the muscle courses around the third molar to the medial side of the mandibular ramus. Deep to the ramus, the posterior edge is attached to a tendinous raphe (pterygomandibular raphe), which is also connected to the anterior edge of the superior pharyngeal constrictor muscle (see Fig. 24–21). Fibers within the anterior end of the buccinator muscle converge toward the modiolus and then continue into the oral region as fibers of the orbicularis oris muscle (see above). The buccinator muscle is innervated by buccal branches of the facial nerve. It acts to compress the cheeks against the teeth in mastication (see Fig. 24–23*L*). The muscle is also used to expel air from the mouth in forced expiration.

BOX 24–6

SPECIAL VISCERAL AFFERENT BRANCHES OF THE FACIAL NERVE

Distal segments of special visceral afferent (SVA) fibers of the facial nerve are carried by branches of the maxillary and mandibular divisions of the trigeminal nerve to innervate taste buds of the tongue and palate

The basic anatomy of the facial nerve is described in Box 24–5. The reader should recall, however, that branches of the trigeminal nerve ultimately carry distal segments of the SVA (taste) fibers of the facial nerve to the taste buds of the soft palate and tongue (see Box 24–2). For example, taste fibers of cranial nerve VII, which innervate the soft palate, are carried by palatine branches of the maxillary division of the trigeminal nerve (see Fig. 24–20 and a detailed description below). The anatomy and course of the palatine nerves are described in Box 24–2. On the other hand, taste fibers are carried to the anterior two thirds of the tongue first via the facial branch of cranial nerve VII, then via the chorda tympani branches of cranial nerve VII, and finally by the lingual branch of cranial nerve V (see Fig. 24–20 and Box 24–3). The anatomy and course of the facial branch of cranial nerve VII are described in Box 24–5, and the anatomy and course of the lingual nerve, a branch of the mandibular division of the trigeminal nerve, are described in Box 24–3 (see also Fig. 24–20 and a detailed description below.)

The **route of the chorda tympani nerve** is as follows. After the nerve branches from the facial nerve within the vertical part of the facial canal, it courses anteriorly within the petrous part of the temporal bone via a canal and then enters the tympanic cavity (see Fig. 24–20). It continues to course anteriorly between the mucous and fibrous layers of the tympanic membrane, crossing medial to the handle of the malleus. It exits the tympanic cavity via an anterior canal to escape the skull (see Fig. 24–20). The chorda tympani nerve descends within a groove on the posterior surface of the sphenoid spine and passes deep to the lateral pterygoid muscles to join the posterior surface of the lingual branch of the trigeminal nerve. Once the chorda tympani nerve has joined the lingual nerve, its SVA fibers are distributed to the taste buds of the anterior two thirds of the tongue (see below). The GSA fibers of the lingual nerve are distributed to the mucosa of the anterior two thirds of the tongue (see Fig. 24–20).

SVA fibers of the facial nerve travel via the geniculate ganglion

The **geniculate ganglion** not only houses unipolar neurons that function in GSA fibers (see Box 24–5), but it also contains unipolar neurons that function in SVA fibers that innervate taste buds. The centripetal fibers of these unipolar neurons synapse with association neurons deep within the pons at the superior end of an elongated structure called the **tractus solitarius** (see Fig. 24–20). From their synapses within the pons, these fibers are transported via the nervus intermedius (sensory root of the facial nerve). They terminate at an SVA unipolar neuron within the geniculate ganglion. As has been noted above, the centrifugal fibers of these unipolar neurons travel peripherally from the geniculate ganglion via one of two routes.

1. The centrifugal fibers may travel to the pterygoid ganglion by way of the **greater petrosal nerve,** which joins the deep petrosal nerve to become the **nerve of the pterygoid canal.** After coursing through the pterygopalatine ganglion without synapsing, these SVA fibers enter **palatine branches** of the maxillary division of the trigeminal nerve to innervate **taste receptors of the palate** (see discussion of the sensory territories of the maxillary division of the trigeminal nerve above and Fig. 24–20). The proximodistal route of these SVA fibers to the soft palate may be summarized as follows:

Pathway of SVA fibers to taste receptors of palate

Centripetal fibers of unipolar special visceral sensory neurons of the geniculate ganglion originate from their synapses with association neurons of the tractus solitarius. →
They course within the nervus intermedius (sensory root of the facial nerve) to the SVA unipolar neurons of the geniculate ganglion. →
These SVA unipolar neurons emit centrifugal fibers that exit the geniculate ganglion and course within the **greater petrosal nerve** in the pterygoid canal. →
They reach the pterygopalatine ganglion, pass through and, as they exit "hitch a ride" with the palatine nerves of the maxillary division of the trigeminal nerve to innervate **taste receptors of the soft palate.**

2. To innervate the tongue, centrifugal SVA fibers of these unipolar neurons must exit the geniculate ganglion via the **facial nerve.** Within the vertical part of the facial canal, these SVA fibers branch as the **chorda tympani nerve.** These fibers of the chorda tympani nerve then join with the GSA fibers of the **lingual nerve** (mandibular division of the trigeminal nerve), providing innervation for all of the taste buds of the anterior (presulcal) part of the **tongue,** except for those associated with the vallate papillae. The proxi-

BOX 24–6, cont'd
SPECIAL VISCERAL AFFERENT BRANCHES OF THE FACIAL NERVE

modistal route of these SVA fibers to the tongue is summarized as follows:

Centripetal SVA fibers originate from their synapses with association neurons in the tractus solitarius. →
Centripetal SVA fibers are transported via the nervus intermedius (sensory root of the facial nerve) to the unipolar SVA neurons of the geniculate ganglion. →
Centripetal fibers from these unipolar neurons exit the geniculate ganglion via the **facial nerve.** →
Centrifugal fibers then branch from the facial nerve as the **chorda tympani nerve.** →
These taste fibers of the chorda tympani nerve "hitch a ride" with the GSA fibers of the **lingual nerve.** →
The taste fibers of the chorda tympani nerve innervate the **taste buds** (except for the vallate papillae) **of the anterior two thirds of the tongue.**

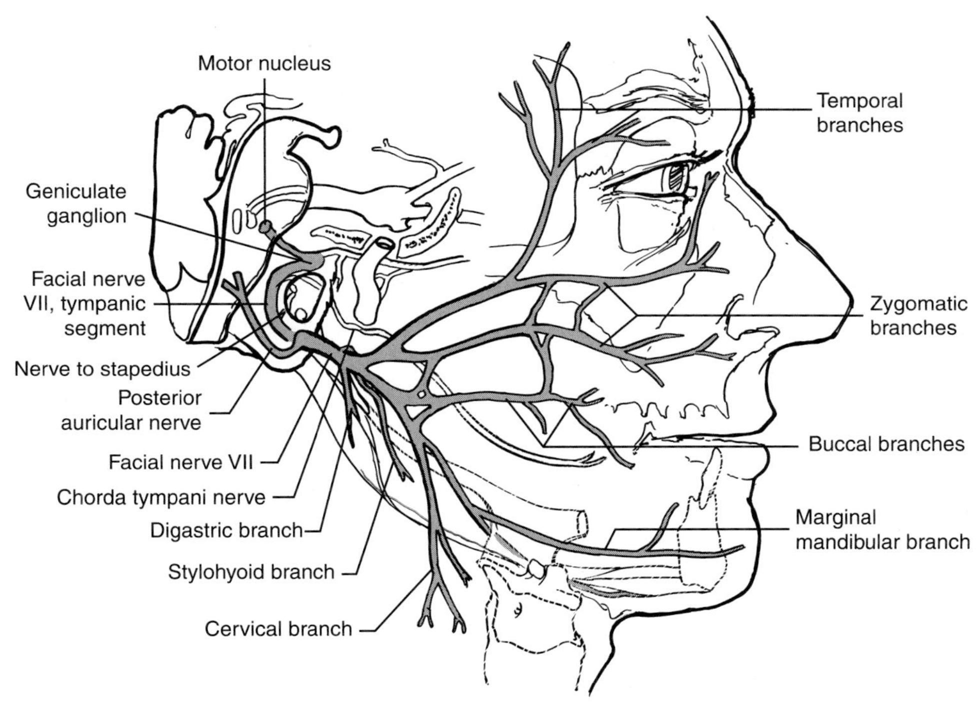

FIGURE 24-24
Facial branchial efferent (BE) nerves (shaded).

Muscles Innervated by Buccal and Marginal Mandibular Branches of the Facial Nerve. The **lower half of the orbicularis oris muscle** consists of two parts: a region intrinsic to the lips called the **pars marginalis inferioris muscle** and a more peripheral region called the **pars peripheralis inferioris muscle,** which extends inferiorly to the mentolabial sulcus (see Fig. 24–21). Specialized fibers of the pars peripheralis inferioris muscle called the **incisivus labii inferioris muscle** arise from the mandible (i.e., from the floor of the mandible's incisive fossa just lateral to the mentalis muscle and inferior to the lateral incisor). These fibers course laterally to blend with other fibers of the muscle and insert into the modiolus (see Fig. 24–21). The lower fibers of the orbicularis oris muscle are innervated primarily by buccal branches of the facial nerve. Its lowest fibers, however, may also be innervated by marginal mandibular branches of the facial nerve. Its acts with the upper half of the orbicularis oris muscle (see above; Fig. 24–23*K*).

BOX 24–7

• BRANCHIAL EFFERENT BRANCHES OF THE FACIAL NERVE

The main branches of the facial nerve serve the muscles of facial expression

Motor axons (branchial efferent [BE] fibers) of the facial nerve grow out from a **motor nucleus** located deep within the pons (see Fig. 24–24). These BE axons form the motor root of the facial nerve. The motor root emanates from the ventral side of the hindbrain (rhombencephalon) just at the caudal boundary of the pons and just medial to the sensory root (see Fig. 24–24). The motor root carries only BE fibers that innervate muscles of facial expression (see below).

The **motor root of the facial nerve** courses anterolaterally within the internal acoustic meatus and terminates in the geniculate ganglion in the horizontal part of the facial canal. Motor fibers then course through the geniculate ganglion without synapsing. These fibers emanate from the inferior surface of the geniculate ganglion within the facial branch of cranial nerve VII along with general somatic afferent (GSA) fibers (which innervate the concha of the auricle), special visceral afferent (SVA) fibers (which form the chorda tympani nerve), and parasympathetic preganglionic general visceral efferent (pGVE) fibers (which innervate the submandibular ganglion) (see Fig. 24–24).

As the facial nerve descends through the vertical part of the facial canal, it gives rise to the **nerve to the stapedius muscle** (BE fibers), chorda tympani nerve (SVA fibers), and ramus to the auricular branch of the vagus nerve (GSA fibers). The remaining motor (BE) fibers and parasympathetic pGVE fibers within the facial nerve continue to course inferiorly before exiting via the stylomastoid foramen (see Fig. 24–24). Upon exiting the facial canal, the facial nerve ramifies into eight major motor branches: **posterior auricular branch, digastric branch, stylohyoid branch, temporal branch, zygomatic branch, buccal branch, marginal mandibular branch,** and **cervical branch.** Their courses and targets are as follows:

1. As soon as the facial nerve exits the stylomastoid foramen, it gives rise to a **posterior auricular branch** (see Fig. 24–24). The posterior auricular nerve courses posteriorly (behind the auricle) and splits into an auricular nerve and an occipital nerve. The **auricular branch** provides motor innervation to the posterior auricular muscle and intrinsic auricular muscles, while the **occipital nerve** courses medially along the superior nuchal line to innervate the occipital part of the occipitofrontal muscle.
2. The short **nerve to the posterior belly of the digastric muscle** branches from the facial nerve close to the stylomastoid foramen to supply the posterior belly of the digastric muscle (see Fig. 24–24). The digastric branch of the facial nerve also communicates with the glossopharyngeal nerve.
3. The **nerve to the stylohyoid muscle** usually branches from the facial nerve near the digastric branch to enter the midregion of the belly of the stylohyoid muscle (see Fig. 24–24).The main trunk of the facial nerve courses anteriorly into the substance of the parotid gland before it gives off its terminal branches, which include the temporal, zygomatic, buccal, marginal mandibular, and cervical nerves (see Fig. 24–24).
4. The **temporal branch of the facial nerve** branches from the main trunk of the facial nerve within the substance of the parotid gland and then quickly branches again to innervate the anterior and superior auricular muscles and lateral intrinsic auricular muscles (see Fig. 24–24). After communicating with the zygomaticotemporal branch of the maxillary nerve (see Box 24–2) and the auriculotemporal branch of the mandibular nerve (see Box 24–3), its main trunk courses superiorly over the zygomatic arch to the temple. The trunk ramifies into branches that innervate the frontal part of the occipitofrontal muscle, superior part of the orbicularis oculi muscle, and corrugator supercilii muscles. Other branches join the lacrimal and supraorbital branches of the ophthalmic nerve (see Fig. 24–24).
5. The **zygomatic branch of the facial nerve** arises from the main trunk of the facial nerve within the substance of the parotid gland (see Fig. 24–24). It then courses anteromedially, crossing the zygomatic arch, to supply the procerus, nasalis, depressor septi, zygomaticus major and minor, levator labii superioris, levator labii superioris alaeque nasi, and levator anguli oris muscles and the superior part of the orbicularis oris muscle (see Table 24–7). The zygomatic branch of the facial nerve also communicates with the lacrimal branch of the ophthalmic nerve and the zygomaticotemporal branch of the maxillary nerve (see Fig. 24–24).
6. The **buccal branch of the facial nerve** arises from the facial nerve within the substance of the parotid gland and courses medially to innervate the superior and inferior parts of the orbicularis oris muscle, including the risorius, depressor anguli oris, and buccinator muscles (see Fig. 24–24). This nerve communicates with buccal branches of the mandibular nerve.
7. The **marginal mandibular branch of the facial nerve** originates from the main trunk of the facial nerve within the substance of the parotid gland. It courses inferiorly, under the angle of the mandible, and then medially, over the body of the mandible (see Fig. 24–24). It provides motor fibers to the inferior part of the orbicularis oris muscle and to the risorius, depressor anguli, depressor labii inferioris, and mentalis muscles. It communicates with the mentalis branch of the mandibular nerve (see Fig. 24–24).
8. The **cervical branch of the facial nerve** arises with the marginal mandibular branch within the substance of the parotid gland (see Fig. 24–24). It sends a branch to the mentalis muscle and courses inferomedially under the platysma muscle, which it innervates (see Fig. 24–24). It also communicates with the transverse cutaneous cervical nerve.

The motor branches and targets of the facial nerve just described are summarized in Table 24–8.

The **risorius muscle** may originate from the zygomatic arch or fascia of the parotid gland, masseter muscle, or platysma muscle. Its fibers converge as they course superiorly from these attachments to insert on the modiolus (see Fig. 24–21). The risorius muscle is innervated by buccal and marginal mandibular branches of the facial nerve. It acts to pull the modiolus and angle of the mouth laterally (Fig. 24–23*M*). The word *risorius* is from the Latin, meaning *laughter* or *grinning*. The risorius muscle is involved not only in these expressions but also in other facial expressions.

The **depressor anguli oris muscle** arises from a broad attachment to the mental tubercle and oblique line of the mandible (see Fig. 24–21). Its fibers converge and ascend to insert into the modiolus at the angle of the mouth. Here, its fibers blend with those of the orbicularis oris and risorius muscles (see below). The depressor anguli oris muscle is innervated by both buccal and mandibular branches of the facial nerve. This muscle acts to depress the modiolus and angles of the mouth, particularly in the expression of sadness (Fig. 24–23*N*).

Muscle Innervated by the Marginal Mandibular Branch of the Facial Nerve. The **depressor labii inferioris muscle** arises from the oblique line of the mandible between the mental symphysis and the mental foramen and from the platysma muscle (see below). The fibers of this quadrilateral muscle ascend to blend with the skin and mucous membrane of the lower lip and with fibers of the pars marginalis inferioris muscle (see Fig. 24–21). It is innervated by mandibular branches of the facial nerve and acts to depress and evert the lower lip, especially in expressions of doubt or grief (see Fig. 24–23*O*).

Muscle Innervated by the Marginal Mandibular and Cervical Branches of the Facial Nerve. The **mentalis muscle** is a small conical muscle that originates from the incisive fossa of the mandible. Its fibers course inferiorly to insert into the mental skin (see Fig. 24–21). The mentalis muscle is innervated by branches of the marginal mandibular branch of the facial nerve. It acts to raise the skin of the chin and to depress the base of the lower lip to assist the depressor labii inferioris muscle in everting the lower lip (see Fig. 24–23*O*).

Muscle Innervated by the Cervical Branch of the Facial Nerve. The **platysma muscle** is a broad thin muscle that originates from fascia of the pectoralis major and deltoid muscles. Its fibers ascend, covering the anterior surface of the neck. Its most medial fibers interdigitate with muscles from the contralateral side. Somewhat more laterally, the fibers ascend to attach to the inferior border of the mandible. Other fibers continue to ascend to insert into the lateral regions of the lower lip. The most lateral fibers ascend over the mandibular body and anterior fascia of the masseter muscle to blend with the skin and subcutaneous connective tissue of the lower face and to insert into the modiolus (see Fig. 24–21). The platysma muscle is innervated by cervical branches of the facial nerve. The muscle acts to tighten the skin of the anterior neck in expressions of terror and astonishment (see Fig. 24–23*P*).

Muscles Innervated by Branches of the Posterior Auricular Nerve. The **occipital muscles** of the occipitofrontal group have been described in the discussion of the scalp above. These muscles are innervated by branches of the posterior auricular nerve. They act to retract the scalp (see above).

The **posterior auricular muscle** arises from the mastoid process of the temporal bone and inserts into the posterior edge of the auricle (see Fig. 24–21). The posterior auricular muscle is innervated by the posterior auricular branch of the facial nerve and acts to pull the auricles posteriorly.

Muscle Innervated by the Digastric Branch of the Facial Nerve. The **posterior belly of the digastric muscle** is a suprahyoid muscle originating from the mastoid notch of the temporal mastoid process. From this point, its fibers course anteriorly just inferior to the mandible (see Fig. 24–22). As it pierces the stylohyoid muscle, it inserts into a tendon that is attached to the anterior belly of the digastric muscle. The **anterior belly of the digastric muscle** originates from the digastric fossa of the mandible (see muscles innervated by the trigeminal nerve above). This tendon is held to the superior edge of the hyoid bone by a fibrous loop. While the anterior belly of the digastric muscle is innervated by a branch of the inferior alveolar nerve, the posterior belly, which is formed within the second pharyngeal arch, is innervated by the digastric branch of the facial nerve. The digastric muscle acts to depress the mandible and elevate the hyoid bone.

Muscle Innervated by the Stylohyoid Branch of the Facial Nerve. The **stylohyoid muscle** is a suprahyoid muscle that originates from the posterior surface of the styloid process of the temporal bone (see Fig. 24–22). Near its insertion, it is pierced by the digastric muscle (see above). It inserts on the hyoid bone at the junction of the bone's body and greater horn. The stylohyoid muscle is innervated by the stylohyoid branch of the facial nerve and acts to pull the hyoid bone posterosuperiorly. This action elongates the floor of the mouth in mastication and vocalization.

Muscle Innervated by the Stapedial Branch of the Facial Nerve. The **stapedius muscle** originates from a cavity within the pyramidal eminence (see Fig. 24–22 and discussion of the ear below). Its tendon escapes from the tip of the pyramid and, from this point, its fibers course anteriorly to insert on the neck of the stapes bone. The stapedius muscle is innervated by the stapedial branch of the facial nerve and acts reflexively to dampen the effects of high-intensity sound on the tympanic membrane. The stapedius muscle directly opposes the action of the tensor tympani muscle, which pulls the tympanic membrane inward.

Abnormal acuteness of hearing **(hyperacusis)** results from paralysis of the stapedius muscle.

A

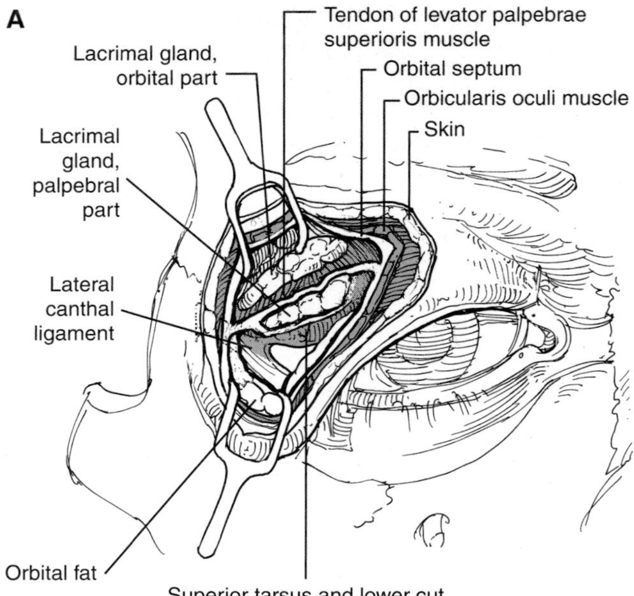

B

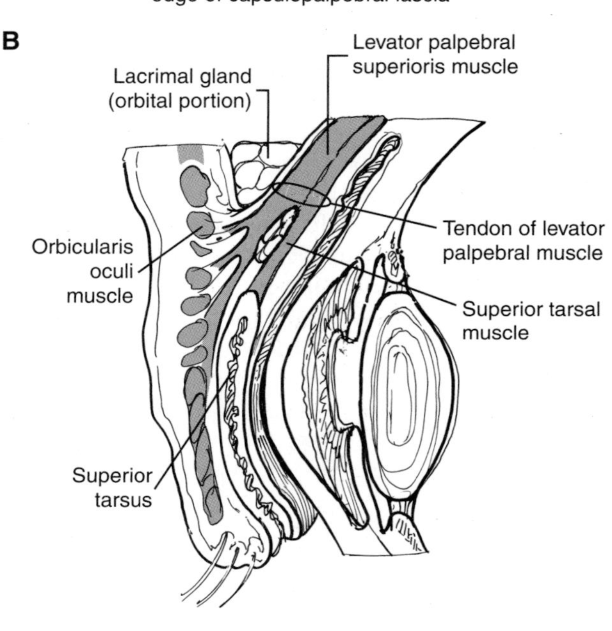

FIGURE 24-25
Lacrimal gland.

Autonomic Targets of the Facial Nerve. *The facial nerve contains parasympathetic secretomotor (pGVE) fibers, which innervate a variety of glands.* In addition to the facial nerve's GSA, SVA, and BE functions described above, the nerve also performs parasympathetic (pGVE) functions by innervating a variety of glands of the face and nasal and oral cavities. These include the lacrimal gland; the mucous glands of the nasal cavity and palatine mucosa; the submandibular and sublingual salivary glands; and the labial, buccal, and palatal glands. As has been described above, however, the distal segments of these fibers are mainly carried by different branches of the trigeminal nerve. In addition, these trigeminal nerves also carry postganglionic sympathetic fibers to these same targets.

Although the **parotid gland** is a parasympathetic target of cranial nerve IX (glossopharyngeal nerve), it is introduced in the following paragraph with other salivary glands.

Lacrimal Gland. The human lacrimal gland has two parts: a large peripheral orbital part and a smaller central palpebral part (Fig. 24–25). Both parts wrap around the concave surface of the aponeurosis of the levator palpebra superioris muscle(a muscle that raises the upper eyelid. The orbital part occupies the lacrimal fossa in the medial aspect of the zygomatic process of the frontal bone. The palpebral part projects below the aponeurosis into the lateral region of the upper eyelid. The four or five ducts of the orbital part of the gland course through the substance of the palpebral part, which has six to eight ducts. All of these ducts empty their secretions (tears) independently into the conjunctival sac. The tears wash across the eyeball, along a groove in the edge of the lower eyelid, into the lacrimal canaliculi (in the edges of the upper and lower eyelids near the medial angle of the eye), and into the lacrimal sac and nasolacrimal duct (see Chapter 25 for a more detailed description of the lacrimal gland). Tears are then transported to the inferior meatus of the nose where they pass posteriorly into the nasopharynx and are swallowed. Innervation of the lacrimal gland is by postganglionic parasympathetic and sympathetic fibers. The course of these fibers is described in the discussion

TABLE 24–8
Autonomic Targets of Facial Nerve Branches

Target	Function
Lacrimal gland	Secretions moisten and lubricate eyeball
Mucous glands of nasal cavity and palatine mucosa	Secrete mucous that captures dust and debris in inspired air for removal to oral pharynx, where it is swallowed
Submandibular, sublingual, and parotid salivary glands	Secretions (mucous and serous) include enzymes that initiate digestion of masticated food in buccal cavity
Accessory salivary glands	Secretions are mainly of the mucous variety

of the maxillary division of the trigeminal nerve above and is reviewed in Box 24–8.

Effects of Rheumatoid Arthritis on Lacrimal Secretion. Normal ongoing lacrimal secretion is reduced in individuals with rheumatoid arthritis. This results in drying of the cornea and increases its vulnerability to ulceration. Nonetheless, emotional distress or irritants that lodge on the cornea may stimulate effusive secretions in these patients. Drying of the cornea is prevented by administration of artificial tears.

Mucous Glands of the Nasal Cavity, Paranasal Sinuses, and Palate. Many mucous glands with branching ducts open onto the epithelial surface of the mucous membrane of the nasal cavity, the paranasal sinuses, the posterior part of the oral side of the hard palate, and the soft palate. The mucous glands secrete a sticky substance that captures debris, which is swept into the pharynx and swallowed. Mucous glands of the nasal cavity and paranasal sinuses are provided with parasympathetic (pGVE) fibers from the facial nerve and sympathetic (sGVE) fibers from the internal carotid plexus via branches of the maxillary division of the trigeminal nerve (see Boxes 24–2 and 24–8).

Salivary Glands. The **submandibular gland** has a superficial large part and a small deep part. The two parts are continuous. The gland is located just medial to the angle of the mandible and medial to the digastric muscle at the posterior border of the mylohyoid muscle (Fig. 24–26*A*). The anterior end of the gland is lateral to the mylohyoid muscle, mylohyoid nerve and vessels, and submental vessels. Its posterior end is just lateral to the styloglossus muscle, stylohyoid ligament, glossopharyngeal nerve, and wall of the pharynx. Inferiorly, the gland is covered by fascia, the platysma muscle, and integument. Numerous small ducts of the superficial part of the gland converge anteriorly to form a single submandibular duct that courses through the deep part of the gland and emerges to course anteriorly between the mylohyoid and hyoglossus muscles (Fig. 24–26*B*). The duct opens in the floor of the oral cavity within a sublingual papilla at the side of the frenulum (Fig. 24–26*C* and see discussion of the tongue in Chapter 26). The submandibular salivary gland produces a mucous and serous secretion, which forms an enzyme-rich saliva used in the initial digestion of food. The secretion is regulated by parasympathetic and sympathetic activity. Postganglionic parasympathetic fibers are obtained from the submandibular ganglion, which is innervated by preganglionic parasympathetic fibers from the facial nerve. These fibers reach the submandibular ganglion via the chorda tympani, the lingual nerve, and a short communicating ramus. Postganglionic sympathetic fibers are obtained through short rami directly from a facial nerve plexus. Postganglionic parasympathetic and sympathetic fibers are then relayed to the submandibular gland and its duct via short branches that emanate from its inferior surface (Fig. 24–26).

The **sublingual salivary glands** are small, elongated glands that lie under the mucosa of the floor of the mouth on either side of the tongue (Fig. 24–26). The two glands meet at their anterior ends, while their posterior ends abut the submandibular salivary glands. The mylohyoid muscle lies immediately beneath the sublingual salivary glands. The mandible is lateral and the genioglossus muscle, submandibular duct, and lingual nerve are medial to the gland (Fig. 24–26*A*). Eight to twenty sublingual ducts open into the floor of the buccal cavity. The sublingual gland obtains its preganglionic parasympathetic fibers from the facial nerve via the chorda tympani, the lingual nerve, and a short communicating ramus. These fibers synapse with peripheral neurons in the submandibular ganglion. An anterior ramus emanating from the ganglion carries the postganglionic parasympathetic fibers to the lingual nerve, which conveys them directly to the sublingual gland. Sympathetic innervation is obtained from a facial nerve plexus by small branches that connect to the submandibular ganglion. These postganglionic sympathetic fibers pass through the submandibular ganglion and are conveyed to the sublingual gland by the same anterior ramus and terminal lingual nerve branches that carry the postsynaptic parasympathetic fibers to the gland (Fig. 24–26).

Several small **accessory salivary glands** are covered by mucosa associated with the lips, palatine tonsils, tongue, and cheeks. These glands are innervated in the same manner as the sublingual gland (see above). Other accessory salivary glands are located in the soft palate and posterior part of the hard palate.

Although the **parotid gland** is a target of cranial nerve IX (glossopharyngeal nerve), it is introduced here because it is such an important structure of the face and is intimately related to several important structures described in this chapter. The parotid gland is the largest of the three major salivary glands. It is located just anterior to the ear (Fig. 24–26*A*). It develops as an outpouching of the cheek. The parotid gland is embedded in cervical fascia and lies deep to the skin and superficial fascia, which contain superficial parotid lymph nodes and facial branches of the great auricular nerve (fibers from spinal nerves C2 and C3). Anteriorly, the gland lies superficial to the medial pterygoid muscle, ramus of the mandible, and temporomandibular joint. Posteriorly, it is superficial to the posterior belly of the digastric muscle, the sternocleidomastoid muscle, the styloid process, the styloid muscles, and the mastoid process.

Many nonglandular structures course through the parotid gland

The parotid gland is especially important in facial anatomy because many nonglandular structures pass through it or ramify within its substance (Fig. 24–27). For example, the external carotid artery enters its pos-

BOX 24–8

PARASYMPATHETIC PREGANGLIONIC VISCERAL EFFERENT FIBERS OF THE FACIAL NERVE

Parasympathetic fibers of the facial nerve are carried to their targets by proximal segments of facial nerve branches and by distal segments of trigeminal nerve branches

The presynaptic parasympathetic preganglionic general visceral efferent (pGVE) fibers of the facial nerve originate from a visceral efferent nucleus within the pons called the **superior salivatory nucleus.** The fibers enter the sensory root of the facial nerve (nervus intermedius) and course into and through the geniculate ganglion without synapsing. They exit the geniculate ganglion with the greater petrosal nerve or with the facial nerve in the following manner:

1. Fibers that exit with the **greater petrosal nerve** join with the deep petrosal nerve (sympathetic general visceral efferent [sGVE] fibers from the internal carotid plexus) to form the **nerve of the pterygoid canal.** These fibers enter the **pterygopalatine ganglion** where they synapse.

   Some pGVE fibers exit to first join the maxillary division of the trigeminal nerve, then the zygomatic branch of the maxillary nerve, and, finally, the zygomaticofacial branch. From this point, a communicating ramus carries these parasympathetic secretomotor fibers to the lacrimal nerve where they innervate the **lacrimal gland** (Fig. 24–28). This parasympathetic pathway can be summarized as follows:

Parasympathetic pathway to lacrimal gland
Central parasympathetic neurons in superior salivatory nucleus emit preganglionic fibers. →
These fibers travel to sensory root of facial nerve (nervus intermedius), →
then are transported through the geniculate ganglion without synapsing, →
to the greater petrosal nerve → to the nerve of the pterygoid canal →
to the pterygopalatine ganglion where they synapse with peripheral
parasympathetic neurons. → The postganglionic rami travel →
to the maxillary nerve → to the zygomatic nerve →to the zygomaticofacial nerve →
to the communicating ramus → to the lacrimal nerve and →
to the lacrimal gland.

It should also be noted that postganglionic sGVE fibers from the internal carotid plexus form the deep petrosal nerve, which joins with the greater petrosal nerve to form the nerve of the pterygoid canal. These sGVE fibers follow the same pathway as parasympathetic fibers that exit the pterygopalatine ganglion to innervate the lacrimal gland. Parasympathetic stimulation produces copious secretions, while sympathetic stimulation results in the reduction of secretions.

Other preganglionic fibers of the greater petrosal nerve synapse with peripheral parasympathetic neurons within the pterygoid ganglion, which emit postganglionic fibers that join with nasal, palatine, and pharyngeal nerves of the trigeminal nerve to innervate the **mucous glands of the nasal cavity** and **palate** and the **mucosa of a small region behind the auditory tube** (Fig. 24–28 and see description of branches of the mandibular division of the trigeminal nerve above). These pathways are summarized as follows:

Parasympathetic pathways to mucous glands of the nasal cavity, palate, and region of pharynx just behind auditory tube begin identically
Central parasympathetic neurons in superior salivatory nucleus emit a preganglionic fibers. →
These fibers travel to sensory root of facial nerve (nervus intermedius), →
then are transported through the geniculate ganglion without synapsing, →
to the greater petrosal nerve → to the nerve of pterygoid canal →
to the pterygopalatine ganglion where they synapse with peripheral parasympathetic neurons. →
Then these postganglionic rami of the pterygopalatine ganglion
target the nasal cavity mucous glands →
via a posterior superior brach of the palatine nerve and lateral posterior superior, medial posterior superior, and nasopalatine braches of the nasal nerve.
target the palate mucous glands →
via greater and lesser palatine braches of the palatine nerve and nasopalatine branches of the nasal nerve or target mucous glands in region of pharynx just behind auditory tube →
via a pharyngeal branch.

mucous glands in nasal cavity via a posterior superior branch of the palatine nerve and lateral posterior superior, medial posterior superior, and nasopalatine branches of the nasal nerve of the pterygopalatine ganglion

mucous glands of palate via greater (hard palate) and lesser (soft palate) palatine branches of the palatine nerve and nasopalatine branch of the nasal nerve (anterior hard palate) of the pterygopalatine ganglion

mucous glands in region of pharynx just behind auditory tube via a pharyngeal branch of the pterygopalatine ganglion

2. Preganglionic parasympathetic fibers also exit the geniculate ganglion with the **facial nerve.** These fibers enter the **chorda tympani nerve** as it branches from the facial nerve and joins the **lingual nerve.** A short communicating branch from the lingual nerve carries these presynaptic parasympathetic fibers to the **submandibular ganglion** where they synapse with peripheral parasympathetic neurons. Postganglionic fibers from these neurons in the submandibular ganglion innervate the **submandibular** and **sublingual salivary glands** (Fig. 24–28). The parasympathetic pathway to both the submandibular and sublingual glands is summarized as follows:

Parasympathetic patway to submandibular and sublingual salivary glands
Central parasympathetic neurons in the superior

BOX 24–8, cont'd

PARASYMPATHETIC PREGANGLIONIC VISCERAL EFFERENT FIBERS OF THE FACIAL NERVE

salivatory nucleus emit preganglionic fibers ⟶
These fibers to to the sensory root of facial nerve ⟶
then course through geniculate ganglion without synapsing ⟶
to the facial nerve ⟶
to the chorda tympani branch of facial nerve ⟶
to the lingual nerve (branch of mandibular division of trigeminal nerve) ⟶
to communicating rami ⟶
synapse with peripheral parasympathetic neurons in the submandibular ganglion to either postganglionic fibers ⟶ to the **submandibular salivary gland** ⟶ or to postganglionic fibers ⟶
to communicating rami ⟶ to lingual nerve ⟶
to **sublingual salivary gland.**

3. **Accessory salivary glands** of the buccal cavity are provided with parasympathetic innervation by the facial nerve (see above). Innervation of the lingual and labial glands (except for the most terminal branches) is by the pathway described for the sublingual salivary gland.
4. Innervation of the **parotid salivary gland** is via the otic ganglion by way of the glossopharyngeal nerve (see discussion of the glossopharyngeal nerve in Chapter 26).

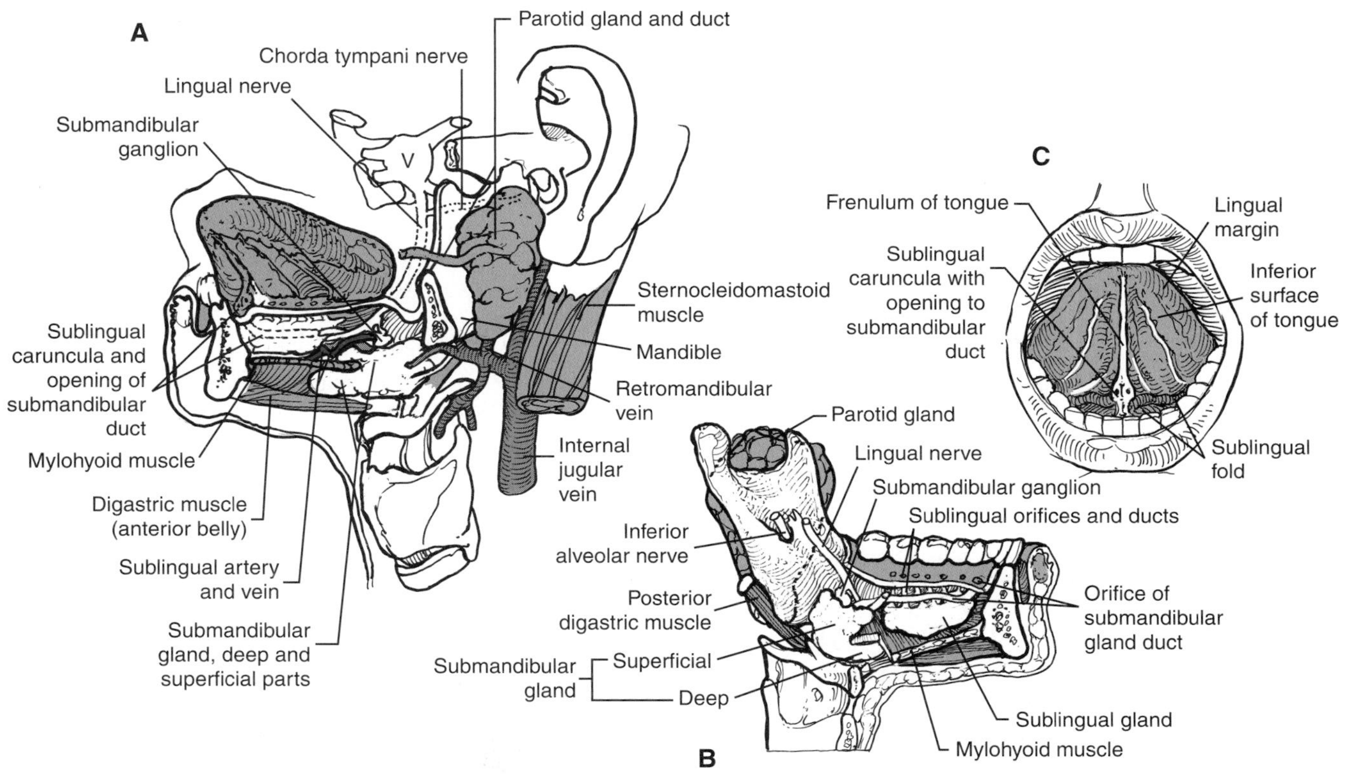

FIGURE 24-26
Salivary glands and submandibular ganglion. **A.** Lateral view of the parotid, submandibular, and sublingual glands (mandible removed). **B.** Medial view of submandibular and sublingual glands showing ducts. **C.** Undersurface of tongue showing sublingual folds and opening for submandibular duct.

teromedial surface and then, within the substance of the gland, divides into two major branches: the maxillary artery and superficial temporal artery. The maxillary artery exits from the anteromedial surface of the gland. The superficial temporal artery first gives off a transverse facial artery and then exits from the superior border of the gland. In some cases, the posterior auricular artery branches from the external carotid artery after it enters the substance of the gland and exits the gland via its posteromedial surface. The maxillary and superficial temporal veins join together to form the retromandibular vein within the substance of the upper part of the

Transverse facial artery
Temporal branch
Superficial temporal artery and vein
Temporal branch
Posterior auricular artery and vein
Zygomatic branch
Masseter muscle
Buccal branch
Occipital nerve
Maxillary artery and vein
Temporofacial division
Cervicofacial division
Buccal branch
Parotid gland
Marginal mandibular branch
External jugular vein (forms from posterior auricular vein and retromandibular vein)
Facial artery and vein
Internal jugular vein
Cervical branch
External carotid artery
Retromandibular vein
Internal carotid artery
Lingual vein
Lingual artery
Common carotid artery
Superior hyoid artery
Common trunk facial, retromandibular, and lingual veins

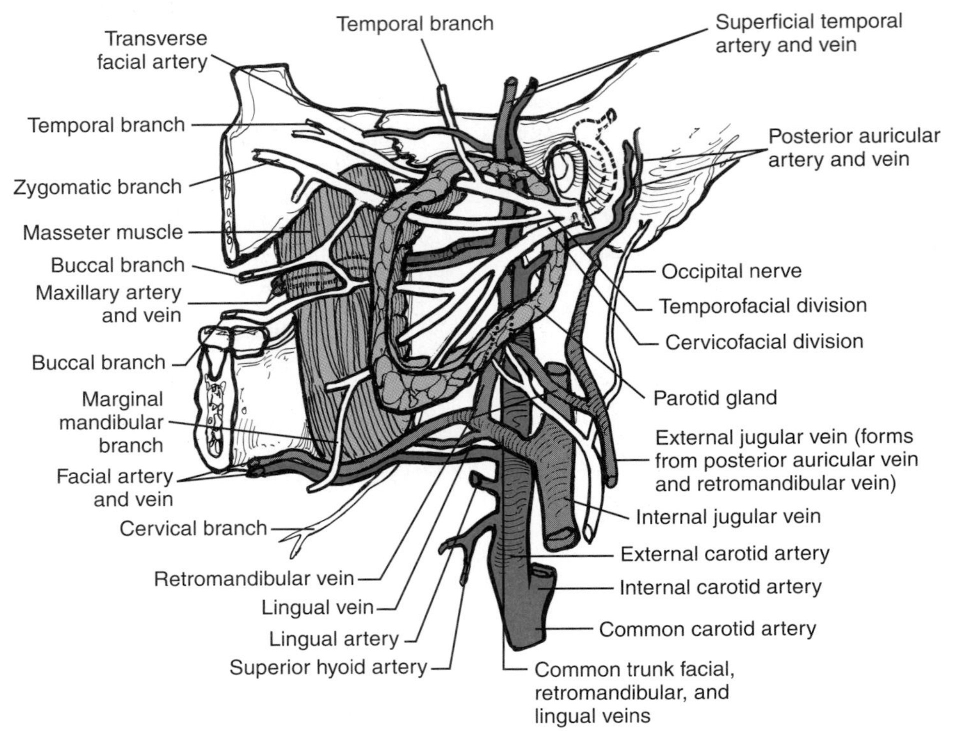

FIGURE 24-27
Relation of the parotid salivary gland to structures within it.

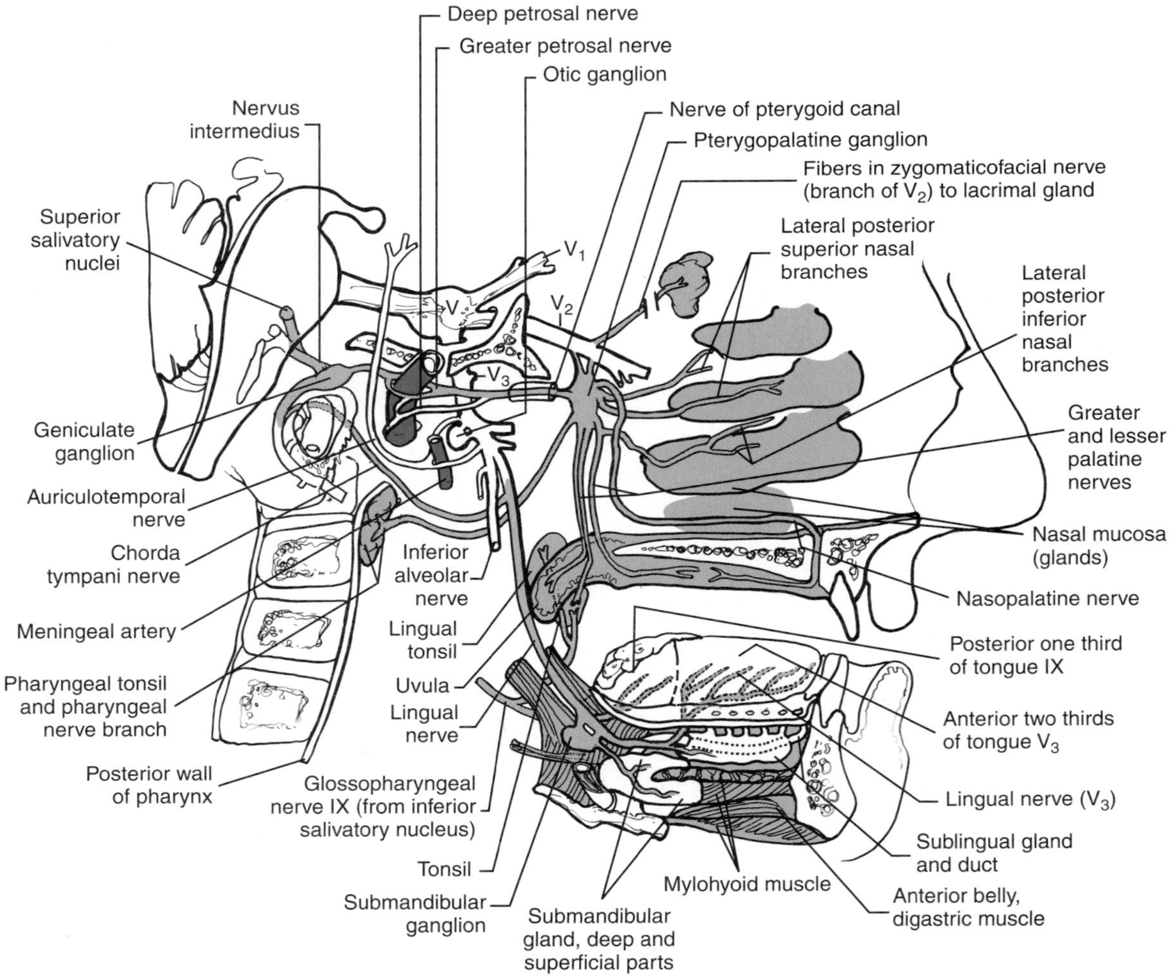

Deep petrosal nerve
Greater petrosal nerve
Otic ganglion
Nervus intermedius
Nerve of pterygoid canal
Pterygopalatine ganglion
Fibers in zygomaticofacial nerve (branch of V_2) to lacrimal gland
Superior salivatory nuclei
Lateral posterior superior nasal branches
V_1
Lateral posterior inferior nasal branches
V
V_2
V_3
Geniculate ganglion
Greater and lesser palatine nerves
Auriculotemporal nerve
Nasal mucosa (glands)
Chorda tympani nerve
Inferior alveolar nerve
Nasopalatine nerve
Meningeal artery
Lingual tonsil
Posterior one third of tongue IX
Pharyngeal tonsil and pharyngeal nerve branch
Uvula
Lingual nerve
Anterior two thirds of tongue V_3
Posterior wall of pharynx
Glossopharyngeal nerve IX (from inferior salivatory nucleus)
Lingual nerve (V_3)
Sublingual gland and duct
Tonsil
Mylohyoid muscle
Anterior belly, digastric muscle
Submandibular ganglion
Submandibular gland, deep and superficial parts

FIGURE 24-28
Parasympathetic targets of the facial nerve.

gland. The retromandibular vein then exits the inferior border of the gland and joins the posterior auricular vein to form the internal jugular vein (see Chapter 27). The facial nerve ramifies within the substance of the parotid gland in a plane that is superficial to the embedded arteries and veins. It enters the posteromedial surface and then ramifies into its terminal branches, which exit the substance of the gland at its anteromedial surface.

The **parotid duct** exits the anterior border of the parotid gland, passes over the masseter muscle where it receives a duct from the accessory lobe, and turns sharply inward to pierce the buccinator muscle. The duct then opens into the oral mucosa just opposite the crown of the second upper molar tooth. A small accessory parotid gland may lie upon the superior surface of the parotid duct just anterior to the main part of the gland where its duct joins the main parotid duct as it crosses the masseter muscle.

The parotid gland is discussed further as a target of the glossopharyngeal nerve in Chapter 26.

Clinical Disorders of the Salivary Glands. Infection and inflammation may occur in any of the salivary glands but is most commonly detected in the parotid gland. This may, in part, be due to the apparent swelling and pain that occurs with viral infections such as **mumps,** which cause expansion of the gland within its tight connective tissue investment. In addition, the enlarged gland may be pinched between the mandible and the mastoid process when a person is chewing. General inflammation of the parotid gland is called **parotiditis.** Bacterial infections causing an **abscess of the parotid gland** are common. They typically result from poor dental hygiene, which causes infection to spread from a tooth into the parotid duct. **Inflammation of the parotid gland** in the absence of dental caries may be diagnosed by early redness of the raised region around the opening of the parotid duct (parotid papilla) within the oral cavity. The parotid duct may be blocked by a calcium deposit called a **sialolith** (from the Greek "sialo," meaning *saliva,* and "lith," meaning *stone*). The patient will feel pain when eating as a consequence of salivary secretion. In certain cases, **excision of the submandibular gland** may be required because of **blockage of the submandibular duct** or the presence of a **tumor** in the gland.

The parotid and submandibular glands may show up more clearly in x-rays if a contrast medium is introduced into their ducts **(sialography).** This technique is useful in examining the diameter of these ducts and their branches to determine whether they are abnormally dilated or constricted. The large number of sublingual ducts and the small bore of their openings excludes them from examination by sialography.

Autonomic Regulation of Salivary Gland Secretions. Salivary secretion by all three major salivary glands and accessory glands occurs almost continuously. However, when a person puts food into his or her mouth, smells food, or has conscious thoughts of food, the salivary secretions rapidly increase. At first the increase occurs primarily through contraction of myoepithelial cells that surround acinar cells of the glands, presumably as a consequence of direct parasympathetic innervation of the myoepithelial cells. The flow of secretions is maintained through direct parasympathetic innervation of the acinar cells. Under parasympathetic control, the secretions are copious and rich in mucus and enzymes. Under sympathetic control, secretions are diminished and watery (see descriptions of the individual glands, above, for information about their sympathetic innervation). It is thought that some additional regulation of secretions may occur through sympathetic vasomotor control of the blood supply to the glands.

Clinical Conditions of the Facial Nerve. *Lesions of the facial nerve pathway may occur at almost any point along it.* The function of the facial nerve may be comprised by strokes, which affect the corticonuclear nerve pathways (between the frontal lobe of the cerebral cortex and the facial nucleus) (supranuclear injury), injury of the facial nerve motor nuclear injury), or injury to the facial neve branches (infranuclear injury).

Supranuclear lesions within the corticobulbar tract (fibers that course from the cortex to the medulla) tend to affect lower facial muscles on the side of the face opposite the lesion because the affected fibers cross over to the contralateral side and because upper facial muscles are regulated by both sides of the cortex. These lesions typically result from a hemiplegia (stroke). The voluntary activities of the facial muscles are usually weakened, but the response to electrical stimulation is not affected. In addition, movements resulting from emotional stimuli remain intact.

Nuclear or **infranuclear lesions** affecting the facial nerve have variable effects, depending upon the point at which the injury occurs. Moreover, injuries to the facial nucleus tend to occur in association with injuries to nearby structures, such as the abducens nerve (with paralysis of the lateral rectus muscle), sensory and motor nuclei of the trigeminal nerve (with sensory loss in the face and anterior scalp and paralysis of the muscles of mastication), and corticospinal tract (leading to paralysis of muscles of the upper or lower limbs). Injuries in the posterior cranial fossa in the vicinity of the internal acoustic meatus or fractures of the petrous part of the temporal bone may affect the chorda tympani branch of the facial nerve and the vestibulocochlear nerve (cranial nerve VIII), resulting in loss of taste in the anterior two thirds of the tongue and deafness. Injuries that result in lesions of the facial nerve in the facial canal proximal to the branching of the chorda tympani result in paralysis of all facial muscles, loss of taste in the anterior two thirds of the tongue, and loss of copious salivary secretions. Sensory innervation to the anterior two-thirds of the tongue is not affected. However, lesions of the lingual nerve just distal to its connection with the chorda tympani result in loss of taste, salivary secretion, and GSA innervation of the anterior two thirds of the tongue.

In contrast to supranuclear injuries, nuclear or infranuclear injuries affect both upper and lower facial muscles on the side of the face where the lesion occurs. The most common condition of this type is **Bell's paralysis,** or **Bell's palsy.** Bell's palsy typically results from inflammation in the vicinity of the stylomastoid foramen, which causes edema and compression of the facial nerve. If all fibers of the nerve are affected, both voluntary and emotional movements of the facial muscles are abolished. The affected side of the face is completely immobile. In addition, all reactions of facial muscles to electrical stimuli are absent. Specifically, the eyebrow droops, the palpebral fissure is wide, and the eye cannot be closed so that tears often dribble from the lower eyelid. The ala of the nose do not flare. Although the oral fissure can be completely closed, the patient cannot form an embrasure or raise the angle of the mouth on the affected side while smiling. Paralysis of the buccinator and orbicularis oris muscles results in dribbling of saliva from the corner of the mouth on the affected side and in retention of food between the teeth and the cheek. Food must be removed with a finger.

Causes of Bell's palsy are typically unknown (idiopathic). Paralysis of the facial nerve may result from surgery of the parotid gland (see above), infections of the middle ear (see Chapter 25), Lyme disease, HIV infection, pregnancy, or dental surgery. In many cases, the symptoms of Bell's paralysis completely disappear.

25 The Orbit and Ear

ANATOMY OF THE ORBIT AND EYE

Review of the Orbit and Eye

A review of the bony orbit and its foramina helps to organize the study of the orbital contents

The **orbit** is the deep bony socket that encloses the **globe of the eye (eyeball)** (see introduction to the orbit in Chapter 22). The orbit protects the eyeball and its associated structures from injury by enclosing them in a bony armor. The orbit also serves as a rigid framework that holds each eyeball securely in place. This security helps the eyes to coordinate their movements in binocular and stereoscopic vision (see discussion of actions of the extrinsic muscles below). The boundaries of the orbit include the roof, floor, medial and lateral walls, apex (most posterior point), and base (anterior opening). The quick review of the bony orbit and its foramina immediately below will serve as a useful framework for organizing the study of the contents of the orbit.

Bony Boundaries and Foramina of the Orbit

The bony boundaries of the orbit include the following:

- **superior wall (roof)** of the orbit, which is formed by the frontal bone and a small part of the lesser wing of the sphenoid bone;
- **inferior wall (floor),** formed by the maxillary process of the zygomatic bone, zygomatic process of the maxillary bone, and part of the palatine process of the maxillary bone;
- **lateral wall,** formed by the frontal process of the zygomatic bone and the greater wing of the sphenoid bone; and
- **medial wall,** formed by the lacrimal bone, orbital plate of the ethmoid bone, and body of the sphenoid bone.

As noted in Chapter 22, numerous foramina in the bones of the orbit provide conduits for the transport of structures between the orbit and the cranial cavity, sinuses, nasal cavity, pterygopalatine and infratemporal fossae, and face. Openings in the walls of the orbit include the following:

- **zygomatic-orbital foramen,**
- **lacrimal foramen,**
- **superior orbital fissure,**
- **inferior orbital fissure,**
- **optic canal,**
- **infraorbital foramen,**
- **supraorbital foramen,** or **notch,**
- **anterior ethmoidal foramen,**
- **posterior ethmoidal foramen,**
- **lacrimal groove,** and
- **nasolacrimal canal.**

These foramina, fissures, grooves, canals, and notches and their functions are illustrated in Fig. 25–1 and summarized in Table 25–1.

Contents of the Orbit

Globe (Eyeball)

The most conspicuous feature of the orbit is the globe (eyeball)

Virtually all living organisms have a sensory device that can respond to light. The vertebrate eye is among the most intricate and perceptive of these devices. The human eye, however, can respond only to a relatively narrow **visible spectrum** of electromagnetic radiation (400–760 nm). Some other organisms can perceive radiation beyond this spectrum, including that in the ultraviolet or infrared spectrums. Light is perceived by visual pigments in visual receptors. In humans, these

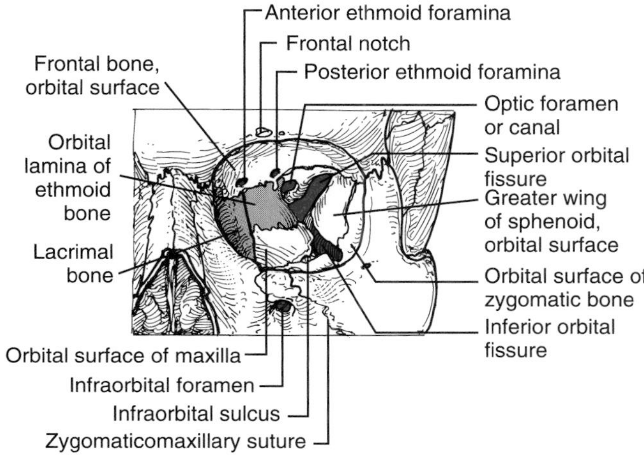

FIGURE 25–1
Bony boundaries and foramina of the orbit of the eye.

TABLE 25-1
Foramina of Bones of the Orbit

Region of Orbit	Bone	Foramen	Structures Passing Through Foramen
Superior wall (roof)	Frontal bone	Anterior ethmoidal foramen Posterior ethmoidal foramen Supraorbital foramen or notch	Anterior ethmoidal vessels and nerve Posterior ethmoidal vessels and nerve Supraorbital nerve
Lateral wall	Zygomatic bone	Zygomatico-orbital foramen	Leads to zygomatic foramen (transporting zygomaticotemporal nerve) and zygomaticofacial foramen (transporting zygomaticofacial nerve)
	Greater wing of sphenoid bone	Lacrimal foramen	Anastomosis of lacrimal and middle meningeal arteries
Between roof and lateral wall	Between greater and lesser wings of ophthalmic sphenoid bone	Inferior orbital fissure	Maxillary nerve, infraorbital vessels, zygomatic nerve, rami of pterygopalatine ganglion
	Maxillary bone	Infraorbital foramen	Infraorbital nerve
Medial wall	Lacrimal bone	Lacrimal groove and canal	Drains tears from conjunctival sac to nasal cavity
	Between body of ophthalmic bone and sphenoid bone and frontal plate	Optic canal	Optic nerve and artery

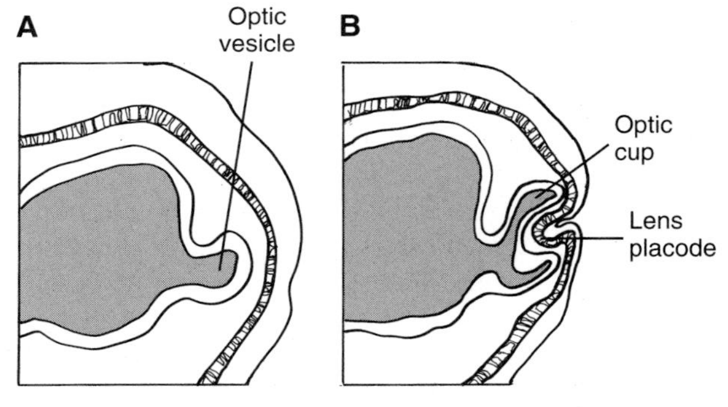

FIGURE 25–2
Development of the globe and lens. **A.** Optic vesicle. **B.** Optic cup with invaginating lens placode.

pigments in the rods and cones of the eye have limitations, which allow them to respond only to a narrow spectrum of wavelengths of light.

Accessory Visual Structures

Accessory visual structures are required for normal function of the globe

In addition to the globe, the orbit contains the following structures:

- **several connective tissue specializations,** including orbital fat, a fascial (bulbar) sheath, an orbital septum, and the periosteum of the orbit (see below);
- **seven extrinsic muscles,** which control the position of the eyeball with respect to the orbit or which raise the upper eyelid (i.e., four rectus muscles, two oblique muscles, and the levator palpebrae superioris muscle) (see below); and
- the **eyelids** and their **conjunctival linings** along with the **lacrimal gland, lacrimal sac,** and **nasolacrimal duct,** which protect the surface of the cornea from bacterial infection, abrasions by debris, and other injuries and which also moisten the globe.

Development of the Globe and Accessory Visual Structures

The globe arises as a diverticulum of the forebrain and a mesenchymal capsule; the lens is derived from surface ectoderm

Early in week 4 of embryologic development, the neural epithelium of the neural plate begins to evaginate in the region of the presumptive diencephalon, a vesicle of the forebrain. The epithelium forms a balloon-shaped structure called the **optic vesicle** (Fig. 25–2*A*). By the fifth week, the apex of the optic vesicle invaginates to form an **optic cup** and **optic stalk** (Fig. 25–2*B*). The inferior side of the optic stalk is marked by the **choroidal fissure** (Fig. 25–3). The walls of the optic cup have two layers: the **neural retina (inner layer)** and the **outer layer.**

The neural retina contains the **rods** and **cones,** which are the photoreceptors of the retina, and the primary and secondary neurons of the retina. Axons of the secondary neurons course back through the stalk of the optic cup to form the **optic nerve.** The outer layer of the

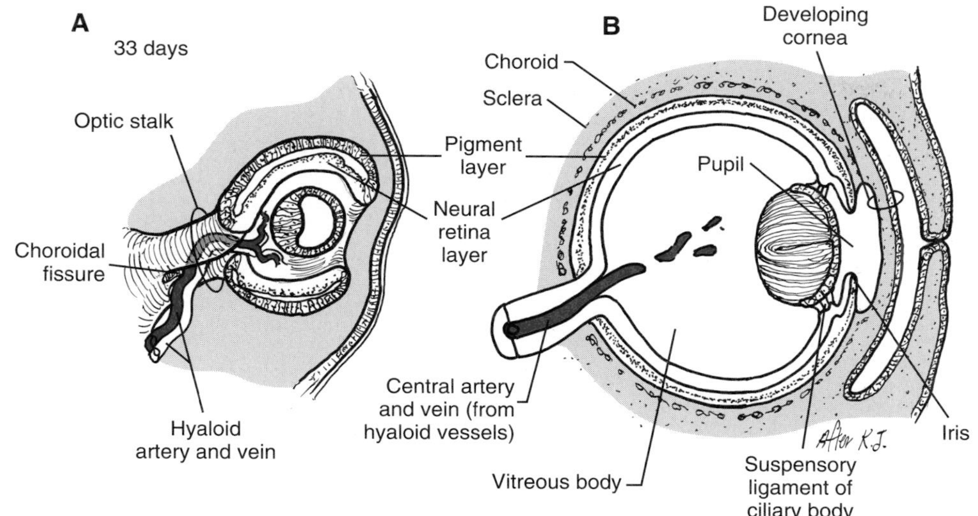

FIGURE 25–3
Development of the central artery and vein of the retina. **A.** Hyaloid vessels in the choroidal fissure. **B.** Proximal segments of hyaloid vessels become the central artery and vein of the retina.

optic cup gives rise to the **pigment retina,** which ultimately forms the middle tunic of the globe, along with the vascularized choroid layer (Fig. 25–3 and see below). The intraretinal space between the pigment retina and neural retina disappears during the seventh week as the two retinal layers fuse loosely.

As the optic cup grows outward during the fifth week, it approaches the surface ectoderm, which has been thickening at the same time to form the **lens placode** (Fig. 25–2*B*). The lens placode invaginates into the optic cup and detaches from the surface ectoderm to form the **lens vesicle,** which ultimately gives rise to the definitive **lens** of the globe. At first, the newly formed lens is vascularized by **hyaloid vessels,** which gain access to it via the choroidal fissure and a **hyaloid canal** in the vitreous body of the optic cup (Fig. 25–3*A*). During fetal life, however, the distal segments of the hyaloid vessels break down, leaving the hyaloid canal empty within the vitreous body. In contrast, the proximal segments of the hyaloid vessels are retained within the stalk of the optic cup as the **central artery** and **vein of the retina** (Fig. 25–3*B*).

By late in the sixth week, the optic cup is surrounded by a **mesenchymal capsule** consisting of cells of the cranial paraxial mesoderm and ectomesenchymal cells originating from the neural crest. The paraxial mesoderm gives rise to the **connective tissue components** of the **wall of the globe** (choroid, sclera, and deep layers of the cornea) and also forms the **meningeal layers** of the optic stalk and optic nerve. These meningeal coverings of the optic stalk remain and are continuous with the meningeal coverings of the brain and with the sclera and choroid of the globe. The sclera of the globe is homologous to the dura mater. The vascularized choroid is homologous to the arachnoid mater and pia mater of the optic stalk and brain.

Because of these anatomic relationships, the optic nerve may become compressed if cerebrospinal fluid accumulates in the subarachnoid space within the meninges of the brain and, consequently, in the subarachnoid space of the meninges investing the optic nerve (see clinical disorders of the neural retina below).

The mesoderm of the mesenchymal capsule also gives rise to the striated **extrinsic muscles** of the globe. In contrast, the neural crest cells of the mesenchymal capsule give rise to smooth muscle fibers of the **intrinsic muscles** of the iris and the ciliary body as well as the tendons of the extrinsic muscles (see below).

During the sixth week, the **eyelids** and their ectodermal linings form. The surface ectoderm that lines the cornea becomes the **conjunctiva** of the lids and the anterior surface of the globe. The space between the globe and this inner lining is the **conjunctival sac.** At about the same time, an invagination of surface ectoderm in the superolateral corner of the orbit gives rise to the **lacrimal gland** (see below). The lacrimal gland is derived from two evolutionary precursors that were originally separate: one that produced a serous secretion and one an oily secretion.

Definitive Anatomy of the Globe

Wall of the Globe. The wall of the definitive globe has an irregular spherical shape. It consists of anterior and posterior parts (Fig. 25–4). The anterior part con-

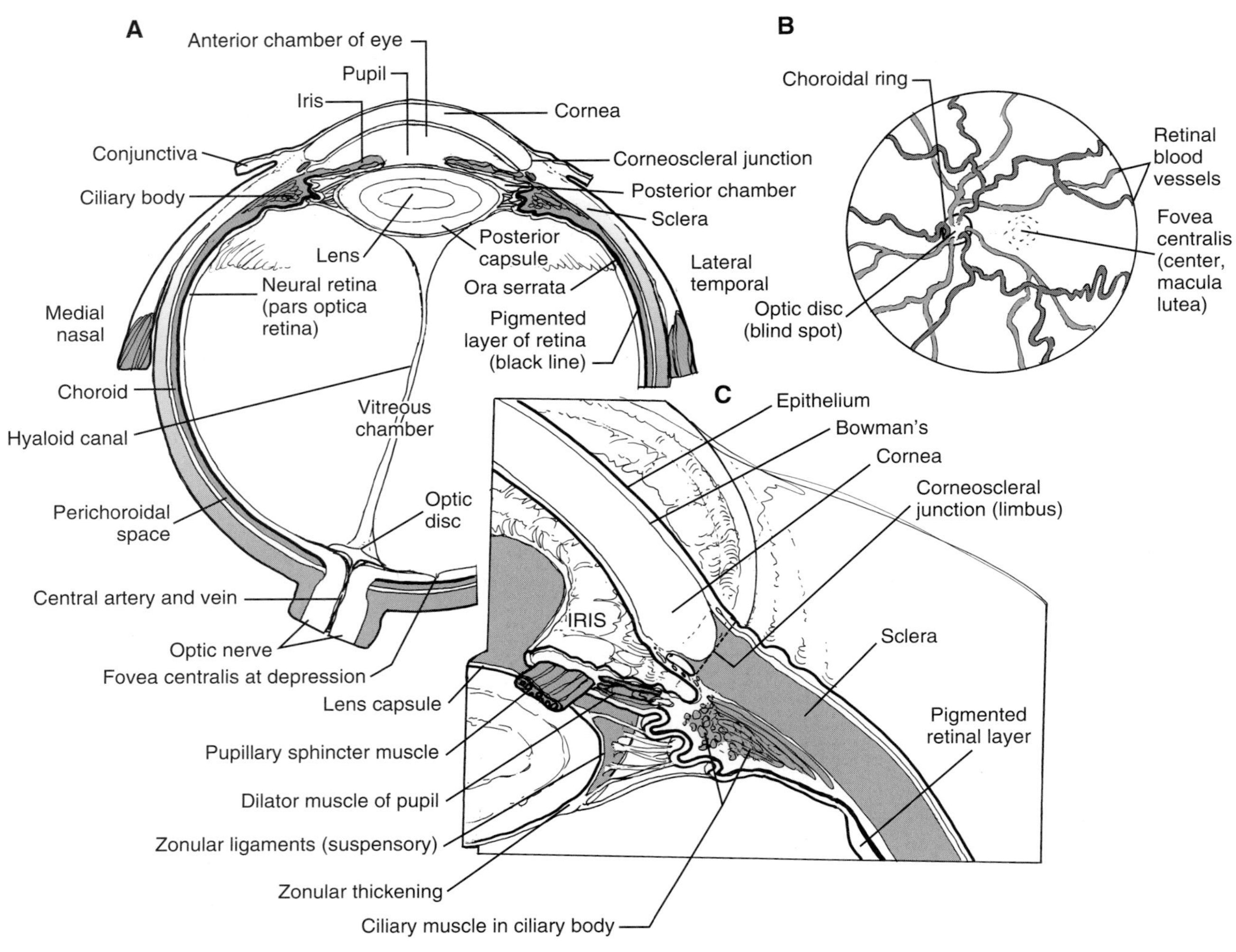

FIGURE 25–4
Definitive anatomy of the globe. **A.** Cross section of globe with detail of the iris. **B.** Ophthalmoscopic view of posterior retinal wall (fundus) of left eye. **C.** Cross section of iris.

stitutes approximately one sixth of the globe. The curvature of the anterior part is more pronounced than the posterior five sixths of the globe. The vertical diameter of the globe is smaller than the transverse diameter.

The wall of the **anterior part** of the globe has only one layer: the transparent **cornea.** The wall of the **posterior part** has three distinct layers: the outermost layer, which is the opaque, white avascular **sclera;** the middle layer, a **vascularized pigmented layer;** and the innermost layer, a **neural layer.**

The vascularized pigmented layer is formed from the vascular **choroid** of the optic capsule and the **pigment retina** of the optic cup (see description of embryologic origins above). The **neural retina** is the innermost layer of the optic cup and is formed by the neural layer (see above). The cornea of the anterior one sixth of the globe and the sclera of the posterior five sixths of the globe are continuous, meeting at the **corneoscleral junction** (Fig. 25–4). The pigmented part of the second layer of the posterior part of the globe, however, is separated from the cornea anteriorly as it forms the **ciliary body** and **iris** of the eye (Fig. 25–4C).

Neural Retina and Its Innervation by the Optic Nerve. The neural retina is the inner layer of the optic cup. The neural layer of the optic cup gives rise to the rods, cones, ganglion, and supporting cells of the neural retina. The rods and cones develop within the outer layer of the neural retina, which is apposed to the pigment retina, and the ganglion and supporting cells form at the inner layer of the neural retina (see Fig. 25–4). Nerve fibers from secondary neurons in this ganglion cell layer sprout axons that grow along the retinal surface back to a region of the posterior retinal wall (fundus) called the **optic disc** (see Fig. 25–4). Here, the axons enter the optic stalk and traverse it to reach the lateral geniculate bodies of the diencephalon (Box 25–1). These fibers of the secondary retinal neurons transform the hollow optic stalk into the definitive **optic nerve** (Fig. 25–5). The

BOX 25–1
THE OPTIC NERVE (CRANIAL NERVE II)

The **optic nerve** facilitates the special sensation of vision. Unlike all other cranial nerves, the optic nerve originates as an outpocketing of the brain, the **optic cup.** It carries special sensory afferent fibers that serve the special sensory function of vision. As has been noted, the optic nerve is formed as axons grow out from secondary neurons of the ganglion layer of the neural retina and then converge at the optic disc where they turn posteriorly to penetrate layers of the neural retina and meninges to enter the optic stalk. Once formed, the resulting bundle of nerve fibers from each globe is called an optic nerve. An optic nerve courses posteriorly from each globe and penetrates a bony **optic canal** between the frontal plate and sphenoid bone of the medial wall of each orbit (see Fig. 25–5 and Table 25–1). Within the skull, both optic nerves course posteromedially, meeting at a "crossroad" called the **optic chiasma.** The optic chiasma is a quadrangular structure in which nerve fibers originating in the nasal (medial) half of each retina (including fibers from the nasal half of the macula lutea) cross over to the contralateral (opposite) side of the chiasma where they exit posterolaterally with fibers from the temporal (lateral) retina of the contralateral eye (see Fig. 25–5). Thus, two fiber tracts emerge from the posterolateral angles of the chiasma. Each carries nasal fibers from the contralateral side and temporal fibers from the ipsilateral (same) side. These fiber tracts are called **optic tracts** (see Fig. 25–5). The optic chiasma lies just anterior to the pituitary gland, posterior and inferior to the jugum and middle clinoid process of the sphenoid bone, and just between the left and right foramen rotundum. Most of the axons within the optic tracts course posterolaterally, entering the brain to synapse with neurons of the **lateral geniculate body** of the thalamus of the diencephalon. From this point, the tertiary neurons of the lateral geniculate bodies emit axons that sweep dorsomedially to the **visual cortex** of the **occipital lobe** of the cerebrum (see Fig. 25–5). Other fibers within the optic tracts course medially to synapse with neurons of the **superior colliculus.** Interestingly, the spatial organization of neurons in the lateral geniculate bodies, superior colliculi, and visual cortex forms an approximation of a point-to-point visual map of the neural retina.

central arteries and veins of the retina also course into the optic stalk via the optic disc.

The retina is the only region of the body in which blood vessels can be viewed directly and are, therefore, accessible for clinical examination. This is accomplished with an **ophthalmoscope,** which allows the examiner to view the retina through the dilated pupil.

Near the center of the retina (just *lateral* to the optic disc) is a small yellowish area called the **macula lutea,** and in its center is a depression called the **fovea centralis.** The fovea centralis is devoid of rod cells and several other layers of the neural retina but contains numerous specialized cones, which give the fovea heightened visual acuity and discriminatory capabilities.

Clinical Disorders of the Neural Retina. **Retinoblastoma** is an embryonic cancer of the photoreceptor cell lineage of the neural retina. It is almost always detected in childhood and is often bilateral. Its incidence is about 1 in 20,000 live-born infants. This disease results from disruption of the RB1 gene at 13q14.1-q14.2. The disease follows an autosomal recessive pattern of inheritance. It typically leads to death in the absence of treatment.

Retinitis pigmentosa is actually a class of inherited degenerative diseases resulting from mutations of photoreceptor proteins, including rhodopsin and the intermediate filament protein peripherin. These diseases are characterized by constriction of the visual field and night blindness, among other symptoms. About 2.5 million individuals are affected worldwide, 84% from autosomal recessive mutations of rhodopsin and other photoreceptor proteins, 10% from autosomal-dominant mutations of rhodopsin or peripherin, and 6% from an X-linked recessive mutation.

Age-related macular degeneration is a major form of irreversible vision loss in the Western world. Initial evidence of the disease may include degenerative changes in the pigment retina and neovascularization of the choroid. These symptoms are followed by the progressive death of photoreceptors (rods and cones) and other cells within the neural retina. The fovea is usually spared until late in the course of the disease. Although causes of the disease are unclear, both cigarette smoking and a complex pattern of inheritance involving one or more genes have been implicated.

The **intraretinal space** between the neural retina and pigment retina is apparent in the newly formed optic cup. The two retinal layers fuse during embryonic life, obliterating the intraretinal space. However, the neural and pigment layers do not fuse tightly, and, thus, various types of trauma, including mild blows to the head, may result in **detachment of the neural retina** from the pigment retina and underlying choroid layers.

Blockage of the central retinal artery results in rapid onset of blindness. The blockage is usually an **embolus** (i.e.,

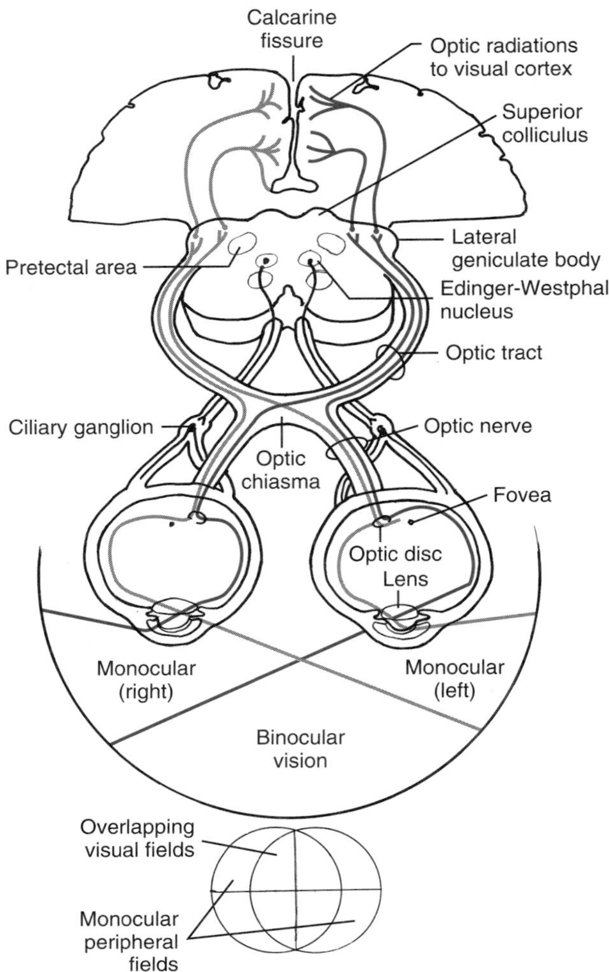

FIGURE 25–5
The optic nerve (cranial nerve II) showing the optic chiasma.

a mass of foreign material such as a blood clot, lipid debris, or fat) that becomes lodged within the artery. This tends to occur more often in elderly individuals. Blockage of the central retinal vein by thrombi (blood clots) may lead to gradual, painless loss of vision.

Edema of the optic disc (papilledema) may occur in conjunction with increased intracranial pressure, which is typically caused by a buildup of cerebrospinal fluid in the subarachnoid space. Since the subarachnoid space of the optic nerve is continuous with the subarachnoid space of the cranial meninges, the increased pressure causes compression of the optic nerve and consequent compression of its central vein. The resulting blockage causes fluid to build up in the globe and a raised papilla to form in the region of the optic disc. The papilla can be seen with an ophthalmoscope. The development of papilledema may be a cause for concern because the underlying increased pressure may indicate that a tumor is blocking the drainage of cerebrospinal fluid from the cranium (see Chapter 27).

The Iris and Pupil and Their Muscles and Nerves

The iris regulates the amount of light cast on the retina

The **iris** (from the Greek for "rainbow") projects into the cavity of the anterior part of the globe and forms an incomplete septum between the **anterior chamber** and the **posterior chamber.** The anterior chamber is located just anterior to the iris, and the posterior chamber is located just posterior to the iris and anterior to the lens (see Figs. 25–3*B* and 25–4*A*). The anterior and posterior chambers contain a fluid called the **aqueous humor,** which is a dialysate of blood containing nutrients for avascular layers of the cornea and for the lens. Most importantly, the aqueous humor is responsible for maintaining the appropriate intraocular pressure, shape, and rigidity of the globe. The aqueous humor enters the posterior chamber as a dialysate of blood through capillaries of the ciliary processes of the ciliary body. It then circulates to the anterior chamber through the hole in the center of the iris called the **pupil** and drains back into the circulation via anterior ciliary veins.

Under normal conditions, the aqueous humor is replaced constantly. If its drainage is blocked, however, the intraocular volume of aqueous humor may increase, causing the intraocular pressure to increase. This condition is called **glaucoma.** The increased pressure leads to "cupping" of the optic disc, blockage of the retinal blood supply, and retinal degeneration. If the blockage occurs between the posterior and anterior chambers because the iris has adhered to the lens, **iridectomy** may alleviate the condition.

Under normal conditions, the size of the pupil varies from 1 to 8 mm as the diaphragmatic iris adjusts to the intensity of ambient light. The intrinsic **sphincter pupillae muscle** of the iris constricts the pupil (miosis), and the **intrinsic dilator pupillae muscle** of the iris enlarges the pupil (mydriasis). The sphincter pupillae muscle consists of myoepithelial cells that form an annular ring at the inner edge of the iris, while the dilator pupillae muscle consists of radially oriented myoepithelial cells at the outer edge of the posterior surface of the iris (see Fig. 25–5C). The fibers of the dilator pupillae muscle extend from the outer edge of the iris to blend with fibers of the outer edge of the sphincter pupillae muscle.

The sphincter pupillae muscle is innervated by **pGVE fibers of cranial nerve III (oculomotor nerve),** and the dilator pupillae muscle by **sGVE fibers of the internal carotid plexus.** The preganglionic (pGVE) fibers of the oculomotor nerves are emitted by central neurons of the parasympathetic **Edinger-Westphal nucleus** of the midbrain (Fig. 25–6 and Box 25–2). These preganglionic fibers project to the parasympathetic ciliary ganglion, where they synapse (see below). Postganglionic fibers arise from peripheral neurons of the cil-

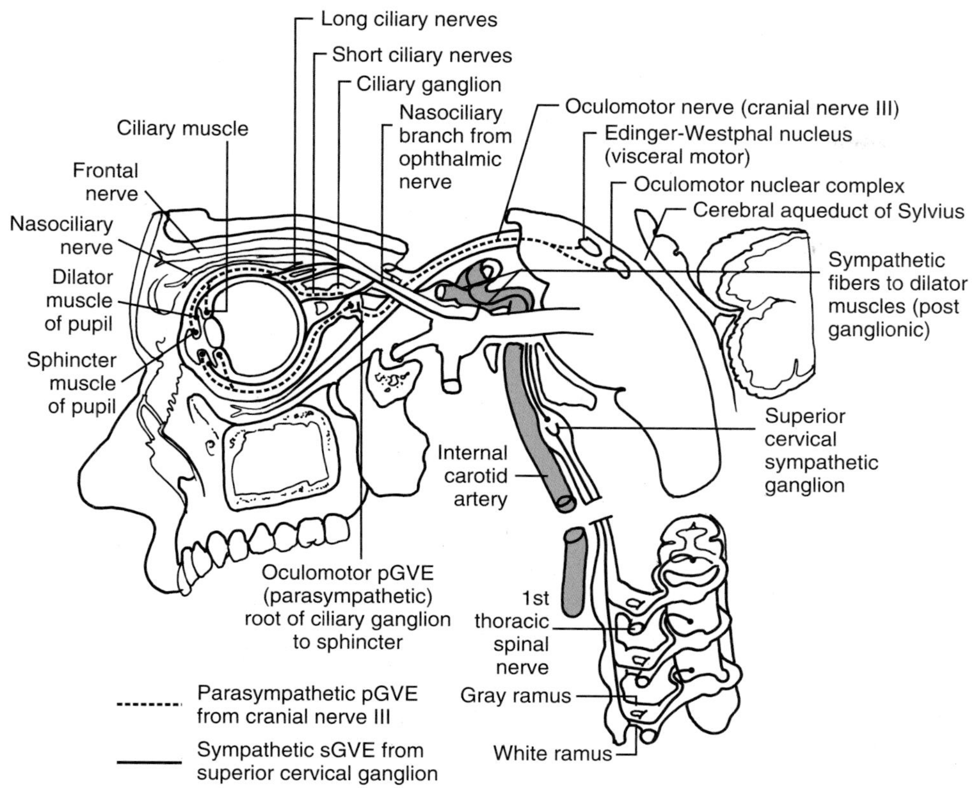

FIGURE 25–6
Innervation of the sphincter and dilator muscles of the iris.

iary ganglion and travel to the sphincter pupillae muscles via short ciliary nerves of the ciliary ganglion of the oculomotor nerve (Box 25–2). In contrast, the postganglionic (sGVE) fibers that innervate the dilator pupillae muscles arise in the superior cervical ganglion, ascend to the internal carotid plexus, and course to the dilator muscle via the ciliary ganglion and short ciliary branches of the oculomotor nerve. The pupil is relatively small during periods of peace and relaxation (if sufficient levels of ambient light are present). However, if a fight-and-flight response is needed, the pupil enlarges to let more light strike the retina. As has been noted in Chapter 24, the sphincter and dilator pupillae muscles are also supplied by afferent (GSA) fibers, which course from the muscles to the ciliary ganglion via short ciliary nerves. However, these centrifugal fibers do not synapse in the ciliary ganglion but, instead, cross over to the nasociliary branch of the ophthalmic division of the trigeminal nerve where they course posteriorly to sensory neurons in the semilunar ganglion (see Box 24–1).

Pupillary Light Reflex. The pupillary light reflex maintains optimal illumination of the retina by regulating the size of the pupil. Retinal ganglion cells respond linearly to luminescence levels. (This means that cells respond in direct proportion to the amount of light received.) Their axons travel to the midbrain via fibers coursing in the optic nerve, optic chiasma, and optic tracts (see Box 25–1). These fibers ultimately synapse with neurons in the olivary pretectal nucleus. Fibers emitted by neurons of the olivary pretectal nucleus, in turn, innervate the central parasympathetic nuclei (Edinger-Westphal nuclei) of cranial nerve III (oculomotor nerve) (Fig. 25–7 and Box 25–2). Central parasympathetic neurons of the Edinger-Westphal nuclei emit preganglionic axons that travel with the oculomotor nerves to innervate neurons in the ciliary ganglia. These neurons emit postganglionic parasympathetic fibers that innervate the iris. In the pupillary light reflex, retinal ganglion cells are activated as luminescence levels increase and impulses travel to the olivary pretectal nucleus, Edinger-Westphal nucleus, and ciliary ganglion. The consequent activity of the cholinergic endings of the postganglionic parasympathetic fibers emitted by the ciliary ganglion excites the constrictor pupillae muscle and inhibits the dilator pupillae muscle, reducing the size of the pupil (Fig. 25–7).

The pupillary light reflex is used in ophthalmologic examination of the retina. Cholinergic blocking agents are administered to dilate the pupils.

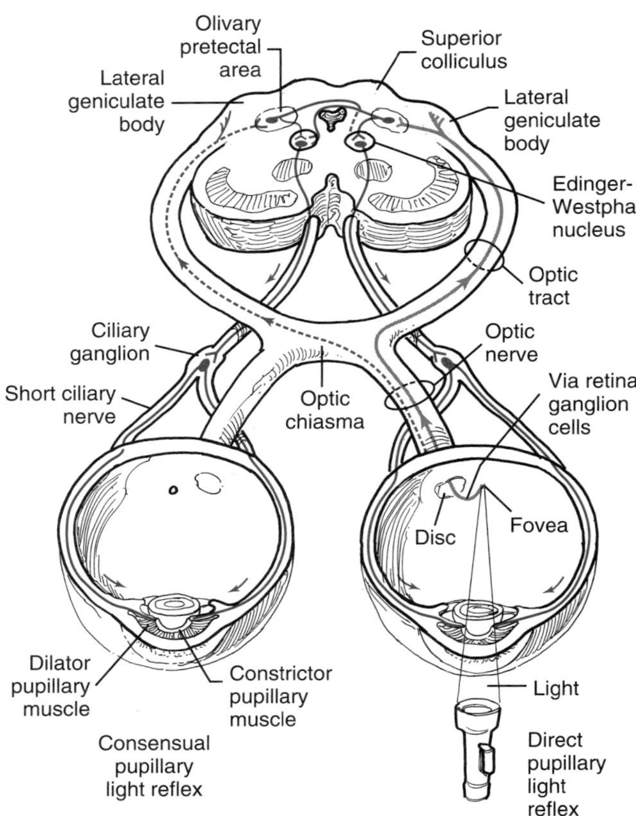

FIGURE 25–7
Pupillary light reflex.

As is the case for axons of secondary neurons in the visual pathway (see Box 25–1), the axons of retinal ganglion cells in the nasal retina cross over to the contralateral (opposite) optic tract at the optic chiasma, while the axons of temporal retinal ganglion cells remain in the optic tract on the ipsilateral (same) side. In addition, the neurons of both pretectal olivary nuclei in the midbrain send neurons to both left and right Edinger-Westphal nuclei. As a consequence, an increase in illumination seen by one eye affects the diameter of both the pupil of the illuminated eye (direct response) and the pupil of the nonilluminated eye (consensual response) (Fig. 25–7). The actions of the iris in each eye are, therefore, defined as being **yoked.**

The pupils may also respond to changes in **emotional status.** For example, as sexual desire is aroused, the dilator pupillae muscles are activated by postganglionic sympathetic fibers of the internal carotid plexus (see above), resulting in dilatation of the pupils.

Clinical Disorders of the Iris. Clinical testing of the pupillary light response is typically carried out with a small penlight. Testing is useful for the analysis of both cranial nerve and brainstem function. Because the pupillary fibers are superficially located in the oculomotor nerve, they are particularly susceptible to **compression by dislocation of parts of the brainstem.** Such dislocations may be caused by a space-occupying tumor, or by edema or bleeding following trauma. The initial evidence of compression of the oculomotor nerve is slowness of the pupillary light response on the illuminated side or of complete dilatation of the pupil. The latter condition may occur when the dilator pupillae muscle is no longer opposed by action of the constrictor pupillae muscle and may indicate dangerous compression of the brainstem.

The Lens and Ciliary Body and Their Muscles and Nerves

The ciliary body adjusts the shape of the lens

The **ciliary body** is a thickened annular ring within the wall of the globe just posterior to the iris (see Fig. 25–8*B*). It is attached to the lens by **zonular ligaments (suspensory fibers of the lens),** which, when tightened by the action of smooth muscle fibers within the ciliary body **(ciliary muscle),** change the shape of the lens and, thus, cause the **dioptric (refractive) power** of the lens to vary. It should be noted that the cornea has a far greater capacity to refract and focus light on the retina than does the lens.

Clinical Disorders of the Lens. The refractive power of the lens is reduced by half by age 40 years and to less than one-tenth by age 60 years. In addition, vision may be impaired with advancing age by opacities of the lens called **cataracts.** Mutations of a gap junction protein, connexin50, have recently been linked to inherited congenital cataract of the lens. Since the lens fibers are linked by gap junctions comprised of connexin50 and connexin46, it is thought that the maintenance of junctional contacts between lens fibers is necessary for normal transparency of the lens.

Innervation of Muscles of the Ciliary Body; Accommodation Reflex. *The ciliary muscle of the ciliary body is innervated by oculomotor postganglionic parasympathetic fibers emitted from the ciliary ganglion within the short ciliary nerves.* The **accommodation reflex** is typically operative when a person attempts to view objects close to the eye. Impulses from the retina course to the lateral geniculate bodies via the optic nerves and optic tracts (cranial nerve II) and from the lateral geniculate bodies to the visual cortex (Fig. 25–8). Long association fibers then carry impulses to frontal visual areas, which are connected to the oculomotor Edinger-Westphal nuclei (cranial nerve III) by descending pathways. From this point, impulses travel along preganglionic parasympathetic fibers of the oculomotor nerve to the ciliary ganglion and then along postganglionic fibers of the short ciliary nerves to the ciliary and constrictor pupillae muscles (Fig. 25–8). As a consequence, the lens is flattened and the pupil constricts to increase the depth of focus. Other fibers from the Edinger-Westphal nuclei innervate the medial recti

BOX 25–2

INTRODUCTION TO THE OCULOMOTOR NERVE AND PARASYMPATHETIC GENERAL VISCERAL EFFERENT INNERVATION OF INTRINSIC MUSCLES OF THE EYE

General somatic efferent (GSE) fibers of the oculomotor, trochlear, and abducent nerves control the movements of the eyeballs through actions of the extrinsic eye muscles. These three nerves, therefore, are regulated coordinately by higher cortical centers. The GSE functions of the three nerves are described together in Box 25–3. The oculomotor nerve, however, stands out as the most important of the three nerves. It innervates four of the six extrinsic muscles as well as the muscle that raises the upper eyelid. It is also distinguished by a parasympathetic component that innervates intrinsic muscles of the eye. Therefore, a general introduction to the oculomotor nerve and its parasympathetic function is provided here.

The oculomotor nerve is typically described as having only motor (GSE) and parasympathetic general visceral efferent (pGVE) functions (see Chapter 23). General somatic afferent fibers innervating proprioceptive endings of the five extrinsic muscles innervated by the oculomotor nerve, however, are also present in distal segments of the nerve. These fibers eventually cross over to the ophthalmic branch of the trigeminal nerve.

The **motor nucleus** of the oculomotor nerve is located in the midbrain at the level of the superior colliculi, near the midline and just anterior to the cerebral aqueduct of Sylvius (see Fig. 25–6). Motor neurons within the nucleus are clustered into groups that innervate each of the extrinsic muscles served by the oculomotor nerve. The GSE fibers of the oculomotor nerve join with parasympathetic fibers from the parasympathetic **Edinger-Westphal nucleus** to form the **oculomotor nerve.** The oculomotor nerve emanates from the midbrain at the junction of the midbrain and the pons within the middle cranial fossa (see Fig. 25–6). From this point, the oculomotor nerve courses anteriorly between the superior cerebral and posterior cerebellar arteries and enters the cavernous sinus. It exits the cranium via the superior orbital fissure, immediately passes through the common annular ring, and splits into superior and inferior branches. The distribution of motor fibers from this point is described in Box 25–3.

The sphincter pupillae and ciliary muscles of the eye are innervated by postganglionic pGVE fibers of the ciliary ganglion. As has been noted in the text, the Edinger-Westphal nucleus provides the preganglionic pGVE fibers of the oculomotor nerve. The Edinger-Westphal nucleus is located in the midbrain just dorsal to the oculomotor nucleus. Preganglionic parasympathetic fibers emitted from the Edinger-Westphal nucleus course anteriorly, joining with motor fibers of the motor nucleus to form the oculomotor nerve, which exits the brain between the midbrain and the pons (see Fig. 25–6). These preganglionic parasympathetic fibers course anteriorly via the oculomotor nerve into the orbit. For a short distance, the fibers course via the inferior division of the nerve and then with the nerve to the inferior oblique muscle. These preganglionic parasympathetic fibers, however, quickly exit from the nerve to the inferior oblique muscle to enter the peripheral parasympathetic ganglion of the oculomotor nerve, the **ciliary ganglion.** The preganglionic fibers synapse with the peripheral parasympathetic neurons in the ciliary ganglion, which then emits postganglionic fibers that exit the ciliary ganglion via 6–10 **short ciliary nerves.** These short ciliary nerves innervate the ciliary muscle of the ciliary body and the sphincter pupillae muscle of the iris. When the sphincter pupillae muscle contracts, it reduces the size of the pupil and thus protects the retina from excessive light.

The dilator pupillae muscles are innervated by postganglionic sympathetic general visceral efferent (sGVE) fibers from the superior cervical ganglion. The dilator pupillae muscle of the eye is innervated by a sympathetic pathway originating from central sympathetic neurons located in upper thoracic levels of the spinal cord. These neurons emit preganglionic sGVE fibers via the ventral rami, which enter their respective thoracic ganglia via a white ramus communicantes. The fibers then immediately leave the thoracic chain ganglion, ascending via the cervical region of the sympathetic trunk to synapse with peripheral sympathetic neurons in the superior cervical ganglion. These peripheral neurons emit fibers that ascend into the skull via the internal carotid artery where they form an internal carotid plexus. These postganglionic sGVE fibers follow the ophthalmic artery into the orbit, pass through the ciliary ganglion, and travel to the dilator pupillae muscles via short and long ciliary nerves. The dilator pupillae muscle acts during conditions of fight and flight.

---

muscles of the eyes so that the eyes can converge to focus on an object within close range (see discussion of extrinsic muscles of the eyes below).

Vitreous Chamber

The **vitreous chamber** is just posterior to the lens and the posterior chamber of the globe (see Fig. 25–4). It comprises approximately four fifths of the total volume of the globe and is filled with a hyaluronan-rich gel called the **vitreous body.** The vitreous body has an anterior depression called the **hyaloid fossa,** which accommodates the lens. A slender **hyaloid canal** courses within the vitreous body along an anteroposterior axis between the center of the posterior surface of the lens and the posterior wall of the globe (see Fig. 25–4). During embryonic and fetal life, the hyaloid canal transmits

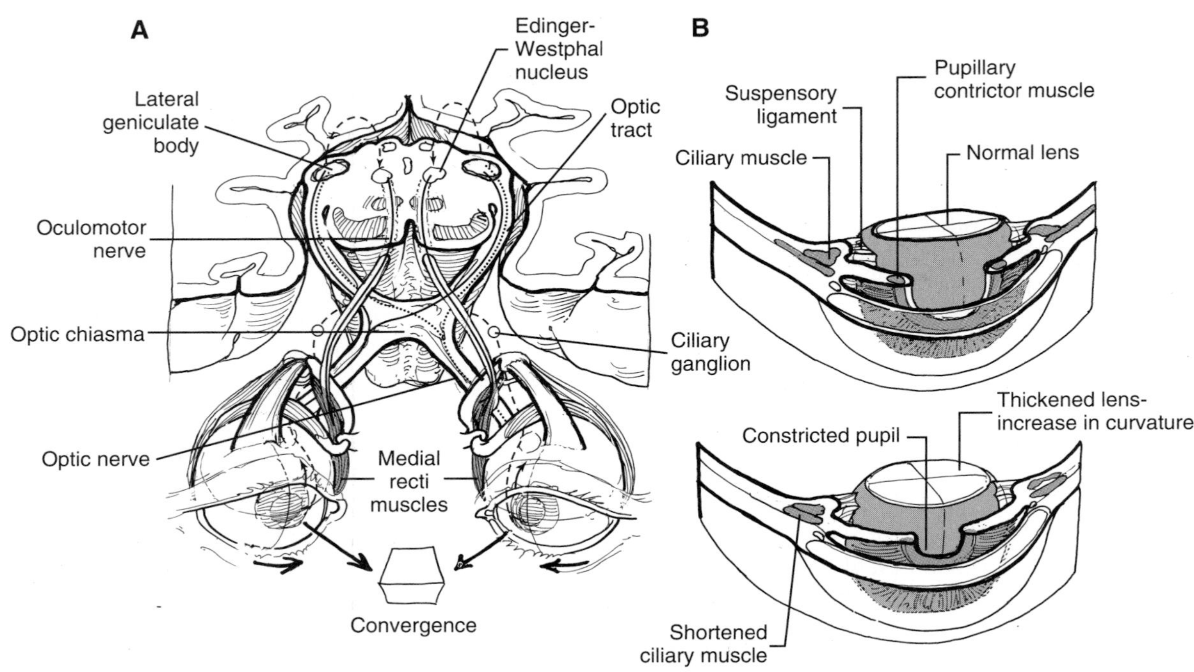

FIGURE 25–8
Accommodation reflex. **A.** Nerve pathways that control the accommodation reflex. **B.** Normal and increased curvature of the lens.

the hyaloid artery and vein, which vascularize the developing lens.

▲ Anatomy of Accessory Structures of the Orbit

Orbital Fat, Fascial (Bulbar) Sheath, and Orbital Fascia

The globe does not fill the entire orbit. It is embedded within an investment of **orbital fat.** However, a thin **fascial (bulbar) sheath** separates the globe from the orbital fat (Fig. 25–9). Anterior boundaries of the sheath blend with the sclera just posterior to the corneoscleral junction. Posteriorly, however, the fascial sheath invests the globe loosely and is separated from it by an **episcleral space,** which is traversed by delicate strands of connective tissue. Thus, the globe is free to rotate within the orbit through the actions of the extrinsic muscles of the eye (see below). These muscles penetrate the fascial sheath to attach to the sclera and are invested to varying degrees by reflections of the bulbar sheath. In addition, a lateral thickening of the bulbar sheath is attached to the zygomatic bone and a medial thickening is attached to the maxilla. These **medial** and **lateral palpebral ligaments** may check the transverse movements of the eyeball. An inferior thickening of the bulbar sheath called the **suspensory ligament of the eye,** along with fascial connections to the periorbit (see below), are thought to support the eyeball within the orbit.

The bony surface of the orbit is covered by **connective tissue (periosteum of the orbit,** or **periorbit).** This thin layer of orbital fascia covers the trochlea and lines the fossa for the lacrimal sac (see below). Posteriorly, the periorbit is continuous with the sheath of the optic nerve, which, in turn, is continuous with the dura mater of the brain (Fig. 25–9).

A thin membrane called the **orbital septum** is attached to the periosteum around the anterior circumference of the orbit. This delicate sheet courses centripetally to blend with the aponeurosis of the muscle that raises the upper lid (levator palpebrae superioris muscle) or into the connective tissue of the lower lid (Fig. 25–9).

Lacrimal Apparatus (Including the Eyelid and Conjunctival Sac)

The lacrimal apparatus includes the lacrimal gland, lacrimal canaliculi, lacrimal sac, nasolacrimal duct, and eyelid

As has been noted in Chapter 24, the **lacrimal glands** of humans have two parts: a larger orbital part and a smaller palpebral part (Fig. 25–10).

The **orbital part** of the lacrimal gland rests in the **lacrimal fossa** of the zygomatic process of the frontal bone. Its superior edge is connected to the orbital periosteum, its inferior edge is connected to the sheath of the levator palpebrae superioris muscle (see below), and its anterior surface to the orbital septum. The **palpebral part** of the lacrimal gland is just inferior to the orbital part. It extends somewhat into the lateral part of the upper eyelid. Both parts of the human lacrimal gland contain cells that produce both serous and mucous secretions, which are elaborated through

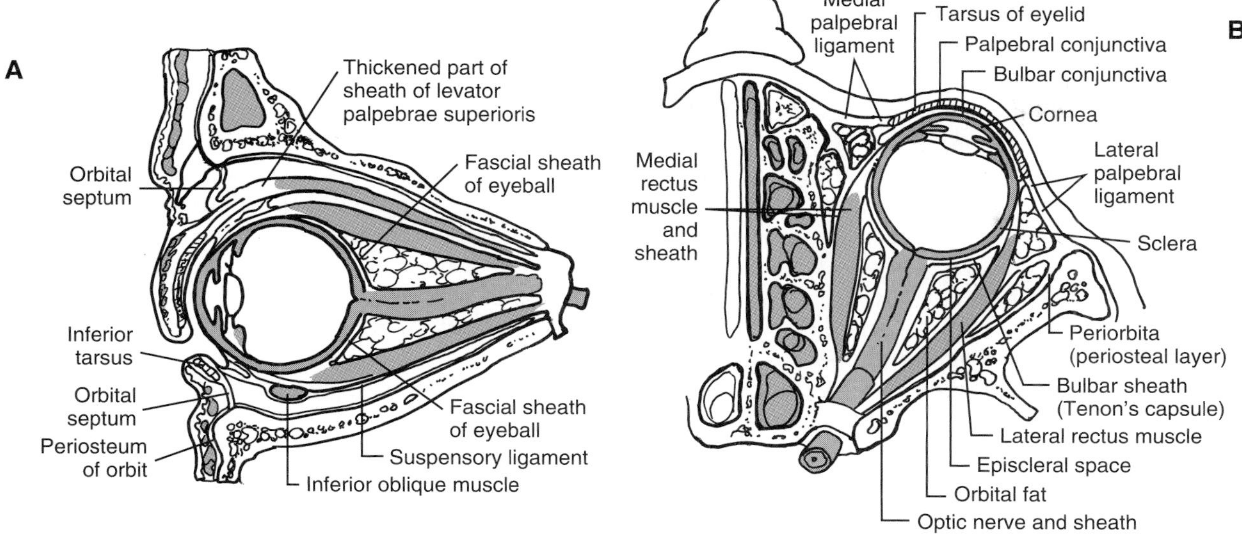

FIGURE 25–9
Connective tissue of the orbit. **A.** Lateral view. **B.** Superior view.

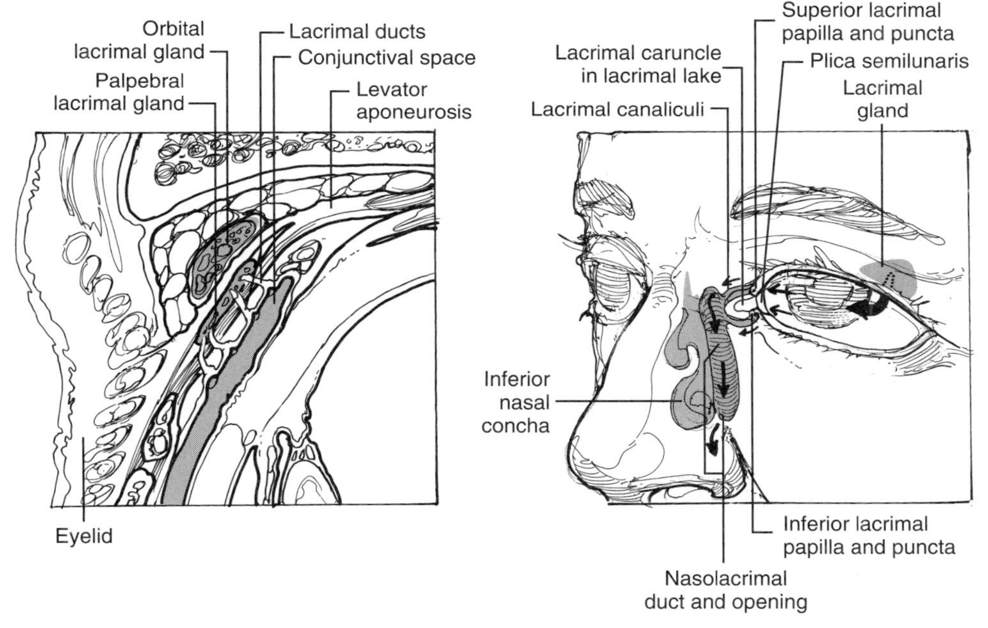

FIGURE 25–10
Lacrimal gland and apparatus.

16 or 17 **lacrimal ducts.** The four to five lacrimal ducts of the orbital part of the gland pass through the substance of the palpebral part, so that removal of the palpebral part effectively disrupts the function of the entire gland. The eyeball, however, is also moistened by tears from small accessory lacrimal glands within the eyelid, and these continue to function even if the main body of the lacrimal gland has been removed.

The inner surface of the eyelid and outer surface of the cornea are covered by a thin membrane called the **conjunctiva.** The enclosed space between the eyeball and inner surface of the eyelid is thus called the **conjunctival space.** The conjunctiva is derived from the surface ectoderm of the embryo. The tears secreted by the lacrimal gland are elaborated into the conjunctival space and eventually enter an orifice at the edge of the

eyelid near the medial canthus: the **superior** and **inferior lacrimal puncta** (Fig. 25–10). The lacrimal puncta are the orifices of the **lacrimal canaliculi,** which are short ducts that lead into an expansion called the **lacrimal sac.** The lacrimal sac lies in a fossa of the lacrimal bone (see above) and should not be confused with the **lacrimal caruncle,** which is a small mound of skin visible in a small triangular region of the conjunctival sac at the medial angle of the eye called the **lacrimal lake.** The lacrimal sac is continuous with the **nasolacrimal duct,** a long vertical conduit that empties tears into the inferior meatus of the nasal cavity.

The Eyelid. *The eyelid is an accessory to the lacrimal apparatus.* The eyelid plays an important role in spreading tears over the cornea and transporting and removing tears from the conjunctival sac (see above). The eyelid is a thin derivative of the superior and inferior folds of embryonic ectoderm that enclose a mesodermal core (Fig. 25–11). In the definitive condition, the eyelid has several layers, including, from outside to inside, the following:

- **skin,**
- **loose connective tissue,**
- **fibers of the orbicularis oculi muscle,**
- **fibers of the levator palpebrae superioris muscle in the upper lid,**
- **tarsus,**
- **orbital septum,**
- **tarsal glands,** and
- **conjunctiva.**

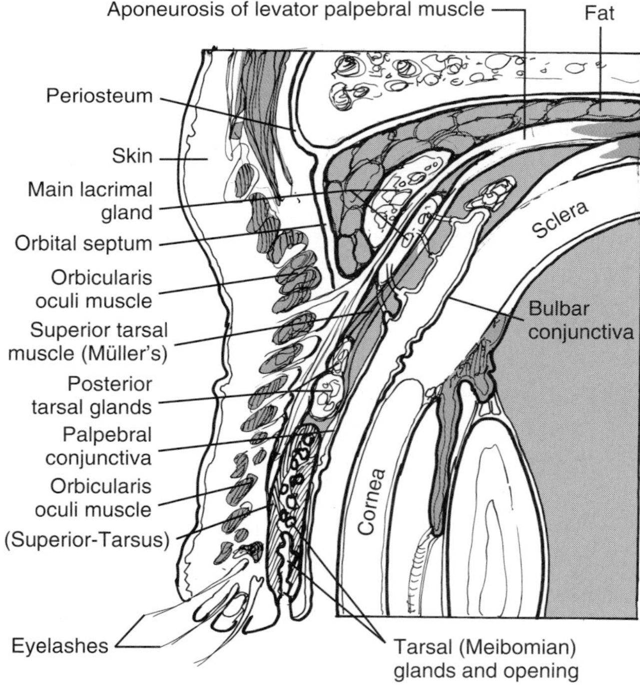

FIGURE 25–11
Layers of eyelids.

The orbital septum is described above and the orbicularis oculi muscle in Chapter 24. The levator palpebrae superioris muscle is described below. The **tarsi** of the upper and lower eyelids are elongated plates of dense connective tissue, which give rigidity and shape to the lids. The upper tarsus is wider than the lower tarsus. The outer surface of the upper tarsus is connected to distal filaments of the levator palpebrae superioris muscle (see below). The outer edges of both the upper and lower tarsi are attached to the orbital septum, and their lateral edges are connected by **lateral palpebral ligaments** to a tubercle of the zygomatic bone. The medial edge of each tarsus is connected by a **medial palpebral ligament** to the superior part of the lacrimal crest. The **tarsal glands** are modified sebaceous glands with ducts that empty at the free margins of the lids. These glands produce an oily secretion that helps to retain tears within the conjunctival sac.

Innervation and Function of the Lacrimal Gland. Parasympathetic fibers of the facial nerve innervate the lacrimal glands via a complex pathway incorporating short segments of the trigeminal nerve as well as facial nerve branches (see discussion of the lacrimal gland and its innervation by facial nerve autonomic fibers in Box 24–8). Parasympathetic stimulation of the serous and mucous cells of the lacrimal gland result in the release of a watery fluid resembling plasma. As has been noted above, this teary secretion is released into the conjunctival sac by the 16 or 17 lacrimal ducts of the orbital and palpebral parts of the lacrimal gland. Tears wash across the eyeball, along a groove in the edge of the lower eyelid, into the lacrimal canaliculi near the medial angle of the eye (through puncta in the edges of the upper and lower eyelids), into the lacrimal sac, and into the nasolacrimal duct. Tears are transported within the nasolacrimal duct to the inferior meatus of the nose from which they pass posteriorly into the nasopharynx and are swallowed. The function of postganglionic sympathetic innervation of the lacrimal gland is not understood.

Eyelid Protection of the Globe; Corneal and Conjunctival Innervation and Reflexes. The fragile contents of the globe are protected by the eyelids, particularly through the **blink reflex.** The blink reflex may be initiated by irritation of the **cornea (corneal reflex)** or **conjunctiva (conjunctival reflex).** The general somatic afferent innervation of the cornea is primarily by branches of **long ciliary nerves** (branches of the ophthalmic division of the trigeminal nerve; see Chapter 24). The distal segments of these nerves are organized radially in an **annular plexus** as they enter the cornea. They ramify both under and between the corneal epithelial cells (Fig. 25–12). In addition, the lateral conjunctiva of the upper eyelid is provided with GSA fibers by the **lacrimal nerve** (originating in the ophthalmic division of the trigeminal nerve), and the medial conjunctiva is supplied with GSA fibers by the **infratrochlear nerve** (from the ophthalmic division of the trigeminal nerve). The conjunctiva of the lower lid is provided with GSA fibers by **palpebral branches of the infraorbital nerve,** which, in turn, are provided by the maxillary nerve (see discussions of the ophthalmic and maxillary divisions of the trigeminal nerve in Chapter 24). These afferent trigeminal nerve branches innervating the cornea and conjunctiva (see Boxes 24–1 and 24–2) project back to the trigeminal sensory nucleus via the semilunar ganglion. From this nucleus, trigeminal neurons project to the motor facial nucleus. The neurons innervate the orbicularis oculi muscle via the temporal and zygomatic branches of the facial nerve (Fig. 25–12 and see Box 24–7). When the blink reflex is activated, irritation of the cornea and conjunctiva results in the propagation of impulses back through centrifugal afferent fibers of trigeminal nerve branches to the trigeminal (semilunar) ganglion and then via centripetal fibers to the sensory trigeminal nucleus. From this point, impulses are conducted to the facial motor nucleus, the temporal and zygomatic branches of the facial nerve, and the orbicularis oculi muscle, which rapidly closes the eyelid.

Corneal or conjunctival irritation also initiates a reflex that suppresses activity of the oculomotor nerve and consequent activation of the levator palpebrae superioris muscle to prevent raising of the upper eyelid. This reflex arc involves the same ophthalmic and maxillary branches and paths described above, that is, the semilunar ganglion and trigeminal sensory nucleus. However, secondary projections go to the oculomotor nucleus with projections of oculomotor fibers to the levator palpebrae superioris muscle (see Box 25–3).

Clinical Disorders of the Cornea. Disruption of the corneal reflex may occur through trauma to sensory branches of the trigeminal nerve that provide GSA innervation to the cornea. Such disruptions may be caused by laceration of the cornea by a sharp object or abrasion of the cornea by small particles of detritus. The consequent development of **ulcers** and permanent **scarring of the cornea** may require corneal transplants (from human donors) or corneal repair with synthetic membranes.

Extrinsic Ocular Muscles: Targets of Cranial Nerves III, IV, and VI

In humans, one muscle elevates the upper eyelid and six muscles rotate the globe

Each orbit contains seven striated extrinsic muscles: a single **levator palpebrae superioris muscle,** four **rectus muscles,** and two **oblique muscles.** The innervation of these muscles is easy to remember. Cranial nerve VI

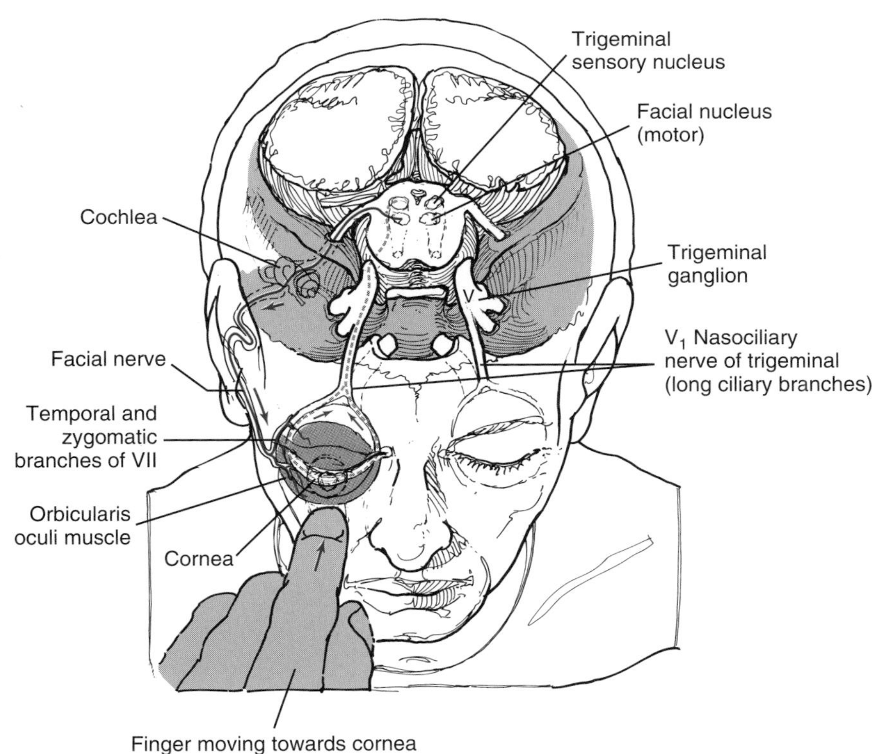

FIGURE 25–12
Blink reflex.

(abducent nerve) innervates the lateral rectus muscle, which abducts the pupil of the eyeball. Cranial nerve IV (trochlear nerve) innervates the superior oblique muscle, which passes through a pulley called the trochlea. The remaining five muscles are innervated by cranial nerve III (oculomotor nerve).

The **levator palpebrae superioris muscle** originates from the inferior surface of the lesser wing of the sphenoid bone (Fig. 25–13*A*). The connective tissue at its proximal end on its inferior surface is fused to connective tissue at the proximal end of the rectus superior muscle (see below). The levator palpebrae superioris muscle courses anteriorly and fans out to attach to the lateral and medial orbital walls as well as the tarsus of the upper eyelid (Fig. 25–14*C*). The muscle is innervated by cranial nerve III (oculomotor nerve) (see Fig. 25–13*A*). Its action is to raise the upper eyelid. It is antagonized by the action of the orbicularis oculi muscle (see Chapter 24) and checked by the orbital septum (see above). The levator palpebrae superioris muscle arose during evolution by delamination from the superior rectus muscle.

The most inferior layer (lamella) of the levator palpebrae superioris muscle consists of smooth muscle fibers that insert into the superior tarsus. These nonstriated myocytes are often referred to as the **superior tarsal muscle,** or **Mueller's muscle,** and are innervated by sympathetic fibers from the superior cervical ganglion (see below).

> Denervation of the superior tarsal muscle at any point along the pathway from the superior cervical ganglion to the superior tarsal muscle results in **Horner's syndrome.** One symptom is drooping of the eyelid **(ptosis).** Other symptoms from sGVE disruption include **miosis** (constriction of the pupil) caused by inability of the intrinsic dilator pupillae muscle to antagonize the parasympathetic-mediated action of the sphincter pupillae muscle (see below) and **anhidrosis** (loss of facial sweating).

The origin of the **superior rectus muscle** is a **common annular tendon (annulus tendineous communis)** of the orbit (Fig. 25–14*A* and *B*). The attachment of the superior rectus muscle to this annular tendon is just superior and somewhat lateral to the optic canal. The ring-shaped common annular tendon surrounds the optic nerve and canal and is attached to the body and lesser wing of the sphenoid bone near the apex of the orbit. This tendinous ring serves as the origin for all four rectus muscles of the orbit (see below). From their sites of origin, the fibers of the superior rectus muscle course anteriorly, just inferior to the levator palpebrae superioris muscle. The muscle penetrates the bulbar sheath and passes within the episcleral space above the superior oblique muscle to insert into the sclera of the eyeball just superoposterior to the sclerocorneal junction (Fig. 25–14*D*). The superior rectus muscle is innervated by the superior branch of cranial nerve III, oculomotor nerve (Fig. 25–13*A*). Its action is to rotate the eyeball superiorly and somewhat medially (Fig. 25–15*A*).

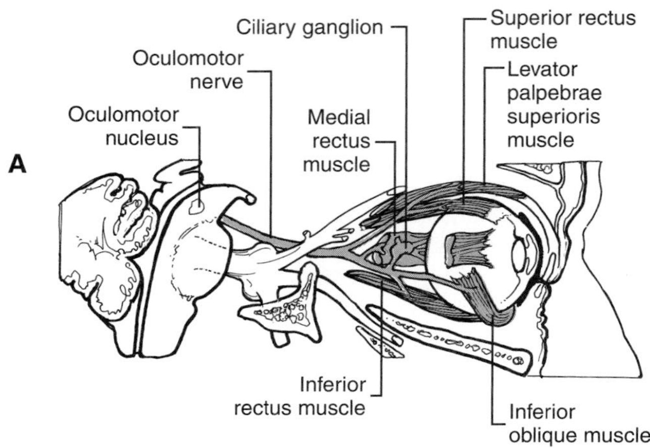

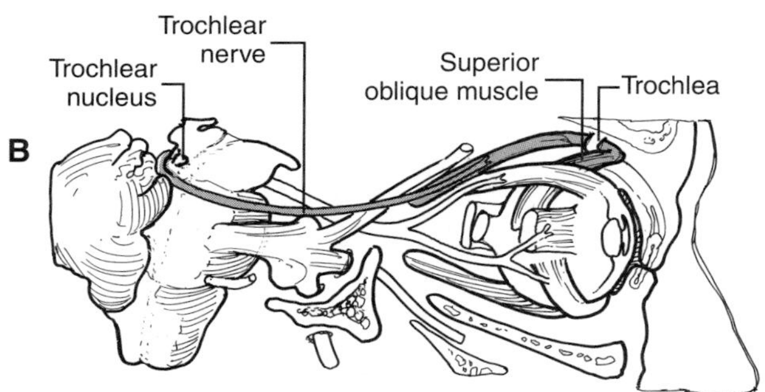

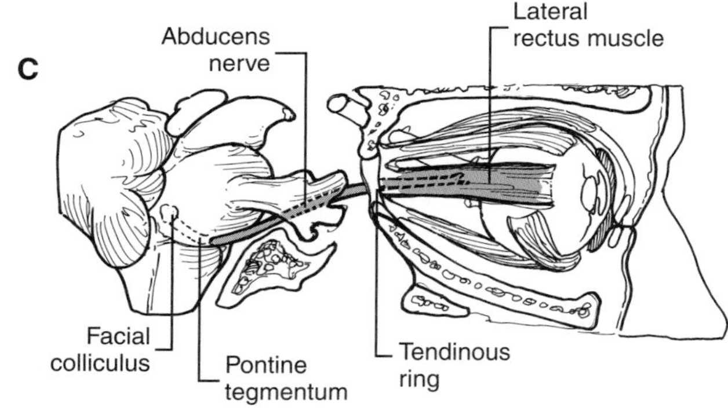

FIGURE 25–13
Innervation of extrinsic muscles of the eye. **A.** Oculomotor innervation of levator palpebrae superioris, superior rectus, inferior rectus, medial rectus, and inferior oblique muscles. **B.** Trochlear innervation of superior oblique muscle. **C.** Abducent innervation of lateral rectus muscle.

The **inferior rectus muscle** arises from the inferior part of the common annular ring just inferior to the optic canal (Fig. 25–14A and B). Its fibers course anteriorly, penetrate the bulbar sheath, and course within the episcleral space just superior to the inferior oblique muscle (see below). Its distal tendon inserts onto the

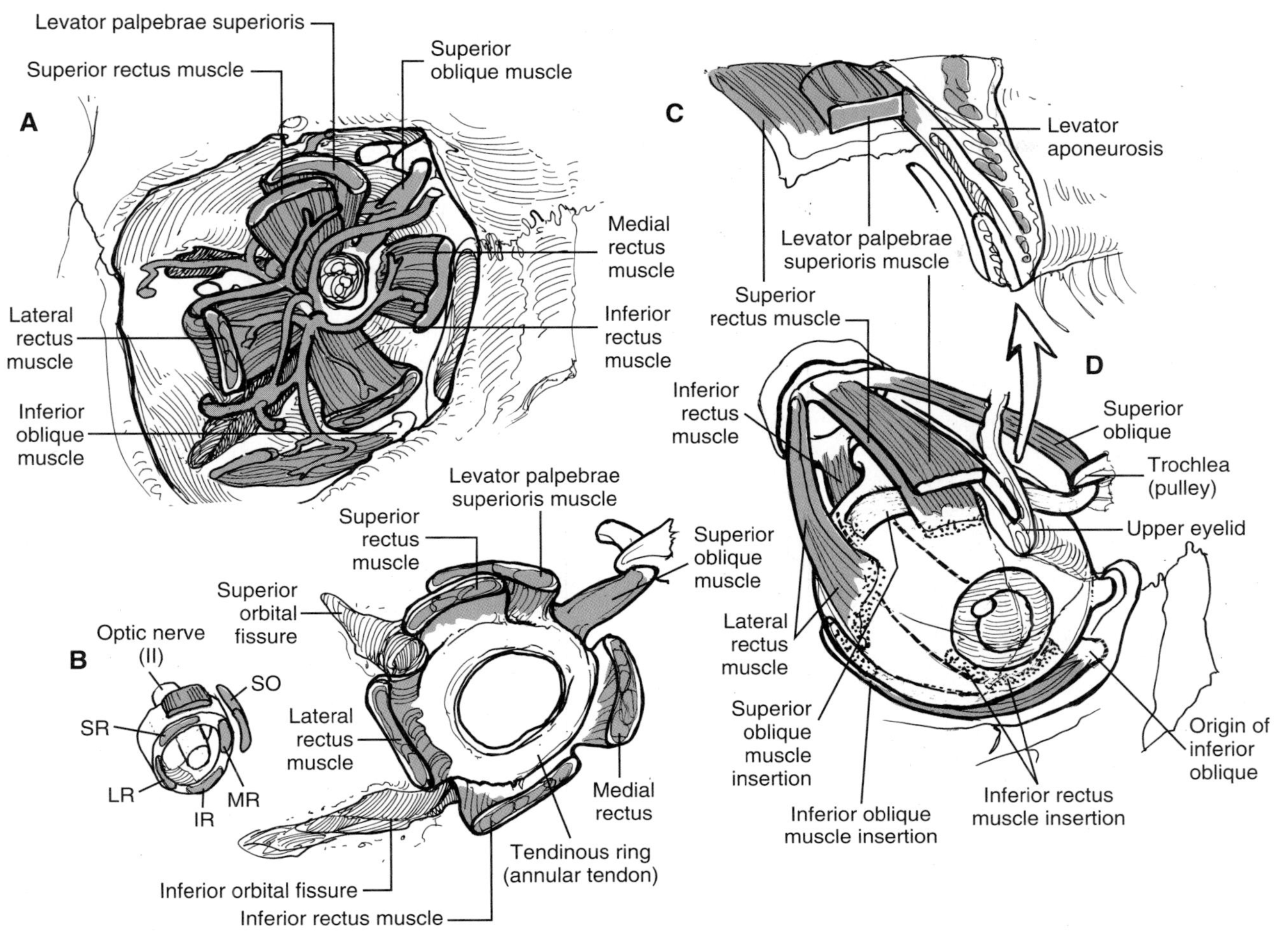

FIGURE 25–14
Origins and insertions of extrinsic muscles of the eye. **A.** Posterior view of the orbit with the globe removed. **B.** Muscles arising from the common annular ring. **C.** Muscles in relation to the eyelid. **D.** Insertion of muscles into the eye.

sclera just posterior to the sclerocorneal junction (Fig. 25–14*D*). The inferior rectus muscle is innervated by the inferior branch of the oculomotor nerve (Fig. 25–13*A*). Its action is to rotate the eyeball inferiorly and somewhat medially (Fig. 25–15*B*).

The **lateral rectus muscle** arises from the inferolateral part of the common annular ring (Fig. 25–14*A* and *B*). Its fibers course anteriorly, but, before the muscle penetrates the bulbar sheath, its fascial sheath gives off a "lateral check ligament," which inserts into the lateral wall of the orbit. Fibers of the lateral rectus muscle then proceed anteriorly to insert onto the lateral side of the eyeball just posterior to the corneoscleral junction (Fig. 25–14*D*). The lateral rectus muscle is innervated by cranial nerve VI, abducent nerve (Fig. 25–13*C*). Its action is to rotate the eyeball laterally (Fig. 25–15*C*).

The **medial rectus muscle** arises from the superomedial region of the common annular ring (Fig. 25–14*A* and *B*). It courses anteriorly underneath the levator palpebrae superioris muscle, penetrates the bulbar sheath, and enters the episcleral space to insert into the sclera just posterior to the sclerocorneal junction. In addition, just prior to its penetration of the bulbar sheath, the fascial sheath of the medial rectus muscle gives off a small "medial check ligament," which attaches to the medial wall of the orbit. The medial rectus muscle is innervated by the inferior branch of the oculomotor nerve (Fig. 25–13*A*). Its action is to rotate the eyeball **medially** (Fig. 25–15*D*).

The **superior oblique muscle** arises from the inferior surface of the lesser wing of the sphenoid bone, just medial and inferior to the origin of the levator palpebrae superioris muscle (Fig. 25–14*A*). Its fibers then course anteriorly, becoming tendinous in the anterior region of the orbit. This tendon passes through a loop of connective tissue fastened to the frontal bone at the upper medial wall of the orbit. This loop-shaped **trochlea** and enclosed synovial sheath serve as a pulley that reverses the direction of the tendon so that it passes posteriorly to penetrate the bulbar sheath just medial to

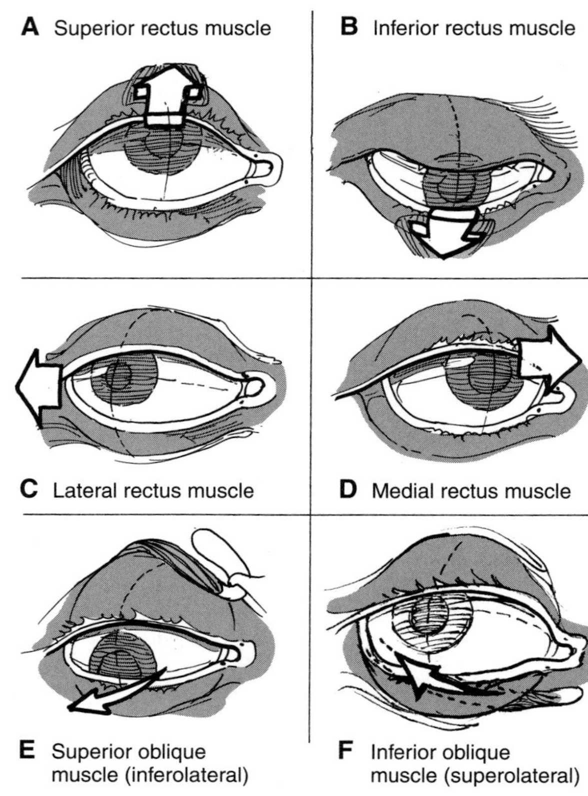

FIGURE 25–15
Movement of the globe by extrinsic muscles. **A.** Superior rectus muscle. **B.** Inferior rectus muscle. **C.** Lateral rectus muscle. **D.** Medial rectus muscle. **E.** Superior oblique muscle. **F.** Inferior oblique muscle.

the superior rectus muscle. The tendon courses within the episcleral space and attaches to the eyeball just superolateral to the optic nerve in the upper lateral quadrant of the posterior surface of the eyeball (Fig. 25–14*D*). The superior oblique muscle is innervated by cranial nerve IV, trochlear nerve (Fig. 25–13*B*). Its action is to rotate the eyeball so that the pupil turns **inferolaterally** (Fig. 25–15*E*).

The **inferior oblique muscle** arises from the anteromedial floor of the **orbit** (Fig. 25–14*A*). Its fibers course lateroposteriorly below the inferior rectus muscle, penetrate the bulbar sheath, course through the episcleral space, and insert onto the posterior surface of the globe in its inferolateral quadrant (just lateral to the optic nerve) (Fig. 25–14*D*). As the muscle penetrates the bulbar sheath, its thickened fascia also courses mediolaterally to form a "suspensory ligament," which provides some support for the globe (see above). The inferior oblique muscle is innervated by the inferior branch of the oculomotor nerve (25–13*A*). Its action is to rotate the eyeball so that the pupil points superolaterally (Fig. 25–15*F*).

Coordinated Actions and Normal Functions of the Extrinsic Muscles. The rectus muscles regulate three major classes of movements of the eyeball. Two of these movements involve coordinated actions of both eyeballs: the **saccade movements** in which the eyeballs rapidly fix on each new target, and the **smooth pursuit movements** in which the eyeballs track slowly moving targets. In the third type of movement, disconjugated **vergence movement,** the angle between the eyeballs adjusts for target distance. While these movements may be initiated as voluntary actions, **compensatory reflex actions** of the extrinsic muscles of the eyes keep the eyes on target when the body or head is moving or rotating.

The organization of the extrinsic muscles with regard to their attachments to the bony orbit provides an anatomic basis for these coordinated, finely regulated movements because the six extrinsic muscles of the eye are organized into three pairs of antagonistic muscles:

- the **lateral** and **medial rectus muscles,**
- **superior** and **inferior rectus muscles,** and
- **superior** and **inferior oblique muscles** (see Fig. 25–15).

As with other striated muscles of the body, the respective dynamic and tonic activities of the apposed muscles contribute to the smooth, graded eyeball movements.

The eyeballs rotate about three axes:

- a **vertical axis,**
- **horizontal axis,** and
- **dorsoventral axis.**

All three axes run through the center of the eyeball. **Horizontal movements** about the vertical axis are controlled by the lateral rectus muscle, which abducts the pupil of the globe (see Fig. 25–15*C*), and by the medial rectus muscle, which adducts the pupil (see Fig. 25–15*D*). **Vertical movements** about the horizontal axis and **torsional movements** about the dorsoventral axis are controlled by the superior rectus muscle, which rotates the pupil superolaterally (elevates and abducts the pupil) (see Fig. 25–15*A*); the inferior rectus muscle, which rotates the pupil inferomedially (depresses and adducts the pupil) (see Fig. 25–15*B*); the superior oblique muscle, which depresses and abducts the pupil (see Fig. 25–15*E*); and the inferior oblique muscle, which elevates and adducts the pupil (see Fig. 25–15*F*).

Clinical Disorders of the Extrinsic Ocular Muscles and Their Nerves. Physical trauma, vascular injuries, or **tumors** involving the oculomotor, trochlear, or abducent nerves or extrinsic muscles may produce specific deficits in movements of the eyeballs. Evidence of a unilateral lesion is often indicated by **strabismus,** or **misalignment of the two eyeballs.** The result of this condition is double vision. The brain may compensate for double vision by simply ignoring the input from one eye. Eventually, this eye may fail to focus **(amblyopia)** or orient itself at all. Depending upon the cause, strabismus may be successfully treated.

Functional deficits of the extraocular muscles may be found by instructing the patient to look in a particular direction. The function of the lateral rectus muscle is tested by having the patient look in a lateral direction (i.e., outward), and the function of the medial rectus muscle by having the patient look in a medial direction (i.e., inward). The superior rectus muscle is tested by having the patient first look in a lateral direction and then upward, and the inferior rectus muscle by having the patient first look in a medial direction and then downward. The function of the superior oblique muscle is tested by having the patient look in a lateral direction and then downward, while the inferior oblique muscle is tested by asking the patient to first look in a medial direction and then upward.

The **nerves of the extrinsic muscles** may be **severed** or **injured.** Interruption of the **oculomotor nerve** leads to several predictable symptoms, including ptosis (paralysis of the levator palpebrae superioris muscle), lateral strabismus (paralysis of the medial rectus muscle), pupillary dilatation and loss of the pupillary reflex (paralysis of the sphincter pupillae muscle), loss of the accommodation reflex (paralysis of the ciliary muscle), proptosis (protrusion of the eyeball) resulting from relaxation of five of the seven extraocular muscles, and diplopia (double vision).

Irritation of or more serious damage to each branch of the oculomotor nerve results in spasm or paralysis of the specific muscle innervated by that nerve.

Injury of the **trochlear nerve** results in paralysis of the superior oblique muscle. The affected eye rotates in a medial direction, causing the patient to have double vision (diplopia) when he or she gazes downward.

Interruption of the **abducent nerve** leads to paralysis of the lateral rectus muscle and consequent medial rotation of the affected eye and diplopia.

ANATOMY OF THE EAR AND VESTIBULAR APPARATUS

General Organization and Function of the Ear

The outer, middle, and inner ear all function in hearing; the inner ear functions in balance as well

The human ear is composed of the following parts:

- an **outer (external) ear,** with a pinna (auricle) and an external acoustic meatus;
- a **middle ear** consisting of a tympanic cavity, tympanic membrane, auditory ossicles and associated muscles; and
- an **inner (internal) ear,** including an auditory and vestibular apparatus.

The **fundamental auditory function** of the ear is to collect, conduct, and amplify sound waves; carry out transduction and signal analysis; and transmit this information to higher centers in the brain (where interpretation of the direction, intensity, frequency, and phases of vibration occurs). This function is carried out by the external and middle ear, and the cochlear portion of the internal ear, and the cochlear or auditory portion of cranial nerve VIII. The **fundamental vestibular function** of the ear is to inform the brain of the head's position in space and its relative rate of movement in space. This function is carried out by sensory nerve terminals in the utricle, saccule, and ampullae of the internal ear, along with the vestibular part of cranial nerve VIII.

The development of the inner, middle, and external ear will be discussed first, and then the bony skeleton of the ear will be reviewed. These two sections will serve as organizing frameworks for the discussion of the definitive anatomy of the internal, middle, and external ear. This latter discussion will include references to the cranial nerve innervation of each part of the ear.

Development of the Internal, Middle, and External Ear

Inner Ear Development

The inner ear arises from a specialized ectodermal placode

A thickened **otic placode,** or **otic disc,** appears in the region of the rhombencephalon (future hindbrain) early in the fourth week of embryonic development (Fig. 25–16*A* and *B*). Within a few days, the otic placode invaginates into the mesenchyme of the head to form the **otic vesicle** and the primordium of the **vestibulocochlear ganglion** (SSA fibers) **of the vestibulocochlear nerve** (cranial nerve VIII; see below). The otic vesicle then develops into the **membranous labyrinth** of the internal ear—a structure that consists of an **endolymphatic sac** and **duct** and expanded **utricular** and **saccular regions,** which become joined by a narrow **utriculosaccular duct** (Fig. 25–16*C*). The endolymphatic sac and duct may regulate the level of endolymphatic fluid within the internal ear by serving as an absorption site for excess endolymphatic fluid. The central embryonic utricular region of the internal ear gives rise to the **anterior, posterior,** and **lateral semicircular ducts** of the vestibular apparatus (see Fig. 25–17*D* and *E*). The ventral tip of the saccule begins to elongate and coil, forming the **cochlear duct,** the auditory part of the internal ear. The saccule and cochlear duct are joined by a narrow **ductus reuniens** (see Fig. 25–25*F*).

Middle Ear Development

The middle ear arises from the first pharyngeal pouch

The pharyngeal arches are separated externally by deep ectoderm-lined clefts called *pharyngeal clefts* (see Chapter 23). Opposing the pharyngeal clefts are endoderm-lined indentations called *pharyngeal pouches.* The pharyngeal pouch between the first and second pharyngeal arches elongates in the fifth week of development to form a **tubotympanic recess,** which ultimately gives rise to the **tympanic cavity** (see Fig. 25–16*C* to *E*). In the following week, the external acoustic meatus begins to develop from the first pharyngeal cleft. During the seventh week, three auditory ossicles differentiate

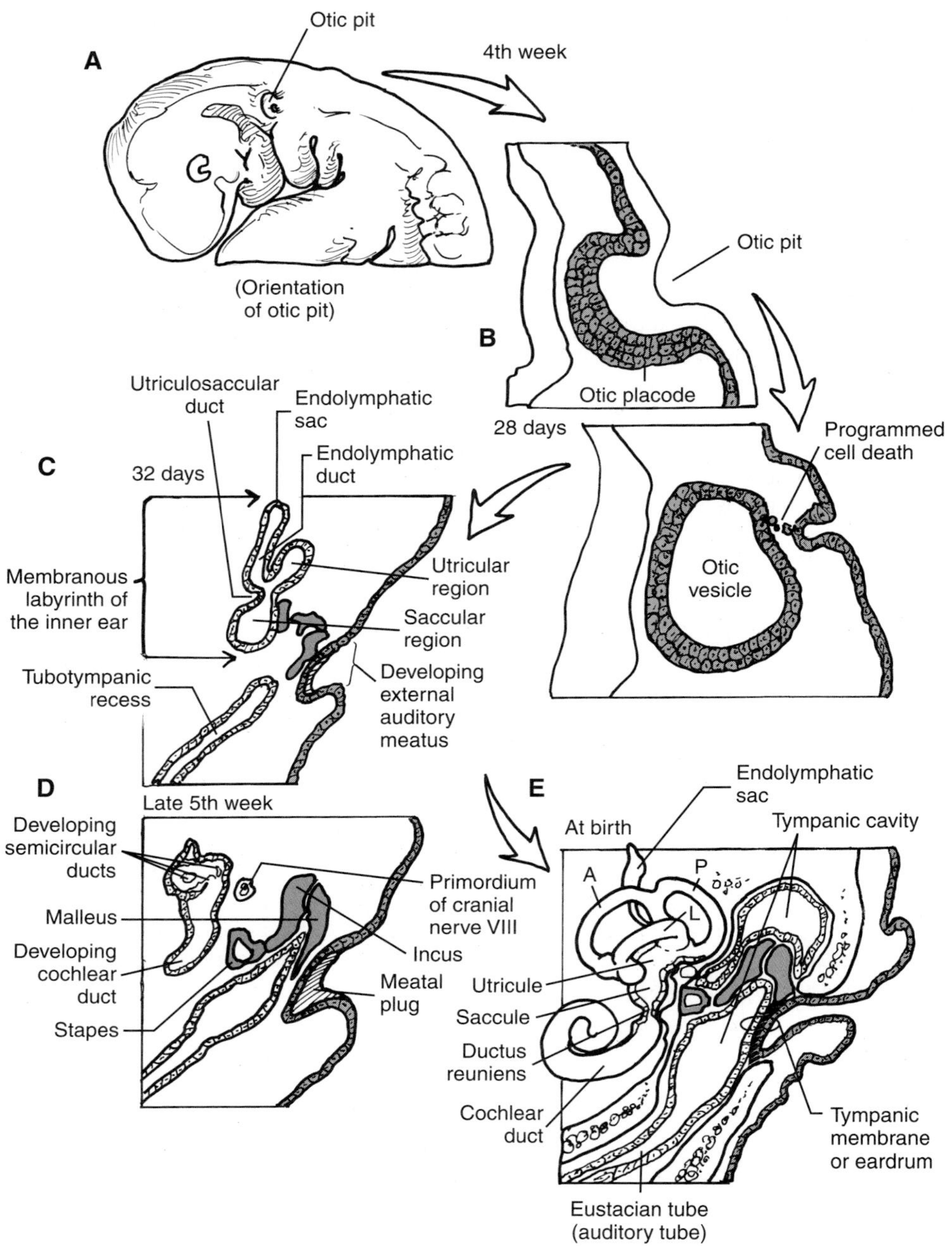

FIGURE 25–16
Development of the ear. **A.** Inner ear. Invagination of the otic placode. **B.** Otic vesicle. **C.** Membranous labyrinth of the internal ear. **D.** Tubotympanic recess of the middle ear. **E.** Ear at birth.

within the mesenchyme in the vicinity of the elongating tubotympanic recess. These are the **incus, malleus,** and **stapes.** The incus and malleus are derived from neural crest cells of the first pharyngeal arch and the stapes from neural crest cells of the second pharyngeal arch. Likewise the tensor tympani muscle associated with the malleus arises from mesenchyme of the first pharyngeal arch, and the stapedius muscle arises from mesenchyme of the second pharyngeal arch. The three auditory ossicles and their associated muscles do not become enclosed within the tympanic cavity until the ninth month of fetal development (see Fig. 25–16*E*).

External Ear Development

The external ear arises from the first pharyngeal cleft and from six auricular hillocks, which arise from surface ectoderm of the first and second pharyngeal arches

The first pharyngeal cleft deepens during the sixth week to form the embryonic **external acoustic meatus.** Proliferation of the ectodermal lining of this canal

BOX 25–3

MOTOR GENERAL EFFERENT BRANCHES OF THE OCULOMOTOR (III), TROCHLEAR (IV), AND ABDUCENT (VI) NERVES

The parasympathetic function of the oculomotor nerve is discussed in Box 25–2. The remaining function of this nerve is to supply motor (general somatic efferent [GSE]) fibers to five of the seven extrinsic muscles of the eye. Likewise, the trochlear nerve (cranial nerve IV) provides motor (GSE) fibers to the superior oblique muscle, while the abducent nerve (cranial nerve VI) supplies motor (GSE) fibers to the lateral rectus muscle. For this reason, the motor function of all three nerves is described in this box.

MOTOR BRANCHES OF THE OCULOMOTOR NERVE

As has been noted in Box 25–2, once the oculomotor nerve emerges from the brain, it courses anteriorly between the superior cerebellar and posterior cerebral arteries. It pierces the dura of the cavernous sinus (see Chapter 27) to run along its lateral wall. It exits the cranium via the superior orbital fissure, passing through the common annular tendon of the orbit and emerging just lateral to the optic nerve. At this point, the nerve splits into superior and inferior divisions. The superior division courses superiorly to innervate the levator palpebrae superioris and superior rectus muscles. The inferior division at first courses inferiorly but then splits into divergent branches that innervate the medial rectus, inferior oblique, and inferior rectus muscles (see Fig. 25–16*A*).

TROCHLEAR NERVE AND ITS MOTOR BRANCHES

The motor nucleus of the trochlear nerve is located in the floor of the cerebral aqueduct at the level of the inferior colliculus in the midbrain (see Fig. 25–16*B*). The axons emitted from the trochlear nuclei follow an unusual route to the orbit. They first course dorsally and then decussate (cross with fibers from the contralateral side as each passes to the opposite side of the brain). The nerve emerges from the dorsal surface of the brain, the only cranial nerve to do so. The trochlear nerve courses around the cerebral peduncle and joins with the oculomotor nerve between the posterior cerebral and superior cerebellar arteries. The trochlear nerve then penetrates the dura of the tentorium cerebelli, courses within the lateral wall of the cavernous sinus with the oculomotor, ophthalmic, maxillary, and abducent nerves, and enters the orbit via the superior orbital fissure. The trochlear nerve passes above the common tendinous ring and then typically splits into three branches to innervate the superior oblique muscle.

ABDUCENT NERVE AND ITS MOTOR BRANCHES

The motor nucleus of the abducent nerve is located in the pontine tegmentum just anterior to the fourth ventricle (see Fig. 25–16*C*). Axons emitted by the abducent motor nucleus course ventrally to emerge from the ventral surface of the brainstem between the pons and the pyramid of the medulla. The abducent nerve courses anteriorly within the subarachnoid space of the posterior cranial fossa and pierces the dura just lateral to the dorsum sellae. The abducent nerve then passes anteriorly to join the oculomotor, trochlear, ophthalmic, and maxillary nerves within the lateral wall of the cavernous sinus. The abducent nerve enters the orbit via the superior orbital fissure, passes through the common tendinous ring, and innervates the lateral rectus muscle.

forms a **meatal plug,** which completely fills the medial end of the canal by week 26. Canalization of the meatal plug in the medial two thirds of the definitive external acoustic meatus occurs by the ninth month of fetal development (see Fig. 25–16*D* and *E*). At this time, the tympanic cavity of the middle ear is separated from the external acoustic meatus by the **tympanic membrane,** or **eardrum.** The tympanic membrane represents the juncture of the pharyngeal cleft from the exterior and the pharyngeal pouch from the interior (the "pharyngeal membrane" between the first and second pharyngeal arches) and is, therefore, comprised of all three germ layers: ectoderm, mesoderm, and endoderm (see Fig. 25–16*E*).

The **auricle,** or **pinna,** of the external ear arises from condensations of surface ectoderm called **auricular hillocks,** which are associated with the first and second pharyngeal arches. The three hillocks of the first pharyngeal arch are the **tragus, helix,** and **cymba conchae auriculae.** The three hillocks of the second pharyngeal arch are the **antitragus, antihelix,** and **concha** (Fig. 25–17). These hillocks grow and fuse during the seventh week to form the definitive auricle of the ear, which is slowly translocated from the neck to a more cranial site.

Congenital Disorders of the Ear. **Goldenhar's syndrome** is a severe example of a group of abnormalities known as **hemifacial microstomia** (from the Greek for "small body") in which both the outer and middle ear may be underdeveloped and there may also be deformities of the temporomandibular joint and mandible. These deformities may arise by a vascular mechanism, for example, a hematoma arising in arteries serving the stapedius muscle (a muscle which acts on the stapes).

A deficit of mesenchyme in the first and second pharyngeal arches causes **mandibulofacial dysostosis,** a group of deformities similar to those of hemifacial microstomia.

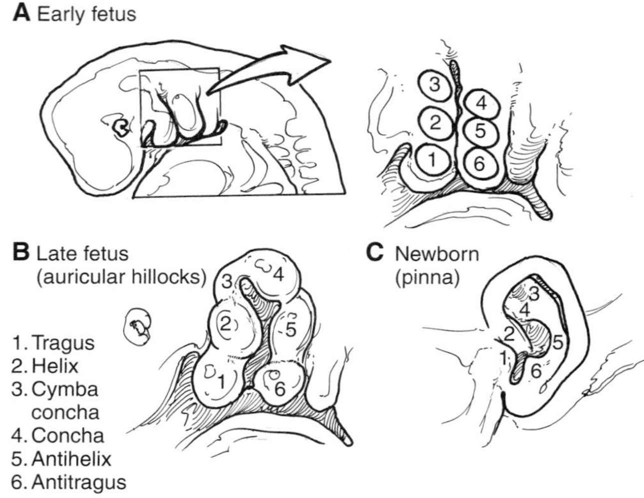

FIGURE 25–17
Development of the auricle (pinna) of the external ear. **A.** Position of the auricular hillocks on apposed surfaces of the first and second pharyngeal arches. **B.** Auricular hillocks. **C.** Pinna of a newborn infant.

Treacher Collins syndrome and **Hallermann-Streiff syndrome** are two examples linked to a genetic cause. It is thought that the former may be caused by the autosomal dominant form, and the latter by the autosomal recessive form of the same gene cluster. Other cases of mandibulofacial dysostosis arise through diverse etiologies. One example is administration of the oral anti-acne drug isotretinoin, which may cause these syndromes in the embryo if the drug is taken during the first month of pregnancy.

Low-set ears and auricular abnormalities are one consequence of the complex of congenital malformations known as **DiGeorge syndrome.** The syndrome is usually associated with partial monosomy of chromosome 22. It also occurs in offspring of alcoholic women.

Anomalies of the inner ear may be caused by mutations of the gap junction protein connexin26. Such mutations, including those resulting in missense, frameshift, or premature stop codons, may be the cause of both autosomal recessive and autosomal dominant **hearing loss** in humans. It is likely that these mutations affect the formation of gap junctions in fibrocytes of the spiral ligament that underlies the striavascularis of the cochlear duct (see below) leading to disruptions of ionic and endolymphatic circulation in the cochlear duct.

Lesions of the middle ear, such as a small benign growth in the tympanic cavity called a **cholesteatoma,** may lead to hearing loss. A cholesteatoma is an endodermal tumor that may arise from a normal epidermoid thickening of the tympanic cavity lining that fails to regress.

Malformations of the external ear (auricle, or **pinna)** may result from abnormal growth of the auricular hillocks. Reduced growth of the hillocks may result in **microtia,** while complete suppression of growth may result in **anotia.** The development of accessory hillocks may produce ectopic **auricular tags.**

Skeletal Framework of the Ear

The bony framework of the internal and middle ear arises from mesenchyme derived from primitive otic capsule ossification centers, which fuse and ossify as a single **periotic (petromastoid) bone** between weeks 16 and 23 of development (see Chapter 22). The **bony labyrinth** of the internal ear is the petrous portion of the temporal bone. The **tympanic cavity** of the middle ear expands into the mastoid part of the temporal bone (Fig. 25–18). A separate **auricular cartilage** develops within the auricular hillocks to form the external ear.

Bony (Osseous) Labyrinth of the Internal Ear

Mesenchyme adjacent to the membranous labyrinth is first transformed to a cartilaginous otic capsule and then ossified to form the **bony labyrinth,** a cavity that encloses the membranous labyrinth. The bony labyrinth is generally considered to consist of three subcavities:

- the **semicircular canals** (housing the semicircular ducts),
- **vestibule** (containing the utricle and saccule), and
- **cochlea** (enclosing the cochlear duct).

The **semicircular canals** (the most posterior region of the bony labyrinth) enclose the semicircular ducts. Each of the semicircular canals (anterior, posterior, and lateral) has a terminal swelling at its base called an **ampulla.** Each ampulla communicates directly with the vestibule (Fig. 25–19). The anterior and posterior semicircular canals are united at the posterior canal's upper end by the **crus commune.** The crus commune opens into the medial vestibule. The posterior end of the lateral semicircular canal communicates independently with the vestibule.

The **vestibule** is the central region of the bony labyrinth posterior to the cochlea, anterior to the semicircular canals, and medial to the tympanic cavity. The vestibule contains the utricle and saccule of the vestibular apparatus, utriculosaccular duct, and ductus reuniens. An extension of the vestibule called the **aqueduct of the vestibule** contains the endolymphatic duct and sac (Fig. 25–18 and see below). Thus, the posterior wall of the vestibule bears the five orifices of the semicircular canals and the root of the vestibular aqueduct. The anterior wall of the vestibule opens into the scala vestibuli of the cochlea. In addition, the lateral wall of the vestibule bears an opening called the **fenestra vestibuli,** or **oval window,** which is closed by the base of the stapedius muscle and its annular ligament.

The most anterior portion of the bony labyrinth is the **cochlea** (from the Latin for "snail shell") (Figs. 25–18 and 25–19). This cone-shaped spiral of bone is comprised of three channels. The **modiolus** is the bony

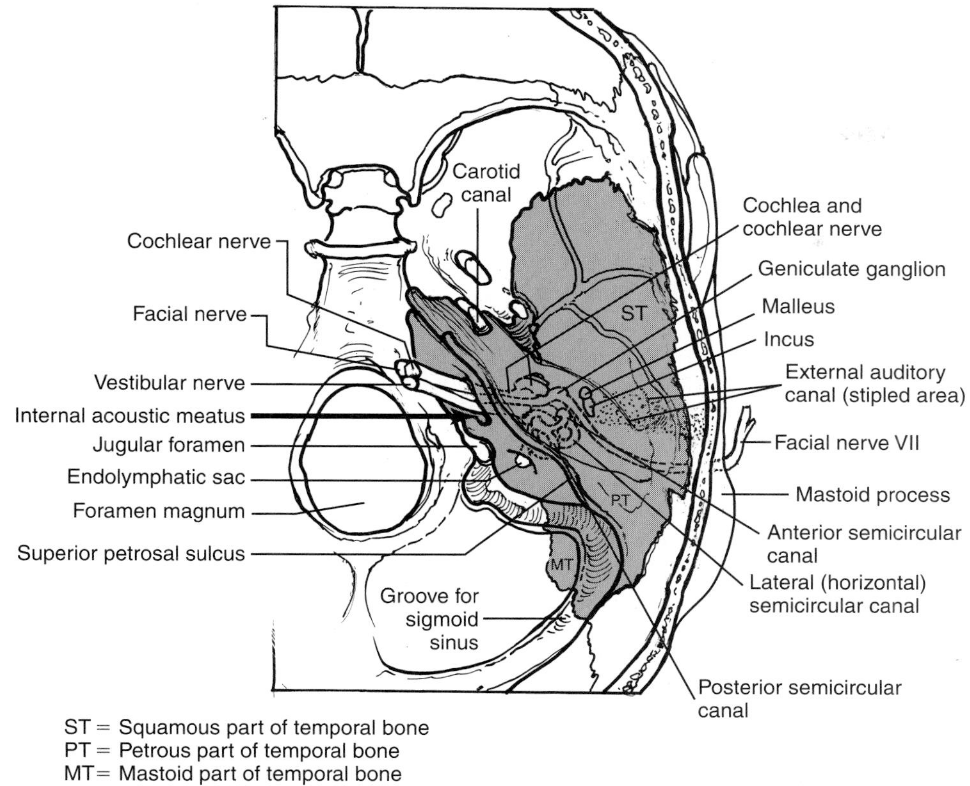

FIGURE 25–18

The skeletal framework of the inner ear. The cochlea and semicircular canal are in position, showing the internal acoustic meatus passageway for the vestibulocochlear and facial nerves.

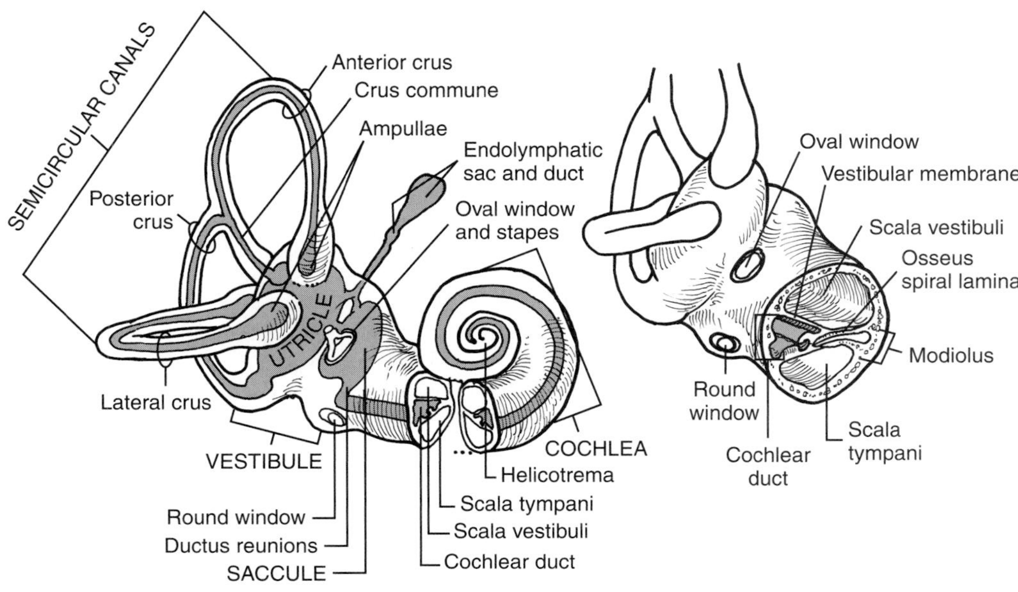

FIGURE 25–19

Osseus labyrinth of the inner ear (semicircular canals, vestibule, and cochlea) with enclosed membranous labyrinth (semicircular ducts, utricle, saccule, endolymphatic sac, and cochlear duct).

core of the cochlea. A delicate ledge, the **osseous spiral lamina,** projects from the modiolus into the osseus canal like the thread of a screw and provides part of the division of the cochlea into its three spiraling channels. The middle channel of the three is the **cochlear duct,** which contains the sensory apparatus responsible for audition. (As noted above, the cochlear duct communicates with the saccule via the ductus reuniens.) The other two channels are perilymphatic channels called the **scala vestibuli** and **scala tympani.** Just inferior to the oval window at the base of the cochlea is the **fenestra cochleae,** or **round window,** which is closed by the secondary tympanic membrane (Figs. 25–19 and 25–20).

Skeletal Framework of the Tympanic Cavity of the Middle Ear

The middle ear consists of the **tympanic cavity,** which contains the **auditory ossicles** and **auditory (pharyngotympanic) tube.** The tympanic cavity is an irregularly shaped cavity filled with air that extends within the temporal bone between the tympanic membrane (eardrum) and the inner ear. The area known as the **tympanic cavity proper** is directly opposite the tympanic membrane. The area above the membrane is called the **epitympanic recess.** In clinical practice, the recess is sometimes referred to as the "attic" (Fig. 25–20).

A compact platelike bone, the **tegmen tympani,** forms the roof of the tympanic cavity, stretching from the roof of the mastoid antrum posteriorly to the roof of the canal for the tensor tympani muscle. At the floor of the cavity, a thin, convex bony plate separates the cavity from the internal jugular vein. The cavity's lateral wall is formed mainly by the tympanic membrane with its surrounding bony border, which is sometimes referred to as the "tympanic ring" (Fig. 25–20). This ring is notched superiorly, and near this area are the petrotympanic fissure and the anterior and posterior openings of the canaliculi (little channels) for the chorda tympani nerve. The upper portion of the posterior wall of the tympanic cavity contains the **aditus** (from the Latin for "entrance to a channel"), leading to the **mastoid antrum,** an air sinus in the petrous part of the temporal bone. The antrum borders the area of the mastoid bone filled with **mastoid air cells** of varying shapes and sizes. The posterior portion of the tympanic cavity, therefore, communicates with the mastoid air cells. The mastoid area is particularly prone to infection because of its connection with the middle ear.

The medial wall of the tympanic cavity is the boundary between the middle ear and inner ear. On this wall are found the oval window, the promontory, the round

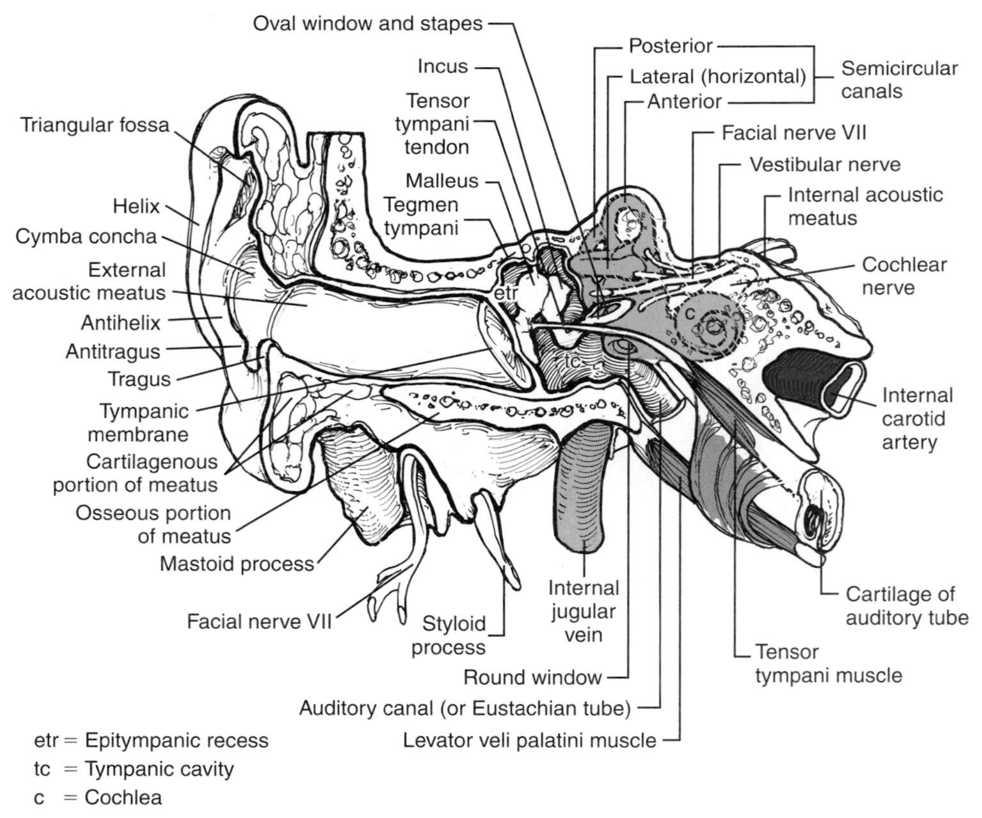

FIGURE 25–20
Schematic overview of the external, middle, and inner ear.

window, and the facial canal. The oval window transmits vibrations from the middle ear, via the base of the stapes, through the vestibule area of the inner ear to the cochlea (Figs. 25-20 and 25–21). The **promontory** is a bulge in the anterior portion of the medial wall of the tympanic cavity, which overlays the basal turn of the cochlea. The **round window** is posteroinferior to the oval window and lies completely under the overhanging promontory. Above the oval window two additional prominences are apparent. One is the **facial canal** through which the facial nerve travels. The other is formed by the prominence of the lateral semicircular canal (Fig. 25–21).

The upper portion of the anterior tympanic wall contains the opening to the **auditory canal** or tube (also referred to as the Eustachian or pharyngotympanic tube). This canal inclines anterormedially downward and provides a connecting air passage between the tympanic cavity and the nasopharynx. The osseus part of the auditory tube extends to the junction of the squamous and petrous parts of the temporal bone (Fig. 25–20). From this point on, the canal is bordered on three sides by a fold of cartilage with fibrous tissues completing the tube. Above the osseus part of the auditory tube is the canal for the **tensor tympani muscle,** which also runs anteromedially. The inferior portion of the anterior tympanic wall is a thin lamina forming the posterior wall of the carotid canal.

Vibrations produced by sound are transmitted across the air-filled tympanic cavity to the fluid-filled inner ear by a chain of three auditory ossicles:

- the **malleus (hammer),**
- **incus (anvil),** and
- **stapes (stirrup)** (Fig. 25–22).

Skeleton of the External Ear

The external ear includes the auricle (pinna) and the external acoustic meatus

The **auricle,** or **pinna,** is a single piece of elastic fibrocartilage covered with skin (see Fig. 25–20). This fibrocartilage is continuous with the cartilage of the external acoustic meatus. Cartilage is absent from the softer lobule, which consists only of fibrous and adipose tissue. The pinna projects from the side of the head to collect sound waves. It is immediately lateral to the supermeatal triangle of the temporal bone, which can be felt through the concave upper part of the pinna.

The **external acoustic meatus** extends in an S-shaped curve from the auricle to the tympanic membrane. The cartilaginous lateral third of this canal is continuous with the auricular cartilage, while the me-

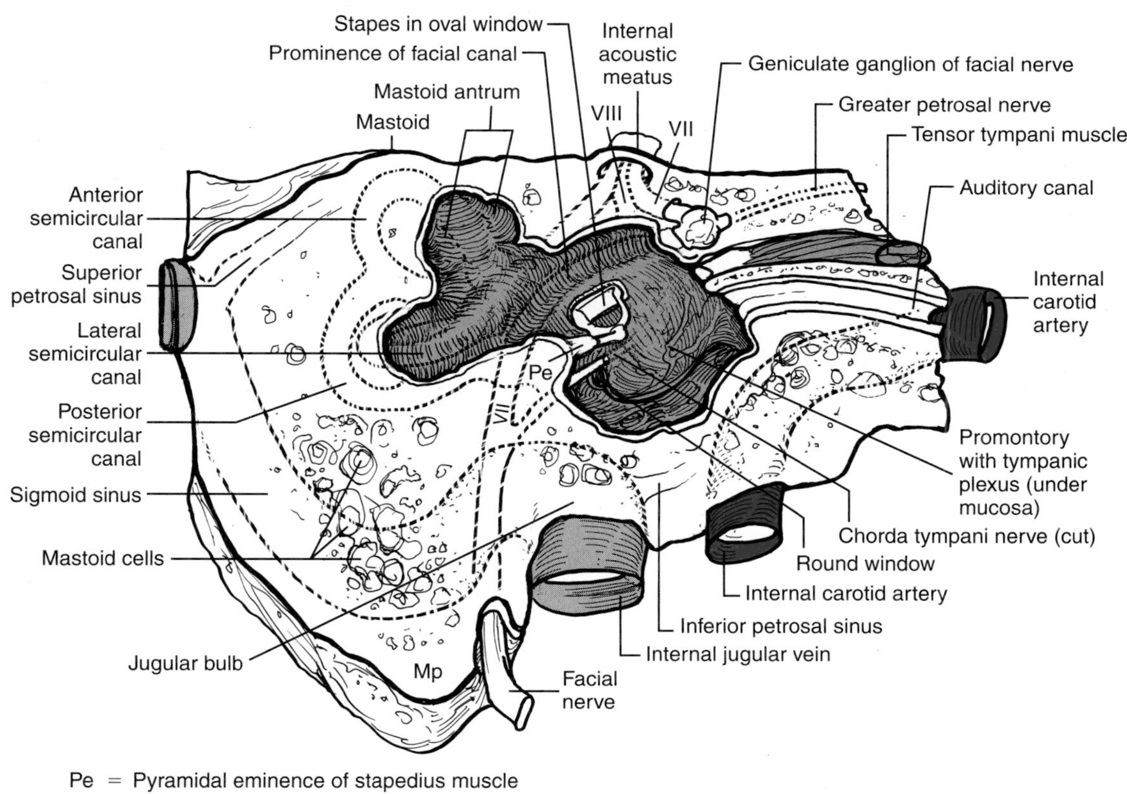

FIGURE 25–21
Lateral view (schematic) of the medial wall of the tympanic cavity of the middle ear.

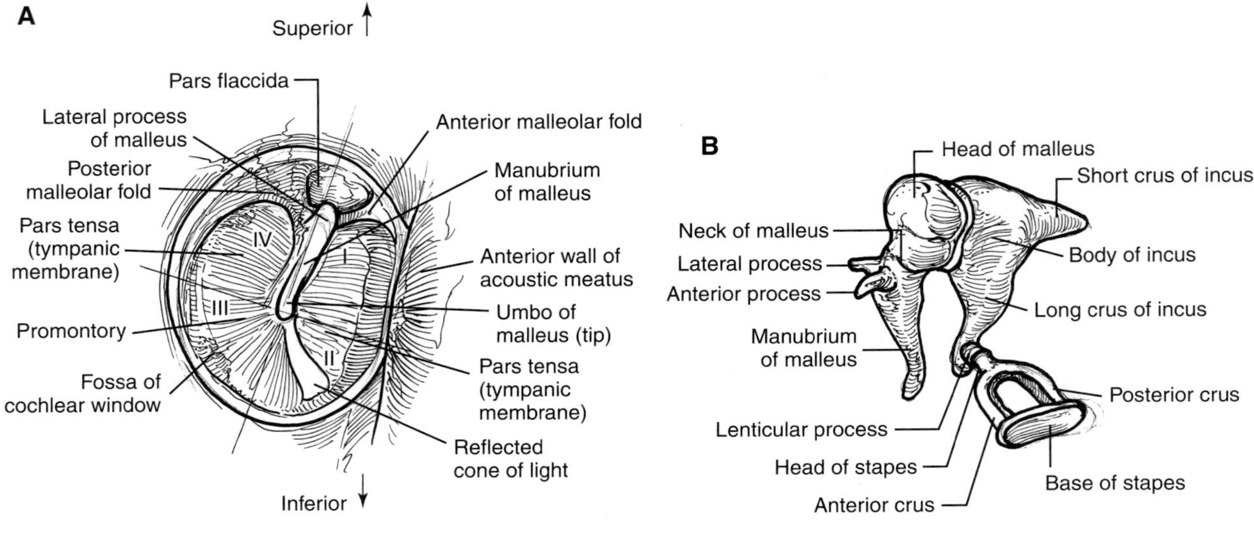

FIGURE 25–22
Auditory ossicles and tympanic membrane. **A.** External view of tympanic membrane. **B.** Auditory ossicles.

dial two-thirds is osseous (see Fig. 25-20). The cartilaginous part is attached to the circumference of the osseus part by fibrous tissue. The anterior, inferior, and most of the posterior osseus meatus is derived from the tympanic portion of the temporal bone, while the squamous temporal bone forms the posterosuperior roof.

▲ Definitive Anatomy, Musculature, and Innervation of the Ear

The Auricle or Projecting Pinna of the External Ear

Regions of the auricle are named for their shape or function

The coiled **helix** forms the curved rim of the pinna while the **antihelix,** a curved prominence, is parallel and anterior to the helix. The antihelix divides anteriorly and superiorly into two bands that border a small concave area called the **triangular fossa** (see Fig. 25–20). The deep **concha** (named for the shell-like shape of the auricle) is encircled by the helix and leads to the external acoustic meatus. It is divided medially by the most anterior projection of the helix into a superior **cymba conchae** and a main cavity. The small curved flap in front of the concha is the **tragus** (from the Greek for "goat"), which derives its name from the fact that hair grows on it. The prominence opposite from the tragus, which also has hair growing on it, is called the **antitragus** (see Figs. 25–17 and 25–20). Extrinsic ligaments connect the auricle to the temporal bone and its zygomatic process. Intrinsic ligaments connect the tragus and antitragus to the helix.

Extrinsic muscles of the auricle are the **anterior, superior,** and **posterior auriculares muscles.** The anterior and superior muscles are supplied by temporal branches of the facial nerve (cranial nerve VII) and the auricularis posterior muscle by the posterior auricular branch of the trigeminal (cranial nerve V). The three muscles move the auricle forward, elevate it, or draw it back, but in humans these actions have little obvious effect.

The skin covering the auricle continues through the external auditory meatus and over the outer surface of the tympanic membrane. The skin adheres tightly to the both the cartilaginous and bony parts of the tube.

Inflammation in the external ear area is, therefore, especially painful because of the tension this skin can exert on adjacent tissues.

Several clinical conditions affecting the external auditory meatus are explained by its innervation. Vagus innervation of the posterior and inferior walls is responsible for a cough reflex when the meatus is irritated (such as by earwax removal). Innervation by the mandibular branch of the trigeminal can cause an earache to be associated with a toothache or a lingual carcinoma.

In order to inspect the external auditory meatus and tympanic membrane, the clinician must pull the auricle up, back, and slightly laterally. When seen in the light from an otoscope, the tympanic membrane appears to be a glistening pearly gray color. A vertical streak midway between the anterior and posterior margins marks the area where the handle of the malleus is attached internally (see Fig. 25–22*A*). The point of attachment, a central depression where the membrane is drawn in toward the tympanic cavity, is called the **umbo.** At the proximal end of the handle of the malleus, above the umbo, anterior and posterior malleolar folds can be seen. Below these folds, the tympanic membrane contains medial and circular fibers and is taut: the **pars tensa membranae tympanicae.** Above the folds the membrane is thin and slack: the **pars flaccida membranae tympanicae.** A bright triangular area of reflected light called the **cone of light** is often seen extending from the umbo in the anterior inferior portion of the membrane.

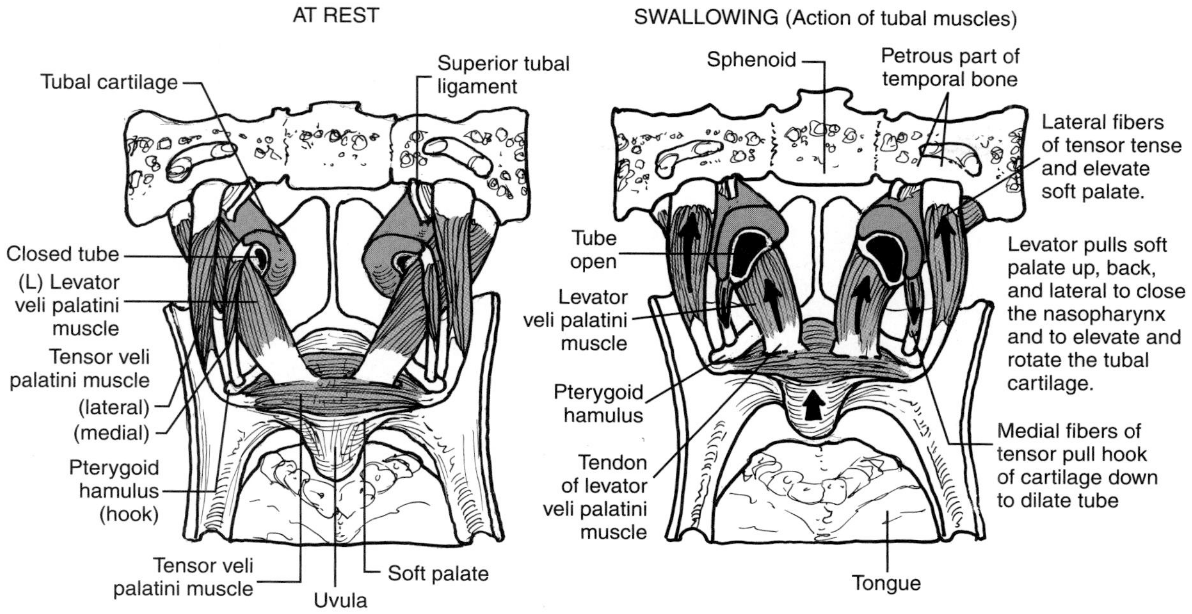

FIGURE 25–23
Muscles involved in equalization of air pressure between the tympanic cavity and the nasopharynx.

Structures Bridging the Tympanic Cavity

As described above, the tympanic membrane marks the border between the outer and middle ear. Beginning at the medial side of this membrane, the chain of auditory ossicles transmits the sound waves across the tympanic cavity to the inner ear. The malleus (mallet) is the largest ossicle. It has a large head, a neck from which anterior and lateral processes project, and a **manubrium** or handle (see Fig. 25–22*B*). Both the lateral process and the manubrium attach to the medial side of the tympanic membrane. The head of the malleus articulates via a synovial joint with the incus (anvil) bone. From the body of the incus bone, a short extension, the **short crus,** attaches by ligamentous fibers to the posterior wall of the tympanic cavity. The **long crus** parallels the manubrium of the malleus at first but, at its tip, bends in a medial direction to articulate with the final auditory ossicle, the stapes (stirrup). The anterior and posterior crura of the stapes join at an oval **base** that fits into the vestibular window, the **fenestra vestibuli** or **oval window** (see Figs. 25–20 and 25–21).

Movements of the ossicles are restricted or dampened by two muscles. The **tensor tympani** arises from the superior surface of the cartilaginous part of the auditory tube and occupies a bony canal superior to the auditory tube. Its tendon crosses the tympanic cavity to insert on the malleus handle near its root (see Fig. 25–20). It acts to pull the malleus medially, tensing the tympanic membrane and reducing its oscillations. This action prevents damage to the ear from loud sounds. The tensor tympani muscle is innervated by a branch of the nerve to the medial pterygoid from the mandibular portion of the trigeminal nerve.

The very small **stapedius** muscle arises from within the **pyramidal eminence** or cone-shaped prominence on the posterior wall of the tympanic cavity (see Fig. 25–21). Its tendon inserts into the posterior neck of the stapes. The stapedius acts to pull the stapes posteriorly, which tilts its base in the oval window and tightens the annular ligament, thus reducing the oscillatory range. The stapedius is innervated by a small branch of the facial nerve.

The **chorda tympani** nerve, a branch of the facial nerve, crosses the tympanic cavity, emerging from a posterior canaliculus to pass medial to the malleus. It leaves the cavity through the petrotympanic fissure anteriorly, eventually joining with the lingual branch of the mandibular nerve (see Fig. 25–21). A delicate network of nerves called the **tympanic plexus** covers the medial wall promontory. This plexus is composed mainly of general sensory tympanic branches of the glossopharyngeal nerve and general visceral motor branches (sympathetic) from the internal carotid plexus. The plexus supplies branches to the auditory tube, the mucosa of the middle ear, and the mastoid air cells. One branch joins the greater petrosal nerve. Another branch, the lesser petrosal nerve, can be considered a continuation of the tympanic branch of the glossopharyngeal nerve.

Equalization of Air Pressure Between the Tympanic Cavity and the Nasopharynx. The auditory tube, which leads from the anterior wall of the tympanic cavity, is normally closed at its pharyngeal end (Fig. 25–23*A*). However, during swallowing or yawning activities, three mus-

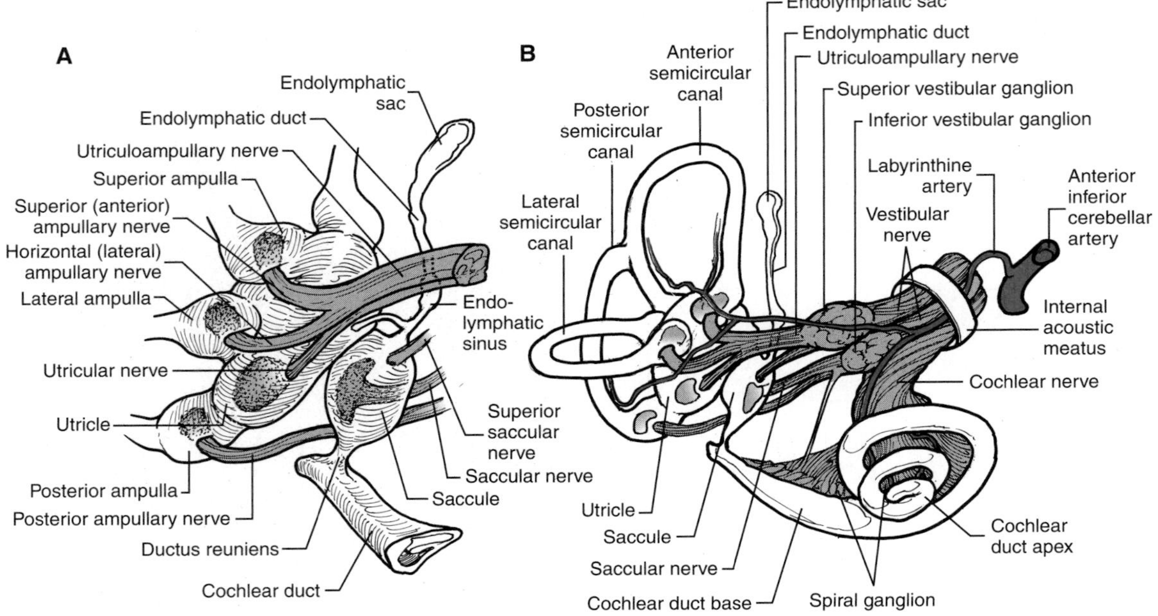

FIGURE 25–24
Vestibulocochlear nerve. **A.** Vestibular fibers. **B.** Vestibulocochlear nerve.

cles associated with the soft palate, the **tensor veli palatini, levator veli palatini,** and the **salpingopharyngeus,** act in combination to open the tube. This provides a natural mechanism for periodic equalization of the pressure on both sides of the tympanic membrane and explains why swallowing or yawning often helps alleviate ear pressure discomfort sometimes experienced during changes in ambient air pressure encountered on plane flights. One suggestion for the way the tensor and levator muscles act in conjunction is shown in Fig. 25–23*B*.

Injury to the Middle Ear. If the floor of the middle cranial fossa is fractured, there is almost always associated fracture of the tympanic cavity roof and crushing of the bony portion of the external acoustic meatus leading to rupture of the eardrum. The risks include extensive bleeding from the ear and escape of cerebrospinal fluid.

Vestibulocochlear Organ of the Inner Ear

The vestibulocochlear organ of the inner ear functions in hearing and maintenance of balance

The membranous labyrinth of the vestibulocochlear organ is a closed system of interconnected, fluid-filled tubes and sacs filled with endolymph. It is suspended in perilymphatic fluid within an osseus or bony labyrinth. The subcavities of the membranous labyrinth are the semicircular ducts, utricle, saccule, endolymphatic duct, and cochlear duct (see Fig. 25–19). Of these, the semicircular ducts, utricle, and saccule are part of the vestibular system, while the cochlear duct is the source of auditory function.

Function of the Semicircular Ducts, Utricle, and Saccule

The structure and position of the semicircular ducts, the utricle, and the saccule enable their mechanoreceptors to detect movement and motion

The semicircular canals are orientated in three planes: horizontal (lateral), posterior, and anterior. These planes record rotational head movements (Fig. 25–24 and see Fig. 25–19). The base of the ampulla of each semicircular duct contains a sensory area, the **crista ampullaris,** that appears as a saddle-shaped ridge in which hair cells with stereocilia are embedded. Completely enveloping the hair cells on the free edge of the crista is a covering of gelatinous material called the **cupula.** Movement of the head in the plane of the duct displaces the fluid endolymph and deflects the cupula and stereocilia of the sensory cells that project into it. This movement sends sensory information to the brain via the vestibular part of cranial nerve VIII (Box 25–4).

The utricle and the saccule contain **maculae,** areas of specialized sensory epithelium analogous to the crista containing terminal fibers of the vestibular nerve, which innervate hair cells. The utricular macula lies horizontally parallel to the base of the skull, while the saccular macula is oriented vertically on its medial wall. Above the gelatinous coating covering the hair cells are calcium carbonate particles (otolith, from the Greek for "ear stones"). Forward-backward or upward-downward movements of the head position relative to gravity (linear acceleration) move these otoliths, bending the stereocilia of the underlying hair cells. Information from the hair cells is sent back to the central nervous system via the vestibular nerve. Because these two maculae are set

BOX 25–4
THE VESTIBULOCOCHLEAR NERVE (CRANIAL NERVE VIII)

The vestibulocochlear nerve is one of only three cranial nerves that function entirely as special sensory afferent (SSA) nerves. The other two are the olfactory nerve (cranial nerve I) and the optic nerve (cranial nerve II). The vestibulocochlear nerve develops from an ectodermal otic placode in the rhombencephalon portion of the brain with some contribution from neural crest cells in the vestibular portion. The nerve has two major sets of fibers, both originating from the inner ear, which serve two different sensory functions. The vestibular fibers carry sensory input about the position and movement of the head in space to facilitate balance. The cochlear fibers carry auditory information. The vestibular fibers from the semicircular canals and the cochlear fibers from the cochlea come together at the internal acoustic meatus. Traveling with the facial nerve (cranial nerve VII) through the internal acoustic meatus, the vestibulocochlear nerve enters the pons-medulla junction in the brain.

Information regarding movement and position transmitted by vestibular nerve fibers is processed by four vestibular nuclei within the brain and distributed to specific efferent targets that control visual and postural reflexes to maintain equilibrium. The bipolar neurons of the vestibular nerve lie in the **vestibular ganglion of Scarpa** in the outer part of the internal auditory meatus. Three afferent (sensory) fiber tracts enter the ganglion, the **utricular nerve, saccular nerve,** and **posterior canal nerve,** which innervate the ampullae of the semicircular ducts and the maculae of the saccule and utricle. The maculae are sometimes referred to as the organs of static balance, while the ampullae relay information about angular acceleration or rotation of the head. Information from the maculae and ampullae about the position of the head travels to four **vestibular nuclei** in the caudal pons-medullar region via the afferent fibers from the vestibular ganglion. These nuclei act as "relay stations" for information received from the semicircular ducts and as "distribution stations" for motor responses. From the nuclei, information is relayed to the cerebellum, vestibulospinal tract, spinal cord, and oculomotor nuclei via descending and ascending paths of the medial longitudinal fasciculus. A few fibers from the vestibular nerve enter the cerebellum directly. Vestibular information sent from vestibular nuclei also reaches several cortical areas of the brain.

Auditory information is carried to the brain via multiple crossed pathways, maintaining a point-to-point "tontopic map." The cochlear nerve joins the vestibular nerve lateral to the internal auditory meatus (see Fig. 25–25). It is derived from many afferent fibers from bipolar cells found in the spiral ganglion within the modiolus of the cochlea. Afferent fibers bringing sensory input from hair cells all along the spiral coil of the cochlear duct reach the spiral ganglion via the osseous spiral lamina (see Fig. 25-24*B*). As previously described, the basilar membrane within the organ of Corti vibrates in response to sound waves, stimulating the hair cells. Two types of bipolar cells are present in the spiral ganglion, recording auditory information from two types of hair cells. Type I ganglion cells, in which many nerve processes synapse with one inner hair cell, respond to a narrow frequency range. Type II ganglion cells, which synapse with more than 10 outer hair cells, are less precisely tuned to frequency but are more sensitive to low-intensity sounds. Of the bipolar neurons, 95% are type I and have myelinated central axons; 5% are type II and have unmyelinated central axons.

Although fibers from the cochlear nerve synapse in the cochlear nuclei at the pons-medulla junction, auditory impulses are relayed through brainstem nuclei in a complex pattern, which includes the crossing over of information at several different levels. Monaural information (from each ear individually) is sent to the contralateral side. Binaural information (from both ears simultaneously) is sent to both ipsilateral and contralateral locations. The first decussation (crossover) point for information is the trapezoid body. This is sometimes referred to as a *functional acoustic chiasma,* since it is similar in function to the optic chiasma. The next level, the superior olivary complex, is the first place where information from both ears converges. Crossover also takes place at the level of the inferior colliculus. From there, information goes through the medial geniculate nucleus, finally reaching the auditory cortex located in the transverse gyri of Heschl. At the cortical level, the corpus callosum provides an additional crossover connection.

Because information crosses over at many points, damage to the ear at or above the superior olivary complex will leave some information paths intact and will not result in monaural deafness.

At all levels, including the auditory cortex, the synaptic contacts retain a point-to-point distribution from high to low frequencies.

---

at right angles to each other, the system is very sensitive to orientation of the head.

The combined sensory information from the vestibular organs on both sides of the head increases the sensitivity of the system. Neurons at the level of the vestibular nucleus in the brainstem receive information from the left and right sides of the head. Since corresponding semicircular canals on opposite sides of the head always respond oppositely to head motion, vestibular nuclei in the rostral medulla and caudal pons effectively "compare" relative discharge rates from the left and right canals.

Movements such as the rocking of a boat in rough water or the shaking of a plane in turbulent air may cause a heightening of the vestibular response, which may result in dizziness or nausea (motion sickness).

Structure of the Cochlear Duct and Its Function in Hearing

Sound waves collected in the outer ear are amplified in the air-filled middle ear for transmission to the fluid-filled cochlea of the inner ear (Fig.25–25*A* and see Fig. 25–19). As indicated earlier, two entirely different fluids are found within the inner ear. The fluid within the membranous labyrinth (in the cochlear duct, utricle, saccule, semicircular ducts and endolymphatic sac) is endolymph, similar in composition to extracellular fluid, with a high concentration of K^+. In contrast, the fluid surrounding the membranous labyrinth (in the vestibule, scala vestibuli, scala tympani, and the semicircular canals) is perilymph, which is similar in composition to cerebrospinal fluid, with a high concentration of Na^+. The ionic differences between these two fluids are crucial for the mechanoelectrical responses required for hearing.

Vibrations transmitted by the base of the stapes to the perilymph of the vestibule results in waves of hydraulic pressure that rise to the apex of the cochlea via the scala vestibuli. These waves then pass through a communication between the scala vestibuli and the scala tympani, the **helicotrema,** and then descend to the basal turn of the cochlea. The waves end as vibrations once again at the secondary tympanic membrane that covers the round window and dissipate in the tympanic cavity (see Fig. 25–19).

The central canal, the cochlear duct, which is roughly triangular in section, is separated from the scala vestibuli by the **vestibular** (or **Reissner's) membrane** and from the scala tympani by the **basilar membrane** (Fig. 25–25*B*). The external boundary of the triangle is the **stria vascularis** (the cells and rich capillary bed involved in the production of endolymph fluid). This central cochlear duct houses the spiral **organ of Corti,** the specialized sensory receptors responsible for hearing, which rests on the basilar membrane (Fig. 25–25*B*). A gelatinous **tectorial membrane** extends over the sensory epithelium. When hydraulic waves ascend and descend, respectively, in the adjacent scala vestibula and scala tympani displacing the basilar membrane, the tips of the hair cells of the organ of Corti embedded in the tectorial membrane are bent. This causes the depolarization of the hair cells (mechanical force is converted into an electrical signal) and sensory information is transmitted along the cochlear nerve fibers.

A schematic look at the cochlear duct illustrates the ways sound waves are analyzed within it (Fig 25–25*A*). High frequencies produce waves with the most amplitude in the stiffer, narrow base, and lower frequencies have waves with the most amplitude in the wider, more flexible apex. Hair cells respond to areas of maximal stimulation by sending sensory information via the cochlear portion of cranial nerve VIII (Fig. 25–25 and see Fig. 25–24). Added to this broad discrimination between frequencies is the "fine tuning" property of individual hair cells that allows them to respond to particular tones. The organization of responses to frequencies at specific places within the cochlea is sometimes referred to as the "place theory of cochlear tuning."

As the information from the cochlear nerve ascends to the auditory cortex, it retains the place nature of sound information as it passes through several synaptic sites ("tonotopic" organization). This means that information about high and low frequencies remains sorted out in higher auditory connections. For example, lower frequencies may be represented in one area and higher frequencies in another. All fibers synapse in the **cochlear nuclei.** They then pass on to the **trapezoid body** or the **superior olivary nucleus** and to the **inferior colliculus.** From there they pass on to the **medial geniculate nuclei** and finally reach the **auditory cortex.** At several levels along the way (particularly within the trapezoid body), information from one ear is sent both to the same side and to the contralateral side. This creates a situation functionally similar to the optic chiasma (see Box 25–4).

Injury or Lesions of the Peripheral Auditory System. Partial or total deafness can result from either conductive or sensorineural disorders. Injury or lesions of the peripheral auditory system can cause hearing loss, vertigo, or tinnitus (a buzzing or ringing in the ear).

External or middle ear pathologies can result in **conduction deafness.** Anything that adversely affects the movement of the tympanic membrane, auditory ossicles, or oval and round windows can reduce hearing.

In the middle ear, inflammatory infections such as **otitis media** typically produce purulent (pus-containing) material that can put pressure on, or even rupture, the tympanic membrane. Repeated rupture of the membrane can cause scarring or hearing loss. If infections recur frequently, a surgical procedure called *tympanotomy* is often employed, which allows the insertion of a small tube into the tympanic membrane to provide a pathway for drainage of fluid from the middle ear.

The function of auditory ossicles can be impaired in several ways. For example, a lesion of the facial nerve can result in paralysis of the stapedius, eliminating the dampening effect of the stapedius muscle in response to loud noises. A state of excessively acute hearing **(hyperacusis)** results. Diseases such as **otosclerosis** can directly affect the freedom of ossicle movement.

Sensorineural hearing loss (nerve deafness) can occur in the inner ear if cranial nerve VIII is damaged. For example if an **acoustic neuroma,** a tumor, grows within the internal auditory meatus (the entrance of the vestibulocochlear nerve), a patient could experience both loss of balance and cochlear

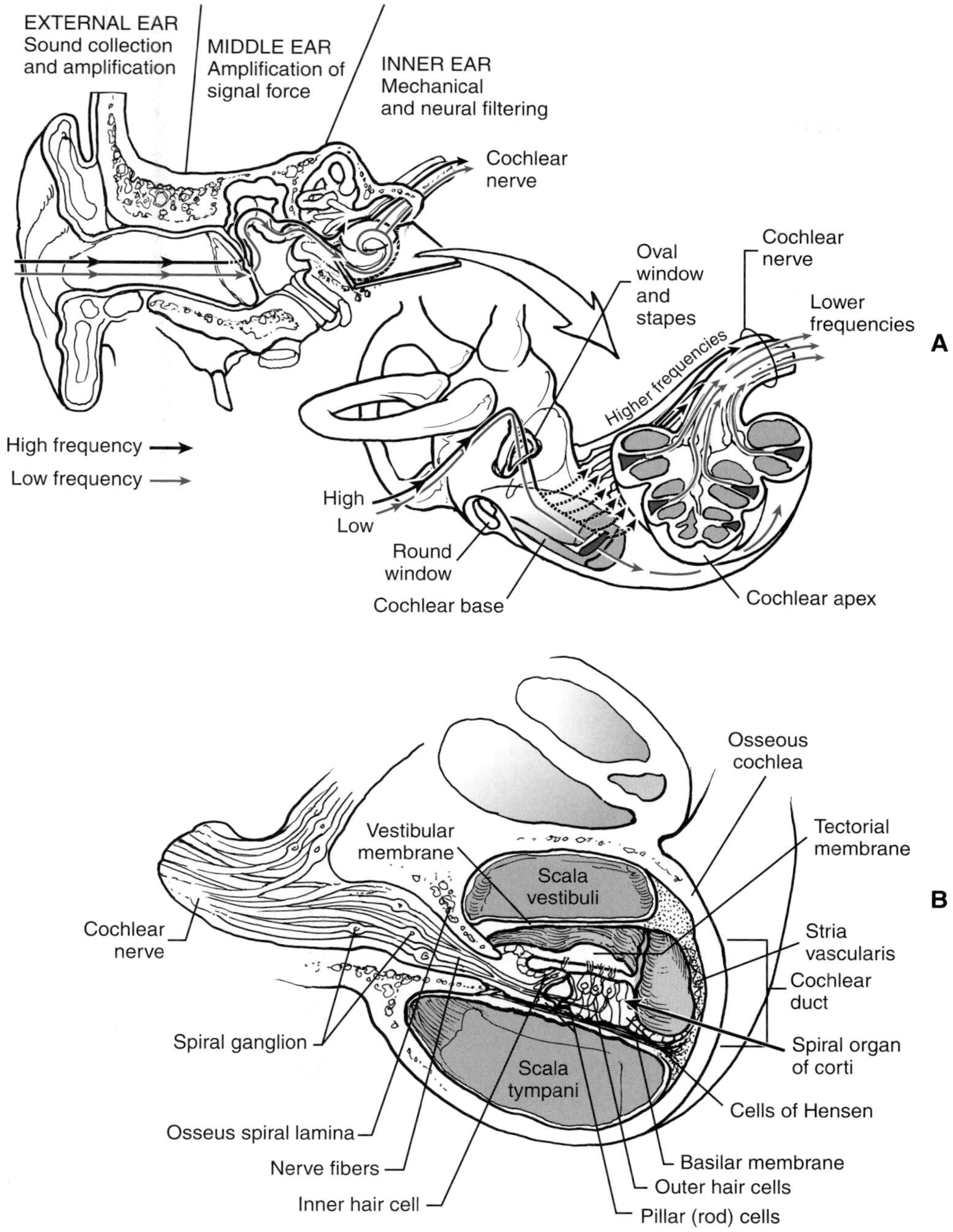

FIGURE 25–25

Structure of the cochlear duct and its function in hearing. **A.** Schematic representation of sound waves processing from the entrance of the ear to the cochlea. **B.** Cross section of the cochlear duct.

hearing impairment. Specific damage to the spiral organ within the cochlea can occur from **exposure to excessively loud sounds.** This kind of damage is seen in people who work around jet engines or very loud machinery without ear protection and results in high-tone deafness.

Meniere syndrome increases endolymphatic volume within the cochlear duct, utricle and saccule, resulting in a sense of pressure in the ear, distortion of sounds, and heightened sensitivity to noise.

In some cases of cochlear hearing loss, implants of fine wire electrodes responsive to a range of frequencies may help a person regain some auditory sensation.

In addition, central auditory pathways may be defective, resulting in apparent loss of hearing or **central deafness.** Because information from the cochlear nerve of each ear crosses over to the other ear, unilateral damage within the central auditory nuclei or the auditory cortex generally affects the hearing capabilities in both ears.

26 Sinuses and Cavities of the Head and Introduction to the Brain

Throughout this chapter, the cavities and sinuses of the head will serve as a framework for anatomic description. These cavities include the nasal cavity, paranasal sinuses, oral cavity, and cranial cavity, which is the largest single cavity in the head.

The senses of smell and taste will be described, as well as the cranial nerves that contribute to these senses: the olfactory nerve (cranial nerve I) and the glossopharyngeal, vagus, and hypoglossal nerves (cranial nerves IX, X, and XII, respectively).

A short description of the anatomy of the brain will follow. The brain receives all of the sensory information and coordinates all of the responses for the body. A brief discussion of the relationship between the endocrine system and the nervous system is also included.

The final chapter, Chapter 27, will present the structures within the neck, including the highly specialized laryngeal apparatus, which allows a human being to communicate in complex ways with other living beings. The accessory nerve (cranial nerve XI) and the musculature of the neck will also be introduced. The vasculature of the head and neck arises from major vessels in the root of the neck, and, therefore, this vasculature will be discussed in Chapter 27 to serve as a review of all interconnected structures within the head.

DEFINITIVE ANATOMY OF THE NASAL CAVITY

Skeletal Structure of the Nasal Cavity

The roof of the **nasal cavity** is formed anteriorly by the frontal nasal spine and the nasal bones. The central roof boundary is the cribriform (sievelike, or perforated) plate through which branches of the olfactory nerves are distributed to the olfactory mucosa. The sphenoid bone and openings to the sphenoid sinuses are found posteriorly. The palatine process of the maxilla and the horizontal plates of the palatine bones form the base of the cavity (Fig. 26–1 and see Fig. 22–10).

The left and right nasal cavities are divided by a **medial vertical septum.** Anteriorly, this septum is composed of the **septal cartilage,** which supports the external nose. Posteriorly, the upper septum is composed of the **perpendicular plate of the ethmoid bone.** The inferior posterior portion is made up of the **vomer** with some contributions from the nasal crests of the maxilla and palatine bones (Fig. 26–1).

The anterior region of the lateral wall of the nasal cavity is made up of the nasal bone, frontal process of the maxillary bone, and the lacrimal bone. Posterior and inferior portions of the wall are irregular because of three projecting curved elevations of mucosa-covered bone called **conchae** ("shell") (Fig. 26–2). The bones are sometimes called **turbinates,** a term that refers to their scrolllike shapes. The conchae curve inferiorly, forming the roof of a groove or meatus that functions as a passageway within the nasal cavity. This structural configuration greatly increases the respiratory surface area within the nose.

The conchae are named **inferior, middle,** and **superior,** according to their positions. The superior and middle conchae are processes of the ethmoidal labyrinth. Below the root of the middle concha is a rounded bulge formed by ethmoid air cells called the **ethmoid bulla** ("bubble"). Below the bulla is another thinner process called the **uncinate process.** The opening to the maxillary sinus, the **semilunar hiatus,** is found in the gap between the bulla and the uncinate processes (Fig. 26–2*B*). The semilunar hiatus leads anteriorly into a curved groove, the **ethmoid infundibulum,** into which the maxillary sinus opens. Above the superior concha at the back, a small projection called the **supreme concha** is sometimes seen. The **nasolacrimal duct** from the lacrimal gland travels in an osseous canal formed by the maxilla, lacrimal bone, and inferior nasal concha and then enters the inferior meatus (Fig. 26–2*B*). The lacrimal duct drains excessive tears from the conjunctiva of the eye into the nasal cavity. Behind the middle and inferior conchae is an area called the **nasopharyngeal meatus,** which ends in the **choana,** or opening into the nasopharynx (Fig. 26–2*A*).

Structure of the External Nose

The external nose is pyramidal in shape, with its root at the forehead and its apex at the tip, where the nostrils, or **external nares,** are found (Fig. 26–3). The flared portions of the lower nose are called **alae**

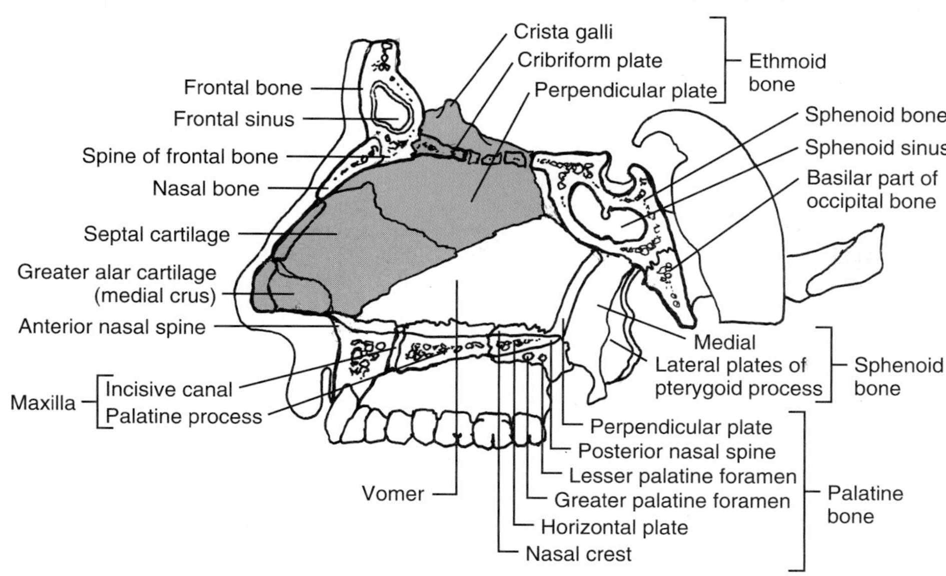

FIGURE 26–1
Skeletal structure of the nasal cavity at the medial nasal wall.

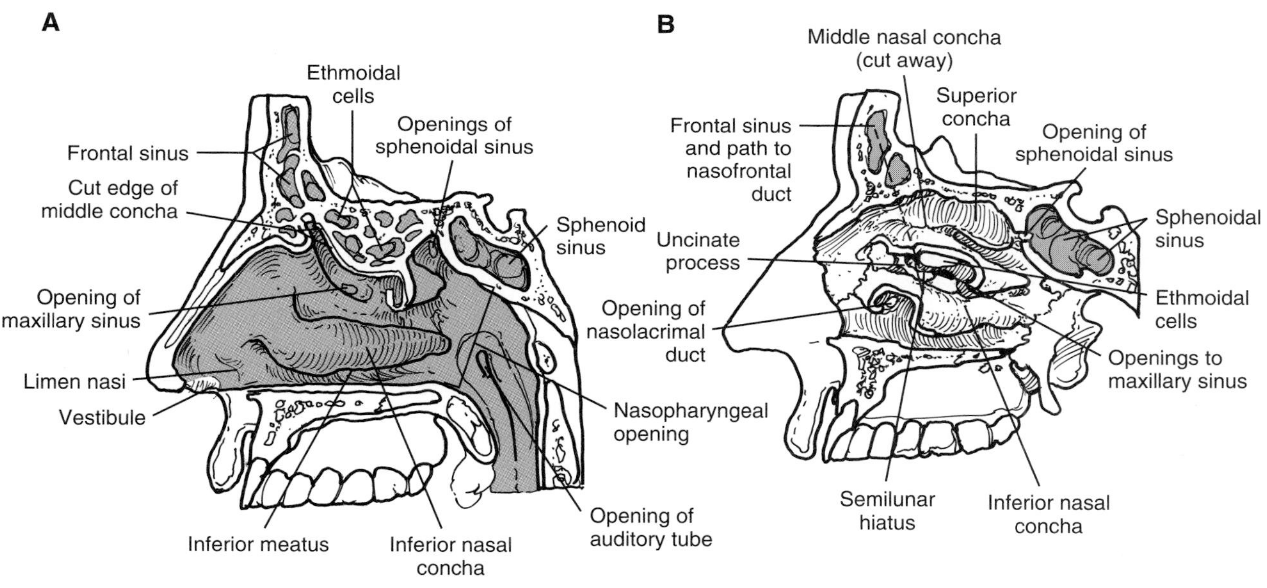

FIGURE 26–2
Internal cavity of the nose. **A.** Lateral nasal wall. **B.** Concha has been removed to show openings from sinuses.

("wings"). In addition to the osseous framework, a system of interlocking cartilages gives flexible support to the nose. A **septal cartilage** forms the anterior segment of the nasal septum and connects to the bony septum. At its medial surface, the septal cartilage is attached to the triangular **lateral nasal cartilages.** The major **alar cartilages** lie below the lateral cartilages (Fig. 26–3). It is possible to palpate the notch, separating the two major alar cartilages at the tip of the nose. All of these cartilages are joined by dense connective tissue.

Each internal cavity of the nose begins at the **naris** and ends posteriorly at the **choana,** or opening to the pharynx (see Fig. 26–2). The entrance to each cavity is a skin-covered area with protective hairs called the **vestibule** (see Fig. 26–2A). An upper lateral limit of the vestibule, the **limen nasi,** can be identified by a crescent-shaped infolding of the lower border of the lateral cartilage. The **agger nasi** is the most anterosuperior projection of the middle nasal concha.

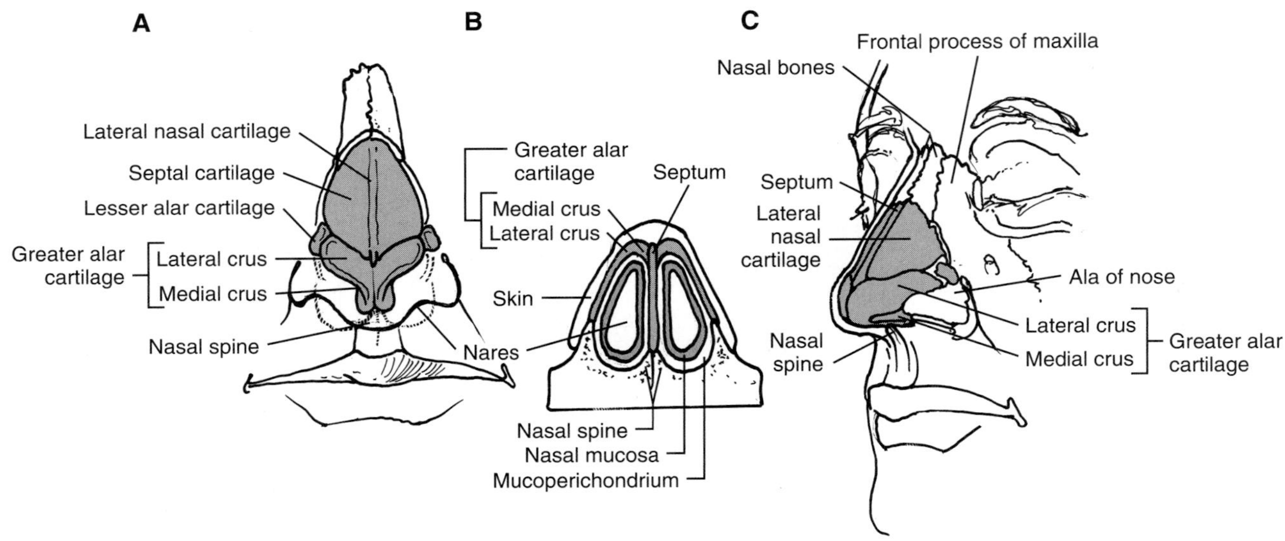

FIGURE 26–3
External nose showing major cartilages. **A.** Anterior view. **B.** Inferior view. **C.** Lateral view.

The **olfactory region** of the nasal cavity is in the narrow roof of the nose. The **respiratory region** of the nasal cavity, including all of the medial and lateral nasal walls, is comprised of glandular and mucous membranes covered with cilia.

This surface is highly vascularized, so that it easily becomes swollen if vasodilation occurs. Treatments for nasal congestion, therefore, often contain epinephrine-like compounds, which decrease secretion of mucus and produce vasoconstriction of the arterioles.

Respiratory Function of the Nose

The ciliated epithelium within the nonolfactory regions (respiratory areas) of the nose contains secretory goblet cells, nonciliated columnar cells, and basal cells. Beneath the basilar lamina are many serous or mucous glands. The combined secretions from goblet cells and mucous glands within the nose make the surface quite sticky. The stickiness traps dust that is carried in the air and also warms and humidifies the air. The cilia move mucus in a posterior direction within the nasal cavity toward the oropharynx, where it is swallowed. Nasal secretions are known to contain antibacterial agents such as immunoglobulins that may inhibit growth of microbes within the nasal cavity.

Sensory Function of the Nose and the First Cranial Nerve

The sensory, or **olfactory, epithelium** of the nose is located within the roof of the nasal cavity. It lies on the superior surface of the nasal septum and medial wall of the superior concha (Fig. 26–4). The olfactory epithelium differs from the nearby nasal respiratory epithelium in that it is thicker and appears slightly yellowish rather than pink. Three different cell types are present: olfactory receptor neurons, supporting cells, and basal cells. Each bipolar receptor neuron has a single apical dendrite and an unmyelinated axon. The apical dendrite ends in a knoblike olfactory vesicle with 10 to 30 olfactory cilia that protrude into the mucus layer. The unmyelinated axons (which are only 0.2 μ in diameter, nearly the smallest in the nervous system) group together to form **olfactory fila** or central processes, which make up the **olfactory nerve** (Fig. 26–4). Olfactory neurons are unusual for two reasons:

1. They are primary sensory neurons with cell bodies next to the sensory surface, unusual in vertebrates.
2. They are the only mammalian neurons that turn over, being replaced by the basal stem cells every 30 to 60 days.

Despite this turnover, up to 1% of olfactory receptors are lost each year of life, causing gradual loss of olfactory sense.

The epithelium is pseudostratified, with supporting cell nuclei at the surface, sensory neuron somata (cell bodies) in the middle region, and basal cell nuclei farthest from the surface. Beneath the olfactory epithelium are tubular **olfactory glands** (of **Bowman**) that secrete the fluid that surrounds the receptor endings on the surface.

Olfactory fila terminate in a forebrain structure located on the ventral surface of the frontal lobe, the **olfactory bulb** (Fig. 26–4). Unlike other sensory systems that are relayed through the thalamus to reach the cortex, the olfactory bulb projects directly to the olfactory cortex on the ventral surface of the telencephalon. Box 26–1 provides a discussion of the olfactory nerve.

Because humans depend less on the sense of smell than other mammals to locate food, detect predators,

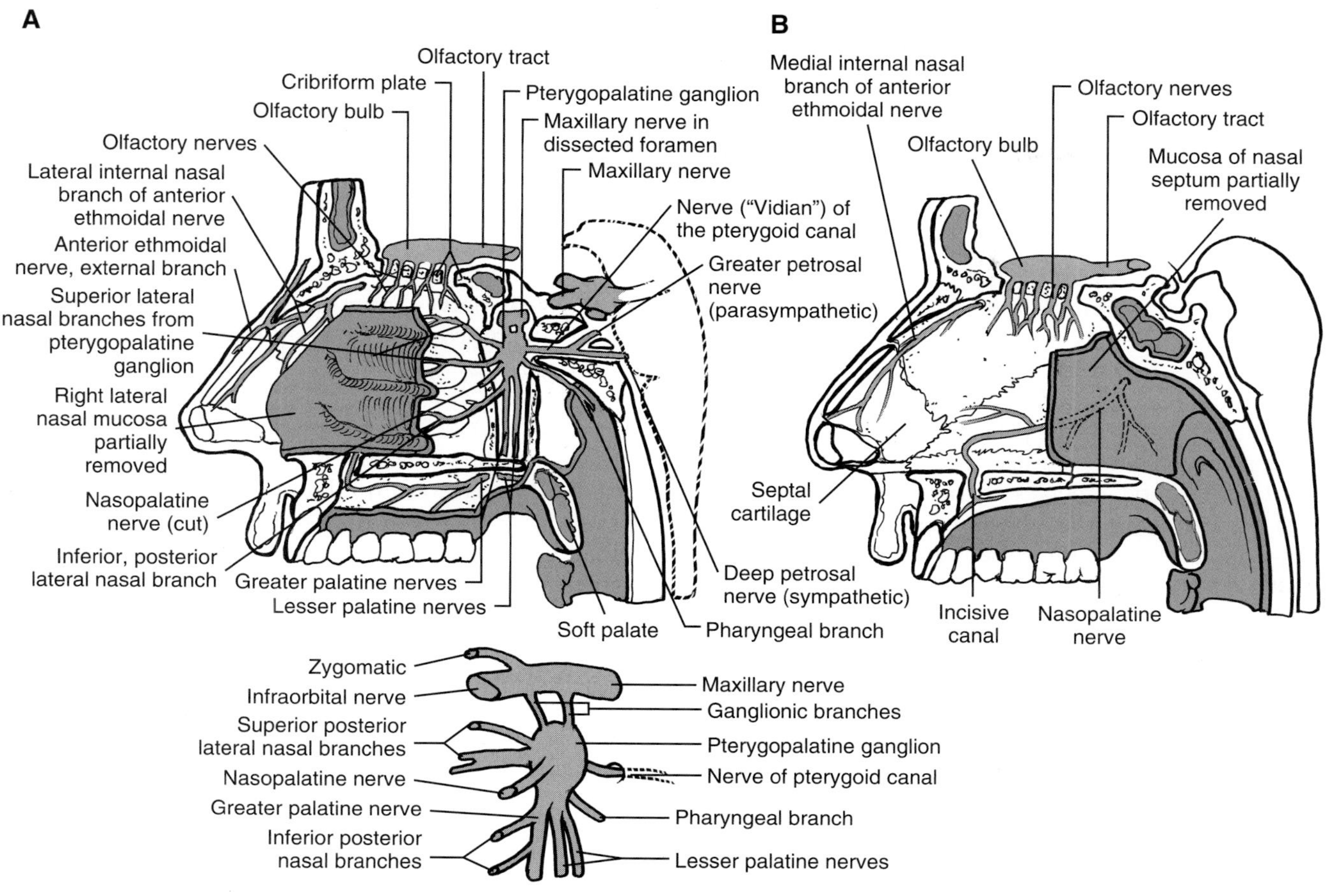

FIGURE 26–4
Nerves of the nasal cavity. **A.** Lateral wall with detail of pterygopalatine ganglion. **B.** Medial nerves.

and select mates, their sensory system is not as well developed. Even so, humans can distinguish thousands of different odors. In contrast, human taste receptors can distinguish only salty, sweet, sour, and bitter tastes. The olfactory system thus plays an important role in facilitating the perception of complex tastes and flavors.

BOX 26–1
THE OLFACTORY NERVE

The olfactory nerve develops from the ectodermal nasal placode at the anterior end of the telencephalon and remains within the epithelium of the nasal mucous membrane. It is entirely sensory in function. Primary neurosensory cells produce axons that grow into the olfactory bulb. Within the bulb, they synapse with secondary olfactory neurons that form the olfactory tract (see Fig. 26–4). The olfactory bulb differs from other sensory systems because it projects directly to the olfactory cortex. Many reciprocal connections occur between separate areas within the olfactory cortex, including connections to nuclei from the contralateral side. Projections outward from the olfactory cortex reach the contralateral olfactory bulb and olfactory cortex. Olfactory information is also relayed to the neocortex, particularly the orbitofrontal and insular cortices. It is thought that neocortical representation is important for discriminating odors. Since some taste sensory input reaches the same neocortical areas, these areas in the neocortex may hold the key to interaction between taste and olfaction for perception of flavor.

Clinical Conditions Affecting the Sense of Smell. Nasal and paranasal upper respiratory infections **(sinusitis)** and allergies **(rhinitis)** can cause the nasal mucosa to become inflamed and swollen. This can block the olfactory epithelium and reduce sensitivity to smells. Permanent damage sometimes results from infections, which can spread to the anterior cranial fossa and nasopharynx.

Neurodegenerative diseases such as **Alzheimer's syndrome, Parkinson's disease,** and **Huntington's chorea** can affect central olfactory pathways and reduce olfactory functions. Olfactory problems often occur early in the course of neurodegenerative diseases and may, in fact, be one of the first symptoms exhibited.

Epilepsy and a variety of psychiatric disorders can create **parosmia,** or distortion of olfactory function, in which smells may be perceived when no stimulus is present.

Trauma to the head can damage central olfactory pathways. In particular, **shearing movements** to the olfactory bulb at its junction with the cribriform plate can break the thin axons from the olfactory neurons. For this reason, boxers often experience **anosmia** (loss of smell) or **hyposmia** (reduced olfactory sensitivity).

General Innervation of the Nose and Nasal Cavity

Innervation of the nose and anterior nasal region is supplied mainly by branches of the **anterior ethmoidal nerve** (a branch of the nasociliary nerve from the trigeminal nerve's ophthalmic division). The anterior ethmoidal nerve travels under the dura mater in a groove along the cribriform plate, entering the nasal cavity through a slit lateral to the crista galli. It continues along a groove on the inside of the nasal bones, dividing into external and internal nasal branches. The **external nasal nerve** emerges at the lower border of the nasal bone and supplies the skin of the nasal ala and apex—the dorsum of the nose. Cutaneous innervation of the side of the nose and the movable portion of the nasal septum are provided by small nasal branches of the maxillary infraorbital nerve. Internally, branches of the **internal nasal nerve** serve the anterior portions of the lateral wall and the medial septum.

More posteriorly, the lateral nasal walls and the central nasal septum are innervated by fibers from the **pterygopalatine ganglion,** which is located in the pterygopalatine fossa directly posterior to the middle nasal concha. The parasympathetic fibers from the facial nerve (cranial nerve VII) synapse at this ganglion (see Box 24–2 for a full discussion). However, the ganglion also serves as a point of convergence for a number of nerves that simply travel through it and emerge, recombined, as the "nerves of the pterygopalatine ganglion." Each of these emerging nerves, therefore, carries contributions from several sources. In addition to postganglionic parasympathetic fibers from the facial nerve (pGVE fibers), these include

- special visceral afferent (SVA) sensory fibers from the nervus intermedius, a branch of the facial nerve;
- general somatic afferent (GSA) sensory fibers from the maxillary nerve (V2); and
- sympathetic general visceral efferent (sGVE) sympathetic fibers from the internal carotid plexus.

Postganglionic parasympathetic fibers control secretion and vasodilation and, as a consequence, can quickly produce a "stuffed-up nose."

Specifically, the nerves from the pterygopalatine ganglion that innervate the nasal cavity include **nasal** and **palatine branches.** These branches enter the nasal cavity through the sphenopalatine foramen. **Superior posterior lateral** and **superior posterior medial nasal branches** innervate the mucosa of the roof of the nasal cavity, the upper two nasal conchae laterally, the nasal septum medially, and the lining of the posterior ethmoidal air sinuses (see Fig. 26–4). A large **nasopalatine nerve** serves the nasal septum, coursing obliquely downward in a groove in the nasal septum to penetrate the hard palate via the nasopalatine foramen. This nerve supplies the mucosa that covers the anterior region of the hard palate. The **greater palatine nerve** gives off **inferior posterior nasal branches** that innervate the posterior area of the inferior nasal concha on its way to the oral cavity (see Fig. 26–4). The greater palatine nerve then continues on to serve the hard palate, while the lesser palatine nerves serve the soft palate, uvula, and upper aspect of the tonsils. Finally, **pharyngeal nerves** from the pterygopalatine ganglion supply the mucosa of the nasopharynx posterior to the auditory tube.

Vascularization of the Nose and Nasal Cavity

The arteries of the nose travel with the larger nerves. **Posterior ethmoidal arteries** and **anterior ethmoidal arteries** from the ophthalmic artery reach the nasal cavity through its roof and supply both the medial septal areas and the lateral walls of the nose (Fig. 26–5). A branch of the maxillary artery, the **sphenopalatine artery,** enters the nasal cavity through the sphenopalatine foramen and divides into lateral and septal posterior nasal arteries to supply posterior inferior areas. Small branches of the facial artery supply the region of the vestibule (Fig. 26–5).

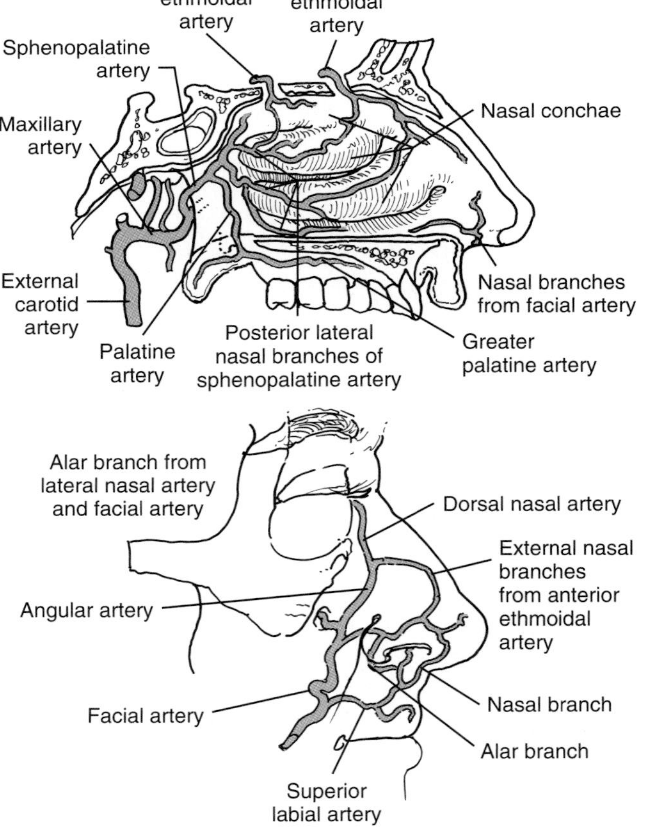

FIGURE 26–5
Vascularization of the nose and nasal cavity. **A.** Lateral nasal wall. **B.** Superficial vascularization.

ANATOMY OF THE PARANASAL SINUSES

The paranasal sinuses are air-filled diverticula of the nasal cavity that grow into adjacent frontal, ethmoid, sphenoid, and maxillary bones

Variations in size and shape of each one of the four paired sinuses are common. The **frontal, maxillary,** and **sphenoid sinuses** are typically large, paired structures (Fig. 26–6). The remaining sinus, the **ethmoidal sinus,** is made up of numerous smaller cavities called **ethmoid cells** (Fig. 26–6). (See Chapter 22 and Fig. 22–16 for more detailed information about the position of the paranasal sinuses within the skull.) All of the sinuses are lined with mucosa, which is continuous with the mucosa of the naval cavity. Mucus secreted by the mucosal lining of the sinuses is swept into the nasal cavity by cilia. The frontal, maxillary, and sphenoid sinuses are also drained by gravity, depending on the position of the head. Because all the sinuses connect to the nasal cavity, infection spreads easily through them.

Although the maxillary and ethmoid sinuses appear by the fifth fetal month, full development of all of the sinuses does not occur until puberty. The postnatal development of the air sinuses significantly alters the relative sizes of the face and cranial vault; this process accounts for the changes that occur in a child's facial features between infancy and puberty. The sinuses add resonance to the voice and, to some extent, may function to lighten the skull.

Frontal, Maxillary, Ethmoidal, and Sphenoid Sinuses

The **frontal sinuses** are found within the frontal bone of the skull (Fig. 26–6 and see Fig. 26–2). They are rarely symmetrical and may even overlap each other but are generally triangular in shape. They open into the nasal cavity under the anterior end of the middle concha through a foramen, which may form a duct. The frontal sinus is innervated by the supraorbital nerve.

The **maxillary sinuses** are the largest accessory air sinuses, reaching full size after development of the permanent teeth. The base of each pyramidal sinus forms the lateral walls of the nasal cavity, the orbit of the eye, and the alveolar process of the maxilla (Fig. 26–6). The apex extends into the zygomatic process of the maxilla. The opening into the nasal cavity is in the region of the hiatus close to the roof of the sinus. Innervation of the upper portion is by the infraorbital nerve; innervation of the anterior, middle, and lower portions is by the posterior superior alveolar nerve.

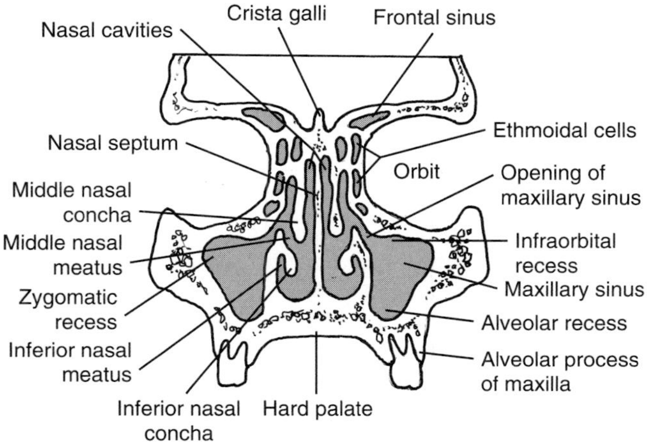

Nasal cavities
Crista galli
Frontal sinus
Ethmoidal cells
Nasal septum
Orbit
Opening of maxillary sinus
Middle nasal concha
Middle nasal meatus
Infraorbital recess
Maxillary sinus
Zygomatic recess
Alveolar recess
Inferior nasal meatus
Alveolar process of maxilla
Inferior nasal concha
Hard palate

FIGURE 26–6
Paranasal sinuses, coronal section. Sphenoid sinuses would be posterior to the plane of this section behind ethmoidal cells.

The small **ethmoidal sinuses** begin as invaginations from the nasal passages into the ethmoidal labyrinth in the space between the upper part of the nasal cavity and the orbits of the eyes (Fig. 26–6 and see Fig. 26–2). The sinuses may be made up of different numbers of subunits, ranging from 3 to 18 on each side. These small sinuses are usually grouped into anterior, medial, and posterior clusters and have three independent sites of communication with the nasal cavity: the anterior and middle regions of the middle meatus and the superior meatus, respectively.

The size and shape of the **sphenoid sinuses** may also vary significantly. One of the pair is occasionally much larger than the other and may extend over the median line behind the other sinus. They are found posterior to the upper part of the nasal cavity within the body of the sphenoid bone (see Fig. 26–2). They are served by the posterior ethmoidal nerves and orbital branches of the pterygopalatine ganglion. Each sinus opens through its anterior wall into the sphenoethmoid recess of the nasal cavity. The sphenoid sinuses are intimately related to a number of important anatomic structures. They lie immediately below the sella turcica and, therefore, the pituitary gland. The carotid sinus, carotid artery, and ophthalmic and maxillary branches of the trigeminal nerve are on either side of the sinuses, and the nerve of the pterygoid canal runs through the anterior floor. The sphenoid sinuses may also extend laterally far enough to be directly related to the optic canal.

Clinical Problems of the Paranasal Sinuses. As mentioned above, the paranasal sinuses are continuous with the nasal cavities, and, therefore, painful infections causing inflammation and swelling (sinusitis) can easily spread from the nasal cavities to any or all of the separate sinuses. Congestion within the sinuses is compounded by the fact that nasal drainage is often blocked. Only the frontal sinuses have ostia that can drain by gravity when one is standing upright (Fig. 26–6 and see Fig. 26–2). The openings to the maxillary sinuses, for example, are at the top of the cavities. Draining of the maxillary sinuses, therefore, requires that a person lie first on one side and then the other. Because of the thin wall between the ethmoidal sinuses and the orbit and the close proximity of ethmoidal cells to the optic canal, ethmoidal sinus infections may have especially serious consequences. Infection in the ethmoidal sinuses may cause optic neuritis or, in severe cases, may even damage the optic nerve and cause blindness.

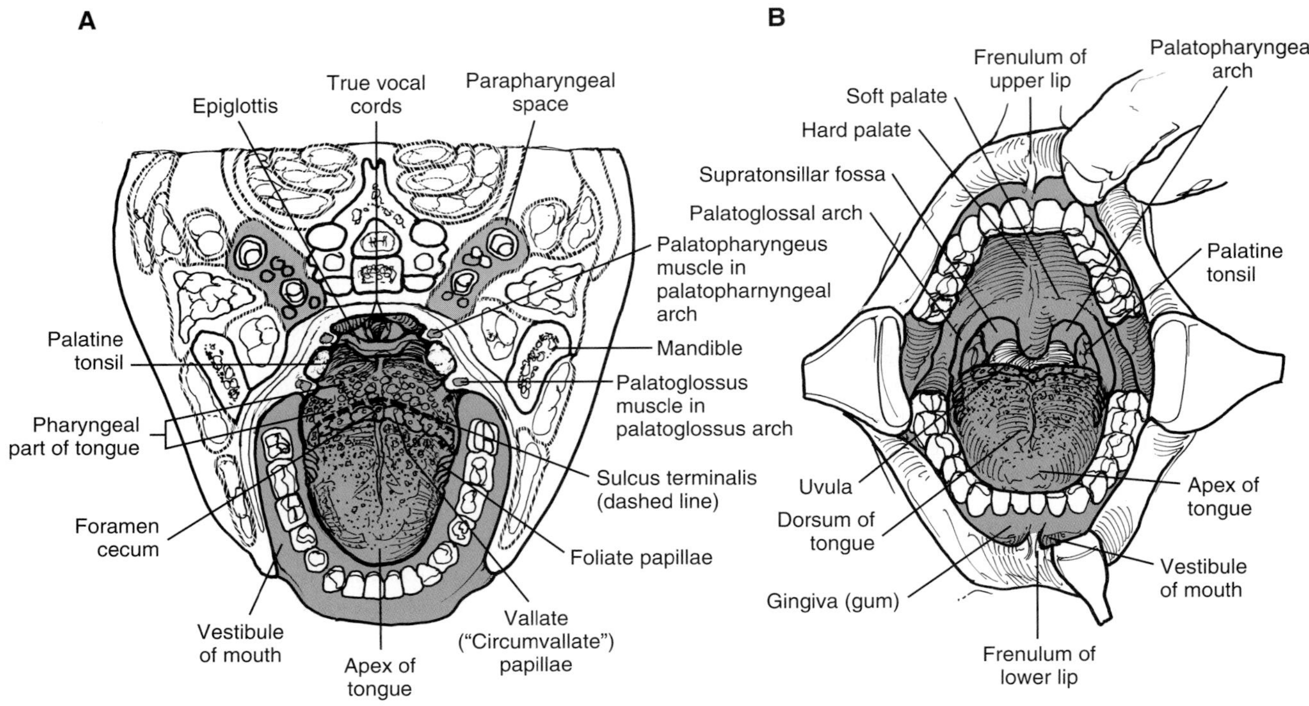

FIGURE 26–7
The oral cavity. **A.** Superior view. **B.** Anterior view.

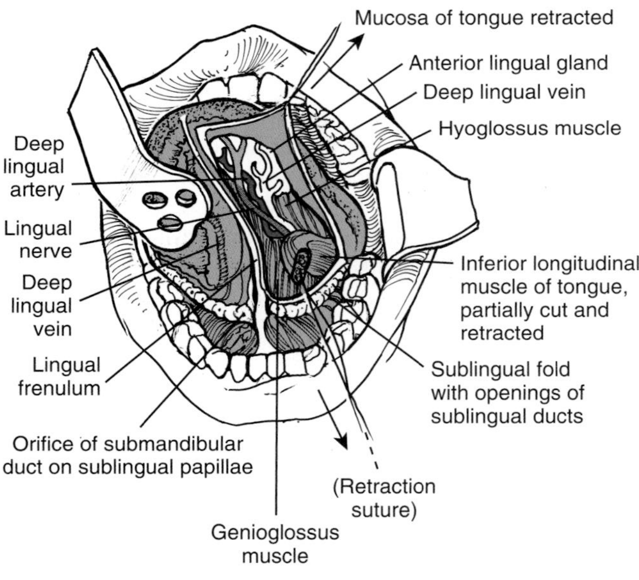

FIGURE 26–8
Inferior lingual surface.

THE ORAL CAVITY AND THE TONGUE

Definitive Anatomy of the Oral Cavity

The mouth, or oral cavity, is divided into two parts. The **vestibule** is the narrow space between the inside of the cheeks and the teeth; the **oral cavity proper** is the cavity inside the teeth and gums that houses the tongue (Fig. 26–7). Within the vestibule, a midline fold called the **frenulum** connects the upper lip to the gum; a similar frenulum exists for the lower lip. At the level of the upper second molar is the **parotid papilla,** the opening from the parotid gland. Other small glands, including **buccal glands** and **sebaceous glands** of the lips, also open into the vestibule. Within the oral cavity proper, the tongue, or **lingua,** forms most of the floor of the cavity (Fig. 26–7). On the lower back surface of the tongue, a median **frenulum** connects the tongue with the oral floor (Fig. 26–8). On each side of the posterior inferior part of the frenulum is found a **sublingual papilla,** which houses the end of the duct from the submandibular salivary gland. From that point at the floor of the mouth, a pair of **sublingual folds** extends diagonally toward the sides of the mouth. Small ducts from the sublingual salivary gland open in this region (Fig. 26–8). The **palatoglossus muscle** extends from the soft palate anterior to the tonsils to the side of the tongue and functions to lift the root of the tongue to close off the oral cavity from the oropharynx.

The roof of the oral cavity proper is formed by the **hard** and **soft palates** (Fig. 26–7*B*). The hard palate in the front is formed by palatine processes of the maxillae bones and horizontal plates of the palatine bones. The soft palate begins at the posterior border of the hard palate and continues back to form a mobile flap between the mouth and the nasal part of the pharynx. It is composed of a fold of mucosa enclosing muscle, vessels, nerves, and lymphoid tissue. The thin expanded tendon of the tensor veli palatini muscle, the **palatine aponeu-**

rosis, covers the first two thirds of the soft palate and provides attachment for all other palatine muscles. A conical process called the **uvula** projects from the middle of the posterior surface of the soft palate (Fig. 26–7*B*).

Facial cleft defects can occur when facial swellings fail to fuse during development

If the two palatine shelves do not fuse along the midline, a condition called **cleft palate** occurs. This can result from a wide range of developmental errors, including inadequate growth of the palatine shelves. Failure of the maxillary swellings to fuse with the intermaxillary process causes **cleft lip,** a condition that can occur on one or both sides. The resulting cleft may range in length from a minor notch just lateral to the philtrum to a cleft that completely separates the lateral lip from the philtrum and nasal cavity. Although cleft lip and cleft palate often occur together, they are not always linked, and the distribution differs with respect to gender, familial association, race, and geographic region of the world. Both defects are multifactorial in etiology, but a number of common drugs, including the anticonvulsant phenytoin and some vitamin A analogs, have been shown to induce cleft lip in experimental animals. Vitamin A, phenytoin, and corticosteroid antiinflammatory drugs may also be a cause of cleft palate in sensitive individuals. Vitamin A and its analogs apparently have particularly deleterious effects on the development of the frontonasal process mesenchyme and, consequently, on the development of the nasal processes. (See Chapter 22 for other facial developmental abnormalities.)

The oral cavity is bounded by the cheeks **(buccae)** and lips **(labia).** Dense fibrous tissue covered with squamous epithelium makes up the gums or **gingivae.** The mucous membrane of the gums is continuous between the inner and outer portions of the teeth and the mucosa of the lips, cheek, floor of the mouth, and hard palate.

A complete set of permanent teeth, the **dentes,** includes a total of 32 teeth, 8 on each side of the upper and lower jaws. Starting at the middle and moving outward, a full set of teeth includes, on each side, two incisors, one canine tooth, two premolars, and three molars. The upper incisor teeth are larger than the lower, or mandibular, incisor teeth. Of these, the upper canine tooth has the longest root of the entire set. The third molar is the last to erupt. In many adults it does not fully erupt or must be removed because it interferes with the development of neighboring molars. In some individuals, roots from the second and third molars can come close to, or even penetrate, the bony floor of the maxillary sinus.

▲ Structure and Function of the Tongue

The highly muscular tongue facilitates mastication, deglutition (swallowing), taste, and speech

The front two thirds of the tongue lies in the oral cavity, while its posterior third forms the anterior wall of the **oropharynx** (the oral part of the pharynx). The oral and pharyngeal parts differ in development and have different types of mucosa and innervation (see below). The dividing line between the two portions is the V-shaped **sulcus terminalis,** which runs diagonally in an anterolateral direction from the central **foramen cecum,** a small blind pit indicating the origin of the thyroglossal duct (see Fig. 26–7 and the discussion of the duct with the thyroid in Chapter 27). The **palatopharyngeal arches** extend from the lateral borders to the sides of the mouth.

The pharyngeal portion of the tongue does not have any papillae. Accumulations of lymphoid tissues called the **lingual tonsil** are found under the surface mucosa of the posterior dorsum of the tongue (see Fig. 26–7). This mucosa also covers the palatine tonsils and extends backward to the epiglottic folds.

Within the oral cavity, the apex of the tongue is at the tip. Its root is attached to the hyoid bone, the mandible, the styloid process, and the palatine aponeurosis of the soft palate. On the underside of the tongue on either side of the frenulum linguae, the deep lingual vein can be seen (Fig. 26–8). The convex **dorsum** (upper surface) of the tongue is covered with numerous projections called **papillae.** In general, papillae are raised epithelial modifications of the mucous membrane that increase the contact area between the tongue and the contents of the mouth. One type, threadlike **filiform papillae,** has keratinized epithelium that helps move particles within the mouth. These are arranged in rows parallel to the sulcus terminalis and are sensitive to touch.

Gustatory Functions of the Tongue

The tongue records sweet, sour, salty, and bitter taste sensations. Receptor cells for taste are located in sensory organs called **taste buds.** Microvilli from 40 to 60 receptor cells extend into a taste pore, sending information through afferent fibers at its base. Taste buds are found not only on the tongue, but also on the palate, pharynx, and larynx. On the tongue, they are associated exclusively with three different types of papillae. Eight to ten large, cone-shaped **vallate papillae** (sometime called **circumvallate,** meaning a circular vallus or wall because they are encircled by a groove) are found at the back of the tongue in front of the sulcus terminalis. **Fungiform** (mushroom shaped) **papillae** are found scattered throughout the dorsal surface. Two **foliate papillae** are leaflike projections at the edge of the tongue with taste buds located within the clefts (see Fig. 26–7).

Sensory Innervation of the Tongue

The mucosal covering of the tongue is derived from several pharyngeal arch precursors and occipital somites and, consequently, is innervated by the sensory branches of four different cranial nerves

The development of the tongue helps explain its complex innervation. The anterior two thirds of the tongue mucosa is derived primarily from first-arch swellings (with some underlying second-arch tissue), whereas the posterior one third is contributed by the third and fourth arches. Sensory fibers from cranial nerves V and VII, therefore, serve the anterior two thirds of the mucosa, and fibers from cranial nerves IX and X innervate the posterior two thirds. The intrinsic muscles of the tongue, on the other hand, arise from occipital somites (served by motor fibers of cranial nerve XII). For this reason, motor and sensory nerve fibers of the tongue are carried by separate sets of cranial nerves.

SVA fibers are carried by two facial nerve branches: the chorda tympani nerve from the anterior two thirds of the tongue and the greater petrosal nerve from the soft palate

The **chorda tympani nerve** (traveling in the sheath of the lingual nerve) carries taste sensation from the tongue's fungiform papillae taste buds, while the greater petrosal nerve (traveling via the trigeminal's palatine nerves) serves taste buds of the soft palate (Fig. 26–9).

Loss of taste perception in the anterior two thirds of the tongue on the ipsilateral side can result from lesions to the seventh cranial nerve or a tumor in the internal auditory meatus (an acoustic neuroma). This impairment would be accompanied by ipsilateral paralysis of facial and stapedius muscles and secretion damage to the nasal and lacrimal glands and the submandibular and sublingual salivary glands.

Sensory innervation from cranial nerve V is nongustatory

General sensation from the mucous membrane of the anterior two thirds of the tongue, as well as the floor of the mouth and the mandibular portion of the gums, is mediated by the afferent fibers of the **lingual nerve,** a sensory branch of the mandibular portion of the trigeminal nerve (cranial nerve V) (Fig. 26–9).

Sensory fibers for both taste and general sensation from the posterior portion of the tongue are supplied by branches of cranial nerves IX (glossopharyngeal nerve) and X (vagus nerve)

The **lingual-tonsillar branch** of the glossopharyngeal nerve (cranial nerve IX) innervates the vallate papillae, the posterior foliate papillae, and the postsulcal mucosa. The **internal laryngeal nerve** from the vagus nerve (cranial nerve X) innervates the taste buds on the epiglottis and esophagus (Fig. 26–9).

Table 26–1 lists structures innervated by cranial nerves IX, X, and XI, that is, structures formed from the third, fourth, and sixth pharyngeal arches. Sensory innervation of the tongue by branches from cranial nerves V and VII (the lingual and chorda tympani nerves, respectively) is included in the discussion of these nerves in Chapter 24.

Both branchial efferent (BE) and GSE nerve fibers carry impulses away from the central nervous system. In clinical practice, it is useful to know that BE fibers in-

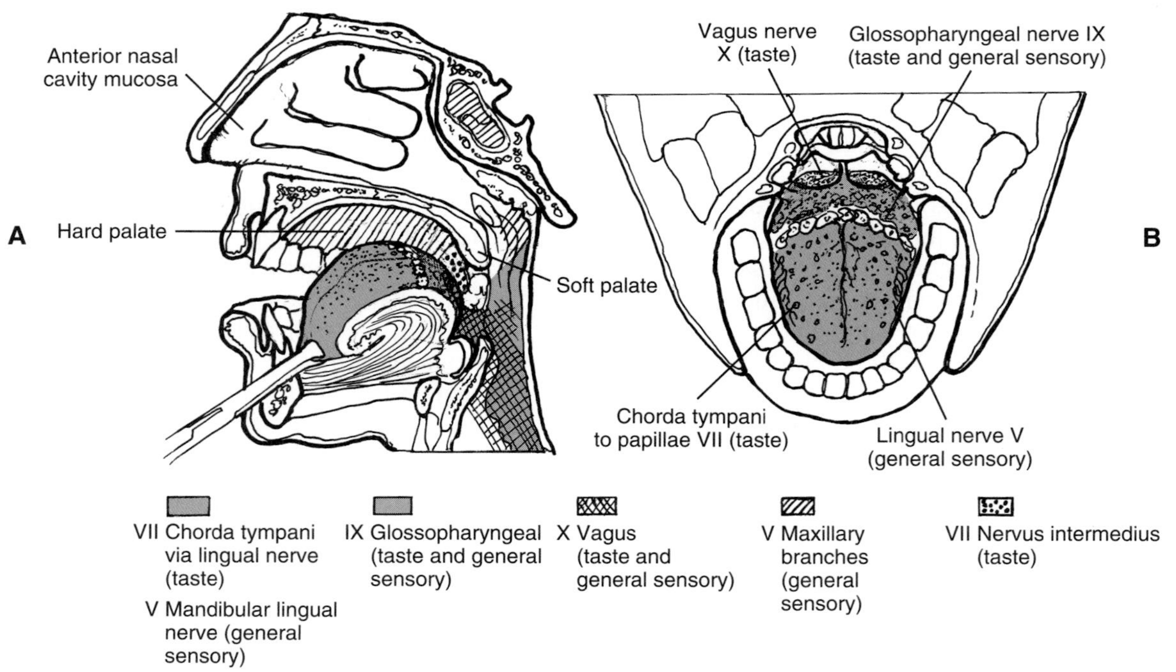

FIGURE 26–9
Sensory innervation of the mouth and pharynx. **A.** Pharynx. Nervous intermedius sensory fibers reach the palate via the greater petrosal nerve, "hitching a ride" on palatine branches of the trigeminal nerve. **B.** Tongue anterior view.

nervate structures derived from the pharyngeal arches and GSE fibers innervate somatic muscles. This knowledge is helpful when one is treating defects associated with abnormal development of the pharyngeal arches.

The principal visceral afferent nucleus of the brain stem is the solitary nucleus

The geniculate ganglion is the location for the cell bodies from the taste fibers in the chorda tympani nerve (cranial nerve VII). The intermediate nerve (part of the facial nerve that travels through the internal auditory meatus) then carries gustatory information to the pons-medulla junction of the brainstem, where the fibers enter the solitary tract and rostral part of the solitary nucleus.

Sensory fibers in the glossopharyngeal nerve (cranial nerve IX) have their cell bodies in the inferior petrosal ganglion, while cell bodies from sensory taste fibers from the vagus nerve (cranial nerve X) are in the nodose ganglion. As with the facial nerve, the central processes of these SVA nerves terminate in the medulla and descend in the solitary tract to the rostral portion of the solitary nucleus. General visceral afferent (GVA) sensation fibers of cranial nerves IX and X terminate in the caudal portion of the solitary nucleus, assisting in the control of certain aspects of swallowing. Table 26–2 provides additional specific targets of fibers from cranial nerves IX and X.

Muscles of the Tongue

A median septum divides muscles of the tongue into two separate groups of intrinsic and extrinsic muscles; intrinsic muscles within the tongue allow it to change shape

Acting singly or in various combinations, the muscles of the tongue orchestrate a great variety of precise movements that facilitate both alimentary functions and speech. The intrinsic muscles are named for their positions: **transverse, vertical, superior longitudinal,** and **inferior longitudinal** (Fig. 26–10). The superior

TABLE 26–1
Innervation of Structures Formed from the Third, Fourth, and Sixth Pharyngeal Arches

Pharyngeal Arch	Cranial Nerve	Nerve Function
THIRD PHARYNGEAL ARCH		
Stylopharyngeus muscle	Glossopharyngeal nerve (IX)	BE
Parotid gland	Glossopharyngeal nerve (IX)	GVE
Mucosa of posterior third of tongue, skin of pinna, and internal surface of tympanic membrane; proprioceptors of stylopharyngeus muscles	Glossopharyngeal nerve (IX)	GSA
Carotid sinus and bodies	Glossopharyngeal nerve (IX)	GVA
Taste receptors of posterior third of tongue	Glossopharyngeal nerve (IX)	SVA
FOURTH PHARYNGEAL ARCH		
Pharyngeal constrictors, cricothyroid and levator veli palatini muscles	Superior laryngeal branch of vagus nerve (X)	BE
Mucosa of pharynx, including epiglottis above vocal folds; proprioceptors of constrictors of pharynx, cricothyroid and levator veli palatini muscles	Superior laryngeal branch of vagus nerve (X)	GSA
Mucous glands of pharynx and larynx above vocal folds	Superior laryngeal branch of vagus nerve (X)	GVE
Taste receptors (epiglottis) of small posterior tongue region	Superior laryngeal branch of vagus nerve (X)	SVA
Interoreceptors (chemoreceptors) of aortic body; stretch receptors in aortic arch; viscera of pharynx	Communicating branch of vagus nerve (X)	GVA
SIXTH PHARYNGEAL ARCH		
Intrinsic muscles of larynx	Recurrent laryngeal branch of vagus nerve (X)	BE (SVE)
Mucosa of larynx below vocal folds	Recurrent laryngeal branch of vagus nerve (X)	GVA
Proprioceptors of intrinsic laryngeal muscles	Recurrent laryngeal branch of vagus nerve (X)	GSA

BE, Branchial efferent (special visceral efferent); *GVE,* general visceral efferent; *GSA,* general somatic afferent; *GVA,* general visceral afferent; *SVA,* special visceral afferent (taste); *SVE,* special visceral efferent.

TABLE 26–2
OVERVIEW OF CRANIAL NERVES IX AND X

Nerve	CNS Nucleus or Nerve Branch	Nerve Function	Branch or Target
Cranial nerve IX (glossopharyngeal nerve)	Ambiguus	BE	Branch to stylopharyngeus muscle (motor)
	Solitarius	SVA	Taste buds (sensory) (taste: posterior third of tongue)
	Spinal nucleus of trigeminal	GSA	External ear—sensory
	Inferior salivatory	GVE	Parasympathetic—lesser petrosal nerve through otic ganglion to parotid gland
	Dorsal nucleus of X	GVA; GVE	General sensation—posterior third of tongue (gag reflex), auditory tube, tonsil, pharynx, carotid sinus
Cranial nerve X vagus	Ambiguus	BE	Levator veli palatini, muscles of larynx and pharynx (from third and fourth pharyngeal arches)
	Solitarius	SVA	Taste fibers from cranial nerves VII, IX and X
	Spinal nucleus of trigeminal	GSA	Location of GSA from many cranial nerves
	Dorsal nucleus	GVE	Preganglionic parasympathetic fibers to thoracic and abdominal viscera
		GVA	Incoming visceral sensory fibers
Branches of the vagus nerve (cranial nerve X)	Meningeal	GSA	Dura mater, posterior cranial fossa
	Auricular	GSA	External acoustic meatus (cough reflex)
	Pharyngeal plexus	GSA	Motor to pharynx (aids swallowing)
	Superior cardiac	GVE	Parasympathetic (slows heart)
	Inferior cardiac	GVA	Regulates reflexes (monitors oxygen and blood pressure)
	Superior laryngeal external	BE	To cricothyroid muscle (produces high pitches)
	Superior laryngeal internal	GVA	Mucosa of upper larynx, above vocal cords (cough reflex)
	Cardiac, thoracic, pulmonary	GVA	Regulate reflexes (respiratory reflexes)
	Recurrent	BE	All laryngeal muscles but laryngeal cricothyroid
	Inferior laryngeal	GVA	Mucous membrane of larynx below vocal cords
	Inferior esophageal	GVE	Smooth muscle parasympathetic fibers (peristalsis, opening of sphincters)
	Anterior and posterior gastric	GVE	Secretion of gastric glands, relaxation of sphincter

BE, Branchial efferent; *SVA*, special visceral afferent; *GSA*, general somatic afferent; *GVE*, general visceral efferent; *GVA*, general visceral afferent.

longitudinal muscle lies beneath the dorsal mucosa and extends from the epiglottis and median lingual septum to the margin of the tongue. The inferior longitudinal muscle is a narrow band of muscle running from root to apex close to the inferior lingual surface. These two muscle groups both function to shorten the tongue. However, the superior longitudinal muscle causes the edges and tip to elevate, creating a concave dorsum of the tongue, while the inferior longitudinal muscle pulls the tip down to create a convex dorsum. The transverse muscles connect the median fibrous septum to the margin of the tongue, acting to narrow and lengthen the tongue. The vertical muscles range from the dorsal to the ventral parts of the anterior section of the tongue and flatten and widen the tongue.

Extrinsic muscles, the four glossal muscles, act on the tongue from the outside

The extrinsic muscles include the genioglossus, the hyoglossus, the styloglossus, and the palatoglossus muscles. The **palatoglossus muscle** (discussed with the definitive anatomy of the oral cavity) acts to elevate the posterior part of the tongue. The **hyoglossus muscle** arises from the whole length of the greater cornu and is attached to the body of the hyoid bone. It extends vertically to enter the side of the tongue (Fig. 26–11). A small

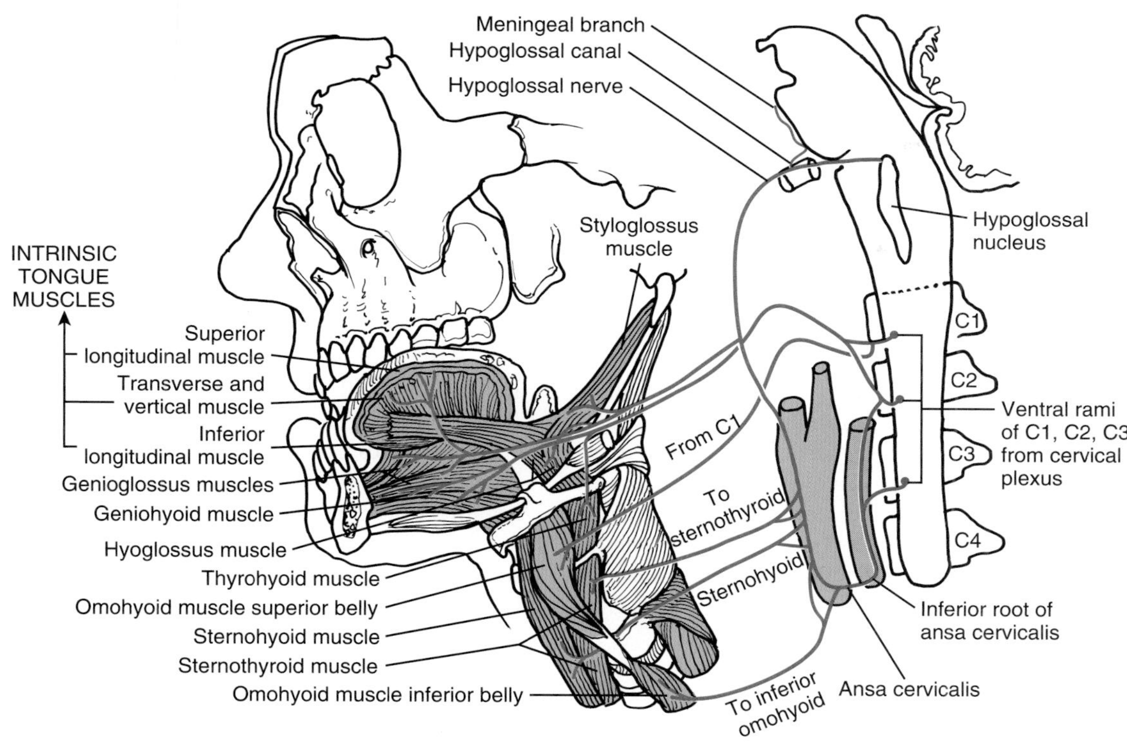

FIGURE 26–10
Intrinsic muscles of the tongue and motor innervation by hypoglossal nerve, cranial nerve XII.

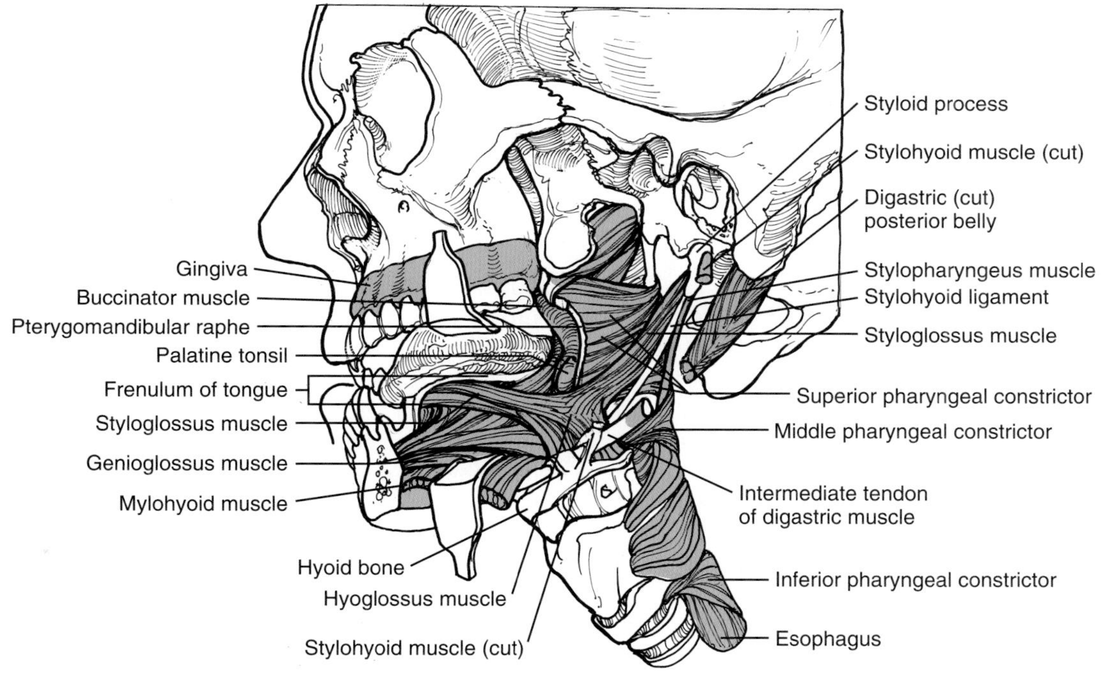

FIGURE 26–11
Extrinsic muscles of the tongue.

muscle arising from the medial side of the lesser cornu, called the **chondroglossus muscle,** is sometimes considered part of the hyoglossus muscle and passes into the tongue with that muscle. The hyoglossus and chondroglossus muscles act to depress and retract the tongue. The **styloglossus muscle** arises from the anterior border of the styloid process near the apex and from the styloid end of the stylomandibular ligament. It runs downward and medially to enter the side of the tongue (Fig. 26–11). It draws the tongue up and backward. The **genioglossus muscle** arises from the superior genial tubercle behind the mandibular synthesis and above the origin of the geniohyoid muscle. It runs backward in a plane parallel to the midline, fanning out to form a triangular shape (Fig. 26–11). The most posteroinferior fibers insert into the body of the hyoid bone. Medial and superior fibers run upward and posteriorly to blend with intrinsic muscles throughout the body of the tongue from root to apex. It moves the tongue forward, allowing the apex to protrude. Acting unilaterally, these muscles cause the tongue to diverge to the opposite side.

Accessory muscles of the floor of the mouth, the suprahyoid muscles, elevate the floor during swallowing

The suprahyoid muscles are the stylohyoid, mylohyoid, geniohyoid, and digastric muscles. These muscles connect the hyoid to the mandible, pharynx, and larynx (Figs. 26–10 and 26–11). Their structure and innervation will be discussed in more detail with musculature of the neck in Chapter 27.

Motor Innervation of the Muscles of the Tongue

All the intrinsic and extrinsic muscles of the tongue, except the palatoglossus muscle, arise from mesoderm of the occipital somites and are innervated by the hypoglossal nerve (cranial nerve XII), which is associated with those somites (Fig. 26–10 and Box 26-2)

Clinical Conditions Affecting the Tongue. Since muscles of the tongue are divided into two functional units at the midline, both sides must cooperate to allow the tongue to protrude. A unilateral paralysis affecting one branch of the **hypoglossal nerve,** therefore, is easily perceived. If a patient is asked to "stick out" his or her tongue, the nerve acts on only one side and the tongue moves toward the side served by the injured nerve. Injuries to the hypoglossal nerve resulting in paralysis can occur through trauma such as fracture of the mandible.

Paralysis of the **genioglossus muscle** allows the tongue to fall backward, obstructing the airway. Because general anesthesia procedures totally relax this muscle, an airway must be inserted during such procedures to prevent the tongue from relapsing.

Afferent branches of the glossopharyngeal nerve in the posterior part of the tongue trigger the gag reflex. When the back of the tongue is touched, branches from cranial nerves IX and X cause the muscles of both sides of the pharynx to contract.

A condition in which the lingual frenulum is either unusually large or short can interfere with tongue movements and speech. Rarely, a short frenulum must be cut (frenectomy) in infants to free the tongue for speech.

Because the deep lingual veins are near the surface under the tongue, drugs can be absorbed quickly in this region. A pill placed under the tongue can be absorbed in less than a minute (see Fig. 26–8).

Salivary Glands in Relation to the Oral Cavity. By definition, any cell or organ that secretes a substance into the oral cavity is a salivary gland. Collectively these secretory bodies or salivary glands assist in providing lubrication for processing and swallowing food, moistening the buccal mucosa, and aiding speech. They also provide an aqueous medium necessary for the functioning of the taste buds and secrete digestive enzymes, hormones, and, possibly, antimicrobial agents. Accessory salivary glands found in the submucosa and mucosa of the palate, tongue, lips, and teeth open directly into the oral cavity. The major salivary glands in humans lie outside the oral mucosa and connect to the oral cavity by ducts. They are the paired **parotid, sublingual,** and **submandibular glands.**

The **parotid glands** are the largest pair of glands, covering the area between the ramus of the mandible and the styloid process of the temporal bone. The duct begins at the anterior border of the gland, crosses the masseter muscle, and turns medially to pass between the oral mucosa and the buccinator muscle (Fig. 26–14). It opens in a small papilla opposite the second molar. The duct can be felt by pressing back on the front edge of the masseter in the vestibule when the teeth are clenched.

There are a number of nerves intimately related to, but not necessarily innervating, the parotid gland. The most important of these is the facial nerve, which branches within the substance of the gland (see Figs. 24–24 and 24–27). Parasympathetic secretomotor innervation of the parotid gland comes from the glossopharyngeal nerve (cranial nerve IX). Preganglionic fibers synapse in the otic ganglion and reach the gland via the auriculotemporal nerve. Postganglionic sympathetic fibers from the superior cervical ganglion reach the parotid gland via the external carotid plexus. Sensory fibers from the gland travel with the great auricular and auriculotemporal nerves.

The parotid gland and its duct are supplied by branches of the external carotid and superficial temporal arteries.

The **submandibular glands** are comprised of superficial and deep sections wrapped around the posterior border of the mylohyoid muscle. The irregularly shaped gland is about the size of a walnut. The superfi-

BOX 26–2
CRANIAL NERVES IX, X, AND XII

Of cranial nerves IX, X, and XII, only cranial nerve XII (the hypoglossal nerve) is exclusively motor (GSE) in function

The **hypoglossal nerve** innervates all of the intrinsic and extrinsic muscles of the tongue except the palatoglossus muscle (see Fig. 26–10). From the hypoglossal nucleus in the floor of the fourth ventricle, the nerve extends caudally, emerging as a series of rootlets between the fourth ventricle and the medulla oblongata and exiting the dura mater at the hypoglossal canal. The hypoglossal nerve descends to the level of the mandibular angle, emerging between the internal jugular vein and internal carotid artery. It runs forward lateral to the external and internal carotid arteries and the hyoglossus muscle and runs inferior to the submandibular gland, duct, and lingual nerve. Moving to the genioglossus muscle, it continues forward to the tip of the tongue. Branches include the **meningeal, descending,** and **thyrohyoid-geniohyoid branches.** The meningeal branch supplies the spongy portion of the occipital bone, the floor and anterior wall of the posterior cranial fossa, and the inferior petrosal sinuses. The descending branch is joined by fibers from the first (and often the second) cervical spinal nerve and supplies the superior belly of the omohyoid muscle. This descending branch is then joined by lower roots of the second and third cervical nerves from the ansa cervicalis to supply the sternothyroid and sternohyoid muscles and the inferior belly of the omohyoid muscle (see Fig. 26–10). Originating near the posterior border of the hyoglossus muscle, the thyrohyoid and geniohyoid branches supply the thyrohyoid and geniohyoid muscles, respectively (see Fig. 26–10). **Muscular branches** reach the styloglossus, hyoglossus, and genioglossus muscles (see Fig. 26–10). The hypoglossal branch supplies structures that develop from occipital somitomeres and somites.

Cranial nerves IX (glossopharyngeal nerve) and X (vagus nerve) include sensory, motor, and parasympathetic fibers

As its name implies, the **glossopharyngeal nerve** serves mainly the tongue and pharynx (Fig. 26–12). *Sensory fibers* (GSA) of the glossopharyngeal nerve innervate the posterior third of the tongue and fibers for taste (SVA) from the vallate papillae. Sensory fibers (GSA) from the vagus nerve also serve this area. As the glossopharyngeal nerve runs downward between the internal and external carotid arteries, it gives off a carotid branch that serves the carotid sinus and carotid body and pharyngeal branches that supply the pharyngeal plexus (GVA) (Fig. 26–12). Both branches, again, are joined by communicating branches from the vagus nerve. Tonsillar branches supply the walls of the pharynx lateral to the tonsils. Finally, the nerve turns upward to supply GSA and SVA fibers to the posterior part of the tongue. A single muscular *motor* branch (BE) supplies the stylopharyngeal muscle (Fig. 26–12). Preganglionic *parasympathetic* fibers from the glossopharyngeal nerve (GVE) travel via the tympanic nerve to the tympanic plexus and then via the lesser petrosal nerve to synapse in the otic ganglion. From there, postganglionic fibers serve the parotid gland (Fig. 26–12). Structures from the third pharyngeal arch innervated by the glossopharyngeal nerve are summarized in Table 26–1.

The **vagus nerve** gets its name from the Latin word for "wandering," since it covers a large area within the body. Its multiple roots leave the medulla and combine to pass through the jugular foramen with the glossopharyngeal nerve (IX) and accessory nerve (XI) (Fig. 26–13). Targets in the head include the dura of the posterior cranial fossa, the tympanic membrane, and the skin behind the ear. A small auricular branch supplies the external auditory meatus. Within the external auditory meatus the nerve functions to provide a cough reflex if a foreign substance enters the outer ear canal (Fig. 26–13). *Sensory* branches reach the larynx and posterior third of the mouth, recording both taste (SVA) and general sensation (GVA). *Motor* branches in the neck and pharynx innervate muscles of the pharynx and soft palate. In the head and neck region, the vagus nerve travels between the common carotid artery and internal jugular vein. Its first major branch is the **superior laryngeal nerve** (Fig. 26–13). An **internal branch** of this nerve supplies all of the laryngeal mucosa superior to the vocal cords. An **external branch** serves the cricothyroid muscle. A major branch is the **recurrent laryngeal nerve,** which serves all the intrinsic muscles of the larynx except the cricothyroid muscle. **Superior** and **inferior cardiac branches** are given off in the neck. These run downward and eventually join the cardiac plexus. After entering the thorax, the vagus nerve is comprised of only *parasympathetic* (pGVE) and general visceral afferent (GVA) fibers, which serve smooth muscles and glands. Other branches of the vagus nerve target the heart, lungs, esophagus, stomach, and liver and approximately two-thirds of the transverse colon (Fig. 26–13). Table 26–1 provides a summary of structures that arise from the fourth pharyngeal arch and that are served by the vagus nerve.

There is a close association between cranial nerves IX and X in the head and neck

The glossopharyngeal and vagus nerves both exit through the jugular foramen. Communicating branches of the glossopharyngeal and vagus nerves together serve the external ear (auricular branches) and the carotid sinus (carotid sinus branches). Both send pharyngeal branches to the pharyngeal plexus. Cranial nerve XI (accessory nerve) also exits through the jugular foramen and is functionally tied to the vagus nerve. A discussion of this nerve will occur with descriptions of the anatomy of the neck in Chapter 27.

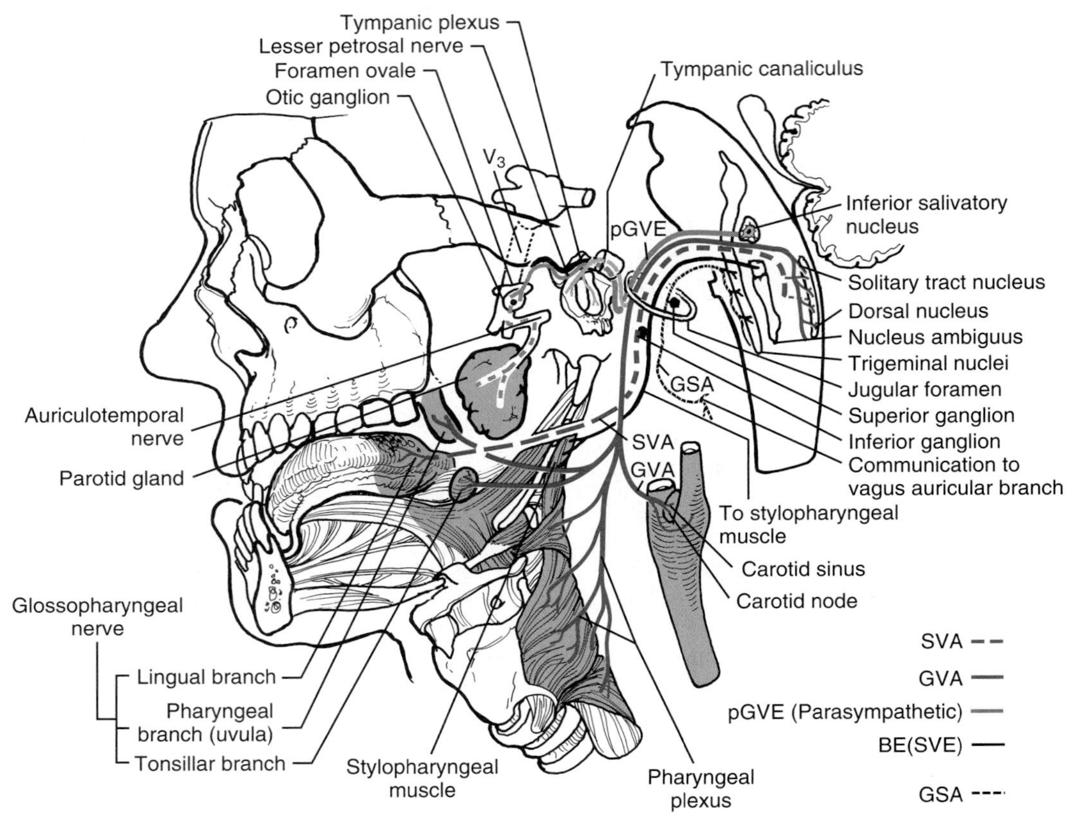

FIGURE 26–12
Glossopharyngeal nerve, cranial nerve IX.

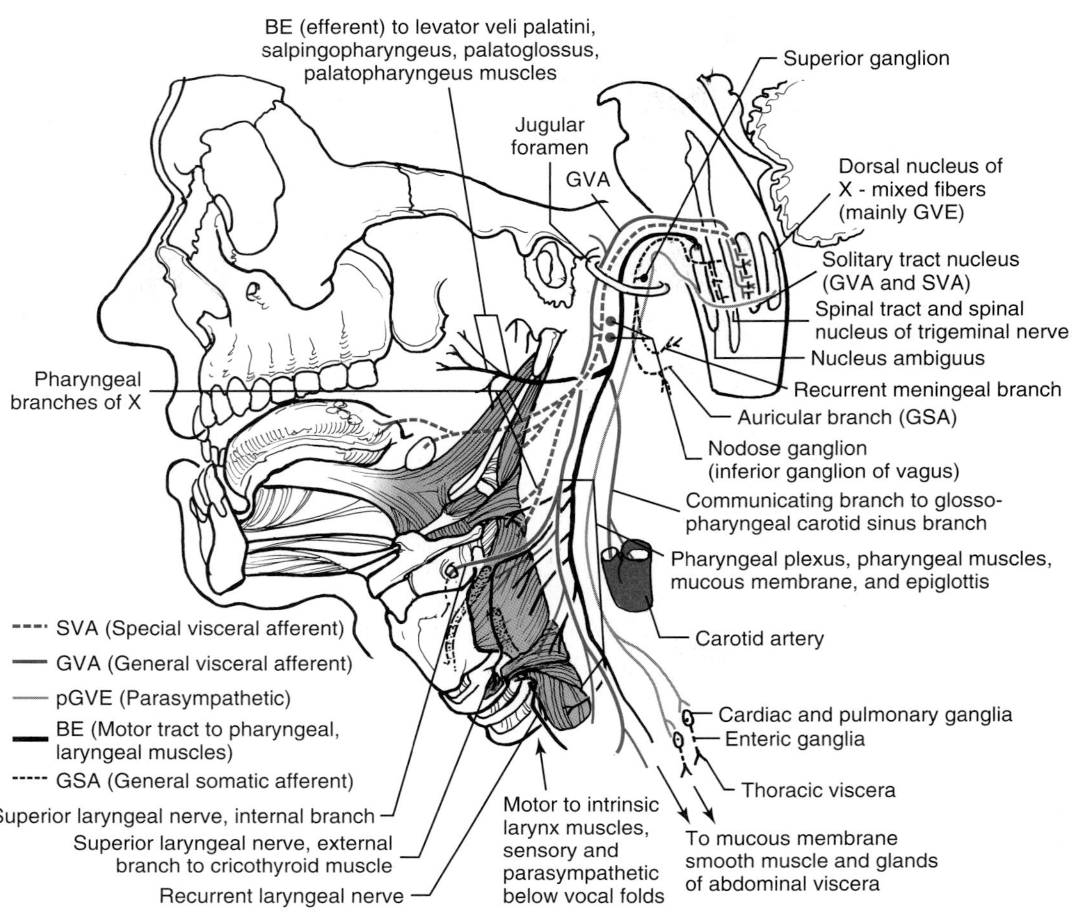

FIGURE 26–13
Summary of vagus nerve innervation, cranial nerve X.

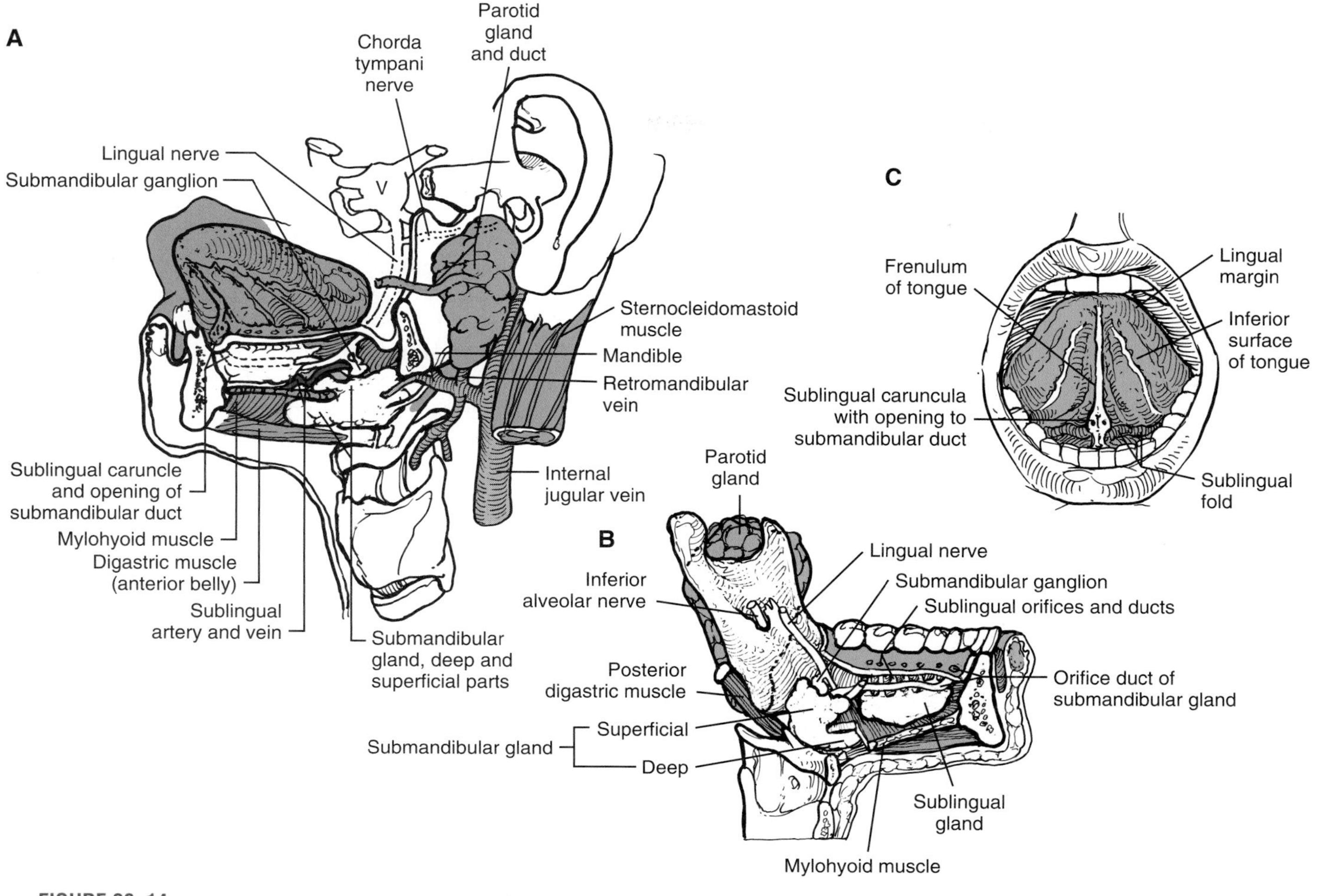

FIGURE 26–14
Salivary glands and submandibular ganglion. **A.** Lateral view of the parotid, submandibular, and sublingual glands (mandible removed). **B.** Medial view of submandibular and sublingual glands showing ducts. **C.** Under surface of the tongue showing sublingual folds and opening for submandibular duct.

cial part extends anteriorly to the anterior belly of the digastric muscle (Fig. 26–14). The submandibular duct is 15.5 cm long. It opens via one to three orifices on the sublingual papilla found on either side of the frenulum under the tongue (Fig. 26–14C).

The smallest of the major salivary glands are the **sublingual glands,** which are found in the floor of the mouth lying beneath the sublingual folds of oral mucosa and above the mylohyoid muscle. These two glands are about the size of almonds (Fig. 26–14). Instead of a single duct, there are generally more than 10 small ducts that empty on the upper surface of the gland through the mucous membrane above the gland. Occasionally, an anterior duct may open into the submandibular duct.

Innervation of both the submandibular and sublingual glands is autonomic. Presynaptic secretomotor parasympathetic fibers are carried by the facial nerve to the lingual nerve via the chorda tympani nerve and synapse with postsynaptic neurons in the submandibular ganglion, which then innervate the glands. The postsynaptic parasympathetic fibers accompany arteries to reach these glands, along with vasoconstrictive postsynaptic sympathetic fibers from the superior cervical ganglion.

The arterial supply of the submandibular and sublingual glands is the submental branch of the facial artery. The sublingual branch of the lingual artery also supplies the sublingual gland.

Clinical Conditions Related to the Salivary Glands. Enlargement of the salivary glands from an acute viral infection is called **mumps.** The increase in size of the parotid gland in particular is quite painful because the gland is tightly encased in a fibrous capsule. Inflammation of the parotid gland alone is called **parotiditis.**

A swollen cheek may also indicate the presence of an **abscess** in the parotid gland. This can be caused by a local infection or a dental bacterial infection carried to the gland by the parotid ducts. For a more in-depth discussion, see the section on clinical disorders of the salivary glands in Chapter 24.

INTRODUCTION TO THE PHARYNX

Organization and Skeletal Framework of the Three Divisions of the Pharynx: Nasopharynx, Oropharynx, and Laryngopharynx

The interconnected nasopharynx, oropharynx, and laryngopharynx are differentiated by their relative locations within the head and neck

The **pharynx** is a membranous tube that extends from the cranial base of the skull to the inferior border of the cricoid cartilage at the level of the sixth cervical vertebra. It is an important structure linking sensory, respiratory, and digestive areas within the head. Anteriorly it opens into the posterior portion of the nasal cavity, or the choanae, and the oral cavity, and anteroinferiorly, it opens into the larynx (Fig. 26–15). Laterally it communicates with the tympanic cavity of the ear through the auditory tube. Inferiorly it is continuous with the esophagus (Fig. 26–15). The internal layer of mucous membrane lining the pharynx is, in fact, continuous with that in the auditory tubes, the nasal and oral cavities, and the larynx.

▲ Anatomical Structure of the Nasopharynx

The nasopharynx lies posterior to the nasal cavity and above the soft palate. It is roofed by the occipital bone posteriorly and by the posterior part of the sphenoid bone anteriorly (Fig. 26–15). It is in direct communication with the nasal cavities by their posterior openings, or choanae. Between the nasal and oral parts there is a connecting passage called the **pharyngeal isthmus.** During swallowing, this is closed by elevation of the palate and contraction of the palatopharyngeal wall. Closure of the isthmus also facilitates the pronunciation of consonants for speech. The entrances of the auditory tubes are found in the lateral wall of the nasopharynx (Fig. 26–15).

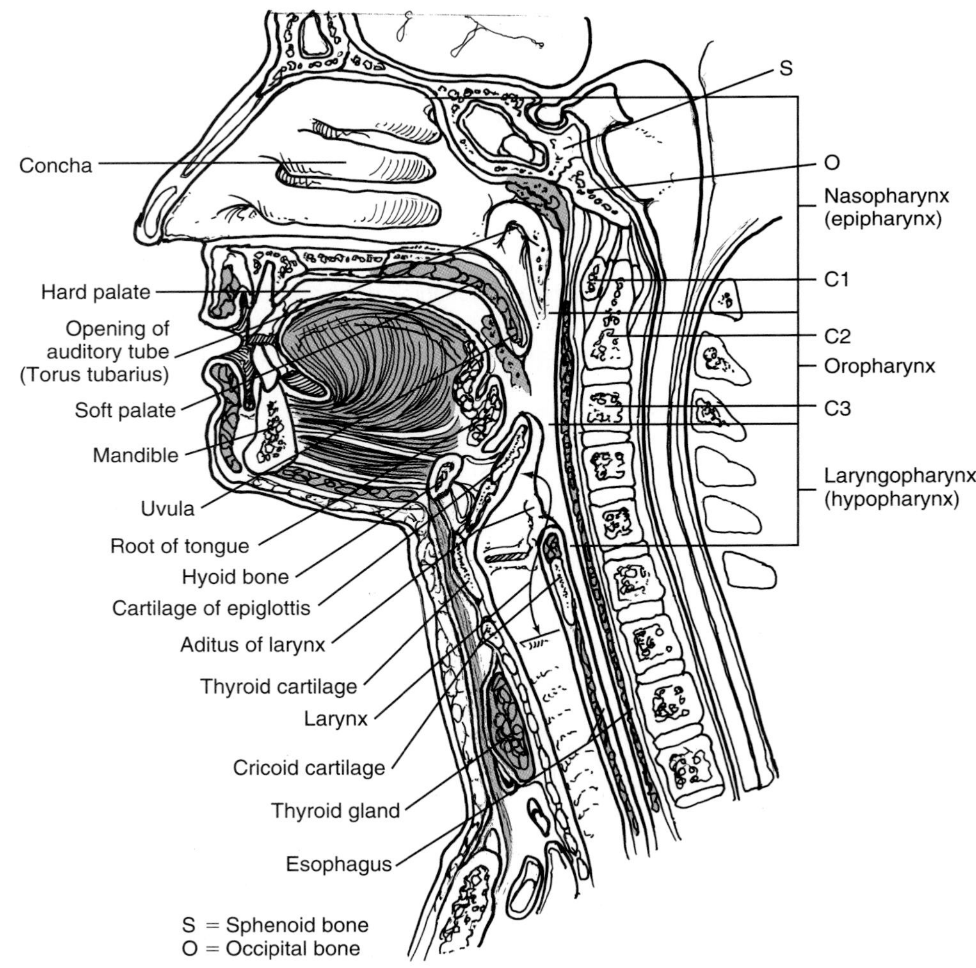

FIGURE 26–15
Regions of the nasopharynx, oropharynx, and laryngopharynx.

Oral Part of the Pharynx

The **oropharynx** is defined as the area from the soft palate to the upper border of the epiglottis at the level of the second cervical vertebra (Fig. 26–15). The lateral borders of the opening from the mouth to the pharynx are made up of two folds, which, together, form the anterior **palatoglossal arch** from the soft palate to the tongue and the posterior **palatopharyngeal arch** along the wall of the pharynx (see Fig. 26–7).

The **epiglottis** is a heart-shaped cartilage covered by mucous membrane that is located posterior to the root of the tongue and hyoid bone and anterior to the laryngeal inlet (Fig. 26–15). The epiglottis is connected to the body of the tongue by two folds, the **median** and **lateral glossoepiglottic folds.** Paired depressions between these folds are called the **epiglottic valleculae.**

Tonsillar Ring

A **pharyngeal tonsil** composed of lymphoid tissue is found near the apex of the nasal septum in children. Although pharyngeal tonsils are prominent in children, they disappear by the time adulthood is reached. Tubal tonsils of similar tissue are found in the ostium of the auditory tube in children.

> If enlarged, tubal and pharyngeal tonsils are referred to as adenoids. Enlargement can cause difficulty in nasal breathing or in hearing if the auditory tube is obstructed.

Between the palatoglossal and palatopharyngeal arches are found the palatine tonsils (see Fig. 26–7), which are supplied by a branch of the facial artery and innervated by the glossopharyngeal nerve. Completing the tonsillar ring is the lingual tonsillar tissue of the tongue. This ring of tonsillar tissue, thus, provides a barrier to infection, particularly in children. If the tonsils become enlarged, however, their function as a defensive barrier is impaired.

Laryngopharynx

The laryngopharynx is located between the epiglottis and the level of the **cricoid cartilage** of the larynx. At that point, the pharynx becomes continuous with the esophagus. The larynx forms the anterior wall of the laryngopharynx.

The posterior and lateral walls of the laryngopharynx are formed by the middle and inferior constrictor muscles. The pharynx also extends lateral to the larynx in extensions called the **piriform recesses,** which are bounded superiorly by the aryepiglottic folds. As the larynx narrows inferiorly, these recesses disappear.

Hyoid Bone and Larynx

The **hyoid bone** is a U-shaped bone consisting of a **body,** two **greater horns (cornua),** and two **lesser horns (cornua).** The upper half of the body and lesser horns are derived from the cartilage of the second pharyngeal arch, and the lower part of the body and greater horns are derived from the cartilage of the third pharyngeal arch. The hyoid bone is suspended and stabilized just under the jaw by stylohyoid ligaments (from the bilateral styloid processes) and by several muscles that connect the hyoid to the mandible, tongue, pharynx, and larynx (Fig. 26–16 and see Fig. 24–22). Hyoid bone function in swallowing and vocalization is discussed in Chapter 27.

The **larynx,** which forms the anterior surface of the pharynx, is part of the respiratory system, continuing on as the trachea. It opens both posteriorly and superiorly into the pharynx. It is supported by four major cartilages: the thyroid, cricoid, arytenoid, and epiglottic cartilages. Structures of the larynx will be discussed more fully in Chapter 27, along with the anatomy of the neck.

Musculature of the Pharynx

Because openings from the nose, mouth, and larynx are on the anterior side of the pharynx, pharyngeal muscles are primarily found on its posterior and lateral sides. Three pairs of constrictor muscles (inferior, middle, and superior constrictors) overlap one another on the posterior side (see Fig. 26–16). A fourth pair of long, thin muscles, the stylopharyngeus muscles, arises from the medial side of the styloid process. They extend downward, entering the gap between the superior and middle constrictors. Each stylopharyngeus muscle continues on, following the inner surface of the constrictor and finally attaching to the upper thyroid cartilage.

Muscles of the Tongue and Pharynx Work Together in Swallowing

Food is chewed with the aid of muscles of mastication, tongue muscles, suprahyoid muscles, and the buccinator muscle. During this phase of eating, salivary glands moisten the food and begin the digestion process. Muscles of the tongue initiate the **voluntary** stage of swallowing by pushing a bolus of food back against the soft palate and closing off the passage to the nasal pharynx. Swallowing movements involving the tongue are primarily controlled by its intrinsic muscles. Following this initiation of the swallowing act, the hyoid bone is moved up and forward. Then the internal muscles of the pharynx (the palatopharyngeus, salpingopharyngeus, and stylopharyngeus muscles) move up the larynx, widening the pharynx. These actions initiate an **involuntary** chain of actions in the oropharynx beginning with contraction of the constrictor muscles of the pharynx. The muscles constrict, in order, from the superior constrictor downward to move the bolus in a posterior direction. When the food reaches the border of the esophagus, it is pushed along by the peristalsis of the esophagus. The pharyngeal plexus nerves from the vagus, glossopharyngeal, and accessory nerves and sympathetic branches from the superior cervical ganglion innervate the constrictor muscles.

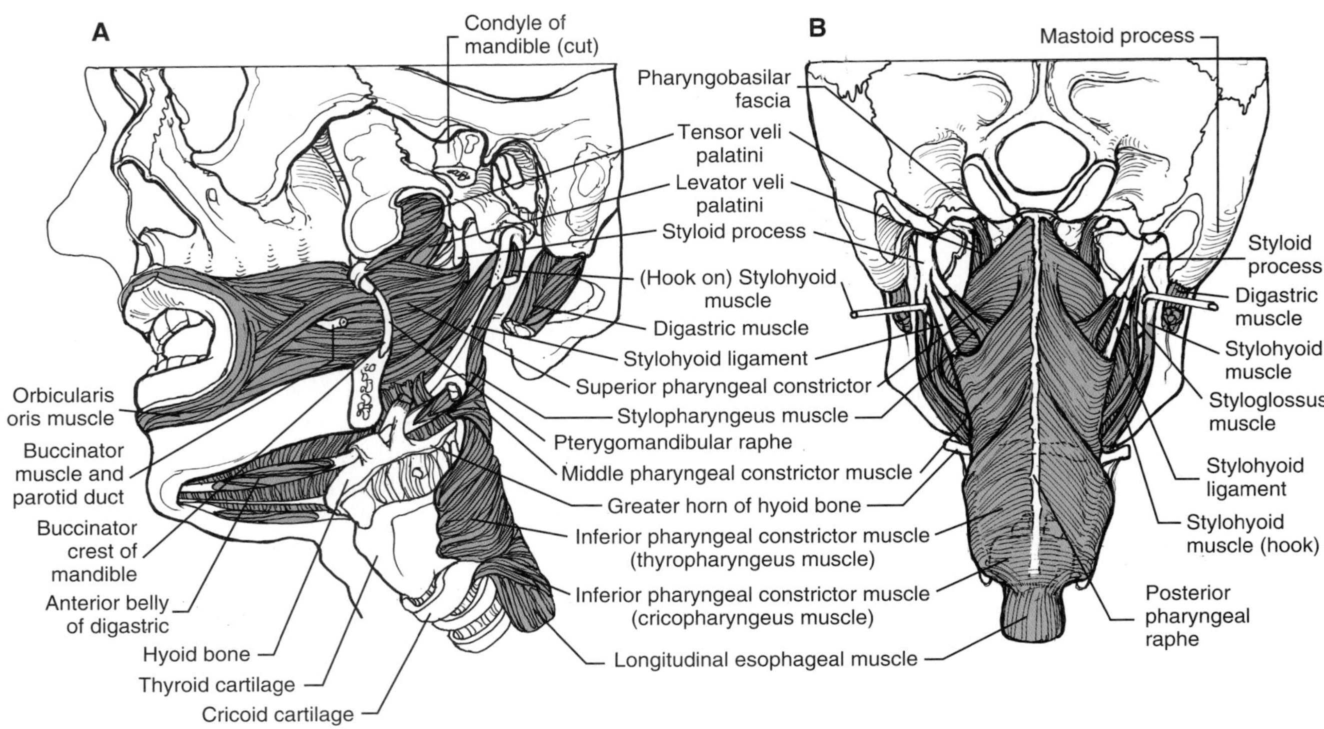

FIGURE 26–16
Musculature of the pharynx. **A.** Lateral view. **B.** Posterior view.

INTRODUCTION TO THE STRUCTURE AND FUNCTION OF THE BRAIN

Development of the Brain

Development of the spinal cord and the brain from surface ectoderm begins very early in embryonic life

By the third week of embryonic life, surface ectoderm cells have already differentiated into the **neuroepithelium** of the **neural plate.** Within the next week, the lateral edges of this plate begin to fold dorsally in a process known as **neurulation.** The two edges meet to form a hollow neural tube, closing first in the midregion; next, superiorly (at the **cranial neuropore**) on day 24; and finally, inferiorly (at the **caudal neuropore**) by day 26. This cavity within the neural tube is called the **neural canal.** The neural canal becomes the central canal of the spinal cord and lumen of the ventricles of the brain. Neuroepithelial cells in the innermost layer of the neural canal produce:

- future neurons of the central nervous system (whose cell bodies form the **gray matter** and cell fibers form the **white matter**),
- future **glial** cells that provide metabolic and structural support to neurons of the central nervous system, and
- specialized **ependymal cells** lining the cerebral ventricles, which, together with blood vessels from the vascularized pia mater, form the **choroid plexuses** that produce cerebrospinal fluid.

By day 26, it is possible to see new structures at the cranial end of the neural tube, including the primary vesicles of the brain and two flexures that divide the brain into the **prosencephalon** (or forebrain), **mesencephalon** (or midbrain), and **rhombencephalon** (or hindbrain). The anterior flexure is called the **mesencephalic** (or **cranial) flexure,** and the more caudal bend is termed the **cervical flexure** (Fig. 26–17*A*). Slight constrictions of the hindbrain (**rhombomeres**), present for just a few weeks at this stage in development, are the only suggestions of segmentation in the brain. Recent discoveries, however, have suggested new ways to consider **metamerism** in the head and neck (i.e., development from a fundamental pattern of repeating units). Interrelationships are being studied between

- homeotic genes that regulate segmentation in the hindbrain rhombomeres of mammals,
- pharyngeal arch formation, and
- cranial somitomeres (mesenchymal structures, which, in more caudal areas, differentiate into somites) (see Fig. 23–3).

By the fifth week, further subdivision of the brain vesicles creates five secondary vesicles:

- the cranial **telencephalon** and caudal **diencephalon,** which are formed by division of the prosencephalon;
- the cranial **metencephalon** and caudal **myelencephalon** (with the dorsal folding of the **pontine**

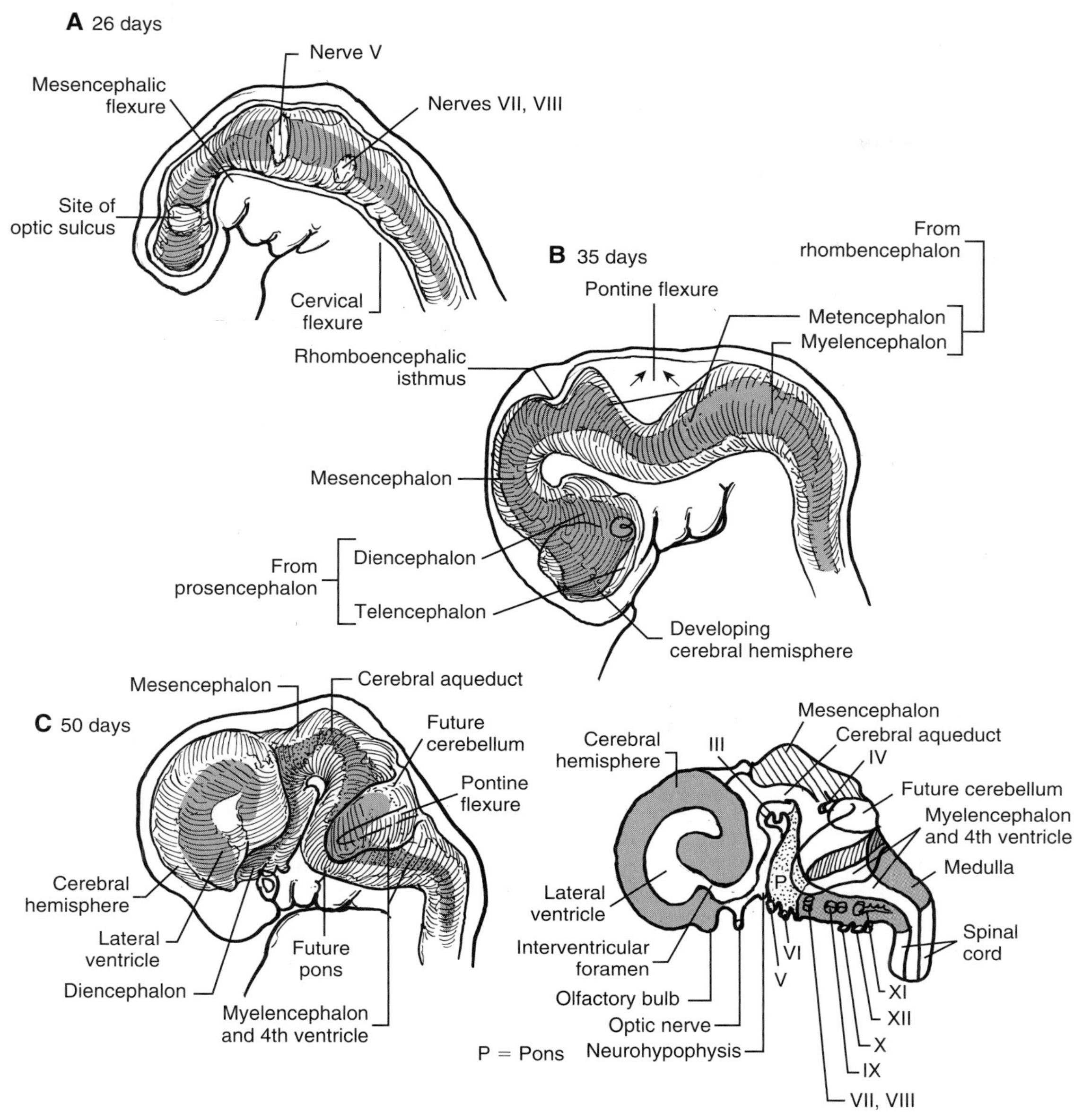

FIGURE 26–17
Early development of the brain. **A.** Position of mesencephalic and cervical flexures. **B.** Three brain vesicles divide into five secondary vesicles. **C.** Structures of the definitive brain and ventricles as they are formed. The cerebral hemispheres and cerebellum expand.

flexure), which are formed by division of the rhombencephalon; and

- the **mesencephalon** (or midbrain), which remains undivided.

Each of these five secondary vesicles gives rise to the definitive structures and ventricles of the brain. From the spinal cord upward, the following structures form:

- The myelencephalon becomes the **medulla oblongata** and its cavity, the **fourth ventricle.**
- The metencephalon gives rise to the **pons** and **cerebellum.**
- The midbrain roof plate gives rise to the **superior** and **inferior colliculi,** and its neural canal forms the narrow **cerebral aqueduct (of Sylvius),** which connects the third and fourth ventricles.
- The walls of the diencephalon form the **thalamus, hypothalamus, epithalamus, pineal gland,** and **pituitary gland.** Its cavity becomes the **third ventricle.**
- The telencephalon forms the **cerebral hemispheres,** their **connecting commissures,** and the **olfactory bulbs** and tracts. Its cavity becomes the paired lateral ventricles of the cerebral hemispheres.

After the closure of the caudal neuropore, the developing brain ventricles and the central canal of the spinal cord are filled with cerebrospinal fluid, a specialized dialysate of blood plasma produced by choroid plexuses in the ventricles. The early development of the brain is summarized in Fig. 26–17, which shows the flexures, formation of the ventricles from the original neural canal, and expanded growth of the cerebral hemispheres and cerebellum.

At birth, the brain is about 25% of its adult volume. Some of the postnatal growth is due to increase in the size of neuronal cell bodies. Most of the growth, however, results from the myelination of nerve fibers, which form the substance of the white matter of the brain. Synaptic connections between neurons continue to form throughout life.

Developmental Abnormalities of the Central Nervous System. Abnormalities of cranial neuropore closure can produce a brain that is an exposed dorsal mass of undifferentiated neural tissue. This defect is known as **anencephaly, exencephaly,** or **craniorachischisis.** The surrounding meninges and skull are absent. Facial abnormalities are usually present. Anencephalic embryos often survive late or full-term fetal life but invariably die within a few hours or days of birth. Since the organs of anencephalic infants are often normal and healthy, the option of using these organs in organ transplants has frequently been considered, particularly since infant or child organ donors are always in short supply. Many arguments pro and con have been expressed, and there is reluctance to initiate such programs on a wide scale.

Obstruction of the flow of cerebrospinal fluid from the forebrain through the cerebral aqueduct in the midbrain to the fourth ventricle during fetal development can cause a condition called **hydrocephalus** in which the third and lateral ventricles are swollen with fluid. The cerebral cortex is abnormally thin, and sutures of the skull are forced apart. Infants born with this condition may also be retarded. Fortunately, ultrasound usually detects hydrocephaly during pregnancy. The disorder can be corrected by inserting a pressure valve to drain the excess cerebrospinal fluid into the amniotic cavity.

Fetal Alcohol Syndrome. Consumption of alcohol during the third week of pregnancy—the sensitive time that the forebrain induction is taking place—is the most common cause of holoprosencephaly (deformities of the forebrain, frontonasal process, calvaria, and midfacial structures).

Although chronic consumption of alcohol later in pregnancy can result in additional, less destructive effects and should be avoided, it is important to counsel prospective parents about this crucial early period, since it occurs during a time when a woman may not yet realize that she is pregnant.

▲ Structures Protecting the Brain

The brain is a highly protected structure enveloped by a bony case, meninges, and cerebrospinal fluid

The Skull

The brain (cerebrum, cerebellum, and hindbrain) is entirely encased within the **cranium** of the skull. The dorsal bones of the skull (the frontal, parietal, and occipital bones and the dorsal portion of the temporal bones) form the roof, whereas the ventral bones of the chondrocranium (ventrolateral portions of the frontal, parietal and occipital bones and the ethmoid, sphenoid, and temporal bones) provide the supporting floor. Fig. 22–4 in the introductory chapter on the skull provides a superior view of the bones of both the calvaria and the brain case floor. The structure and interrelationships of the bones of the skull that protect the brain are described in detail within that chapter.

Cranial Meninges

Inside the skull, three layers of cranial meninges (membranes) cover the brain

The three meningeal layers include the dura mater, the arachnoid mater, and the pia mater.

The Dura Mater. *The dura mater covers the surface of the brain, folds inward to divide regions of the brain, and houses the venous sinuses.* The **dura mater** ("tough mother") is the outermost layer of the meninges that adhere to the inside surface of the skull. It is composed primarily of fibrous collagen fibers, but also has some elastic fibers. Since the dura separates into two layers in areas where it encloses large venous ducts or sinuses, it is often described as having two sublayers (Fig. 26–18). The external portion of the dura mater, next to the inner surface of the skull, is called the **endosteal** (or **periosteal**) **layer,** whereas the inner portion is called the **meningeal layer.** The fibrous inner meningeal layer is continuous with the dura mater that covers the spinal cord. In the calvaria, the dura mater can be separated from the overlying bones; however, in the cranial base, the dura mater tightly adheres to the bones. Consequently, cranial base fractures can tear the dura mater and result in leakage of cerebrospinal fluid.

The inner meningeal layer of the dura mater folds inward to divide the regions of the brain and to provide some support to the different sections of the brain. These meningeal folds are called the **falx cerebri,** the **tentorium cerebelli,** and the **diaphragm sellae.**

The crescent-shaped, middorsal infolding is called the **falx** (sickle-shaped) **cerebri** (Fig. 26–19). Attaching anteriorly to the front crest of the frontal bone and posteriorly to the internal occipital protuberance, the falx cerebri separates the right and left cerebral hemispheres. The **superior sagittal sinus,** which collects blood from veins on the surface of the brain, follows along the dorsal groove formed by the infolding of the cerebral falx (Fig. 26–19). The relationship of the dura mater to the venous drainage of the brain will be dis-

Coronal section through center of skull (superior sagittal sinus)
Arachnoid granulation
Granular foveola
Calvaria
Superior sagittal sinus
Dura mater (two layers)
Pericranium
Fat
Emissary vein
Diploic vein
Skin
Tributary of superficial temporal vein
Galea aponeurotica
Emissary vein
Epidural and subdural "spaces"
Cerebral sulcus
Cerebral gyrus
Gray matter or cerebral cortex
White matter
Subarachnoid space
Vacuos lacunae
Cerebral artery
Arachnoid layer
Pia mater
Falx cerebri
Cerebral hemisphere
Superior cerebral vein

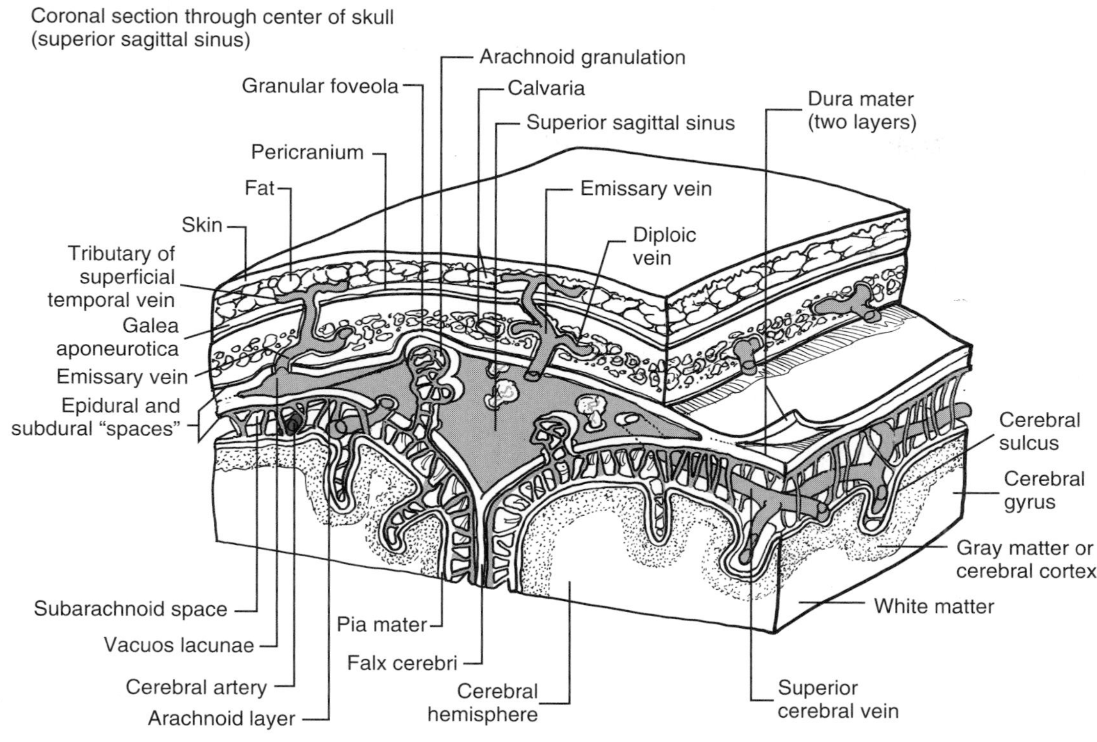

FIGURE 26–18
Meningeal layers and superficial cerebral veins.

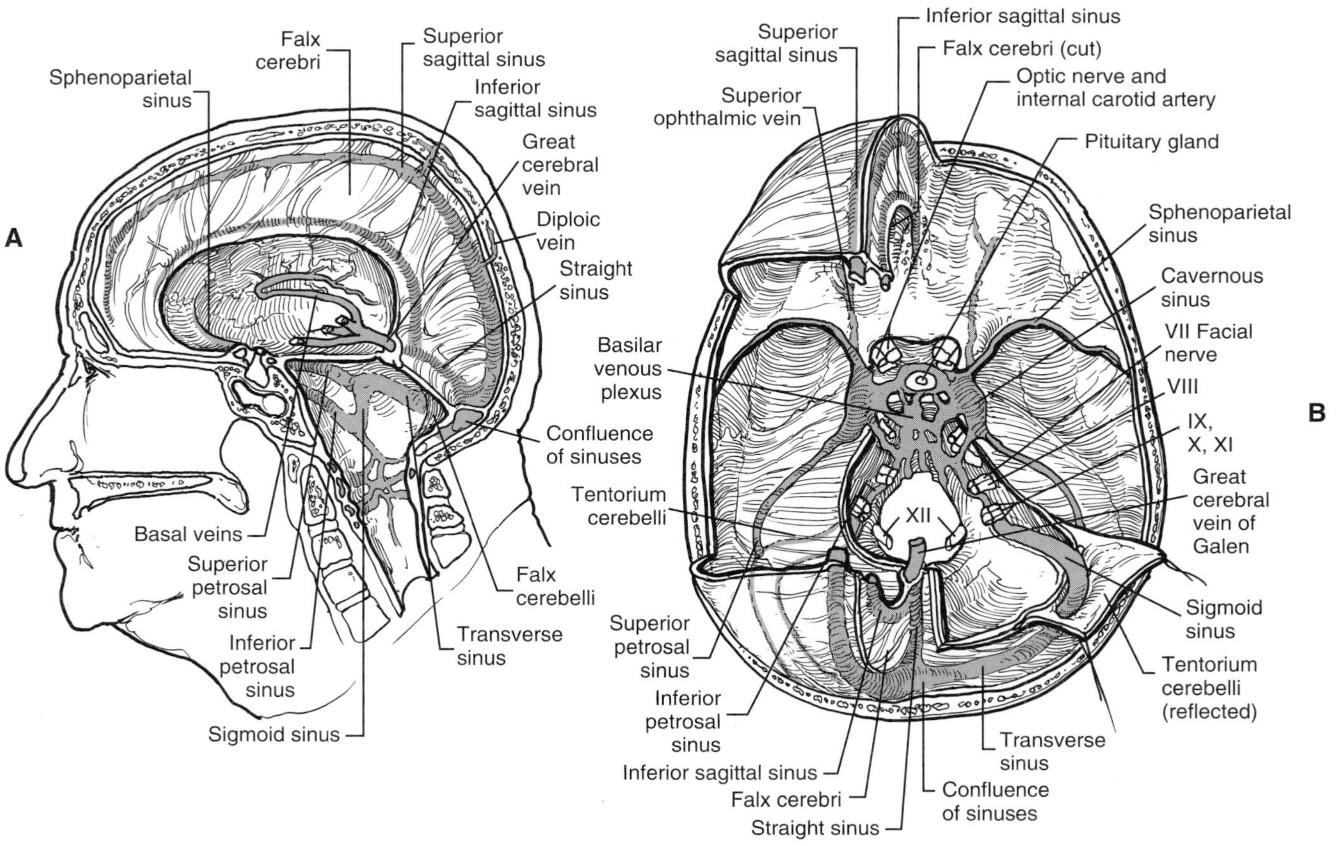

A
Sphenoparietal sinus
Falx cerebri
Superior sagittal sinus
Inferior sagittal sinus
Great cerebral vein
Diploic vein
Straight sinus
Confluence of sinuses
Basal veins
Superior petrosal sinus
Inferior petrosal sinus
Sigmoid sinus
Transverse sinus
Falx cerebelli
B
Superior sagittal sinus
Inferior sagittal sinus
Falx cerebri (cut)
Superior ophthalmic vein
Optic nerve and internal carotid artery
Pituitary gland
Sphenoparietal sinus
Cavernous sinus
VII Facial nerve
VIII
IX, X, XI
Basilar venous plexus
Tentorium cerebelli
XII
Great cerebral vein of Galen
Sigmoid sinus
Tentorium cerebelli (reflected)
Superior petrosal sinus
Inferior petrosal sinus
Inferior sagittal sinus
Falx cerebri
Straight sinus
Transverse sinus
Confluence of sinuses

FIGURE 26–19
The dura mater folds within the brain, showing the venous sinuses.

cussed further in Chapter 27 with the vasculature of the head and neck.

The **tentorium cerebelli** is a more horizontally oriented inward fold of the dural membrane that separates the cerebellum from the occipital lobes of the cerebrum (Fig. 26–19*B*). It attaches to the clinoid processes of the sphenoid bone, the petrous part of the temporal bone, and the internal surface of the occipital bone. An attachment of the falx cerebri to the tentorium cerebelli gives it a tentlike appearance; hence, its name. Inferior to the cerebellar tentorium, a small, vertical fold, the **falx cerebri,** separates the cerebellum into two hemispheres (Fig. 26–19*A*).

The smallest dural infolding is the horizontal **diaphragm sellae,** which forms a roof over the hypophyseal fossa at the sella turcica.

The Arachnoid Mater and Pia Mater Meningeal Layers. *The brain becomes suspended within the subarachnoid space.* The remaining two lower membranes of the meninges, directly below the dura mater, are the **arachnoid mater** and **pia mater.** The two are so closely related that they are sometimes described together as the **pia-arachnoid** or **leptomeninges layer** (Fig. 26–18). The delicate membrane of the **arachnoid** portion is not vascularized. Instead, it contains fibroblasts, collagen fibers, and elastic fibers. It follows the inner surface of the dura mater. **Arachnoid granulations** (tufts of arachnoid tissue or villi that project from the superior surface) extend into the dura mater and, in some cases, form indentations in the bones of the skull (**granular foveola).** These arachnoid granulations reabsorb cerebrospinal fluid and return it to the venous system.

The even thinner **pia layer** is a highly vascularized membrane that covers and attaches to the surface of the brain. Between the arachnoid and pia layers, arachnoid **trabeculae** (flattened irregular fibroblasts) form a spider weblike net. This is, in fact, the origin of the name arachnoid (Greek for "resembling a spider's web") (Fig. 26–18). Cerebrospinal fluid produced by the choroid plexuses of the ventricles fills this weblike space **(subarachnoid space)** between the arachnoid and pia layers (Fig. 26–18). The subarachnoid space varies in size, being larger in areas where the pia mater dips down into the sulci of the brain. Areas with the largest amount of cerebrospinal fluid are called **cisterns.** Names given these cisterns vary, but all describe their anatomic positions (e.g., the cistern cerebellomedullaris at the interface between the inferior cerebellum and the medulla; the cistern chiasmatis above the optic chiasma) (see Fig. 26–23 and the discussion below). The brain loses as much as 97% of its weight because it is suspended within cerebrospinal fluid.

Meningeal Layers and Trauma to the Head. In addition to the subarachnoid space between the arachnoid and pia layers, two other points where meningeal layers interface are given descriptive anatomic names. Neither of these interfaces is considered an actual space, however, except when trauma to the head causes blood to accumulate within these areas. The dura-skull interface is often called the *epidural space.* In similar fashion, the dura-arachnoid interface is termed the *subdural space* (see Fig. 26–18). In an **epidural hemorrhage,** or **hematoma,** arterial blood collects between the external dura layer and the calvaria. This is caused by serious head trauma. In a **subdural hematoma,** trauma may cause a cerebral vein to break. Blood released from this vein forces border cells of the dural layer to come apart from the arachnoid layer. The blood fills this newly formed space.

Although the subarachnoid space provides a protective cushion for the brain, its trabeculae are flexible, and, therefore, a sudden blow to the head may result in some movement of the brain within this space, causing a momentary blackout and a minor injury such as a concussion or contusion. **Subarachnoid hemorrhage** may also be caused by trauma or the leakage of blood (usually arterial blood) from an intracranial aneurysm.

▲ The Cerebrum: The Highest Level of the Brain

The cerebrum comprises the cerebral hemispheres and the diencephalon

Cerebral Hemispheres

Within the cerebrum are found the **cerebral hemispheres,** which make up the largest portion of the brain involved in the highest processing and coordination of sensory information. The cerebral hemispheres extend posteriorly over the cerebellum and fill the anterior and middle cranial fossae. The longitudinal cerebral fissure separates the hemispheres completely into right and left portions. They are connected at the base of the fissure by a bundle of connecting fibers called the **corpus callosum** (Fig. 26–20).

The surface of the brain is highly convoluted, with multiple folds or **gyri** separated by grooves or **sulci** (Fig. 26–20*A*). Major sulci serve as visible markers to somewhat arbitrarily divide each hemisphere of the brain into four lobes. The lobes take their names from the adjacent cranial skeletal bones. The **frontal lobe** extends from the area of the frontal bone back to the **central sulcus** (Fig. 26–20). (The central sulcus lies posterior to the coronal suture.) A **lateral sulcus** forms the lower lateral border of each frontal lobe. Beneath the lateral sulcus on either side lies the **temporal lobe** (Fig. 26–20). The temporal lobes extend back and are continuous with the posterior **occipital lobes.** A small **preoccipital notch** marks the division point (Fig. 26–20). Both of these lobes lie on the tentorium cerebelli, which covers the cerebellum. Often a moderately prominent sulcus, the **parieto-occipital sulcus,** can be found marking the anterior edge of the occipital lobe. The remaining area of the brain is called the **parietal lobe** (Fig. 26–20*A*).

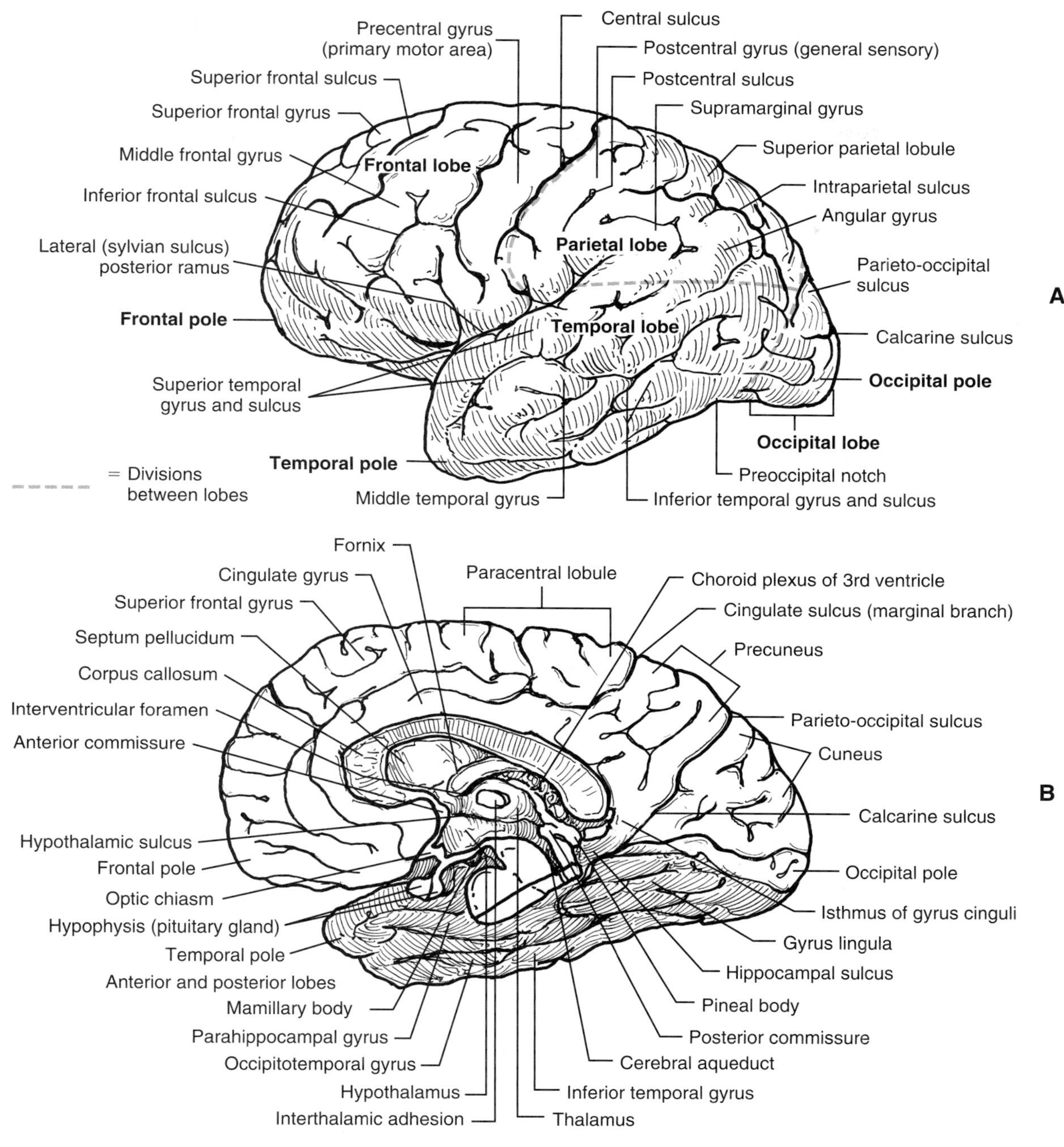

FIGURE 26–20
The cerebrum. **A.** Lateral view showing major sulci and divisions. **B.** Medial view showing the fiber tract (corpus callosum), which connects the two hemispheres and structures of the diencephalon.

In addition to marking the division between the frontal and parietal lobes of the cerebrum, the central sulcus is also an important functional marker. The postcentral gyrus behind this sulcus is the **general sensory area** of the brain (Fig. 26–20). Within this sensory gyrus area, the portion of the sensory cortex devoted to a particular part of the body varies, depending upon the density of sensory receptors in that part of the body. For example, a large portion of this postcentral gyrus is devoted to the face and the hands, while much smaller areas are devoted to the midback region (see Fig. 20–24). The precentral gyrus directly in front of the central sulcus is the **primary motor area** (Fig. 26–20). **Visual function** is found primarily in the occipital lobe, and the **auditory areas** are located in the temporal lobes. **Speech areas** are found in lateral parts of both the frontal and temporal lobes.

A cross section of the cerebral hemispheres shows

an outer gray matter or the cerebral cortex **(pallium)** made up of nerve cells and an inner white matter composed of nerve fibers (see Fig. 26–18). This is in contrast to the relative positions of nerve cells and their fibers in the spinal cord.

The only cranial nerve associated with the cerebral hemispheres is the first, the olfactory nerve (see Box 26–1 and discussions of the olfactory sense).

The Diencephalon

The **diencephalon,** which is the central core of the cerebrum, is completely covered by the cerebral hemispheres. (As a side note, because of its close physical association to structures of the midbrain, some anatomic textbooks refer to the diencephalon as the most rostral part of the brainstem.) The diencephalon is composed of two major areas: the (dorsal) **thalamus** and **hypothalamus** and two smaller portions, the **epithalamus** (containing the pineal body) and **ventral thalamus,** or **subthalamus.**

The diencephalon lies anterior to the tentorium cerebelli. Since it is entirely overlaid by the cerebral hemispheres of the brain, it is best seen in cross sections of the brain. Fig. 26–20*B* shows a sagittal section through the median ventricle of the diencephalon. The **interthalamic adhesion** connects the right and left halves. A sulcus, termed the **hypothalamic sulcus,** can be seen extending from the interventricular foramen to the mid-dorsocaudal surface of the optic chiasm (see Fig. 26–20). The area dorsal to this sulcus is called the **dorsal thalamus,** usually referred to simply as **thalamus,** while the area below it is the **hypothalamus.** The caudal border of the diencephalon approximates a line drawn from the posterior portion of the mamillary bodies to the posterior commissure (see Fig. 26–20*B*). The hypothalamus lies directly over the hypophyseal fossa, or sella turcica ("Turkish saddle"), which contains the **hypophysis cerebri** (pituitary gland).

The **thalamus** acts primarily as a relay center for the cerebral cortex. It receives information from subcortical structures and relays it to the appropriate cortical areas. Within the thalamus, the sense of sight is handled by the lateral geniculate bodies and the sense of hearing by the medial geniculate bodies. The **hypothalamus** regulates the endocrine activity of the pituitary gland, influences the intake of food and water and sexual behavior, and takes part in many autonomic responses such as temperature regulation (see discussion of endocrine functions below). It also participates in the limbic and prefrontal cortex system that controls emotion. During the development of the brain, part of the **epithalamus** evaginates to form a diverticulum that differentiates into the endocrine pineal gland. The roof of the diencephalon becomes the epithelial roof of the third ventricle and forms the paired choroid plexuses of that ventricle within the brain (see Fig. 26–20*B*). The cavity of the third ventricle is a narrow, vertically oriented space located between the two sides of the thalamus and hypothalamus.

In the anterior floor of the third ventricle are the **optic chiasma** and **optic tracts** of the optic nerve, the only cranial nerve associated with the diencephalon (Fig. 26–21). Lying at the posterior portion of the diencephalon floor in the interpeduncular fossa are two **mamillary bodies,** which are approximately the shape and size of peas. It should be noted that in this view of the brain, ventral structures from the midbrain or mesencephalon are also visible. A large pair of axon bundles called the **crura cerebri** can be seen emerging caudal to the optic tracts (Fig. 26–21). These tracts converge medially, disappearing into the pons near the area where the oculomotor nerves exit from the midbrain. In this same area, posterior to the mamillary bodies, the **posterior perforated substance** containing apertures for the posterior cerebral arteries can be seen. (A similarly perforated area that provides arterial access to the forebrain, the **anterior perforated substance,** is also visible.) Between the optic chiasma and the mamillary bodies is a small convex area called the **tuber cinereum,** from which arises the **infundibulum,** or stalk, to the **pituitary gland.**

▲ A Brief Introduction to the Endocrine System

Both the autonomic nervous system and the endocrine system act to regulate and maintain a stable internal environment within the body. They differ in mode of transmission, speed at which they operate, and specificity or localization of targets. In the autonomic system, information is conducted swiftly by nerves, and neurotransmitters are released that cause fast localized responses. In the endocrine system, chemical hormones travel more slowly through the bloodstream to less localized targets, resulting in more prolonged responses.

From an anatomic point of view, several characteristics are shared by all **endocrine glands.** All are ductless. Their secretions are discharged into the blood and lymph. As a consequence, endocrine glands are served by well-developed vascular tissue (e.g., the thyroid gland has extensive vascularization; see Chapter 27). The close link of these glands to the bloodstream is evident even at the cellular level. The endothelial layer of cells of capillaries serving these glands is fenestrated (i.e., the cells have thin walls perforated by microscopic "pores"), which facilitates the diffusion of hormones into the blood.

Endocrine glands are dispersed throughout the entire body. Some are distinct anatomic structures; others are simply clusters of endocrine cells within other organs. They all produce hormones crucial to the development and maintenance of the body. As part of the overall system of regulation, many of these glands act on other endocrine glands. A brief summary of three of these glands follows.

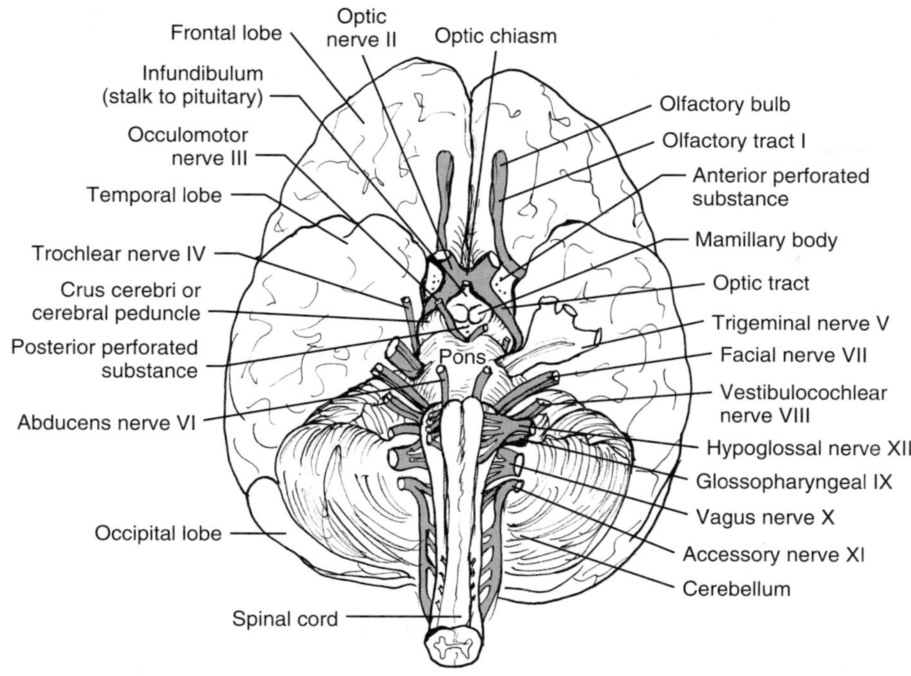

FIGURE 26–21
Ventral view of brain partially dissected to reveal structures of the midbrain as well as the diencephalon.

The paired **suprarenal (adrenal) glands** on the anterior superior pole of each kidney are essential to life, producing a wide range of hormones regulating water balance, carbohydrate balance, and sex hormone production (see Chapter 13).

The **thyroid gland** in the neck produces thyroxine, which stimulates the cellular metabolic rate (see Chapter 27).

The **parathyroid glands** embedded within the thyroid gland control the level and distribution of calcium and phosphorus (see Chapter 27).

Also, numerous small pockets of hormone-producing cells have regulatory roles within various systems of the body. The **pancreatic islet cells** (of Langerhans) within the pancreas produce insulin in response to glucose in intercellular fluids. Two other examples are **gastroenteroendocrine cells** in the stomach and intestine (see Chapter 12) and the carotid bodies within the carotid sinus. The gonads also have significant endocrine functions.

Central Controls and the Interrelationship of Nervous and Endocrine Functions

Two endocrine glands found within the diencephalon, the hypophysis and the pineal gland, serve important roles in the regulation of the other glands

Endocrine secretions of the **pineal gland** have a mostly inhibitory role, reducing both the synthesis and release of hormones in other endocrine glands. The **hypophysis cerebri,** however, has a more far-reaching effect on other glands, a fact that explains its common designation as the "master gland."

An understanding of the dual origin of the **hypophysis** helps explain the different functions of its anterior and posterior lobes. As indicated above in the discussion of the diencephalon, the posterior lobe or **neurohypophysis** forms from an outgrowth of the diencephalic floor called the **infundibulum** (see Fig. 26–20*B*). However, the anterior lobe, or **adenohypophysis,** forms from an evagination of the ectodermal roof of the future mouth (Rathke's pouch) that detaches from the pharyngeal area and becomes attached to the posterior lobe. An extension from the adenohypophysis also forms part of the infundibulum, the **pars tuberalis.** Between these two lobes is a rudimentary vestige from the development of the adenohypophysis termed the **pars intermedia,** which usually disappears during childhood.

The **neurohypophysis** secretes antidiuretic hormone, also known as vasopressin, and oxytocin, which promotes contraction of the uterus. The hormones produced by the **adenohypophysis,** or anterior glandular lobe, affect hormone production in many other endocrine tissues. Adenohypophysis hormones that target other endocrine glands include adrenocorticotropin, which stimulates hormone production in the adrenal glands, thyrotropic hormone to the thyroid gland (a growth hormone), and gonadotropic hormones.

The hypophysis illustrates the close association between regulation of the body via the nervous system and hormonal regulation via the endocrine glands. The most obvious connection is that the posterior lobe of the pituitary gland, the neurohypophysis, is directly connected with the diencephalon. Axons from hypothalamic neurons are carried by the infundibulum (pituitary stalk) from the diencephalon directly into this posterior lobe of the gland. Research suggests that hormones released by the neurohypophysis are actually produced by nerve cells in the brain. Coordination between neural and hormonal activity is also evident in the anterior adenohypophysis. Secretory activity in that lobe (which has far-reaching effects on the endocrine system as a whole) responds to releasing factors from neurons in the hypothalamic nuclei.

Because of the pituitary gland's proximity to the optic chiasm, tumors of the gland often damage vision. A pituitary tumor can affect the crossing fibers in the optic chiasm and damage the temporal portion of visual fields in both eyes, a condition called **bitemporal hemianopsia.** Less commonly, a tumor will affect a lateral portion of the chiasm, damaging only the nasal visual field on the same side (right or left **ipsilateral nasal hemianopsia**).

A Brief Summary of Sympathetic and Parasympathetic Autonomic Systems in the Head

Sympathetic Fibers Associated with Cranial Nerves

All sympathetic fibers traveling with cranial nerves are postganglionic and have cell bodies in the superior cervical ganglion. They are generally associated with plexuses around major blood vessels, such as the internal and external carotid arteries, and join cranial nerves that pass in close proximity. The preganglionic cell bodies are found in the lateral horn of the upper thoracic spinal cord. Their axons travel in the sympathetic trunk to the superior cervical ganglion where they synapse. The postsynaptic fibers pass from the ganglion to the internal carotid artery and other arteries directly via arterial rami. Sympathetic fibers from the internal carotid plexus communicate with the trigeminal and pterygopalatine ganglia and pass through the ciliary ganglion without synapsing (see Chapters 24 and 25). Sympathetic fibers join numerous cranial nerves, including the abducent, oculomotor, trochlear, trigeminal, and glossopharyngeal nerves.

Sympathetic innervation of cranial structures elicits characteristic autonomic responses (fight or flight). For example, activation of the sympathetic innervation of the dilator pupillae muscle of the eye via the long ciliary nerves (from the nasociliary branch of cranial nerve V) dilates the pupil (see Chapter 25).

The Cranial Parasympathetic System

Parasympathetic ganglia in the head include the otic, ciliary, pterygopalatine, and submandibular ganglia

The otic, ciliary, pterygopalatine, and submandibular ganglia are near the viscera that they supply; therefore, postganglionic fibers leaving the ganglia are relatively short compared with sympathetic fibers. Preganglionic parasympathetic fibers are carried to

- the otic ganglion by the tympanic branch of the glossopharyngeal nerve (see Fig. 26–12),
- the ciliary ganglion by the oculomotor nerve (see Fig. 25–6),
- the pterygopalatine ganglion by the nervous intermedius part of the facial nerve (via the greater petrosal nerve and nerve of the pterygoid canal) (see Fig. 24–28), and
- the submandibular ganglion by the nervous intermedius part of the facial nerve (via the chorda tympani and lingual nerves) (see Figs. 24–12 and 24–28).

The vagus nerve (cranial nerve X) also carries preganglionic parasympathetic fibers, but it targets mainly structures in the thorax and portions of the abdomen.

In general, parasympathetic activity results in responses that relax the body and conserve energy. Within the head, glands such as the lacrimal, submandibular, sublingual, and parotid glands are affected, as well as muscles around the pupil of the eye.

The Cerebellum and Brainstem

The Cerebellum

Although the cerebellum ("little brain") arises from the same region of the brain as the pons, it is not part of the brainstem. As it grows, it bulges dorsally, and processes of fissuration and foliation vastly increase the surface area. The definitive **cerebellum** consists of two lateral hemispheres united by a narrow connection, the vermis (Fig. 26–22). It is located under the cerebellar tentorium membrane, ventral to the posterior part of the cerebrum but dorsal to the pons and medulla of the brainstem. It fills much of the posterior fossa. It has no interior ventricle but forms a portion of the roof of the fourth ventricle. The cerebellum controls balance and posture. It also coordinates the contraction of voluntary muscles, allowing for the smooth execution of movements.

The Brainstem

The **brainstem** includes the midbrain, pons, and medulla oblongata. All of the 12 cranial nerves except the first (olfactory nerve) and second (optic nerve) arise from nuclei located in the brainstem (see Fig. 26–21). See Chapter 23 for an overview of the cranial nerves.

The rostral portion of the brainstem is the **midbrain,** or **mesencephalon.** Much of the mesencephalon is composed of white matter, massive fiber tracts that connect the forebrain with the hindbrain and spinal cord. The superior and inferior colliculi, important relay stations for sight and hearing, respectively, are prominent swellings on the dorsal surface of the midbrain (see Fig. 26–22).

The cavity of the midbrain forms the narrow **cerebral aqueduct** (of Sylvius), which allows cerebrospinal fluid to be transported from the lateral and third ventricles to the fourth ventricle (see Fig. 26–22). The aqueduct is located at the juncture between the middle and posterior cranial fossae.

The **pons** (from the Latin meaning *bridge*) is primarily an expansion of the massive fiber tracts serving the cerebellum. It relays signals between the spinal cord and cerebral and cerebellar cortices. It lies between the midbrain and the more caudal medulla oblongata and ventral to the cerebellum (see Fig. 26–22). Its dorsal surface, the **pontine tegmentum,** forms the superior portion of the floor of the fourth ventricle (see Fig. 26–22).

The **medulla oblongata** is the most caudal portion of the brainstem, lying in the posterior cranial fossa between the hemispheres of the cerebellum. It extends from the lower border of the pons to the point where the first pair of spinal nerves emerge (see Fig. 26–21). It is continuous with the spinal cord and retains some organizational similarities with it. The internal structure of the medulla, however, changes gradually as it becomes more distant from the spinal cord (see Fig. 23–5). The central canal of the spinal cord continues into the lower half of the medulla.

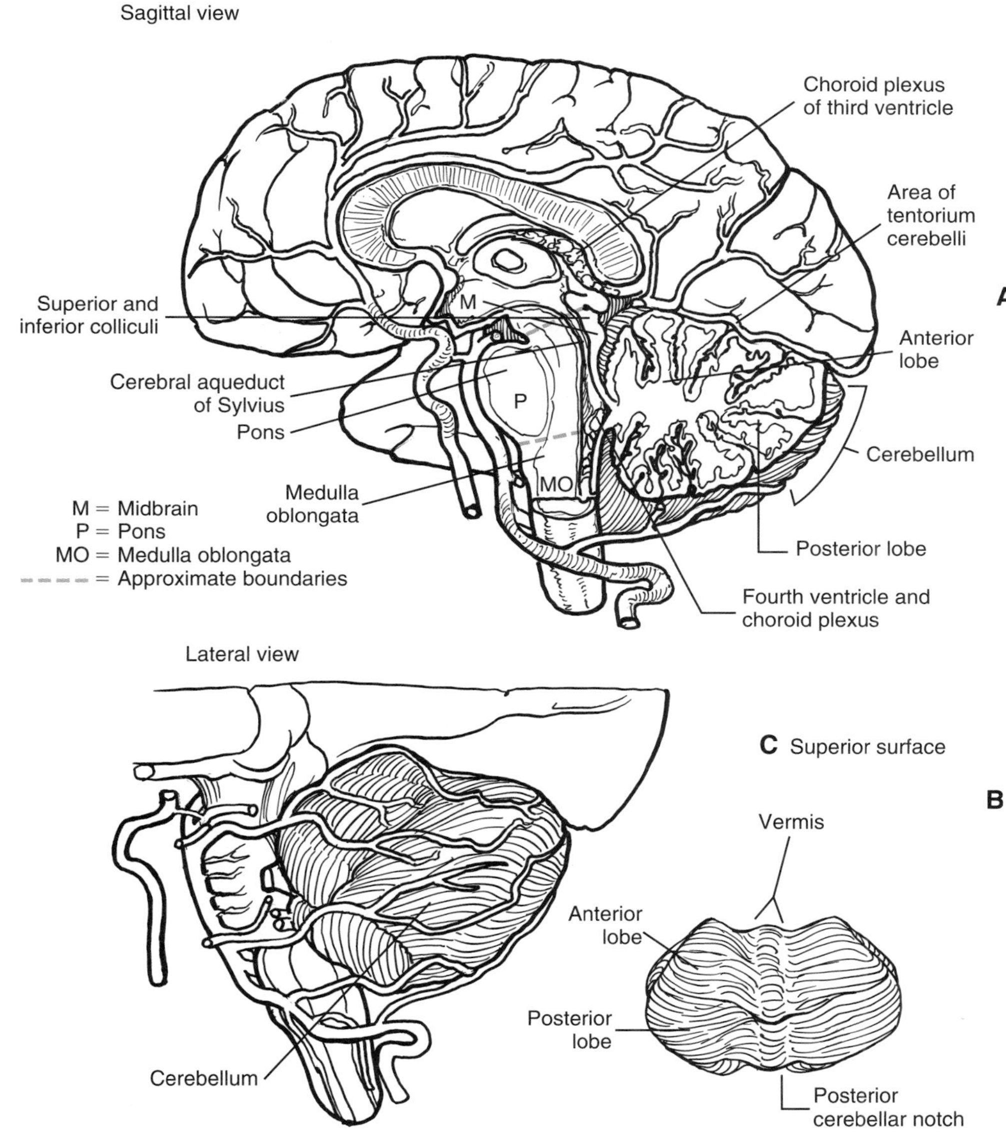

FIGURE 26–22
The cerebellum. **A.** Sagittal view. **B.** Lateral view. **C.** Superior surface.

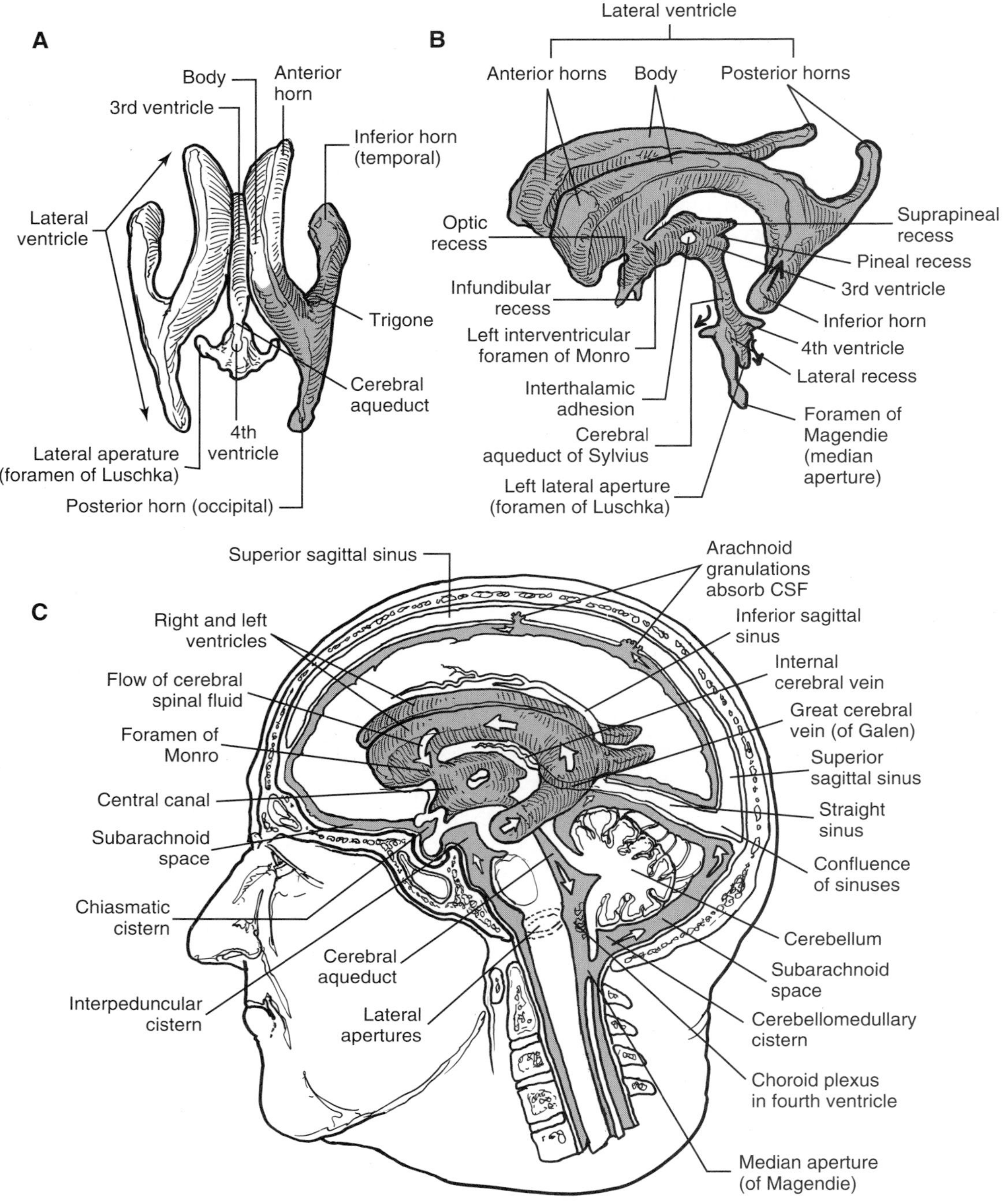

FIGURE 26–23
Ventricles of the brain and circulation of cerebrospinal fluid.

This cavity opens dorsally and expands to form the inferior part of the fourth ventricle (see Figs. 26–22 and 26–23).

▲ Ventricles of the Brain

The ventricles of the brain and subarachnoid spaces are filled with circulating cerebrospinal fluid

Fig. 26–23 shows the direction of flow of the cerebrospinal fluid within the brain and the relationship of the lateral, third, and fourth ventricles.

Within each cerebral hemisphere is a lateral ventricle, derived from the original neural canal, which extends into the frontal lobe and curves around to occupy the temporal lobe (see the developmental sequence in Figs. 26–17 and 26–23). The anterior horns extend into the frontal lobes, the inferior horns into the temporal lobes, and the posterior horns into the occipital lobes. The two lateral ventricles of the cerebrum open into the third ventricle (cavity of the diencephalon) by an interventricular foramen (of Monro) (Fig. 26–23*B*).

The third ventricle communicates with the cerebral aqueduct, which connects the third and fourth ventricles (Fig. 26–23*A* and *B*). The fourth ventricle (extending between the rostral pons and the cerebellum to the caudal medulla) is continuous with the central canal of the spinal cord (Fig. 26–23*C*). These ventricles are filled with circulating cerebrospinal fluid secreted by the choroid plexuses in the lateral, third, and fourth ventricles. The area of the choroid plexus of the fourth ventricle is shown in Fig. 26–23*C*.

Cerebrospinal fluid enters the subarachnoid space only through three apertures in the fourth ventricle. They are the median aperture (foramen) of Magendie and the two lateral apertures (foramina) of Luschka (Fig. 26–23).

If these apertures are blocked, a dangerous condition occurs in which the cerebrospinal fluid distends the ventricles and compresses the cerebral hemispheres. Negative consequences of an increase in cerebrospinal fluid can also occur at other sites. If pressure rises in the subarachnoid space surrounding the optic nerve, fluid can accumulate and cause the optic disc to swell **(papilledema).** This condition can be seen with an ophthalmoscopic examination of the retina.

Cerebrospinal fluid circulation is continuous with that in the subarachnoid space surrounding the spinal cord. This is the space into which spinal anesthesia is administered. After circulating around the brain and spinal cord, cerebrospinal fluid reenters the vascular system through absorption by the arachnoid granulations.

Subarachnoid Cisterns

Some areas of the brain **(cisterns)** contain "pools" of cerebrospinal fluid that separate the arachnoid and pia layers. Cisterns contain arteries, veins, and, rarely, a cranial nerve. The names of these subarachnoid cisterns come from structures in close proximity (see Fig. 26–23 for positions):

- **posterior cerebellomedullary cistern** located between the cerebellum and the medulla (sometimes called the *cisterna magna*);
- **pontine cistern** located ventral to the pons;
- **interpeduncular cistern** (basal cistern) located between the cerebral **interpeduncular fossa** of the midbrain, which contains the oculomotor nerves and upper part of the basilar artery (part of the cerebral arterial circle of Willis);
- **chiasmatic cistern,** the point of crossing for the optic nerve fibers; and
- **quadrigeminal cistern** located between the posterior part of the corpus callosum and the superior surface of the cerebellum.

The posterior cerebellomedullary cistern may be used as a site for obtaining cerebrospinal fluid (as an alternative to using the lumbar cistern). A needle is introduced into the cistern through the atlanto-occipital membrane. The cerebromedullary cistern can also be used for injecting antibiotics or contrast media for medical imaging.

27 The Neck and Vasculature of the Head and Neck

INTRODUCTION TO THE NECK

Three types of structures will be used as a framework for presenting the anatomy of the neck: the anterior and posterior triangles, fascial planes, and nerves and vasculature of the head and neck.

The first structures, the **anterior and posterior triangles,** are significant because they can be viewed on the surface of the neck and are bordered by major muscles and bones of the neck. Therefore, the triangles are used as markers for major cervical structures. Neither the anterior nor the posterior triangle is a flat, planar surface. Each spirals around the cylindrical neck column. Some anatomists argue that the designation of these triangles is arbitrary, since blood vessels, nerves, and even viscera extend across the boundaries between the triangles. The designations remain useful, however, because the triangles and their subdivisions can often be identified visually or by palpation and, therefore, are invaluable in clinical examinations.

Fascial planes are fascial laminae that separate functional areas of the neck. They will be used to describe the complex three-dimensional relationships of cervical structures. The fasciae are clinically important in localizing nerves and blood vessels that are crucial in surgery. Fascial planes also outline compartments within which infection is likely to spread. Structures encircled by the middle fascial layer, the larynx, the thyroid and parathyroid glands, and the esophagus, will be discussed in this section.

Nerves and muscles integrate the neck and will make up the last group of organizing structures. The general **innervation** of the neck will be presented. Functional integration of structures in the neck is accomplished by cranial nerves IX, X, XI, and XII and by cervical spinal nerves of the **cervical plexus.**

The **vasculature** of the head and neck will be used to help integrate all of the systems within the head that are covered in Chapters 22 through 27.

SKELETAL LANDMARKS AND SUPERFICIAL MUSCLES OF THE NECK

Skeletal Structure of the Neck

The neck arises mainly from cervical segments of the trunk, although elements are also derived from the second, third, fourth, and sixth pharyngeal arches (see Chapter 26). The seven cervical vertebrae of the **axial skeleton** provide the internal support for the neck; the manubrium serves as the anterior inferior boundary; the U-shaped hyoid bone maintains an open airway and provides an attachment point for anterior neck muscles; and the clavicles from the **superior appendicular skeleton** serve as the neck's lateral inferior border (Fig. 27–1).

The hyoid bone is attached to the thyroid cartilage via the thyrohyoid membrane and to the styloid processes of the temporal bones by the stylohyoid ligaments. It does not articulate directly with any other bone and, consequently, has a fairly wide range of movement. The hyoid bone can be felt moving upward as a person swallows (Fig. 27–1).

Superficial Muscles of the Neck

Major superficial muscles in the neck are the unpaired platysma muscle and the paired sternocleidomastoid and trapezius muscles

An exceedingly thin, broad muscle, the **platysma muscle** (from the Greek for "flat plate"), lies just beneath the skin and covers the anterolateral sides of the neck. It arises in the tela subcutanea over the upper part of the thorax, runs over the clavicles, and blends with the facial muscles over the mandible. This muscle has no significant action, although as a muscle of facial expression, its tension conveys stress and can help open the mouth (see Chapter 24, especially Fig. 24–23*P*). The platysma muscle frequently contracts strongly in moments of sudden violent exertion. Because the platysma muscle is derived from the second pharyngeal arch, it is innervated by the cervical branch of the facial nerve (cranial nerve VII).

Within the investing (superficial) layer of the cervical fascia are two pairs of muscles, the sternocleidomastoid and trapezius muscles. These muscles are important markers for identifying structures in the neck. The **sternocleidomastoid muscle** is named for its two attachments, the clavicle and the mastoid process of the temporal bone. Inferiorly, the muscle has two points of origin, one from the manubrium and the other from the

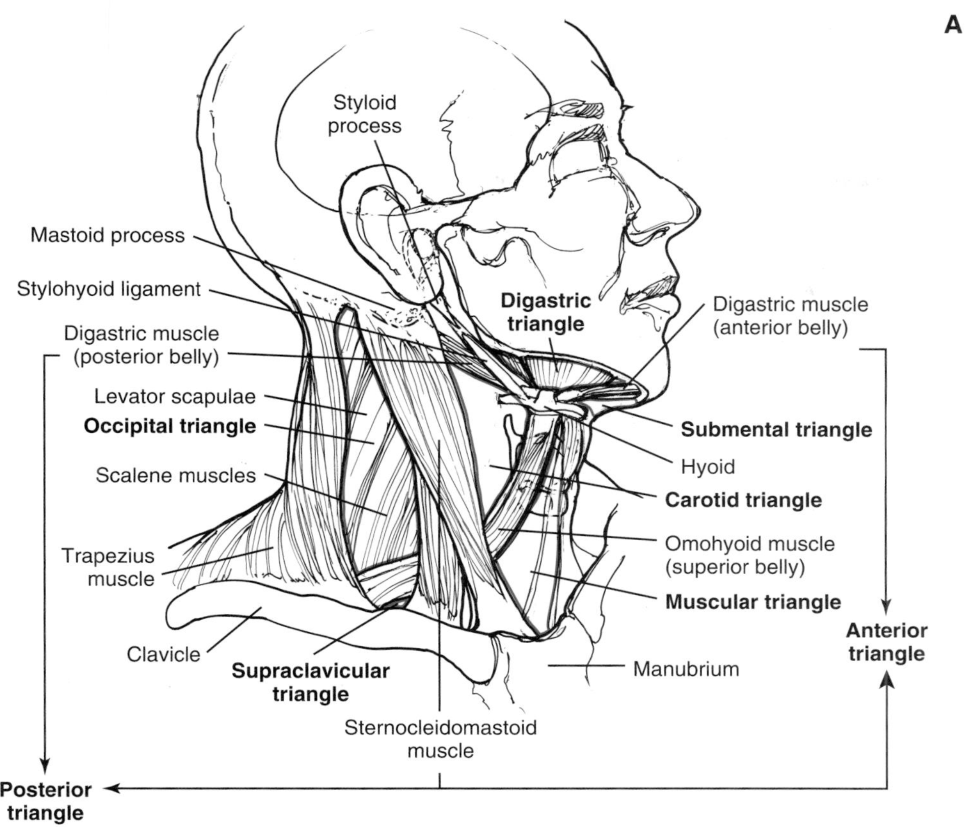

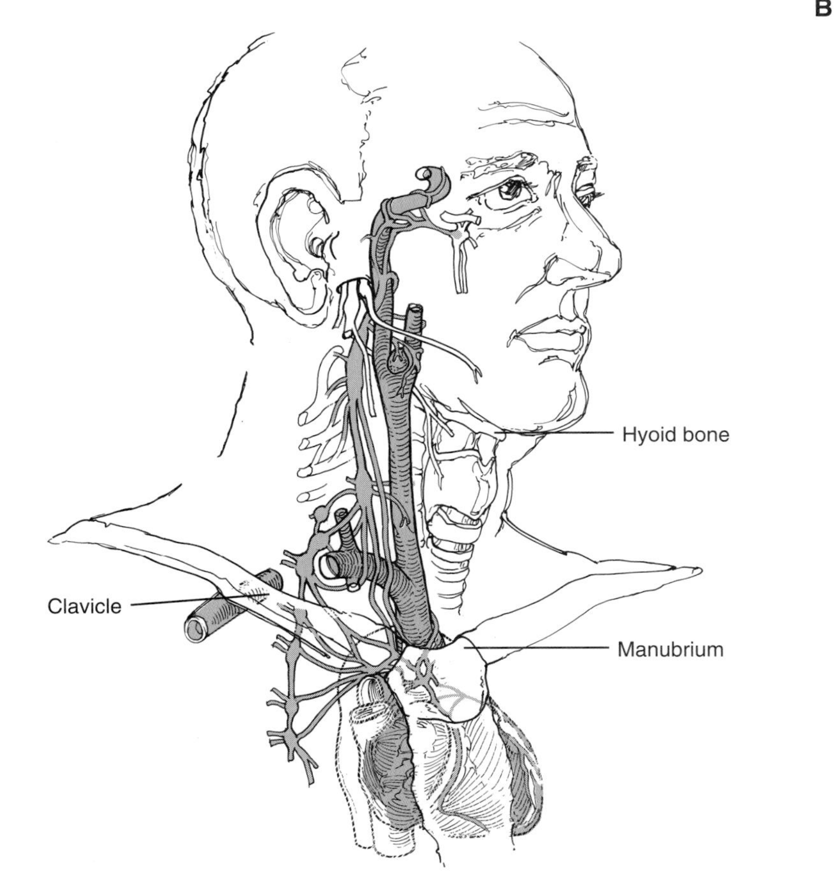

FIGURE 27–1
Triangles and superficial muscles of the neck.

medial clavicle (*cleid* is the Latin term for "clavicle") (Fig. 27–1). Superiorly, the muscle inserts on the mastoid process behind the ear and on the lateral portion of the superior nuchal line of the temporal bone. When both sternocleidomastoid muscles contract together, they *act* to forcibly flex the head and neck and can lift the head from the supine position. When each muscle acts alone, it flexes the neck and tilts the head toward the ipsilateral side while it rotates the face toward the contralateral side (e.g., when a person glances to the side and upward).

Torticollis is a clinical condition that occurs from spasmatic or chronic contracture of the sternocleidomastoid muscle.

The **trapezius muscle** is a large, triangular muscle serving the back and shoulder as well as the neck (Fig. 27–1). It originates from the superior nuchal line, external occipital protuberance, ligamentum nuchae from the skull to vertebra C7 and the spinous process of vertebra C7, and all of the thoracic vertebrae and their supraspinous ligaments. Its uppermost fibers run downward to insert on the distal clavicle; its middle fibers insert on the acromion; and its fibers from the thoracic region run superolaterally to insert on the spine of the scapula. Since it connects the pectoral girdle with the skull and axial skeleton, it moves the head and neck as well as the scapula and clavicle. When the shoulder is fixed, it can act to bend the head and neck posterolaterally. (See Chapters 5 and 20 for further illustrations of its anatomic position and actions.)

TRIANGLES OF THE NECK

Traditionally, the sternocleidomastoid muscle marks the boundary between the anterior and posterior triangles of the neck; the anterior triangles lie in front of the muscle, and the posterior triangles lie behind it

▲ Anterior Triangles

The paired anterior triangles angle outward (superolaterally) from an apex at the anterior median line. The boundaries of the three sides are the mandible (above), anterior median line or cervical midline (medially), and anterior border of the sternocleidomastoid muscle (laterally) (Fig. 27–1). The floor of the anterior cervical compartment is formed by the pharynx, larynx, and thyroid gland.

Subregions Within the Anterior Triangle

Within the anterior triangle are the following subregions:

- digastric (submandibular) triangle;
- carotid triangle;
- submental triangle; and
- muscular triangle (Fig. 27–1).

The glandular **digastric (submandibular) triangle** contains the submandibular gland and its surrounding lymph nodes. It is the area directly inferior to the mandible but above the hyoid bone, between the anterior and posterior digastric muscles and the associated stylohyoid muscle (Fig. 27–1). The mylohyoid and hypoglossus muscles are below it.

The vascular **carotid triangle** is bounded by the anterior border of the sternocleidomastoid muscle posteriorly, superior belly of the omohyoid muscle anteriorly, and stylohyoid muscle and posterior belly of the digastric muscle superiorly (Fig. 27–1). It contains the carotid sheath and the structures within it, which are the internal jugular vein, common carotid artery, and vagus nerve, as well as the carotid sinus and carotid body (see below). A clinician examining a patient can usually see the carotid triangle as a small depression.

The unpaired **submental triangle** is found directly under the chin, anterior to the submandibular triangles. The left and right anterior digastric muscles form the sides, and the hyoid bone forms the inferior border of the triangle (Fig. 27–1).

Finally, the **muscular triangle** lies between the carotid triangle and the anterior midline of the neck, below the hyoid bone. It is bounded anteriorly by the median line of the neck from the hyoid bone to the sternum, posteriorly by the anterior border of the sternocleidomastoid muscle, and posterosuperiorly by the superior belly of the omohyoid muscle (Fig. 27–1). Within this triangle are found the thyroid and parathyroid glands and the infrahyoid muscles.

Infrahyoid and Suprahyoid Muscles

Together, the suprahyoid and infrahyoid muscles support and move the hyoid bone and the larynx

The suprahyoid and infrahyoid muscles are important in swallowing, chewing, vocalization, and respiration. The general functions of the suprahyoid muscles are to elevate the hyoid bone and also the tongue and floor of the mouth, while the antagonistic infrahyoid group depresses the hyoid bone and lowers the larynx. Individual muscle pairs, however, have specific capabilities. For example, the suprahyoid digastric muscles act together to depress the mandible and the infrahyoid omohyoid muscles act together to depress the hyoid bone and larynx to allow prolonged inspiratory efforts (or the singing of a low note). The infrahyoid and suprahyoid muscles may also work together to fix the hyoid bone, providing a firm base for movements of the tongue, or may cooperate to perform more complex movements.

The **suprahyoid muscles,** superior to the hyoid bone, include the

- digastric muscle,
- mylohyoid muscle,
- geniohyoid muscle, and
- stylohyoid muscle.

These are muscles of the neck, but the mylohyoid muscle also contributes to the floor of the mouth. The

digastric muscle has two bellies connected by a tendon in the middle that is attached to the hyoid body by a fibrous loop (Fig. 27–2). The posterior belly of the muscle extends from the mastoid process to the hyoid bone and the anterior belly from the hyoid bone to the chin. The two **mylohyoid muscles** form the floor of the submental triangle (part of the anterior triangle) and fill much of the space between the two sides of the body of the mandible (Fig. 27–2). The narrow **geniohyoid muscle** is found directly above the medial portion of the mylohyoid muscle, extending from the mental spine downward to the hyoid bone. Together, the geniohyoid and mylohyoid muscles provide a movable but firm floor of the mouth. The **stylohyoid muscle** arises from the styloid process and passes downward and forward, parallel to the posterior belly of the digastric muscle. It inserts on the hyoid bone, splitting to pass on either side of the digastric tendon (Fig. 27–2).

The **infrahyoid muscles,** inferior to the hyoid bone, are often referred to as **strap muscles** because of their ribbonlike appearance. They include the

- sternohyoid muscle,
- omohyoid muscle,
- sternothyroid muscle, and
- thyrohyoid muscle.

As a group, they cover the front and most of the sides of the larynx, trachea, and thyroid gland. Together, they steady the hyoid bone and depress the hyoid bone and larynx during vocalization and deglutition. The **sternohyoid muscle** is the most medial, running from the manubrium of the sternum and medial end of the clavicle to the body of the hyoid bone (Fig. 27–2).

The **omohyoid muscle,** like the digastric muscle, has two bellies joined by a central tendon. The superior belly lies lateral to the sternohyoid muscle and attaches lateral to it on the hyoid bone. As the superior belly runs inferiorly, it parallels the sternohyoid muscle, deviating inferiorly to pass in front of the carotid sheath. Its muscle fibers then give way to a tendon between the superior and inferior bellies, which is held down to the clavicle by a fascial sling. The muscle's central tendon is deep to the sternocleidomastoid muscle and close to the internal jugular vein (Fig. 27–2). The omohyoid muscle's inferior belly runs posteriorly across the posterior triangle, dividing it into the upper occipital and lower subclavicular triangles (Fig. 27–2). After disappearing deep to the trapezius muscle, it attaches to the superior border of the scapula, medial to the scapular notch.

Underlying the sternohyoid muscle is the **sternothyroid muscle,** which, like the sternohyoid muscle,

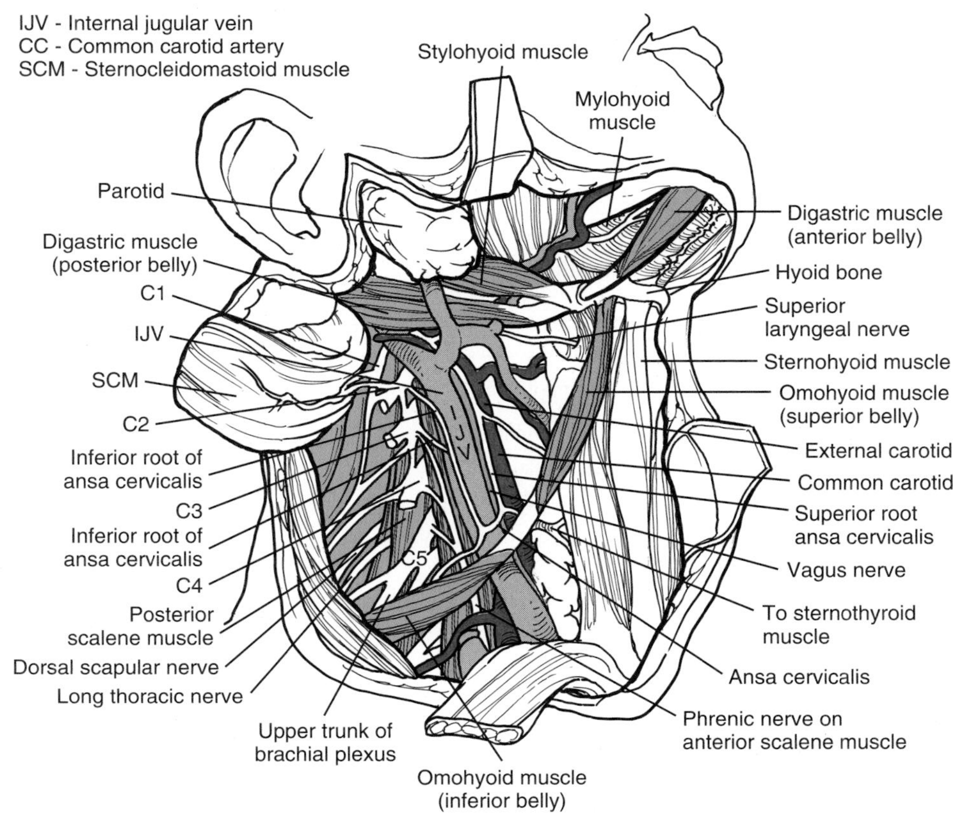

FIGURE 27–2
The infrahyoid and suprahyoid muscles.

originates from the posterior surface of the manubrium (Fig. 27–2). The sternothyroid muscle covers the thyroid gland and inserts on an oblique line on the thyroid cartilage. The closely related **thyrohyoid muscle** begins at the oblique line of thyroid cartilage and inserts on the hyoid bone (Fig. 27–2). Table 27–1 lists the hyoid and extrahyoid attachments of these muscles.

▲ Posterior Triangle

The **posterior triangle** spirals around the lateral surface of the neck posterior to the sternocleidomastoid muscle. Boundaries of the paired posterior cervical triangles of the neck include the middle third of the clavicle inferiorly, posterior border of the sternocleidomastoid muscle anteriorly, and anterior border of the trapezius muscle posteriorly (see Fig. 27–1).

The deep fascia that covers the space between the sternocleidomastoid and trapezius muscles forms the roof of the triangle. The floor is formed by four lateral prevertebral muscles: the splenius capitis, levator scapulae, scalenus medius, and scalenus posterior muscles (see Fig. 27–1). These muscles will be discussed below.

The external jugular vein crosses the posterior triangle from its anterior border to the inferior posterior area, terminating in the subclavian vein.

Subsidiary Triangles (Occipital and Supraclavicular Triangles) Within the Posterior Triangle

The **occipital triangle** has the same upper borders as the posterior triangle but is bounded at its lowest point by the omohyoid muscle (see Fig. 27–1). Its name comes from the fact that the occipital artery is found at its apex. The accessory nerve (cranial nerve XI) crosses the area.

The very small **supraclavicular triangle** has the same general borders as the posterior triangle but is bounded superiorly by the inferior belly of the omohyoid muscle (see Fig. 27–1). The floor of this triangle is the first rib, a scalenus muscle, and the first digitation of the serratus anterior muscle. Since the subclavian artery crosses this area deep to the triangle, this region is sometimes called the **subclavian triangle.** In a living person, a depression called the *supraclavicular fossa* can be seen in this area; it is sometimes nicknamed the "salt cellar."

> The position of the subclavian artery in this triangle is clinically important. Blood flow can be controlled by compressing the artery retroclavicularly against the first rib.

Prevertebral Muscles. *Prevertebral muscles are deep muscles of the neck that lie within the prevertebral fascia and form the floor of the anterior and posterior triangles.* The **anterior vertebral muscles** are all flexors of the head. They include the longus capitis muscle (long muscle of the head) and the longus colli muscle (long muscle of the neck), as well as the rectus capitis anterior and rectus capitis lateralis muscles. The **longus capitis muscle** runs from vertebra C6 to the base of the occipital bone. The **longus colli muscle** has three parts, the superior oblique, inferior oblique, and intermediate vertical parts. These are attached by tendinous slips to vertebrae from the atlas to the third thoracic vertebrae. The **rectus capitis anterior** and **rectus capitis lateralis muscles** both lie posterior to the longus capitis muscle and extend from the atlas to points on the occipital bone (Fig. 27–3).

The **lateral vertebral muscles** extend obliquely, like scaling ladders, from the upper two ribs to the transverse processes of cervical vertebrae. They include

TABLE 27–1
Muscles and Ligaments Attached to the Hyoid Bone

Muscle or Ligament	Extrahyoid Attachment	Hyoid Attachment
Stylohyoid ligament	Styloid process of temporal bone	Apices of lesser horns
Stylohyoid muscle	Styloid process of temporal bone	Junction of body and greater horn
Geniohyoid muscle	Lower mental spine of mandible	Upper anterior surface of body
Mylohyoid muscle	Mylohyoid line on inner surface of mandible	Lower anterior surface of body
Omohyoid muscle	Superior border of scapula	Lower anterior surface of lateral body
Sternohyoid muscle	Manubrium and sternal head of clavicle	Lower anterior surface of medial body
Thyrohyoid muscle	Oblique line of thyroid cartilage	Lower border of body greater horns
Hyoglossus muscle	Tongue	Upper surface of greater and lesser horns
Genioglossus muscle	Tongue	Upper surface of body (lowest fibers)
Fibrous loop for digastric tendon	Digastric muscle connects digastric fossa of mandible and mastoid notch of temporal bone	Near and posterior to the junction of the body and greater horn
Thyrohyoid membrane	Thyroid cartilage of larynx	Medial border of greater horn

the **anterior, medius,** and **posterior scalene muscles.** The scalene muscles are found deep to the sternocleidomastoid muscle and are part of the floor of the posterior triangle. The **anterior scalene muscle** arises from the anterior tubercles of the transverse processes of vertebrae C3 or C4, C5, and C6. It then runs inferolaterally to insert on the first rib (Fig. 27–3). This muscle is related to several important structures: the phrenic nerve lies on its anterior surface; it is crossed anteriorly by branches of the thyrocervical vascular trunk; and the thoracic duct turns laterally in front of the anterior scalene muscle to enter the subclavian vein at the angle of its juncture with the internal jugular vein. The subclavian vein passes anterior to the anterior scalene muscle, while the subclavian artery passes behind it. The **middle scalene muscle** is the largest of the three and originates from the transverse processes of all the cervical vertebrae except the atlas. It travels inferolaterally to insert behind the anterior scalene muscle on the first rib. The subclavian artery and most of the components of the brachial plexus emerge from between the anterior scalene and middle scalene muscles. These structures are sometimes compressed as they cross the first rib. Two nerves from the brachial plexus (the dorsal scapular nerve, which innervates the rhomboid muscles, and the long thoracic nerve, which innervates the serratus anterior muscle) usually run through the middle scalene muscle. The **posterior scalene muscle** is small. It arises from the posterior tubercles of vertebrae C4, C5, and C6 and descends in front of the levator scapulae muscle to insert on the second rib.

Two other muscles in this area, the **splenius capitis** and **levator scapulae muscles,** also form part of the floor of the posterior triangle. The levator scapulae mus-

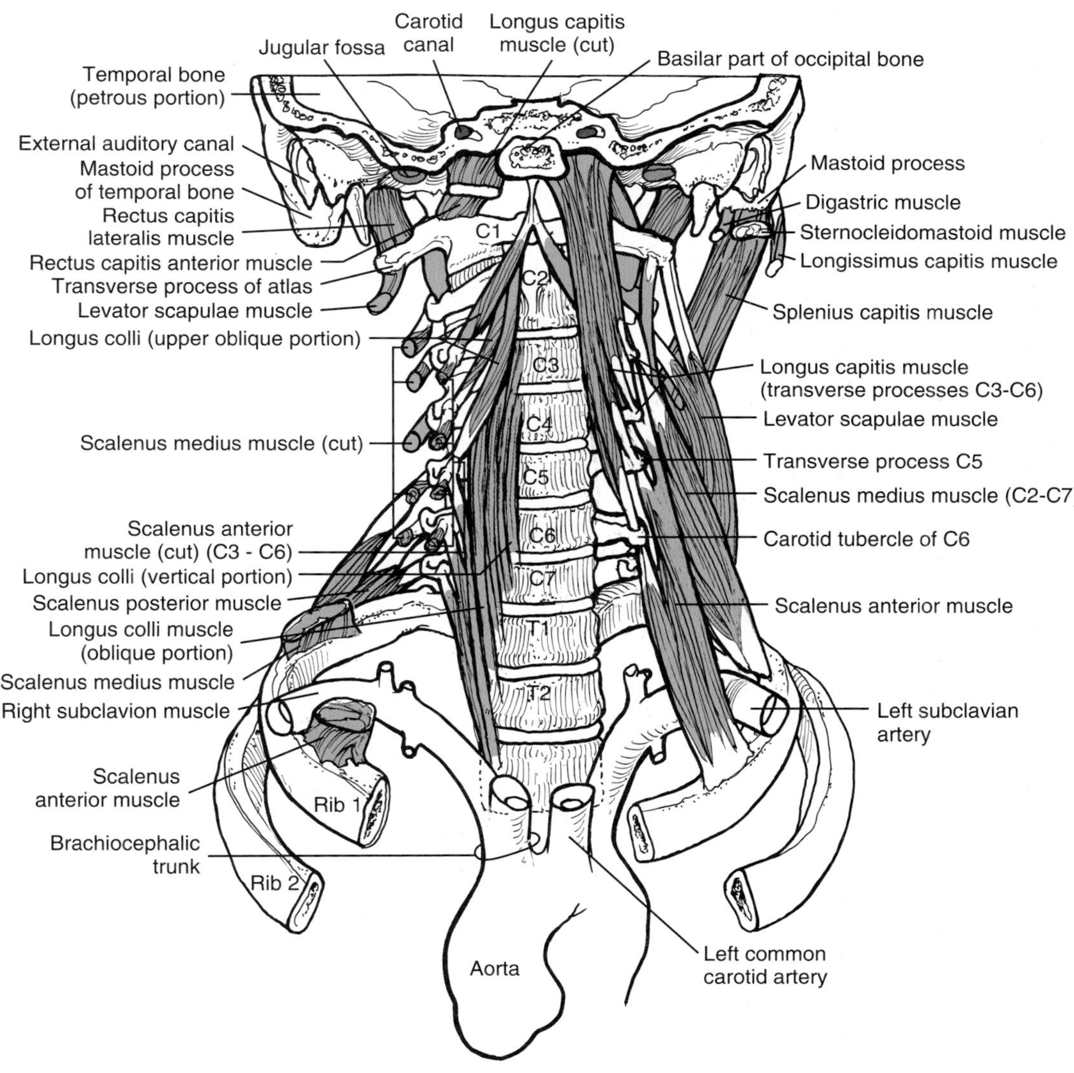

FIGURE 27–3
Prevertebral muscles.

TABLE 27–2
Summary of Structures Within the Anterior and Posterior Triangles of the Neck

- Anterior triangle
  - Submandibular triangle
    - Submandibular gland and duct
    - Submandibular lymph nodes
    - Hypoglossal nerve (cranial nerve XII)
    - Nerve to mylohyoid muscle
    - Facial artery and vein
    - Submental artery
  - Submental triangle
    - Submental lymph nodes
    - Branches of anterior jugular vein
  - Carotid triangle
    - Carotid sheath with common carotid artery, carotid sinus, carotid body
    - Internal jugular vein
    - Vagus nerve (cranial nerve X)
    - Hypoglossal nerve (cranial nerve XII)
    - Accessory nerve (cranial nerve XI)
    - Thyroid gland, larynx, pharynx
    - Branches of cervical plexus
    - Deep cervical lymph nodes
  - Muscular triangle
    - Sternohyoid and sternothyroid muscles
    - Thyroid and parathyroid glands
- Posterior Triangle
  - Occipital triangle
    - Occipital artery at apex
    - Accessory nerve (cranial nerve XI)
    - Posterior branches of cervical plexus of nerves
    - Trunks of brachial plexus
    - Transverse cervical artery
    - Cervical lymph nodes
  - Supraclavicular triangle
    - External jugular vein
    - Suprascapular artery
    - Subclavian artery (third part)

cle, as its name implies, acts with other muscles to rotate or elevate the scapula. Therefore, it is described with muscles of the upper limb (see Figs. 27–1 and 27–3.)

Table 27–2 summarizes structures within the anterior and posterior triangles.

STRUCTURES THAT INTEGRATE THE NECK: THE FASCIAL PLANES

Beneath the superficial skin of the neck, there are three deep cervical fascial layers, as well as neurovascular compartments called the carotid sheaths

Some cervical fascial layers are well-defined fibrous sheaths, whereas others are thinner or less well-organized fibrous sheaths around structures. Areas of loose connective tissue between layers are often described as fascial "spaces" of the neck.

There is some variability in the anatomic nomenclature used for particular layers. The skin, with its accompanying subcutaneous lymph nodes, fatty tissue, superficial nerves and blood vessels, and the platysma muscle comprise what is often described as the **superficial fascial layer.** Inside this perimeter, the **deep cervical fascia** has three layers: one encircling the neck and two enclosing two inner compartments. Their names and functions are as follows:

- the **superficial investing layer** completely surrounds the neck;
- the **middle pretracheal (visceral) layer** encloses cervical viscera such as the trachea and esophagus; and
- the **deep prevertebral layer** encircles the vertebral column and muscles associated with the vertebrae (Fig. 27–4).

In the anterolateral areas on either side of the neck, these three layers blend with a fibrous lamina called the **carotid sheath,** creating a neurovascular compartment. The carotid sheath, which surrounds the internal jugular, common carotid, and vagus nerves, is also considered part of the deep cervical fascia (Fig. 27–4).

The layers of fascia in the neck afford a small degree of protection against sharp, penetrating objects and allow structures to glide past one another during functions such as swallowing or turning of the head. The separation of fascial planes by the fascia may limit the spread of infection from one plane to another. The laminar divisions can be separated during surgical procedures.

▲ Divisions of the Deep Cervical Fascia Layers

The **investing layer of fascia** encircles the neck just underneath the dermis. It splits into superficial and deep layers to enclose the trapezius muscles at the sides of the neck and the sternal portion of the sternocleidomastoid muscles (Fig. 27–4). The superficial layer attaches to the anterior manubrium and the deep layer to the posterior manubrium.

The investing layer extends superiorly from the manubrium, clavicles, and acromium of the scapula to the skull. It has attachments to the hyoid bone and the anteroinferior border of the mandible and, more laterally, to the zygomatic arches and mastoid processes of the temporal bones. Posteriorly, it is continuous with the nuchal ligament, which is a medial fibrous septum between the muscles on either side of the neck.

The **pretracheal layer** of deep cervical fascia, immediately behind (and sometimes including) the infrahyoid muscles, surrounds the trachea, thyroid gland, and esophagus in a space described as the visceral compartment (Fig. 27–4). This fascial layer blends laterally with the carotid sheaths, is continuous posteriorly with the buccopharyngeal fascia of the pharynx, and extends inferiorly from the hyoid bone to blend with the fibrous pericardium.

The **prevertebral layer** is the innermost layer of deep cervical fascia, enclosing the vertebral column and

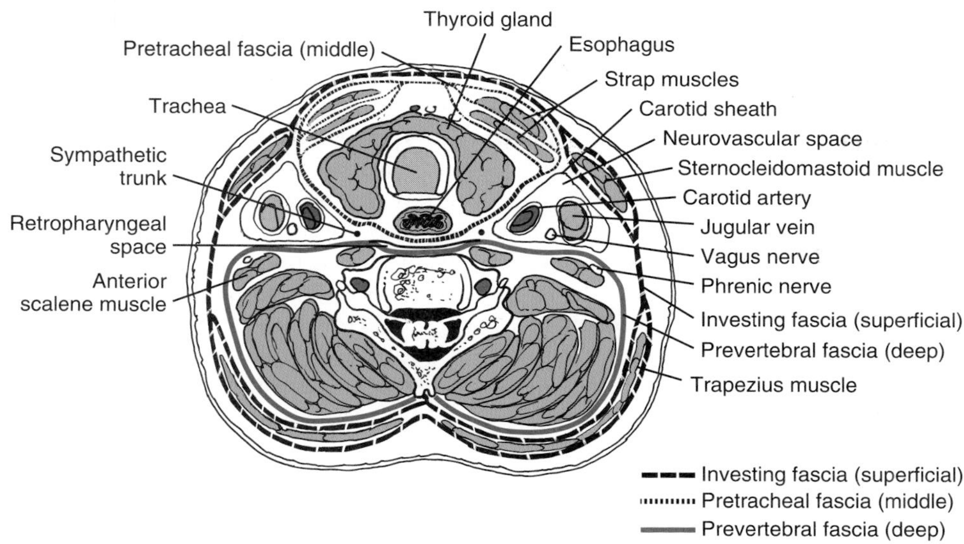

FIGURE 27–4
Cervical fascial layers.

muscles associated with it from the skull down to vertebra T3. Its lateral extension encloses the brachial plexus, axillary vessels, and sympathetic trunks. In the area directly anterior to the vertebral column, the prevertebral fascia splits into two layers. The anterior portion is sometimes given a separate name, the **alar fascia.** The area between the buccopharyngeal fascia and the prevertebral fascia is the **retropharyngeal space.** (Some anatomists apply this term more narrowly to describe just the area between the two prevertebral layers.)

Although the fascial layers compartmentalize and separate the structures within the neck, they communicate freely with other cavities of the body. For example, the carotid sheath and pretracheal fascia communicate inferiorly with the mediastinum of the thorax and superiorly with the cranial cavity, providing a pathway for the spread of infection to these areas.

Spaces between some of the fascial layers can also be important for function. For example, the retropharyngeal space between the prevertebral fascia and the buccopharyngeal fascia allows movement of the pharynx, esophagus, larynx, and trachea during actions such as swallowing.

▲ Endocrine Viscera of the Neck

Two ductless hormone-secreting glands, the thyroid and parathyroid glands, are enclosed within the pretracheal (visceral) layer of deep cervical fascia

Development of the Thyroid and Parathyroid Glands

The thyroid and parathyroid glands begin to develop by the fifth week and migrate to their adult positions by week seven

The **thyroid gland** develops from an invagination of the tongue endoderm at the position of the foramen cecum (see Fig. 26–7). The gland primordium migrates ventrocaudally at the end of a slender thyroglossal duct. This duct normally breaks down by the fifth week of development, and the glandular structure, already composed of lateral lobes connected by a well-defined isthmus, descends to its final position inferior to the cricoid cartilage by the seventh week. Studies show that it begins to function within the embryo, incorporating iodine into thyroid hormone, as early as week 10 to 12.

C cells within the thyroid gland that produce calcitonin originate from a separate source. During development, small paired invaginations behind the fourth pharyngeal pouches become populated by epithelial cells and form **ultimobranchial bodies.** These bodies detach and migrate mediocaudally to implant within the dorsal wall of the thyroid gland.

Knowing how the thyroid gland develops helps explain the occurrence of several abnormal conditions. Occasionally, a portion of the thyroglossal duct persists, resulting in a self-contained thyroglossal cyst or thyroglossal sinus, which may communicate with the surface of the neck. If present, cysts are most commonly found in the anterior part of the neck, near the body of the hyoid bone. Rarely, a fragment of the thyroid gland becomes detached during descent and forms a patch of ectopic thyroid tissue. This may be the only thyroid gland tissue present in the individual.

By the fifth week of development, rudiments for both the inferior and **superior parathyroid glands** have formed in the third and fourth pharyngeal pouches, respectively. Both rudiments detach from the pharynx and migrate inferomedially, coming to rest by the seventh week at their final superior and inferior positions on the dorsal side of the thyroid gland.

Thyroid Gland

The **thyroid gland** is the largest endocrine gland in the body, and its major product, thyroid hormone (thyroxin), affects all parts of the body except the thyroid gland itself, the brain, the spleen, the testes, and the uterus. Thyroid hormone regulates the rate of metabolism, while another of its hormones, calcitonin, affects calcium metabolism.

The gland is bilobed, lying deep to the sternothyroid and sternohyoid muscles and just anterior to the larynx and trachea at the level of vertebrae C5 through T1. The right and left lobes are united anteriorly by an isthmus (Fig. 27–5*A*). The thyroid gland has a thin fibrous capsule and is enclosed by the pretracheal deep cervical fascia. Dense connective tissue from the posterior of the thyroid gland attaches its capsule to the cricoid cartilage and superior border tracheal rings (Fig. 27–5*B*).

The thyroid gland is highly vascularized by the inferior and superior thyroid arteries. The superior thyroid arteries are branches of the external carotid arteries, which pierce the visceral pretracheal fascia to supply the superior pole of each lobe of the gland. An anterior branch descends on either side and anastomoses across the midline. A posterior branch of the superior thyroid artery supplies the posterior side of the gland and anastomoses with the inferior thyroid artery. The inferior thyroid artery is a branch of the thyrocervical trunk, which arises from the subclavian artery. It supplies the inferior pole of the gland.

In a small percentage of individuals, an additional artery is found, the **thyroid ima artery.** This artery normally arises from the brachiocephalic trunk and ascends on the anterior surface of the trachea to reach the isthmus of the gland that it supplies.

Because of the possibility that this arterial variation might be present, care must be taken in surgical procedures such as tracheostomies to avoid severing it and causing unnecessary bleeding. The cricothyroid membrane is the preferred point of access for emergency airway procedures.

Three pairs of veins, the superior, middle, and inferior veins, serve the superior, middle, and inferior parts of the gland. The two upper pairs drain into the internal jugular vein, and the inferior thyroid vein drains into the brachiocephalic vein.

Innervation of the thyroid gland is from the superior, middle, and inferior sympathetic ganglia. These

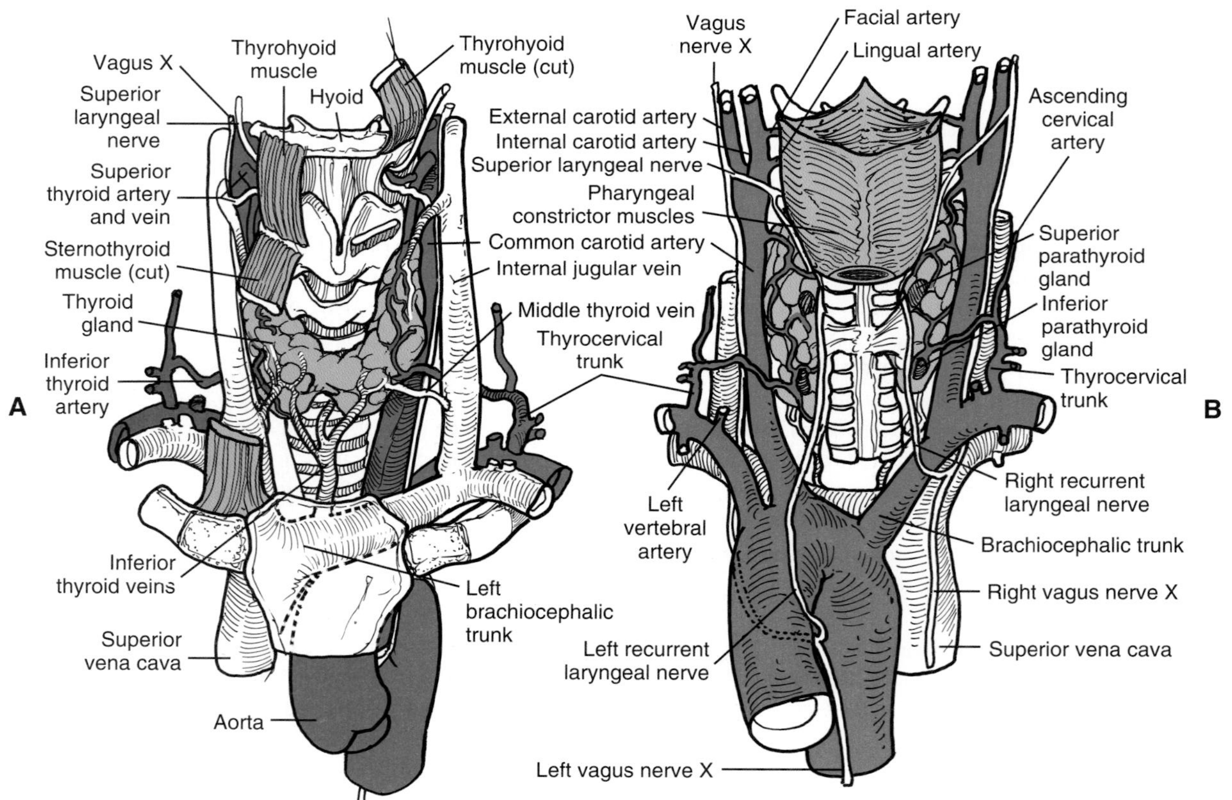

FIGURE 27–5
Thyroid and parathyroid glands. **A.** Anterior view. **B.** Posterior view. Inferior constrictor muscles are shown in a cutaway view, and the esophagus has been removed to show the connection of the thyroid gland to the trachea.

nerve fibers are vasomotor fibers, causing constriction of blood vessels, and travel primarily with plexuses surrounding the thyroid arteries. Secretomotor control of the gland is hormonally regulated by the pituitary gland.

It is normal for the thyroid gland to enlarge somewhat in females during periods of menstruation and pregnancy. Any other enlargement of the gland is termed a **goiter.** This condition can be common in people living in areas of the world where iodine is lacking in the diet. Enlargement of the thyroid gland can have other causes, including a disorder in which excessive thyroid hormone is produced. One symptom of this disease, termed **exophthalmic goiter,** is bulging eyeballs. Any form of goiter has the potential to compress the trachea, esophagus, and recurrent laryngeal nerve.

Parathyroid Glands

Most people have two pairs of small oval **parathyroid glands** (Fig. 27–5*B*). They are generally found on the posteromedial sides of the thyroid gland within its sheath, but the exact location and even the number of glands vary (e.g., about 5% of people have more than four parathyroid glands). The superior pair is generally found at the inferior border of the cricoid cartilage, above the entrance level of the inferior thyroid arteries. The inferior pair is often found on the inferior pole of the thyroid gland, below the arterial entry level.

Because the location of the parathyroid lobes varies, care must be taken to avoid inadvertent removal of the glands during thyroid surgery.

The parathyroid hormone, **parathormone,** controls the metabolism of phosphorus and calcium in the blood. The main target organs are the skeleton, kidneys, intestine, and muscle. Atrophy or inadvertent removal of the glands can quickly lead to convulsive muscle spasms.

The parathyroid glands can be served by the inferior or superior thyroid arteries or the laryngeal or tracheal arteries, depending on their positions relative to the thyroid gland.

Innervation of the parathyroid glands is from thyroid branches of the cervical sympathetic ganglia.

▲ Respiratory Viscera of the Neck: Larynx and Trachea

The larynx and trachea function together to provide an airway and produce vocalization

Specifically, the musculocartilaginous larynx, which connects the oropharynx with the trachea, functions to close off the airway during swallowing, to regulate air entering or leaving the lungs, to help vary intraabdominal pressure (e.g., building up pressure to facilitate coughing), and to allow vocalization. Vocalization is so important, in fact, that phonation (the uttering of sound by the vocal cords) is usually considered the larynx's prime function. These highly complex functions are possible because of articulations between the parts of the cartilaginous skeleton and the system of fibroelastic ligaments and membranes controlled by the intrinsic muscles.

Cartilaginous Structure of the Larynx

The cartilaginous skeleton of the larynx helps protect the air passages during swallowing

The **larynx** is at the inferior end of the oropharynx. It extends from the tongue to the trachea. In males, its position is level with the third to sixth vertebrae. The adult female larynx is smaller and slightly higher in position.

Nine cartilages make up the skeleton of the larynx, with the hyoid bone at its superior edge. The three largest cartilages are unpaired: the epiglottic, thyroid, and cricoid cartilages. The six remaining cartilages are paired: the arytenoid, corniculate, and cuneiform cartilages. All nine are joined by ligaments and membranes.

The heart-shaped **epiglottic cartilage** sits at the junction between the mouth and the laryngeal inlet (Figs. 27–6 and 27–7 and see Fig. 26–15). It is posterior to the root of the tongue and anterior to the laryngeal tract. It forms the superior part of the laryngeal inlet. Anteriorly, it is attached to the hyoid bone by the hyoepiglottic ligament (Fig. 27–7*C* and *D*). Its narrow posterior stalk attaches to the angle formed by the thyroid laminae by the thyroepiglottic ligament. It is covered by a thin layer of connective tissue on both its anterior and posterior surfaces.

The **thyroid cartilage** is the largest unpaired cartilage and forms the main body of the larynx. The prominence at the midline, where two platelike laminae fuse, is commonly known as the laryngeal prominence (Adam's apple). Superior to this prominence, the two laminae diverge to form a V-shaped notch called the **superior thyroid notch.** Oblique diagonal lines across the laminae serve as attachment sites for muscles. The cartilage has upward extensions called **superior horns** posteriorly. The entire upper edge of the cartilage attaches to the hyoid bone by the **thyrohyoid membrane** (Fig. 27–6). The thyroid cartilage also has side extensions, the **inferior horns,** at its inferior end. These horns articulate with the lateral surfaces of the cricoid cartilage. The articulations are called the **cricothyroid joints.** They allow movements of the larynx that change the length of the vocal cords. The inferior portion of the thyroid cartilage also attaches to cricoid cartilage at its medial surface by the median cricothyroid ligament.

The **cricoid cartilage** is the only cartilage to completely encircle the airway passage. It is shaped like a signet ring, with a smaller anterior band called the **arch** and a wider posterior (signet) portion called the **lamina** (Fig. 27–6*B*). At its inferior end, it attaches to the first

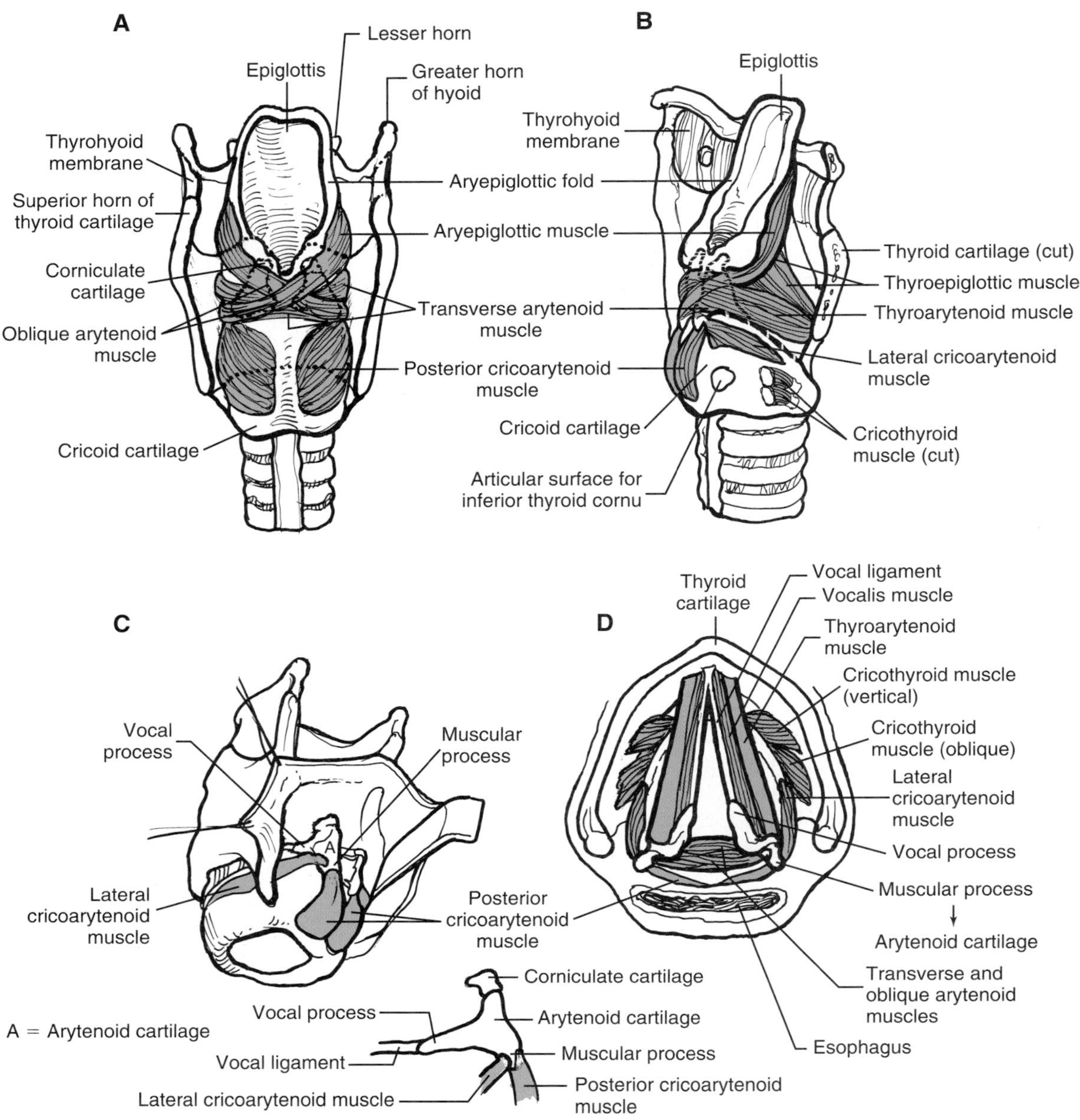

FIGURE 27–6

Cartilages and intrinsic muscles of the larynx. **A.** Posterior view. The arytenoid and thyroid cartilages are outlined with dotted lines. **B.** Right oblique, lateral view. **C.** Posterior detail featuring arytenoid cartilage. **D.** Superior view showing the relationship of muscles to vocal ligaments and arytenoid cartilages.

tracheal "ring" by the cricotracheal ligament. Superiorly, it attaches to the inferior margin of the thyroid cartilage by the median cricothyroid ligament.

The three paired cartilages are the arytenoid, corniculate, and cuneiform cartilages

Inferior to the thyroid cartilage are found the pair of **arytenoid cartilages,** which are important for approximating, tensing, and relaxing the vocal cords (Fig. 27–6C, detail). The arytenoid cartilages are pyramidal in shape. Their bases articulate with the superolateral laminal surfaces of the cricoid cartilage. These cricoarytenoid joints allow the arytenoid cartilages to slide together or apart, tilt, or rotate. These actions approximate, tense, or relax the vocal folds.

A **muscular process** projects laterally from the base of each arytenoid cartilage. This process acts as a lever, since it is the attachment site for the posterior and lat-

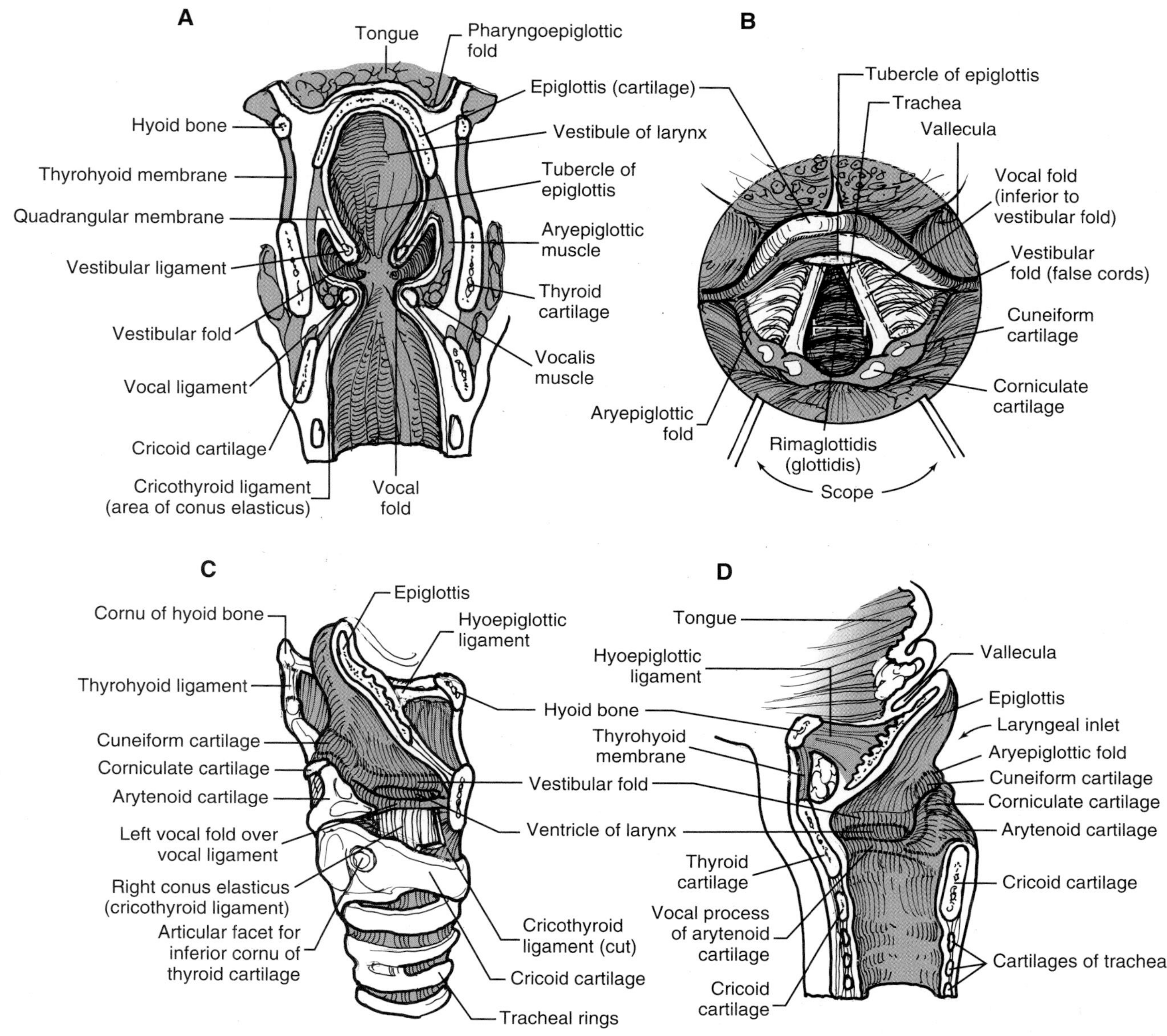

FIGURE 27–7
A. Coronal section of the larynx. **B.** Laryngoscopic view. **C.** Partial sagittal section. **D.** Complete sagittal section.

eral cricoarytenoid muscles. Anteriorly, the arytenoid cartilage has the **vocal process**, which provides the posterior attachment for the vocal ligament.

Each arytenoid cartilage has a superior apex on which is found the **corniculate cartilage** and an attachment to the epiglottic cartilage via the aryepiglottic fold (Fig. 27–7*D*).

The **cuneiform cartilages** are small elastic fibrocartilages appearing as small nodules slightly superoanterior to the corniculate cartilages on the aryepiglottic folds (Figs. 27–6*C* and 27–7*D*).

Articulations and Ligaments of the Larynx

Synovial joints permit rotation and gliding movements between the thyroid and cricoid cartilages and between the cricoid cartilage and the bases of the arytenoid cartilages.

Extrinsic ligaments connect the larynx to extralaryngeal structures (Fig. 27–7*C* and *D*), which include

- **thyrohyoid membrane** (connecting the thyroid cartilage to the hyoid bone),
- **hyoepiglottic ligament** (connecting the anterior epiglottis to the hyoid bone), and

- **cricotracheal ligament** (connecting the cricoid cartilage to the first tracheal cartilage).

The intrinsic ligaments of the larynx are fibroelastic membranes beneath the laryngeal mucosa that connect laryngeal cartilages to one another (Fig. 27–7). These include the

- **thyroepiglottic ligament** (connecting the epiglottis to the thyroid cartilage),
- **quadrangular membrane** (connecting the arytenoid cartilages and the epiglottis), and
- **cricothyroid ligament** (connecting the thyroid, cricoid, and arytenoid cartilages).

The superior margin of the quadrangular membrane, a thin sheet of connective tissue, is covered by mucosa to form the aryepiglottic fold.

The vocal ligaments that support the vocal folds are the medial, free edges of the cricothyroid ligament, the conus elasticus

The **conus elasticus** (comprised of the cricothyroid ligament, which is sometimes referred to as the **cricovocal membrane)** is a fibroelastic membrane that arises from the entire upper border of the arch of the cricoid cartilage. Its free, thickened medial edges attach anteriorly to the mid-dorsal surface of the thyroid cartilage and posteriorly to the vocal processes of the arytenoid cartilages. These upward-projecting thickened edges form the vocal ligaments. The vocalis muscles insert onto the vocal ligaments, and, together with the overlying mucous membrane, they form the vocal folds.

Interior of the Larynx

The anterior inlet to the larynx is bounded by the upper portion of the epiglottis, with the aryepiglottic folds forming the lateral sides and mucosa of the arytenoid cartilages at the back. Paired folds of mucosa, the superior **vestibular folds** (false vocal folds) and the inferior **vocal folds** (vocal cords), partially divide the space within the laryngeal cavity (Fig. 27–7*A*). The space midway between the vocal folds is the **rima glottidis** (Fig. 27–7*B*). (*Rima* is from the Latin for "slit" or "fissure." *Glottis* technically applies to the vocal folds and entire vocal apparatus, but it is sometimes used in a general way to describe the aperture alone.) The area from the inlet to the vestibular folds is called the **laryngeal vestibule;** the lateral pocket between the vestibular folds and the vocal folds is called the **ventricle;** and the region from the vocal folds to the trachea is called the **infraglottic cavity** (Fig. 27–7*A*).

Intrinsic Muscles of the Larynx and their Functions

Intrinsic muscles that connect structures entirely within the larynx can be grouped by their main functions, which are to modify the laryngeal inlet and regulate the glottis during respiration and vocalization

In addition to the basic function of the human larynx as a sphincter, which prevents swallowed materials from entering the trachea, closes off the airway to build pressure for coughing, and facilitates strenuous muscular effort, the larynx is highly specialized to perform complex actions. Muscles acting on the rima glottidis allow a person to have voluntary control of respiratory functions so that a person can hold his or her breath or breathe deeply. These muscles also control vocal production by bringing the vocal folds together and tensing them so that air vibrates as it passes through the rima glottidis. Some have suggested that the capacity for speech, with its accompanying written symbolism, has been fundamental to the development of human intelligence.

Muscles that modify the laryngeal inlet are protective during swallowing

The muscles that modify the laryngeal inlet are the

- oblique arytenoid,
- aryepiglottic, and
- thyroepiglottic muscles.

The **oblique arytenoid muscles** are two bands that arise from the muscular processes of the arytenoid cartilages and cross one another to reach the apex of the arytenoid cartilages on the opposite side. Some fibers continue beyond the arytenoid cartilages within the aryepiglottic fold to form the **aryepiglottic muscles** (see Fig. 27–6*A* and *B*). The **thyroepiglottic muscles** are formed from muscle fibers of the upper portion of the thyroarytenoid muscle. These fibers extend upward toward the aryepiglottic fold and insert into both the quadrangular membrane and the epiglottic margin (see Fig. 27–6*B*). The thyroarytenoid muscle originates from the inner surface of the thyroid angle. Its lower portion inserts on the lateral border of the arytenoid cartilage and regulates the vocal ligaments (see discussion below).

The oblique arytenoid and aryepiglottic muscles *act* as sphincter muscles, while the thyroepiglottic muscles widen the inlet by their actions on the aryepiglottic folds.

Muscles controlling the glottis that function in respiration are the posterior cricoarytenoids (abductors) and the lateral cricoarytenoids and transverse and oblique arytenoids (adductors).

Only one muscle pair, the posterior cricoarytenoid muscles, abducts the vocal folds. Intrinsic muscles that adduct the vocal folds include the lateral cricoarytenoid and transverse and oblique arytenoid muscles (see Fig. 27–6*A* and *B*).

The **posterior cricoarytenoid muscles** arise from either side of the midline of the posterior surface of the cricoid cartilage and ascend laterally to the muscular processes of the arytenoid cartilages, covering most of the cricoid cartilage's posterior lamina (see Fig. 27–6*A* and *D*). They increase the size of the respiratory orifice during breathing, abducting the vocal folds to open the rima glottidis (Fig. 27–8*C*). Their role in vocalization is discussed below.

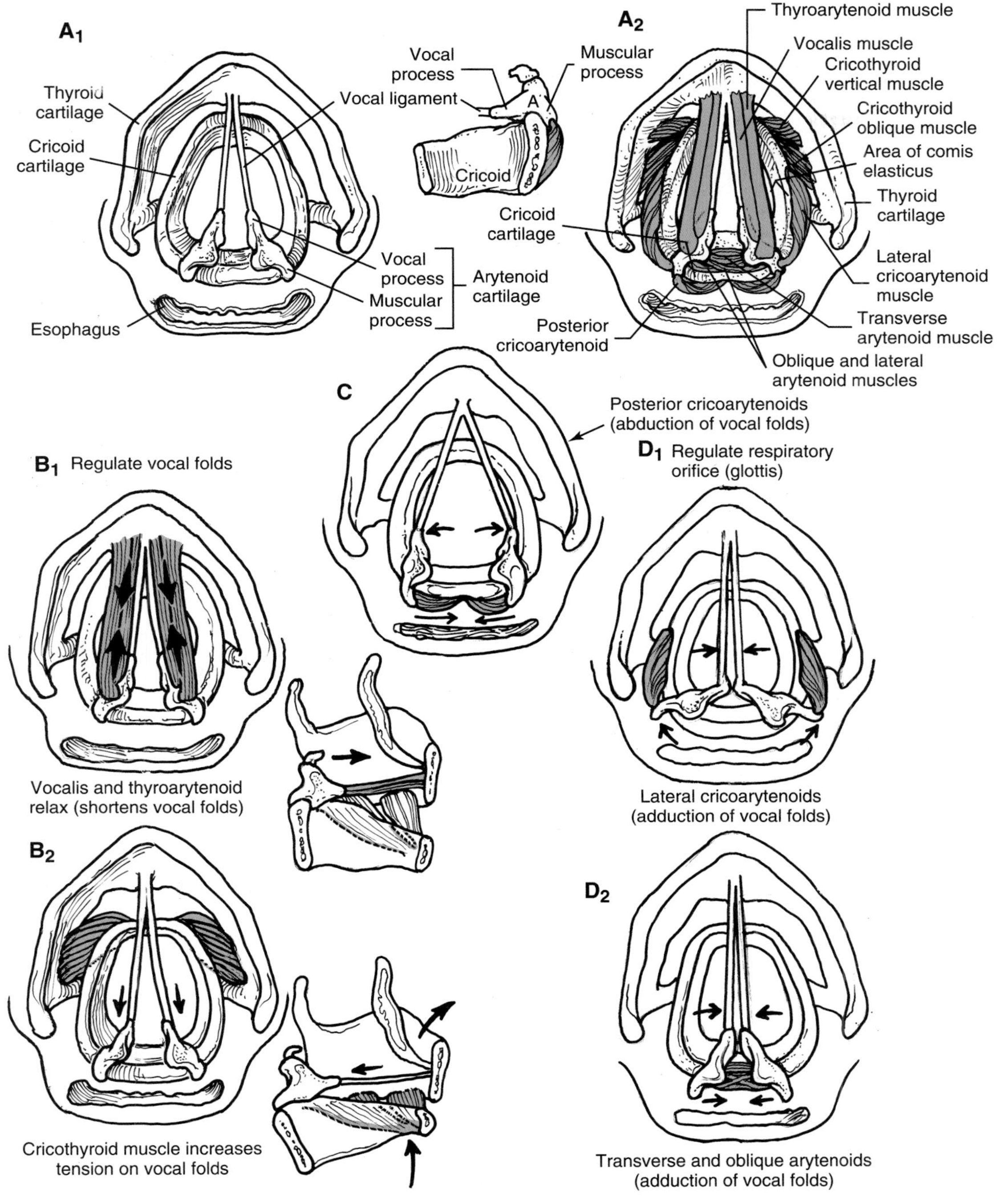

FIGURE 27–8

Laryngeal muscle function in vocalization and respiration. **A.** Superior view of cartilages alone *(1)* and with muscles *(2)*. **B₁** and **B₂**. Muscles regulating tension of the vocal folds. The vocalis, thyroarytenoid, and cricothyroid muscles are shown. **C.** Cricoarytenoid muscles abduct the vocal folds for breathing and vocalization. **D₁** and **D₂**. Muscles regulating the respiratory orifice (glottis) are the cricoarytenoid transverse and oblique arytenoid muscles.

The **lateral cricoarytenoid muscles** are smaller than the posterior muscles. They extend backward from the upper cricoid arch border to the arytenoid muscular processes (see Fig. 27–6*B* and *D*). They decrease the size of the rima glottidis during speech, swallowing, or increased intraabdominal pressure (straining) by adducting the vocal folds (Fig. 27–8*D*).

The only unpaired muscle of the larynx, the **transverse arytenoid muscle,** connects the muscular processes of the two arytenoid cartilages (see Fig. 26–6*A* and *D*). When the muscle contracts, along with some lower fibers of the **oblique arytenoid muscle,** the two arytenoid muscles move closer together and the glottis closes (Fig. 27–8*D*).

Muscles controlling the glottis that regulate the tension of the vocal ligaments during vocalization are the vocalis, thyroarytenoid, cricothyroid, and posterior cricoarytenoid muscles.

The **vocalis muscle** and lower portion of the **thyroarytenoid muscle** are both closely associated with the conus elasticus and the vocal ligament. Both originate from the inner surface of the lower half of the thyroid angle and insert on the anterolateral surface of the arytenoid cartilage (see Fig. 27–6*D*). The vocalis muscle inserts on the lateral surface of the vocal process. Its deeper fibers run lateral to the vocal ligament and along the conus elasticus below the ligament. The insertion of the thyroarytenoid muscle on the arytenoid surface is slightly lateral to the insertion of the vocalis muscle. Some fibers of the thyroarytenoid muscle continue upward toward the aryepiglottic fold (see discussion of thyroepiglottic muscles above).

The **cricothyroid muscle** originates from the external surface of the arch of cricoid cartilage and covers the cricothyroid ligament (see Fig. 27–6*A* and *D*). Fibers travel in an oblique path to the inferior cornu of the thyroid cartilage and in a straighter path to the lower posterior border of the thyroid cartilage.

The **thyroarytenoid muscles** draw the arytenoid muscles toward the thyroid cartilage, shortening and relaxing the vocal ligaments. The deeper **vocalis muscles** selectively tense or relax parts of the vocal folds, producing slight adjustments during speech and singing (Fig. 27–8*B*).

The **cricothyroid muscles** tilt the cricoid cartilage, effectively pulling the thyroid cartilage anteriorly. This increases the distance between the vocal processes of the arytenoid cartilages and their attachments on the thyroid cartilage, stretching the vocal ligaments (Fig. 27–8*B*).

The abducting action of the **posterior cricoarytenoid muscles** also retracts the arytenoid cartilages, thereby assisting the cricothyroid muscles in tensing the vocal folds (Fig. 27–8*C*).

Innervation of the Larynx by Superior Laryngeal and Recurrent Laryngeal Branches of the Vagus Nerve

The **superior laryngeal nerve** from the inferior ganglion of the vagus nerve descends in the neck along the pharynx and medial to the internal carotid artery. It sends two branches to the larynx. The larger **internal branch** crosses the posterior part of the thyrohyoid membrane and penetrates it above the superior laryngeal artery. It provides sensory innervation to the mucosal surface of the larynx above the vocal folds, as well as both epiglottic surfaces. The **external branch** curves forward below the thyroid cartilage to supply motor innervation to the cricothyroid muscle (see Fig. 26–13). The superior laryngeal nerve also carries parasympathetic fibers to the mucous glands of the larynx and pharynx.

The **recurrent laryngeal branch** of the vagus nerve reaches the larynx from the ventral side, dividing into motor and sensory branches. The motor branch supplies all the intrinsic muscles of the larynx except the cricothyroid. Below the vocal folds, the sensory branch provides sensory innervation to the laryngeal lining and parasympathetic fibers to mucous glands of the larynx.

The path of the recurrent laryngeal nerve is different on the two sides of the body because of the asymmetric development of the aortic arches. On the left side, the nerve branches from the vagus nerve near the aortic arch, curves backward beneath it, and ascends along the groove between the trachea and the esophagus. On the right side, it branches from the vagus nerve anterior to the subclavian artery, curves around it posteriorly, and turns obliquely toward the trachea, where it ascends behind the common carotid artery (see Fig. 27–5). Fibers from the recurrent laryngeal nerve also join descending branches from the superior laryngeal nerve.

Cough Reflex

If a foreign substance enters the laryngeal outlet, the internal branch of the superior laryngeal nerve of the vagus nerve is the afferent limb of the cough reflex. Efferent motor fibers from the vagus nerve, along with spinal nerves and the phrenic nerve, first abduct the vocal cords by the posterior cricoarytenoid muscles, so the person can gasp for breath, and then close the larynx as the vestibular folds come together. When pressure increases in the thorax, the folds open, letting air out rapidly in a cough to expel the foreign substance.

Paralysis of Recurrent Laryngeal Nerve. Since posterior and anterior branches of the vagus nerve's recurrent laryngeal nerve innervate all the muscles concerned with active movement of the vocal cords, paralysis of either recurrent laryngeal nerve causes severe impairment of vocalization. Over time, the paralyzed vocal cord may move toward the midline, resulting in some improvement in the production of sound. Because the inferior laryngeal nerve is very close to the thyroid gland at the point where it enters the larynx, there is a serious risk of injury to the nerve during a thyroidectomy.

▲ Connections of the Esophagus to the Pharyngeal Muscles and Larynx

The **esophagus,** a tubal continuation of the pharynx, begins at the lower portion of the larynx and provides a passageway from the oropharynx to the stomach. It has both an outer longitudinal layer of muscles and an inner circular layer. Both are innervated by the recurrent laryngeal nerve from the vagus nerve. Since these muscle layers are striated, the branches from the vagus nerve are branchial efferent nerves rather than visceral efferent nerves. Branches from the inferior thyroid artery provide the blood supply. These nerves and blood vessels enter through a gap below the lateral attachment of the inferior constrictor muscle to the side of the cricoid cartilage (see Fig. 26–13).

The posterior portion of the outer longitudinal muscle layer divides into two bands around the lower border of the cricoid cartilage, exposing a small portion of the inner circular muscle. This portion of the circular musculature is continuous with the **cricopharyngeal muscle,** which is part of the inferior pharyngeal constrictor muscle of the pharynx (see Fig. 26–16). The two separate bands of longitudinal muscle pass forward around the esophagus and combine to form the **cricoesophageal tendon,** which connects the esophagus to the posterior cricoid cartilage of the larynx.

In the cervical area, the esophagus is a closed tube, unless food or liquid is passing through it.

NERVES INTEGRATING STRUCTURES WITHIN THE NECK

Functional distributions of cranial nerves IX through XII and the first four cervical spinal nerves are closely interrelated in the neck

Cranial Nerves

In addition to the cervical spinal nerves, four cranial nerves pass through and innervate structures in the neck: the glossopharyngeal nerve (cranial nerve IX), vagus nerve (cranial nerve X), hypoglossal nerve (cranial nerve XII), and accessory nerve (cranial nerve XI). Table 23–1 lists innervation targets and motor, sensory, and autonomic functions for these four (and all other) cranial nerves. Fig. 26–21 shows all cranial nerves emerging from the ventral side of the brain.

Cranial nerves IX, X, and XII were discussed in detail with the structures of the oropharynx and the sensation of taste in Chapter 26. (Branches of these nerves within the head and cervical region are shown in Figures 26–11 through 26–13.) In this chapter the anatomical structure and function of the only cranial nerve as yet undescribed, the accessory nerve (cranial nerve XI), will be introduced (Box 27–1). In addition, specific instances within the neck region where cranial nerves IX through XII interact with each other or with cervical nerves will be pointed out.

The hypoglossal nerve is joined by fibers from the ventral rami of the first or second cervical nerves (or both). These fibers later leave the hypoglossal nerve to form the superior loop of the ansa cervicalis (see the cervical plexus below).

The accessory nerve (cranial nerve XI) serves the sternocleidomastoid and trapezius muscles. It has a dual origin, from cranial and spinal roots. Its pathway is coordinated with that of other nerves serving the neck, both the vagus nerve and branches of the cervical spinal nerves (Box 27–1).

Cervical Spinal Nerves

Eight cervical nerves serve the neck. The first, spinal nerve C1, emerges from the vertebral canal between the occipital bone and the atlas and is therefore often termed the **suboccipital nerve.** The last, spinal nerve C8, emerges between vertebrae C7 and T1.

As has been described in Chapter 4, each spinal nerve is formed by a dorsal sensory root and a ventral motor root. The roots join, and the nerve then splits into a dorsal primary ramus and a ventral primary ramus. Each ramus contains all the fibers found in the entire nerve: sensory, motor, sympathetic efferent, and visceral afferent fibers. (See Figures 4–3, 4–6, and 4–12.) Dorsal rami supply deep back muscles and the skin on the back of the neck and scalp. Ventral rami

BOX 27–1

THE ACCESSORY NERVE

The **accessory nerve** (cranial nerve XI) is formed from both cranial and spinal roots. The cranial root emerges from the nucleus ambiguus in the medulla oblongata as four or five small rootlets (Fig. 27–9). As the cranial root travels through the jugular foramen, it is briefly joined by the spinal root but then divides into cranial and spinal portions. The **cranial division** joins the vagus nerve at the inferior vagal ganglion. This portion of the nerve travels with the recurrent laryngeal nerve to the larynx. The **spinal division** arises from fibers that emerge between the cervical dorsal and ventral spinal roots. The trunk formed by these fibers ascends toward the foramen magnum of the skull and turns in a lateral direction to pass through the jugular foramen. After it exits the jugular foramen, the spinal division travels posterior to the internal jugular vein. It descends obliquely, medial to the styloid process, to reach the upper part of the sternocleidomastoid muscle's deep surface, joining branches of the **second** and **third cervical spinal nerves** that also supply that muscle. The accessory nerve's spinal root supplies motor innervation, while the second and third cervical spinal nerves carry proprioceptive information back to the central nervous system (Fig. 27–9).

As the **accessory spinal root** emerges from the sternocleidomastoid muscle's posterior border, it crosses the posterior triangle. Here it receives fibers from **spinal nerves C3** and **C4.** These three nerves innervate the trapezius muscle. The accessory nerve again provides motor innervation, while spinal nerves C3 and C4 send proprioceptive fibers and some motor fibers to the muscle (Fig. 27–9).

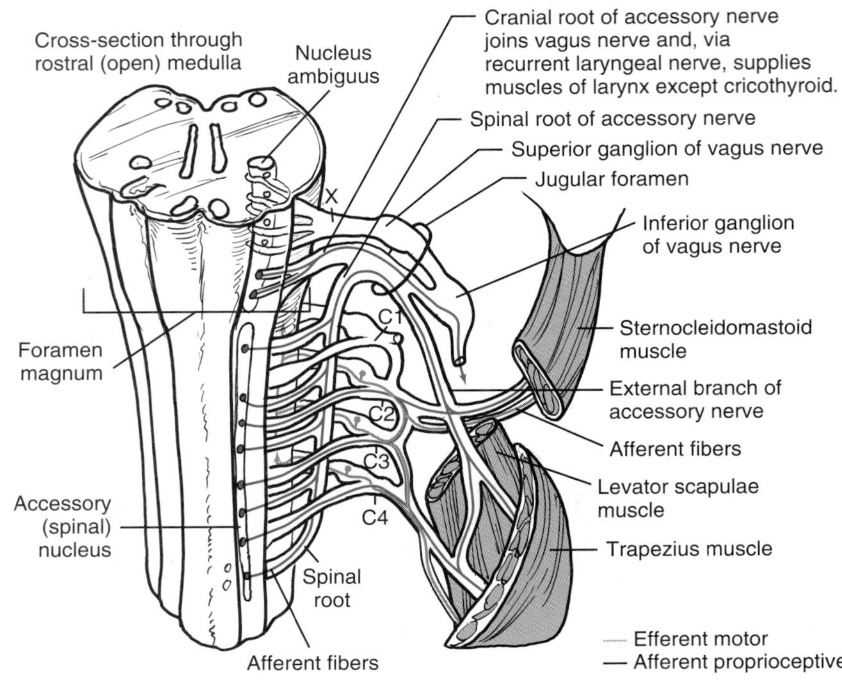

FIGURE 27–9
Accessory nerve (cranial nerve XI).

supply motor innervation to the anterolateral musculature of the neck and sensory innervation to the skin overlying these muscles. The ventral rami of the cervical nerves connect near their points of origin to form the cervical and brachial plexuses. Dorsal rami of the cervical nerves remain independent and do not unite to form a plexus.

Dorsal Rami of the Cervical Nerves

Cervical dorsal rami supply the muscles and skin of the posterior regions of the neck and upper trunk

The first cervical dorsal ramus **(suboccipital nerve)** emerges superior to the posterior arch of the atlas and enters the suboccipital triangle to supply muscles of the back of the neck, which are the rectus capitis posterior major and minor, superior and inferior oblique capitis, and semispinalis capitis muscles (see Fig. 5–8).

The second cervical dorsal ramus emerges between the atlas and the axis and divides into two branches. The medial branch **(greater occipital nerve)** supplies the skin of the back of the scalp, the trapezius muscle, and the semispinalis capitis muscles (see Fig. 24–4*B* and *C*). It is joined by a branch from the third cervical dorsal ramus. The lateral branch supplies the longissimus capitis and semispinalis capitis muscles.

The third cervical dorsal ramus has a medial branch that supplies the skin at the back of the neck at the level of the splenius capitis muscle. A portion of the ramus, the **third occipital nerve,** supplies the skin of the lower occipital region (see Fig. 24–4*C*).

The fourth and fifth dorsal rami innervate the muscles and skin at the level of the splenius and trapezius muscles. The lowest three rami are small, with medial branches serving muscles at the back of the neck.

Innervation by the Cervical Plexus (Ventral Rami of the Cervical Nerves)

Cervical plexus nerves include sensory cutaneous branches and motor branches to the infrahyoid and prevertebral muscles

The **cervical plexus** is formed by the ventral rami of cervical nerves 1 to 4. (The lower four cervical nerves and the first thoracic ventral ramus form the brachial plexus.) The cervical plexus lies directly under the sternocleidomastoid muscle of the neck. All rami except the first one emerge between the anterior and posterior intertransverse muscles. Four major branches are cutaneous nerves, all sensory in function. They are the

- ♦ lesser occipital nerve,
- ♦ great auricular nerve,
- ♦ transverse cervical nerve, and
- ♦ supraclavicular nerve.

Generally originating from the ventral rami of the second cervical nerve, the **lesser occipital nerve** runs vertically upward over the sternocleidomastoid muscle to serve the skin and scalp behind the ear. Directly below it, formed from portions of the second and third cervical nerves, the **great auricular nerve** follows the path of the external jugular vein and innervates the ear and skin around it. The **transverse cervical nerve (transverse cutaneous nerve),** which also branches

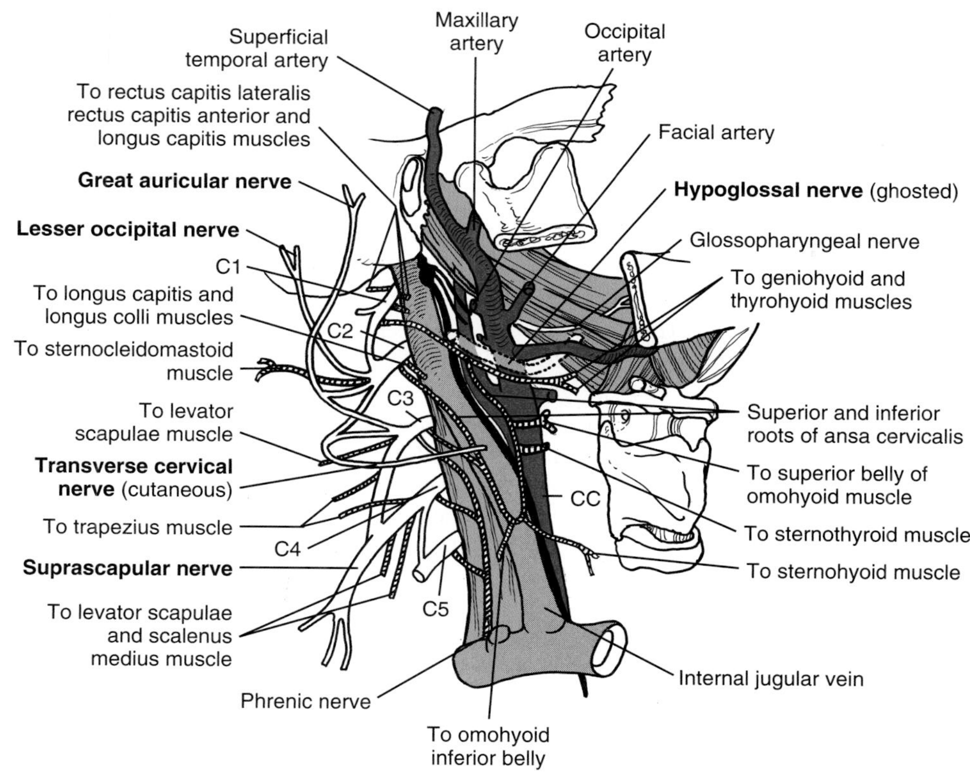

FIGURE 27–10

Nerves of the cervical plexus. C1 to C4 indicate ventral rami of cervical spinal nerves; muscular branches are striped; and the path of the hypoglossal nerve is shown by dotted lines. Cutaneous sensory branches are the great auricular nerves (C2, C3), lesser occipital nerves (C2, C3), transverse cervical nerves (C2, C3), and supraclavicular nerves (C3, C4). *CC,* Common carotid.

from the second and third cervical nerves, crosses over the sternocleidomastoid muscle to the front of the neck. It divides into two branches, which serve superior and inferior portions of the skin on the front of the neck (Fig. 27–10 and see Fig. 24–4). Branches of the lowest **supraclavicular nerve** (with fibers from the third and fourth cervical nerves) emerge within the cervical fascia in the posterior triangle and supply the skin on the anterior base of the neck, superior portion of the thorax, and top of the shoulder (Fig. 27–10).

Smaller efferent nerves from the cervical plexus innervate the prevertebral and infrahyoid muscles

The **prevertebral muscles** are innervated by small branches directly from the ventral rami of cervical nerves. The longus capitis and rectus capitis muscles are supplied superiorly, and the scalenus medius and levator scapulae muscles are supplied laterally. A muscle may be innervated by one or several cervical nerves. For example, nerve C1 sends branches to the rectus capitis lateralis muscle, but it also joins nerve C2 to innervate the longus capitis and rectus capitis anterior muscles. Direct branches to the sternocleidomastoid and trapezius muscles may also be present. Figure 27–10 is a schematic drawing of a sample of these muscular branches.

Infrahyoid muscles are innervated by branches from the **ansa cervicalis** (*ansa* means "loop") formed by fibers from nerves C1 through C3 (Fig. 27–10). The **superior root** of the ansa cervicalis is usually formed of the fibers from nerves C1 and C2 that "join" the hypoglossal nerve (cranial nerve XII). Some of these fibers travel with the hypoglossal nerve to innervate the thyrohyoid and geniohyoid muscles. Others descend as the superior root of the ansa cervicalis, some branching off to the superior belly of the omohyoid muscle. The **inferior root** of the ansa cervicalis, made up of fibers from nerves C2 and C3, descends in close proximity to the internal jugular vein. At the bottom of the loop (ansa cervicalis), efferent branches to the sternothyroid muscle, sternohyoid muscle, and inferior belly of the omohyoid muscle are given off (Fig. 27–10).

The **phrenic nerve** originates primarily from the fourth cervical ramus but also from the third and fifth rami. It travels along the scalene muscle directly underneath the muscle's prevertebral fascial layer. The phrenic nerve carries some sensory fibers, but its motor fibers are crucial because they are the only motor fibers supplying the diaphragm. See Chapter 10 for the phrenic nerve's function in regulating the diaphragm.

Nerves C5 through C8 become part of the brachial plexus (see Chapter 21, especially Fig. 21–26).

VASCULATURE SERVING THE NECK AND HEAD

Development of the Major Arteries

Asymmetric remodeling of the aortic arches during development results in asymmetry of the major vessels leaving the heart

All aortic arches except the fifth begin to develop between days 26 and 29 of fetal life. However, the first two arch pairs regress as the later pairs form and never become part of the major vessels from the heart. The third pair of aortic arches continues developing and eventually become the paired **common carotid arteries** and proximal portions of the **internal carotid arteries.** The fourth and sixth pairs of aortic arches undergo asymmetric remodeling during development.

On the right side, connections from the sixth arch are lost. The fourth arch acquires a branch, the right seventh cervical intersegmental artery, which grows into the right upper limb bud and becomes the **right subclavian artery.** The base of this vessel develops into the **brachiocephalic artery,** the first major branch of the dorsal aorta on the right side of the body (Fig. 27–11).

On the left side, the fourth aortic arch remains connected to the fused dorsal aorta and develops into part of the **aortic arch** and the most cranial portion of the **dorsal aorta.** The left seventh cervical intersegmental artery sprouts directly from the left dorsal aorta and gives rise to the **left subclavian artery** (Fig. 27–11). Consequently, on the left side of the heart, both the left subclavian artery and the common carotid artery branch directly from the dorsal aorta. The subclavian arteries from both sides, however, have similar pathways within the lower portion of the neck.

In contrast to the right side, the sixth aortic arch on the left side remains complete. Its distal portion forms the **ductus arteriosus,** which allows blood to shunt from the pulmonary trunk to the descending aorta throughout gestation. This bypass closes at birth and is later transformed into the **ligamentum arteriosum,** which attaches the pulmonary trunk to the aorta (Fig. 27–11).

Arteries in the Root of the Neck

Arteries that serve the head all originate from major branches emerging from the arch of the aorta

As has been shown above, during embryologic development the left common carotid artery branches directly from the arch of the aorta, while the right common carotid artery emerges from the brachiocephalic trunk. The common carotid arteries on both sides travel superiorly on either side of the trachea (Fig. 27–12). The thick fascia **(carotid sheath)** surrounding the carotid artery in the neck also encloses the internal jugular vein and vagus nerve. Slightly above the level of the superior border of the thyroid gland, the common carotid arteries branch into the **internal** and **external carotid arteries** (Fig. 27–13).

At the point where the common carotid artery splits, there is a somewhat dilated area called the **carotid sinus** (Fig. 27–13). Nerve endings in this por-

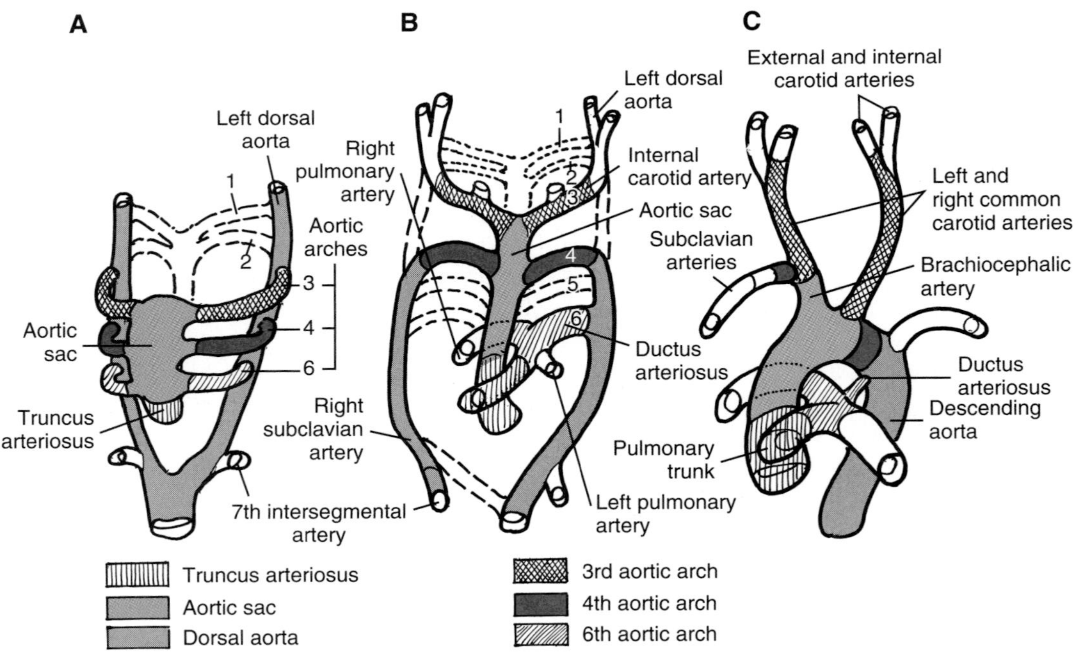

FIGURE 27–11
Embryological development of aortic arches.

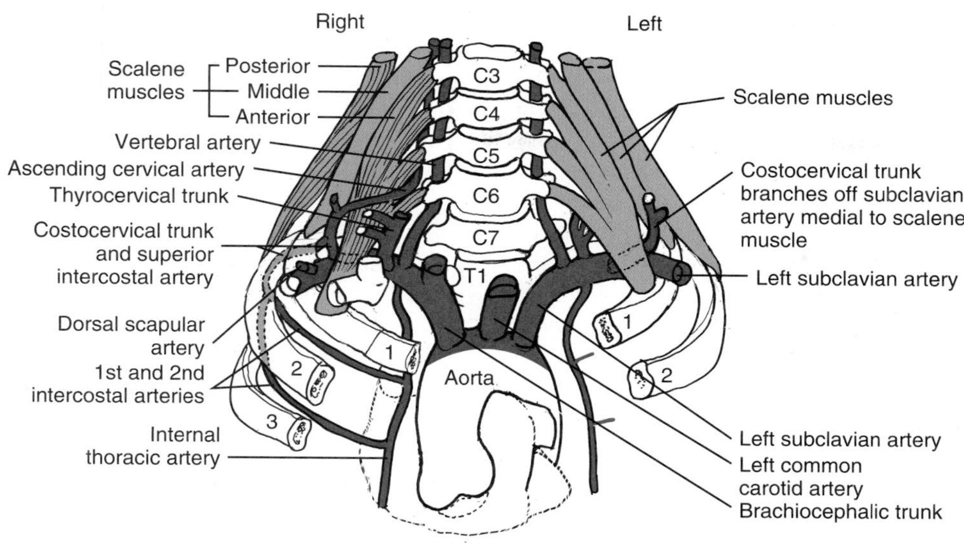

FIGURE 27–12
Pattern of branching of major vessels from the aorta.

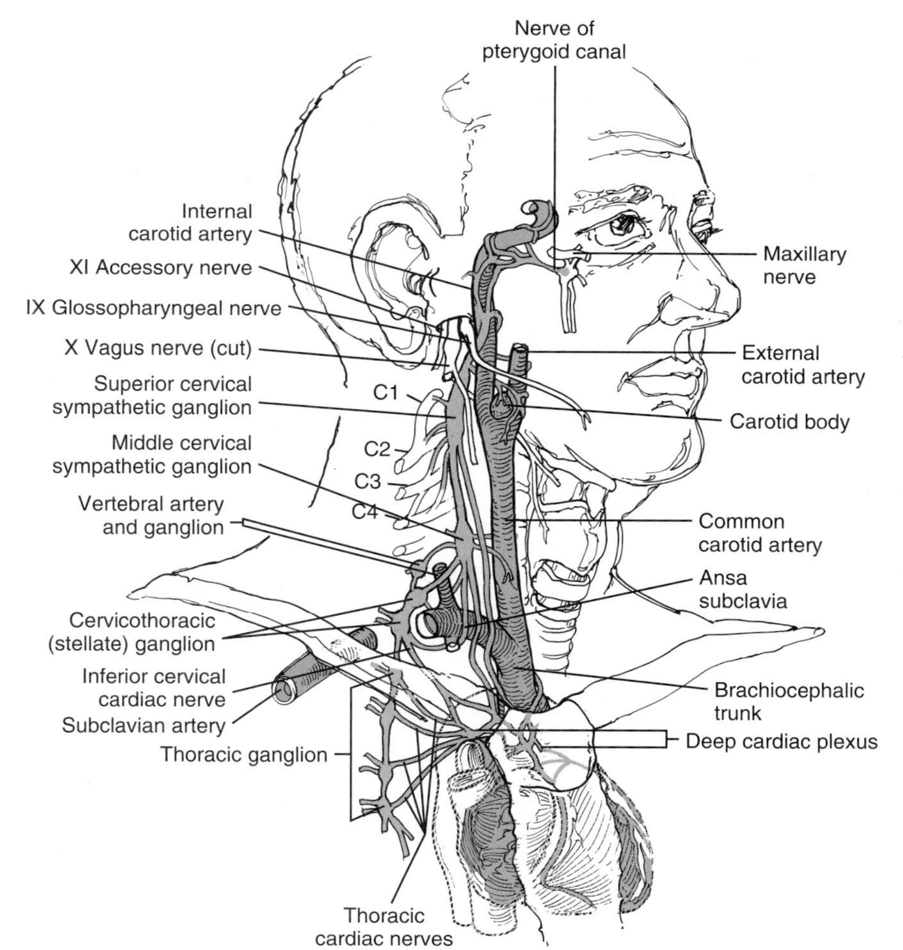

FIGURE 27–13
Branching of the common carotid artery, showing the carotid sinus.

tion of the vessel detect increases in blood pressure and initiate impulses that reflexively lower the blood pressure. In the same area where the carotid artery bifurcates, there is a small disc-shaped structure called the **carotid body,** which contains special nerve fibers that detect chemical changes in the blood, such as reductions in oxygen level. In response, the **carotid body** initiates reflex actions that may include increased rate of breathing, increased pulse rate, and elevation of blood pressure. Innervation of both the carotid sinus and the carotid body is primarily by the glossopharyngeal nerve (cranial nerve IX), with branches from the vagus nerve (cranial nerve X) (Fig. 26–13). Both the internal and external carotid arteries receive sympathetic nerve fibers from the superior cervical ganglion. The fibers form the internal and external carotid plexuses.

The internal carotid artery initially travels posterolaterally to the external carotid artery but turns in a medial direction as it flows upward. It has no branches in the neck. The external carotid artery, however, has numerous cervical branches that "rebranch" extensively to serve structures in the neck. Superior branches of the external carotid artery serve all regions of the head as well, with the exception of the orbit and brain. Branches in the neck include the superior thyroid, lingual, ascending pharyngeal, occipital, facial, posterior auricular, maxillary, and superficial temporal arteries. Variations in the branching patterns of these vessels are common.

▲ *Branches of the External Carotid Artery*

The **superior thyroid artery** is usually the first anterior branch of the external carotid artery. It is directed toward the upper portion of the thyroid gland, traveling deep to the infrahyoid muscles (Fig. 27–14). In addition to the thyroid gland, it supplies a portion of the sternocleidomastoid muscle and the larynx.

The **ascending pharyngeal artery** is the smallest branch of the external carotid artery, exiting at about the same level as the superior thyroid artery. It supplies muscles of the pharynx and palate and the palatine tonsil (Fig. 27–14).

The **lingual artery** is also an anterior branch, originating just above the superior thyroid artery at about the level of the hyoid bone. It runs forward along the surface of the middle constrictor muscle, passes be-

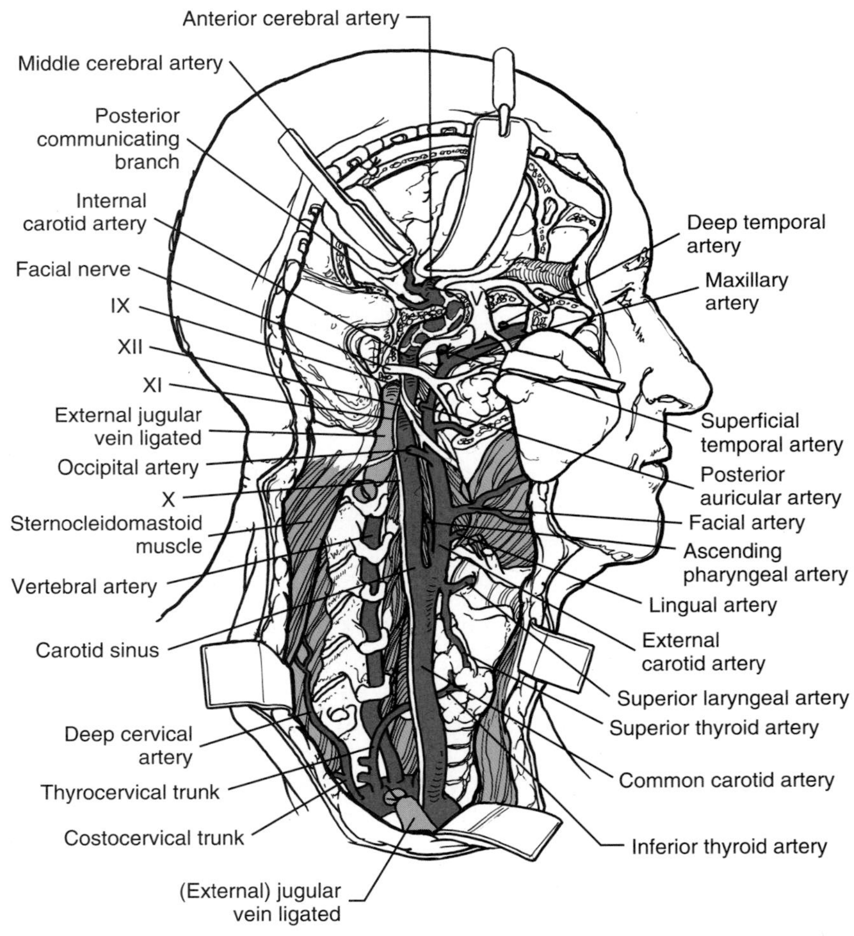

FIGURE 27–14
Internal carotid, external carotid, and vertebral arteries.

neath the hyoglossus muscle, and enters the tongue, where it terminates as the deep lingual artery (Fig. 27–14).

The **facial artery** may arise from the same trunk as the lingual artery or may branch directly from the external carotid artery superior to the lingual artery. It runs forward and upward, emerging at the lower border of the mandible, where it turns upward to supply the face (Fig. 27–14).

The **occipital artery** exits the external carotid artery posteriorly, below the level of the hyoid bone. It gives off a branch to the sternocleidomastoid muscle, passing through the posterior triangle of the neck (Fig. 27–14).

After the external carotid artery passes under the posterior belly of the digastric muscle, three branches arise from it to serve the cervical region: the **posterior auricular artery** and two terminal branches, the **maxillary** and **superficial temporal arteries.** The posterior auricular branch arises below the ear and supplies the area behind the ear. The maxillary artery supplies the jaws, palate, and inside of the nose. Finally, the superficial temporal artery supplies the side of the head (Fig. 27–14). It can be palpated in front of the upper part of the ear.

▲ Subclavian Artery Branches to the Neck and Head

Arteries to the neck that arise from the first segment of the subclavian artery include paired vertebral arteries, the thyrocervical trunks, the internal thoracic artery, and the costocervical trunks. The vertebral arteries and superior branch of the thyrocervical trunk will be described here. (The internal thoracic and costocervical trunks serve the upper thorax.) (see Chapter 21.)

The **vertebral arteries** are the most medial branches of the subclavian artery. The arteries run upward and in a slightly posterior direction, entering the transverse foramen of the sixth vertebra and continuing up through successive foramina to the base of the brain (Fig. 27–14). The arteries turn medially to enter the vertebral canal through the atlanto-occipital membrane. Here they enter the subarachnoid space and pass through the foramen magnum into the cranial cavity, eventually uniting to form the basilar artery. At the juncture of the vertebral artery and the base of the brain is found the small **occipital venous plexus,** which collects blood from occipital veins. The occipital sinus joins the internal vertebral plexuses and eventually ends in the confluence of sinuses.

The **thyrocervical trunk** branches from the upper anterior part of the subclavian artery. After giving off the transverse cervical and suprascapular arteries, it ends in the **inferior thyroid artery** (Fig. 27–14).

Lateral to the thyrocervical trunk, the costocervical trunk from the subclavian artery gives off a **deep cervical artery,** which ascends in the posterior portion of the neck. At its superior end, it anastomoses with the occipital artery, a branch of the external carotid artery (Fig. 27–14).

▲ Blood Supply to the Brain

The paired internal carotid arteries and paired vertebral arteries provide the blood supply to the brain, joining together in the circle of Willis on the ventral surface of the brain

Internal Carotid Artery

From the point at which the internal carotid artery divides from the common carotid artery to the point at which it enters the carotid canal in the petrous temporal bone, it ascends in a nearly straight line and gives off no branches. From that point on, however, the internal carotid artery makes a series of bends as it traverses foramina and curves around bony processes of the skull to supply structures in the head and the brain (Fig. 27–14). This path has prompted anatomists to name sections of the artery according to their locations as the artery ascends into the head. The lowermost segment is the **cervical segment;** the portion within the carotid canal is the **petrous segment;** the section near the cavernous sinus is the **cavernous segment,** and the uppermost segment is the **cerebral segment.** Recently, it has been suggested that the neurosurgical clinical significance of particular areas may warrant additions to this traditional terminology. For example, the **lacerum segment** would designate the portion of the internal carotid artery that traverses the foramen, an area important in transfacial surgical approaches; and the **ophthalmic segment** would describe a portion that is important in understanding the development of aneurysms relating to the eye and for developing surgical procedures. As an introduction to the basic anatomy of the internal carotid artery within the head, however, this textbook will concentrate on the artery's branches and its general course through the neck and head. Students will probably encounter more detailed classifications of arterial segments in future clinical studies.

The internal carotid artery ascends posterolaterally to the wall of the pharynx and enters the carotid canal anterior to the jugular foramen. Within the bone, this canal turns horizontally and medially toward the apex of the petrous bone, above the foramen lacerum (Fig. 27–14). The internal carotid artery runs anteriorly across the foramen lacerum and along the sella turcica in the cavernous sinus. Just before it reaches the anterior clinoid process, it gives off the **ophthalmic artery** (see Fig. 27–17 for a diagrammatic illustration of internal carotid artery branches). The internal carotid artery gives off two more branches before ending in the terminal **middle cerebral arteries** and **anterior cerebral arteries.** One branch is the **anterior choroid artery** to the choroid plexus in the lateral ventricle (Fig. 27–15*B*). The other is the **posterior communicating artery,** which connects the internal carotid artery with the basilar artery, which is formed from the two vertebral artery branches.

The **middle cerebral artery** runs upward between the temporal and frontal lobes to supply blood to the lower lateral surfaces of the cerebral hemisphere. Its dis-

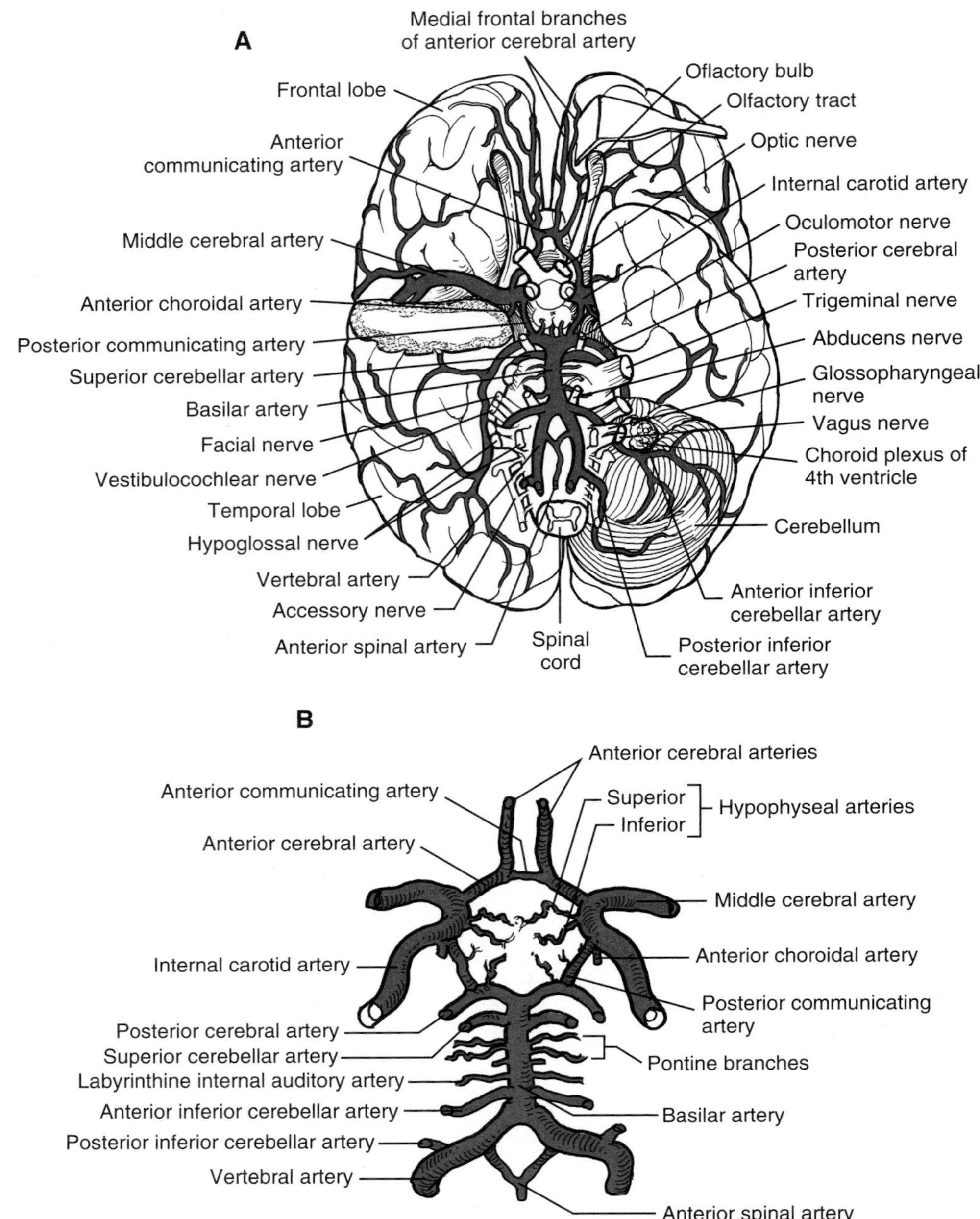

FIGURE 27–15
Arteries of the ventral brain. **A.** Ventral arteries of the brain. **B.** Detail of the circle of Willis.

tribution extends back toward the area served by the posterior cerebral branch of the vertebral artery (Figs. 27–15 and 27–16). The middle cerebral artery also gives off small branches to the brain and the corpus striatum near the internal carotid artery. Hemorrhage or occlusion of the small vessels that serve this bundle of fibers from the cerebral hemisphere causes a common type of stroke.

Branches of the **anterior cerebral arteries** supply the medial surfaces of the cerebral hemispheres, as well as the upper and lateral parts. They ultimately anastomose with branches of middle cerebral arteries from the internal carotid artery and the posterior cerebral arteries from the basilar artery (Figs. 27–15 and 27–16).

Vertebral Arteries and Vascularization of the Cerebellum

After the vertebral arteries enter the cranial cavity, they provide branches to the anterior spinal cord. These branches unite to form a single trunk, the **anterior spinal artery,** which descends ventrally to supply the spinal cord (Fig. 27–17). The anterior spinal artery also receives cervical branches from the ascending cervical and vertebral arteries, which enter the vertebral canal through intervertebral foramina (Fig. 27–17).

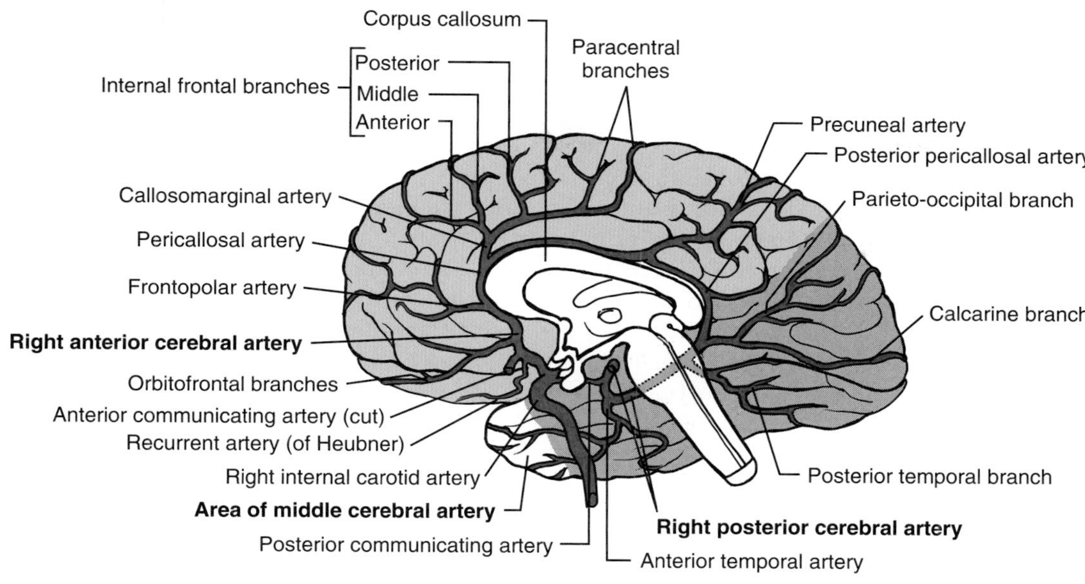

FIGURE 27–16
Medial arteries of the cerebral hemisphere.

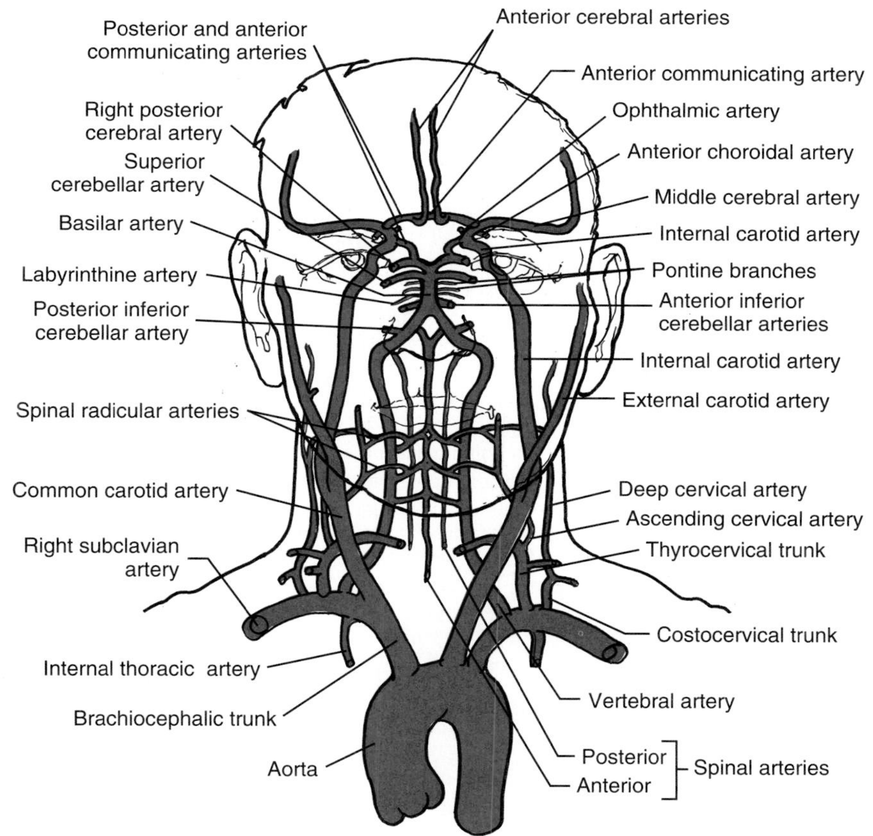

FIGURE 27–17
Schematic overview of arteries of the head and neck.

The **posterior inferior cerebellar artery** is the largest branch of the vertebral arteries supplying the cerebellar hemisphere, inferior vermis, inferior cerebellar surface, and medulla oblongata (Figs. 27–17 and 27–18). The two vertebral arteries join at the lower pontine border to form a midline **basilar artery** (Figs. 27–15, 27–17, and 27–18). Small **pontine branches** leave the basilar artery to supply the pons and adjacent structures. The **anterior inferior cerebellar artery** forms a loop into the internal acoustic meatus below cranial nerves VI, VII, and VIII (Fig. 27–18). The **superior cerebellar artery** arises near the end of the basilar artery and divides into branches that supply the superior cerebellar surface as well as the pons, pineal body, and tela choroidea of the third ventricle. The **posterior cerebral artery** arises near the superior cerebellar artery and travels around the cerebral peduncle to reach the tentorial cerebral surface (Fig. 26–18). The distribution of this artery is extensive. Fig. 26–16 shows only the medial cerebral distribution. A central branch of this artery supplies the anterior thalamus, the lateral wall of the third ventricle, and the globus pallidus. Smaller divisions of the central branch also supply the choroid plexuses of the third and lateral ventricles and also the fornix, posterior thalamus, colliculi, pineal gland, and medial geniculate body.

Cortical branches of the posterior cerebral artery reach the uncus, parahippocampus, medial and lateral occipitotemporal gyri, posterolateral surface of the occipital lobe, and visual area and other structures in the visual pathway.

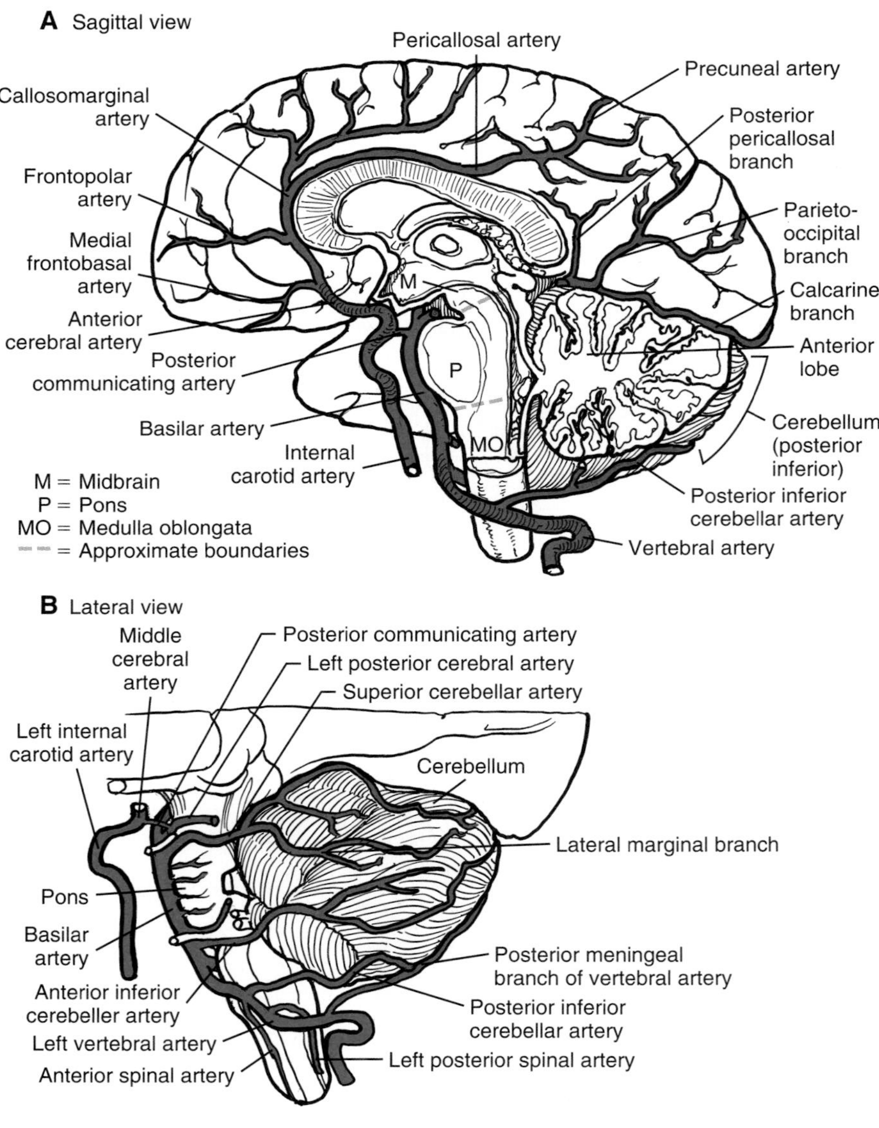

FIGURE 27–18

Arterial circulation of the cerebellum. **A.** Sagittal section. **B.** Superficial arteries.

Arterial Circle of Willis

Branches of the internal carotid arteries and the basilar artery anastomose into the central **arterial circle (of Willis)** via two communicating branches from the internal carotid artery. Anteriorly, the **anterior communicating artery** connects the two anterior cerebral arteries, and posteriorly, the **posterior communicating artery** joins the two posterior cerebral arteries from the basilar artery to the internal carotid artery (see Figs. 27–15 and 27–17). The resulting "circle" is actually more like a polygon in shape, framing the optic chiasm and neural infundibular stem of the hypophysis cerebri.

▲ Veins of the Head and Neck

The venous drainage of the head and neck will be presented from superior to inferior and from superficial to deep

Superficial Veins of the Head

Patterns of individual superficial veins vary considerably from one individual to the next. One common pattern is shown in Fig. 24–4. Starting at the scalp, five different veins collect blood from an extensive venous network: the superficial temporal, supratrochlear, supraorbital, posterior auricular, and occipital veins, all of which drain the same area.

The **supratrochlear** and **supraorbital** veins from the forehead descend near the midline and join to form a common vein, which becomes the facial vein. The **facial vein** continues on to drain into the internal jugular vein in the upper angle of the carotid triangle near the hyoid bone (Fig. 27–19). The **superficial temporal vein** enters the parotid gland to join the maxillary vein, forming the **retromandibular vein** (Fig. 27–19). The **posterior auricular vein** descends directly behind the auricle and joins the retromandibular vein to form the external jugular vein. The **occipital vein** usually follows the occipital artery into the internal jugular vein but may, instead, drain into the external jugular vein.

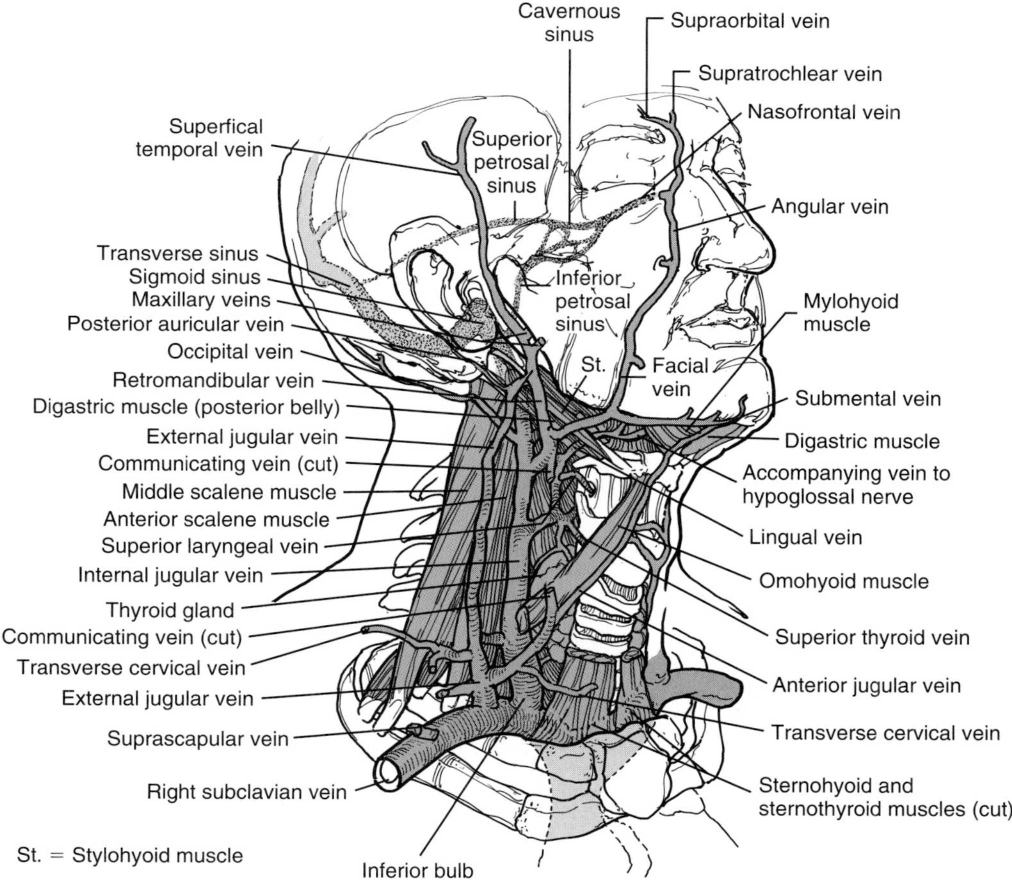

FIGURE 27–19

Superficial veins of the neck. Drainage of superficial veins from the surface of the head is shown with the sternocleidomastoid muscle removed. The external jugular vein is superficial to the sternocleidomastoid muscle, but the posterior portion of the anterior jugular vein and all of the internal jugular vein would be covered by the muscle.

Veins of the Skull and Brain: Diploic, Meningeal, Cerebral, and Cerebellar Veins

Veins in the head communicate extensively, have thin walls with no valves, and usually drain into cranial sinuses

Diploic veins collect blood within the diploë of cranial bones (see Fig. 26–18). They communicate via emissary veins with veins of the scalp and with the dural venous sinuses. Although there is great variety in branching patterns of these veins, several fairly regular channels have been observed, all of which open into venous sinuses in the dura mater. The anterior branches within the frontal bone end in the **sphenoparietal sinus** (Fig. 26–19A). Posterior temporal branches join the **transverse sinus.** An occipital diploë vein opens into the occipital veins or the transverse sinus. A number of the diploic veins emerge near the **superior sagittal sinus** and drain directly into it.

There is no arterial equivalent to the diploic veins. Arterial blood is provided to this area by meningeal and pericranial arteries.

Meningeal veins originate in the dura mater and drain into vessels that connect with lacunae of the superior sagittal sinus and other cranial sinuses. They also connect with the diploë veins.

Venous drainage of the exterior and medial surfaces of the brain is by superficial veins (superior, middle, and inferior cerebral veins), which empty into the venous sinuses in the dura mater. **Superior cerebral veins** follow the sulci of the superolateral and medial surfaces of each hemisphere of the brain and drain into the superior sagittal sinus (Fig. 27–20A).

The **superficial middle cerebral vein** collects blood from the lateral surface of the cerebrum and empties into the cavernous sinus (Fig. 27–20A)

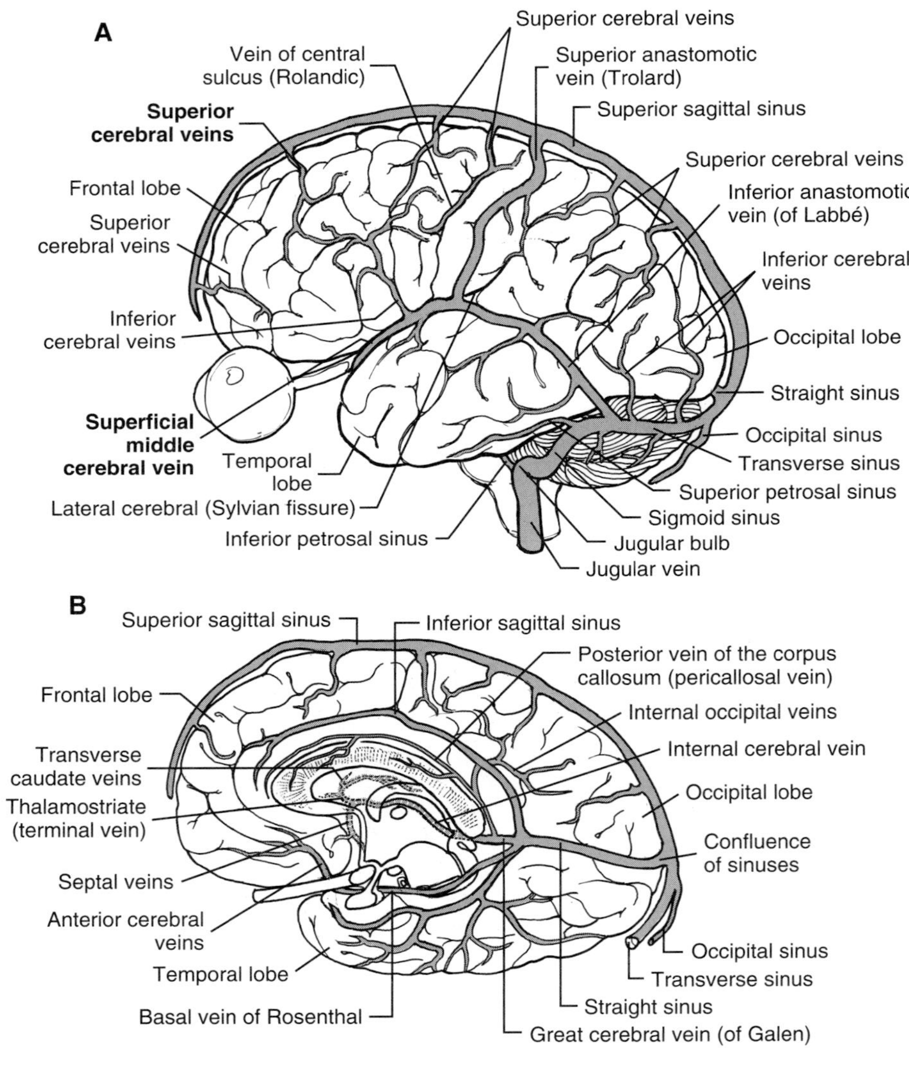

FIGURE 27–20

Venous drainage of the cerebrum. **A.** Superficial veins of the cerebrum. **B.** Sagittal view of veins of the cerebrum.

Inferior cerebral veins draining the lower portions of the hemispheres are quite small. They empty into sinuses at the base of the skull.

Deep cerebral veins drain deep parts of the hemisphere, receiving veins from the caudate nucleus and thalamus. The thalamostriate and choroid plexuses on each side of the brain unite to form paired **internal cerebral veins** (Fig. 27–20). The union of the two internal cerebral veins then forms the **great cerebral vein (of Galen).** This vein receives branches from the basal veins and opens into the anterior end of the straight sinus (Fig. 27–20*B*).

Superior and inferior branches of the **cerebellar veins** drain all sides of the cerebellum (Fig. 27–20). Depending on the direction of the veins, they open into the straight sinus, great cerebral vein, superior petrosal sinus, sigmoid sinus, or inferior petrosal and occipital sinuses.

Major Veins of the Neck

The external and internal jugular veins collect blood from the head and neck, emptying into the right and left subclavian veins

The **external jugular vein** drains primarily the scalp and the face. As has been described above, it originates at the juncture of the retromandibular and posterior auricular veins, just below the parotid gland near the mandibular angle. As it descends obliquely toward the midclavicle (through the subclavian triangle), it lies deep to the platysma muscle and superficial fascial layers and superior to the sternocleidomastoid muscle. It traverses the deep fascia to enter the subclavian vein (see Fig. 27–19). The vein is often visible on the surface of the neck in the area where it crosses the sternocleidomastoid muscle. Near the point where it enters the subclavian vein, the external jugular vein receives a branch from the **anterior jugular vein** that collects blood from the submandibular veins in the area of the hyoid bone (see Fig. 27–19).

The **internal jugular vein** collects blood from superficial parts of the face but also drains the skull, brain, and neck. At its origin at the base of the cranium, it is continuous with the sigmoid sinus (Fig. 27–21). Descending in the carotid sheath lateral to the carotid arteries, it joins the subclavian vein to form the brachiocephalic vein. The internal jugular vein is covered by the sternocleidomastoid muscle. Superiorly, the posterior belly of the digastric muscle overlaps the vein, and inferiorly, the superior belly of the omohyoid muscle overlaps it (Fig. 27–19 and see Fig. 27–2 for the position of the internal jugular vein within surrounding structures in the neck). At the end where it meets the brachiocephalic vein, it is dilated in a structure called the **inferior bulb** (see Fig. 27–19). In the area where the bulb extends into the depression between the sternal and clavicular heads of the sternocleidomastoid muscle is a site that can be used for precise insertion of a needle.

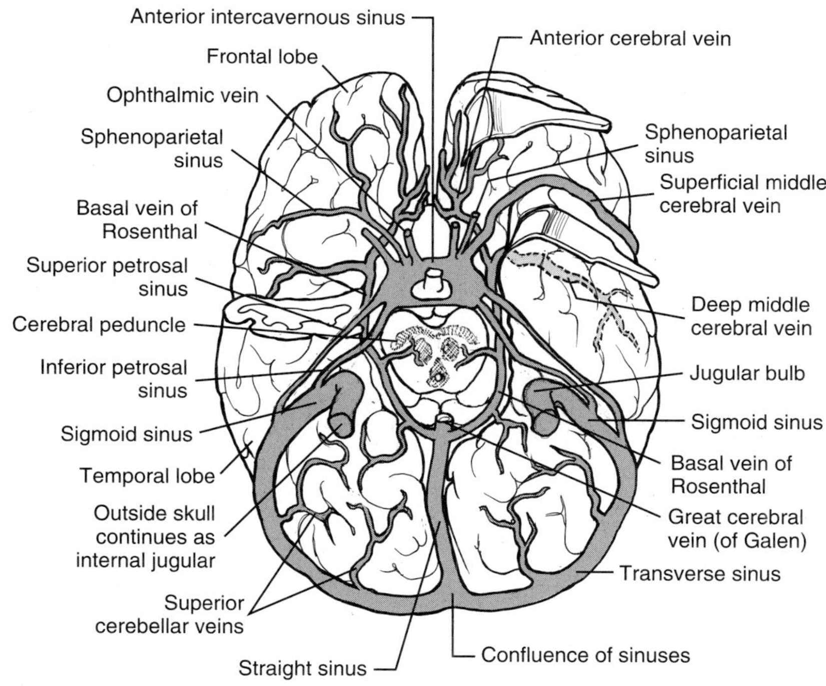

FIGURE 27–21
Ventral view of venous drainage of the brain.

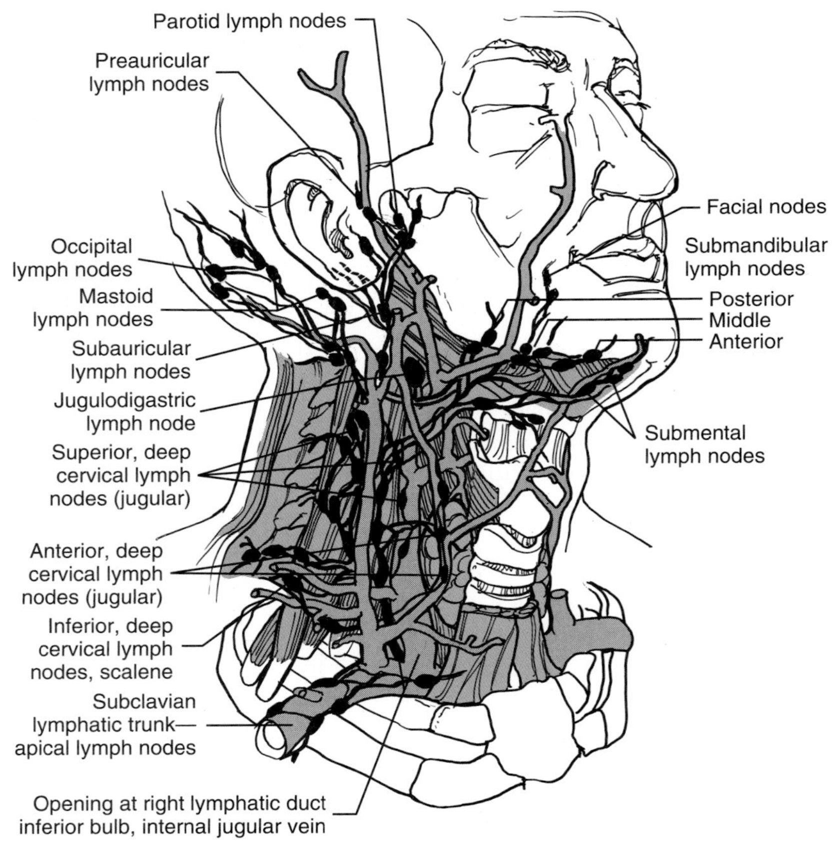

FIGURE 27–22
Lymphatic system of the head and neck.

The internal jugular vein collects blood from many tributaries and sinuses:

- the inferior petrosal sinus from the anterior part of the jugular foramen,
- the lingual veins from the dorsal and inferior regions of the tongue,
- the pharyngeal veins from a pharyngeal plexus external to the pharynx, and
- the superior and middle thyroid veins.

Venous drainage of the vertebral canal is carried out by the vertebral vein, which descends lateral to the vertebral artery and behind the internal carotid artery and opens into the brachiocephalic vein. Additional branches from the neck include the anterior vertebral vein and deep cervical vein.

Lymphatic Drainage of the Head and Neck

Cervical lymph vessels return lymph to the venous system near the junction of the internal jugular and subclavian veins. Outlying groups of lymphatics from the head and neck include vessels and nodes from the

- occipital region,
- retroauricular and mastoid regions,
- parotid area,
- facial (buccal) regions, and
- submandibular and submental areas (Fig. 27–22).

All of these outlying groups from the head and neck, as well as lymph vessels from tissues of the head and neck internal to the deep fascia, drain into a collecting group, the **deep cervical lymph nodes,** which run along the internal jugular vein. Efferents from these deep cervical lymph nodes form the **jugular trunk,** which delivers lymph from the head and neck to the brachiocephalic vein (Fig. 27–22).

Other lymphatic collection trunks also converge in this area. The **subclavian trunk** conveys lymph from the upper limb and thoracoabdominal wall, while the **bronchomediastinal trunk** (not shown in figure) brings lymph from deeper portions of the thorax. On the right side of the body, these trunks usually enter the venous system through the **lymphatic duct,** as shown in Fig. 27–22. On the left side, in addition to the three trunks named above, the **thoracic duct** is a fourth collection trunk, which drains all of the remaining regions of the body near the jugulosubclavian junction.

Index

M

N

O